EMT COMPLETE
A Basic Worktext

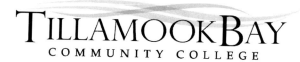
W9-BSE-265

EMT COMPLETE
A Basic Worktext

DANIEL LIMMER

CHRISTOPHER J. LE BAUDOUR

Medical Editor

Edward T. Dickinson, MD, FACEP

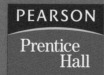

PEARSON

Prentice Hall

BRADY

Upper Saddle River, New Jersey 07458

Library of Congress Cataloging-in-Publication Data

Limmer, Daniel.
  EMT complete : a basic worktext / Daniel Limmer, Christopher J.
Le Baudour ; medical editor, Edward T. Dickinson.
    p. cm.
  Includes bibliographical references and index.
  ISBN 0-13-119265-5
  1. Emergency medical technicians—Outlines, syllabi, etc. 2. Emer-
gency medicine—Outlines, syllabi, etc. I. Le Baudour, Chris.
II. Dickinson, Edward T. III. Title.
  [DNLM: 1. Emergency Treatment—methods—Problems and Exer-
cises. 2. Emergency Medical Services—methods—Problems and
Exercises. 3. Emergency Medical Technicians—Problems and
Exercises. WB 18.2 L441e 2007]
RC86.92.L56 2007
616.02′5—dc22

2006010707

Publisher: Julie Levin Alexander
Publisher's Assistant: Regina Bruno
Executive Editor: Marlene McHugh Pratt
Senior Managing Editor for Development: Lois Berlowitz
Assistant Editor: Matthew Sirinides
Development Editor: Triple SSS Press Media Development, Inc.
Managing Photography Editor: Michal Heron
Director of Marketing: Karen Allman
Executive Marketing Manager: Katrin Beacom
Marketing Coordinator: Michael Sirinides
Managing Editor for Production: Patrick Walsh
Production Liaison: Faye Gemmellaro
Production Editor: Heather Willison, Carlisle Publishing Services

Media Project Manager: John J. Jordan
Manager of Media Production: Amy Peltier
New Media Project Manager: Stephen J. Hartner
Manufacturing Manager: Ilene Sanford
Manufacturing Buyer: Pat Brown
Senior Design Coordinator: Cheryl Asherman/
  Christopher Weigand
Interior and Cover Design: Wee Design/
  Wanda Espana
Cover Image: Getty Images
Composition: Carlisle Publishing Services
Printing/Binding: Courier Kendallville
Cover Printer: Phoenix Color

Studentaid.ed.gov, the U.S. Department of Education's website on college planning assistance, is a valuable tool for anyone intending to pursue higher education. Designed to help students at all stages of schooling, including international students, returning students, and parents, it is a guide to the financial aid process. The website presents information on applying to and attending college as well as on funding your education and repaying loans. It also provides links to useful resources, such as state education agency contact information, assistance in filling out financial aid forms, and an introduction to various forms of student aid.

Pearson Education, Ltd.
Pearson Education Singapore, Pte. Ltd.
Pearson Education, Canada, Ltd.
Pearson Education—Japan
Pearson Education Australia PTY, Limited

Pearson Education North Asia Ltd.
Pearson Educación de Mexico, S.A. de C.V.
Pearson Education Malaysia, Pte. Ltd.
Pearson Education, Upper Saddle River, New Jersey

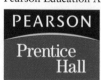

10 9 8 7 6 5 4 3 2 1
ISBN: 0-13-119265-5

To Stephanie, Sarah, and Margo. A husband and father is blessed to be surrounded by such love, beauty, support, and smiles.

—D.L.

It is with sincere gratitude and respect that I dedicate this book to the following individuals:

Anne Thompson, my very first educational mentor and the best role model any teacher could ever have. Anne, thank you for believing in me from the very beginning.

To my friends Erin Eachus Reed, Art Gartisar, Kelly Bates, and Diane Codding. You all made the ultimate sacrifice by giving your lives so that others could live. We will forever remember your shining examples and are comforted knowing that you are our angels in flight.

And last but not least to Audrey, Kaitlyn, and Jordan for your unwavering support in allowing me to live my passion.

—C.J.L.

To Debbie, Stephen, and Alex for their endless love and extraordinary patience throughout this and many other projects.

—E.T.D.

CONTENTS

CHAPTER 3   LEGAL AND ETHICAL CONSIDERATIONS OF PROVIDING CARE   56

CHAPTER 4   BASIC HUMAN ANATOMY   83

MODULE 3   Patient Assessment   224

CHAPTER 10   OBTAINING VITAL SIGNS AND A MEDICAL HISTORY   250

CHAPTER 14   PERFORMING AN ONGOING ASSESSMENT   364

CHAPTER 15   COMMUNICATIONS IN EMS   377

CHAPTER 16   DOCUMENTING YOUR ASSESSMENT AND CARE   399

CHAPTER 17   MODULE REVIEW AND PRACTICE EXAMINATION   420

MODULE 4   Medical Emergencies   426

MODULE 5   Trauma   664

CHAPTER 28   CONTROLLING BLEEDING   688

CHAPTER 29   PATIENTS WITH SOFT-TISSUE INJURIES   717

CHAPTER 31   PATIENTS WITH INJURIES TO THE CHEST AND ABDOMEN   776

CHAPTER 32   PATIENTS WITH MUSCULOSKELETAL INJURIES   796

CHAPTER 35 MODULE REVIEW AND PRACTICE EXAMINATION

MODULE 6 Pediatrics and Geriatrics

CHAPTER 36 CARING FOR PEDIATRIC PATIENTS

CHAPTER 44   RESPONSES INVOLVING TERRORISM   1103

CHAPTER 45   MODULE REVIEW AND PRACTICE EXAMINATION   1122

MODULE 8   Advanced Airway   1128

CHAPTER 46   ADVANCED AIRWAY   1130

There are two things that Brady Publishing understands very well—EMS students and EMS education. *EMT Complete: A Basic Worktext* is a product of that understanding. What you hold in your hands is the result of over two years and many thousands of hours of labor. *EMT Complete: A Basic Worktext* is the next *evolution* in EMS education.

Rest assured that the foundation for the content of this new textbook is the most current DOT National Standard Curriculum for EMT-Basic and includes pertinent changes in science and practice, including new AHA recommendations affecting EMS. Our goal is simply to assist in the evolutionary process of EMS education by placing a greater focus on you, the student, and the development of critical thinking skills that will affect you, your EMT colleagues, and your patients.

We are introducing several new features in this book as well as including several well-established features that you have come to expect from Brady.

It's NOT just another Textbook. . .

First and foremost this textbook serves as both a *textbook AND a workbook*, hence the name "Worktext." As a textbook it represents the same high-quality content for which Brady is well known. This project was conceived, developed, written, and reviewed by some of the most dedicated and leading professionals in EMS education today. You will find that the content is well-organized, easy to read, and based on current EMS research and practice.

It's NOT just another Workbook. . .

Embedded in each chapter are elements traditionally found in EMS workbooks. We have integrated workbook elements throughout each chapter to challenge and encourage you to test your understanding of the material and concepts as they are being presented rather than by using a separate workbook.

We have created a process whereby you read a section of content and the content is then reinforced with each *Stop, Review, Remember!* section. This cycle repeats throughout each chapter and is summarized in a chapter review. Each *Stop, Review, Remember!* feature contains a minimum of three workbook elements: multiple choice questions, an activity, and critical thinking questions. In most chapters, case studies are also included. Each of these elements is designed to engage you in the learning process and encourage you to apply the content being presented.

EMERGENCY DISPATCH

A familiar Brady feature that you will see following the introduction of each chapter is the *Emergency Dispatch*. The objective of this chapter-opening scenario is to thrust you into the mindset of an EMT or EMT partners who have just been dispatched to an emergency. The *Emergency Dispatch* sets the stage for the context of the chapter. It also allows you to begin the all-important, "what-would-I-do" critical-thinking process.

PERSPECTIVES

Working in EMS is about people caring for other people and how our actions affect those for whom we care and with whom we work. Being successful in EMS means being able to "see" a situation from more than one perspective or from another person's viewpoint. It also means developing an understanding of the values, feelings, attitudes, and beliefs of those around you. Woven throughout each chapter—and continuing the scenario introduced in the Emergency Dispatch—is the key feature *Perspectives*. Each *Perspective* is narrated by one of the many "characters" commonly encountered on an emergency scene. We take you inside the minds of frightened patients, angry and anxious family members, and nosy neighbors. You go inside the thoughts of EMTs and their partners, fire captains, and other rescue personnel on the scene. It is through these insightful *Perspectives* that you begin to glimpse how an emergency call can affect you and how your words and actions can affect not just the patient but also others around you.

DISPATCH SUMMARY

Each scenario wraps up at the end of each chapter with the *Dispatch Summary.* Here you learn the outcome of the *Emergency Dispatch* that opened the chapter and that continued as *Perspectives* throughout the chapter. As you will see when reading these scenarios, people don't always say and do the "right" thing. Many of the scenarios—the *Dispatches* and the *Perspectives*—are based on actual events involving actual people. We, therefore, have allowed the human side to show through, even when it does not always model the recommended behavior.

MODULE REVIEW AND PRACTICE EXAMINATIONS

The content and organization of this Worktext is based on the seven modules of the DOT EMT-Basic National Standard Curriculum. At the end of each learning module, you can take a practice multiple-choice exam modeled after both state- and national-style certification exams that will provide valuable practice for your own certification exam.

Appendix A offers more review in the format of a 150-question Practice Review.

In total, you will have approximately *1,800* different questions and exercises in this text to help reinforce your knowledge.

NEW AND EXPANDED CHAPTERS

We are very proud to include several expanded topics. The first is "Caring for Geriatric Patients." The geriatric population of America is growing at a significant rate. As an EMT who will be caring for these older patients, you will need to develop a clear understanding of their individual needs. This chapter outlines the unique ways these patients present and provides tips for a thorough and accurate assessment.

The chapter on shock has been expanded to include a new feature that takes you through the development of shock step by step, sign by sign, and symptom by symptom, using "Richard," a simulated trauma patient.

Several new chapters address topics related to large-scale incidents that, in some other texts, are combined into one or two chapters. The key to an appropriate response is preparation, and the key to preparation is knowledge. The likelihood of a large-scale incident with many casualties is greater now than ever. To help you understand your potential role during such an incident, we have included the following chapters: "Overview of the Incident Command System," "Responses Involving a Multiple-Casualty Incident," "Responses Involving Hazardous Materials," and "Responses Involving Terrorism."

We have added a chapter to the line-up that we think will provide real value as you consider a career in EMS. The chapter "Your Successful Career in EMS" is full of valuable tips from career EMS professionals and is designed to provide you with an overview of the many options available to you as a new EMT. Being an EMT is not just about working on an ambulance. Today the options available to you are many and varied. Even though this chapter appears at the end of the book, we think you will benefit by reading it early and referring to it frequently throughout your training.

COMPANION CD-ROMs

Consistent with the Brady tradition, this book would not be complete without the high-tech resources available on the companion CD-ROMs found inside the back cover. They are packed full of state-of-the-art 3D animations, as well as interactive exercises, and lessons that will engage you and further reinforce the core content.

This Is EMS

Now that we have provided a glimpse of what's inside this new learning package and its new approach to EMS education, sit back, lace up your boots, and hang on as you begin the incredible journey of becoming an EMT. We, as your authors, are honored and excited to be a part of your training. Collectively with Edward T. Dickinson, M.D., the Medical Editor, we have been fortunate enough to call EMS our career for nearly 82 years and want to share our experiences with you. We want to share the highs and the lows, the successful resuscitations as well as the loss of life, because this is *our* life. . . . *This is EMS*!

Dan Limmer
Chris Le Baudour

✳ ACKNOWLEDGMENTS

CONTENT CONTRIBUTORS

The authors would like to thank the following contributors:

Melissa R. Alexander, NREMT-P, who authored the Module Review, Practice Examinations, and Appendix A. In addition, Melissa provided the content for chapter 37.

Brian D. Bricker, EMT-B, NREMT, EMSA, Oklahoma City, Oklahoma, who is the author of the Perspectives feature in each chapter. Brian did a fantastic job using his creative writing skills and EMS knowledge to bring the EMTs, patients, family members, and bystanders to life. In addition, Brian was a contributor to several Stop, Review, Remember! sections and Chapter Review questions.

Bruce Evans, MPA, Fire Captain, Henderson Fire Department, Henderson, Nevada, and Fire Programs Coordinator, Community College of Southern Nevada, Las Vegas, Nevada, who is the author of chapters 40, 42, 43, and 44. Bruce's specialized knowledge of these topics enabled this book to include each chapter as a separate learning unit, where other texts combined the topics into one chapter.

Laura Gittleman, BSN, CEN, who is the author of chapter 36. We appreciate her diligence in creating this chapter and expanding this content.

Eric T. Mayhew, NREMT-P, Training Officer Pender Emergency Medical Services, Pender County, North Carolina, for his technical editing and organization of five chapters as well as the writing of exercises for these chapters.

Will Krost, EMT-P, for his contributions to chapter 46.

Chris Suprun for his contributions to chapter 39.

REVIEWERS

We wish to thank the following reviewers for providing invaluable feedback, insight, and suggestions in the preparation of *EMT Complete: A Basic Worktext.*

Maria Aliftiras
NREMT-Paramedic

David K. Anderson, BS, EMT-P
Paramedic Program Director
NW Regional Training Center
Vancouver, WA

Woody Ball
Danville Fire Department
Danville, KY

Barbara Boonton, NREMT-P, EMS-IC
Emergency Education
Brookings, SD

Brian D. Bricker, EMT-B
EMSA
Oklahoma City, OK

Maureen L. Bruce, APRN, FNP-BC,
    EMT-P, MSN, CAS
Charlotte Hungerford Hospital
Torrington, CT

Gary Bonewald, MEd, LP
Associate Department Chair
Houston Community College
EMS Program
Houston, TX

Major Raymond W. Burton, Retired
Plymouth Academy
Plymouth, MA

Paul H. Coffey, EMT-I
MDPH-OEMS & Holliston Fire EMS
Holliston, MA

Steven A. Cohen, NREMT-P
Education Coordinator
EMS Department
Jersey City Medical Center
Jersey City, NJ

Steven Creech, NC EMT-P
  EMS Instructor
Training Officer
Washington County EMS
Plymouth, NC

Tony Crystal, Director
Emergency Medical Services
Lake Land College
Mattoon, IL

Heather Davis, MS, NREMT-P

Bruce Evans, MPA, NREMT-P
Fire Captain
Henderson Fire Department
Henderson, NV
Fire Programs Coordinator
Community College of Southern Nevada
Las Vegas, NV

James W. Fox, EMT-P, EMS Instructor
Adjunct Faculty Des Moines Area
  Community College (DMACC),
  Ankeny campus
Emergency Medical Services (EMS)
  Assistant Coordinator
Des Moines Fire Department
Des Moines, IA

Bruce L. Gadol, NREMT, CCT EMS I/C
Director of Education
Southeastern School of Allied Health
  Medicine
Miami, FL

Rudy Garrett, NREMT-P
Somerset, OK

Kevin M. Garvey
Adjunct Professor
Greenfield Community College,
  Williams College,
  Mount Holyoke College
  University of Massachusetts
Boston, MA

Jaime S. Greene
Instructor
Lake City Community College
Lake City, FL

Michael Grill
Sierra Vista, AZ

Rod Hackwith, BS, NREMT-P
EMS Program Director
Community College of Southern Nevada
Las Vegas, NV

Michael Hastings MS, NREMT-P
EMS Program Director
Central Piedmont Community College
Charlotte, NC

Rick Heironimus
EMS Continuing Education Instructor
Columbus, OH

Attila J. Hertelendy, MHSM, CCEMT-P,
  NREMT-P
Department of Emergency Medical
  Technology
School of Health Related Professions
University of Mississippi Medical Center
Jackson, MS

Don E. Hess, NREMT-P
EMS Coordinator
St. Anthony Medical Center
Crown Point, IN

Joseph A. Holmbo, NREMT-P, EMS-I
Eastern Iowa Community College District
Clinton, IA

Christopher Jones
Youngstown State University
Rural/Metro Ambulance
Youngstown, OH

Gregory R. LeMay, BS, NREMT-P
TEEX WMD EMS Instructor
College Station, TX

James S. Lion, Jr.
AEMT- I, EMS Lieutenent
Williamsville Fire Department
Williamsville, NY

William Locke
EMS Instructor/Coordinator
Moraine Park Technical College
Fond du Lac, WI

J.J. Magyar, MS, NREMT-P
Magyar Consulting and Training
Montgomery, PA

Ryan Maloney, BS, EMT-P
University of New Mexico Health Sciences
  Center Emergency Medical Services
  Academy
Santa Fe, NM

Eric T. Mayhew, AAS, NREMT-P
Training Officer
Pender Emergency Services
Pender County, NC

Ned M. McElfresh, BA, EMSI, FSI
Paramedic Program
Instructor/Coordinator
EHOVE Ghrist Adult Career Center
Milan, OH

Michael Morgan, NREMT-Paramedic
Fort Sam Houston, TX

Helen Newland
Hocking College
Nelsonville, OH

Gus Pappas, BS, EMT-P
FDNY/EMS Chief Retired
New York, NY

Jeffrey L. Pellegrino, PhD
Indianapolis, IN

Bernadette A. Royce, BA, FF/EMT-P
Osceola County Fire Rescue
Valencia Community College
Orlando, FL

John N. Schupra
BS, CCEMTP, EMS I/C
EMS Faculty, Kellogg Community College
Battle Creek, MI

Beth Sheeran, MA, EMT-B
Montgomery County Community College
Montgomery, PA

Terry A. Taylor, II
Rochester, NY

Larry Thompson, Engineer/Paramedic
Marin County Fire Department
Santa Rosa Junior College-Instructor
Windsor, CA

Jimmy VanCleve
Industrial Training Coordinator
KCTCS—State Fire Rescue Training
Kansas City, KS

Cheri Volta
Paramedic
Capital Ambulance
Bangor, ME

Sandy Waggoner
EMT-P
Milan, OH

Annette G. Young, EMT-B (I)
Bergen County Law & Public Safety
  Institute
EMS Academy
Mahwah, NJ

Jason P. Zielewicz, MS, BS, NREMT-P
EMS Instructor/Supervisor
Pennsylvania State University Office of
  EMS
University Park, PA

Mark S. Zinn, NREMT-P
Baltimore City Fire Department
Baltmore, MD

PHOTO CREDITS

All photographs not credited adjacent to the photograph or in the photo credit section below were photographed on assignment for Brady/Prentice Hall.

ORGANIZATIONS

We wish to thank the following organizations for their valuable assistance in creating the photo program for this edition:

American Medical Response
Eric Polan, Director of Operations
Dean Anderson, Operations Manager
Sonoma/Marin, CA

REACH Air Medical Services
Jim Adams, CEO
Santa Rosa, CA

Santa Rosa Junior College
Ken Bradford, Director of EMC Programs
Santa Rosa, CA

Sonoma County Sheriffs Department
Sgt. Scott Dunn
Sonoma County, CA

Rincon Valley Fire Department
Chief Doug Williams
Santa Rosa, CA

veriHealth Ambulance Service
Gary Tennyson, CEO
Sean Sullivan, Operations Manager
Petaluma, CA

Windsor Fire Department
Chief Ron Collier
Windsor, CA

Windsor Golf Club
Windsor, CA

TECHNICAL ADVISORS

Thanks to the following people for providing valuable technical support during the photo shoots:

John Martin, EMT-B
Sonoma County Search and Rescue
Sonoma County, CA

Scott Snyder, EMT-P
Folsom, CA

Ted Williams, EMT-B
Sonoma Life Support
Santa Rosa, CA

Photo assistant: Sam Willard, Berkeley, CA

Assistant model coordinator: Audrey Le Baudour

Digital post-production: Sam Willard, Berkeley, CA

MODELS

Thanks to the following people who provided locations and/or portrayed patients and EMS providers in our photographs.

Christian Abballo
James Adams
Jarrett Bagliato
Abigail Barajas
Rafael Bautista
Rachael Berey-Phillips
Lance Bollens
Kenderick Braal
Jessica Brucato
Colleen Cahill
David W. Cassetta
Cameron Cornelssen
Robert de Lambert
James DeMoss
Darin P. Divita
Allyson Emery
Jacob Feickert
Cayden Fleming
Thera Fleming
Amber Gentry
Dan Grevious
Hannah Grevious
Kobi Grevious
Frank A. Harrah

Diane Hayes
Paul Hentz
Hope L. Hunt
Lynn Hunt
Jennifer Imboden
Jeton B. Ireland
Kurt Masami Kawamoto
Jim Kegerreis
Robert Latham
Audrey Le Baudour
Jordan Le Baudour
Kaitlyn Le Baudour
Fred Leuenberger
Kathy Logee
Lena Lorenzoni
Kelsey D. Louden
Paul Louden
John W. Martin
Jane Martin-Leach
Gary McCalla
Mary Anne Helen Elizabeth Meier
Ronald Meints
Joshua Menzies
Gina Monraz

Kevin C. Morrow
Wendy Morrow
Roya Nikzad
Monique O'Dell
Ryan Osborne
Joseph Perez
Tony Peters
Steven Powers
Greg Quacchia
Deanna Schutz
Christal Seubert
William Seubert
Scott Snyder
Katie Steiss
Jennifer Stuart
Leah Taylor
Matthew A. Taylor
Larry Thompson
Bill Vandisne
Nora Villagomez
Mason Wagner
Sam Willard
Ted Williams

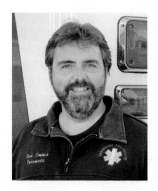

Daniel Limmer

Daniel Limmer, EMT-P, has been involved in EMS for more than 27 years. He remains active as a paramedic with Kennebunk Fire Rescue in Kennebunk, Maine, and the Kennebunkport EMS (KEMS) in Kennebunkport, Maine. A passionate educator, Limmer teaches EMT and paramedic courses at the Southern Maine Community College in South Portland, Maine, and has taught at The George Washington University in Washington, DC, and the Hudson Valley Community College in Troy, New York. He is a charter member of the National Association of EMS Educators and a member of the National Association of EMTs (NAEMT), for which he serves on the Advanced Medical Life Support Committee.

Limmer was formerly involved in law enforcement, beginning as a dispatcher and retiring as a police officer in Colonie, New York, where he received three command recognition awards as well as the distinguished service award (Officer of the Year) in 1987. During his 20-year law enforcement career he served in the communications, patrol, juvenile, narcotics, and training units.

In addition to authoring several EMS journal articles, Limmer is co-author of a number of EMS textbooks for Brady, including *Emergency Care, First Responder: A Skills Approach*, and *Advanced Medical Life Support*. He speaks frequently at regional, state, and national EMS conferences.

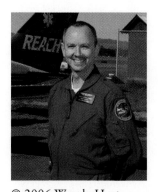

Christopher J. Le Baudour

Christopher Le Baudour has been working in the EMS field since 1978. He has worked as an EMT-I and an EMT-II in both the field and clinical settings. In 1984 he began his teaching career in the Department of Public Safety—EMS Division at Santa Rosa Junior College in Santa Rosa, California.

Le Baudour holds a Master's Degree in Education with an emphasis in online teaching and learning as well as numerous certifications. He has spent the past 22 years mastering the art of experiential learning in EMS and is well known for his innovative classroom techniques and his passion for teaching and learning in both traditional and online classrooms.

© 2006 Woody Hurt Photography

Le Baudour is very involved in EMS education at the national level as a member of the Distributed Learning Subcommittee of the National Association of EMS Educators. He is a frequent presenter at both state and national conferences and a prolific EMS writer. He currently serves as the Fixed-Wing Business Manager for REACH Air Medical Services in Santa Rosa, California.

Le Baudour is also author, co-author, or contributor to these other Brady texts:

✳ *First Responder*, 7th Edition
✳ *First Responder Workbook*, 7th Edition
✳ *Emergency Care 360*—Online EMT Program

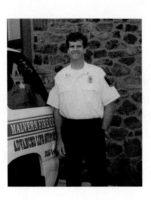

Edward T. Dickinson, Medical Editor

Edward T. Dickinson, MD, NREMT-P, FACEP, is currently Associate Professor and Director of EMS Field Operations in the Department of Emergency Medicine of the University of Pennsylvania School of Medicine in Philadelphia. He is Medical Director of the Malvern Fire Company, the Berwyn Fire Company, and the Township of Haverford paramedics in Pennsylvania. He is a residency-trained, board-certified emergency medicine physician who is a Fellow of the American College of Emergency Physicians.

Dr. Dickinson began his career in emergency services in 1979 as a firefighter-EMT in upstate New York. He has remained active in fire service and EMS for the past 26 years. He frequently rides with EMS units and has maintained his certification as a National Registry EMT-Paramedic.

He has served as medical editor for numerous Brady EMT-B and First Responder texts and is the author of *Fire Service Emergency Care* and co-author of *Emergency Care, Fire Service Edition*, and *Emergency Incident Rehabilitation*. He is co-editor of *ALS Case Studies in Emergency Care*.

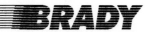

Brady
Prentice Hall Health
Upper Saddle River, NJ 07458

Dear Instructor:

Brady, your partner for life, is pleased to present a new solution for your EMT course. As the #1 publisher in EMS, we feel it's our responsibility to remain in front of the curve when it comes to providing better ways to teach and learn. Based on years of success in EMS, our experience in educational publishing across many disciplines, and extensive feedback from our customers, we identified a new approach to teaching your EMT course. This approach focuses on two ideas: 1) a combination text/workbook enables students to instantly apply knowledge learned—throughout a chapter, not just at the end; 2) understanding the perspectives of all individuals on scene makes for better judgment and decisionmaking.

EMT Complete was conceived through comprehensive surveys and focus groups and listening to customers' changing needs. It brings together two key authors—Dan Limmer and Chris Le Baudour—whose combined experience, philosophies, and perspectives make for one of the most exciting new books to enter the EMT market in quite a while. It also brings together feedback and direction from hundreds of instructors, all crafted into an easy-to-use, timely, and effective solution for EMT training.

The following Walkthrough outlines the features found in each chapter and provides information for each of *EMT Complete*'s student and instructor supplements. Also, we introduce several related products that can be used to make your program the best it can be.

Our mission and message remain simple: We're your partner for life. We remain as committed to EMS publishing as we did when we began over 30 years ago. We have helped millions of providers save the lives of millions more. With this privilege comes responsibility—a responsibility to continue to innovate and create solutions that make all of us better at what we do. We hope you'll allow us to do so for many years to come.

Sincerely,

Julie Levin Alexander
VP/Publisher

Katrin Beacom
Executive Marketing Manager

Marlene McHugh Pratt
Executive Editor

Thomas Kennally
National Sales Manager

Lois Berlowitz
Senior Managing Editor

Matthew Sirinides
Assistant Editor

✳ A Guide to Key Features

CHAPTER OBJECTIVES ▶

Divided into Cognitive, Affective, and Psychomotor sections, objectives correspond to their individual DOT numbers and the text pages on which they appear.

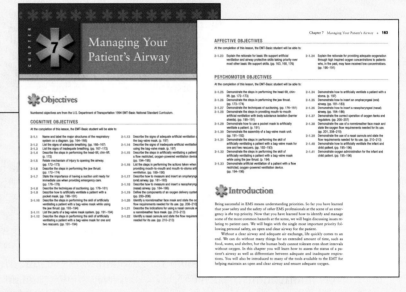

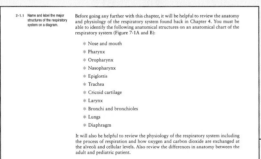

◀ RUNNING OBJECTIVES

Objectives are repeated next to the text in which they're first covered.

EMERGENCY DISPATCH ▶

Each chapter begins with a dispatch describing the scenario that will be followed throughout the chapter's *Perspectives*.

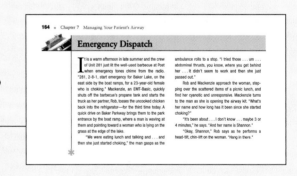

Perspective

Shannon—The Patient

"I woke up with a mask on my face and I was being forced to breathe. It was a totally unnatural feeling . . . and a pretty frightening one! I can remember taking a bite of my sandwich and laughing, and then suddenly I couldn't get a breath. I've never been so scared in my life! I was looking at my boyfriend and trying so hard to breathe. I really thought that I was going to die."

◀ PERSPECTIVE

Points of view from people on the scene, whether it be the EMT, the EMT's partner, the patient, other rescuers, bystanders, family members, or the ER doctor. These show the reader what may be going on in the minds of all participants at a call. This helps him to get a greater understanding of his impact on the scene overall, making for better patient care.

STOP, REVIEW, REMEMBER! ▶

The "work" part of the Worktext, these are integrated throughout chapters. They stop at several key places, enabling readers to instantly assess their learning before going on. Write-in multiple choice, fill in the blank, matching, and critical thinking questions provide readers with immediate feedback.

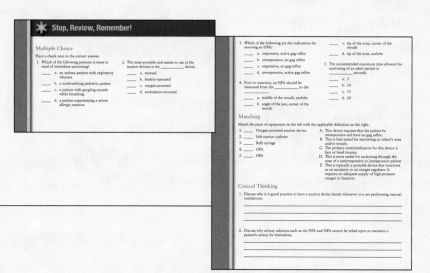

THE USE OF AIRWAY ADJUNCTS

EMTs have two mechanical devices (airway adjuncts) they can use to assist in maintaining a patent airway. They are the **oropharyngeal airway**, sometimes referred to as the "oral" airway or OPA, and the **nasopharyngeal airway**, commonly referred to as the "nasal" airway or NPA. It must be clearly understood that both of these devices only *assist* the EMT in maintaining a patent airway. Simply placing either device does not ensure a patent airway. These devices should be used in conjunction with good airway management techniques, such as continuous monitoring for adequate chest rise and fall, head-tilt, chin-lift, and jaw-thrust maneuvers, and appropriate suctioning when indicated.

* **oropharyngeal airway**
  a curved device inserted into the patient's mouth and the pharynx to help maintain an open airway.

* **nasopharyngeal airway**
  a soft flexible breathing tube inserted through the patient's nose into the pharynx to help maintain an open airway.

◀ RUNNING GLOSSARY

Definitions for key terms are provided in margins, next to the text in which they're first introduced.

CLINICAL CLUES ▶

These provide need-to-know information regarding contraindications, criteria, safety, tips, etc.—things that will help the practitioner make decisions in the field.

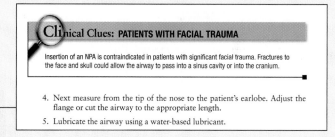

Clinical Clues: PATIENTS WITH FACIAL TRAUMA

Insertion of an NPA is contraindicated in patients with significant facial trauma. Fractures to the face and skull could allow the airway to pass into a sinus cavity or into the cranium.

4. Next measure from the tip of the nose to the patient's earlobe. Adjust the flange or cut the airway to the appropriate length.
5. Lubricate the airway using a water-based lubricant.

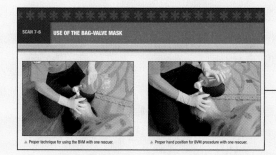

SCAN 7-6   **USE OF THE BAG-VALVE MASK**

▲ Proper technique for using the BVM with one rescuer.   ▲ Proper hand position for BVM procedure with one rescuer.

◀ SCANS

Procedures performed step by step with explanations and photographs.

DISPATCH SUMMARY ▶

Completion of the call that began at the beginning of the chapter. This allows the reader to see resolution and follow-up care, as appropriate.

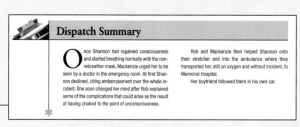

Dispatch Summary

Once Shannon had regained consciousness and started breathing normally with the non-rebreather mask, Mackenzie urged her to be seen by a doctor in the emergency room. At first Shannon declined, citing embarrassment over the whole incident. She soon changed her mind after Rob explained some of the complications that could arise as the result of having choked to the point of unconsciousness.

Rob and Mackenzie then helped Shannon onto their stretcher and into the ambulance where they transported her, still on oxygen and without incident, to Memorial Hospital.

Her boyfriend followed them in his own car.

THE LAST WORD ▶

A summary of the important points learned in each chapter.

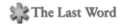

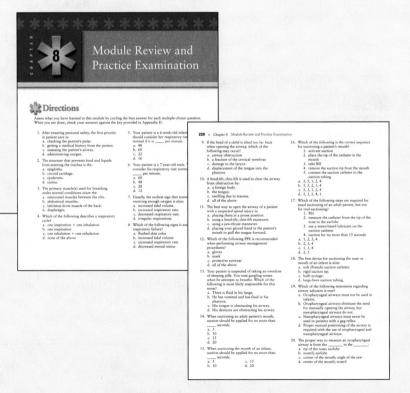

◀ CHAPTER REVIEW

Each chapter ends with a review containing multiple choice, labeling, and critical thinking questions and case studies.

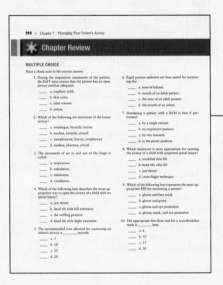

MODULE REVIEW AND PRACTICE EXAMINATION ▶

After each of eight modules, a test is provided to ensure that learning is cumulative throughout the text.

✳ Student CDs

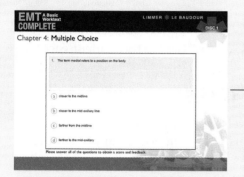

◀ MULTIPLE CHOICE QUESTIONS

Each chapter offers self-testing in a multiple choice format. Upon completion, a score and feedback are provided for post-assessment.

ANIMATIONS ▶

Newly created 3D, animated movies offer a deeper understanding and graphical view of difficult concepts and procedures.

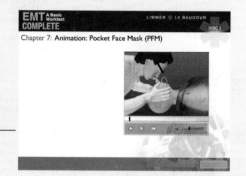

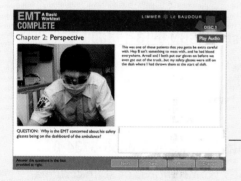

◀ PERSPECTIVES

An extension of the Perspectives found in the book, text and audio exercises ask you to comment on how you would handle certain thoughts and concerns on scene. "Expert" answers appear.

RESUME BUILDER ▶

This easy-to-use program helps you to create professional resumes and supporting documents. Includes four different resume styles, cover letters, reference lists, post interview letters, and much more!

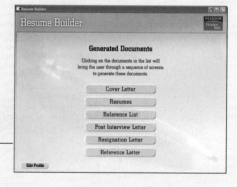

◀ HAZMAT EXERCISE

This interactive exercise aids in the quick and accurate identification of Hazmat placards. Use the binoculars to get a closer look, reference the associated Hazmat manual pages and NFPA placard document, answer the questions, and see how you do.

✳ Resources, Review, and Reference

Companion Website

Free site offering additional assessment, links, and resources for student success.

Active Learning Manual ISBN 0-13-113629-1

Go beyond the text and get active! The *Active Learning Manual* reinforces classroom presentations, allowing you to approach material in a hands-on manner.

Audio Lecture & Study Guide: EMT-B ISBN 0-13-177713-0

This new resource enables you to study and review anytime, anywhere. It supports the core concepts learned in class in an engaging, easy-to-use format. Top EMS authors and instructors present material in a consistent, relevant, and entertaining style.

EMT Achieve: Basic Test Preparation ISBN 0-13-113609-7

This online test preparation program allows you to practice taking national- and state-type tests and quizzes. Rationale and remediation is included. Check it out at www.prenhall.com/emtachieve.

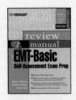

EMT-Basic Self-Assessment Exam Prep ISBN 0-8359-5134-0

This is the resource to help you pass your national or state certification exam. All items are written and reviewed by educators and offer proven, authoritative information. In-book CD contains practice tests.

EMT-B National Standards Self-Test, 3rd Ed. ISBN 0-13-170787-6

This is the highly motivated EMT's ultimate tool for test preparation. Based on the EMT-B National Standard Curriculum, it uses the self-test format to target the areas you need to study further and contains a section on preparing for any practical exam.

Basic Life Support Skills ISBN 0-13-193865-3

This highly visual manual guides you through 50 practical skills in detail. Step-by-step procedures are shown in full-color and are accompanied by rationales. This accessible, easy-to-follow format helps you understand what, how, and why each skill is performed.

BLS Skills Review CD ISBN 0-13-152965-X

More than 150 minutes of video show 50 skills close-up, step-by-step for thorough review, so that you can see exactly how skills should be performed. A companion to the *Basic Life Support Skills* text, this powerful package is all you need to study for your practical exam.

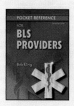

Pocket Reference for the BLS Providers, 3rd Ed. ISBN 0-13-173730-9

This handy field reference is on water-resistant paper and includes skills checklists, common medications, abbreviations and acronyms, anatomy charts, and much more.

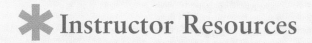

❋ Instructor Resources

Instructor's Resource Manual ISBN 0-13-226974-0

This important resource helps instructors utilize and integrate *EMT Complete* to its best effect. Features include more than 200 handouts, objectives checklists, chapter quizzes, scenarios, and unique exercises such as "Changing Shoes," which correlate to each chapter's Perspectives; "Hit the Street" role-playing exercises; and "Keeping It in Perspective"—designed to enhance understanding by applying and extending concepts to real people and situations.

PowerPoint Presentation ISBN 0-13-173955-7

2,500 customizable slides for classroom presentation.

TestGen Program ISBN 0-13-221884-4

Contains 800 multiple-choice and scenario-based questions to prepare students for their national or state exams.

Instructor's Resource CD ISBN 0-13-119267-1

CD package containing all instructor resources, including all text images and Word and PDF downloads for the Instructor's Resource Manual.

EMT COMPLETE
A Basic Worktext

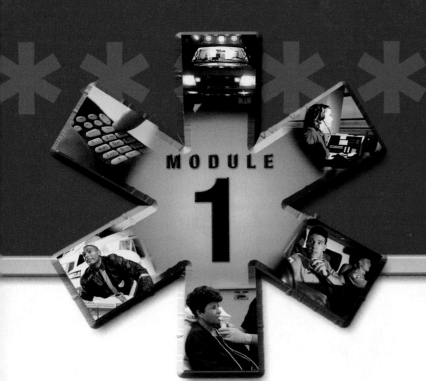

MODULE

1

Introductory Module

> "I just couldn't seem to get anyone to understand me. My right hip and shoulder were pretty sore, but when I tried to tell the ambulance people the words were coming out all wrong. I just wanted someone to help and to find out what was wrong with me."

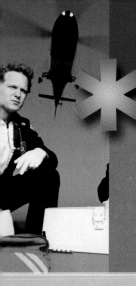

Module Outline

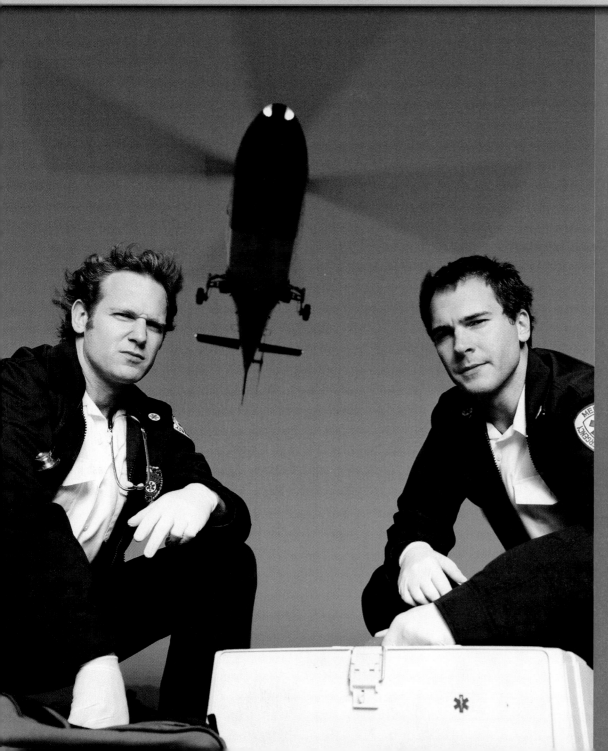

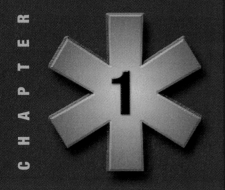

You and the EMS System

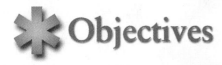

Objectives

Numbered objectives are from the U.S. Department of Transportation 1994 EMT-Basic National Standard Curriculum.

COGNITIVE OBJECTIVES

At the completion of this lesson, the EMT-Basic student will be able to:

1-1.1 Define Emergency Medical Services (EMS) systems. (pp. 9–12)

1-1.2 Differentiate the roles and responsibilities of the EMT-Basic from other prehospital care providers. (pp. 12–13)

1-1.3 Describe the roles and responsibilities related to personal safety. (p. 18)

1-1.4 Discuss the roles and responsibilities of the EMT-Basic towards the safety of the crew, the patient, and bystanders. (pp. 18–20)

1-1.5 Define quality improvement and discuss the EMT-Basic's role in the process. (p. 20)

1-1.6 Define medical direction and discuss the EMT-Basic's role in the process. (pp. 16–18)

1-1.7 State the specific statutes and regulations in your state regarding the EMS system. (p. 20)

AFFECTIVE OBJECTIVES

At the completion of this lesson, the EMT-Basic student will be able to:

1-1.8 Assess areas of personal attitude and conduct of the EMT-Basic. (p. 20)

1-1.9 Characterize the various methods used to access the EMS system in your community. (p. 20)

PSYCHOMOTOR OBJECTIVES

No psychomotor objectives identified.

✳ Introduction

Congratulations on your decision to enter the world of EMS and become an Emergency Medical Technician. Whether this is a choice you made all on your own or one that someone else made for you, becoming an EMT will provide you with knowledge and skills that will carry over into all aspects of your life for many years to come. Not everyone who takes this course intends on working on an ambulance or in an emergency department at a local hospital. Some of you might be taking this course because you will be working as a camp counselor, lifeguard, firefighter, or perhaps a police officer. What is common to everyone who learns the skills of an EMT is that they are willing to serve those in need. Albert Schweitzer once said, *"One thing I know: The only ones among you who will be really happy are those who will have sought and found how to serve."* Serving others in their time of need is an honor, a privilege, and not something everyone desires to do.

Make no mistake, making decisions about another person's care during a sudden illness or injury can be very stressful and sometimes may even involve life-and-death decisions. Your choice to take this course and become a part of the team of people who are called to assist an ill or injured person brings with it great responsibility. With that responsibility also come great rewards including the opportunity to save a life.

This chapter will introduce you to the evolution of the modern-day Emergency Medical Services (EMS) system and the many components that work together to ensure a safer world for all of us.

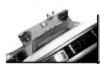

Emergency Dispatch

"**D**addy, why is there a fire truck out front?"

Mark Bennett stopped trying to find his daughter Amy's favorite Dr. Seuss bedtime book and joined her at the window. A large red fire truck was parked across the street, its emergency strobe lights flashing rhythmically, bouncing off the houses up and down the street.

"It's at Hansons' house." Mark's son, Jared, was now at the window next to them.

"Well, I don't see any signs of a fire," Mark said, peering into the dark evening sky. "I'm sure everything is okay."

Just then, several sirens screamed into range and rapidly grew louder. More emergency lights careened around the neighborhood as an ambulance and a police car joined the fire truck over at the Hansons'.

The Evolution of Modern EMS

Illness and injury have existed since the dawn of humankind. What has not always existed is an organized and efficient means of caring for those illnesses and injuries. Our ability to care for one another has evolved slowly over many thousands of years and began with simple care provided by those closest to the ill or injured person. Family members provided shelter and necessities such as warmth, food, and water to the person who needed care. This simple care would be given until the injury healed or the illness ran its course. There was little if any care that directly affected the specific illness or injury.

Through trial and error certain individuals became especially skilled at caring for others. Eventually, either an ill or injured person would be taken to one of these skilled people or the skilled caregiver would be brought to the patient. These early caregivers were the forerunners of our modern medical professionals, including EMTs. Much of the emergency medical experience throughout history was gained during wars (Figure 1-1A and B). For example, early Greeks and Romans would transport the injured by chariot from the battlefield to waiting physicians.

The first formal ambulance system in the United States was developed during the Civil War when the Union army began training soldiers to provide first aid to the wounded on the battlefield. These "corpsmen" were trained to care for the most immediate life threats, such as bleeding. After initial care, the injured were transported by horse-drawn wagon to waiting physicians.

At the turn of the twentieth century, the few ambulance services that existed were mostly operated by hospitals and staffed by medical interns. Those who drove the vehicles had little or no formal training and generally did not assist with medical care. It was around 1909 when the American Red Cross began offering first-aid classes to the general public. In 1928 Julian Stanley Wise founded the nation's first official rescue squad, the Roanoke Life Saving and First Aid Crew (Figure 1-2). Mr. Wise dedicated much of his life to spreading the concept of the volunteer rescue squad around the nation and is credited with starting the first-aid and rescue movement in the United States.

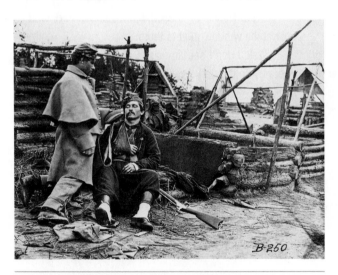

FIGURE 1-1A Wars and battles played an early role in the development of modern emergency medical services. The American Civil War. (National Archives and Records Administration) (Bettmann/CORBIS.)

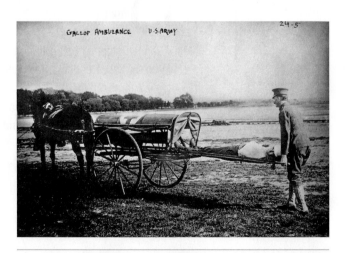

FIGURE 1-1B World War I. (© CORBIS.)

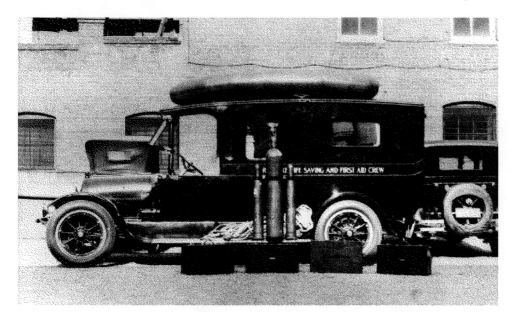

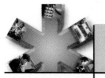

Perspective

Pat Hanson—The Patient's Wife

"Oh my heavens! A fire truck, the police, and the ambulance? I just don't get why so many people showed up. I only called 9-1-1 because Bill fell and cut his head real good. You would've thought that we were gettin' invaded or something! They probably woke up the whole darn neighborhood. And now what'll everyone think? I can just hear it now, 'Did you see that police car over at Pat's house? I wonder what's really going on over there?' This was all so embarrassing!"

While the rescue-squad and first-aid movement gained momentum, little emphasis was placed on training the rescuers. Their primary job was to reach the patients as quickly as possible and return them to the hospital for care. In fact, many funeral home vehicles doubled as ambulances during this time.

It was not until the late 1950s and early '60s that an emphasis on improving prehospital care began. It was during this period that oxygen made its first appearance on ambulances, and cardiopulmonary resuscitation (CPR) was introduced as a life-saving measure. In 1966 the National Academy of Sciences published a report titled *Accidental Death and Disability: The Neglected Disease of Modern Society.* This report detailed many weaknesses in the nation's ability to prevent and manage injuries from accidents. In the prior year, nearly 50,000 Americans had died on the nation's roads and highways, more casualties than occurred during the entire 8 years of the Vietnam War. The report also offered many recommendations, including standards for ambulance construction and the preparation of nationally accepted texts and training programs for fire, police, and ambulance personnel. That same year Congress passed the Highway Safety Act, which led to the formation of the National Highway Traffic Safety Administration

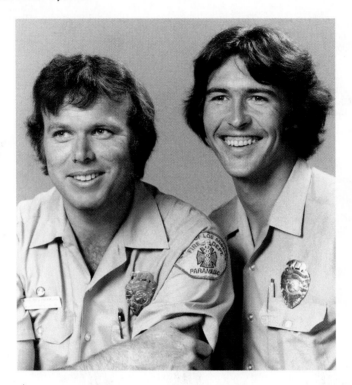

FIGURE 1-3 The television series *Emergency* created an awareness of paramedic programs. (Kobal Collection NBC/TV.)

(NHTSA). NHTSA has since helped many communities plant the seeds of their own coordinated EMS programs.

In 1972 the television series *Emergency* made the word *paramedic* a household term. Based on the real-life paramedic program started in Los Angeles, California, in 1969, the television program created an awareness and demand that is credited in great part with the rapid increase in paramedic programs across the nation (Figure 1-3). In 1973 Congress passed the Emergency Medical Services Systems (EMSS) Act, which provided federal funding for the establishment of EMS systems all across the nation. The Department of Transportation developed training and equipment standards for EMS personnel, and state EMS offices began to spring up around the country.

The 1980s and '90s saw the formation of several national organizations such as the National Association of State EMS Directors and the National Association of EMS Physicians. These organizations were formed to develop and improve EMS systems throughout the nation. Similarly, the National Association of EMS Educators was formed to enhance the quality and content of EMS education on a national level. The '90s also saw the further development of EMS education with the revision of the DOT national standard curricula for all levels of prehospital care. In 1996 the *EMS Agenda for the Future* was released, creating for the first time a vision for EMS that industry leaders, educators, and field personnel could embrace.

WHAT DOES THE FUTURE HOLD?

A specialized task force led by the National Association of State EMS Directors and the National Council of State EMS Training Coordinators has been tasked with redefining *The National Scope of Practice Model*. The purpose of the task force is to look closely at our current national EMS model and make suggestions for change that will reflect the future of EMS in the United States and how EMS systems can best meet the needs of the populations we serve. *The National Scope of Practice Model,* as it has been revised, represents the integration of health services and the second of five steps outlined by the *EMS Agenda for the Future.*

The Vision of EMS as Written in the EMS Agenda for the Future

Emergency medical services (EMS) of the future will be community-based health management that is fully integrated with the overall health care system. It will have the ability to identify and modify illness and injury risks, provide acute illness and injury care and follow-up, and contribute to treatment of chronic conditions and community health monitoring. This new entity will be developed from redistribution of existing health care resources and will be integrated with other health care providers and public health and public safety agencies. It will improve community health and result in more appropriate use of acute health care resources. EMS will remain the public's emergency medical safety net. To learn more about the EMS Agenda for the Future, go to: http://www.nhtsa.dot.gov/people/injury/ems/agenda/emsman.html. To reach the National Scope of Practice Model, go to http://emsscopeofpractice.org/

By completing this EMT course, you are about to become a vital part of the EMS of the future.

A Systematic Approach to Saving Lives

You may have heard it before and will likely hear it again and again throughout your training as an EMT: Injury is the leading cause of death in the United States for persons age 1 to 35. It is also the most common cause of hospitalizations for persons under the age of 40. Each year approximately 40,000 people lose their lives on the nation's roads with approximately 56 percent of those deaths occurring on rural highways.

The cost of these deaths to society is staggering in hard dollars as well as in the emotional suffering that families who have lost a loved one must endure. The federal agency charged with reducing accidental injury and deaths on the nation's highways is the National Highway Traffic Safety Administration (NHTSA), which was formed out of the Highway Safety Act revision of 1970. Among its many programs are the EMS Technical Assistance Program and the development of the National Standard Curricula for all four levels of EMS providers. The four levels of EMS providers will be discussed further later in this chapter.

An **Emergency Medical Services (EMS)** system is a highly specialized chain of resources designed to minimize the impact of sudden injury and illness on our society. Figure 1-4A–G on pages 10–11 shows how this chain can work.

To make best use of its limited resources, NHTSA's EMS Technical Assistance Program focuses on helping individual states with the development and evaluation of their emergency medical services. NHTSA has also identified ten key components of an integrated EMS system and assists states in developing and assessing these components. The ten components are listed below along with a brief description of each (Figure 1-5 on page 11):

* **Regulation and policy**—To provide a high-quality, effective system of emergency medical care, each state must have in place legislation that identifies and supports a lead EMS agency. This agency has the authority to plan and implement an effective EMS system and to create appropriate rules and regulations for each recognized component of the EMS system.

* **Resource management**—Each state must have in place a centralized method to coordinate all system resources.

1-1.1 Define Emergency Medical Services (EMS) systems.

* **Emergency Medical Services (EMS)**

a highly specialized chain of resources designed to minimize the impact of sudden injury and illness on our society.

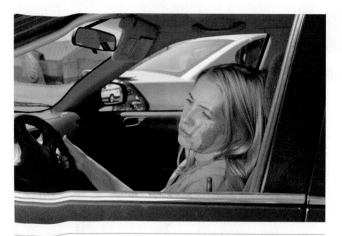

FIGURE 1-4A Emergency Medical Services (EMS) is made up of a highly specialized chain of resources. A crash scene.

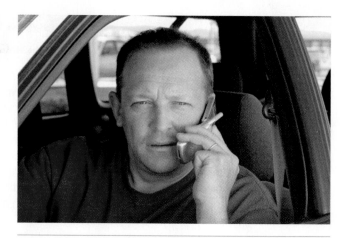

FIGURE 1-4B A citizen calls 9-1-1.

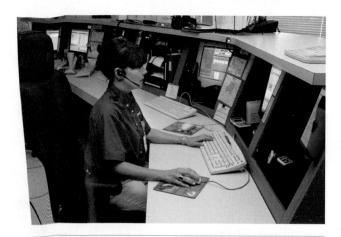

FIGURE 1-4C The Emergency Medical Dispatcher allocates resources. (© 2005 Scott Metcalfe LLC. All Rights Reserved.)

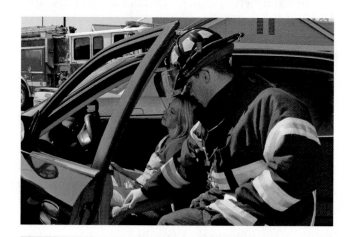

FIGURE 1-4D A First Responder (Emergency Responder) assists the patient.

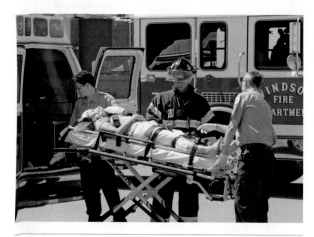

FIGURE 1-4E EMTs continue treatment en route to the hospital.

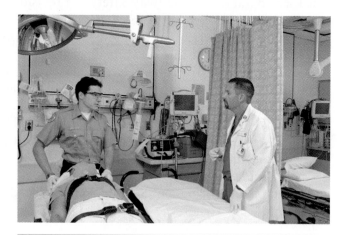

FIGURE 1-4F The patient is transferred to the care of Emergency Department personnel.

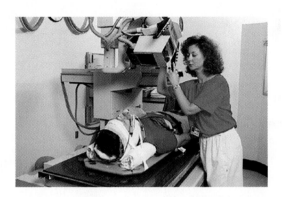

FIGURE 1-4G The continuum of care continues at the hospital.

The National Highway Traffic Safety Administration's
Ten standards for EMS system

1. Regulation and policy	6. Communication
2. Resource management	7. Public information and education
3. Human resources and training	8. Medical direction
4. Transportation	9. Trauma systems
5. Facilities	10. Evaluation

FIGURE 1-5 NHTSA has identified ten key components of an integrated EMS system.

* **Human resources and training**—The lead state EMS agency must have a mechanism to assess current human resource needs and establish a comprehensive plan for stable and consistent EMS training programs. EMS training programs and instructors must be routinely monitored to ensure that instructors meet certain requirements, the curriculum is standardized throughout the state, and valid and reliable testing procedures are utilized.

* **Transportation**—Each state must have a comprehensive transportation plan that includes provisions for uniform coverage, including a protocol for air medical dispatch and a mutual aid plan.

* **Facilities**—It is imperative that the seriously ill patient be delivered in a timely manner to the closest appropriate facility. The lead agency must have a system for categorizing the functional capabilities of all individual health care facilities that receive patients from the out-of-hospital emergency medical care setting.

* **Communications**—The lead agency in each state is responsible for the central coordination of EMS communications. The public must be able to access the EMS system with a single, universal emergency phone number, such as 9-1-1, and the communications system must provide for prioritized dispatch.

* **Public information and education**—Each state must develop and implement an EMS public information and education (PI&E) program. The PI&E component of the state EMS plan ensures that consistent, structured PI&E programs are in place that enhance the public's knowledge of the EMS system, support appropriate EMS system access, demonstrate essential self-help and appropriate bystander care actions, and encourage injury prevention.

* **Medical Direction**—Each state must ensure that physicians are involved in all aspects of the patient care system. The role of the EMS **Medical Director** must be clearly defined, with legislative authority and responsibility for EMS system standards, protocols, and evaluation of patient care. A

* **Medical Director**

a physician who assumes ultimate responsibility for the patient care aspects of the EMS system.

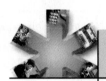

Perspective

Mark—The Neighbor

"I was wondering if I should call over to the Hansons' and ask if there was anything that I could do. I mean, with all of those cops, firemen and stuff, it had to be pretty major. And speaking of the cops . . . don't they only show up if there's a crime? I really hope everything's okay with Pat and Bill."

comprehensive system of medical direction for all out-of-hospital emergency medical care providers must be utilized to evaluate the provision of medical care as it relates to patient outcome, appropriateness of training programs, and medical direction.

✳ **Trauma systems**—To provide a high-quality, effective system of trauma care, each state must have trauma care components that are clearly integrated with the overall EMS system. Legislation should be in place for the development and implementation of the trauma care component of the EMS system. This should include trauma center designation, triage and transfer guidelines for trauma patients, data collection and trauma registry definitions and mechanisms, mandatory autopsies, and quality improvement for trauma patients. In many systems, it is the EMT who determines which patients go to which hospitals by following local policies and protocols.

✳ **Evaluation**—Each state EMS system is responsible for evaluating the effectiveness of services provided to victims of medical or trauma emergencies. A uniform, statewide data-collection system must exist to capture the minimum data necessary to measure compliance with standards. It must also ensure that data are consistently and routinely provided to the lead agency by all EMS providers and that the lead agency performs routine analysis of this data. Your participation in the evaluation process will help drive the improvement of the EMS system and the care that patients receive.

In addition to complying with the ten components just listed, many states are also implementing and evaluating their own disaster systems in order to be better prepared to respond to large-scale events within their borders.

1-1.2 Differentiate the roles and responsibilities of the EMT-Basic from other prehospital care providers.

NATIONAL LEVELS OF EMS TRAINING

At the present time there are four nationally recognized levels of care as defined by the Department of Transportation (DOT), the parent agency for NHTSA. As part of the redefinition of *The National Scope of Practice Model* mentioned earlier, these four levels of care are currently undergoing a detailed review and may emerge at some future date with different names and duties (Figure 1-6). For example, the term First Responder will become Emergency Responder. In addition, many states have further divided these four levels of training to meet the unique and specific needs of their systems. We will not attempt to describe all of these differences, but we want you to be aware of their existence. Each of the following four levels of training is supported by a document known as the National Stan-

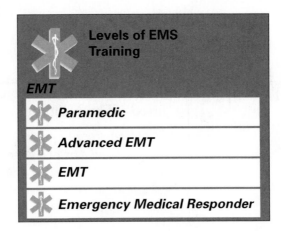

FIGURE 1-6 The four levels of training in EMS are First Responder, EMT-Basic, EMT-Intermediate, and EMT-Paramedic.

* **Emergency Medical Responder, formerly First Responder**

  this level of training is designed for the person who is often first at the scene. The emphasis is on activating the EMS system and providing immediate care for life-threatening injuries or illnesses, controlling the scene, and preparing for the arrival of the ambulance.

* **Emergency Medical Technician, formerly EMT-Basic**

  the curriculum for the EMT deals with the assessment and care of the ill or injured patient and in most areas is considered the minimum level of certification for ambulance personnel. Certification as an EMT requires successful completion of a state approved EMT Training Program or its equivalent and approval by a state EMS program or other authorizing agency.

* **Advanced EMT, formerly EMT-Intermediate**

  this level of EMT has completed additional training in order to provide a minimum level of advanced life support, such as the initiation of intravenous (IV) lines, advanced airway techniques, and administration of some medications beyond those the EMT is permitted to administer.

* **Paramedic, formerly EMT-Paramedic**

  the paramedic receives significant additional training in advanced life support procedures. Paramedics are trained to perform invasive procedures such as the insertion of endotracheal tubes, initiation of IV lines, administration of a variety of medications, interpretation of electrocardiograms, and cardiac defibrillation.

dard Curriculum (NSC). Each level of training has its own curriculum, which defines the scope of practice for each level of care. The concept of scope of practice will be discussed more in Chapter 3.

* **Emergency Medical Responder**—This is the most basic level of nationally recognized care and the NSC for this level represents approximately 40 hours of training. **Emergency Medical Responders** are most often the first people on the scene of an emergency and are trained to identify potential hazards, identify and treat immediate life threats, and assist other EMS personnel at the scene. Emergency Mecical Responders are trained to function with a minimum of equipment.

* **Emergency Medical Technician**—The NSC for the **EMT** represents approximately 110 hours of training and in nearly all areas of the United States is the minimum level of training for someone providing care on an ambulance. The EMT receives training in the assessment and care of many of the most common injuries and illnesses and will provide care for patients while at the scene and during transport to an appropriate receiving facility. The level of care provided by EMTs is known as Basic Life Support or BLS.

* **Advanced EMT**—The NSC for the **Advanced EMT** represents between 300 and 400 hours of instruction and is the first level that is referred to as Advanced Life Support or ALS. In addition to all the BLS skills of an EMT, the Intermediate can administer certain medications, start intravenous lines, interpret and shock specific heart rhythms, and provide more advanced airway management.

* **Paramedic**—The NSC for the Paramedic level of training represents between 1,000 and 1,200 hours and is currently the most advanced level of nationally recognized EMS care. Performing ALS skills in addition to BLS skills, the **Paramedic** can administer a wide variety of medications, initiate intravenous lines, interpret and shock specific heart rhythms, insert advanced airway devices and perform a variety of other advanced procedures.

In most EMS systems around the country it is common to find two or more of these levels of providers working closely together. A typical system will have firefighters trained as First Responders arriving first at the scene, followed closely behind by an ambulance staffed with an EMT and a paramedic. Regardless of your level of training, you must remember that you are an important link in the EMS chain.

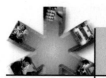

Perspective

Jared—The Neighbor's Child

"It's really scary when those lights are flashing everywhere. Everything turns red and blue and it looks like the people are moving in slow motion. It can probably give you a headache if you watch too long. I could see our neighbors all up and down the street looking out their windows. I don't ever want the police and firemen to come to our house!"

Stop, Review, Remember!

Multiple Choice

Place a check next to the correct answer.

1. This is one of the 10 essential elements of an EMS system and deals specifically with the creation of appropriate rules and regulations for each recognized component of the EMS system.

   _____ a. communication

   _____ b. regulation and policy

   _____ c. human resources

   _____ d. evaluation

2. Which of the following essential components of an EMS system deals with categorizing the functional capabilities of all individual health care facilities?

   _____ a. trauma systems

   _____ b. evaluation

   _____ c. facilities

   _____ d. human resources

3. Which of the following levels of care is considered Basic Life Support (BLS)?

   _____ a. Advanced Practice Paramedic

   _____ b. Paramedic

   _____ c. Advanced EMT

   _____ d. EMT

Fill in the Blank

1. Using a minimal amount of equipment, the _____ must identify and care for immediate life threats and assist other EMS personnel.

2. The _____ is responsible for developing the standards for each level of training.

3. An _____ is a highly specialized chain of resources designed to minimize the impact of sudden injury and illness on our society.

4. The _____ receives training at the BLS level on the assessment and care of patients while at the scene and during transport.

5. _____ has identified ten key components of an integrated EMS system and assists states in developing and assessing these components.

Critical Thinking

The following questions are designed to help develop your awareness and understanding of the EMS system where you live or plan on working:

1. Identify and list as many components as you can that make up the EMS system where you live or plan to work.

   _____

   _____

   _____

   _____

2. What is the fundamental difference between the First Responder level of training and the three other levels?

   _____

   _____

   _____

   _____

3. To what level are firefighters and law enforcement personnel trained in your system?

   _____

   _____

   _____

EMS and the Health Care System

The EMS system is just one small component of a much larger health care system designed to manage and care for patients over a longer period of time. Can you imagine an EMS system without hospitals or emergency rooms? We would just drive the ambulance around with our patients until they either got better or died and we delivered them to a mortuary. Fortunately that is not the case, and the EMS system is able to deliver patients to appropriate facilities staffed with skilled professionals who can continue to deliver the care they need.

Our health care system is constantly becoming more specialized, and many of our larger metropolitan areas now have hospitals with personnel specifically trained and equipped to manage such things as major trauma, burns, pediatric emergencies, and spinal-cord injuries.

MEDICAL DIRECTION

1-1.6 Define medical direction and discuss the EMT-Basic's role in the process.

✳ **Medical Direction**
oversight of the patient-care aspects of an EMS system by the Medical Director.

✳ **protocols**
written guidelines or treatment plans for patient care to help the EMT provide the most appropriate care. Protocols are approved by the Medical Director of an EMS system.

One of the ten essential components of an EMS system and certainly one that is vital to quality patient care is **Medical Direction.** Simply stated, Medical Direction is the oversight of all patient care aspects of an EMS system by the physician designated as the Medical Director (Figure 1-7).

As an EMT you will be acting as an "agent" of the Medical Director while you are caring for patients in the prehospital setting. You will have completed a training program and must follow written guidelines or **protocols** that have been approved by the Medical Director. Protocols are written guidelines or treatment plans for patient care that help the EMT provide the most appropriate care for the patient. In essence, you are providing care under the authority of the physician Medical Director, and the extent and nature of this authority can vary from state to state and region to region. In most EMS systems, EMTs rarely interact directly

FIGURE 1-7 Oversight of all aspects of patient care belongs to a designated physician called the Medical Director.

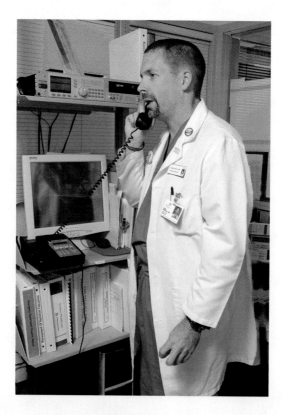

with the Medical Director but simply provide care based on written protocols or **standing orders.** Standing orders are written directives from the Medical Director that allow the EMT to provide specific types of treatment for certain patients without first contacting the Medical Director. For instance, an EMS system may have a standing order that allows EMTs to administer epinephrine for all patients presenting with a severe allergic reaction. These written protocols and standing orders guide the EMT and assist in determining how care should be delivered. They are referred to as **off-line medical direction** because there is no real-time direct interaction with the Medical Director. When an EMT must interact directly with medical direction, such as by radio or telephone regarding patient care, this is known as **on-line medical direction.** In on-line medical direction, the physician or his designee is providing real-time instructions regarding care for the patient. EMT-Intermediates and paramedics in many EMS systems routinely consult medical direction from the field because they often provide advanced care not covered by the system's protocols and standing orders.

In addition to establishing the minimum standards for patient care within their city, county, region, or state, Medical Directors are responsible for the continued quality assurance of their EMS systems.

ACCESS TO THE EMS SYSTEM

Accessing emergency services has not always been as easy as dialing 9-1-1. In fact it is only within the past 20 years that most 9-1-1 systems became operational around the country. It wasn't until 1999 that President Bill Clinton signed into law Senate Bill 800 designating 9-1-1 as the official nationwide emergency number (Figure 1-8). To this day, approximately 10 to 15 percent of the nation is not covered by 9-1-1 service and must access emergency services the old-fashioned way by dialing the appropriate seven-digit number.

The agencies responsible for answering 9-1-1 calls are referred to as **Public Safety Answering Points (PSAPs).** They are typically, but not always, law enforcement dispatch centers and are staffed 24/7 by trained emergency dispatchers. Like everything else in EMS, the training some of these dispatchers receive is evolving and becoming more and more specialized. A special designation of dispatcher is the **Emergency Medical Dispatcher** (EMD) who is trained to take calls for medical assistance, determine the most appropriate resources, and provide pre-arrival care instructions over the phone until EMS arrives.

The technology behind 9-1-1 systems continues to evolve and improve as well. Even today, there are two main types of 9-1-1 systems in place, standard and enhanced. The standard system is capable of routing all calls to the most appropriate

* **standing orders**

a written order issued by a Medical Director that authorizes EMTs and others to perform particular skills in certain situations without medical direction contact.

* **off-line medical direction**

consists of standing orders issued by the Medical Director that allow EMTs to give certain medications or perform certain procedures without speaking to the Medical Director or another physician.

* **on-line medical direction**

consists of orders from the on-duty physician or their designee given directly to an EMT in the field by radio or telephone.

* **Public Safety Answering Point (PSAP)**

the agency responsible for answering 9-1-1 calls.

* **Emergency Medical Dispatcher (EMD)**

specially trained dispatchers who not only obtain the appropriate information from callers but also provide medical instructions for emergency care, including instructions for CPR, artificial ventilation, bleeding control, and more.

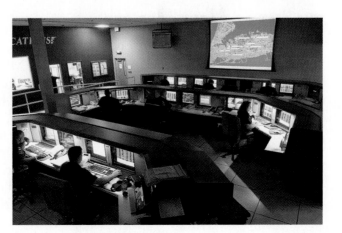

FIGURE 1-8   A 9-1-1 dispatch center.

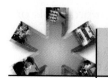

Perspective

Police Officer

"Man . . . that lady demanded to know why I showed up. She had called for an ambulance and, apparently, only wanted an ambulance. I tried to explain that in a lot of communities, fire crews and law enforcement show up to medical calls. Believe me! These calls can be so odd and unpredictable at times that it's a help to have a lot of people available! Plus, we're all in these professions because we want to help people out. That's all I was trying to do."

PSAP, where an emergency dispatcher must take the information from the caller. With the enhanced systems, the address and phone number of the caller are automatically displayed on the 9-1-1 terminal screen, making it less likely that information will be lost or errors made during the subsequent dispatch.

The introduction of the cell phone has created more problems than solutions for many of the busiest 9-1-1 systems around the country. In most areas of the country, cell phone calls are funneled through a central dispatch center, which often covers a large geographical area. This makes it difficult for dispatchers to accurately locate the caller and the emergency. In the not too distant future, a new technology will be able to route cell phone calls to the most appropriate PSAP, as with a standard (landline) telephone. Global positioning system (GPS) technology has also entered the cellular world and will soon allow 9-1-1 dispatchers to pinpoint a caller's exact location.

Roles and Responsibilities of the EMT

As an EMT, you will be required to fulfill many roles. Safety officer, patient care provider, quality assurance officer, patient advocate, and record keeper are just a few of the many hats an EMT is likely to wear. To be as effective as possible, you must have a basic understanding of each of these roles and the responsibilities that go along with it.

THE EMT AS SAFETY OFFICER

1-1.3 Describe the roles and responsibilities related to personal safety.

1-1.4 Discuss the roles and responsibilities of the EMT-Basic towards the safety of the crew, the patient, and bystanders.

The importance of safety in EMS cannot be overstated. To be able to do the job safely and effectively, every member of the EMS team must continually have safety in mind. It is not enough to ensure that the scene is safe for you personally; you must constantly be concerned for the safety of everyone else at the scene, including your team members, patients, and bystanders. Emergency scenes are dynamic, and the safety status of an emergency scene can change in an instant.

As an EMS professional, you have no obligation, legal or otherwise, to put yourself at unreasonable risk to assist someone who is ill or injured. Later in this course, you will learn some of the more common risks associated with managing emergency scenes and how best to minimize them.

THE EMT AS CARE PROVIDER

Providing appropriate emergency care promptly and effectively is the core of an EMT's job. You have a responsibility to provide the best care possible based on a thorough assessment of the patient. You are responsible for safely moving the patient from the scene to the ambulance and then transporting the patient to the most appropriate medical facility. Once at the hospital, you must transfer the care of the patient to the hospital staff by way of a detailed verbal report followed by a written report. You have a responsibility to be clear, concise, and as objective as possible to ensure that the patient continues to receive the best possible care.

THE EMT AS RECORD KEEPER

Everything you do and see pertaining to the care you provide must be accurately documented. You have a responsibility to document all details of every patient contact in an accurate and timely manner. These records serve many purposes, including data collection for statistical analysis and quality improvement, and may also serve as evidence in a court of law.

THE EMT AS PATIENT ADVOCATE

One of your most important roles as a member of the EMS team is that of patient advocate (Figure 1-9). To truly serve another person means to put their needs before your own, excluding personal safety. This means that you have a responsibility to see that your patients receive the best care possible, even if it interrupts your meals or wakes you during the night. Many patients are not immediately aware of their own needs and therefore must rely on you to make the right decision concerning their well-being. As an EMT you will see patients at their most vulnerable, frightened, and angry moments, when even the most "composed" person may behave irrationally or become incapable of making a rational decision. EMTs are often called upon to assist the patient in making appropriate choices regarding his immediate care and well-being.

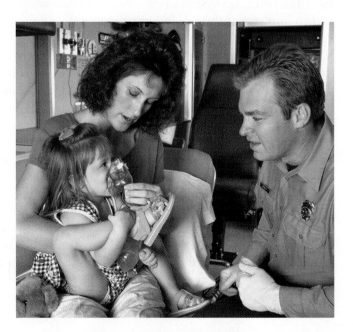

FIGURE 1-9   Reassuring the patient is part of patient advocacy. If at all possible, let a young child sit in the parent's lap during assessment and care. (During transport, the child should be in a car seat or immobilized to a backboard.)

FIGURE 1-10 As an EMT, you will interact with other public service agencies, such as the fire service and law enforcement.

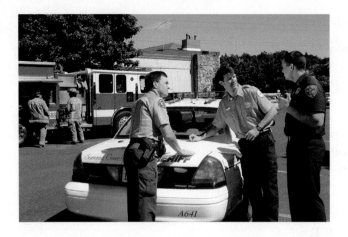

THE EMT AS AN EMS PROFESSIONAL

As an EMT, you are a highly visible symbol of the EMS profession and will be interacting with all aspects of your community. It is essential that you present in a professional manner at all times. You have a responsibility to your agency as well as to the profession to appear neat and well groomed at all times and maintain a caring and respectful attitude.

You will be interacting on a regular basis with the other professions related to public safety, law enforcement, and the fire service. It is important to remember that you are just one part of a larger public safety team and that you must consider yourself an ambassador for EMS when interacting with these other agencies (Figure 1-10).

Another responsibility of being an EMS professional means staying abreast of the most current laws and issues affecting your job as an EMT. You have a responsibility to maintain both your knowledge and skills relating to the job and attend all required training to maintain your certification or license to practice.

THE EMT AS QUALITY IMPROVEMENT OFFICER

1-1.5 Define quality improvement and discuss the EMT-Basic's role in the process.

✳ **Quality Improvement (QI)**

a process of continuous self-review with the purpose of identifying and correcting aspects of the system that require improvement.

Quality Improvement is a complex system of internal and external reviews of all aspects of an EMS system. It is designed to identify aspects that need improvement and to implement the needed improvements, all in an effort to assure that the public receives the highest quality prehospital care.

Each and every member of the EMS team plays an important role in the quality improvement process. By fulfilling your responsibility to maintain accurate documentation, attending formal reviews of recent calls, participating in the gathering of feedback from patients and other health care professionals, maintaining your equipment in top operating condition, attending required continuing education sessions and keeping up on less-frequently used skills, you will ensure the continued quality improvement of the system in which you work.

1-1.7 State the specific statutes and regulations in your state regarding the EMS system.

Knowing Your EMS System   As a member of the EMS team, you have a responsibility to learn and understand the unique qualities of the system in which you work. Your instructor will likely address specific aspects of your system, but you must not rely entirely on what you learn during your formal training. You must take responsibility for learning the laws, guidelines, and protocols that govern the functions of EMTs in your system. You must also take responsibility for learning all of the available resources within your system, such as specialty rescue teams, HazMat teams, air ambulances, and specialty hospitals.

Stop, Review, Remember!

Multiple Choice

Place a check next to the correct answer.

1. Which of the following is NOT a typical emergency specialty hospital?

   _____ a. trauma

   _____ b. neurosurgery

   _____ c. pediatrics

   _____ d. geriatrics

2. An EMS Medical Director must be a _____.

   _____ a. physician

   _____ b. trauma surgeon

   _____ c. former paramedic

   _____ d. registered nurse

3. Which of the following is the best example of 'off-line' medical direction?

   _____ a. orders given via radio

   _____ b. orders given via telephone

   _____ c. orders given via fax

   _____ d. written protocols

4. 9-1-1 dispatchers who are trained to provide pre-arrival instructions are referred to as _____ Dispatchers.

   _____ a. Pre-arrival

   _____ b. Emergency Medical

   _____ c. Advice

   _____ d. Advanced Directive

5. Maintaining accurate documentation, attending formal reviews of recent calls, attending required continuing education sessions, and keeping up on less-frequently used skills fall under which of the following EMT responsibilities?

   _____ a. safety

   _____ b. care provider

   _____ c. quality improvement

   _____ d. patient advocate

Matching

Match the description on the left with the applicable term on the right.

1. _____ The oversight of all patient care aspects of an EMS system by a specifically designated physician

2. _____ Written guidelines or treatment plans for patient care

3. _____ Written directives that allow the EMT to provide specific types of treatment for certain patients

4. _____ Medical direction involving no real time direct interaction with the Medical Director

5. _____ Agencies responsible for answering 9-1-1 calls

6. _____ Specially trained dispatchers who determine the most appropriate resources and provide pre-arrival care instructions over the phone until EMS arrives

A. Standing orders
B. Medical direction
C. Protocols
D. Emergency medical dispatchers
E. Public safety answering point (PSAP)
F. Off-line medical direction

Critical Thinking

1. What hospitals in your city, region, or state can you identify that have specific treatment specialties such as trauma, burns, or pediatrics?

   _____

   _____

   _____

   _____

2. Which of the responsibilities of the EMT mentioned previously do you feel might be the most difficult for you to learn, and why?

   _____

   _____

   _____

   _____

3. As an EMT there are specific requirements for you to maintain and renew your EMT license or certification. What are those requirements in your state or region?

   _____

   _____

   _____

   _____

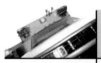

Dispatch Summary

The EMTs on scene controlled Bill's bleeding and bandaged his head before transporting him to the Glenfield Medical Center in Iverton. After 23 stitches and a series of tests, he was released home in good spirits.

Over the next several days, the Hansons' neighbors knocked on their door in ones and twos, asking if there was any way to be of help.

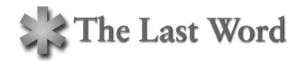

The Last Word

EMS systems have been evolving for many years and will continue to evolve for many more. Find a way that you can make a difference in each of the 10 core areas of your EMS system. Once you have been an EMT for awhile, seek to *learn* more about the next levels of providers such as Advanced EMT and Paramedics.

* Keep an open mind and always be willing to *learn*, even from those who you might think have less experience than you.

* *Learn* as much about your local EMS system as possible. Make a point to learn something new about it every day.

Chapter Review

MULTIPLE CHOICE

Place a check next to the correct answer.

1. Which of the following is NOT typically a component of an EMS system?

    _____ a. ground ambulances

    _____ b. dispatchers

    _____ c. air ambulances

    _____ d. doctors offices

2. Which of the following best describes an EMS system?

    _____ a. a specialized chain of resources designed to minimize the impact of sudden injury and illness

    _____ b. the communication systems that connect dispatchers with field personnel

    _____ c. the chain of resources contained within a major hospital

    _____ d. ambulance and emergency room personnel

3. Which of the following levels of EMT are able to start an IV on an ill or injured patient?

    _____ a. EMT

    _____ b. EMT and Paramedic

    _____ c. Advanced EMT and Paramedic

    _____ d. EMT and Advanced EMT

4. Which of the following is the EMT's primary role at the scene of any emergency?

    _____ a. patient care

    _____ b. safety

    _____ c. transportation

    _____ d. extrication

5. Which of the following best defines the term *quality improvement* as it pertains to the EMT?

    _____ a. lifelong learning

    _____ b. participation in continuing education

    _____ c. a complex system of internal and external reviews

    _____ d. the process of asking patients for feedback

6. The 10 standards for EMS systems as defined by NHTSA address all of the following EXCEPT:

_____ a. transportation and resource management.

_____ b. regulation and policy.

_____ c. communications.

_____ d. organ donor programs.

7. One whose training emphasizes care of immediate life threats and assisting other EMS providers is a(n):

_____ a. Emergency Medical Responder.

_____ b. EMT.

_____ c. Advanced EMT.

_____ d. Paramedic.

8. Which of the following is NOT a responsibility of an EMT?

_____ a. participation in quality improvement programs

_____ b. design of patient care protocols

_____ c. assuring the safety of the crew, bystanders, and patient

_____ d. consulting with medical direction

9. The EMT acts as an agent of the _____ when providing care in the prehospital setting.

_____ a. paramedic partner

_____ b. EMS Director

_____ c. Medical Director

_____ d. base station hospital

10. _____ are written guidelines or treatment plans for patient care.

_____ a. Advance directives

_____ b. Standing orders

_____ c. Online direction

_____ d. Protocols

MATCHING

Match the definition on the left with the applicable term on the right.

1. _____ Specially trained personnel who answer calls for help and provide pre-arrival instructions to callers

2. _____ Written protocols or directives from the Medical Director that allow the EMT to provide specific types of treatment for certain patients

3. _____ The complex system of internal and external reviews of all aspects of the EMS system to identify areas of weakness and recommend ways to improve

4. _____ The highest level of EMS training

5. _____ Written guidelines or treatment plans for patient care

A. Paramedic
B. Emergency Medical Dispatcher
C. Standing orders
D. Protocols
E. Quality Improvement

CRITICAL THINKING

1. Prioritize the 10 essential elements of an EMS system in order of importance, and be prepared to discuss your reasoning.

_____

_____

_____

2. As an EMT, how might you begin to play a part in the education of the public about what EMS is and how it functions?

_____

_____

_____

3. In what ways does the job of the EMT differ from that of the Emergency Medical Responder? How about from that of the Advanced EMT or Paramedic?

_____

_____

_____

4. List at least 4 types of specialty hospitals that might be available to receive patients on an emergency basis.

_____

_____

_____

5. Medical direction can exist in a variety of forms. List as many examples of medical direction as you can think of.

_____

_____

_____

6. What is the difference between a traditional dispatcher and one designated as an Emergency Medical Dispatcher (EMD)?

_____

_____

_____

CASE STUDIES

Case Study 1

You are an EMT with a local ambulance company and are working standby at the local fair when an obese woman in her 60s approaches you and asks that you help her with some blisters that have formed on her feet. You have her sit down at the first aid station and take a look. You see several good-size blisters on the sides and bottom of both feet. She asks that you please just pop them so that she can go about her way.

1. Since draining blisters is not within the scope of practice for an EMT, how will you respond to this woman's request?

   _____

   _____

   _____

   _____

2. If you were not sure how to appropriately care for this woman, who would you consult?

   _____

   _____

   _____

   _____

3. Why would it be important to carefully document any care that you might provide for this patient?

   _____

   _____

   _____

   _____

Case Study 2

It's 2100 hrs and you are in the ambulance on your way back to the station following mutual aid training at one of the local fire departments when you happen upon a two-car collision with injuries. The collision has occurred at a blind curve on a well-traveled two-lane highway. You and your partner are the first ones on scene.

1. What will be your primary concern at this scene?

   _____

   _____

   _____

   _____

2. What are the immediate hazards at this scene and how will you mitigate them?

_____

_____

_____

_____

3. Is it ethical to deal with safety issues before caring for the injured?

_____

_____

_____

_____

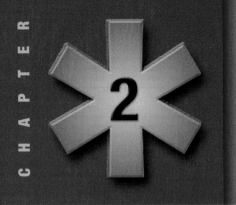

CHAPTER 2

Staying Safe
and Well in EMS

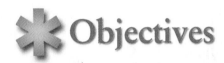

Objectives

Numbered objectives are from the U.S. Department of Transportation 1994 EMT-Basic National Standard Curriculum.

COGNITIVE OBJECTIVES

At the completion of this lesson, the EMT-Basic student will be able to:

1-2.1 List possible emotional reactions that the EMT-Basic may experience when faced with trauma, illness, death, and dying. (p. 32)

1-2.2 Discuss the possible reactions that a family member may exhibit when confronted with death and dying. (p. 39)

1-2.3 State the steps in the EMT-Basic's approach to the family confronted with death and dying. (pp. 39–41)

1-2.4 State the possible reactions that the family of the EMT-Basic may exhibit due to their outside involvement in EMS. (p. 31)

1-2.5 Recognize the signs and symptoms of critical incident stress. (pp. 32–33)

1-2.6 State possible steps that the EMT-Basic may take to help reduce/alleviate stress. (pp. 35–38)

1-2.7 Explain the need to determine scene safety. (p. 43)

1-2.8 Discuss the importance of body substance isolation (BSI). (p. 43)

1-2.9 Describe the steps the EMT-Basic should take for personal protection from airborne and bloodborne pathogens. (pp. 43–47)

1-2.10 List the personal protective equipment necessary for each of the following situations:
- Hazardous materials (pp. 48–49)
- Rescue operations (p. 49)
- Violent scenes (p. 50)
- Crime scenes (p. 50)

AFFECTIVE OBJECTIVES

At the completion of this lesson, the EMT-Basic student will be able to:

1-2.11 Explain the rationale for serving as an advocate for the use of appropriate protective equipment. (pp. 43–47)

PSYCHOMOTOR OBJECTIVES

At the completion of this lesson, the EMT-Basic student will be able to:

1-2.12   Given a scenario with potential infectious exposure, the EMT-Basic will use appropriate personal protective equipment. At the completion of the scenario, the EMT-Basic will properly remove and discard the protective garments. (pp. 48–49)

1-2.13   Given the above scenario, the EMT-Basic will complete disinfection/cleaning and all reporting documentation. (pp. 48–50)

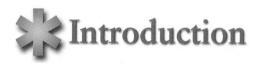 # Introduction

Responding to other people's emergencies can be both risky and stressful, regardless of your level of training or experience. Many lay persons are reluctant to receive even the most basic training in first aid and CPR because they fear that they will not be able to respond appropriately during a medical emergency. In short, people are afraid of making a mistake or making the wrong decision during an emergency. For most people, emergencies are few and far between, but for the EMT they are quite often a daily routine. The stress associated with the responsibility of responding to and caring for victims of all types of emergencies can be overwhelming. In addition, you will face many hazards when responding to emergency scenes, not the least of which is exposure to infectious disease. Without a thorough understanding of these risks and stressors and the mechanisms for minimizing their effects, you can quickly become overwhelmed or injured.

In this chapter we will discuss some of the more common stressors that the EMT faces as well as many of the hazards encountered in the prehospital setting. We will also discuss several methods for coping with job stress and ways for staying safe and minimizing exposure to risk while caring for victims of illness and injury.

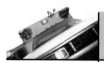

Emergency Dispatch

"**U**nit ninety-nine, headquarters." The dispatcher's voice exploded from the speakers, startling the two EMTs after almost five hours of absolute silence.

"Oh, my gosh, that scared me," Arnell grinned as he picked up the microphone. "Go ahead to ninety-nine."

"Ninety-nine, respond priority one to 2001 Wildwood Lane for an adult male vomiting blood."

"Ten-four, show us en route to 2001 Wildwood," Arnell took a deep breath and slid the ambulance into gear.

Several minutes later, Arnell and his partner, Jeff, were met at the front door by a sobbing woman who identified herself as Natasha.

"Come quick," she said, grabbing at Arnell's uniform shirt. "My uncle's back here. He's been sick for a few months, but now he. . . he started throwing up blood. I think he's dying!"

In the back room they found an approximately 50-year-old man named Raymond lying on a hospital bed. The sheets and pillow were soiled red and a small bowl on the night stand contained fresh blood.

(continued on p. 30)

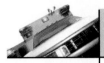

Emergency Dispatch

(continued)

While Arnell began preparing the man for transport, Jeff quickly gathered medical information from Natasha. Her uncle suffers from end-stage liver disease, has been on a transplant list for almost a year, is HBV positive and has a do-not-resuscitate order.

"Can't you just give me somethin' for the pain?" Raymond said through clenched teeth. "You gotta help."

Emotional Aspects of Emergency Care

Emotions are a fact of life. Everyone experiences them many times each and every day. Like most things in life, there are both positive and negative emotions, healthy emotions and not-so-healthy emotions. Think for a moment of a recent time when you were very happy and excited. Perhaps it was a birthday party or the birth of a child. The emotions you felt were likely strong feelings of happiness and joy. Now think back to your most recent bad customer-service experience. Perhaps it was at a restaurant when nothing seemed to go right and the server didn't seem to care, or maybe it was when you tried to get something fixed that should have been covered under warranty and the salesperson insisted he or she could do nothing to help you. Both of these situations are burned into memory by the emotions they aroused.

✳ **stress**

any event or situation that places extraordinary demands on a person's mental or emotional resources.

Stress can be defined as any event or an accumulation of events that places extraordinary demands on a person's mental or emotional resources.

It's no secret; the job of the EMS professional is stressful. Being an EMT can be an emotional rollercoaster as you attempt to manage your own emotions as well as those of patients and their loved ones. Many of these emotions are caused by the day-to-day stress of responding to emergencies and caring for ill and injured patients (Figure 2-1).

Over time, the job can take its toll on mental and emotional resources, leaving the EMT unable to cope with the job as well as with the normal activities of life.

FIGURE 2-1 Dealing with patients and family members is often stressful.

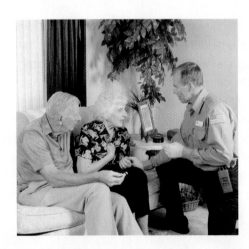

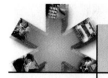

Perspective

Natasha—The Niece

"No one ever warned us that this kind of thing could happen! We were just watching TV and all of a sudden Uncle Raymond started throwing up blood. Could his liver problem cause this? Was he dying? I didn't know and I just wanted someone to help him."

Recognizing the aspects of the job that cause stress and learning to manage that stress is an essential skill that every EMS professional must learn early on.

COMMON CAUSES OF STRESS IN EMS

It may seem ironic, but many of the factors that attract people to EMS are the very factors that are likely to cause job stress. Such things as responding to other people's emergencies, long hours, driving fast with lights and siren, and working independently can all be stressors.

The following is a partial list of some of the situations that an EMT may respond to that are both stressful and emotional:

* A first encounter with the death of another human being

* Mass casualty incidents (multiple patients)

* Emergencies involving infants and children

* Incidents involving major trauma, such as an amputation

* Incidents involving abuse and/or neglect

* The death or injury of a co-worker or colleague

It is possible for an EMT to become overwhelmed by stress following a single event, such as a plane crash or the terrorist attacks on September 11, 2001. More commonly, stress is cumulative and builds gradually over time. If the build-up of stress is not managed properly along the way, it can result in an emotional breakdown (Figure 2-2A and B on page 32).

THE EFFECTS ON FAMILY AND LOVED ONES

More than many typical jobs, the job of an EMS professional can cause unexpected stress at home. EMS can be addicting; responding to emergencies and caring for others in their time of need is very satisfying, and most of us cannot get enough, especially when we are new to the job. For this reason, we tend to spend as much time as possible at the station and working extra hours. Our friends and family don't always understand our passion for EMS and may experience anger and frustration when we are always at work or volunteering our time.

Shift work causes many EMTs to be away from home for 24 and 48 hours at a time, leaving others to pick up the slack around the house. Being on call also

1-2.4 State the possible reactions that the family of the EMT-Basic may exhibit due to their outside involvement in EMS.

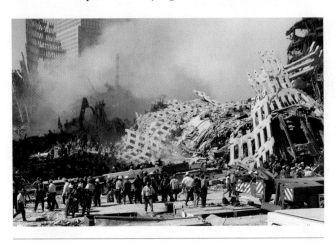

FIGURE 2-2A   Rescue workers stand near the rubble of the fallen World Trade Center towers in New York, September 13, 2001. (© Reuters/CORBIS.)

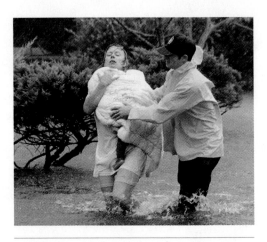

FIGURE 2-2B   Dealing with pediatric patients can be very stressful for the EMT.

causes tension when family members may be left alone on a moment's notice while you respond to someone else's emergency. While this may seem fun and exciting for friends and family in the beginning, the novelty may soon wear off and cause feelings of anger, resentment, abandonment, and jealously.

1-2.1   List possible emotional reactions that the EMT-Basic may experience when faced with trauma, illness, death, and dying.

1-2.5   Recognize the signs and symptoms of critical incident stress.

SIGNS AND SYMPTOMS OF STRESS

Although everyone responds to stress a little differently, most people will display at least a few signs that stress is present in their lives. The following is a list of some of the more common warning signs of stress:

* Increased irritability
* Inability to concentrate
* Increased levels of anxiety
* Difficulty sleeping
* Nightmares
* Increased indecisiveness
* Decreased appetite
* Feelings of guilt
* Decreased sex drive
* Wanting to be alone more
* Lack of interest in work
* Increased negative attitude

We all know people who may display at least a few of these characteristics on a normal basis. Perhaps you just chalked it up to who they were and never considered that these traits may be caused by stress.

It is important to remember that not all stress is caused by a person's job. People carry the effects of stress from one aspect of their lives to another. They will bring the effects of stress from school, home, relationships, and other jobs with them to their job as an EMT.

THREE COMMON REACTIONS TO STRESS

When we encounter stress we respond by changing our behavior in predictable ways. In other words, stress causes a normal response to an abnormal event. Response to stress can be divided into three categories: acute, delayed, and cumulative.

* **Acute stress response**—Acute stress reactions are most commonly linked to sudden, unexpected catastrophic events such as large earthquakes, plane crashes, or the line-of-duty death of a coworker. The signs and symptoms of an acute stress response occur almost immediately following the event and, in some cases, may require immediate intervention.

* **Delayed stress response**—The triggers for a delayed stress reaction are similar to those for an acute stress reaction; however the signs and symptoms may not appear until days, months, or even years later. Because of the delay in the onset of symptoms, victims are often confused as to why they are feeling the way that they are. This confusion often leads to a delay in treatment and can result in years of drug and alcohol abuse. Delayed stress can be diagnosed as a condition called posttraumatic stress disorder and often requires professional treatment.

* **Cumulative stress response**—Unlike the other categories of stress response, cumulative stress is not caused by a single event. Instead it results from the accumulation of recurring low-level stressors over many years. Commonly called "burnout," cumulative stress is usually the result of stress from more than one aspect of the person's life.

 Stop, Review, Remember!

Multiple Choice

Place a check next to the correct answer.

1. Which of the following is the best definition of stress?

_____ a. any response for which you are not prepared

_____ b. any event or situation that places extraordinary demands on a person's mental or emotional resources

_____ c. the uncontrolled increase in vital signs as a result of seeing something traumatic

_____ d. any event that causes high emotions

2. The stress of being an EMT can extend to family and friends. These people may exhibit stress in all of the following ways EXCEPT:

_____ a. jealousy.

_____ b. resentment.

_____ c. anger.

_____ d. elation.

3. Which of the following most accurately depicts the common signs and symptoms of stress in an EMT?

_____ a. irritability, insomnia, loss of appetite

_____ b. irritability, sleepiness, hunger

_____ c. inability to concentrate, hunger, desire to exercise

_____ d. inability to concentrate, insomnia, desire to be with others

4. The term *burnout* is associated with which type of stress reaction?

_____ a. acute   _____ c. cumulative

_____ b. delayed   _____ d. severe

5. _____ stress responses are commonly linked to sudden, unexpected catastrophic events.

_____ a. Acute

_____ b. Delayed

_____ c. Cumulative

_____ d. Sudden

Matching

Match the description on the left with the applicable type of response on the right.

1. _____ Any event or situation that places extraordinary demands on a person's mental or emotional resources

2. _____ Commonly linked to sudden, unexpected catastrophic events

3. _____ Stress reactions that may not appear for days, months, or even years after the stressful event

4. _____ Results from the accumulation of recurring low-level stressors over many years

A. Delayed stress response
B. Stressor
C. Cumulative stress response
D. Acute stress response

Critical Thinking

1. Describe the most stressful moment in your entire life. What emotions can you remember feeling at the time? How did you deal with the stress at the time?

_____

_____

_____

_____

_____

2. List some of the stressors that you face in your life. How do you deal with those stressors when they appear?

_____

_____

_____

_____

_____

3. What is your biggest fear about becoming an EMT? What can you do in advance to help overcome or deal with that fear should it become a reality?

_____

_____

_____

_____

_____

Learning to Manage the Effects of Stress

The proper management of stress, regardless of the cause, must be a proactive process and not just a reactive one. You must make lifestyle changes to minimize the effects of stress before the signs and symptoms appear. As you will see, these changes are not specific to the EMS profession and could be considered universal for a happy, healthy life regardless of your chosen profession.

1-2.6. State possible steps that the EMT-Basic may take to help reduce or alleviate stress.

IMPROVING DIET

A healthy diet is essential to a healthy mind and body. As the old saying goes, "You are what you eat," and many of us wouldn't want to admit what we eat sometimes. Change is difficult for most people. However, if change is made in small steps, it is far less painful. Some of the important first steps for improving one's diet are to reduce sugar, caffeine, and alcohol consumption. All we have to do to get started is to eliminate one or two sodas, coffee drinks, or beers from our daily routine (Figure 2-3 on page 36).

Minimizing foods high in saturated fats (most fast food) is another step toward a healthy diet. It may be difficult for the busiest of us to eliminate fatty foods altogether, but choosing a salad instead of a burger or not ordering fries with each meal are easy first steps.

Staying well hydrated is another area where many of us fall short in our daily routine. Keeping a good supply of fresh water handy while on duty and drinking small amounts throughout the shift will help to ensure that you keep plenty of water in your system.

FIGURE 2-3 A healthy diet is essential to a healthy mind and body.

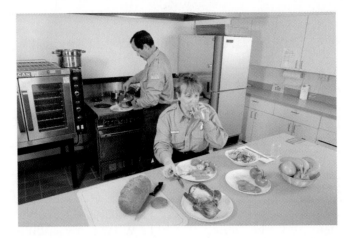

DEVELOPING A DAILY EXERCISE ROUTINE

A good diet is only part of a well-balanced life. Exercise is just as important and, to maximize its benefits, must become part of a daily routine. Like most things that take up time in our day, exercise must be scheduled into your daily routine. Twenty to thirty minutes of moderate exercise is all that is needed, but exercise can be more extreme, depending on your level of fitness. Taking time to walk, jog, or bicycle a mile or two a few times a week will do wonders for your ability to work long shifts, miss meals, and still maintain a positive attitude (Figure 2-4).

Another aspect of an effective exercise routine is allowing personal time for relaxation or meditation. Scheduling personal time to relax and do nothing is as important to a well-balanced life as diet and exercise (Figure 2-5).

BALANCE IS THE KEY

If something in our lives becomes a focal point and we become obsessed, it can create stress and imbalance. Our lives are made up of many aspects that, when balanced, work together to create an enjoyable and joy-filled life. You must bring this new profession into your life and the lives of your friends and family in a balanced manner.

Learning to become an EMT may take you away from some of the other aspects of your life while you are in school, and that is okay. Just do not allow your

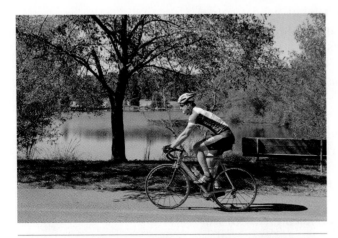

FIGURE 2-4 A daily exercise program is an important part of a well-balanced life.

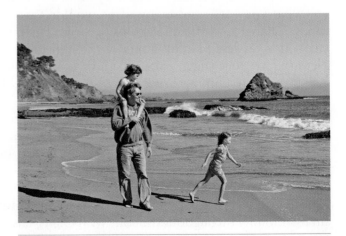

FIGURE 2-5 Allow time for relaxation.

schooling to become the only priority in your life. Balance school with your job, spiritual life, family, personal time, and exercise. When you are out of school and working as an EMT, do your best to adjust your scale of activities as often as necessary to maintain a healthy balance.

Once you are working in EMS there are several small things you can do to help maintain that balance. Not working as much overtime, requesting shifts that allow for more time with family, and requesting an assignment in a less busy area are just a few examples. When all of these things fail to provide the balance that you are trying to achieve and you find yourself displaying some of the signs and symptoms of stress, it may be time to seek outside assistance. Many employers offer assistance in the form of informal peer counselors as well as more formal professional counseling. It is not a sign of weakness but of wisdom when one seeks outside assistance for coping with stress. Like so many of the things an EMT learns, stress management is just another skill that takes practice in order to manage it well.

Critical Incident Stress Management

According to the International Critical Incident Stress Foundation, **Critical Incident Stress Management (CISM)** is a comprehensive, integrated, multi-component crisis intervention system comprised of seven core components (Table 2-1). It includes resources for all phases of a crisis including the pre-crisis, crisis, and

* **Critical Incident Stress Management (CISM)**

a comprehensive, integrated, multi-component crisis intervention system comprised of seven core components: pre-crisis preparation, support programs, defusing, debriefing, one-on-one intervention, family crisis intervention, and follow-up.

TABLE 2-1	SEVEN CORE COMPONENTS OF A CRITICAL INCIDENT STRESS MANAGEMENT SYSTEM
1. **Pre-Crisis Preparation**	Stress avoidance and management education and crisis management training for both individuals and agencies.
2. **Support Programs**	Community support programs for large-scale incidents and disasters.
3. **Defusings**	Structured small-group discussions that are provided within hours following a critical incident. Designed to address acute symptoms of stress.
4. **Debriefings**	Structured group discussions typically provided 1 to 10 days post crisis. Designed to address acute symptoms of stress, assess the need for follow-up, and provide a sense of post crisis psychological closure.
5. **One-on-One Intervention**	Intervention and counseling support for individuals throughout the entire crisis process.
6. **Family Crisis Intervention**	Intervention and counseling support for entire families.
7. **Follow-Up**	Assessment and referral mechanisms for continued treatment of symptoms as needed.

post-crisis phases. While many EMS systems and large agencies have a CISM system in place, most use only select components.

A **defusing** is a small-group discussion held within hours of a critical incident, designed to address acute symptoms of stress.

The term **Critical Incident Stress Debriefing (CISD)** is used frequently in EMS to describe any form of crisis intervention. It is important to point out that the terms CISM and CISD are not interchangeable. CISD is only one component of a multi-component CISM system designed to help people cope with their feelings before, during, and following a critical incident. If CISD is the only component used, some experts feel that the likelihood of a successful outcome for those involved is minimized.

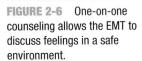

∗ **defusing**

small-group discussion held within hours of a critical incident, designed to address acute symptoms of stress.

∗ **Critical Incident Stress Debriefing (CISD)**

a process in which teams of professional and peer counselors provide emotional and psychological support to EMS personnel who are or have been involved in a critical (highly stressful) incident.

THE CRITICAL INCIDENT STRESS DEBRIEFING

The most commonly used component of a CISM system is the Critical Incident Stress Debriefing or CISD. A CISD is designed to accelerate the normal recovery process following a critical incident. It is recommended that a CISD be held between 1 and 10 days following a critical incident (in most cases a CISD is held between 24 and 72 hours after such an incident) and is facilitated by trained peer counselors and/or mental health professionals. In most cases, all individuals who were involved in the critical event are invited to participate in the CISD.

Timing is important for a successful CISD. Too soon after an event and some people will not have had time to experience the effects or begun to process their feelings, too late and it is much more difficult to begin the healing process. Individuals need to know that they have been affected by the event and then be allowed to vent their feelings in a safe environment.

A skilled facilitator will establish important ground rules for the debriefing, including emphasizing that all discussions remain confidential and should not be shared with others not in attendance. It is also explained that the debriefing is NOT an investigation or an interrogation. Facilitators are there to encourage an open discussion of the event and allow those involved to share their feelings, fears, and reactions in a nonthreatening environment. The ultimate objective for the facilitators is to evaluate the information and responses shared during the CISD and offer suggestions for coping with and eventually overcoming the stress caused by the event. One-on-one counseling may also be helpful in restoring emotional health (Figure 2-6).

As an EMT you must become familiar with the CISM system that may be in place in your EMS system and know how to access it. Your instructor can assist you in this process. You are also encouraged to participate in ongoing training and

FIGURE 2-6 One-on-one counseling allows the EMT to discuss feelings in a safe environment.

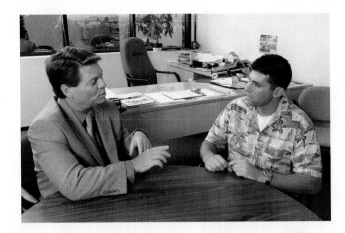

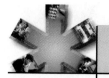

Perspective

Uncle Raymond—The Patient

"The pain was killing me! Why couldn't they give me something for it? I'll tell you what was worse, though. . . puking blood. Nothing like that has ever happened to me before. Can your liver make you do that? I'm waiting for a new one, you know, but if I'm throwing up blood and feeling pain like that, I doubt if I'll ever live long enough to get one. Actually I'd rather die than go through that again."

preplanning as well as to get involved in peer support groups before a crisis occurs. The better prepared you are in advance, the easier it will be to assist others or to overcome the effects of stress yourself.

NOTE: *It is important to mention that recent research is suggesting that group debriefings such as those conducted during a traditional CISD may not be as helpful as once thought. There is little data to suggest that post-event group debriefings are helpful. Instead, data suggest that personal, symptom-driven support is more successful. A new strategy called the "resiliency model" of stress management is emerging that is based on prevention. It focuses on the development of preexisting personal stress management strategies (strategies that promote resiliency).*

Reactions to Death and Dying

You have probably heard it said: "The only sure things in life are death and taxes." As an EMT you are sure at least to get more than your fair share of the former. Death is as much a part of life as birth. However, as a society we tend to insulate ourselves from that which is painful, and therefore most people have very little experience with death. As an EMT you will likely encounter death many times throughout your career. While it is not something we expect you will ever get used to, it is something you must learn to cope with. Successful coping takes knowledge and skills that must be developed over time.

Research has revealed that human beings go through predictable emotional stages as they attempt to cope with death, whether it is one's own impending death or the death of a loved one. Dr. Elizabeth Kübler-Ross identified five stages of dying in terminal patients (Table 2-2 on page 40). Although these stages provide a helpful framework to understand the cycle of grief, it must be kept in mind, that the stages of grief are not necessarily a step-by-step or orderly process. Furthermore, a person may experience more than one stage of grief at the same time, and not everyone goes through all the stages.

1-2.2 Discuss the possible reactions that a family member may exhibit when confronted with death and dying.

HELPING THE PATIENT AND LOVED ONES COPE

There is just no telling when you may encounter death as an EMT. It could be the sudden death of a child struck by a car or the loss of a grandmother after a long

1-2.3 State the steps in the EMT-Basic's approach to the family confronted with death and dying.

TABLE 2-2	KÜBLER-ROSS 5 STAGES OF DEATH
1. **Denial**	This is sometimes called the "not me" stage and is a defense mechanism against the thought of dying.
2. **Anger**	Patients may become outwardly angry at those around them. An attitude of "why me?" is common during this stage.
3. **Bargaining**	This is the beginning of acceptance and patients may attempt to bargain with themselves, God, or others. An attitude of, "Okay, but let me first . . . ." is common during this stage of coping.
4. **Depression**	Patients often slip into deep mourning depression, often unwilling to communicate with others.
5. **Acceptance**	Patients appear to have come to accept their fate. In some situations the patient reaches this stage before loved ones, who may need more support at this time.

and fruitful life. Whatever the circumstances, you must be prepared to offer both the patient and the patient's loved ones a dignified and compassionate response. The following key points will help:

✳ **Assess the Situation**—Identify those most in need of support, given the specific circumstances. In most cases, providing patients with the utmost respect and preserving their dignity will help their loved ones as well. Acknowledge the patient directly and avoid talking about the patient to others in his presence.

✳ **Be Tolerant**—You may encounter patients or their loved ones in various stages of coping. Do not take anger that appears to be directed at you personally, and, most important, do not become defensive.

✳ **Listen with Compassion**—Listen carefully and empathetically and be mindful of your body language. Look people in the eyes when speaking to them. You may not be able to fix the situation, but you can offer emotional support. Speak in a confident and compassionate tone (Figure 2-7).

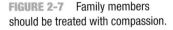

FIGURE 2-7 Family members should be treated with compassion.

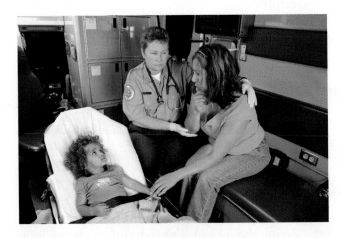

*   **Offer Honesty and Comfort**—Let the family know that everything that can be done will be done. If appropriate, a reassuring touch may be helpful in gaining their confidence. Provide as much comfort and support as you can for both patient and loved ones. Offer to contact additional resources such as hospice support or a clergyperson if it is appropriate. Most of all, show that you care.

 Stop, Review, Remember!

Multiple Choice

Place a check next to the correct answer.

1. Which of the following is the best definition of CISM?

    _____   a. a group of peer counselors who are on call to assist following a critical incident

    _____   b. a comprehensive crisis intervention system that includes resources for all phases of a crisis

    _____   c. a structured small group discussion that is provided within hours following a critical incident

    _____   d. a structured group discussion typically provided 1 to 10 days post crisis

2. It is recommended that a CISD be conducted between _____ following a critical incident.

    _____   a. 1 and 10 hours

    _____   b. 2 and 4 days

    _____   c. 1 and 10 days

    _____   d. 7 and 14 days

3. According to Kübler Ross's five stages of dying, this stage is expressed by withdrawal from others and a desire to be alone. Communication becomes difficult for the patient during this stage.

    _____   a. denial   _____   c. bargaining

    _____   b. anger   _____   d. depression

4. Which of the following is NOT a technique the EMT should use when helping loved ones cope with loss?

    _____   a. Remain focused on the patient and do not be distracted by loved ones.

    _____   b. Remain tolerant of others' feelings and emotions.

    _____   c. Listen with compassion.

    _____   d. Be honest and do your best to comfort those in need.

5. In this stage of the dying process, patients appear to have come to accept their fate.

    _____   a. denial

    _____   b. anger

    _____   c. acceptance

    _____   d. depression

Matching

Match the description on the left with the applicable term on the right.

1. _____ A comprehensive, integrated, multi-component crisis intervention system

2. _____ A forum held between 1 and 10 days following a critical incident, facilitated by trained peer counselors and/or mental health professionals

3. _____ A structured small-group discussion that is provided within hours following a critical incident

4. _____ Sometimes called the "not me" stage, it is a defense mechanism against the thought of dying

5. _____ An attitude of, "Okay, but let me first. . . ." is common during this stage of coping with dying

A. Defusing
B. CISM
C. CISD
D. Bargaining stage
E. Denial stage

Critical Thinking

1. On a scale of 1 to 10, 10 being totally balanced, how would you rate your life at this point in time? What is the single factor causing the most imbalance?

_____

_____

_____

_____

_____

2. What does it mean to be "proactive" versus "reactive" concerning stress in your life?

_____

_____

_____

_____

3. What does the word "resiliency" mean to you and how does it apply to coping with the affects of stress?

_____

_____

_____

_____

_____

Personal Safety During Emergencies

As an EMT you will be responding to those who are injured and ill in a wide variety of situations and environments. Remaining safe must be your top priority. The exposure or potential exposure to body substances such as blood and vomit is one of the biggest hazards you will face. To assist health care professionals in minimizing exposure to infectious disease, the Centers for Disease Control and Prevention (CDC) have established guidelines and practices known as **standard precautions**. The foundation of standard precautions (also called *universal precautions*) is an awareness that all patients are potentially infectious regardless of diagnosis or presumed infection.

One of the most important aspects of standard precautions is a practice called **body substance isolation precautions (BSI)**. Body fluids can contain organisms known as **pathogens**. Pathogens are organisms such as viruses and bacteria that are capable of causing disease. While it is not realistic to expect that you can perform your duties as an EMT and avoid all contact with body fluids, there are things you can do to greatly minimize your chances of becoming exposed.

At the core of proper BSI precautions is appropriate **personal protective equipment (PPE)**. PPE includes anything the EMT might use or wear to minimize risk of illness or injury. The PPE necessary for appropriate BSI precautions are:

* Gloves

* Eye protection

* Masks

* Disposable clothing

GLOVES

Proper BSI begins with wearing appropriate gloves for all patient contacts (Figure 2-8). Now more than ever, the EMT has a choice in the type and material of gloves worn in the field. The most common gloves are the nonsterile latex type found in most health care settings. As more and more health care professionals are finding they are sensitive to latex, however, they are switching to gloves made of nonlatex materials such as Nitrile or vinyl.

Gloves must be donned prior to patient contact when there is an expectation that there will be contact with blood or body fluids. Eye and facial protection and a disposable gown should be donned prior to patient contact when there is

1-2.7   Explain the need to determine scene safety.

1-2.8   Discuss the importance of body substance isolation (BSI).

1-2.9   Describe the steps the EMT-Basic should take for personal protection from airborne and bloodborne pathogens.

* **standard precautions**

  Centers for Disease Control and Prevention (CDC) guidelines and practices based on the awareness that all patients are potentially infectious regardless of diagnosis or presumed infection. Also called *universal precautions*.

* **body substance isolation (BSI) precautions**

  the practice of using appropriate barriers to infection at the emergency scene, such as gloves, masks, gowns, and protective eyewear.

* **pathogens**

  organisms that cause infection, such as viruses and bacteria.

* **personal protective equipment (PPE)**

  equipment that protects the EMS worker from infection and/or exposure to the dangers of rescue operations.

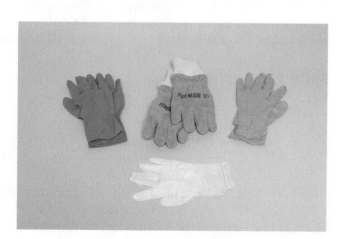

FIGURE 2-8   Proper BSI includes wearing the appropriate gloves.

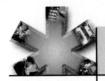

Perspective

Jeff—The EMT

"This was one of those patients that you gotta be extra careful with. Hep B ain't something to mess with, and he had blood everywhere. Arnell and I both put our gloves on before we even got out of the truck, but my safety glasses were still on the dash where I had thrown them at the start of shift. Have you ever worn those things? They can be uncomfortable and sometimes they fog up, and they'll never make anyone's fashion list! But Arnell made me go out and get them. It's more important to be safe than have that guy vomit blood in my eyes. I'm no good to anyone if I'm messed up."

reasonable expectation of uncontrolled bleeding or the presence of body fluids such as uncontrolled vomiting. Gloves should also be changed between contacts with different patients. Utility gloves, which are thicker and nondisposable, should be worn when decontaminating the ambulance or nondisposable equipment used during the care of the patient.

Microorganisms and bacteria multiply fast in the warm moist environment inside the gloves. It is important to wash hands thoroughly following the removal of protective gloves.

EYE PROTECTION

The eyes and their surrounding membranes are highly vascular (contain many blood vessels) and are susceptible to exposure to outside elements such as the splatter and spray that accompany many patient contacts. Body fluids from a patient that make contact with the eyes and surrounding tissue can be absorbed into the bloodstream and potentially cause an infection. For this reason, the EMT should wear appropriate eye protection for any patient who presents a reasonable risk of infection. Eyewear should be readily available and worn whenever a potential risk is evident (Figure 2-9).

Appropriate eye wear should provide protection against spray and splatter from the front and the sides. If prescription glasses or sunglasses are used as PPE, they should include snap-on side pieces for added protection (Figure 2-10). In most situations, full goggles are not required but should be available just in case.

FACE PROTECTION

The mucous membranes of the nose and mouth are vulnerable, much like the exposed tissues of the eyes. For this reason, it may be necessary in some situations to shield these areas against the splatter of body fluids. A simple surgical mask worn by the EMT is appropriate for most situations (Figure 2-11A and B). In situations where it is known or suspected that the patient may have an airborne disease such as tuberculosis, a specialized mask is required. The masks referred to as high efficiency particulate air (HEPA) respirators and N-95 masks have been approved for this purpose by the National Institute for Occupational Safety and Health (NIOSH).

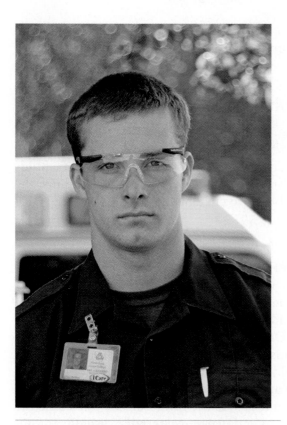

FIGURE 2-9 Proper eyewear is an important part of BSI.

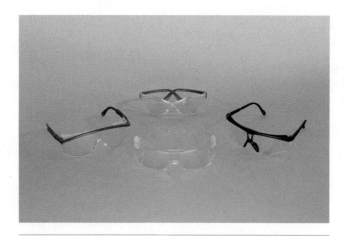

FIGURE 2-10 To provide protection, a selection of protective eyewear is available.

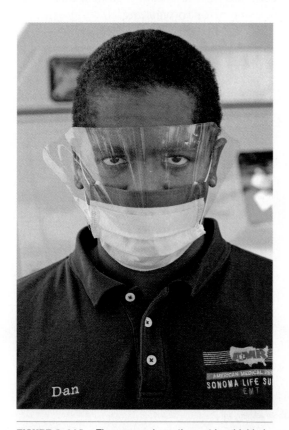

FIGURE 2-11A The eyes and mouth must be shielded against the splatter of body fluids. Simple surgical mask with eye shield.

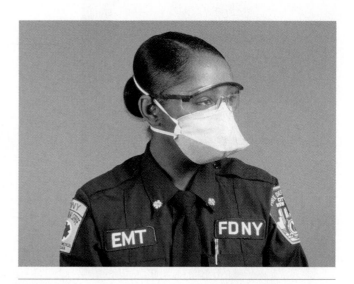

FIGURE 2-11B N-95 mask offers a higher level of protection against airborne pathogens.

In cases where you are caring for a patient with a known or suspected airborne infection, it is also helpful to place a similar mask on the patient to further minimize exposure.

DISPOSABLE CLOTHING OR GOWNS

In rare cases of serious arterial bleeding, such as major trauma or field delivery of an infant, the EMT should have access to and consider donning a full disposable clothing (Figure 2-12). This will provide extra protection against bodily fluids soaking through street clothing to unprotected skin, and will also minimize the chances of a soiled uniform that would require changing.

HAND WASHING

In addition to considering the use of PPE, it is necessary to understand the importance of proper hand washing. The CDC states that "hand washing is the single most important means of preventing the spread of infection." Whether or not we want to admit it, we carry both good and bad organisms on our hands all the time. Simply wearing gloves is not enough. Once we remove the gloves, we must wash our hands to cleanse them of the organisms that multiplied in the hot damp environment inside the glove. Hands should be washed between patient contacts, after removing gloves, and anytime they are visibly soiled (Figure 2-13).

In the field, there are essentially two methods the EMT can use to cleanse the hands. The preferred method utilizes soap and warm water and is usually accomplished while at the hospital. Vigorous rubbing with soap and warm water for at least 15 to 30 seconds is adequate. Concentrate on the cuticles, ridges, under the nails, and between the fingers. Remove jewelry prior to washing.

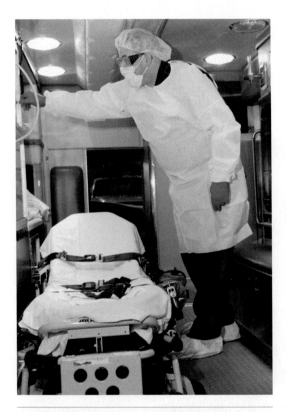

FIGURE 2-12 A gown should be worn in cases of major trauma or childbirth.

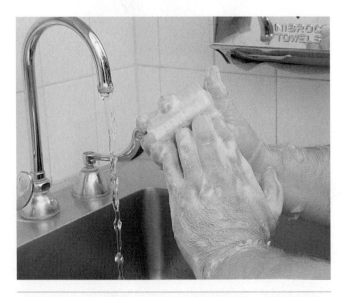

FIGURE 2-13 Hand washing is the single most important means of preventing the spread of infection.

When an adequate supply of water and soap are not available, alcohol-based waterless hand cleaners that are commercially available serve as a good alternative to traditional hand washing. Most alcohol-based cleansers are less effective when they come in contact with visible contaminants. For these hand cleaners to be most effective, the hands must first be cleansed of any visible contamination, such as blood or dirt. This may require that you cleanse your hands twice, once to remove the visible blood, dirt, or other substances and a second time to decontaminate your hands. Place a dime-sized amount of alcohol-based cleanser in the palm of one hand and rub vigorously for several seconds to cover both hands entirely. DO NOT dry your hands but instead allow them to air dry as the alcohol evaporates.

OSHA LOOKING OUT FOR YOU

The Occupational Safety and Health Administration (OSHA) has one primary focus: to ensure the safety and health of the nation's workforce, and this includes you. OSHA has well-established policies and guidelines that employers must follow to ensure a safe workplace. It is in your best interest to become familiar with these guidelines, follow them, and be sure your employer follows them.

Some states have established their own standards and have created even more stringent guidelines pertaining to infection control. Your instructor can provide the specifics of the guidelines established for your state or region. Most if not all states have laws or statutes that require the reporting of a known exposure to an infectious disease. If you think you may have been exposed to a patient's body fluids and you have any reason to suspect the patient could have carried an infectious disease, notify your supervisor immediately and follow your agency's procedure for postexposure follow up.

IMMUNIZATIONS

One of the requirements that OSHA has established to minimize the transmission of communicable disease is that employers must offer voluntary, no-cost immunizations. Any employee who has a reasonable risk of being exposed to an infectious disease in the course of normal duties must be offered a free immunization. Of course, EMS professionals fit into this category. The following is a list of recommended immunizations for the EMS professional:

* Tetanus

* Hepatitis B

* Measles

* Mumps

* Rubella

More and more of the recommended immunizations are being given as part of the normal childhood immunization series but do not feel you don't need them because you had them when you were a child. Check with a doctor as to which ones should be repeated and how often during your adult years (Figure 2-14 on page 48).

Many agencies are accepting test results that confirm the immune status of the individual. The tuberculin purified protein derivative (PPD), indicating whether or

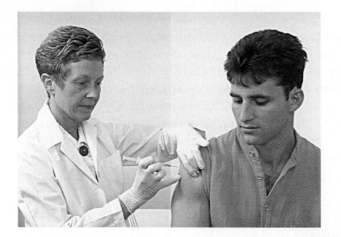

not the person has been exposed to tuberculosis, is such a test. In cases where the individual is certain that he has had a prior immunization, such as for hepatitis or measles, but cannot produce adequate documentation to support it, he may opt for a blood test that can verify his immune status.

1-2.10 List the personal protective equipment necessary for each of the following situations:
- Hazardous materials
- Rescue operations

Protection for Specific Emergencies

As mentioned earlier, PPE includes anything the EMT might use or wear to minimize the risk of illness or injury. So far we have only discussed exposure to body fluids. As an EMT you will be responding to many different types of emergencies that will expose you to additional hazards that will need to be identified and likely require specific types of PPE. The following sections discuss types of emergencies that expose the EMT to increased levels of risk. For each of these emergency situations, we offer suggestions for identifying the potential hazards as well as ways the EMT can minimize exposure to the risks at the scene.

HAZARDOUS MATERIALS INCIDENTS

As you have learned, confirming that the scene is safe is one of the very first tasks you will perform when arriving on the scene of an emergency. Of course if you know in advance that you are responding to a hazardous materials (HazMat) scene, you should remain at a safe distance until trained HazMat personnel have cleared you for entry into the scene. There are times when it is not known in advance that a spill or release has occurred. For this reason have a high index of suspicion when responding to scenes with the potential for hazardous materials. Chapter 42 covers this topic.

Observe from a distance for any evidence of a spill or vapor release. Use binoculars, if you have them, to try to identify any placards that may indicate what has been spilled. A great resource that should be carried in all emergency vehicles is the *Emergency Response Guidebook,* developed jointly by the U.S. Department of Transportation, Transport Canada, and the Secretariat of Communications and Transportation of Mexico (SCT), and updated regularly, for use by firefighters, police, and other emergency services personnel who may be the first to arrive at the scene of a transportation incident involving a hazardous material. It is primarily a guide to aid first responders in (1) quickly identifying the specific or generic classification of the material(s) involved in the incident, and (2) protecting themselves and the general public during this initial response phase of the incident. More information, including electronic copies of the guidebook and recent updates, can be found at http://hazmat.dot.gov/pubs/erg/gydebook.htm (Figure 2-15).

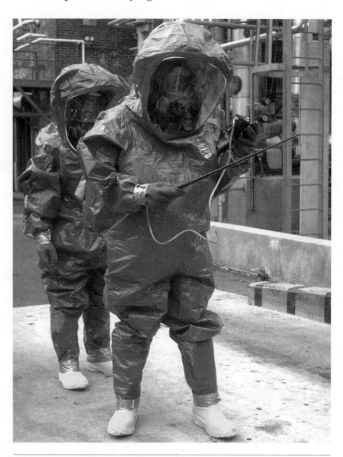

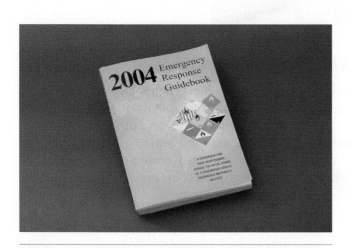

FIGURE 2-15 The *Emergency Response Guidebook* should be carried in all emergency vehicles.

FIGURE 2-16 Entering a HazMat scene requires specific training and equipment.

Do not attempt to enter a HazMat scene unless you are specifically trained and equipped (Figure 2-16). Many HazMat scenes require the donning of specialized suits and self-contained breathing apparatus (SCBA) prior to entry. As an EMT your primary role will be one of patient care. In most cases you will have to wait until patients have been removed from the scene and safely decontaminated before you will be allowed to provide emergency care. Rely on those with specialized HazMat training to provide direction and guidance at the scene.

RESCUE OPERATIONS

Emergency scenes involving rescue operations also involve a higher degree of risk than most other types of calls to which an EMT may respond. Rescue operations may involve vehicle extrications, live electrical wires, and fire and explosion hazards as well as hazardous materials. As with HazMat responses, incidents involving rescue operations require specialized training and equipment (Figure 2-17 on page 50). It is, however, quite common for an EMT to work side by side with the rescuers providing patient care during the rescue process. These situations may require additional PPE not typically found on an ambulance. In addition to protective eye wear, the EMT may want to utilize firefighter style "turnout" clothing as well as puncture-resistant gloves and a helmet.

In most cases, once you have arrived on scene and identified the need for additional resources, you will only do what is safe until a specialized rescue team can bring the patient to safety. Chapters 40–44 will cover this information in more detail.

FIGURE 2-17 The Jaws of Life is used for extrication from an automobile.

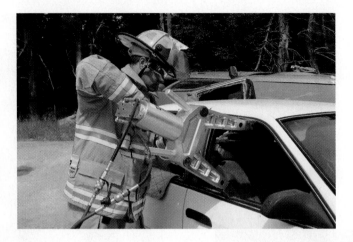

SCENES INVOLVING VIOLENCE AND CRIME SCENES

As an EMT you will be responding to all types of emergencies, including those involving violence. You may respond to the victim of an assault or shooting where the perpetrator is still at large and potentially a risk to you and others at the scene. Bystanders and family members can become violent and begin to lash out at those trying to care for their loved ones. Any time you have any reason to suspect a crime has been committed or that your safety is threatened by another person at the scene, immediately retreat and request law enforcement.

There may be times when you are asked to respond to an incident and "stage" or stand by some distance away until you are cleared by law enforcement to enter. This is usually because they have reason to suspect that additional injuries may occur before the incident is over. Do not enter until you have been specifically requested to do so by law enforcement at the scene. Even after you have been cleared to enter, you should remain very alert for potential hazards.

If you are called to enter a crime scene to care for a patient, be respectful of any potential evidence in or around the scene. Once it is safe for you to enter, the patient is always your top priority. However, be careful to disturb only what is necessary to provide excellent patient care. Do not throw anything away or transport materials with the patient from the scene that may be needed by law enforcement as evidence.

Stop, Review, Remember!

Multiple Choice

Place a check next to the correct answer.

1. Which of the following is the best description of BSI precautions?

   _____ a. always wearing gloves when contacting patients

   _____ b. wearing proper PPE only when blood is present

   _____ c. using proper PPE whenever there is a reasonable expectation that exposure to body fluids is present

   _____ d. using proper PPE only when body fluids such as blood and vomit are present

2. Which of the following forms of PPE is best for minimizing the exposure to an airborne disease?

_____ a. HEPA mask

_____ b. gloves

_____ c. eye glasses

_____ d. surgical mask

3. Which of the following represents the greatest risk of exposure for the EMT?

_____ a. vomit on a gloved hand

_____ b. splatter of blood in the eyes

_____ c. blood exposure over intact skin

_____ d. saliva splatter in the ear

4. The foundation of standard precautions is:

_____ a. an awareness that all patients are potentially infectious regardless of diagnosis or presumed infection.

_____ b. that only patients with a known infectious status pose any real threat.

_____ c. based on good hand washing.

_____ d. based on getting all immunizations before being exposed.

5. According to the CDC, _____ is/are the single most effective means of preventing the spread of infection.

_____ a. immunizations

_____ b. awareness

_____ c. hand washing

_____ d. protective gloves

Critical Thinking

1. Discuss the relationship between body substance isolation precautions and personal protective equipment.

_____

_____

_____

_____

_____

_____

2. List the PPE you would want to wear if you were caring for victims following a hazardous materials spill.

_____

_____

_____

_____

_____

_____

3. What are some ways you could help preserve potential evidence when caring for a patient from the scene of a crime?

_____

_____

_____

_____

_____

4.

Guide to Proper BSI Precautions—Given the different situations below, choose the appropriate PPE. (Place a check in the appropriate column or columns.)

Situation	Gloves	Glasses	Mask	Gown
Minor bleed to the left hand				
Suctioning a vomiting patient				
Assisting with a birth				
Cleaning a bloody backboard				
Taking a blood pressure on a medical patient				
Major bleed of the lower leg with spurting blood				
Cleaning the back of the ambulance after a call				

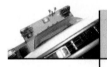

Dispatch Summary

Raymond was transported to Sutter Memorial Hospital where he underwent a procedure to repair a broken vessel in his esophagus. He is recovering well from that, but his liver continues to weaken and, due to a widespread shortage of organ donors, his chances for survival decline each day.

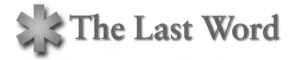 The Last Word

The primary goal of this chapter has been to begin preparing you to properly manage the stressors and other hazards that are so much a part of a career as an EMS professional. A long and successful career in EMS begins with three steps:

1. Developing an awareness of the stressors and hazards that exist in EMS
2. Learning to recognize the signs and symptoms caused by stress
3. Learning to manage the effects of stress by being prepared and developing a resiliency to its effects.

Balance is the key to managing life's stresses and the stress of EMS is no exception. Establishing a well-balanced diet, an adequate amount of sleep, and a regular exercise routine will do wonders toward preparing us for stress as well as helping us to manage its effects after the fact.

The top priority for all EMS professionals is personal safety. If the scene is not safe, DO NOT enter. Proper BSI precautions are recommended for all patient contacts and include such PPE as gloves, eye protection, and face masks.

✳ Chapter Review

MULTIPLE CHOICE

Place a check next to the correct answer.

1. As an EMT you must remain as uninvolved emotionally as possible if you expect to do a good job.

    _____ a. true

    _____ b. false

2. The five stages that most dying patients experience are denial, anger, _____, depression, and acceptance.

    _____ a. resentment

    _____ b. frustration

    _____ c. bargaining

    _____ d. anticipation

3. Irritability with coworkers, inability to concentrate, indecisiveness, and loss of appetite are all warning signs of:

    _____ a. psychosis.

    _____ b. stress.

    _____ c. anxiety.

    _____ d. isolation.

4. You receive a dispatch for a possible assault victim. What additional resources will you want to respond as well?

    _____ a. fire department

    _____ b. additional ambulance

    _____ c. field supervisor

    _____ d. law enforcement

5. One of the best techniques for helping comfort a person who has lost a loved one is to:

    _____ a. just listen.

    _____ b. offer a drink.

    _____ c. suggest a nap.

    _____ d. avoid eye contact.

CRITICAL THINKING

1. How do you deal with acute stress? How have you reacted to acute stress in the past and did you react appropriately?

_____

_____

_____

_____

2. What are you doing in your current lifestyle that will help you deal with stress? What areas can you improve?

_____

_____

_____

_____

3. Imagine yourself attending a CISD following a critical incident. Would you be willing or able to talk about your thoughts and feelings in front of your peers?

_____

_____

_____

_____

CASE STUDIES

Case Study 1

You have arrived at work to find that your regular partner, Tim, has called in sick for the shift and that your new partner for the day is Will. You find out from your supervisor that both Will and Tim were on a double fatality a couple of days earlier that involved two pediatric patients. Your supervisor asks you to be sensitive to the issue and to please alert him if you see any unusual behavior in Will during your shift together. As you and Will begin the shift and complete the ambulance inspection, you notice that Will is definitely not his usual outgoing self.

1. Is it appropriate for you to engage Will in a conversation regarding the call?

_____

_____

_____

_____

2. Describe the typical behavior of someone such as Will who has experienced a traumatic event.

_____

_____

_____

_____

3. What can you do as Will's partner to help him deal with the stress he is under?

_____

_____

_____

_____

Case Study 2

You have been working as an EMT for about a year and taking all the overtime shifts that you could get your hands on. At one point you even pulled a 96-hour shift without a break, but most have been 24s and 48s. You are finding it more and more difficult to find the energy to make it to the next call and your partners have been avoiding you while on duty because of your negative attitude. Clearly, stress is taking its toll on you.

1. In what other ways might you find that stress is affecting your life?

_____

_____

_____

_____

2. If you do nothing to change the situation, how will this buildup of stress probably end up affecting you?

_____

_____

_____

_____

3. List at least 3 things you can you do to ease the stress and keep from getting burned out?

_____

_____

_____

_____

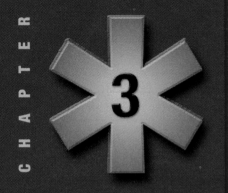

CHAPTER

3

Legal and Ethical Considerations of Providing Care

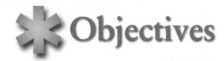

Objectives

Numbered objectives are from the U.S. Department of Transportation 1994 EMT-Basic National Standard Curriculum.

COGNITIVE OBJECTIVES

At the completion of this lesson, the EMT-Basic student will be able to:

1-3.1 Define the EMT-Basic scope of practice. (pp. 57–60)

1-3.2 Discuss the importance of do not resuscitate [DNR] (advance directives) and local or state provisions regarding EMS application. (pp. 69–71)

1-3.3 Define consent and discuss the methods of obtaining consent. (p. 64)

1-3.4 Differentiate between expressed and implied consent. (pp. 64–67)

1-3.5 Explain the role of consent of minors in providing care. (pp. 65–67)

1-3.6 Discuss the implications for the EMT-Basic in patient refusal of transport. (p. 67)

1-3.7 Discuss the issues of abandonment, negligence, and battery and their implications to the EMT-Basic. (pp. 67–69)

1-3.8 State the conditions necessary for the EMT-Basic to have a duty to act. (p. 61)

1-3.9 Explain the importance, necessity, and legality of patient confidentiality. (pp. 74–75)

1-3.10 Discuss the considerations of the EMT-Basic in issues of organ retrieval. (p. 76)

1-3.11 Differentiate the actions that an EMT-Basic should take to assist in the preservation of a crime scene. (pp. 75–76)

1-3.12 State the conditions that require an EMT-Basic to notify local law enforcement officials. (pp. 75–76)

AFFECTIVE OBJECTIVES

At the completion of this lesson, the EMT-Basic student will be able to:

1-3.13 Explain the role of EMS and the EMT-Basic regarding patients with DNR orders. (pp. 70–71)

1-3.14 Explain the rationale for the needs, benefits, and usage of advance directives. (p. 69)

1-3.15 Explain the rationale for the concept of varying degrees of DNR. (pp. 70–71)

PSYCHOMOTOR OBJECTIVES

No psychomotor objectives identified.

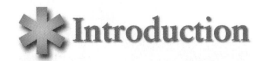

Introduction

There is simply no way around it: We live, work, and play in a litigious society. Everywhere we turn we either hear or read about another lawsuit. The reasons go beyond the scope of this text, but your actions can greatly reduce your chances of being litigated against. Suffice it to say that, no matter where we live or what our job is, much of our daily lives are influenced in some way by the legal system. This is especially true in EMS.

It is not that the rules are really any different in the world of EMS. It is that EMS is a relatively high-profile job, and many pairs of eyes are on us as we deliver patient care. One of your first responsibilities as an EMT is to learn the laws as they pertain to providing patient care at the scene of an emergency. It's no different than learning the rules of the road when first learning to drive. Common sense provides much of what we need to know, while training and experience fill in the remaining requisite knowledge.

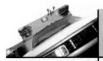

Emergency Dispatch

"I think this is it right here," EMT Brandon Gervais said, searching the dilapidated duplex for an address. "I don't see a number, but 212 . . . 214 . . . this has to be 216."

As Brandon and his partner, Jewel, were pulling the cot from the back of the ambulance, a young woman emerged from the house and walked quickly up to them.

"Oh great, you're here." She glanced at her watch and placed her hand on the cot. "But you won't need this."

"Who are you?" Brandon said, pulling the cot from her hand.

"I'm Janine," the woman said, "Mr. Flowers's caretaker. Look, I just need you guys to help me get him back into bed. He fell onto the floor, I can't lift him, and I'm late for my next appointment."

The house was a mess. Old newspapers, mail, and clothes were strewn everywhere, and the stench of urine was almost caustic. Janine led them back to the only bedroom in the small house. There on the floor next to the bed was Henry Flowers, moaning and clad in nothing but wet undershorts.

"I left about 40 minutes ago to go shopping for him, and when I came back, this is where I found him." She reached down and began pulling on one of his thin arms. "If you'll just help me get him back into bed, we can all go on with our day."

Scope of Practice

The EMT **scope of practice**, sometimes called the *scope of care*, is a detailed description of the specific care and actions EMTs are allowed to perform. It is defined by state legislation and enhanced by medical direction through the use of protocols and standing orders.

1-3.1 Define the EMT-Basic scope of practice.

* **scope of practice**
   a detailed description of the specific care and actions EMTs are allowed to perform.

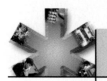

Perspective

Brandon—The EMT

"Something just didn't seem right there. That caregiver woman didn't seem concerned at all about Henry's well-being. Come on! He didn't seem to be aware of his surroundings or anything and all she can think of is getting on to her next appointment! I tell you . . . that's really some standard of care she's providing."

The scope of practice for the EMT is referenced to a document known as the *Emergency Medical Technician-Basic: National Standard Curriculum (NSC)*, which was developed by the **National Highway Traffic Safety Administration (NHTSA)**, a division of the U.S. Department of Transportation (DOT).

STANDARD OF CARE

An EMT's scope of practice that differs from the NSC and is unique to a specific community, region, or state is commonly referred to as a **standard of care.** In other words, a standard of care is a modified scope of practice designed to meet the needs of a specific area or region.

The standard of care for a specific region is established by key stakeholders in the EMS system in accordance with local laws and regulations. These stakeholders are often physician medical directors, EMS administrators and experienced field personnel. The local standard of care is most often defined by protocols and/or standing orders. Protocols are general written guidelines that help direct the EMT in providing the most appropriate care. Standing orders are predetermined treatment directives from a physician that allow the EMT to provide the indicated care in specific situations.

MEDICAL DIRECTION

As an EMT providing care within an EMS system, you are acting as an extension of a physician who acts as Medical Director. As you learned in Chapter 1, all EMS systems are required to have a physician acting as the Medical Director. The Medical Director's job is to oversee all aspects of patient care within the EMS system and to ensure continuous quality improvement of the system.

ETHICAL RESPONSIBILITIES

As an EMT you will be expected to perform your duties in accordance with both legal and ethical guidelines. While the law may be fairly clear cut, sometimes the ethical side of being an EMT can be somewhat cloudy.

Webster's Dictionary defines ethics as *the study of the general nature of morals and the specific moral choices an individual makes in relating to others.* Morals are defined as *rules or habits of conduct with regard to standards of right and wrong.*

✳ *Emergency Medical Technician-Basic: National Standard Curriculum (NSC)*

the Curricululm developed by the U.S. Department of Transportation as the foundation for the scope of practice for all EMTs, formerly EMT-Basics.

✳ **National Highway Traffic Safety Administration (NHTSA)**

a division of the U.S. Department of Transportation (DOT). This agency develops the National Standard Curricula for various levels of EMS providers.

✳ **standard of care**

a modified scope of practice specifically designed to meet the needs of a specific area or region.

EMT Code of Ethics

As Adopted by the National Association of EMTs

Professional status as an Emergency Medical Technician and Emergency Medical Technician-Paramedic is maintained and enriched by the willingness of the individual practitioner to accept and fulfill obligations to society, other medical professionals, and the profession of Emergency Medical Technician. As an Emergency Medical Technician-Paramedic, I solemnly pledge myself to the following code of professional ethics:

A fundamental responsibility of the Emergency Medical Technician is to conserve life, to alleviate suffering, to promote health, to do no harm, and to encourage the quality and equal availability of emergency medical care.

The Emergency Medical Technician provides services based on human need, with respect for human dignity, unrestricted by consideration of nationality, race, creed, color, or status.

The Emergency Medical Technician does not use professional knowledge and skills in any enterprise detrimental to the public well being.

The Emergency Medical Technician respects and holds in confidence all information of a confidential nature obtained in the course of professional work unless required by law to divulge such information.

The Emergency Medical Technician, as a citizen, understands and upholds the law and performs the duties of citizenship; as a professional, the Emergency Medical Technician has the never-ending responsibility to work with concerned citizens and other health care professionals in promoting a high standard of emergency medical care to all people.

The Emergency Medical Technician shall maintain professional competence and demonstrate concern for the competence of other members of the Emergency Medical Services health care team.

An Emergency Medical Technician assumes responsibility in defining and upholding standards of professional practice and education.

The Emergency Medical Technician assumes responsibility for individual professional actions and judgment, both in dependent and independent emergency functions, and knows and upholds the laws which affect the practice of the Emergency Medical Technician.

An Emergency Medical Technician has the responsibility to be aware of and participate in matters of legislation affecting the Emergency Medical Service System.

The Emergency Medical Technician, or groups of Emergency Medical Technicians, who advertise professional service, do so in conformity with the dignity of the profession.

The Emergency Medical Technician has an obligation to protect the public by not delegating to a person less qualified, any service which requires the professional competence of an Emergency Medical Technician.

The Emergency Medical Technician will work harmoniously with and sustain confidence in Emergency Medical Technician associates, the nurses, the physicians, and other members of the Emergency Medical Services health care team.

The Emergency Medical Technician refuses to participate in unethical procedures, and assumes the responsibility to expose incompetence or unethical conduct of others to the appropriate authority in a proper and professional manner.

Written by: Charles Gillespie M.D.

Adopted by: The National Association of Emergency Medical Technicians, 1978.

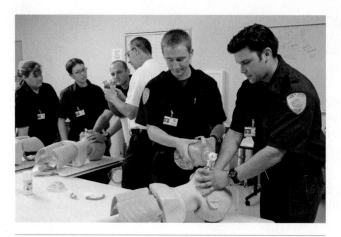

FIGURE 3-1A Quality training promotes a high standard of care for your patients.

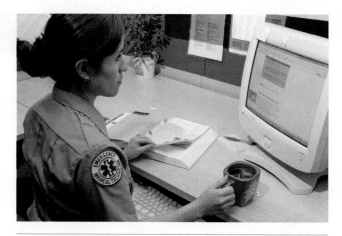

FIGURE 3-1B Maintaining your skills and knowledge is part of the EMT Code of Ethics.

Because ethics are based on morals and morals are somewhat subjective, making good ethical choices is not always the same for everyone. In an effort to develop an ethical standard for all EMTs, the National Association of EMTs adopted the EMT Code of Ethics. This document was adopted in 1978 and has served as an excellent ethical standard for all EMTs.

The EMT Code of Ethics addresses such things as:

* Providing care based on need and without regard for nationality, race, creed, color, religion, or status

* Protecting patient confidentiality

* Respecting patient dignity

* Promoting a high standard of care for all

* Assuming responsibility for personal actions and conduct

* Upholding professional standards of practice and education (Figure 3-1A and B)

As an EMT you have an ethical obligation to place the needs of those you are caring for first, so long as it is safe to do so. You must also maintain your skills and knowledge of your chosen profession in an effort to continually improve yourself and the system. You must also provide accurate and complete documentation of the care you provide.

While it may seem like an impossible responsibility on the surface, making the right choices as an EMT is usually not hard to do, and it is extremely rewarding.

YOUR CORE VALUES

One way to become more aware of your actions as they pertain to ethics is to identify your personal core values. Values are our beliefs and what we consider important as human beings. Your beliefs are what drive your actions and, in turn, they become the example by which people see and judge you. By identifying and embracing core values such as integrity, compassion, accountability, respect, and empathy, EMTs will find it easier to make good decisions and do what is right for the patient as well as others in their life. To find out more about exploring your own personal core values, visit *www.icarevalues.org*.

Legal Aspects of Providing Care

Once you become an EMT and begin working for an EMS provider, you will have a legal obligation to render care to those in need and to do so to an established standard of care. This obligation is referred to as a **duty to act.** You must also obtain consent from those to whom you offer care and must ensure that those who choose to refuse care understand the consequences of their decision.

A LEGAL DUTY TO ACT

An EMT's duty to act can be implied, as in the case of some volunteer rescue and ambulance squads, or it can be contractual, such as when an EMS provider (volunteer or otherwise) has a contract to provide service to an event or a community.

The concept of a duty becomes less obvious when the trained EMT is not associated with an established EMS agency. For instance, in some states the EMT has no legal obligation to stop and render care at the scene of an emergency. An EMT who is off duty or one who received his training simply out of personal interest may have no legal obligation to assist those injured in a vehicle collision, even if he witnessed the incident. The laws pertaining to a duty to act are different in each state, and you must research the laws of your state or region. Your instructor should be able to provide the specifics for your area.

Most states have made it clear that once someone begins to render care to an injured person, a legal duty to act is established and that person must remain at the scene and provide care to the best of his ability and training. Once you have begun to care for the victim of an injury or illness, you MUST remain at the scene and continue to provide care until someone of equal or higher training takes over care. Failure to continue to provide care may be considered **abandonment** and can result in a charge of negligence. More about negligence will be discussed later.

GOOD SAMARITAN LAWS

As we mentioned earlier, passersby in most states are not required by law to stop and render medical assistance to those in need unless there is a preexisting duty to act. For that reason all states now have specific laws to encourage passersby to stop and assist those in need of medical attention. In essence, **Good Samaritan laws** encourage passersby, regardless of training, to stop and provide medical assistance without fear of being held civilly liable for anything they do or do not do while caring for the victim. Good Samaritan laws protect those who "in good faith and not for compensation" render care to those in need and do so as "any prudent man or woman would do" given the same circumstances and training.

Many people state that the reason they would not stop and render care at the scene of an emergency is fear of being sued. The reality is that lawsuits involving passersby who render care are quite rare. Fortunately, the majority of people respond to their ethical and moral obligation to assist a person in need, despite their fear of not knowing exactly what to do.

---

* **duty to act**
  a legal obligation to provide care to a patient.

1-3.8 State the conditions necessary for the EMT-Basic to have a duty to act.

* **abandonment**
  leaving a patient after care has been initiated and before the patient has been transferred to someone with equal or greater medical training.

* **Good Samaritan laws**
  laws, varying in each state, designed to provide limited legal protection for citizens and some health care personnel when they are administering emergency care.

Stop, Review, Remember!

Multiple Choice

Place a check next to the correct answer.

1. Which of the following best describes the term *scope of practice?*

   _____ a. It is established by state laws and regulations.

   _____ b. It is established by local protocols and guidelines.

   _____ c. It is the same for every state.

   _____ d. It is determined by a local physician medical director

2. A standard of care is most often defined by:

   _____ a. national leaders in EMS.

   _____ b. local protocols and guidelines.

   _____ c. national standard curricula.

   _____ d. your on-duty supervisor.

3. The obligation you will have as an EMT providing care to the sick and injured is known as a(n):

   _____ a. legal obligation.

   _____ b. ethical obligation.

   _____ c. duty to act.

   _____ d. moral responsibility.

4. The EMT-Basic National Standard Curriculum was developed by the:

   _____ a. National Association of EMS Educators.

   _____ b. National Association of State EMS Directors.

   _____ c. U.S. Department of Transportation.

   _____ d. National Association of EMS Physicians.

5. Which of the following best describes the purpose of Good Samaritan laws?

   _____ a. They encourage passersby to stop and render care.

   _____ b. They discourage untrained passersby from rendering care.

   _____ c. They hold passersby exempt from having to stop.

   _____ d. They require passersby to stop and render care.

Matching

Match the definition on the left with the applicable term on the right.

1. _____ A detailed description of the specific care and actions EMTs are allowed to perform as defined by state laws and regulations

2. _____ A modified scope of practice specifically designed to meet the needs of a specific area or region

3. _____ The organization responsible for developing the National Standard Curricula and the Scope of Practice for EMS

A. Good Samaritan law
B. Medical direction
C. Ethics
D. Duty to act
E. NHTSA
F. Scope of practice
G. Standard of care

4. _____ The process of overseeing all aspects of patient care within the EMS system and to ensure continuous quality improvement of the system

5. _____ The study of the general nature of morals and the specific moral choices an individual makes in relating to others

6. _____ A legal obligation to render care to those in need and to do so to an established standard of care

7. _____ Specific laws to encourage passersby to stop and assist those in need of medical attention

Critical Thinking

1. Does the scope of practice differ from the standard of care in the system in which you will be working? How might you find this out?

   _____

   _____

   _____

   _____

   _____

2. Describe the difference between and provide an example of a legal duty and an ethical duty as they pertain to the job of an EMT.

   _____

   _____

   _____

   _____

3. Describe the purpose and function of Good Samaritan laws.

   _____

   _____

   _____

   _____

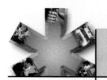

Perspective

Henry—The Patient

"I just couldn't seem to get anyone to understand me. My right hip and shoulder were pretty sore, but when I tried to tell the ambulance people the words were coming out all wrong. I just wanted someone to help and to find out what was wrong with me."

1-3.3 Define consent and discuss the methods of obtaining consent.

✳ **consent**

permission from the patient for care or other action by the EMT. See also expressed consent; implied consent.

1-3.4 Differentiate between expressed and implied consent.

✳ **expressed consent**

consent given by adults who are of legal age and mentally competent to make a rational decision in regard to their medical well-being. See also consent; implied consent.

Obtaining Consent and Patient Refusal

Before you can legally provide care for a patient, you must obtain consent. **Consent,** or permission from the patient to provide care, can take a variety of forms such as verbal, nonverbal, written and implied. Regardless of the form, it is a legal requirement that the EMT receive consent from the patient before providing care.

EXPRESSED CONSENT

Consent that is obtained from alert, competent adult patients who understand the consequences of their choice is referred to as **expressed consent,** also called *informed consent* (Figure 3-2). Expressed consent can be verbal, nonverbal or written and can only be obtained from patients who are of legal age and deemed mentally competent to make informed rational decisions about their own care. In most cases, expressed consent is verbal. That is, you introduce yourself and ask the patient if it is okay for you to help them and they respond verbally. In some instances, you may ask the responsive patient for permission to treat and they offer no verbal response. In these instances, as long as the patient does not refuse care it is considered expressed consent and you may proceed with the appropriate care.

Clinical Clues: CONSENT

It should not be assumed that when you arrive on the scene behind Emergency Responders such as fire or law enforcement personnel that the patient has always provided consent. Observe the entire scene carefully as you approach, and obtain an appropriate briefing from the First Responders before you approach the patient. Is the patient being cooperative or displaying signs of resistance? Observing the interaction between the patient and the Emergency Responders will help determine the best approach for the patient. In most cases when a patient is cooperative, you can simply introduce yourself and inform the patient that you will be caring for them. In situations where there may be some resistance on the part of the patient, a slower approach may be best. Introducing yourself and asking permission to treat will usually be a good way to begin.

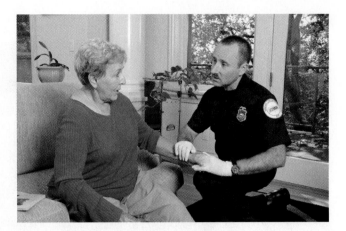

FIGURE 3-2   Before you can legally provide care for a patient, you must obtain consent.

COMPETENCY

A **competent** adult is one who is able to make informed and rational decisions about his own well-being. The concept of competency is somewhat subjective, and it can be difficult at times in an emergency situation for the EMT to determine whether a person is making a rational decision or not. In most cases, you will be called to the scene of an emergency and begin rendering care with no resistance from the patient. Where competency may become an issue is when a patient refuses care. A patient who is ill or injured and refusing your care may not be able to make rational decisions because of the medical condition or injury. For this reason you must use great caution when allowing patients to refuse care. It is also important to understand that a competent adult has the right to refuse care at any time, even after care has been initiated. More on refusal of care will be discussed later.

IMPLIED CONSENT

Implied consent is a legal term used to describe an assumed permission to treat. Permission may be assumed when you are caring for the following types of patients:

∗ Not of legal age (Figure 3-3A on page 66)
∗ Unresponsive (Figure 3-3B on page 66)
∗ Mentally incompetent

∗ **competent**
the ability of an adult to make informed and rational decisions about his own well-being.

1-3.5   Explain the role of consent of minors in providing care.

∗ **implied consent**
the consent it is presumed a patient or patient's parent or guardian would give if they could, such as for an unconscious patient or by a parent who cannot be contacted when care is needed. See also consent; expressed consent.

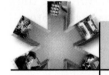

Perspective

Jewel—The EMT

"That poor old guy sure seemed confused, and it wouldn't surprise me at all if he really hurt himself falling out of bed like that. But I'll tell you what, we couldn't just put him back in bed and leave like that lady wanted us to. After all, can't I still take care of a patient even though he couldn't give consent or anything? I think I can. Can't I?"

FIGURE 3-3A Implied consent is assumed when a pediatric patient requires care and a parent or guardian is not immediately available.

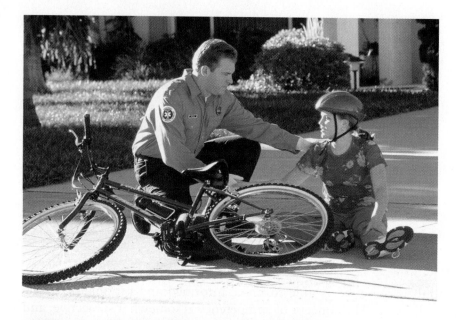

FIGURE 3-3B Patients who are unresponsive can be cared for based on implied consent.

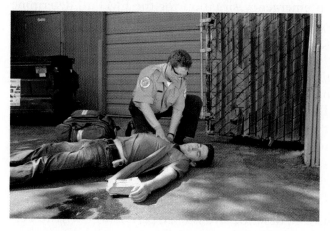

In the case of an unresponsive patient, the EMT may provide care because it is assumed that if the patient were aware of his situation he would consent. In the case of a minor who is ill or injured, it is assumed that the parents would grant permission to treat if they were present.

Even though the standard legal age in the U.S. is 18 years, most states allow persons between the ages of 14 and 18 who meet strict requirements to become emancipated and therefore obtain the full legal rights of an adult. Some of the more common reasons a minor may become emancipated are marriage, preg-

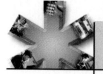

Perspective

Brandon—The EMT

"You know, I'm not sure if that caregiver can legally refuse care for Mr. Flowers. I assume that she's his legal guardian, but does that give her that right? I really felt that he needed to be seen by a doctor, and it wasn't like he seemed to be refusing care."

nancy, and enlistment in the armed forces. In most cases, emancipation requires an action by the courts and is rarely encountered.

Patients who are incompetent because of mental illness or as a result of their illness or injury may also be cared for legally based on implied consent. One of the most common reasons for a patient to be deemed incompetent is intoxication from drugs or alcohol. It is important to understand, however, that although you have the legal right to provide care based on implied consent, the patient may still attempt to refuse your help. In these instances, it is appropriate to call for assistance from law enforcement.

PATIENTS WHO REFUSE CARE

As stated earlier, any patient of legal age who is competent may refuse care at any time. Additionally, this means that parents and legal guardians may refuse care on behalf of those for whom they are responsible. It is also important to understand that competent adults may refuse care even after it has been initiated and they are on the way to the hospital.

As an EMT you have specific responsibilities when dealing with patients who refuse your care. First you must make every effort to convince them that providing consent and allowing you to care for them is in their best interest. You must clearly explain the risks and consequences of their decision to refuse care, and you must feel certain that they understand what you are telling them. If all of these conditions are met and a patient still refuses care, it is common practice to ask the patient to sign a release form. These forms are sometimes referred to against-medical-advice or AMA forms and, in theory, they release the medical team from liability should the patient's condition worsen later (Figure 3-4 on page 68).

If you are ever in doubt as to whether the patient is truly competent or if, in your opinion, they really need further medical attention, you should err on the side of caution. Depending on the situation, you may need to contact Medical Direction, your supervisor or, in extreme cases, law enforcement personnel. In cases where the patient is refusing care but you feel they should receive care or risk serious harm or death, in some jurisdictions a law enforcement officer can place the patient on a legal hold and force them to accept the appropriate medical attention. In all cases of patient refusal, seek a second opinion from your partner or other EMS provider on scene. It is unwise to make an independent decision not to transport.

Proper documentation is always important when providing care for an ill or injured person. It becomes especially important in cases of patient refusal because of the likelihood that their condition may worsen. Be diligent in your documentation of these cases. Include details about your assessment of the patient, your attempts to convince the patient to agree to care, and any witnesses to the patient refusal. When possible, as already discussed, have the patient sign a refusal form. In some cases, the patient will even refuse to sign the form. In these instances, you should have another EMS, fire, or law enforcement official sign the form as a witness to the refusal.

ABANDONMENT

Abandonment is a legal term that the EMT should study and understand thoroughly. Abandonment refers to a situation where an EMT has a legal duty to provide care but leaves or abandons the patient before turning care of the patient over to someone of equal or higher training. For a case involving an accusation of abandonment to hold up, it must first be established that the EMT had a legal duty to care for the patient.

1-3.6 Discuss the implications for the EMT-Basic in patient refusal of transport.

1-3.7 Discuss the issues of abandonment, negligence, and battery and their implications to the EMT-Basic.

∗ **abandonment**

leaving a patient after care has been initiated and before the patient has been transferred to someone with equal or greater medical training.

Coastal Valleys EMS Agency

Applicable for:
✓ Napa County
✓ Sonoma County
✓ Mendocino County

Serving Mendocino, Napa and Sonoma Counties

RAS/AMA FORM

Date _____ ALS # _____ Dispatch # _____

Section I   Release at Scene (RAS)

I understand that any evaluation and/or emergency treatment I have received by these EMS personnel has been on an emergency basis only and is not intended to be a substitute for complete medical assessment and/or care. I understand it appears that further emergency transportation and/or care does not appear to be needed at this time. I understand that I may have an illness or injury that is unforeseen at this time. I understand that if I change my mind or if my condition changes or becomes worse and I need further treatment/transportation by the Emergency Medical Services System, I can call back and they will respond.

Patient Name (print)_____ Patient Signature_____

Patient / Guardian Signature_____ Relationship_____

Paramedic / EMT signature_____ Witness Signature_____

Comments: _____

Section II   Refusal of Evaluation / Treatment / Transportation Against Medical Advice (AMA)

I, _____ acknowledge that on_____
      Patient Name (print)

                                                                                          Date

_____   /_____   /_____   _____
      EMT-Paramedic/EMT   License/Cert #   Service Provider Agency

explained my condition to me and advised me of some of the potential risks and/or complications which could or would arise from refusal of medical care. I have also been advised that other unknown risks and/or complications are possible up to and including the loss of life or limb. Being aware that there are known and unknown potential risks and/or complications, it is still my desire to refuse the advised medical care.

• All Care Refused   • Specific Care Refused:_____

I do hereby release EMS personnel from all liability resulting from any adverse medical condition(s) caused by my refusal of the recommended medical care.

Patient Signature_____Paramedic / EMT Signature_____

Patient / Guardian Signature_____Relationship_____

Witness Name:_____ Witness Signature_____

Comments:_____

FIGURE 3-4   A patient who refuses care should be asked to sign a release form. (Coastal Valleys EMS Agency.)

While on the surface this may seem obvious, most cases of abandonment are much more subtle. For example, you and your partner are working a busy EMS system and are on your third call in a row. As you wheel your chest-pain patient into the busy emergency department, you catch the attention of one of the nurses who tells you to put your patient in Room 3 and that she will be right there. While transferring the patient to the hospital bed, you receive a dispatch over your radio for a vehicle collision on the other side of town. You quickly finish getting the pa-

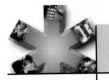

Clinical Clues: RELEASE AT SCENE

In some EMS systems an additional document called a Release at Scene (RAS) is used when both the patient and the EMTs feel that ambulance transport is not necessary. This option respects the rights of a competent adult who wishes to seek medical care but not be transported by ambulance. In most cases, specific criteria must be met before a patient can be appropriately released at the scene. It is important to find out if such a form or policy exists in your EMS system. If in doubt, contact medical direction.

Perspective

Janine—The Caregiver

"I just don't have time for that. I've got fourteen patients that I have to see each and every day. Henry was fine. Heck, I don't even remember how many times he's fallen down. It's not that big of a deal. Those ambulance people must be new or something. Other crews just get him back into bed and go about their day, because then they have the time to help people who really need it."

tient onto the hospital bed, gather up your supplies and, as you are heading out the door, yell to the nurse that you have another call. However, the nurse is so busy that it is 15 minutes before she gets a chance to check on your patient. When she does, she finds him on the bed without respirations or a pulse.

It will not be hard for an attorney to establish that you and your partner had abandoned this patient, because you left him without formally transferring care to someone of equal or higher training. Simply yelling at the nurse that you were leaving on another call is not what most would consider a formal transfer of care. You must provide a detailed verbal report directly to the person who is taking over care. In many instances you will also leave a copy of your written report, which becomes part of the patient's permanent medical record.

Advance Directives

It is becoming increasingly common for patients to provide specific instructions regarding their health care. An **advance directive** is a legal statement of a patient's wishes regarding his own health care. As an EMT it is only a matter of time before you will encounter a patient with one form or another of an advance directive.

Advance directives come in different forms and address a variety of health care issues. One form is a written document known as a *living will*. A living will is a legal document describing in detail the patient's specific instructions. Patients may provide instructions for their care in the event they become too ill to let their wishes be known. The advance directive may describe which treatments and care the patient wants and which they do not want should they be unable to

1-3.2   Discuss the importance of do not resuscitate [DNR] (advance directives) and local or state provisions regarding EMS application.

* **advance directive**

    a legal statement of a patient's wishes regarding his own health care.

communicate. This document is typically signed by the patient and his physician. In most states, an advance directive must be in writing and be in the presence of the patient at all times. Some states will accept an advance directive in the form of medical identification jewelry. Your instructor will provide the details of acceptable advance directives in your state or region.

✳ **do not resuscitate (DNR) order**

a legal document, usually signed by the patient and his physician, which states that the patient has a terminal illness and does not wish to prolong life through resuscitative efforts.

DO NOT RESUSCITATE (DNR) ORDER

Another type of advance directive is the **do not resuscitate (DNR) order** (Figure 3-5). Its purpose is to advise health care professionals that the patient does not want to be resuscitated in the event of a cardiac or respiratory arrest. There are

---

PREHOSPITAL DO NOT RESUSCITATE ORDERS

<u>ATTENDING PHYSICIAN</u>

In completing this prehospital DNR form, please check part A if no intervention by prehospital personnel is indicated. Please check Part A and options from Part B if specific interventions by prehospital personnel are indicated. To give a valid prehospital DNR order, this form must be completed by the patient's attending physician and must be provided to prehospital personnel.

A) _____**Do Not Resuscitate (DNR):**
No Cardiopulmonary Resuscitation or Advanced Cardiac Life Support be performed by prehospital personnel

B) _____**Modified Support:**
Prehospital personnel administer the following checked options:
_____Oxygen administration
_____Full airway support: intubation, airways, bag/valve/mask
_____Venipuncture: IV crystalloids and/or blood draw
_____External cardiac pacing
_____Cardiopulmonary resuscitation
_____Cardiac defibrillator
_____Pneumatic anti-shock garment
_____Ventilator
_____ACLS meds
_____Other interventions/medications (physician specify)
_____

Prehospital personnel are informed that (print patient name)_____
should receive no resuscitation (DNR) or should receive Modified Support as indicated. This directive is medically appropriate and is further documented by a physician's order and a progress note on the patient's permanent medical record. Informed consent from the capacitated patient or the incapacitated patient's legitimate surrogate is documented on the patient's permanent medical record. The DNR order is in full force and effect as of the date indicated below.

_____   _____
Attending Physician's Signature

_____   _____
Print Attending Physician's Name   Print Patient's Name and Location
                                            (Home Address or Health Care Facility)

_____
Attending Physician's Telephone

_____   _____
Date   Expiration Date (6 Mos from Signature)

FIGURE 3-5   An example of an advance directive is the do not resuscitate (DNR) order.

varying degrees of DNR order that indicate specific care that can or cannot be initiated. For instance, a terminally ill patient may wish to continue to receive pain medication as his condition worsens, but should he go into cardiac arrest he does not want anyone to begin CPR. Another patient may state that he would like to be ventilated should he stop breathing on his own, but if his heart stops he does not want anyone initiating CPR.

As an EMT who is called to the scene of a patient with a DNR order, you must insist on seeing a written copy of the order to determine the specific degree and nature of the order. Without documented proof of a DNR order, you will be compelled to begin resuscitative efforts. In any case where there is confusion regarding the presence of a DNR order, it is best to begin care until the DNR order can be confirmed or you have transferred care at the hospital.

 Stop, Review, Remember!

Multiple Choice

Place a check next to the correct answer.

1. Which of the following is the best example of expressed consent?

    _____ a. a drunk 20-year-old who agrees to allow you to provide care

    _____ b. a frightened 6-year-old who just sits there and allows you to help

    _____ c. a wife who provides consent for her unresponsive husband

    _____ d. a 40-year-old who asks for assistance

2. Which of the following statements regarding a competent adult is most accurate?

    _____ a. A competent adult patient may refuse care at any time.

    _____ b. Once care has begun, a patient may not refuse.

    _____ c. Only a law enforcement officer can determine if a patient is competent.

    _____ d. An EMT may restrain any patient who is determined to be incompetent.

3. Which type of consent would be used for an 11-year-old unresponsive patient whose parents are not immediately available?

    _____ a. informed consent

    _____ b. expressed consent

    _____ c. implied consent

    _____ d. assumed consent

4. Before leaving a patient who is refusing care, the EMT must do all of the following EXCEPT:

    _____ a. explain that proper care is in the patient's best interest.

    _____ b. threaten to call the police if the patient doesn't provide consent.

    _____ c. explain the risks of a decision to refuse care.

    _____ d. have the patient sign a release form.

5. Which of the following is the most accurate definition of an advance directive?

_____ a. a legal statement of a patient's wishes regarding health care

_____ b. a family's verbal wishes regarding the care of a loved one

_____ c. a patient's verbal refusal of any further care

_____ d. a patient's wishes regarding funeral arrangements

6. Leaving a patient before formally transferring care to an appropriate health care provider may be considered:

_____ a. within the EMT scope of practice.

_____ b. standard practice.

_____ c. abandonment.

_____ d. part of the duty to act.

Matching

Match the definition on the left with the applicable term on the right.

1. _____ Permission from the patient to provide care

2. _____ Consent that is obtained from alert, competent adult patients

3. _____ A legal term used to describe an assumed permission to treat

4. _____ The term used to describe someone who is able to make informed and rational decisions about their own well-being

5. _____ A situation where an EMT had a legal duty to provide care and left the patient before turning care of the patient over to someone of equal or higher training

6. _____ A legal statement of a patient's wishes regarding his or her own health care

7. _____ A form advising health care professionals that the patient does not want to be resuscitated in the event of a cardiac or respiratory arrest

A. Implied consent
B. Competent
C. Advance directive
D. Abandonment
E. DNR
F. Consent
G. Expressed consent

Critical Thinking

1. In what ways may a responsive adult patient provide consent for treatment? Must it always be verbal?

_____

_____

_____

_____

2. In what situations might it be difficult to determine if a patient is competent enough to refuse care?

_____

_____

_____

_____

3. How might you handle a situation where the family states that there is a DNR but they cannot produce a copy of it?

_____

_____

_____

_____

Assault and Battery

Although it is quite rare, an EMT who attempts to force care on a competent person may be accused of assault and battery. **Assault** is the threat to use force upon another and **battery** is the carrying out of that threat. It is important to understand that assault can be alleged even when no physical contact is made. Simply threatening to inflict physical contact against a patient's wishes can be construed as assault.

An accusation of battery requires that actual unwanted physical contact be made between the EMT and the patient. This can occur when attempting to care for a combative patient whom you feel is not competent. Unless law enforcement is there to assist, it is not wise to make contact with a patient who is refusing care. Even a simple touch, if unwanted, can constitute battery. In cases where the patient has become a threat to himself, the EMT, or others, it may become necessary to restrain the patient for safety. These situations are relatively rare and should be documented thoroughly, including statements from any witnesses at the scene.

* **assault**
  the threat to use force upon another.

* **battery**
  the carrying out of a threat to use force upon another.

Negligence

No discussion of the legal aspects of providing care would be complete without a dialogue on the topic of **negligence**. Negligence is another of those fundamental terms that every EMT must understand thoroughly. *Webster's Dictionary* defines negligence as *the omission or neglect of reasonable care, precaution, or action.* As an EMT you must provide what is considered to be a reasonable standard of care for your patient and make every attempt to minimize any further harm.

* **negligence**
  a finding of failure to act properly in a situation in which there was a duty to act, needed care as would reasonably be expected of the EMT was not provided, and harm was caused to the patient as a result.

For an accusation of negligence to hold up in a court of law, four specific elements must exist. These elements are:

* Duty
* Breach of duty
* Damages
* Causation

DUTY

It must be established that the EMT had a legal duty to provide care to the person making the accusation, in this case the patient.

BREACH OF DUTY

It must be determined that the EMT breached his duty in some form or manner. A breach is a failure to live up to a legal obligation such as the EMT's duty to provide medical care. The case of abandonment discussed earlier (where the chest-pain patient was left in the emergency department with the EMTs simply yelling to the nurse that they were leaving on another call) could easily be deemed a breach of duty. Providing care outside of one's scope of practice may also be considered a breach of duty.

DAMAGES

The next item required for a successful negligence suit is the element of damages. It must be proven that the patient suffered some form of actual physical or emotional damages. In the abandonment case just discussed, the damages would be the death of the chest-pain patient.

CAUSATION

The final and most difficult element is the concept of causation. It must be proven that the actions or lack thereof by the EMT actually caused the damages being alleged. In most unsuccessful negligence suits, this is where the argument falls apart. While it is clear that the EMT crew had a duty, that they breached that duty, and that the man did die, it is another thing altogether to prove that the actions of the EMT crew, in this case leaving the patient, actually caused the man's death.

While we do not expect every EMT to become a virtual lawyer, it is important to develop a good understanding of these key legal terms and concepts. Together with an equal dose of common sense and experience, this knowledge will go a long way to help keep you from being named or convicted in a lawsuit.

1-3.9 Explain the importance, necessity, and legality of patient confidentiality.

✳ **Health Insurance Portability and Accountability Act (HIPAA)**

federal law protecting the privacy of patient-specific health care information and providing the patient with control over how this information is used and distributed.

Patient Confidentiality

More than ever before in the history of EMS, the concept of patient confidentiality is being stressed and enforced. Recent legislation, the **Health Insurance Portability and Accountability Act (HIPAA)**, has imposed a number of restrictions on how health care providers may use and share patient information.

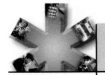

Perspective

Jewel—The EMT

"That whole situation stunk. That old man is definitely not receiving the quality of care that he deserves. Heck . . . his sheets were just plain nasty; he's got bed sores that were obviously infected and he doesn't look like he had eaten in days. That's just plain . . . I mean there's just . . . definitely some neglect going on there in my opinion. Somebody should do something about it!"

As an EMT you have access to a significant amount of personal information about patients. This can include information such as where they live, their age, their medical history, their employment, and their insurance status. You must keep in mind that any information you gather about a patient is considered confidential and must not be shared with others except in very specific circumstances.

You may legally share information with other care providers who will be taking over care of the patient, but you may share only information that directly affects patient care and may not share other, nonmedical information. In order to legally share confidential information with other individuals such as law enforcement officers or attorneys, you may need prior written consent from the patient or receive a legal subpoena for release of the information.

It is important to learn what your agency's policy is regarding patient confidentiality. Just to be on the safe side, it may be best to refer all such requests to your supervisor.

Special Situations

Most states have laws that identify specific situations where an EMT must report what they see or hear. The most common situations involve cases of known or suspected abuse or neglect that involve a child, the elderly, or a spouse. Should you ever care for someone who you suspect is a victim of abuse or neglect, you may be required by law to report it. Immediately discuss any such case with your supervisor, who will probably be more knowledgeable about the reporting laws in your state.

Other mandatory reporting laws regard situations that involve a crime such as sexual assault or injuries sustained from a firearm. It is highly likely that you will be mandated by the laws in your state to report these cases to the proper authorities.

1-3.12 State the conditions that require an EMT-Basic to notify local law enforcement officials.

CRIME SCENES

At times you may be called to provide care for someone injured or ill at a known or suspected crime scene. In these instances, a law enforcement officer will probably be dispatched to the scene ahead of the ambulance. Should you arrive at the scene of an emergency and suspect that it may involve a crime, you should request law enforcement immediately. Remember that you do not have an obligation to put yourself at undue risk to assist an injured or ill person. The scene must be safe before you can enter (Figure 3-6 on page 76).

1-3.11 Differentiate the actions that an EMT-Basic should take to assist in the preservation of a crime scene.

FIGURE 3-6   A law enforcement officer should be requested at a suspected crime scene.

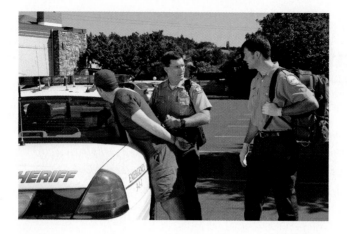

Once you have been called into the scene by law enforcement, your primary duty is to provide excellent patient care to those who need it without disturbing the scene more than absolutely necessary. You may need to document your findings in more detail than usual, since the call may be involved in a future court case. Pay attention to and document as much detail as you can about the scene as you found it. Document where you entered the scene and where you were at all times within the scene. Observe and document anything that may seem unusual about the scene or the patient. Be careful not to disturb potential evidence at the scene or on the patient. If possible when removing clothing from your patient, cut around, not through, obvious bullet or stab holes in the patient's clothing.

1-3.10 Discuss the considerations of the EMT-Basic in issues of organ retrieval.

POTENTIAL ORGAN DONORS

More and more people are becoming educated about organ donation and are choosing to be identified as a potential organ donor should they die. The most common form of identification for an organ donor is the card that accompanies the driver's license. Sometimes there is a small sticker with the word *Donor* on it that is placed on the front of the driver's license, or there may be a check-off section on the back of the license that indicates the person's wish to be an organ donor (Figure 3-7).

As an EMT you are likely to encounter patients who have designated themselves as potential donors. Do not let this information change the way in which you care for the patient. In most instances, the patient is transported to the hospital before death is declared. Continue resuscitative efforts according to your local protocols and advise hospital personnel and/or medical direction of the patient's donor status.

FIGURE 3-7   The driver's license is the most common form of identification as an organ donor.

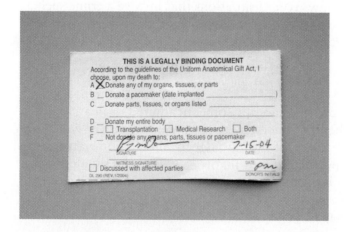

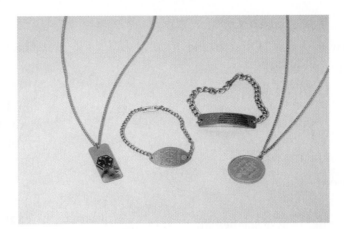

FIGURE 3-8 Medical identification jewelry identifies the wearer's specific needs or conditions.

MEDICAL IDENTIFICATION JEWELRY

A number of private companies manufacture specialized medical identification jewelry. The most common forms of medical jewelry are the necklace and the bracelet (Figure 3-8). Some people prefer to wear their medical jewelry around the ankle so that it is less obvious to the general public. Medical identification also can take other forms, such as a wallet card or small tag placed on a key ring, watchband, or belt.

The purpose of medical identification jewelry or cards is to alert others to the person's existing medical conditions should the wearer become unresponsive. The most commonly identified are conditions such as diabetes, allergies, epilepsy, and heart conditions.

Stop, Review, Remember!

Multiple Choice

Place a check next to the correct answer.

1. Which of the following best describes the term *assault?*

   _____ a. Inflicting physical harm to another person

   _____ b. The verbal threat to use force upon another person

   _____ c. Holding another person against his will

   _____ d. Verbal abuse

2. Which of the following could most likely be considered a breach of duty by an EMT?

   _____ a. Providing high-flow oxygen to an emphysema patient in acute distress

   _____ b. Transporting an unresponsive child without a parent's consent

   _____ c. Leaving the scene of one emergency to respond to another emergency before additional help arrives

   _____ d. Assisting a chest-pain patient with taking his nitro pills

3. Which of the following is NOT one of the four elements of a case of suspected negligence?

_____ a. duty

_____ b. breach of duty

_____ c. abandonment

_____ d. causation

4. Which of the following best describes the EMTs role regarding patient confidentiality?

_____ a. All information obtained by the EMT may be shared with others so long as it is done in private.

_____ b. Only information documented on the patient care report can be shared with others.

_____ c. The EMT may not share any information about the patient with anyone.

_____ d. The EMT may share information with those who are directly involved with the care of the patient.

5. An EMT who goes beyond the scope of practice, for example attempting to start an intravenous line on a chest-pain patient, could be guilty of:

_____ a. breach of duty.

_____ b. abandonment.

_____ c. causation.

_____ d. scopus exceedus.

Matching

Match the definition on the left with the applicable term on the right.

1. _____ The threat to use force upon another

2. _____ The carrying out of a threat to do harm to another

3. _____ The omission or neglect of reasonable care, precaution, or action

4. _____ A legal obligation to provide care

5. _____ A failure to live up to a legal obligation

6. _____ Some form of actual physical or emotional damages

7. _____ The actions or lack thereof that actually caused damage to the patient

A. Causation
B. Negligence
C. Breach of duty
D. Duty
E. Damages
F. Battery
G. Assault

Critical Thinking

1. Describe the difference between the legal terms *assault* and *battery*.

_____

_____

_____

_____

2. Describe a situation whereby an EMT could be accused of negligence.

_____

_____

_____

_____

_____

3. Describe the steps you would take if you were working as an EMT and suspected that a child or elder is being abused or neglected.

_____

_____

_____

_____

_____

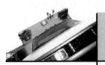

Dispatch Summary

Brandon and Jewel argued with Mr. Flowers's caregiver that he needed to be taken to the hospital. She finally relented and then stormed from the house on her way to the "next appointment."

Further evaluation of Henry revealed an elevated blood pressure and marked weakness on his left side.

Mr. Flowers was placed on high-flow O_2 and transported to Young America Memorial Hospital where he was treated for a stroke, pneumonia, and gangrenous pressure sores.

Sadly, Mr. Flowers died 3 weeks later after being moved to a skilled nursing facility.

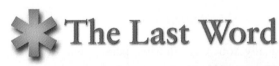

The Last Word

Much of what we do as EMTs is directed or governed by law's, guidelines, protocols, and policies. These will differ from state to state and region to region. Learn and understand those that affect EMT practice in your system. Do not ever forget that, first and foremost, you are there for the patient. If you make decisions based on what is right for the patient, it will be difficult for others to question your motives. What you see and do at work as an EMT should stay there. Respect patient confidentiality at all times.

Chapter Review

MULTIPLE CHOICE

Place a check next to the correct answer.

1. The _____ is a detailed description of the specific care and actions EMTs are allowed to perform based on state laws and regulations.

   _____ a. standard of care

   _____ b. scope of practice

   _____ c. national standard curriculum

   _____ d. national scope of care

2. A do not resuscitate (DNR) order gives the EMT the ability to choose whether or not to attempt resuscitation of the patient, regardless of the patient's wishes.

   _____ a. true

   _____ b. false

3. Which of the following statements about the concept of consent is most accurate?

   _____ a. Verbal consent must be obtained from all patients regardless of age.

   _____ b. Parents do not have the right to refuse care for their children.

   _____ c. Consent can come in many forms such as verbal, nonverbal, and written.

   _____ d. It is not necessary to seek consent for treatment of a minor.

4. An EMT who ceases to provide care for a patient before formally handing the patient off to someone of equal or higher training may be accused of:

   _____ a. abandonment.   _____ c. assault.

   _____ b. battery.   _____ d. causation.

5. EMTs are required to report all suspected cases of _____ and _____ to the appropriate authorities.

   _____ a. abuse, neglect

   _____ b. abuse, Alzheimer's

   _____ c. negligence, neglect

   _____ d. abandonment, negligence

6. Consent to treat an unresponsive patient is referred to as:

   _____ a. parental.

   _____ b. expressed.

   _____ c. implied.

   _____ d. verbal.

7. As an EMT, your care for a patient will not change if it is determined that he is an organ donor.

   _____ a. true

   _____ b. false

8. The primary responsibility of an EMT at a crime scene is:

   _____ a. preservation of evidence.

   _____ b. assisting with the investigation.

   _____ c. patient care.

   _____ d. collection of evidence.

9. Which organization created the EMT-Basic National Standard Curriculum?

   _____ a. U.S. Department of Labor

   _____ b. World Health Organization

   _____ c. Centers for Disease Control and Prevention

   _____ d. U.S. Department of Transportation

10. Physically touching another person without that person's consent can be considered:

    _____ a. assault.

    _____ b. battery.

    _____ c. negligence.

    _____ d. causation.

CRITICAL THINKING

1. Describe a situation when it might be necessary to use force to restrain a patient you are caring for.

_____

_____

_____

2. As a passerby to a motor vehicle collision, are you legally obligated to stop and render care in the state where you live?

_____

_____

_____

_____

3. How might your care change if you discovered that the patient you were caring for was an organ donor?

_____

_____

_____

_____

CASE STUDIES

Case Study 1

You are on your way home from EMT class one evening and are on a remote section of a two-lane highway, when you come across an SUV that has rolled over on the side of the road. The wheels on the overturned vehicle are still spinning as you approach the scene. Your heart begins to race as you consider the prospect of stopping and rendering care. You are only 3 weeks into your EMT class and are very unsure if you will know what to do. As you slowly approach the scene, you see one person lying face down on the opposite side of the road from the vehicle and another person moving about inside the overturned vehicle.

1. Are you obligated by law to stop and render aid to the victims at this scene?

_____

_____

_____

_____

2. What are the legal ramifications if you decide not to stop and just keep going?

_____

_____

_____

_____

3. You have decided to stop and help. Following a brief assessment of the unresponsive victim lying outside the vehicle you are unable to tell if she is breathing or has a pulse. In a moment of panic you decide to get back in your car and leave the scene. What are the legal ramifications of your actions?

_____

_____

_____

_____

Case Study 2

You have been called to a residence for difficulty breathing. Upon arrival you find a 56-year-old male with terminal lung cancer. The patient's respirations are shallow and very labored at a rate of 8 per minute. You begin to ventilate the patient using a bag-valve mask and, after a minute or so, family members advise you that the patient has a DNR order. When you ask to see a copy of the order, they show you a medical alert bracelet on the patient's wrist indicating a DNR.

1. How would you handle this situation?

_____

_____

_____

_____

2. Can a piece of medical jewelry serve as an appropriate DNR?

_____

_____

_____

_____

3. Should you stop ventilating the patient?

_____

_____

_____

_____

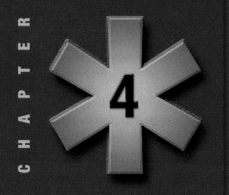
Basic Human Anatomy

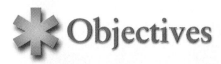

Objectives

Numbered objectives are from the U.S. Department of Transportation 1994 EMT-Basic National Standard Curriculum.

COGNITIVE OBJECTIVES

At the completion of this chapter, the EMT-Basic student will be able to:

1-4.1 Identify the following topographic terms: medial, lateral, proximal, distal, superior, inferior, anterior, posterior, midline, right, left, midclavicular, bilateral, and midaxillary. (pp. 84–86)

1-4.2 Describe the anatomy and function of the following major body systems: respiratory (pp. 92–96), circulatory (pp. 96–102), musculoskeletal (pp. 105–112), nervous (pp. 112–114), and endocrine (pp. 115–117).

AFFECTIVE OBJECTIVES

No affective objectives identified.

PSYCHOMOTOR OBJECTIVES

No psychomotor objectives identified.

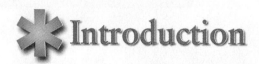

Introduction

Knowledge of human anatomy is essential for the EMT student. It sets a foundation for the remainder of the course. Imagine bandaging an area of the body but not knowing how to refer to it . . . or having a patient point to where his pain is and you are unable to document exactly to what he pointed.

Almost every chapter in this book from this point forward will refer to the material presented here. And every call to which you respond in the future, every patient you treat, every report you write, and every call you make to the hospital will refer to the material in this chapter.

So, yes, knowledge of anatomy is vitally important. You will need to learn, understand, speak, and practice anatomy.

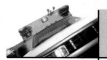

Emergency Dispatch

EMT Heather Hunter and her partner, Josh Mitchell, sat at a small table in front of a coffee shop when the portable radio barked, "Truck eighty-one, respond to the Village Square apartments, number 42, for a patient with abdominal pain."

Heather and Josh already had lids on their drinks, knowing calls frequently interrupt coffee and meals. "To go" is a way of life.

When Heather and Josh arrived at the patient's apartment, they found Jocelyn—a 27-year-old female—

curled into a fetal position on the couch. She was crying and complaining through clenched teeth of pain on both sides of her stomach.

"I'm Josh, and this is my partner, Heather. We're going to help you, OK? Can you tell me about the pain?" Josh asked.

"It's here," Jocelyn said, "my stomach . . . and my back. Like someone is stabbing me."

1-4.1 Identify the following topographic terms: medial, lateral, proximal, distal, superior, inferior, anterior, posterior, midline, right, left, midclavicular, bilateral, and mid-axillary.

✳ **anatomical position**

the standard reference position for the body in the study of anatomy. In this position, the body is standing erect, facing the observer, with arms down at the sides and palms of the hands forward.

Anatomical Terms and Positions

The language of medicine relies on knowledge of anatomy. For you to describe and document complaints, injuries, and examination findings you will need to use exact medical terms. Terms you may be used to such as "around here" or "my stomach hurts" are not appropriate in EMS.

When describing any part of the body, the first point of reference is the **anatomical position** (Figure 4-1). The anatomical position is a person standing, facing forward, with palms facing forward. All descriptions from this point on refer to this position. You will soon see why this is important.

Many descriptions are relative. This means that they can change unless a standard is made. Place your right arm down alongside your body. Place your palm forward. There is an inside surface (closest to your body) and an outside

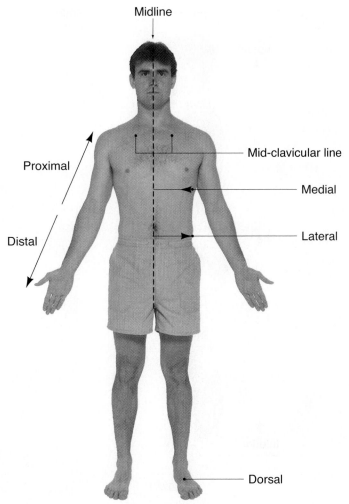

Midline

Proximal

Distal

Mid-clavicular line

Medial

Lateral

Dorsal

FIGURE 4-1   The anatomical position.

surface (farthest away from your body). Now turn your hand so your palm is facing the rear. The side that was previously outside is now inside. The inside is now outside. What if you had to document the location of a wound on that arm? This is why we always refer to anatomical position as the standard point of reference—regardless of how you find the patient. It is a standard among health care professionals.

One other thing to remember. When you refer to **left** or **right,** it is always the patient's left or right—*not yours*.

The body can also be divided into planes (Figure 4-2 on page 86). A **plane** is a straight line or a flat surface that divides something into sections as if slicing through a solid object. For example if you ran a line down from the top of the head, centered on the nose and umbilicus (belly button), you would have the body's **midline.** The plane formed at the midline would divide the body into left and right halves. The midline is also a point of reference for the first terms we will learn: *medial* and *lateral*. Something that is **medial** is closer to the midline. **Lateral** is farther away from the midline. A laceration might be located on "the medial aspect of the left thigh." A bruise might be on "the lateral aspect of the right upper arm."

The term **bilateral** means both sides. If someone has two broken lower legs he would have "bilateral lower leg fractures."

The body can also be divided into a front and back by the **midaxillary** line. This is a vertical line down the side of the body from the armpit to the ankle bone. It divides the body into the **anterior** (front) and **posterior** (rear). If you had a laceration on your shin, it would be on the anterior portion of your leg. If you

* **left**

  referring to the patient's left.

* **right**

  referring to the patient's right.

* **plane**

  a flat surface formed when slicing through a solid object.

* **midline**

  an imaginary line drawn down the center of the body, dividing it into right and left halves.

* **medial**

  toward the midline of the body.

* **lateral**

  to the side, away from the midline of the body.

* **bilateral**

  on both sides.

* **midaxillary**

  line drawn vertically from the middle of the armpit to the ankle.

* **anterior**

  the front of the body or body part. Opposite of *posterior*.

* **posterior**

  the back of the body or body part. Opposite of *anterior*.

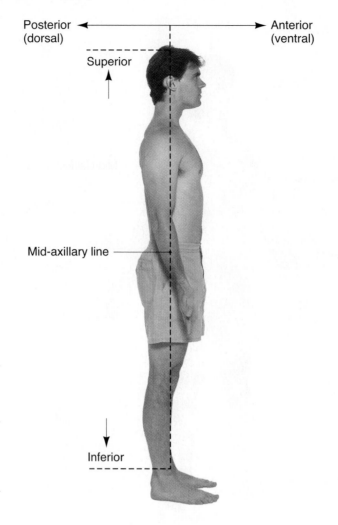

Posterior
(dorsal) ◄————————► Anterior
(ventral)

Superior

Mid-axillary line

Inferior

＊ **ventral**

referring to the front of the body. Synonym for *anterior.*

＊ **dorsal**

referring to the back of the body or the back of the hand or foot. Synonym for *posterior.*

＊ **midclavicular**

the vertical line through the center of each clavicle.

＊ **superior**

toward the head (e.g., the chest is superior to the abdomen). Opposite of *inferior.*

＊ **inferior**

away from the head; usually compared with another structure that is closer to the head (e.g., the lips are inferior to the nose). Opposite of *superior.*

＊ **plantar**

referring to the sole of the foot.

＊ **palmar**

referring to the palm of the hand.

＊ **proximal**

closer to the torso. Opposite of *distal.*

＊ **distal**

farther away from the torso. Opposite of *proximal.*

had a laceration on your lower back, it would be on the posterior of your body. The anterior is sometimes called **ventral** and the posterior may also be called **dorsal.**

The **midclavicular** line is on the anterior surface of the body and runs vertically through the center of the clavicle (collar bone) down through the nipple. There are two clavicles so there are two midclavicular lines, one on each side of the body. If a patient had a wound in this area, it could be described as "on the midclavicular line at the level of the fifth rib."

Superior and *inferior,* simply stated, refer to up and down. **Superior** is up and **inferior** is down. Your ribs are superior to your belly button. Your eyes are inferior to your forehead. **Plantar** refers to the sole of the foot. **Palmar** refers to the palm of the hand.

Two of the most confusing terms (but also two of the most commonly used) are *proximal* and *distal.* **Proximal** means closer to the body (closer to the trunk or heart) while **distal** means farther away. The confusion comes from the fact that a part of the body can be proximal to one part but distal to another. An example is the knee. The knee is distal to the hip (farther away from the torso) but proximal to (closer to the torso than) the ankle. These terms are used frequently. A patient may have a suspected fracture in the proximal third of the femur or a laceration on the distal forearm. You are now able to picture where these injuries are because of your knowledge of anatomy and terms used to describe it.

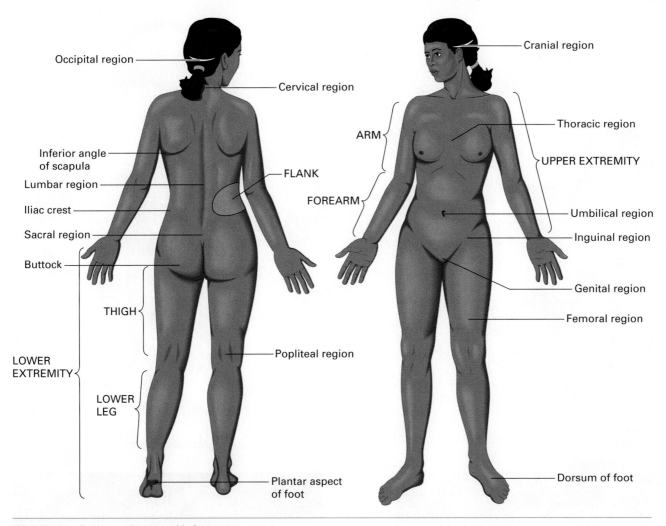

FIGURE 4-3   Regions and topographic features.

ANATOMICAL REGIONS

Locations of the body may also be referred to by region and by topographic features. Some of these are common such as "thigh" or "forearm" while others are a bit more technical. These regions and features are shown in Figure 4-3.

The body also has certain cavities. For example the heart, lungs, and major blood vessels (the "great vessels," including the aorta and venae cavae) lie within the thoracic cavity. Our stomach, intestines, gall bladder, appendix, and other organs lie within the abdominal cavity. The abdomen is divided into four quadrants (Figure 4-4 on page 88). The diaphragm separates the thoracic cavity from the abdominal cavity. Figure 4-5 on page 88 shows the body cavities.

TERMS OF POSITION

There are also terms for the way the patient is positioned. The position may be the way the patient is found or a position in which you place him for care. There are five major positions (Figure 4-6A–E on pages 88 and 89):

 * **Supine** is when a patient is lying on his back.

 * **Prone** refers to the patient lying on his anterior body surface or "front."

* **supine**

lying on the back. Opposite of *prone*.

* **prone**

lying on the stomach. Opposite of *supine*.

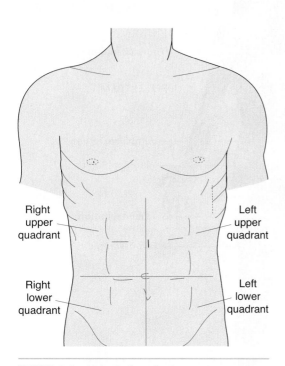

FIGURE 4-4 Abdominal quadrants.

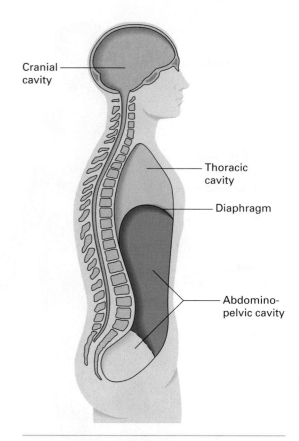

FIGURE 4-5 Main body cavities.

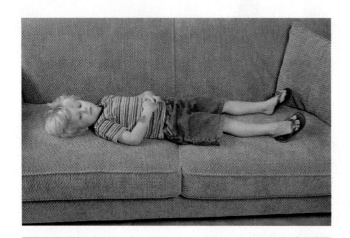

FIGURE 4-6A The supine position.

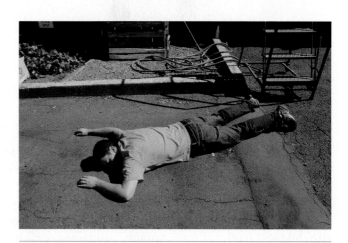

FIGURE 4-6B The prone position.

✳ **laterally recumbent**
lying on the side.

✳ **Fowler's position**
a sitting position.

✳ **Semi-Fowler's**
a semi-sitting position.

✳ **Trendelenburg position**
a position in which the patient's feet and legs are higher than the head. Also called shock position.

✳ **Laterally recumbent** refers to the patient lying on his side. Unconscious or semi-conscious patients who are breathing are often placed in this position to facilitate drainage from the mouth and prevent aspiration of secretions or vomitus into the lungs.

✳ **Fowler's position** refers to a sitting position. **Semi-Fowler's** refers to a semi-sitting position. Patients with difficulty breathing usually prefer a sitting or semi-sitting position.

✳ **Trendelenburg position** refers to the patient lying with his head lower than his feet. This is sometimes used in patients experiencing shock.

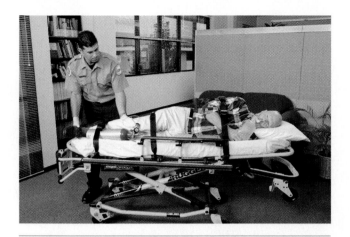

FIGURE 4-6C   The laterally recumbent position.

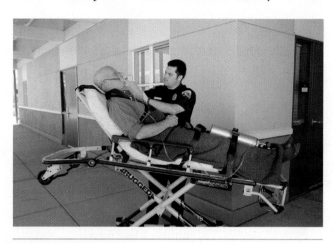

FIGURE 4-6D   The semi-Fowler's position.

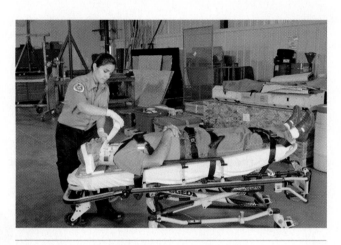

FIGURE 4-6E   The Trendelenburg position.

✳ Stop, Review, Remember!

Multiple Choice

Place a check next to the correct answer.

1. A patient who is supine is lying:

_____ a. face up.

_____ b. face down.

_____ c. on the left side.

_____ d. on the right side.

2. The term *proximal* is best defined as:

_____ a. closer to a joint or extremity.

_____ b. farther away from a joint or extremity.

_____ c. closer to the midline of the body.

_____ d. farther away from the midline of the body.

3. The heart, lungs, and great vessels are found in the:

_____ a. abdominal cavity.

_____ b. peritoneal space.

_____ c. retroperitoneal space.

_____ d. thoracic cavity.

4. Plantar refers to the:

_____ a. palm of the hand.

_____ b. sole of the foot.

_____ c. forehead.

_____ d. buttocks.

5. The midclavicular line passes through the:

_____ a. armpit.

_____ b. umbilicus.

_____ c. nipple.

_____ d. palm.

6. When referring to left and right, you should use your left and right, not the patient's.

_____ a. true

_____ b. false

7. Trendelenburg position is a sitting position.

_____ a. true

_____ b. false

Labeling

On the following photograph, label the listed anatomical terms, regions, or planes:

✳ torso

✳ left leg

✳ right arm

✳ lateral aspect of the right leg

✳ medial aspect of the left chest

✳ mid-clavicular line

✳ midline

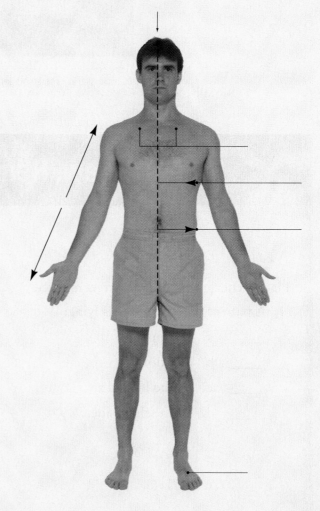

Fill in the Blank

1. The elbow is _____ to the wrist and _____ to the shoulder.

2. A patient found "face down" is said to be in a _____ position.

3. _____ is the line that is drawn downward from the collar bones.

4. _____ is the line drawn through the armpit down through the ankles and divides the body into _____ and _____.

5. _____ means "both sides."

Critical Thinking

Each of the following injuries or complaints is stated in common terms. Describe their locations accurately using the anatomical terms and references you learned in this chapter.

1. Your patient has a cut on his left arm near the wrist. It is right about where the face of his watch would cover.

   _____

   _____

   _____

   _____

2. Your patient has a cut on the back of his leg just below the knee.

   _____

   _____

   _____

3. Your patient complains of pain in his lower abdomen on the right side that shoots toward the center of his belly.

   _____

   _____

   _____

   _____

4. Your patient has a bruise on his forehead above the right eye.

_____

_____

_____

_____

5. Your patient stepped on a nail causing a puncture wound on the bottom of his left foot.

_____

_____

_____

_____

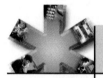

Perspective

Jocelyn—The Patient

"I just couldn't take it any more. I had my friend Sara come over to drive me to the hospital, but when she got there I realized that I couldn't get off of the couch! There was just no way that I was gonna get out of my apartment and the thought of squeezing into that little car of hers! I didn't know what to do. I really didn't want to bother the ambulance people ... plus ... I knew all of my neighbors would come out and stare at me. That would be embarrassing! But, Sara called 9-1-1 anyway. I guess I'm actually glad that she did."

1-4.2 Describe the anatomy and function of the respiratory system.

* **pharynx**

  passageway from nose and mouth to trachea.

* **oropharynx**

  the area directly posterior to the mouth.

* **nasopharynx**

  the area directly posterior to the nose.

* **larynx**

  the structure containing the vocal cords that is connected to the superior portion of the trachea.

Body Systems: The Respiratory System

The respiratory system is responsible for bringing oxygen into the body and delivering this oxygen to the blood so that it can be distributed throughout the body. The respiratory system also receives carbon dioxide from the blood and removes it from the body. Without a constant and efficient respiratory system we wouldn't survive for more than a few minutes.

The respiratory system (Figure 4-7) begins at the nose and mouth. As air enters, it is moved back to the **pharynx.** The area behind the mouth is called the **oropharynx.** The area behind the nose is called the **nasopharynx.** Air then moves through the larynx and the trachea toward the lungs. The **larynx,** commonly called

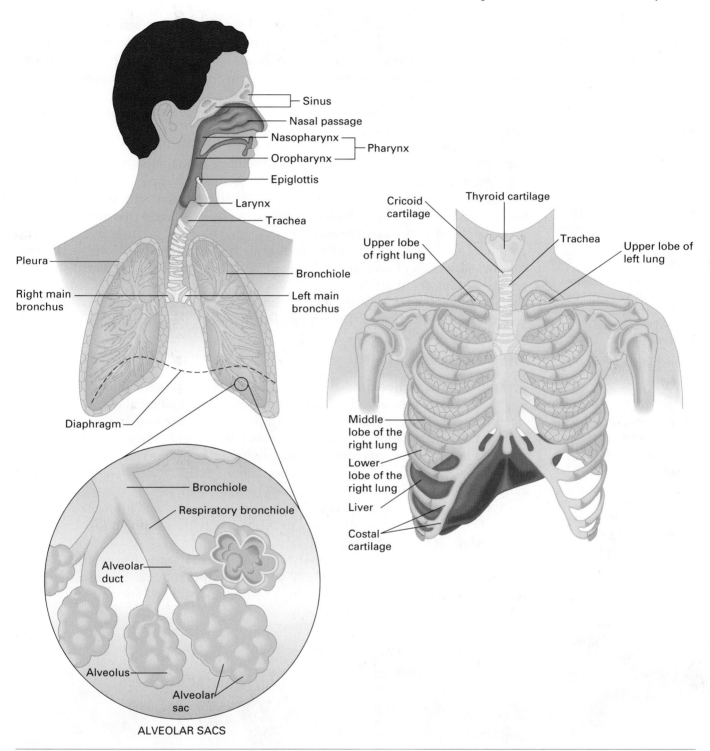

FIGURE 4-7   The respiratory system.

the *voice box,* is the structure that contains the vocal cords and connects to the opening of the trachea. You will note a prominence in the anterior neck of your patients. This is the **thyroid cartilage,** which is commonly referred to as the *Adam's apple*. This cartilage forms the anterior surface of the larynx. The **cricoid cartilage,** which lies just inferior to the thyroid cartilage, forms a complete ring at the distal end of the larynx and the beginning of the trachea.

* **thyroid cartilage**

  prominence in the anterior neck. Also called the *Adam's apple.*

* **cricoid cartilage**

  the ring-shaped structure that circles the trachea at the lower edge of the larynx.

✳ **epiglottis**

a leaf-shaped structure that covers and prevents food and foreign matter from entering the larynx and trachea.

✳ **trachea**

the structure that connects the pharynx to the lungs. Also called the *windpipe.*

✳ **cartilage**

tough tissue that covers the joint ends of bones and helps to form certain body parts such as the ear.

✳ **bronchi**

the two large sets of branches that come off the trachea and enter the lungs. There are right and left bronchi. Singular *bronchus.*

✳ **bronchioles**

smallest branches of bronchi.

✳ **alveoli**

the microscopic sacs of the lungs where gas exchange with the bloodstream takes place.

✳ **capillaries**

thin-walled, microscopic blood vessels where the oxygen/carbon dioxide and nutrient/waste exchange with the body's cells takes place.

✳ **lung**

the primary organ of respiration. There is a left lung and a right lung.

The larynx and trachea are protected by a leaf-shaped structure called the **epiglottis.** The epiglottis folds down over the opening to the larynx and trachea during swallowing to prevent food and liquids from going down that passageway and entering the lungs. When patients are unresponsive, the epiglottis will not close effectively and may allow substances to be breathed (aspirated) into the lungs. *This* is why you will pay so much attention to protecting the airway of unresponsive patients through positioning and suction.

The **trachea,** also called the *windpipe,* is the tube through which air passes to enter the lungs. The trachea has rings of **cartilage** to maintain its shape. The trachea bifurcates (or splits) into two **bronchi,** one traveling to each lung. The bronchi continue to split into smaller and smaller air passages until they reach the smallest level, the **bronchioles.** At the termination of these tiny airways are the **alveoli,** tiny air sacs where the actual exchange of oxygen and carbon dioxide with the blood takes place. This exchange is done between the alveoli and **capillaries,** tiny blood vessels. There are millions of alveoli in the lungs, grouped in small grape-like clusters of air sacs.

The **lung** is the primary organ of respiration. There are two lungs. Each lung is divided into **lobes,** or sections. The left lung has two lobes; the right lung has three lobes.

THE ACT OF BREATHING

Breathing or **respiration** can be described as a two-step process: inhalation and exhalation. We do it thousands of times a day without thinking about it.

Inhalation is an active process: It requires muscle use and energy. During inhalation, the diaphragm contracts and moves downward. The intercostal muscles (muscles between the ribs) contract and move the ribs upward and outward. These movements increase the size of the chest cavity, creating negative pressure and causing air to flow into the lungs.

Exhalation is passive and occurs when the diaphragm and intercostal muscles relax. This causes a reduction in size of the chest cavity, creating positive pressure and forcing air out of the lungs.

One respiratory cycle is an inhalation and an exhalation (Figure 4-8).

An adult breathes, on average, 12 to 20 times per minute. The rate may be a bit slower at rest and a bit faster during exertion and still be "normal." One of the

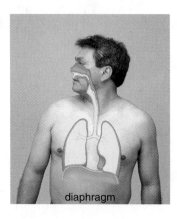

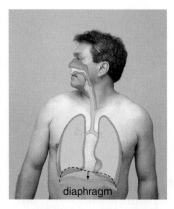

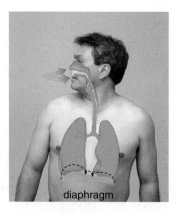

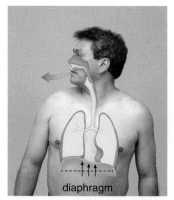

| diaphragm | diaphragm | diaphragm | diaphragm |

RELAXED

CONTRACTION
Inspiration begins

INSPIRATION

RELAXED
Passive expiration begins

FIGURE 4-8   The respiratory cycle.

most important things you will do as an EMT is evaluate a patient's breathing. In this section we will briefly talk about normal and abnormal breathing—but rest assured that it will be covered in much greater detail in Chapter 7.

You will know when your patient is breathing normally by looking at several indicators. The rate of breathing will be within normal ranges and the breathing will be of adequate depth and regular. Air will move in and out of both lungs without excess effort. The patient's color will be good. The patient will also appear normal—not sleepy or anxious. This is called **adequate breathing.** Adequate breathing, simply stated, is breathing that is sufficient to support life.

The opposite of adequate breathing is **inadequate breathing.** As you might expect, this is when breathing is not sufficient to support life. The respiratory rate will be very slow or even very fast, it may be irregular, and it will most likely be shallow. The patient may have poor skin color and be anxious or sleepy in appearance. The patient breathing inadequately may also appear to be having difficulty breathing. The muscles between the ribs and in the neck are used more than usual and have the appearance of "sucking in" or "tugging."

As a patient's breathing deteriorates from adequate to inadequate, **agonal respirations** may develop. These are occasional, gasping attempts at breathing. They are very shallow and slow (sometimes 4 to 8 breaths per minute), literally one step from not breathing at all. **Respiratory arrest** is not breathing at all. It is the total absence of respiratory effort.

ABOUT BREATHING—INFANTS AND CHILDREN

Kids are generally healthy little creatures. If they do suddenly become critically ill, the respiratory system is often the culprit. This means that your attention to an infant or child's respiratory system will be critical—as will your knowledge of the differences between the respiratory structures of children and adults (Figure 4-9).

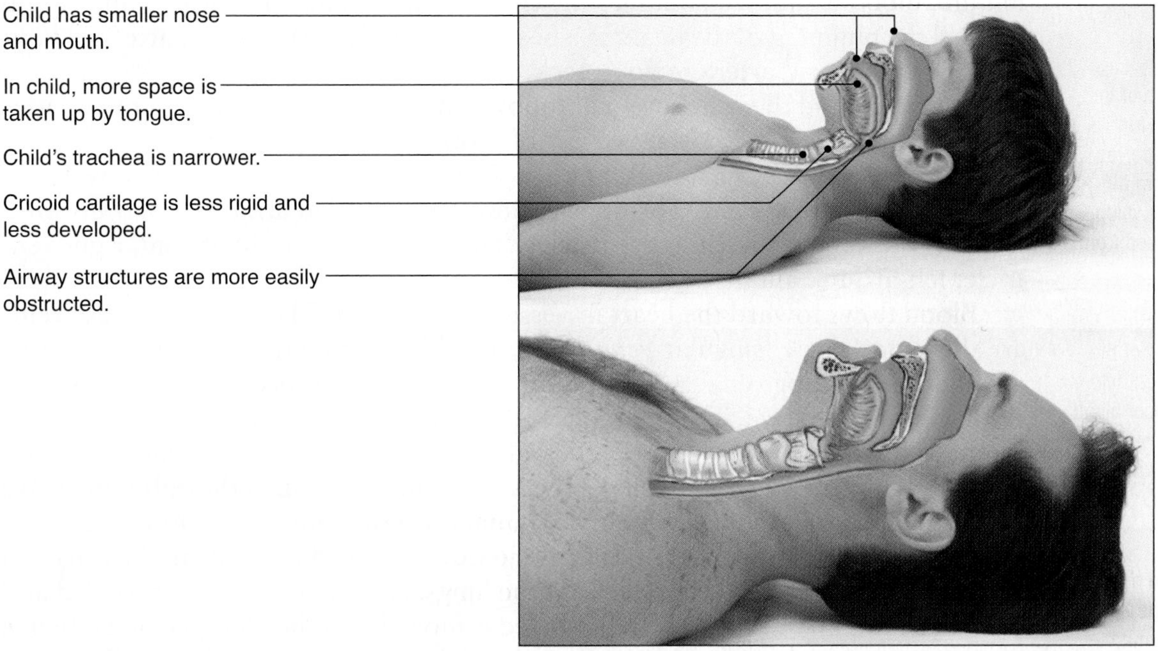

* **lobes**

  sections of the lung. The left lung has two lobes; the right lung has three lobes.

* **respiration**

  inhalation and exhalation. May also be called *ventilation*.

* **inhalation**

  an active process in which the intercostal (rib) muscles and the diaphragm contract, expanding the size of the chest cavity and causing air to flow into the lungs. Also called *inspiration*.

* **exhalation**

  a passive process in which the intercostal (rib) muscles and the diaphragm relax, causing the chest cavity to decrease in size and air to flow out of the lungs. Also called *expiration*.

* **adequate breathing**

  breathing that is sufficient to support life.

* **inadequate breathing**

  breathing that is not sufficient to support life.

* **agonal respirations**

  occasional, gasping attempts at breathing.

* **respiratory arrest**

  when breathing completely stops.

Child has smaller nose and mouth.

In child, more space is taken up by tongue.

Child's trachea is narrower.

Cricoid cartilage is less rigid and less developed.

Airway structures are more easily obstructed.

FIGURE 4-9   A comparison of the adult and child respiratory systems.

Some of these differences include the following:

✳ Children's respiratory structures are smaller. As a consequence, an obstruction, infection, or swelling can cause a reduction in air flow much more quickly than in an adult.

✳ The tongues of infants and children take up proportionally more space in the mouth and pharynx than an adult's, so the tongue is more likely to obstruct the airway.

✳ The trachea is narrower, softer, and more flexible than an adult's. This means the child's trachea will be more easily occluded (blocked) by obstruction or swelling.

✳ The cricoid cartilage is less developed than an adult's, giving less support to the tracheal structure.

✳ The chest wall is softer, so infants and children tend to rely on the diaphragm to move air in and out. Therefore, a degree of diaphragmatic breathing in the child is normal, whereas it would indicate respiratory distress in an adult.

The Cardiovascular System

There are three main components of the **cardiovascular system** (also called the *circulatory system*): the heart, the vessels, and the blood. The purpose of the cardiovascular system is to pump blood to every cell of the body in order to deliver nutrients and remove wastes. Failure to get blood throughout the body or to provide these nutrients and remove wastes can cause serious conditions or even death.

THE HEART

The heart is a pump. It is a well designed, efficient pump tasked with pumping blood to the entire body. It never rests. The heart pumps about 70 times per minute. Blood is squeezed out into the circulation each time the heart pumps. You can feel the pumping of the heart as a beat of your **pulse** at the radial artery in your wrist or the carotid artery in your neck.

To understand the heart, we will follow blood as it travels through the various chambers. Figure 4-10 shows the flow of blood through the heart.

The heart is a four-chambered pump. The chambers are divided into two sides of the heart, left and right. The upper chambers are called **atria** (singular *atrium*); the lower chambers are called **ventricles.** This gives us the right atrium, right ventricle, left atrium, and left ventricle.

Blood flows toward the heart in vessels called veins. The largest of these veins are the venae cavae (singular *vena cava*). The blood from the lower body returns through the inferior vena cava. Blood from the head and neck returns by way of the superior vena cava. These large vessels come together and return blood to the right atrium. Blood is moved from the right atrium through the **tricuspid valve** and into the right ventricle. Blood leaves the right ventricle through the **pulmonic valve** and is pumped to the lungs via the **pulmonary arteries.** Since this blood is coming back from the body it is high in **carbon dioxide** it has picked up from the cells and low in oxygen delivered to the cells. At the lungs, carbon dioxide is off-loaded and exhaled, and oxygen that has been inhaled is moved into the blood. This exchange of oxygen and carbon dioxide is done through the alveoli and the capillaries, as noted in the previous section.

1-4.2 Describe the anatomy and function of the circulatory system.

✳ **cardiovascular system**

the system made up of the heart (*cardio*), the blood vessels (*vascular*) and the blood. Also called the *circulatory system.*

✳ **pulse**

the pumping of the heart as a pressure wave felt over an artery.

✳ **atria**

the two upper chambers of the heart. Singular *atrium.* There is a right atrium (which receives unoxygenated blood from the body) and a left atrium (which receives oxygenated blood from the lungs).

✳ **ventricles**

the two lower chambers of the heart. There is a right ventricle (which sends oxygen-poor blood to the lungs) and a left ventricle (which sends oxygen-rich blood to the body).

✳ **tricuspid valve**

a structure between the right atrium and right ventricle that opens and closes to permit the flow of a fluid in only one direction.

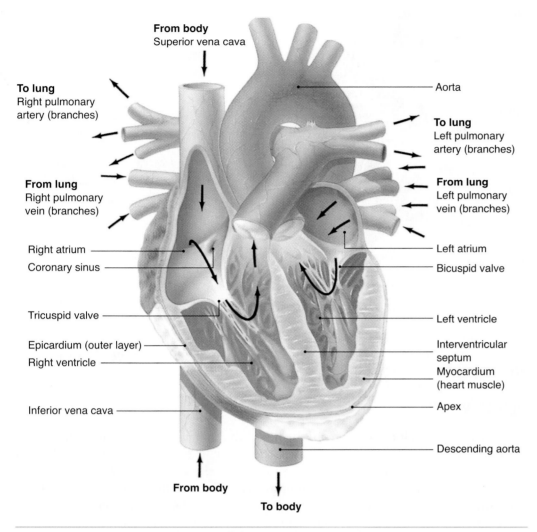

From body
Superior vena cava

Aorta

To lung
Right pulmonary
artery (branches)

To lung
Left pulmonary
artery (branches)

From lung
Right pulmonary
vein (branches)

From lung
Left pulmonary
vein (branches)

Right atrium

Left atrium

Coronary sinus

Bicuspid valve

Tricuspid valve

Left ventricle

Epicardium (outer layer)

Interventricular
septum

Right ventricle

Myocardium
(heart muscle)

Inferior vena cava

Apex

Descending aorta

From body

To body

FIGURE 4-10   The flow of blood through the heart.

* **pulmonic valve**

   a structure between the right ventricle and pulmonary arteries that opens and closes to permit the flow of a fluid in only one direction.

* **pulmonary arteries**

   vessels that carry blood from the right ventricle to the lungs.

* **carbon dioxide**

   waste gas found in the blood. This is exchanged with oxygen in the lungs.

* **pulmonary veins**

   vessels that carry blood from the lungs to the left atrium.

* **mitral valve**

   a structure between the left atrium and left ventricle that opens and closes to permit the flow of a fluid in only one direction.

* **aortic valve**

   a structure between the left ventricle and aorta that opens and closes to permit the flow of a fluid in only one direction.

* **aorta**

   the largest artery in the body. It transports blood from the left ventricle to begin systemic circulation.

* **coronary arteries**

   arteries that branch off the aorta and provide blood supply directly to the heart.

* **myocardial infarction**

   deadening of the heart tissue caused occlusion of one or more of the coronary arteries. Also called a *heart attack*.

* **conduction system**

   specialized tissue that provides the electrical stimulus that makes the heart beat.

* **pacemaker**

   site within the heart that originates an electrical impulse.

* **conductive tissue**

   a system of specialized muscle tissues that conduct the electrical impulses that stimulate the heart to beat.

Blood returns from the lungs to the left atrium through the **pulmonary veins.** The blood is now richly oxygenated and ready to be pumped to the body again. The left atrium receives the blood and pumps it through the **mitral valve** into the left ventricle. The left ventricle is the largest and most muscular chamber of the heart. This is because blood pumped from the left ventricle must reach all parts of the body. Blood from the left ventricle is passed through the **aortic valve** into the **aorta.** From the aorta blood is moved through a series of branching and gradually smaller arteries, then into the tiny capillaries, until every cell in the body is supplied with oxygenated blood.

The heart is a muscle. Although the heart is filled with blood at all times, it does not receive the blood it needs for its own oxygen and nutrients from the blood that passes through it. The heart receives its own blood supply through a series of arteries known as the **coronary arteries.** These arteries branch off the aorta directly to the heart. When a patient has a "heart attack," also known as a **myocardial infarction,** it is caused by the occlusion (blockage) of one or more of the coronary arteries.

The heart also has a specialized **conduction system** (Figure 4-11 on page 98). In addition to the strong muscle tissue within the heart, there is electrical tissue, which provides the electrical stimulus that makes the heart beat. The heart has a normal **pacemaker** site, which originates an electrical impulse. Specialized **conductive tissue** spreads the impulse throughout the heart. When the heart beats,

FIGURE 4-11 The conduction system of the heart.

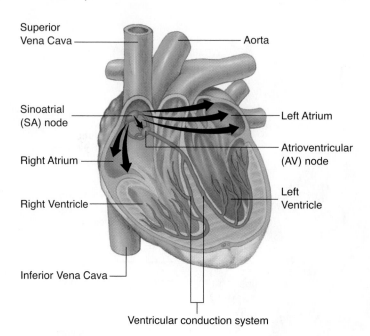

Superior Vena Cava
Aorta
Sinoatrial (SA) node
Left Atrium
Atrioventricular (AV) node
Right Atrium
Right Ventricle
Left Ventricle
Inferior Vena Cava
Ventricular conduction system

both of the upper chambers (atria) squeeze at the same time, followed by the two lower chambers (ventricles).

BLOOD VESSELS

Vessels that carry blood away from the heart are **arteries.** Vessels that return blood to the heart are **veins.** As blood leaves the heart, it enters the aorta, the largest vessel in the body. As blood moves away from the heart—toward the toe, for example—it enters smaller and smaller arteries. Eventually the blood reaches the **arterioles,** the smallest artery branches, which in turn lead to capillaries.

Capillaries are tiny vessels that are found between, and connect, arterioles and venules. Capillaries have very thin walls that allow the exchange of gasses between a cell and the blood in a capillary. After moving through the capillaries, blood begins its return trip through the venous system back to the heart. Capillaries are followed by **venules,** veins and, eventually, the venae cavae, the blood entering larger and larger vessels as it approaches the heart.

Blood in the arteries is under high pressure. This assures that blood is pumped to all parts of the body. Venous blood returning to the heart is under much lower pressure. Veins have valves that prevent blood from backing up through the system.

There are several arteries and veins that will be mentioned specifically because of their relevance to patient assessment and care (Figure 4-12). These include the following:

✳ **Carotid artery.** The major artery of the neck, a primary supplier of blood to the head. It is the artery of choice when checking for a pulse in unresponsive patients.

✳ **Brachial artery.** Artery of the upper arm that is palpated to obtain a pulse in infants that also serves as a pressure point to control bleeding from the arm in all age groups. This is the artery found near the elbow that you listen to when obtaining a blood pressure.

✳ **Femoral artery.** A major supplier of blood to the leg. This pulse is palpated near the crease formed by the abdomen, leg, and groin.

✳ **arteries**

blood vessels that carry blood away from the heart.

✳ **veins**

blood vessels that return blood to the heart.

✳ **arterioles**

the smallest arteries.

✳ **capillaries**

tiny vessels that connect arterioles and venules.

✳ **venules**

the smallest veins.

✳ **carotid artery**

the large neck artery that carries blood from the heart to the head. There is one carotid artery on each side of the neck.

✳ **brachial artery**

the major artery of the upper arm.

✳ **femoral artery**

the major artery supplying the lower extremity.

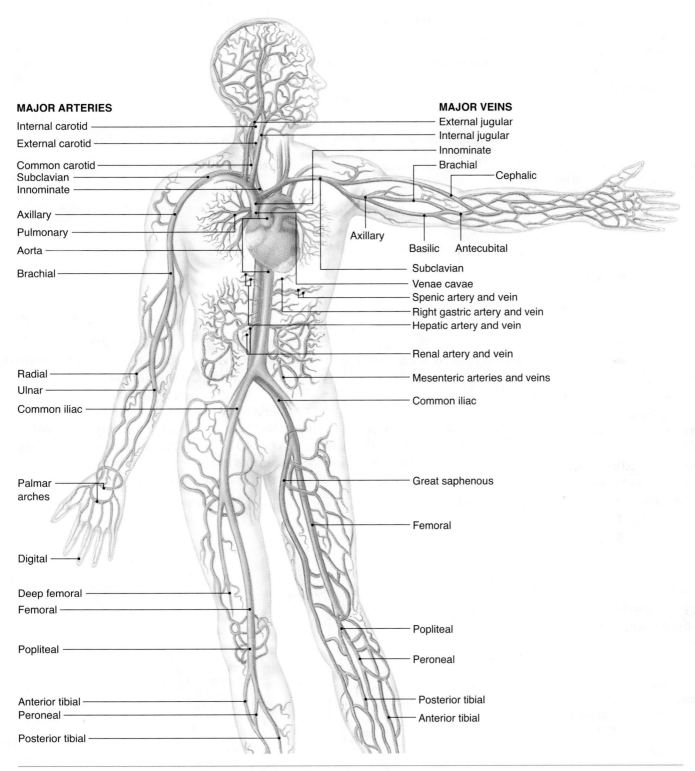

MAJOR ARTERIES

Internal carotid
External carotid
Common carotid
Subclavian
Innominate
Axillary
Pulmonary
Aorta
Brachial
Radial
Ulnar
Common iliac
Palmar arches
Digital
Deep femoral
Femoral
Popliteal
Anterior tibial
Peroneal
Posterior tibial

MAJOR VEINS

External jugular
Internal jugular
Innominate
Brachial
Cephalic
Axillary
Basilic Antecubital
Subclavian
Venae cavae
Spenic artery and vein
Right gastric artery and vein
Hepatic artery and vein
Renal artery and vein
Mesenteric arteries and veins
Common iliac
Great saphenous
Femoral
Popliteal
Peroneal
Posterior tibial
Anterior tibial

FIGURE 4-12 Major arteries and veins of particular importance to patient assessment and care.

* **radial artery**

artery of the lower arm. It is felt when taking the pulse at the wrist.

* **posterior tibial artery**

artery supplying the foot, behind the medial ankle.

* **dorsalis pedis artery**

artery supplying the foot, lateral to the large tendon of the big toe.

* **vena cava**

either of two major veins that carry oxygen-poor blood from the body to the right atrium. The superior vena cava carries blood from the head; the inferior vena cava carries blood from the lower body. Plural *venae cavae.*

* **pulmonary vein**

vessel carrying oxygen-rich blood from the lungs to the left atrium.

* **pulmonary artery**

vessel carrying oxygen-poor blood from the right ventricle to the lungs.

* **red blood cells**

blood cells that contain hemoglobin.

* **hemoglobin**

molecule within the red blood cell that carries oxygen to the cells and carbon dioxide away from the cells.

* **pulse oximeter**

an electronic device for determining the amount of oxygen carried in the blood, known as the oxygen saturation. The pulse oximeter measures the percentage of hemoglobin molecules that are saturated with oxygen.

* **saturated**

filled, as hemoglobin with oxygen.

* **white blood cells**

cells within the blood that produce substances that help fight infection.

* **infection**

invasion and multiplication of foreign microorganisms within the tissues of the body.

* **Radial artery.** Artery that supplies blood to the lower arm. It is palpated on the lateral aspect of the anterior wrist.

* **Posterior tibial artery.** Artery that is palpated on the posterior surface of the medial malleolus. It is sometimes used to determine if there is circulation to the distal areas of the leg.

* **Dorsalis pedis artery.** Artery located on the anterior surface of the foot. Like the posterior tibial artery, it may be palpated to assess distal circulation.

* **Vena cava.** Large vein that carries oxygen-poor blood to the right atrium of the heart.

* **Pulmonary vein.** Vein that carries oxygen-rich blood from the lungs to the heart.

* **Pulmonary artery.** Artery that carries oxygen-poor blood from the heart to the lungs.

THE BLOOD

Blood travels through the circulatory system as the "vehicle" that carries oxygen and nutrients (e.g., glucose) to the cells and that carries waste products away from the cells. There are four basic components in the blood (Figure 4-13):

* **Red blood cells.** In addition to giving the blood its characteristic red color, the red blood cells contain **hemoglobin.** Hemoglobin is the molecule within the red blood cell that carries oxygen to the cells and carbon dioxide away from the cells. When you use a **pulse oximeter** you are measuring the percentage of hemoglobin molecules that are **saturated** (filled with) oxygen.

* **White blood cells.** The white cells provide the body's primary defenses against **infection.**

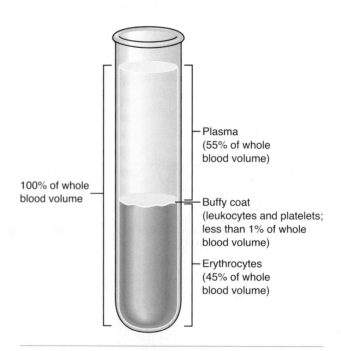

100% of whole blood volume

Plasma (55% of whole blood volume)

Buffy coat (leukocytes and platelets; less than 1% of whole blood volume)

Erythrocytes (45% of whole blood volume)

FIGURE 4-13 Blood is composed of red cells (erythrocytes), plasma, and white cells and platelets.

* **Plasma.** Plasma is the fluid that carries the red and white cells as well as nutrients (e.g., glucose).

* **Platelets.** Platelets play a vital role in the body's ability to form blood clots.

ABOUT CIRCULATION

After learning about the components of the circulatory system, you are probably wondering how these critical concepts will apply to what you do as an EMT. Your evaluation of circulation will be critical to your patient's survival. Without adequate circulating blood, patients become very sick and may die. **Perfusion** is the act of distributing blood to all parts of the body to deliver oxygen and remove waste products.

When the body's tissues are adequately perfused, they appear normal in color, are usually warm and dry, and have pulses in the areas around the tissue.

Hypoperfusion (also known as *shock*) is inadequate perfusion of blood to an organ or organs. When the body is not perfused properly (circulating blood is inadequate), a severe condition results. The patient will appear pale, gray, or blue (cyanotic), the skin will be cool and clammy (moist), the pulse and breathing will increase, the patient may become anxious or restless, and in some cases the patient may have a low blood pressure.

Blood pressure is the pressure exerted by the blood on the walls of an artery. Recall that blood is pumped from the left ventricle under high pressure. When you feel a pulse in the body, the beat you feel corresponds with the compression of the left ventricle sending blood into the aorta.

For each beat of the heart, an average of 70 ml of blood is ejected into the aorta. This is called **stroke volume.** If the heart beats 70 times per minute, 4,900 ml of blood is pumped by the heart each minute.

$$\text{heart rate} \times \text{stroke volume} = \text{cardiac output}$$

or:

$$(\text{HR} \times \text{SV} = \text{CO})$$

For example,

$$70 \text{ (beats per minute)} \times 70 \text{ (ml per beat)} = 4{,}900 \text{ ml/minute}$$

The body strives to maintain a consistent cardiac output. If the stroke volume falls (as happens with serious blood loss), the body compensates by raising the heart rate. An elevated heart rate is a crucial sign of hypoperfusion.

> 4,900 ml is almost 5 liters—equivalent to two
> 2½-liter soda bottles per minute.

Pressure is required to move blood to all parts of the body. The delicate balance of pressure is maintained by the amount of blood in the body, the pumping of the heart, and the size of the blood vessels. Arteries have the ability to increase or decrease their size. When additional blood volume is needed, arteries can expand and allow more blood flow. In the event of blood loss, arteries can constrict to help maintain blood pressure. The constriction of blood vessels that supply the skin causes the cool, clammy skin often encountered in patients with shock.

---

* **plasma**
  the fluid portion of the blood.

* **platelets**
  components of the blood; membrane-enclosed fragments of specialized cells.

* **perfusion**
  distribution of blood to all parts of the body to deliver oxygen and remove waste products.

* **hypoperfusion**
  inadequate distribution of blood to an organ or organs of the body. Also called *shock*.

* **blood pressure**
  the pressure exerted by blood against the walls of blood vessels. Usually arterial blood pressure (the pressure in an artery) is measured. *Systolic blood pressure* is the maximum arterial pressure that occurs during a ventricular contraction. *Diastolic blood pressure* is the minimum arterial pressure that occurs while the heart is at rest between contractions.

* **stroke volume**
  amount of blood ejected into the aorta with each heart beat.

FIGURE 4-14 Three components
are required to maintain blood
pressure.

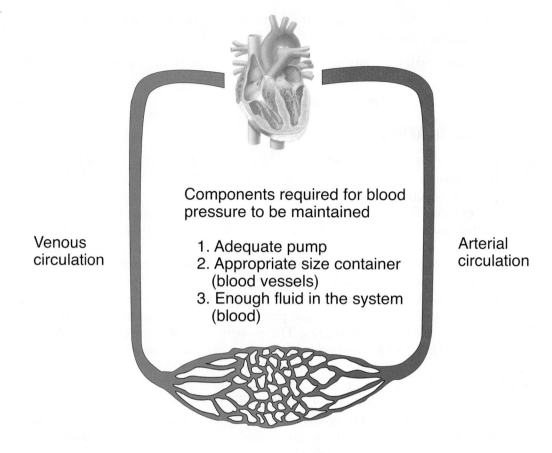

Venous
circulation

Components required for blood
pressure to be maintained

1. Adequate pump
2. Appropriate size container
   (blood vessels)
3. Enough fluid in the system
   (blood)

Arterial
circulation

FIGURE 4-14 Three components are required to maintain blood pressure.

✳ **systemic vascular
resistance**

an indicator of the diameter of
the blood vessels.

Blood pressure is defined as cardiac output (defined earlier) times the resistance or diameter (also called **systemic vascular resistance** or SVR) of the blood vessels (Figure 4-14).

$$\text{cardiac output} \times \text{systemic vascular resistance} = \text{blood pressure}$$

or:

$$(CO \times SVR = BP)$$

If any of the factors in these equations falter, blood pressure falls. If a heart attack causes damage to the left ventricle and cardiac output falls, blood pressure falls. If a patient loses a lot of blood, cardiac output will fall because there will be less blood for the heart to eject. Sometimes the size of the vessels increases. This can be caused by a nervous system disorder or by an allergic reaction. If the vessels (the size of the pipes in the system) suddenly expand, the resistance inside the arteries become less, and the blood pressure drops.

Stop, Review, Remember!

Multiple Choice

Place a check next to the correct answer.

1. The trachea splits into two:

   _____ a. capillaries.

   _____ b. alveoli.

   _____ c. bronchi.

   _____ d. valves.

2. Which of the following is not a valve in the heart?

   _____ a. aortic

   _____ b. pulmonic

   _____ c. tricuspid

   _____ d. ventral

3. The rings of the trachea consist of:

   _____ a. ligaments.   _____ c. cartilage.

   _____ b. bone.   _____ d. muscle.

4. The formula for determining cardiac output (CO) is:

   _____ a. SV × BP = CO

   _____ b. SV × HR = CO

   _____ c. HR × BP = CO

   _____ d. HR × SVR = CO

5. The left lung has _____ lobe(s).

   _____ a. one   _____ c. three

   _____ b. two   _____ d. four

Fill in the Blank

1. The small, grape-like clusters of air sacs in the lungs are called _____.

2. The area posterior to the nose but superior to the larynx is called the _____.

3. _____ carry blood away from the heart.

4. _____ are tiny vessels that connect arterioles and venules.

5. The upper chambers of the heart are called _____ and the lower chambers are called _____.

6. The _____ artery is the artery that produces a pulse in the wrist.

Labeling

On the diagram of the heart below, label each chamber and draw the path of blood as it flows between the chambers, to the lung, and to the body.

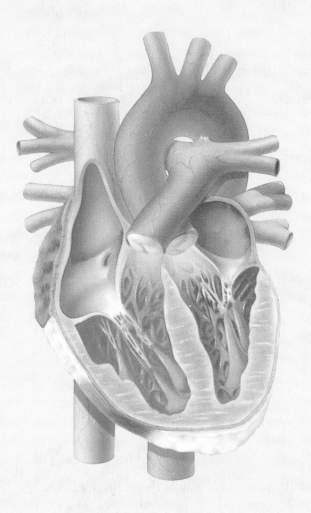

Critical Thinking

1. List three signs of inadequate breathing.

   _____

   _____

   _____

   _____

   _____

2. Differentiate between perfusion and hypoperfusion.

_____

_____

_____

_____

3. List three ways a child's airway is different from an adult's.

_____

_____

_____

_____

The Musculoskeletal System

The musculoskeletal system is comprised of the bones and skeletal muscles of the body. This system has three major functions:

* To give the body shape
* To protect internal organs
* To provide the ability to move

THE SKELETON

The bones of the body literally range from head to toe (Figure 4-15 on page 106). Some of the most important bones for you to know include:

* Head (Figure 4-16 on page 107)—The **cranium** is a series of bones that are fused together to protect the brain within. The **facial bones** and the bones of the jaw, the **mandible** and **maxilla,** combine to give us our facial structure as well as the ability to breathe and eat.

* Upper extremities (Figure 4-17 on page 107)—The upper extremities begin with the **clavicles** (collarbones) and **scapulae** (shoulder blades), the **humerus** (upper arm bone), **radius** and **ulna** (lower arm bones), and the **carpals** and **metacarpals** (bones of the wrist and hand).

* Torso (Figure 4-18 on page 108)—The **sternum** (breastbone) and the **ribs** form the structure of the chest cavity. When you perform CPR, you compress the sternum. There are twelve ribs—one attached to each of the twelve

1-4.2 Describe the anatomy and function of the musculoskeletal system.

∗ **cranium**

the bony structure making up the forehead, top, back, and upper sides of the skull.

∗ **facial bones**

bones combined to give us our facial structure as well as to allow breathing and eating.

∗ **mandible**

the lower jaw bone.

∗ **maxilla**

the two fused bones forming the upper jaw.

∗ **clavicles**

the collarbones.

∗ **scapulae**

the shoulder blades. Singular _scapula._

∗ **humerus**

the bone of the upper arm, between the shoulder and the elbow.

∗ **radius**

the lateral bone of the forearm.

THE SKELETON

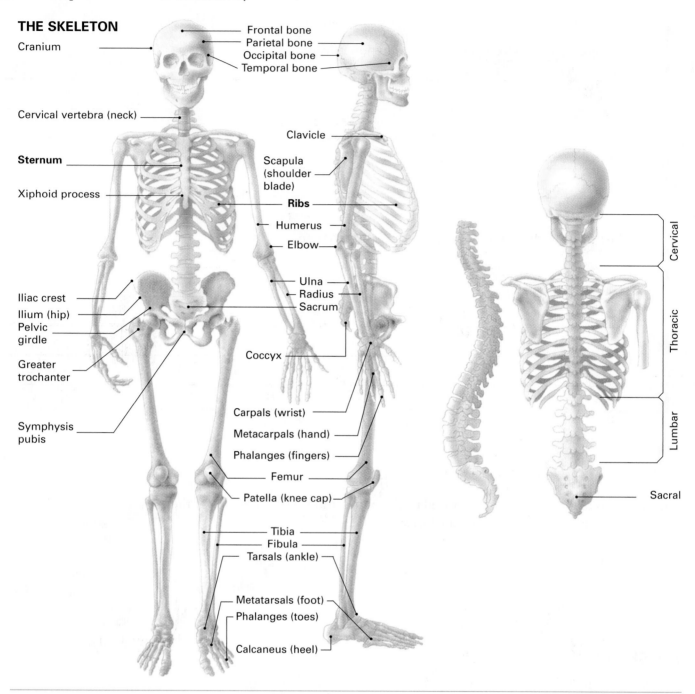

Cranium

Frontal bone
Parietal bone
Occipital bone
Temporal bone

Cervical vertebra (neck)

Clavicle

Sternum

Scapula (shoulder blade)

Xiphoid process

Ribs

Humerus

Elbow

Ulna
Radius
Sacrum

Iliac crest
Ilium (hip)
Pelvic girdle

Greater trochanter

Coccyx

Symphysis pubis

Carpals (wrist)

Metacarpals (hand)

Phalanges (fingers)

Femur

Patella (knee cap)

Tibia
Fibula
Tarsals (ankle)

Metatarsals (foot)
Phalanges (toes)
Calcaneus (heel)

Cervical

Thoracic

Lumbar

Sacral

FIGURE 4-15 The skeletal system.

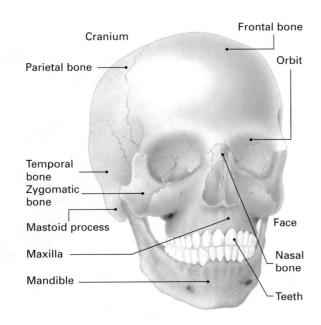

THE SKULL

FIGURE 4-16   The cranium.

✳ **ulna**
the medial bone of the forearm.

✳ **carpals**
the wrist bones.

✳ **metacarpals**
the hand bones.

✳ **sternum**
the breastbone.

✳ **ribs**
twelve pairs of bones that help form the thoracic cavity

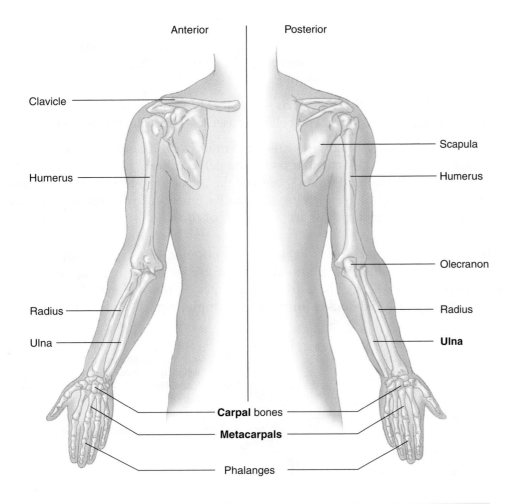

FIGURE 4-17   The upper extremities.

FIGURE 4-18 The torso.

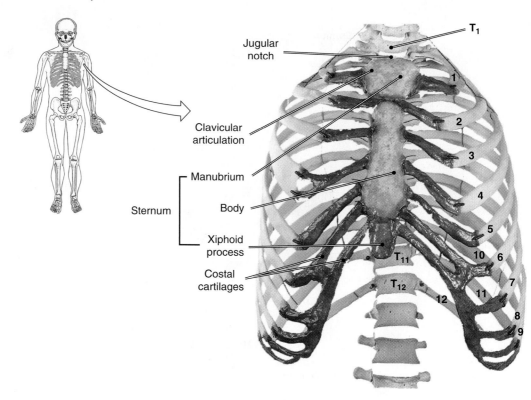

* **pelvis**

  the basin-shaped bony structure that supports the spine and is the point of proximal attachment for the lower extremities.

* **ilium**

  the superior and widest portion of the pelvis.

* **ischium**

  the lower, posterior portions of the pelvis.

* **pubis**

  the medial anterior portion of the pelvis.

* **sacral spine**

  vertebrae that form the posterior pelvis.

* **femur**

  the large bone of the thigh.

* **articulates**

  connects or unites, as bones at a joint.

* **tibia**

  the medial and larger bone of the lower leg.

thoracic vertebrae of the spinal column and curving anteriorly toward the sternum. Ten of the ribs connect to the sternum. The two not attached to the sternum are called "floating ribs."

✳ Pelvis (Figure 4-19)—The **pelvis** is a series of fused bones that include the **ilium, ischium,** and **pubis.** The pelvis is fused with the **sacral spine** posteriorly.

✳ Lower extremities (Figure 4-20)—the **femur** (thigh bone) is the largest long bone in the body. It **articulates** with the pelvis to form the hip joint. The femur and the **tibia** and **fibula** (bones of the lower leg) meet at the knee joint, which is covered anteriorly by the **patella** (kneecap). The **tarsals** form the ankle, and the **metatarsals** are the bones of the foot.

Bones must articulate (connect) with each other at joints to provide the ability to move. Some joints are immovable, some are slightly movable, and others are movable (Figure 4-21). There are several types of joints (Figure 4-22 on page 110), including **ball-and-socket joints** (for example, hip, shoulder), **hinge joints**

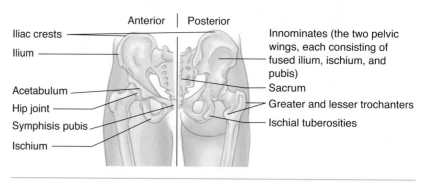

FIGURE 4-19 The pelvis.

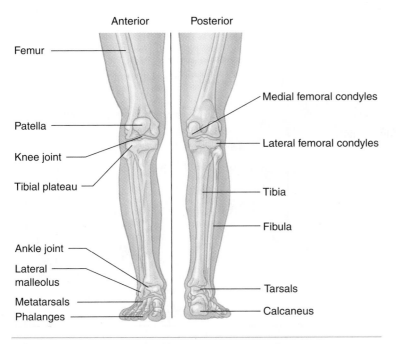

FIGURE 4-20   The lower extremities.

✳ **fibula**

the lateral and smaller bone of the lower leg.

✳ **patella**

the kneecap.

✳ **tarsals**

the ankle bones.

✳ **metatarsals**

the foot bones.

✳ **ball-and-socket joints**

type of joint where the ball-shaped head of one bone fits into a rounded receptacle or socket in another bone; type of joint with the greatest range of motion.

✳ **hinge joints**

type of joint that moves in only one direction.

✳ **gliding joints**

type of joint where one bone end slides upon another.

✳ **fused joints**

type of joint where bones meet but do not move.

✳ **ligaments**

tissues that connect bone to bone.

✳ **tendons**

tissues that connect muscle to bone.

✳ **sprain**

injury to a ligament.

(for example, knee, elbow), and **gliding joints** (for example, wrist and ankle). Some joints are **fused joints** that are not designed to move (for example, the joints or sutures of the skull bones). Some joints allow flexibility but move only minimally (for example, the vertebrae of the spine).

Our bones and joints have two types of connective tissue: ligaments and tendons (Figure 4-23 on page 110). These hold our joints together and allow for movement. **Ligaments** connect bones to bones while **tendons** attach muscle to bone. If you have ever suffered a **sprain** you have injured one or more ligaments.

THE SPINE

The spinal cord is housed within the **spinal column**—sometimes simply called the spine. The spinal column is a series of **vertebrae** that are stacked one on top of the other to form the column. The spinal cord runs through the hollows at the centers of the vertebrae.

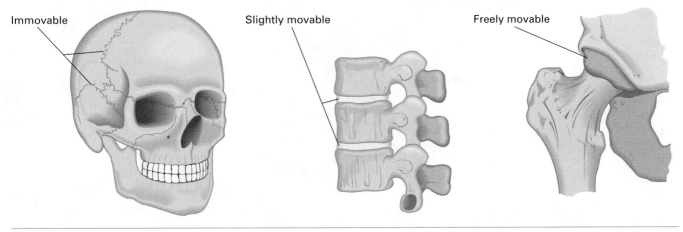

FIGURE 4-21   Types of joints.

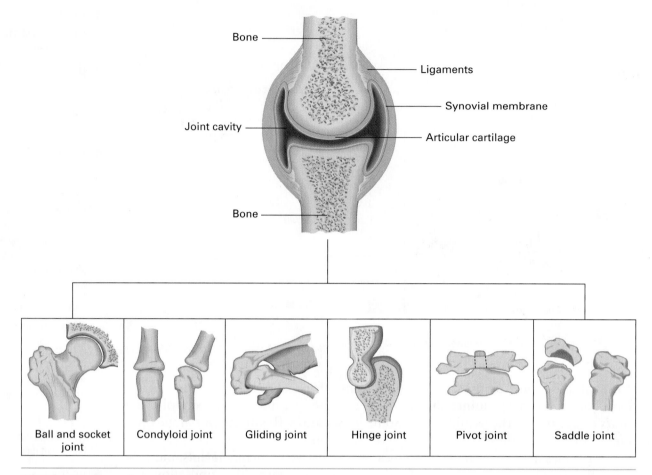

Bone

Ligaments

Synovial membrane

Joint cavity

Articular cartilage

Bone

| Ball and socket joint | Condyloid joint | Gliding joint | Hinge joint | Pivot joint | Saddle joint |

FIGURE 4-22 The anatomy of joint types.

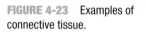 **FIGURE 4-23** Examples of connective tissue.

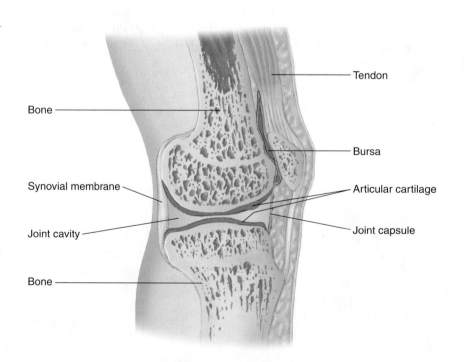

Tendon

Bone

Bursa

Synovial membrane

Articular cartilage

Joint cavity

Joint capsule

Bone

There are:

✳ **7 cervical vertebrae,** which begin at the head and meet the thoracic vertebrae. The slight bony bump you feel at the base of your neck is the seventh cervical vertebra.

✳ **12 thoracic vertebrae** in the upper and mid back. Each rib is attached to a thoracic vertebra.

✳ **5 lumbar vertebrae** in the lower back. These are frequently injured by EMTs when lifting improperly.

✳ **5 sacral vertebrae** (fused) that help to form the pelvis.

✳ **5 coccygeal vertebrae** (fused) that make up the coccyx or tailbone.

MUSCLES

When we think of muscles we think of our ability to walk, run, lift, and breathe. Muscles do this—and more. There are three types of muscle: voluntary, involuntary, and cardiac (Figure 4-24).

Voluntary muscle, also known as **skeletal muscle,** is responsible for movement. It attaches to bones and can be moved by people as they choose (voluntarily).

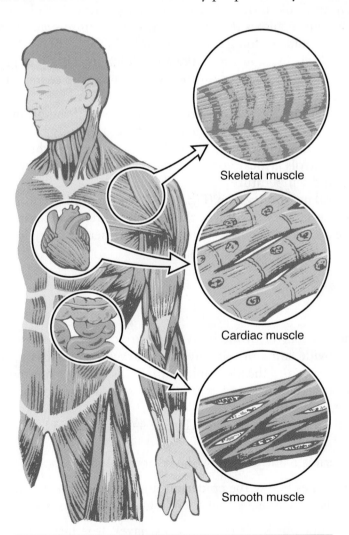

Skeletal muscle

Cardiac muscle

Smooth muscle

FIGURE 4-24   Three types of muscles.

✳ **spinal column**

a series of vertebrae that are stacked one on top of the other to form the column.

✳ **vertebrae**

the 33 bones of the spinal column. Singular *vertebra.*

✳ **cervical vertebrae**

vertebrae that begin at the head and meet the thoracic vertebrae.

✳ **thoracic vertebrae**

vertebrae that help form the thoracic cage. A rib is attached to each thoracic vertebra.

✳ **lumbar vertebrae**

vertebrae that form the lower back.

✳ **sacral vertebrae**

fused vertebrae that help to form the pelvis.

✳ **coccygeal vertebrae**

fused vertebrae that make up the coccyx or tailbone.

✳ **voluntary muscle**

muscle that can be consciously controlled. Also called *skeletal muscle.*

✳ **skeletal muscle**

see voluntary muscle.

* **involuntary muscle**

  muscle that responds automatically to brain signals but cannot be consciously controlled. Also called *smooth muscle.*

* **smooth muscle**

  see involuntary muscle.

* **cardiac muscle**

  specialized involuntary muscle found only in the heart.

* **automaticity**

  the ability of the heart muscle to generate and conduct electrical impulses on its own.

1-4.2 Describe the anatomy and function of the nervous system.

* **central nervous system (CNS)**

  the brain and the spinal cord.

* **peripheral nervous system (PNS)**

  the nerves that enter and leave the spinal cord and that convey impulses to and from the central nervous system.

* **sensory nerves**

  portion of the nervous system that carries information from the body back to the central nervous system.

* **motor**

  portion of the nervous system that carries information from the brain through the spinal cord and to the body.

* **epidermis**

  the outer layer of the skin.

* **dermis**

  the inner (second) layer of the skin, found beneath the epidermis. It is rich in blood vessels and nerves.

* **subcutaneous layer**

  the deepest layer of the skin. It is fatty tissue and provides shock absorption and insulation for the body.

Voluntary muscle forms the majority of the muscle mass of the body and is noticeable in places like the bicep.

Involuntary muscle, also known as **smooth muscle,** is found in the walls of the intestine, blood vessels, and bronchi. These muscles contract and control the flow through the structures. As mentioned earlier, one factor in blood pressure is vascular resistance (size of the container). This is controlled by the smooth muscle in the arteries and arterioles. Smooth muscle contracts and moves food through our intestines. When a patient has an asthma attack, it is the smooth muscle of the bronchioles that contracts and causes wheezing and difficulty breathing.

Cardiac muscle, as the name implies, is found only in the heart. It is involuntary muscle but has the special property of **automaticity.** Automaticity is the ability to stimulate an impulse and contract on its own (without the nervous system). Cardiac muscle is the only muscle in the body that has this ability. The amount of work performed by the heart is truly amazing. As noted earlier, your heart beats an average of 70 beats per minute, faster in times of stress and slower at rest. That is over 4,000 times per hour and 100,000 times per day—every day of your life!

The Nervous System

The nervous system controls the voluntary and involuntary actions of the body. You don't have to think about breathing or tell your heart to beat every second. The nervous system regulates that for you. If you reach to pick up your textbook (something you should be doing frequently in EMT class) or walk to the refrigerator, it is a conscious decision you make and direct your body to perform.

There are two major parts of our nervous system: the central nervous system and the peripheral nervous system.

The **central nervous system** (Figure 4-25) consists of the brain and the spinal cord. It is called central because all the nerves from the body branch off the spinal cord or brain. The brain interprets all of the sensations brought in from the body. The brain also controls critical body functions such as respiratory and pulse rates, consciousness, and temperature.

The **peripheral nervous system** (Figure 4-26 on page 114) contains **sensory** and **motor nerves.** The sensory portion of the nervous system carries information from the body to the central nervous system. The motor nerves carry information from the central nervous system to the body.

The Skin

The skin is the outer layer of the body. It covers our bones, muscles, and organs and helps to provide some of our physical characteristics. It is a first line of defense against bacteria and the environment. It helps regulate our temperature. Our skin contains nerve endings and is used as a sensory organ for heat and cold, touch, pressure, and pain.

There are three layers to the skin (Figure 4-27 on page 115):

* The **epidermis** is the outermost layer of the skin

* The **dermis** lies below the epidermis and contains the sweat and sebaceous (oil) glands, hair follicles, nerve endings, and some blood vessels.

* The **subcutaneous layer** is the deepest layer. It is fatty tissue and provides shock absorption and insulation for the body.

THE BRAIN

DIVISIONS OF THE SPINAL CORD

THE SPINAL CORD

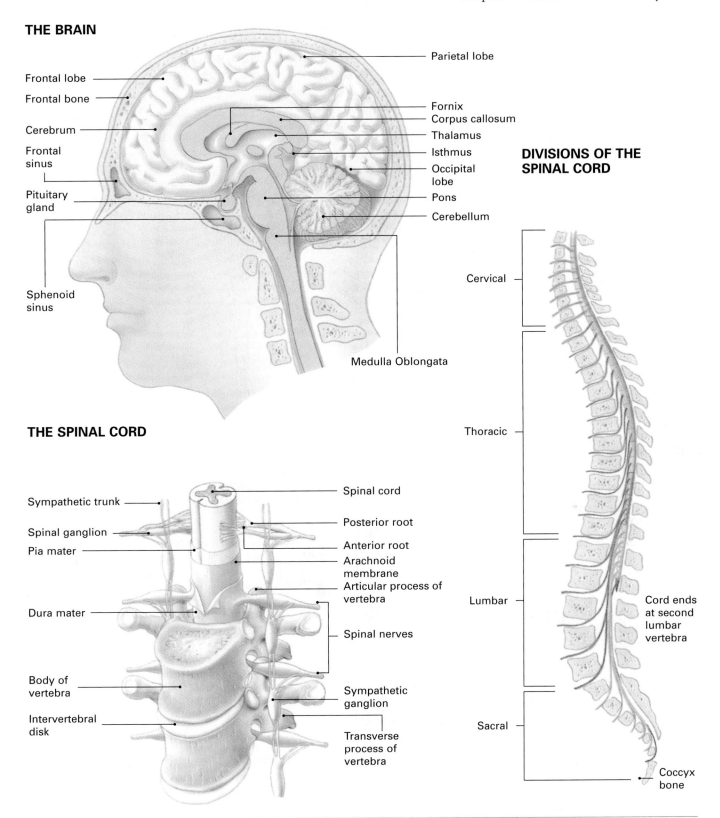

FIGURE 4-25   The central nervous system consists of the brain and spinal cord.

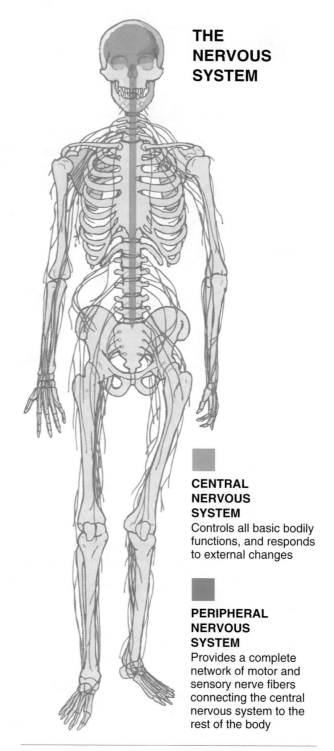

THE NERVOUS SYSTEM

CENTRAL NERVOUS SYSTEM
Controls all basic bodily functions, and responds to external changes

PERIPHERAL NERVOUS SYSTEM
Provides a complete network of motor and sensory nerve fibers connecting the central nervous system to the rest of the body

FIGURE 4-26 The central peripheral nervous systems.

FIGURE 4-27 The layers of the skin.

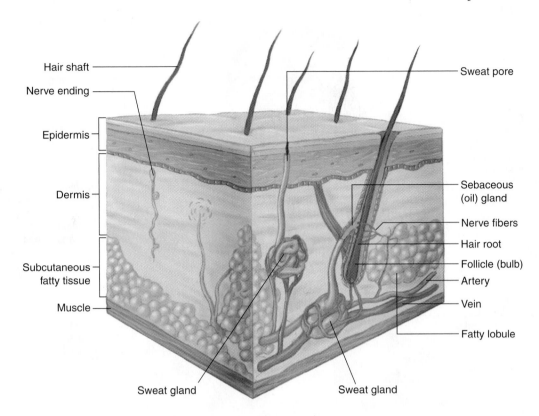

Hair shaft

Nerve ending

Epidermis

Dermis

Subcutaneous fatty tissue

Muscle

Sweat gland

Sweat pore

Sebaceous (oil) gland

Nerve fibers

Hair root

Follicle (bulb)

Artery

Vein

Fatty lobule

Sweat gland

The Endocrine System

The endocrine system (Figure 4-28 on page 116) is involved in regulation of the body. This is done through releases of chemicals called **hormones.** Two hormones you may recognize even without taking this course are **insulin,** which allows the body to use glucose (sugars) as fuel, and **epinephrine** which stimulates the body in response to stress. There are many other hormones, including those that control reproductive functions and metabolism.

The Abdomen

The abdomen is not a body system—it is a body region. The organs in and around the abdomen perform functions of many systems including the digestive, endocrine, urinary, reproductive, and circulatory systems. EMS calls to complaints of pain in this complex region are frequent.

The abdomen can be divided into quadrants. Imaginary vertical and horizontal lines are drawn through the umbilicus (navel) to delineate the four quadrants: upper right quadrant, upper left quadrant, lower right quadrant and lower left quadrant (Figure 4-29 on page 117). These quadrants provide landmarks for identifying the location of organs as well as describing the location of pain or discomfort described by the patient. The abdomen is bordered superiorly by the diaphragm and inferiorly by the floor of the pelvis.

The abdominal cavity is covered by the **peritoneum.** The peritoneum is made up of two thin membranes—one covering the abdominal organs and another attached to the abdominal wall.

1-4.2 Describe the anatomy and function of the endocrine system.

* **hormones**

   chemicals involved in regulation of body functions.

* **insulin**

   a hormone produced by the pancreas or taken as a medication by many diabetics that helps the body to use glucose as fuel.

* **epinephrine**

   chemical that stimulates the body in response to stress. Also called *adrenalin.*

* **adrenalin**

   see epinephrine.

* **peritoneum**

   two thin membranes, one covering the abdominal organs and the other attached to the abdominal wall.

✳ **stomach**

organ that receives food from the esophagus.

✳ **small intestine**

organ that digests solid foods and absorbs nutrients through the intestinal wall. The small intestine has three segments: duodenum, jejunum, and ileum.

✳ **large intestine**

organ that is a muscular tube that removes water from waste products received from the small intestine and removes anything not absorbed by the body toward excretion from the body. Also called the *colon.*

✳ **colon**

see large intestine.

✳ **excretion**

elimination of waste products from the large intestine.

✳ **liver**

produces bile to assist in breakdown of fats and assists in the metabolism of various substances in the body.

✳ **bile**

chemical that assists in the digestion of fat.

✳ **detoxifies**

breaks down harmful substances and renders them harmless.

✳ **glucose**

a simple form of sugar that is required by all cells as fuel for metabolic processes.

✳ **gallbladder**

an organ in the form of a sac on the underside of the liver that stores bile produced by the liver.

✳ **pancreas**

a gland located behind the stomach that produces insulin and produces juices that assist in digestion of food in the duodenum of the small intestine.

✳ **secreting**

releasing of substances.

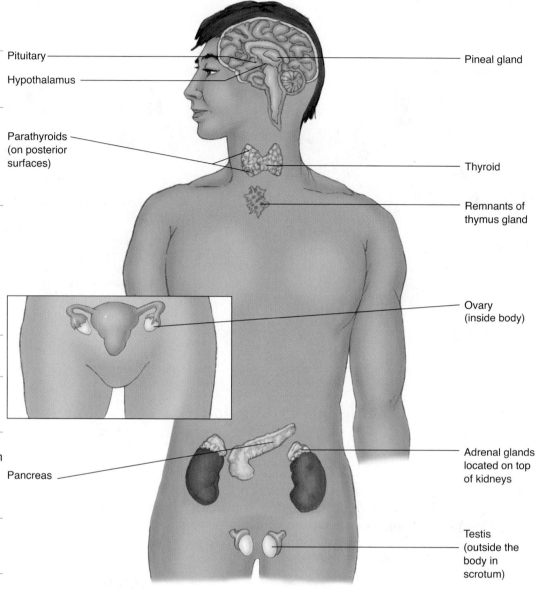

FIGURE 4-28 The endocrine system.

Organs located in the abdomen and their functions include:

✳ **Stomach**—The stomach receives food from the esophagus. It is a tubular organ that expands as it fills with food. Gastric juices work to digest (break down) the food as it moves to the small intestine.

✳ **Small intestine**—The small intestine continues the work of the stomach in digesting solid foods and absorbing nutrients through the intestinal wall. The small intestine has three segments: duodenum, jejunum, and ileum.

✳ **Large intestine**—Also known as the **colon,** the large intestine absorbs water and moves waste products along for **excretion.**

✳ **Liver**—The liver secretes **bile** to the small intestine. Bile assists in the digestion of fat. The liver also **detoxifies** harmful substances (for example, alcohol) and stores a limited amount of **glucose.**

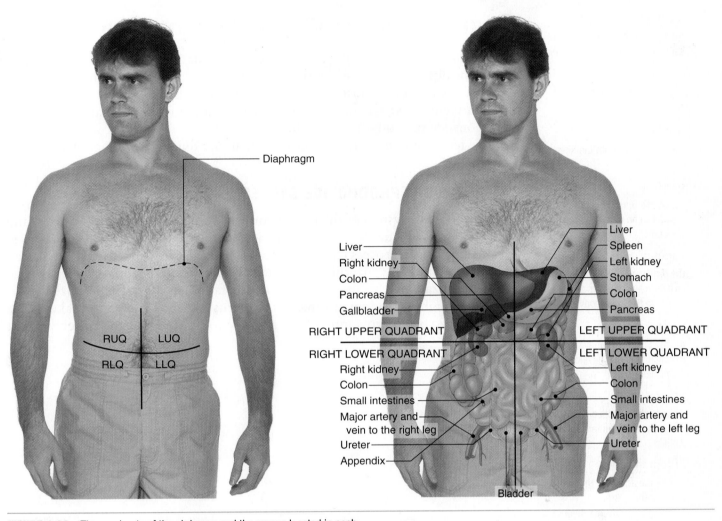

FIGURE 4-29 The quadrants of the abdomen and the organs located in each.

* **Gallbladder**—A small organ located behind the liver, the gallbladder stores bile from the liver.

* **Pancreas**—The pancreas has a digestive function in **secreting** substances that help digest **proteins** and **carbohydrates**. The **islets of Langerhans.** These are cells in the pancreas that secrete insulin and other hormones into the blood.

* **Spleen**—The spleen filters the blood, including the removal of old blood cells. The spleen also creates white blood cells. At any given time, the spleen contains a significant amount of blood, which can be used as a reserve if needed.

Some organs and structures are **retroperitoneal,** meaning "behind the peritoneum" or "outside the abdominal cavity." The **kidneys** are retroperitoneal organs. They provide filtering and waste removal. Water and waste removed by the kidneys are excreted as urine.

The abdominal aorta is also a retroperitoneal structure. This is why patients with an abdominal aortic **aneurysm** may experience back pain.

* **proteins**
  source of amino acids, the building blocks of the body.

* **carbohydrates**
  source of fuel for the body.

* **islets of Langerhans**
  a group of cells in the pancreas that secrete insulin and other hormones into the blood.

* **spleen**
  organ that filters the blood, including the removal of old blood cells. The spleen also creates white blood cells.

* **retroperitoneal**
  referring to the area behind the abdominal cavity.

* **kidneys**
  a pair of organs that filter the blood to remove excess water and waste.

Genitourinary and Reproductive Systems

The urinary systems for males and females are similar interiorly (although we recognize the differences in the external genitalia). The kidneys filter the blood to remove excess water and waste. The waste is moved from the kidneys to the **bladder** through the **ureters**. The **urethra** transports the urine from the bladder to be excreted outside the body (Figure 4-30).

The female and male reproductive systems are illustrated in Figure 4-31.

THE FEMALE REPRODUCTIVE SYSTEM

The reproductive system of the female consists of the **vagina, uterus, ovaries,** and **fallopian tubes** (Figure 4-31). The ovaries contain eggs (**ova**) that are released every 28 days in a process called **ovulation**. The eggs are guided into a fallopian tube by tiny **fimbria** (fingerlike projections). **Sperm** from the male meets the egg during **fertilization.** This usually occurs in the fallopian tube. The fertilized egg is guided through the fallopian tube to the uterus where **implantation** takes place and the **embryo** will grow into a **fetus** and develop through birth. The **cervix** is at

* **aneurysm**

the ballooning of a weakened section of the wall of an artery.

* **bladder**

organ that stores urine until excretion.

* **ureters**

transport urine from the kidneys to the bladder.

* **urethra**

transports urine from the bladder to be excreted outside the body.

* **vagina**

the birth canal. The tubular structure leading from the uterus to the outer body.

* **uterus**

the muscular abdominal organ in which the fetus develops. Also called the *womb.*

* **ovaries**

internal gland producing the ovum. Female counterpart to the testicles.

* **fallopian tubes**

carries the egg from the ovary to the uterus. Female counterpart to the vas deferens.

* **ovum/ova**

female sex cell. Female counterpart to the sperm.

* **ovulation**

the release of an ovum (egg) from the ovary.

* **fimbria**

a fingerlike anatomical part or structure.

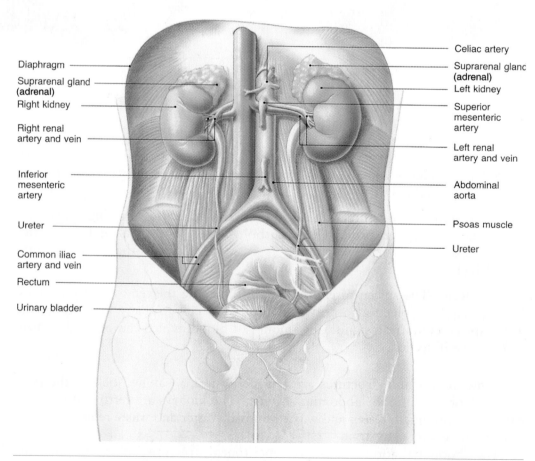

FIGURE 4-30 The organs associated with the urinary system.

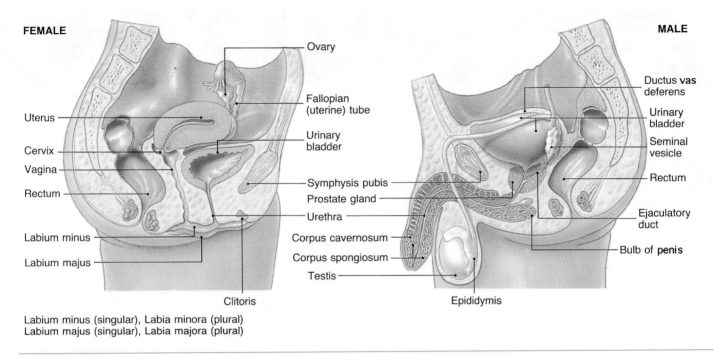

FEMALE   MALE

Ovary

Fallopian
(uterine) tube

Uterus

Urinary
bladder

Cervix

Vagina

Rectum

Symphysis pubis

Prostate gland

Urethra

Labium minus

Corpus cavernosum

Labium majus

Corpus spongiosum

Testis

Clitoris

Epididymis

Ductus **vas**
deferens

Urinary
bladder

Seminal
vesicle

Rectum

Ejaculatory
duct

Bulb of **penis**

Labium minus (singular), Labia minora (plural)
Labium majus (singular), Labia majora (plural)

FIGURE 4-31   The female and male reproductive systems.

the distal end of the uterus. This is the beginning of the birth canal, which extends through the vagina, the exterior opening of the birth canal.

THE MALE REPRODUCTIVE SYSTEM

The male reproductive system consists of the **testicles,** where sperm are created, the **vas deferens,** which transports sperm to the urethra, and the **penis** (Figure 4-31).

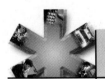

Perspective

Heather—The EMT

"We found Jocelyn on the couch in what is called the 'lateral recumbent' position. It seemed that any movement at all made her pain worse, even turning her head to talk to me made her wince. Now, she kept telling me that it was her 'stomach' that was hurting, but it was actually her abdomen. I learned quickly in this business that patients and EMS people use different words to describe the same thing! What to her was a 'sharp pain on both sides of her stomach that moves around back,' was, to me, a 'sharp, shooting pain across both lower abdominal quadrants, radiating to the back.' I know that it just seems like semantics, but everyone in the EMS system—from first responders to doctors—has to speak the same language. If I had told the ER doc that this girl's 'stomach hurts', would that really tell him anything useful?"

* **sperm**

  male sex cell. Male counterpart to the ovum.

* **fertilization**

  the combining of a sperm and an egg. Usually occurs in the fallopian tube.

* **implantation**

  the attachment of a fertilized egg to the uterine lining.

* **embryo**

  prefetal product of conception from implantation to the eighth week of development.

* **fetus**

  the baby as it develops in the womb.

* **cervix**

  the neck of the uterus at the entrance to the vagina.

* **testicles**

  external gland producing the sperm.

* **vas deferens**

  carries the sperm from the testicles to the urethra.

* **penis**

  external male genitalia that contains the urethra.

✳ Stop, Review, Remember!

Multiple Choice

Place a check next to the correct answer.

1. The _____ carry urine from the kidneys to the bladder.

    _____ a. urethras

    _____ b. capillaries

    _____ c. ureters

    _____ d. uterus

2. The layer of skin that contains blood vessels, nerve endings and hair follicles is called the:

    _____ a. epidermis.

    _____ b. polydermis.

    _____ c. subdermis.

    _____ d. dermis.

3. The organ that secretes insulin and aids in digestion is the:

    _____ a. aorta.

    _____ b. liver.

    _____ c. spleen.

    _____ d. pancreas.

4. The abdominal quadrants are formed by imaginary:

    _____ a. horizontal and vertical lines through the umbilicus.

    _____ b. transecting intermammary and anterior axillary lines.

    _____ c. horizontal and vertical lines through the eighth thoracic vertebrae.

    _____ d. none of the above

5. The endocrine system regulates the body through the use of:

    _____ a. hemoglobin.

    _____ b. hormones.

    _____ c. motor nerves.

    _____ d. hematocrit.

6. The part of the spine most commonly injured while lifting and moving is the:

    _____ a. cervical.

    _____ b. lymphatic.

    _____ c. thoracic.

    _____ d. lumbar.

7. The kneecap is called the:

    _____ a. patella.

    _____ b. tibia.

    _____ c. femur.

    _____ d. periosteum.

Fill in the Blank

1. The bones of the forearm are the _____ and _____.

2. Two ribs are not connected to the sternum. These are called _____ ribs.

3. The elbow is an example of a _____ joint.

4. The vertebrae in the neck are called _____ vertebrae.

5. The muscle lining the bronchioles is known as _____ or _____ muscle.

6. The central nervous system is comprised of the _____ and _____.

Critical Thinking

1. List the three functions of the musculoskeletal system.

   _____

   _____

   _____

   _____

2. List the four abdominal quadrants with one organ found in each.

   _____

   _____

   _____

   _____

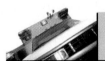

Dispatch Summary

We carefully moved Jocelyn to the stretcher and allowed her to remain in the position of most comfort during transport to the hospital.

Once she was at the ED, the doctor suspected (and then confirmed) that she was suffering from kidney stones. "That explains the pain radiating to the patient's back," the doctor told Heather and Josh. "The kidneys are, after all, retroperitoneal."

The patient was treated at the hospital and has had no further problems.

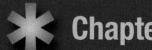

The Last Word

Anatomical descriptors are essential for describing or documenting important facts such as injuries, patient complaints, or positions.

The anatomy of body organs and systems creates critical foundations for the studies you will continue in upcoming weeks. These include:

✳ Airway structures and breathing in the airway module
✳ The respiratory system as you discuss difficulty breathing
✳ The cardiovascular system as you study chest pain, bleeding, and shock
✳ The musculoskeletal system as you learn treatment for suspected fractures
✳ The nervous system as you learn to treat injuries to the head and spine
✳ The endocrine system as you deal with conditions such as diabetes

✳ Chapter Review

MULTIPLE CHOICE

Place a check next to the correct answer.

1. The molecule in the red blood cell that binds with oxygen is:

_____ a. hormone.

_____ b. hemocult.

_____ c. hemoglobin.

_____ d. hematoglobulin.

2. A patient lying on her stomach would be described as lying in a _____ position.

_____ a. supine

_____ b. prone

_____ c. laterally recumbent

_____ d. dorsally-oriented

3. The ankle is _____ to the knee.

_____ a. anterior

_____ b. posterior

_____ c. proximal

_____ d. distal

4. The area that houses the vocal cords and opens into the trachea is known as the:

_____ a. oropharynx.

_____ b. pharynx.

_____ c. larynx.

_____ d. epiglottis.

5. The vessels that carry deoxygenated blood from the heart to the lungs are the:

_____ a. pulmonary arteries.

_____ b. pulmonary veins.

_____ c. pulmonary capillaries.

_____ d. pulmonary emboli.

6. Your patient has a bruise on the thumb side of his forearm. This is called the _____ side of the arm.

_____ a. proximal

_____ b. lateral

_____ c. medial

_____ d. It depends on how the patient is standing.

7. The bones of the lower leg are the:

_____ a. radius and ulna.

_____ b. scapula and clavicle.

_____ c. carpals and tarsals.

_____ d. tibia and fibula.

8. The hormone that allows glucose to be utilized by the cells is:

_____ a. cortisol.

_____ b. hemoglobin.

_____ c. adrenalin.

_____ d. insulin.

9. Which of the following structures is located in the lower right quadrant of the abdomen?

_____ a. spleen

_____ b. liver

_____ c. appendix

_____ d. pancreas

10. Smooth muscle is found in all of the following places except the:

_____ a. bicep.

_____ b. bronchi.

_____ c. intestine.

_____ d. arterioles.

MATCHING

Match the name of the bone on the left with the part of the body it is found in on the right.

1. _____ Femur
2. _____ Cranium
3. _____ Sternum
4. _____ Metatarsal
5. _____ Maxilla
6. _____ Clavicle
7. _____ Fibula
8. _____ Radius
9. _____ Maleolus
10. _____ Metacarpal
11. _____ Patella
12. _____ Ischium
13. _____ Humerus
14. _____ Scapula
15. _____ Vertebra

A. Head
B. Face
C. Anterior shoulder
D. Posterior shoulder
E. Chest
F. Spine
G. Upper arm
H. Forearm/wrist
I. Hand
J. Pelvis
K. Thigh
L. Knee
M. Lower leg
N. Ankle
O. Foot

LABELING

In the diagram below, draw the following areas and organs in their proper location:

Abdominal quadrants
Stomach
Liver
Gallbladder
Pancreas
Spleen
Large intestine
Small intestine
Diaphragm

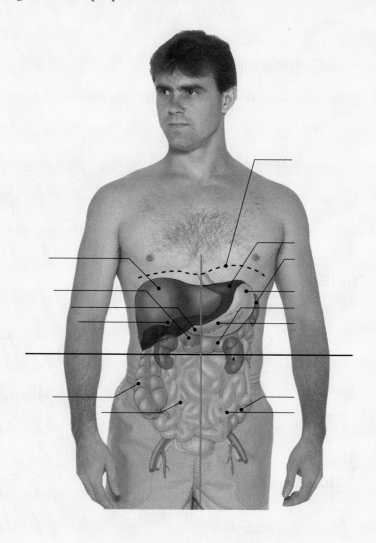

ORDERING

Number the following cardiovascular structures in the order blood flows when entering the heart from the venae cavae.

_____ Mitral valve   _____ Tricuspid valve

_____ Lung   _____ Aorta

_____ Right atrium   _____ Right atrium

_____ Left ventricle   _____ Right ventricle

_____ Pulmonary artery   _____ Pulmonic valve

_____ Pulmonary vein   _____ Aortic valve

CRITICAL THINKING

Describe the following patient complaints using correct anatomical and directional terms:

1. A patient has pain just under his rib cage on the right side.

   _____

   _____

   _____

2. A patient has a deformity on his left arm near the wrist.

   _____

   _____

   _____

3. A patient has a laceration on his left hand across his knuckles.

   _____

   _____

   _____

CASE STUDY

You are called to a motor vehicle collision with injuries. You find one injured patient. He was the passenger in a vehicle that was struck directly into the passenger-side door where the patient was sitting. You notice that the door was pushed about a foot into the passenger compartment.

1. The patient complains of pain to the right side of his rib cage over the lower five or six ribs. If there were internal injuries, what organs may be affected?

   _____

   _____

   _____

2. The patient also complains of some tenderness to palpation in the upper right abdominal quadrant. What organ or organs could be affected there?

   _____

   _____

   _____

3. Do you think either of these complaints/injuries could be serious?

   _____

   _____

   _____

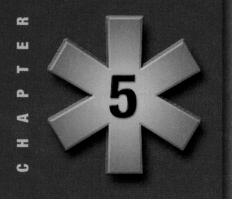

Lifting, Moving, and Positioning Your Patients

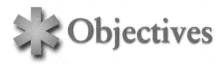 Objectives

Numbered objectives are from the U.S. Department of Transportation 1994 EMT-Basic National Standard Curriculum.

COGNITIVE OBJECTIVES

At the completion of this lesson, the EMT-Basic student will be able to:

1-6.1 Define body mechanics. (p. 128)

1-6.2 Discuss the guidelines and safety precautions that need to be followed when lifting a patient. (pp. 127–127)

1-6.3 Describe the safe lifting of cots and stretchers. (p. 129)

1-6.4 Describe the guidelines and safety precautions for carrying patients and/or equipment. (pp. 127–128)

1-6.5 Discuss one-handed carrying techniques. (pp. 128–129)

1-6.6 Describe correct and safe carrying procedures on stairs. (pp. 131–132)

1-6.7 State the guidelines for reaching and their application. (p. 129)

1-6.8 Describe correct reaching for log rolls. (p. 128)

1-6.9 State the guidelines for pushing and pulling. (p. 130)

1-6.10 Discuss the general considerations of moving patients. (pp. 127–130)

1-6.11 State three situations that may require the use of an emergency move. (p. 139)

1-6.12 Identify the following patient-carrying devices:
- Wheeled ambulance stretcher (pp. 131, 132)
- Portable ambulance stretcher (p. 136)
- Stair chair (pp. 131, 133–134)
- Scoop stretcher (p. 136)
- Long spine board (pp. 134–135)
- Basket stretcher (pp. 135–136)
- Flexible stretcher. (p. 134)

AFFECTIVE OBJECTIVES

At the completion of this lesson, the EMT-Basic student will be able to:

1-6.13 Explain the rationale for properly lifting and moving patients. (pp. 127–128)

PSYCHOMOTOR OBJECTIVES

At the completion of this lesson, the EMT-Basic student will be able to:

1-6.14 Working with a partner, prepare each of the following devices for use, transfer a patient to the device, properly position the patient on the device, move the device to the ambulance, and load the patient into the ambulance:
- Wheeled ambulance stretcher (pp. 131, 132)
- Portable ambulance stretcher (p. 136)
- Stair chair (pp. 131, 133–134)
- Scoop stretcher (p. 136)
- Long spine board (pp. 134–135)
- Basket stretcher (pp. 135–136)
- Flexible stretcher. (p. 134)

1-6.15 Working with a partner, the EMT-Basic will demonstrate techniques for the transfer of a patient from an ambulance stretcher to a hospital stretcher. (pp. 142–144)

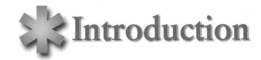

Introduction

Lifting and moving patients may seem easy at first glance. Strong muscles would be the first and most important requirement.

Wrong.

Lifting, moving, and positioning patients is a tremendous responsibility. It depends on the patient's condition and location—even the environment. EMTs of all sizes and shapes can move a wide variety of patients safely through the use of the equipment carried on the ambulance—and some critical thinking. Whether your patient has fallen in the bathtub or out in the woods, had a heart attack on a third floor (no elevator), or is found in a car wreck, the material you learn in this chapter will help you get the job done safely and efficiently while helping the patient's condition.

Emergency Dispatch

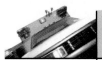

"Rescue 25, Rescue two-five, respond to 14427 South Orleans. That'll be apartment number 302 for a difficulty breathing. Time out 2317 hours."

"Rescue 25 copies," Brent, a new EMT, responds. "Show us en route from Main and Wilmore."

"South Orleans?" Brent's partner, Suki, looks thoughtful for a moment. "Oh wait, I think that's that three-story building where the elevator doesn't work!"

As if on cue, both EMTs sigh and think the same thing: It's been a long, tiring shift. Please don't let this be a big patient!

As Brent navigates the curb in front of the building, he sees that it is the place with the age-faded *Out of Order* sign on the elevator door. They take their equipment off of the stretcher and climb the three flights of winding stairs to Apartment 302.

They find their patient, 44-year-old Julie Ordeen, on a hospital bed that has been set up in the small, dark front room of her apartment. She is a double amputee—thanks to diabetes—and looks like she weighs well over 350 pounds.

As Brent begins talking to Julie, Suki radios dispatch and requests a lift-assist from the local fire crew.

Body Mechanics and Lifting

Lifting is an inevitable part of being an EMT. You will be called on to lift both patients and equipment. Performing these tasks safely and efficiently is vital for your health and well-being.

PRINCIPLES OF SAFE LIFTING

There are certain guidelines that will apply to every lift you make. They will apply whether you are lifting a patient, a stretcher, or even a heavy piece of equipment.

1-6.2 Discuss the guidelines and safety precautions that need to be followed when lifting a patient.

1-6.4 Describe the guidelines and safety precautions for carrying patients and/or equipment.

1-6.10 Discuss the general considerations of moving patients.

There are two main principles to keep in mind when lifting:

✳ Use your legs, not your back.

✳ Keep the person or item you are lifting as close to your body as possible.

One important thing to do before lifting is to plan. When you need to lift a piece of equipment, it will only take a moment to get in a good position close to the object and to lift with your legs. Lifting and moving a patient will usually take more planning. This planning will entail choosing a device with which to move the patient and determining how urgent the move is, the terrain you will be moving over and through (narrow halls or doorways, stairs), and the needs of the patient.

With experience, many of the decisions you will need to make will come naturally as you size up the scene and assess your patient. The following are guidelines to use when lifting any item or person:

1-6.1 Define body mechanics.

✳ Determine the weight to be lifted. Do this as part of the decision-making process before you lift.

✳ Use at least two people.

✳ Use an even number of people to maintain balance. If you have two people on one side of a stretcher and only one on the other, the stretcher may be thrown off balance.

✳ Have enough help available.

✳ Know the weight limitations for your carrying device and what to do when this weight is exceeded.

✳ **body mechanics**

the proper use of one's body to facilitate lifting and moving in such a way as to minimize injury.

✳ **power lift**

a lift from a squatting position with weight to be lifted close to the body, feet apart and flat on the ground, body weight on or just behind balls of feet, back locked in. The upper body is raised before the hips. Also called the *squat-lift position*.

✳ **locked-in technique**

when lifting, locking your back in position, avoiding twisting.

✳ **power grip**

gripping with as much hand surface as possible in contact with the object being lifted, all fingers bent at the same angle, hands at least 10 inches apart.

1-6.5 Discuss one-handed carrying techniques.

BODY MECHANICS

Body mechanics refers to the proper use of the body while lifting. The chief elements of body mechanics are position, grip, and techniques used while lifting.

When lifting, the **power lift** should be used (Figure 5-1). The power lift ensures that the legs and not the back are used to lift. This technique is used when lifting stretchers and other heavy items. When using the power lift:

✳ Your feet should be a comfortable distance apart.

✳ Your back should have a slight inward curve with the abdominal muscles tight and the back kept locked in using the **locked-in technique.**

✳ The weight should be distributed evenly between both feet. The balls of your feet should receive the majority of the weight.

The **power grip** (Figure 5-2) is designed to provide a solid grip for maximum efficiency in the lift. In the power grip, the palm and fingers contact the item being lifted as much as possible. When possible, the hands should be at least 10 inches apart.

At times, you may need to lift and carry a piece of equipment or the end of a stretcher using one hand. To lift with one hand, follow these rules:

✳ Stagger your feet with the forward knee up and the rearward knee pointing toward the ground.

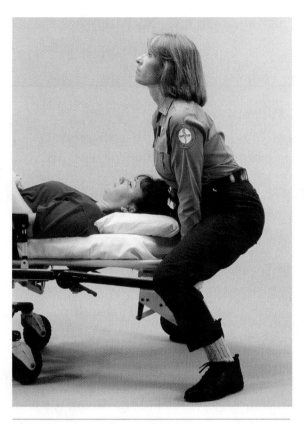

FIGURE 5-1 The power lift position.

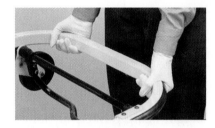

FIGURE 5-2 The power grip.

* Bend at the hips, not the waist, and don't lean your torso forward more than 45 degrees.

* Lift by pushing upward through the arch and heel of the forward foot and the ball of the rearward foot.

To carry a stretcher or piece of equipment using one hand:

* Keep your back locked.

* As much as possible, avoid leaning to the opposite side to compensate for the weight imbalance.

Reaching, pushing, and pulling are movements that frequently cause injury to the EMT. We don't usually think of these as risky moves because they do not always involve direct or heavy lifting.

When reaching (Figure 5-3 on page 130), use the same locked-in technique for your lower back that you would use while lifting. Avoid twisting and prolonged, strenuous reaching (more than a minute). Reaching more than 15 to 20 inches in front of your body may place you in a position with a higher risk of injury.

Use the same guidelines for reaching when you are leaning forward to log roll a patient. Lock your back, avoid twisting, and kneel close to the patient so you do not have to reach more than 20 inches.

When you are in a position where you have a choice between pushing or pulling, keep in mind that pushing poses less risk for injury. In a foot drag, you

1-6.3 Describe the safe lifting of cots and stretchers.

1-6.7 State the guidelines for reaching and their application.

1-6.8 Describe correct reaching for log rolls.

1-6.9 State the guidelines for pushing and pulling.

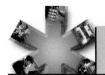

Perspective

Julie Ordeen—The Patient

I hate it when things get so bad that I have to call 9-1-1. Almost as much as I hate being sick. Have you ever had to be dependent on others for everything? Let me tell you; it just plain sucks. You know what I hate most of all though? The looks I get from the ambulance and fire people. I'm not happy that I weigh a little over 400 pounds, but I do. Do I eat too much? Probably. What would you do if you were bedridden, alone in an apartment all of the time, with nothing to do but watch TV? I've also got a thyroid problem. So it's not all my fault. The last time I had to be taken to the hospital, one of you guys from the ambulance made some comment about me "eating too many Twinkies." That made me cry for the better part of two days.

1-6.12 Identify the following patient-carrying devices:
- Wheeled ambulance stretcher
- Portable ambulance stretcher
- Stair chair
- Scoop stretcher
- Long spine board
- Basket stretcher
- Flexible stretcher.

will often need to pull the patient (Figure 5-4). Bend your knees and keep the weight being pushed or pulled close to your body. If the item or person is below waist level, use a kneeling position to push. Keep your elbows bent and close to your sides.

Specific Devices and Situations

The following subsections highlight some of the most common devices and situations EMTs encounter in the field along with some practical information you can use in addition to the general principles we have just discussed.

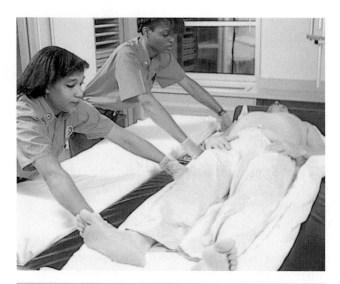

FIGURE 5-3 When reaching, use the locked-in technique for your lower back.

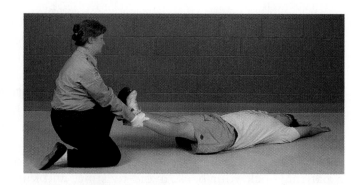

FIGURE 5-4 Pulling poses risk for injury. Instead, pull.

Generally, it is better to wheel patients, rather than carrying them, whenever it is possible and safe to do so. The choice of carrying device depends on many factors, including patient condition, terrain, space considerations, and the weight being carried.

WHEELED AMBULANCE STRETCHER

You will use the **wheeled stretcher** (Figure 5-5), also called the *cot* or *gurney*, on most calls. It is probably the most commonly used device for moving patients (Scan 5-1 on page 132). It should be used on smooth terrain.

The device is moved by pulling the foot end of the stretcher while a second EMT guides the head end of the stretcher (Figure 5-6 on page 133). The stretcher should be moved along the long axis. Avoid sideways or lateral movements. The high center of gravity of the stretcher may cause the stretcher to tip over and injure the patient.

Use an even number of providers when lifting the wheeled stretcher. An odd number (two on one side, three on the other) may cause the stretcher to become off balance and tip. Communicate with your partner and know each other's abilities and limitations. Call for help if necessary.

Some stretchers are referred to as **self-loading** or *auto-loading* (Figure 5-7 on page 133). These stretchers are wheeled up to the ambulance and, once the wheels at the head of the stretcher are securely on the floor of the ambulance, the undercarriage with the ground-level wheels may be collapsed upward and slid into the ambulance with the stretcher. This minimizes lifting. However, there is no such thing as a truly "self-loading" stretcher.

Injuries to patients from accidents involving stretchers is a significant cause of lawsuits against EMS providers. You must be alert and diligent when using the stretcher. Be sure that you or your agency maintains the stretcher according to manufacturer's guidelines. Do not exceed the weight limit of your stretcher.

STAIR CHAIR

As the name implies, the **stair chair** (Figure 5-8 on page 133) can be used to move patients up and down stairs. Wheeled stretchers are too bulky and heavy to move

✳ **wheeled stretcher**

the most commonly used device for moving patients. Also called *cot* or *gurney*.

✳ **self-loading**

stretchers that are wheeled up to the ambulance and, once the wheels are securely on the floor of the ambulance, the wheels may be lifted into the ambulance. Also called *auto-loading*.

1-6.6 Describe correct and safe carrying procedures on stairs.

✳ **stair chair**

a chair-style device used to move patients up and down stairs in a sitting position.

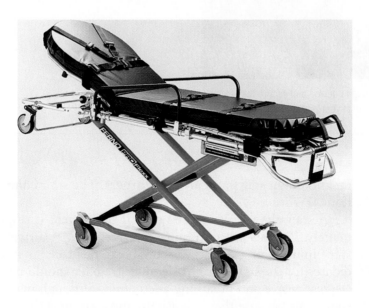

FIGURE 5-5 A wheeled stretcher, lift-in type. (Ferno Corporation)

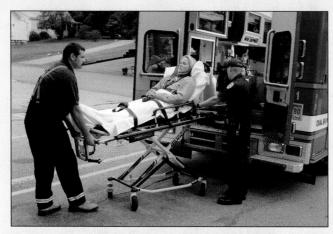

▲ Position the wheels closest to the patient's head at the opening of the ambulance.

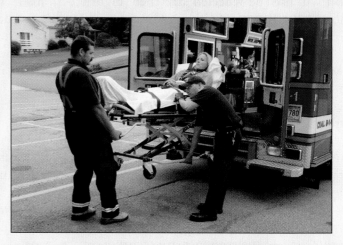

▲ Once the wheels are securely on the ambulance floor, the rescuer at the rear of the stretcher activates the lever to release the wheels. (This may require a slight lift to get the weight off the wheels.) The second rescuer should guide the collapsing carriage, if necessary. *Ferno Corporation.*

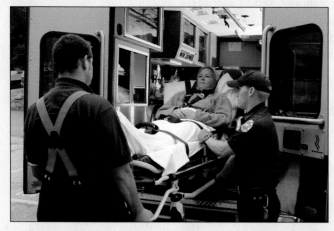

▲ Move the stretcher into the securing device and secure the stretcher in front and rear. Communicate with your partner to achieve balance.

up and down stairs and around corners. The stair chair is excellent in these situations (Figure 5-9).

A stair chair may be used only if the patient is responsive and breathing adequately. Patients who are unresponsive, require airway care or ventilation, have spine injuries, or are otherwise unable to be placed in a sitting position are not candidates for the stair chair. A flexible stretcher should be used instead. Patients who are responsive and breathing adequately, although with difficulty, are ideal for the stair chair because they are usually most comfortable in a sitting position.

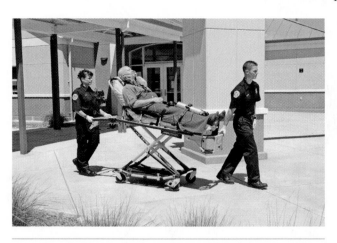

FIGURE 5-6 One EMT pulls the foot end of the stretcher while the second EMT guides the head end of the stretcher.

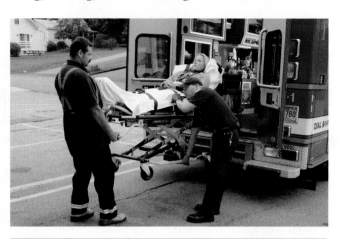

FIGURE 5-7 The self-loading, or auto-loading, stretcher. (Ferno Corporation)

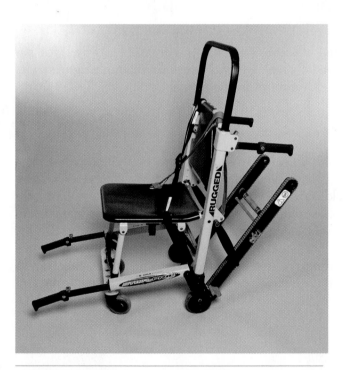

FIGURE 5-8 The stair chair.

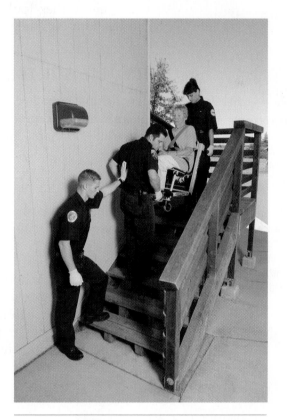

FIGURE 5-9 The stair chair is used to move the patient up and down stairs.

When using the stair chair, be sure to secure the patient to the device and reassure the patient (Figure 5-10 on page 134). The patient may feel awkward or frightened being carried down stairs and may reach out and grab a railing or other object. This can cause the chair to shift, resulting in the patient falling and/or back injury to the EMTs carrying the device. Also, because the stair chair is stored in a folded position, it is critical to ensure that the device is fully expanded and locked in position before you seat the patient.

The EMT going down the stairs first will be going backward. The EMT nearer the patient's head will face forward. Use the proper methods described earlier in

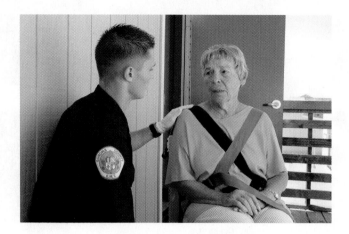

FIGURE 5-10 When using the stair chair, be sure to use the belt to secure the patient to the chair. Reassure the patient before beginning the transport process.

the chapter for lifting. Have someone act as a spotter behind the first EMT to coach him or her, look for dangers and unstable surfaces, and help ensure good footing with each step.

FLEXIBLE STRETCHER

✳ **flexible stretcher**

a lightweight device used for carrying supine patients down stairs or through tight spaces. Also known as a *Reeves stretcher.*

The **flexible stretcher,** also called a *Reeves stretcher* (Figure 5-11), is used for patients who are supine and must be carried down stairs or through tight spaces (Figure 5-12). Some have a rigid aluminum frame for support.

LONG SPINE BOARD

✳ **long backboard**

a rigid device, usually made of a plastic or composite material that is used to stabilize a patient with a suspected spinal injury. Also called a *long spine board.*

The **long backboard** or *long spine board* is a rigid device, usually made of a plastic or composite material, that is used when the patient has a suspected spine injury. At one time, most backboards were made of wood, but concerns for potentially infectious substances soaking into the wood caused most agencies to go to impermeable and more easily cleaned plastics.

The device is called a long backboard because it is designed to support the whole body (although the lower extremities of those over 6 feet tall will hang off the end a bit). This support is designed to restrict motion of the spine and minimize additional spine injury.

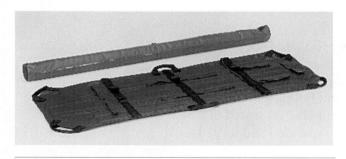

FIGURE 5-11 The flexible or Reeves stretcher.

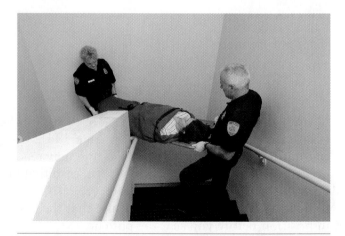

FIGURE 5-12 The flexible stretcher is used to move patients down stairs or through tight spaces.

Research has shown that rigid backboards, while important in minimizing further spine injury, cause significant discomfort to the patient during transport, at the hospital, and for days after the incident. Chapter 34 will describe procedures for applying long and short backboards.

SHORT BACKBOARD

The **short backboard** (Figure 5-13) and the **vest-type extrication device** (Figure 5-14) are primarily used during extrication of a patient from a vehicle that has been involved in a collision (Figure 5-15). When a patient is seated in a vehicle, the short backboard or vest-type device is applied before moving the patient from the vehicle to minimize additional injuries in the moving process.

BASKET STRETCHER

Also called a **Stokes basket,** the *basket stretcher* (Figure 5-16) is designed to move patients over challenging terrain (Figure 5-17 on page 136). The basket is

* **short backboard**
  a flat rigid device primarily used to stabilize the spine of a seated patient during extrication from a vehicle.

* **vest-type extrication device**
  a rigid vest-type device primarily used to stabilize the spine of a seated patient during extrication from a vehicle.

* **Stokes basket**
  a metal or plastic basket designed to move patients over uneven terrain. Also called a *basket stretcher.*

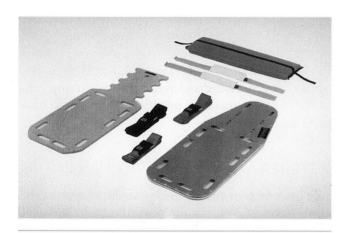

FIGURE 5-13 The short backboard.

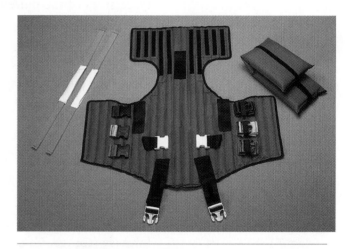

FIGURE 5-14 A vest-type extrication device.

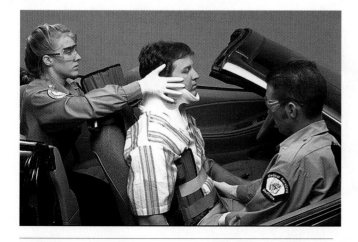

FIGURE 5-15 The vest-type extrication device is used to remove a patient from a vehicle involved in a collision.

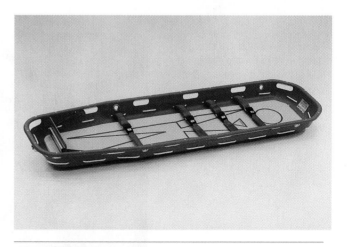

FIGURE 5-16 The Stokes or basket stretcher. (Ferno Corporation.)

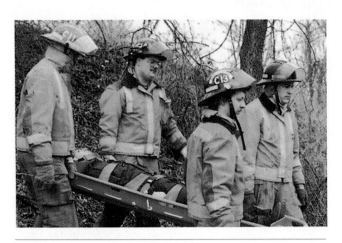

FIGURE 5-17 The basket stretcher is used to move patients over challenging terrain.

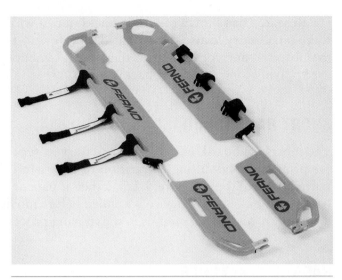

FIGURE 5-18 The scoop or orthopedic stretcher. (Ferno-Washington Inc.)

made of a metal or plastic, which provides protection from hard surfaces on three sides of the patient.

SCOOP STRETCHER

✳ **scoop stretcher**

a device that separates in two and can be used to "scoop" the patient off the ground. Also called an *orthopedic stretcher.*

The **scoop stretcher** (Figure 5-18), also called the *orthopedic stretcher,* is so named because it separates in half and comes back together again to literally "scoop" the patient off the ground (Figure 5-19). This is sometimes used in patients who have suspected hip or pelvic fractures.

PORTABLE AMBULANCE STRETCHER

✳ **portable stretcher**

a lightweight device made of canvas or plastic with two poles extended from each side for easy carrying.

The **portable stretcher** may be made of canvas or plastic and is usually lightweight. Two poles extend from each side for easy carrying. Some portable stretchers fold for easy storage. One common use of portable stretchers is at a multiple-casualty incident.

FIGURE 5-19 The scoop stretcher separates into halves to enable the EMTs to "scoop" the patient off of the ground.

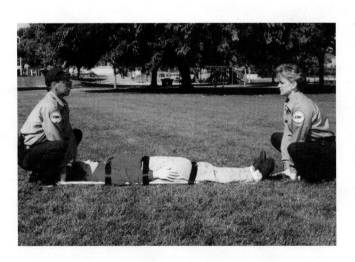

Stop, Review, Remember!

Multiple Choice

Place a check next to the correct answer.

1. Which of the following statements about lifting is incorrect?

_____ a. You should communicate with your partner before lifting.

_____ b. An even number of people should be used.

_____ c. You should use your legs, not your back to lift.

_____ d. When practical and safe, patients should be lifted rather than wheeled.

2. Which of the following would be inappropriate when transporting an unconscious patient?

_____ a. basket stretcher

_____ b. long backboard

_____ c. stair chair

_____ d. wheeled stretcher

3. You are part of a team caring for dehydrated and exhausted patients at a marathon road race. There are many patients. Each of these patients may most appropriately be placed on a:

_____ a. basket stretcher.

_____ b. stair chair.

_____ c. long backboard.

_____ d. portable stretcher.

4. You are called to care for a patient who is experiencing difficulty breathing. You find the patient in a second-floor back bedroom of the house. You examine the patient, find him alert. To get this patient downstairs, you would likely use the:

_____ a. basket stretcher.

_____ b. wheeled stretcher.

_____ c. stair chair.

_____ d. flexible stretcher.

5. The weight you are lifting should be kept as close to your body as possible.

_____ a. true

_____ b. false

6. Pushing is preferred over pulling whenever possible.

_____ a. true

_____ b. false

Matching

Match the piece of equipment on the left with the applicable situation on the right.

1. _____ Reeves stretcher

2. _____ Vest-type extrication device

3. _____ Basket stretcher

4. _____ Stair chair

5. _____ Wheeled stretcher

6. _____ Orthopedic stretcher

A. Moving a patient down a rocky slope

B. Extricating a patient sitting in a vehicle that has crashed

C. Moving an unresponsive patient down a narrow hallway

D. Moving a patient on a long board a short distance to the ambulance

E. Moving a patient with mild trouble breathing from a second-floor bedroom

F. Moving a patient who has fallen in the bathroom and has a possible hip injury

Critical Thinking

1. Describe the following lifting techniques:

    a. Power grip

    _____

    _____

    _____

    _____

    _____

    b. Power lift

    _____

    _____

    _____

    _____

    _____

2. What could happen to you if you didn't use appropriate lifting techniques such as the power lift?

    _____

    _____

    _____

    _____

    _____

3. What could happen to your patient if a move were done without regard to safety?

    _____

    _____

    _____

    _____

    _____

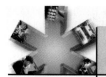

Perspective

Suki—The EMT

"When I walked into the room, my heart just sank. My back started to hurt just thinking about moving that woman down three flights of stairs. It's part of the job, though. This wasn't the first—and won't be the last—time for a patient like this. I honestly can't imagine what it's like for the patient, though. Brent, my new partner, just stared at her. I don't think he'd ever seen anyone so big. I had to get him started on the assessment while I contacted dispatch for help. It actually turned out okay. We started some high-flow oxygen while we waited for fire, and with a heavy-duty stair chair, four carriers, two spotters, and me, we got her to the truck. Ms. Ordeen got safely to the hospital, all of our backs survived, and we were back on the street in no time. I guess planning was the key."

Types of Moves

Patients require movement for a wide variety of reasons. Some may be extreme emergencies while others are simply routine. Earlier in this chapter we mentioned that priorities, devices, and means of movement are determined by a wide range of factors including patient condition and priority for transport, terrain, and environment. This section puts these determining factors into perspective by setting criteria for the various types of patient moves. The types of patient moves are emergent moves, urgent moves, and non-urgent moves.

Emergent moves are performed when there is an immediate risk of death to the patient, when injuries may occur that outweigh any harm that may come to the patient by moving her, or when the patient must be moved to access another patient who needs lifesaving care (Scan 5-2 on page 140). Examples include:

* Fire or threat of fire

* Explosives or other hazardous materials

* Inability to protect the patient from hazards at the scene (e.g., falling debris at a construction site or oncoming traffic)

* Moving one patient in a motor vehicle collision to access a critically injured patient.

Emergent moves do not offer extensive protection for injuries to the spine or other bones. Emergent moves do not have to be reckless, however, and there are ways that these moves can be done quickly, yet with some concern for the spine. One of these methods is called the **long-axis drag**. To drag the patient away from danger, pull from the patient's shoulders while cradling the head. The term *long axis* refers to the head-to-toe axis. By keeping this axis straight during the drag, you minimize the chance of spine injuries that can occur when a patient isn't immobilized on a backboard.

1-6.11 State three situations that may require the use of an emergency move.

* **emergent moves**

a category of patient moves performed when there is an immediate risk of death or serious injury to the patient or another patient.

* **long-axis drag**

a method used to move a patient while maintaining the body's long axis.

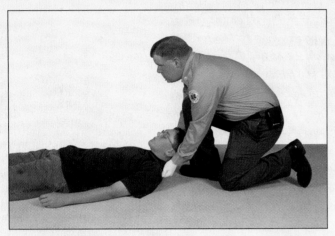

▲ Clothes drag.

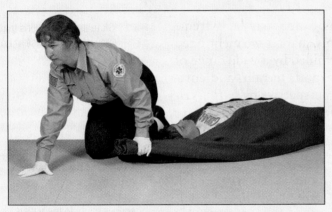

▲ Blanket drag. Gather half of the blanket material up against the patient's side. Roll him toward your knees, place the blanket under him, and gently roll him onto the blanket. During the drag, keep the patient's head as low as possible.

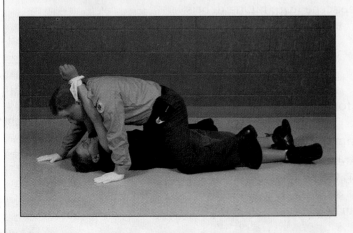

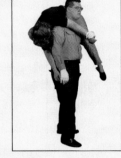

▲ Firefighter's carry. Place your feet against her feet and pull patient toward you. Bend at waist and flex knees. Duck and pull her across your shoulder, keeping hold of one of her wrists. Use your free arm to reach between her legs and grasp her thigh. Weight of patient falls onto your shoulders. Stand up. Transfer your grip on thigh to patient's wrist.

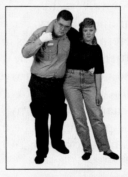

▲ One-rescuer assist. Place patient's arm around your neck, grasping her hand in yours. Place your other arm around the patient's waist. Help patient walk to safety. Be prepared to change movement technique if level of danger increases. Be sure to communicate with patient about obstacles, uneven terrain, and so on.

◀ Firefighter's drag. Place patient on his back and tie his hands together. Straddle him, crouch, and pass your head through his trussed arms. Raise your body, and crawl on your hands and knees. Keep the patient's head as low as possible.

Urgent moves are performed when the patient's condition is serious or is deteriorating and the patient must be moved promptly for treatment and transportation. Examples include:

* Moving a patient to position him or her for airway care

* Performing a **rapid extrication** of a patient from a vehicle.

A note about rapid extrication: When a patient with a spine injury is taken out of a vehicle, the move is normally done with a short backboard or vest-type extrication device to protect the spine. In cases where the patient is in serious condition (e.g., airway problems, severe shock), taking time to attach a short backboard or vest to the patient would allow his condition to worsen. In this situation, a rapid extrication would take place. This is done cautiously but without a short backboard or vest because of the patient's condition. Rapid extrication will be taught in Chapter 34.

Non-urgent moves are exactly what the name implies—not urgent. Non-urgent moves are done when there is nothing about the patient's condition and no hazards at the scene that would require expedited (emergent or urgent) moves.

A wide variety of moves make up the non-urgent category, and which one you use depends on the position in which you find the patient. Remember: You will find patients on the floor, in bed, sitting in chairs or standing, caught between the sink and toilet or in a narrow hallway. Determining the proper move or combination of moves will help you in any of these situations. Keep in mind, however, that patients with spinal injuries, even those who are considered non-urgent, must receive full spinal immobilization.

Non-urgent moves include the direct ground lift (Scan 5-3 on pages 142–143) and the extremity lift, which can be used to transfer a patient from the floor or a chair to the stretcher. Do not use the extremity lift if you suspect injury to any of the extremities.

Some moves are used in transferring the patient from a bed to a stretcher, for example, from the patient's bed at home to the ambulance stretcher or in transfers from the hospital to another health care facility. These moves include the draw-sheet method and the direct carry.

Another transfer situation involves moving the patient from the ambulance stretcher to a bed in the emergency department. When there are only two people to make the move, the transfer is commonly made using the draw-sheet method or the direct carry. When there are four people to make the move (for example, two EMTs and two members of the hospital staff) the stretcher-to-stretcher transfer can be made using a modified draw-sheet method (Scan 5-4 on page 144).

PATIENT POSITIONING

In addition to moving your patient, you will also be responsible for properly positioning your patient. Positioning and transportation go hand-in-hand. The proper position depends on the patient's condition.

The basic positions that you should know include **supine, laterally recumbent,** and **prone** (Figures 5-20A–C on page 145).

Certain positions are preferred in specific medical conditions. These conditions and positions include the following:

* *Unresponsive patients* who do not have a suspected spinal injury are placed in a laterally recumbent position. Usually the patient is placed on the left side. This is also referred to as the *recovery position.*

* *Patients with suspected spinal injuries* are immobilized in the supine position on a backboard. The patient found in a sitting position will also be

---

* **urgent moves**

a category of patient moves performed when the patient's condition is serious or is deteriorating and the patient must be moved promptly for treatment and/or transportation.

* **rapid extrication**

the rapid removal of a patient from a vehicle when the patient's condition or the situation does not permit use of a short backboard or vest-type extrication device.

* **non-urgent moves**

a category of patient moves performed when there is no need to expedite due to the patient's condition or hazards at the scene.

* **supine**

lying face up. Opposite of prone.

* **laterally recumbent**

lying on one side.

* **prone**

lying face down. Opposite of supine.

DIRECT GROUND LIFT

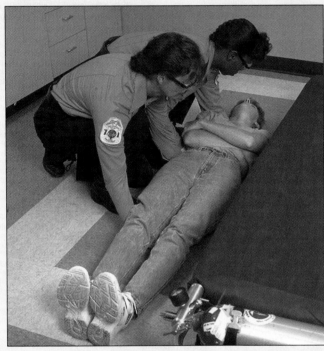

▲ **1.** The stretcher is set in its lowest position and placed on the opposite side of patient. EMTs face patient, drop to one knee, and, if possible, place patient's arms on his chest. The head-end EMT cradles patient's head and neck by sliding one arm under the neck to grasp shoulder, the other arm under patient's back. The foot-end EMT slides one arm under patient's knees and other arm under patient above buttocks.

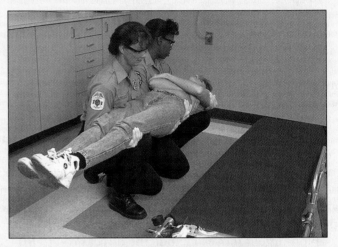

▲ **2.** On signal, the EMTs lift patient to their knees.

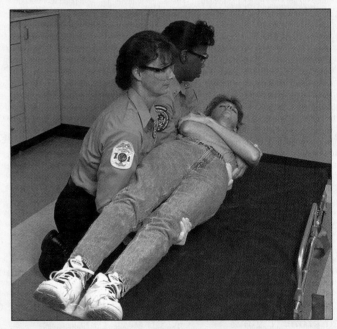

▲ **3.** On signal, the EMTs stand and carry patient to stretcher, drop to one knee, and roll forward to place him onto mattress.

Note: If a third rescuer is available, he should place both arms under patient's waist while the other two slide their arms up to the midback or down to the buttocks, as appropriate.

DIRECT CARRY

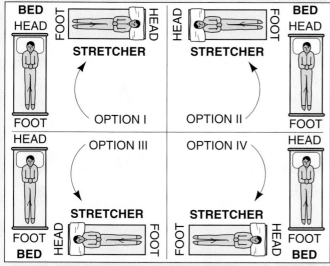

▲ **1.** Stretcher is placed at 90° angle to bed, depending on room configuration. Prepare stretcher by lowering rails, unbuckling straps, and removing other items. Both EMTs stand between stretcher and bed, facing patient.

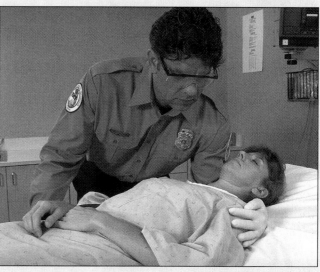

▲ **2.** Head-end EMT cradles patient's head and neck by sliding one arm under patient's neck to grasp shoulder.

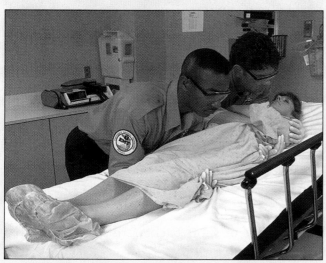

▲ **3.** Foot-end EMT slides hand under patient's hip and lifts slightly. Head-end EMT slides other arm under patient's back. Foot-end EMT places arms under patient's hips and calves.

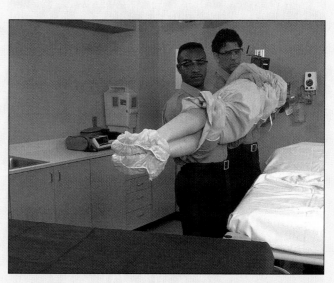

▲ **4.** EMTs slide patient to edge of bed and bend toward her with their knees slightly bent. They lift and curl patient to their chests and return to a standing position. They rotate, then slide patient gently onto stretcher.

✳✳✳✳✳✳✳✳✳✳✳✳✳✳✳✳✳✳✳✳✳

SCAN 5-4   **TRANSFER FROM AMBULANCE STRETCHER TO HOSPITAL STRETCHER**

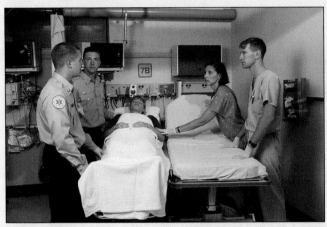

▲ **1.** Position raised ambulance cot next to hospital stretcher. Hospital personnel then adjust stretcher (raise or lower the head) to receive patient.

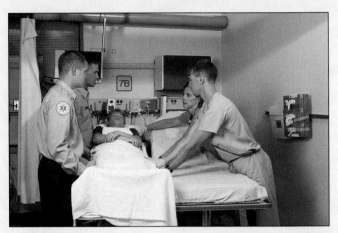

▲ **2.** You and hospital personnel gather the sheet on either side of the patient and pull it taut in order to transfer the patient securely.

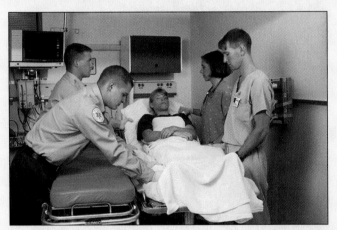

▲ **3.** Holding the gathered sheet at support points near patient's shoulders, midtorso, hips, and knees, you and hospital personnel slide patient in one motion onto hospital stretcher.

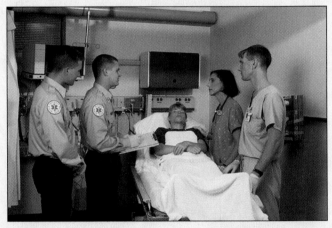

▲ **4.** Make sure patient is centered on stretcher and stretcher rails are raised before turning him over to emergency department staff.

immobilized in a vest-type device or short backboard and then moved to a supine position.

✳ *A patient with chest pain or discomfort or respiratory distress* is allowed to attain a position of comfort. This is usually a sitting position. Patients who are breathing inadequately or are unable to maintain their own airway must be placed in a supine position and provided aggressive airway and ventilatory assistance.

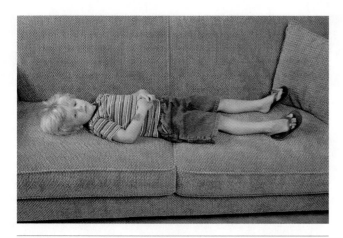

FIGURE 5–20A   The supine position.

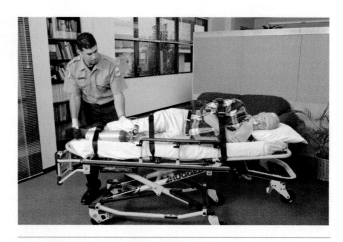

FIGURE 5–20B   The laterally recumbent position.

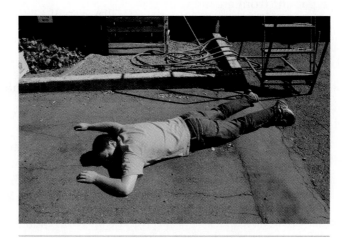

FIGURE 5–20C   A patient found in the prone position.

* *Patients who are in shock (hypoperfusion)* will be placed in the supine position (on a backboard if spine injuries are suspected) with the legs elevated 8 to 12 inches. Do not perform this elevation if you suspect injury to the legs.

* *Patients who are nauseated or vomiting but alert* may be transported in a position of comfort. Monitor the airway carefully and be prepared to suction, especially if the patient's mental status deteriorates.

* *Pregnant patients experiencing hypotension* should be transported on their left side to take pressure off the inferior vena cava. Patients with advanced pregnancy (6 to 9 months) should be transported on their left side during transport unless there are spinal injuries. If spinal injury is suspected, place the patient supine with a towel or blanket under the right side of the board, which will cause the patient to shift to the left.

Stop, Review, Remember!

Multiple Choice

Place a check next to the correct answer.

1. Which of the following would not call for the use of an emergency move?

   _____ a. moving a patient with a confused mental status from a vehicle

   _____ b. removing a patient from a car that is on fire

   _____ c. moving a patient away from a wall that is about to collapse

   _____ d. moving a patient away from a tanker of hazardous materials that may rupture

2. Emergency moves are made using spinal immobilization.

   _____ a. true

   _____ b. false

3. To properly move a patient via a long-axis drag, you would drag the patient by the:

   _____ a. head.

   _____ b. shoulders.

   _____ c. arms.

   _____ d. waist.

4. In using one hand to help lift and carry a patient on a stretcher, you should do all of the following EXCEPT:

   _____ a. stagger your feet.

   _____ b. bend at the hips.

   _____ c. keep your back locked.

   _____ d. lean away from the stretcher.

5. A patient lying on his front (stomach) is said to be:

   _____ a. supine.

   _____ b. prone.

   _____ c. laterally recumbent.

   _____ d. in a position of comfort.

6. You are treating a patient who is unresponsive but breathing adequately. You should position this patient in a _____ position.

   _____ a. supine

   _____ b. prone

   _____ c. laterally recumbent

   _____ d. comfortable

7. You are transporting a patient who is about 33 weeks pregnant. You place her on the stretcher and in a short time she begins to feel weak and dizzy. You should:

   _____ a. place her in a prone position.

   _____ b. roll her to her left side.

   _____ c. roll her to her right side.

   _____ d. do nothing; pregnancy normally cause weakness and dizziness.

8. Which of the following is least likely to determine the patient transport device used?

   _____ a. the terrain over which the patient must be transported

   _____ b. patient priority

   _____ c. patient complaint

   _____ d. EMT's prior back injury

9. Patient movement and transportation methods affect a patient's condition.

   _____ a. true

   _____ b. false

Fill in the Blank

1. A full-term pregnant patient who was involved in a motor vehicle collision is placed on a backboard. You should place a towel under the _____ side of the backboard to cause the patient to roll to the _____.

2. A patient found near spilled gasoline at a motor vehicle collision would require a(n) _____ move.

3. A patient lying face down is said to be in the _____ position.

4. A patient with respiratory distress who is breathing adequately is often transported in a position of _____.

5. An emergent move that is designed to keep the spine in line is called a _____ drag.

Critical Thinking

1. Describe one situation (each) when you would use an emergency move, an urgent move, and a non-urgent move.

   _____

   _____

   _____

   _____

   _____

2. What is the difference between an emergent move and an urgent move?

   _____

   _____

   _____

   _____

   _____

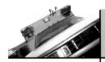

Dispatch Summary

Julie was transported to Physician's Hospital on Fifth Street and treated for a urinary tract infection and several diabetes-related issues and released two days later.

Due to her condition, and those of several other people in the same apartment building, the management company was ordered to repair the elevator—which it did.

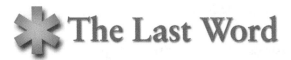

The Last Word

Lifting and moving patients involve much more than strength. Proper lifting and moving ensure EMTs and patients will be kept safe, helps the patient's clinical condition, and reduces effort as well as liability. Improper lifting and moving can do the opposite of all those things. As an EMT you are more likely to be forced to retire because of back injuries than injures received in any other way—including ambulance collisions and violence. Lifting and moving is also about decision making. The decisions you make to be safe, efficient, and correct for your patient are at the core of what lifting and moving are about.

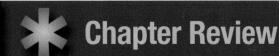

Chapter Review

MULTIPLE CHOICE

Place a check next to the correct answer.

1. Lifting patients generally goes better with an odd number of EMTs.

_____ a. true

_____ b. false

2. The short backboard and vest-type extrication device are used for the same purpose.

_____ a. true

_____ b. false

3. Auto-loading stretchers load without any lifting by the EMT.

_____ a. true

_____ b. false

4. Errors in lifting and moving can cause tremendous liability for EMTs.

_____ a. true

_____ b. false

5. The vest-type extrication device is used when a patient:

_____ a. is transferred from a hospital bed to a stretcher.

_____ b. is involved in a motor vehicle collision.

_____ c. is transported over rough terrain.

_____ d. has rib fractures.

6. Body mechanics refers to the:

_____ a. mechanical workings of the body of the stretcher.

_____ b. use of the patient's body weight to facilitate lifting.

_____ c. use of the EMT's body while lifting.

_____ d. sum lifting potential (in pounds) of all rescuers on scene.

7. An emergency move could be used in which of the following situations?

_____ a. a patient complaining of severe neck pain and partial paralysis in a motor vehicle collision

_____ b. a patient in a motor vehicle collision where the car is on fire and smoke is billowing into the passenger compartment

_____ c. a patient who is found on the ground and appears to have been thrown from a vehicle

_____ d. a patient who pulled to the side of a road while driving a propane truck because he believed he was having a heart attack

8. A patient with a spinal injury from a fall would be placed on a _____ to prevent further injury.

_____ a. stair chair

_____ b. basket stretcher

_____ c. long spine board

_____ d. wheeled stretcher

9. Which of the following is NOT a correct guideline for reaching forward to log roll a patient?

_____ a. Lock your back.

_____ b. Avoid twisting.

_____ c. Kneel close to the patient.

_____ d. Don't reach farther than 36 inches.

10. In transferring a supine patient to a stretcher, which of the following methods would be LEAST appropriate if spinal injuries are suspected?

_____ a. extremity carry

_____ b. direct carry

_____ c. direct ground lift

_____ d. draw-sheet method

MATCHING

Match the patient presentation on the left with the most common position for transport on the right.

1. _____ Patient with spinal injuries

2. _____ Patient with difficulty breathing

3. _____ Pregnant patient with hypotension

4. _____ Patient in shock

5. _____ Vomiting patients

A. Supine position
B. Supine, legs elevated
C. Supine, rolled to left
D. Position of comfort
E. Laterally recumbent

LABELING

1. Write the position in which each patient is shown in the space below the photo.

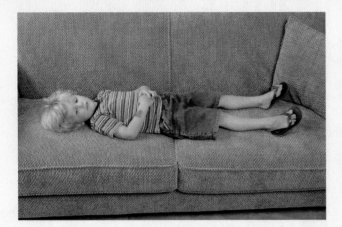

A. _____

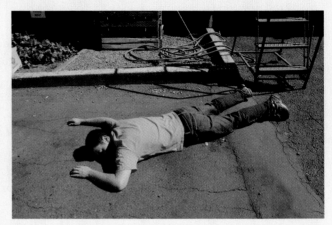

B. _____

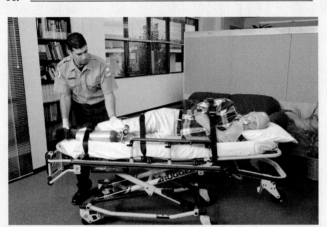

C. _____

2. Write the name of each device in the space below its photo.

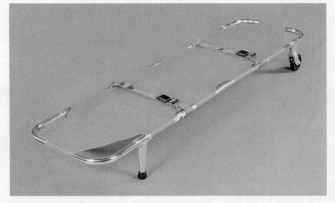

D. _____

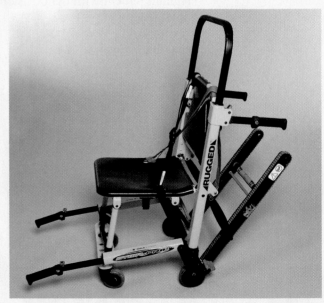

E. _____

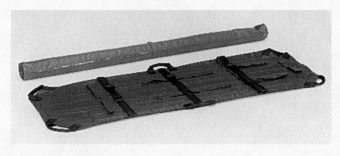

F. _____

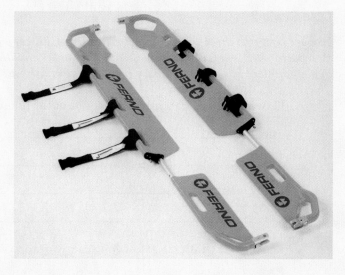

G. _____

CASE STUDIES

Case Study 1

You are called to a motor vehicle collision. You find a badly mangled car with the driver's side wrapped around a tree. You approach the vehicle and find a woman who is alert and able to speak in the front passenger seat. She has an apparent broken arm and no other complaints. You look past her to the driver's seat and observe an apparently unresponsive male with a head injury and bleeding about the mouth and nose.

1. In reference to the female patient which statement is correct?

   _____ a. The female patient would be placed in a vest-type extrication device and moved from the vehicle because she appears stable.

   _____ b. The female patient would be moved from the vehicle via rapid extrication because she is unstable.

   _____ c. The female patient would be moved from the vehicle rapidly, but with a vest-type extrication device because she may be unstable.

   _____ d. The female patient would be moved from the vehicle via rapid extrication to allow access to the male patient.

2. Which statement in reference to the male patient is correct?

   _____ a. The male patient would be placed in a vest-type extrication device and moved from the vehicle because he appears stable.

   _____ b. The male patient would be moved from the vehicle via rapid extrication because he is unstable.

   _____ c. The male patient would be moved from the vehicle rapidly, but with a vest-type extrication device because he may be unstable.

   _____ d. The male patient would be dragged from the vehicle by any means possible because he appears unresponsive.

Case Study 2

You are part of a three-person crew performing CPR on a patient in a living room. The patient is placed on a backboard and CPR continues. You have an automated defibrillator, oxygen, pocket face mask, and two equipment bags that you have brought into the house.

1. How would you carry the patient out of the house and integrate CPR?

_____

_____

_____

_____

2. Recall your CPR class. How long can you stop CPR for moving a patient?

_____

_____

_____

_____

3. How would you get your equipment from the house to the ambulance?

_____

_____

_____

_____

Case Study 3

You are called to a "sick patient" and find a 532-pound man who feels weak, is unable to stand, and must be transported to the hospital. You are part of a two-person crew.

1. How much help would you call for?

_____

_____

_____

_____

2. Would you need any special equipment?

_____

_____

_____

_____

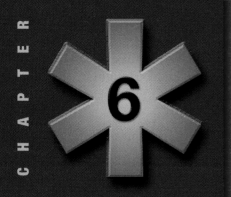

✳ Directions

Assess what you have learned in this module by circling the best answer for each multiple-choice question.
When you are done, check your answers against the key provided in Appendix D.

1. Which of the following most accurately defines
   an EMS system?
   a. a network of injury prevention resources
   b. legislation and regulations that govern
      prehospital care and emergency
      transportation
   c. all of the EMS provider agencies in a
      geographical area
   d. a chain of resources designed to minimize
      the impact of sudden illness and injury

2. Which of the following is an EMS system
   component as defined by NHTSA?
   a. EMS training
   b. ambulance advisory committee
   c. rehabilitation services
   d. bioterrorism preparedness

3. Which of the following is necessary to evaluate
   the effectiveness of an EMS system?
   a. review of records by NHTSA
   b. a state-wide uniform data collection system
   c. sophisticated computer software
   d. a court-order to release patient information

4. Which of the following levels of EMS
   responder is nationally recognized by the
   DOT?
   a. Advanced EMS
   b. Cardiac Technician

c. EMT-Intermediate
d. Paramedic Specialist

5. Which of the following is the minimum level of
   training necessary for providing patient care
   during ambulance transportation?
   a. CPR certification
   b. First Responder (Emergency Responder)
   c. EMT
   d. EMT-Ambulance

6. Of the following, who is responsible for
   overseeing all patient care aspects of an EMS
   system?
   a. the state EMS bureau or agency
   b. a county EMS agency
   c. the chief trauma surgeon of the nearest
      trauma center
   d. the EMS officer

7. Which of the following is an example of "on-
   line" medical direction?
   a. receiving orders from a physician over the
      radio
   b. receiving direction from a nurse bystander
      on the scene
   c. consulting with a paramedic who is
      responding to the scene
   d. following your system's standing orders

8. The EMT must be concerned for the safety of:
    a. patients.
    b. himself.
    c. bystanders.
    d. all of the above

9. The purpose of Quality Improvement processes is to:
    a. identify and discipline individual EMTs for providing inadequate medical care.
    b. reduce the cost of professional liability insurance.
    c. ensure that the public receives the best possible prehospital care.
    d. comply with laws regulating payment for the delivery of medical care.

10. Which of the following is a way in which EMTs can participate in Quality Improvement?
    a. attend continuing education classes.
    b. Practice infrequently used skills.
    c. Document patient care accurately and thoroughly.
    d. all of the above

11. Jan just completed her EMT-Basic course and has been accepted as a member of the volunteer rescue squad in her community. As she increases her amount of time away from her family, which of the following feelings are they likely to experience?
    a. jealousy
    b. satisfaction
    c. novelty
    d. grief

12. A cumulative stress response is also known as:
    a. posttraumatic stress disorder.
    b. burnout.
    c. an "adrenalin rush."
    d. anguish.

13. Which of the following changes in your coworker's behavior should make you suspect that he is suffering from an increased amount of stress?
    a. increased hunger, excessive sleeping, being overly cooperative
    b. increased sleeping, reporting "night sweats," decreased appetite
    c. irritability, decreased appetite, lack of enthusiasm about work
    d. increased social activity, starting a new exercise program, excessive eating

14. The best time to initiate stress management is:
    a. before a stressful event occurs.
    b. during the stressful event.
    c. immediately after the stressful event.
    d. after the immediate "fight or flight" response has subsided.

15. Which of the following is NOT a recommended stress management technique?
    a. regular exercise
    b. a healthy diet
    c. striking a balance between work, family, and recreation
    d. drinking 2–3 alcoholic beverages after each work shift

16. Which of the following is NOT a helpful technique in helping a family member cope with the sudden loss of a loved one?
    a. encouraging denial
    b. being tolerant of their anger
    c. touching in a supportive, empathetic manner
    d. being honest about the fact the loved one has died

17. You have been called to the scene of a possible cardiac arrest. On your arrival you find that Mrs. Thompson obviously died a few hours ago and will not benefit from resuscitation. When you tell Mr. Thompson that his wife has died, he asks, "Will she be admitted to the intensive care unit again?" This is an example of which stage of grief?
    a. bargaining
    b. depression
    c. remorse
    d. denial

18. The term "standard precautions" (universal precautions) applies to the EMT's actions regarding:
    a. traffic hazards.
    b. crime scenes.
    c. combative patients.
    d. exposure to body substances.

19. Which of the following is considered appropriate personal protective equipment for body substance isolation?
    a. firefighting turnout gear
    b. latex, Nitrile, or vinyl gloves
    c. contact lenses
    d. all of the above

20. Your patient is a 15-year-old male who has crashed his scooter into a curb. He has a cut on his forehead and scrapes on his hands and knees. Which of the following is the best choice of PPE in caring for this patient?
    a. HEPA mask, gown, gloves, protective eye wear
    b. gloves
    c. gloves and protective eye wear
    d. protective eye wear and a HEPA mask

21. Which of the following is the most important method by which EMTs can prevent the spread of infection?
    a. wearing gloves for every patient contact
    b. hand washing
    c. maintaining up-to-date immunizations
    d. using all PPE available for every patient

22. The primary agency concerned with the health of the medical workforce is the:
    a. National Association of EMTs.
    b. American Medical Association.
    c. Occupational Safety and Health Administration.
    d. Department of Health and Human Services.

23. The primary role of an EMT in responding to an incident involving hazardous materials is:
    a. identifying the material.
    b. determining whether or not there is a leak or vapor cloud.
    c. evacuating area residents.
    d. providing patient care.

24. You have been dispatched for an assault in a private residence. Law enforcement has been notified and is en route. As you arrive at the scene, you note law enforcement has not yet arrived. Which of the following is the best action for you to take?
    a. Park several houses away and await law enforcement.
    b. Park directly in front of the residence and await law enforcement.
    c. Park several houses away and approach the residence from the side, rather than from the front.
    d. Approach the house, look in windows, and listen carefully to determine whether it is safe to enter.

25. The best action for an EMT in regard to the stress associated with working in EMS is to:
    a. consider EMS to be a short-term occupation and plan on leaving the field within 5 years.
    b. develop proactive coping mechanisms to build resilience.
    c. avoid thinking about stressful events that occur on the job.
    d. participate in regular critical incident stress debriefings.

26. The specific actions that an EMS provider is allowed to perform, based on level of training and state regulations, best describes:
    a. standard of care.
    b. scope of practice.
    c. duty to respond.
    d. limit of liability.

27. Which of the following statements regarding EMS providers' practice is true?
    a. Protocols are national standards that describe the specific actions EMS providers are allowed to perform.
    b. Individual states generally allow more skills than those described by the national standard curriculum.
    c. Standing orders describe the entire standard of care for a given EMS system.
    d. The standard of care is a modified scope of practice that meets the needs of a given region.

28. Which of the following is best described as an ethical, rather than legal, consideration for EMS providers?
    a. scope of practice
    b. licensure
    c. protecting the patient's dignity
    d. duty to act

29. An EMT may NOT have a legal obligation to provide emergency care in which of the following situations?
    a. An off-duty EMT drives up on the scene of a motorcycle collision that has just occurred and no responders have yet arrived at the scene.
    b. An off-duty EMT has stopped to render emergency care but realizes he is now late to work and leaves the patient to avoid being disciplined at work.
    c. An on-duty EMT responds to a call and discovers that the patient is not having an emergency but thinks she will be seen more quickly in the emergency department if she arrives by ambulance.
    d. An on-duty EMT working for a private ambulance service is assigned to provide care at an outdoor concert.

30. Who may be protected by Good Samaritan laws?
    a. untrained bystanders
    b. EMTs
    c. physicians
    d. all of the above

31. In which of the following instances is it necessary to have consent to treat a patient?
    a. The patient is alert and mentally competent.
    b. The patient is alert but appears to be intoxicated with alcohol.
    c. The patient is unresponsive.
    d. all of the above

32. In which of the following instances can you assume that the patient consents to treatment?
    a. The patient is a diabetic who is very confused, does not know what day it is, and does not understand why you are in his home.
    b. The patient has fallen down a flight of stairs and is talking to a First Responder from the fire department when you arrive.
    c. The patient does not answer you, but does not object when you begin to assess him.
    d. Both a and c are correct.

33. Which of the following patients is most likely to have the right to consent to or refuse treatment on his or her own?
    a. a 14-year-old whose parents are out of town for the day and can't be reached by phone
    b. a 16-year-old who is married
    c. a 12-year-old who is pregnant
    d. a 15-year-old attending a military school

34. Mr. Wickett is having chest pain that he describes as "indigestion." He is angry that his wife called EMS and is refusing to allow you to assess or treat him. You should:
    a. leave so as to avoid upsetting him further.
    b. explain that it may be indigestion, but there are also some serious medical problems that feel like indigestion and ask if you can check his pulse and blood pressure.
    c. tell him that you cannot leave unless he signs a form that he is refusing treatment "Against Medical Advice."
    d. explain that most people who think they are having indigestion may be really having heart attacks and he could go into cardiac arrest at any time and needs to go with you immediately.

35. Your patient is a 50-year-old female having severe abdominal cramps. She looks pale and is sweating profusely. Her coworkers called EMS out of concern for her. The patient is alert and answers questions appropriately but is embarrassed and is refusing to be transported. Which one of the following is NOT appropriate at this time?
    a. Contact law enforcement.
    b. Contact medical direction.
    c. Contact your supervisor.
    d. Enlist the assistance of her coworkers in convincing the patient to be transported.

36. You are caring for a 22-year-old male who injured his ankle while ice skating. On arrival at the emergency department, the triage nurse asks you to have your patient sit in a wheelchair and to take the patient to the registration desk. Which of the following is the best action?
    a. Tell the nurse you can only place the patient in a treatment room.
    b. Tell the nurse you cannot leave the patient before he is seen by a physician.
    c. State to the nurse, "I can do that, but I need to give you a report on this patient first."
    d. Transport the patient to a different emergency department.

37. You have arrived at a nursing home where Mr. Jenkins is lying in bed in cardiac arrest. Just as you prepare to perform CPR, the nurse says, "Wait! I think he has a DNR order. Let me go call his doctor." What should you do?
    a. Begin CPR and prepare to transport the patient.
    b. Wait to start CPR and ask the nurse to call Mr. Jenkins's doctor from the room to save time.
    c. Do chest compressions but do not ventilate until you're sure of the patient's DNR status.
    d. Tell the nurse that you cannot honor a DNR under any circumstances.

38. You have just arrived on the scene of a 30-year-old male who reportedly had a seizure. His eyes are closed and he is not responding to requests from the first EMT on the scene to "open your eyes." The first EMT on the scene appears to believe the patient is "faking" the seizure and unresponsiveness. He says to the patient, "You need to open your eyes and talk to me or we're going to stick a tube down your throat." This could be interpreted as:
    a. battery.
    b. assault and battery.
    c. damages.
    d. assault.

39. An EMT is caring for a diabetic patient who is awake but whose blood sugar is low. The EMS service standing orders state that patients such as this should receive oral glucose. The EMT does not give the oral glucose and the patient becomes unresponsive on the way to the hospital. Once at the emergency department, the patient receives an IV and intravenous dextrose to raise the blood sugar. The patient regains consciousness and is released from the emergency department after treatment and observation. The patient would NOT likely be successful in suing the EMT for negligence because:
    a. there are no discernable damages.
    b. there was no breach of duty.
    c. the EMT did not have a duty to act.
    d. only the medical director can be negligent, not the EMT.

40. Mr. Robertson was shot by his neighbor during an argument. Which of the following situations is a violation of patient confidentiality?
    a. You describe the location of the wound to law enforcement on the scene.
    b. You discuss this case with your partner to see if there was something you could have done differently to improve patient care.
    c. You include this information in your documentation, part of which will be used for insurance and billing purposes.
    d. none of the above

41. Which of the following serves as the standard reference for describing the location of human anatomy?
    a. prone position
    b. anatomical position
    c. sagittal plane
    d. physiologic standard

42. The portion of the clavicle (collarbone) that is closest to the sternum (breastbone) is its _____ end.
    a. distal
    b. lateral
    c. medial
    d. plantar

43. The wrist is _____ to the fingers and _____ to the elbow.
    a. proximal, distal
    b. distal, proximal
    c. medial, lateral
    d. lateral, medial

44. The abdominal cavity is separated from the thoracic cavity by the:
    a. mesentery.
    b. ribs.
    c. omentum.
    d. diaphragm.

45. Another name for the voice box is the:
    a. pharynx.
    b. epiglottis.
    c. larynx.
    d. thyroid cartilage.

46. The passageway that transports air from the larynx to the bronchi is the:
    a. pharynx.
    b. trachea.
    c. alveoli.
    d. esophagus.

47. Which of the following is a sign of adequate breathing?
    a. irregular respirations
    b. using muscular activity to exhale
    c. breathing 14 times per minute
    d. agonal respirations

48. Which of the following is true concerning ways in which a child's respiratory system is different than an adult's?
    a. Children rely more on their diaphragms for breathing.
    b. A child's trachea is short and wide compared to an adult's.
    c. A child's tongue takes up much less space in the mouth.
    d. The cricoid cartilage is very pronounced in a child.

49. The cardiovascular system includes all of the following components EXCEPT the:
    a. heart.
    b. blood.
    c. blood vessels.
    d. lungs.

50. The primary function of hemoglobin is to:
    a. help blood clot.
    b. carry oxygen.
    c. carry carbon dioxide.
    d. detoxify waste products.

51. Which of the structures below carries oxygenated blood?
    a. pulmonary arteries
    b. tight atrium
    c. vena cava
    d. pulmonary veins

52. Which of the following directly affect(s) cardiac output?
    a. Tidal volume
    b. Stroke volume
    c. Heart rate
    d. Respiratory rate
    e. b and c

53. Which of the following could you use to assess circulation to the foot?
    a. vena cava
    b. dorsalis pedis artery
    c. brachial artery
    d. femoral vein

54. The skull is made up of the:
    a. cranium and scalp.
    b. cranium and face.
    c. carpals and metacarpals.
    d. carpals and ilium.

55. The largest, strongest bone in the body is the:
    a. sacrum.
    b. sternum.
    c. femur.
    d. mandible.

56. A sprain involves an injury to a:
    a. ligament.
    b. bone.
    c. tendon.
    d. muscle.

57. There are _____ cervical vertebrae in the _____.
    a. 5, lower back
    b. 12, posterior chest
    c. 4, tailbone
    d. 7, neck

58. In which of the following structures would smooth muscle be found?
    a. lungs
    b. bicep
    c. heart
    d. all of the above

59. When a muscle performs its work without conscious thought about it, it is known as a/an _____ muscle.
    a. skeletal
    b. voluntary
    c. involuntary
    d. none of the above

60. Which of the following is part of the central nervous system?
    a. vertebrae
    b. spinal cord
    c. motor nerves
    d. sensory nerves

61. Which of the following is a function of the skin?
    a. temperature regulation
    b. protection against infectious bacteria
    c. provides information about the environment
    d. all of the above

62. The outermost layer of the skin is the:
    a. epidermis.
    b. dermis.
    c. subcutaneous layer.
    d. fascia.

63. By drawing imaginary vertical and horizontal lines that intersect at the umbilicus, the abdomen is divided into the:
    a. right upper lobe, right lower lobe, left upper lobe, left lower lobe.
    b. right upper quadrant, right lower quadrant, left upper quadrant, left lower quadrant.
    c. right epigastric region, left epigastric region, right pubic region, left pubic region.
    d. right peritoneal area, left peritoneal area, right gastric area, left gastric area.

64. The organ that secretes insulin is the:
    a. spleen.
    b. liver.
    c. kidney.
    d. pancreas.

65. Which of the following is NOT a retroperitoneal organ?
    a. right kidney
    b. left kidney
    c. stomach
    d. abdominal aorta

66. Urine moves from the kidneys to the bladder through the:
    a. urethra.
    b. vas deferens.
    c. ureter.
    d. fallopian tube.

67. The "power-lift" position is used to make sure that the muscles of the _____ are used in lifting rather than the muscles of the _____.
    a. arms, legs
    b. legs, arms
    c. arms, back
    d. legs, back

68. Your patient is a 60-year-old man with difficulty breathing. He is conscious and alert and able to cooperate but is in a basement apartment in a building without an elevator. Which of the following would be the best way to get this patient out of his apartment?
    a. stair chair
    b. basket stretcher
    c. long spine board
    d. blanket carry

69. You are on your first ambulance ride-along, and the lead EMT asks you to go to the ambulance and get the gurney. You should get the:
    a. stair chair.
    b. basket stretcher.
    c. wheeled ambulance stretcher.
    d. reeves stretcher.

70. In which of the following situations would the use of a short backboard be appropriate?
    a. Your patient is under 5 feet tall.
    b. Your patient needs to be carried up or down stairs.
    c. Your patient was injured in a vehicle collision and is still seated in the vehicle.
    d. Your patient is sitting in a recliner, complaining of low back pain.

71. Mrs. Johnson fell two days ago in her kitchen and has been unable to get to the phone. When she heard the mail carrier on her porch this morning, she shouted for help and the mail carrier called EMS. You find Mrs. Johnson lying on her back, complaining of pain in her right leg and hip. Which of the following devices would most likely cause Mrs. Johnson the least amount of pain in preparing her for transport?
    a. scoop stretcher
    b. long spine board
    c. Stokes basket
    d. stair chair

72. Your patient is a 29-year-old woman who was driving her vehicle when a large truck coming from the opposite direction crossed the median and struck her vehicle "head-on." The patient is unresponsive and does not have adequate breathing, but the scene is free from additional hazards. Your patient should be moved using a/an _____ move.
    a. emergent
    b. urgent
    c. non-urgent
    d. critical

73. Your patient has a long history of lung problems and has called EMS today because she is having difficulty breathing. She is able to maintain her own airway and is breathing on her own but needs oxygen. Which of the following is the best choice of position for transporting this patient?
    a. left lateral recumbent
    b. supine
    c. supine with legs elevated 8–12 inches
    d. sitting

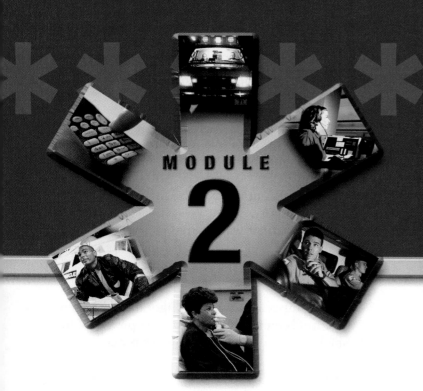

MODULE
2

Airway

“ *. . . here's this person you love more than anything in the world and you're looking into her eyes and all you see is fear, absolute terror. I can't even imagine what it's like to not be able to breathe.* ”

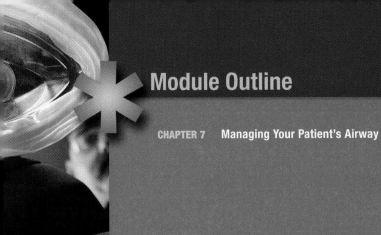

Module Outline

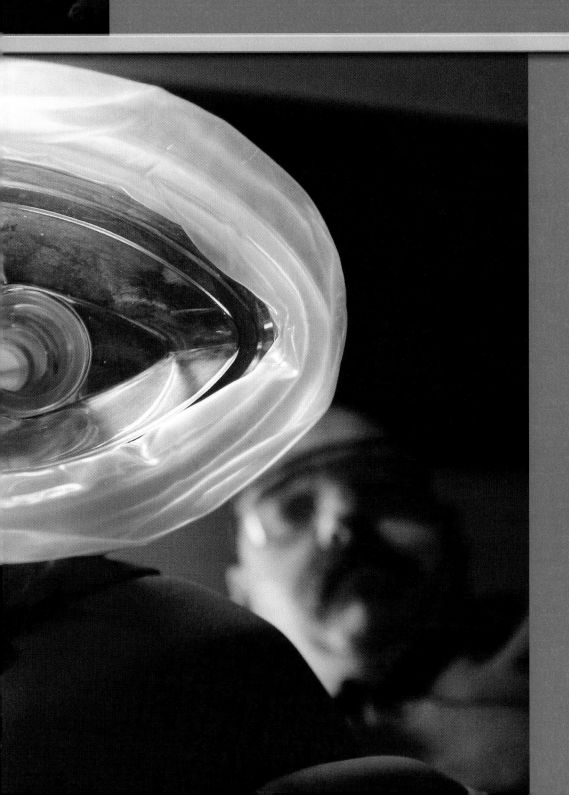

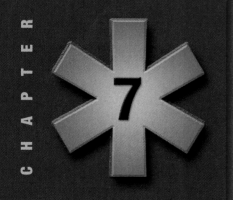

7 Managing Your Patient's Airway

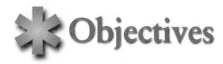 Objectives

Numbered objectives are from the U.S. Department of Transportation 1994 EMT-Basic National Standard Curriculum.

COGNITIVE OBJECTIVES

At the completion of this lesson, the EMT-Basic student will be able to:

2-1.1 Name and label the major structures of the respiratory system on a diagram. (pp. 164–166)

2-1.2 List the signs of adequate breathing. (pp. 166–167)

2-1.3 List the signs of inadequate breathing. (pp. 167–172)

2-1.4 Describe the steps in performing the head-tilt, chin-lift. (p. 172)

2-1.5 Relate mechanism of injury to opening the airway. (pp. 172–173)

2-1.6 Describe the steps in performing the jaw thrust. (pp. 172–174)

2-1.7 State the importance of having a suction unit ready for immediate use when providing emergency care. (pp. 176–178)

2-1.8 Describe the techniques of suctioning. (pp. 178–181)

2-1.9 Describe how to artificially ventilate a patient with a pocket mask. (pp. 190–191)

2-1.10 Describe the steps in performing the skill of artificially ventilating a patient with a bag-valve mask while using the jaw thrust. (pp. 193–194)

2-1.11 List the parts of a bag-valve mask system. (pp. 191–194)

2-1.12 Describe the steps in performing the skill of artificially ventilating a patient with a bag-valve mask for one and two rescuers. (pp. 191–194)

2-1.13 Describe the signs of adequate artificial ventilation using the bag-valve mask. (p. 197)

2-1.14 Describe the signs of inadequate artificial ventilation using the bag-valve mask. (p. 197)

2-1.15 Describe the steps in artificially ventilating a patient with a flow restricted, oxygen-powered ventilation device. (pp. 194–195)

2-1.16 List the steps in performing the actions taken when providing mouth-to-mouth and mouth-to-stoma artificial ventilation. (pp. 189–190)

2-1.17 Describe how to measure and insert an oropharyngeal (oral) airway. (pp. 181–183)

2-1.18 Describe how to measure and insert a nasopharyngeal (nasal) airway. (pp. 184–186)

2-1.19 Define the components of an oxygen delivery system. (pp. 200–208)

2-1.20 Identify a nonrebreather face mask and state the oxygen flow requirements needed for its use. (pp. 208–210)

2-1.21 Describe the indications for using a nasal cannula versus a nonrebreather face mask. (pp. 210–213)

2-1.22 Identify a nasal cannula and state the flow requirements needed for its use. (pp. 210–213)

AFFECTIVE OBJECTIVES

At the completion of this lesson, the EMT-Basic student will be able to:

2-1.23   Explain the rationale for basic life support artificial ventilation and airway protective skills taking priority over most other basic life support skills. (pp. 163, 168, 176)

2-1.24   Explain the rationale for providing adequate oxygenation through high inspired oxygen concentrations to patients who, in the past, may have received low concentrations. (pp. 190–191)

PSYCHOMOTOR OBJECTIVES

At the completion of this lesson, the EMT-Basic student will be able to:

2-1.25   Demonstrate the steps in performing the head-tilt, chin-lift. (pp. 172–173)

2-1.26   Demonstrate the steps in performing the jaw thrust. (pp. 173–174)

2-1.27   Demonstrate the techniques of suctioning. (pp. 176–181)

2-1.28   Demonstrate the steps in providing mouth-to-mouth artificial ventilation with body substance isolation (barrier shields). (pp. 190–191)

2-1.29   Demonstrate how to use a pocket mask to artificially ventilate a patient. (p. 191)

2-1.30   Demonstrate the assembly of a bag-valve mask unit. (pp. 191–192)

2-1.31   Demonstrate the steps in performing the skill of artificially ventilating a patient with a bag-valve mask for one and two rescuers. (pp. 192–193)

2-1.32   Demonstrate the steps in performing the skill of artificially ventilating a patient with a bag-valve mask while using the jaw thrust. (p. 194)

2-1.33   Demonstrate artificial ventilation of a patient with a flow restricted, oxygen-powered ventilation device. (pp. 194–196)

2-1.34   Demonstrate how to artificially ventilate a patient with a stoma. (p. 197)

2-1.35   Demonstrate how to insert an oropharyngeal (oral) airway. (pp. 181–183)

2-1.36   Demonstrate how to insert a nasopharyngeal (nasal) airway. (pp. 184–186)

2-1.37   Demonstrate the correct operation of oxygen tanks and regulators. (pp. 200–207)

2-1.38   Demonstrate the use of a nonrebreather face mask and state the oxygen flow requirements needed for its use. (pp. 201, 208–210)

2-1.39   Demonstrate the use of a nasal cannula and state the flow requirements needed for its use. (pp. 210–213)

2-1.40   Demonstrate how to artificially ventilate the infant and child patient. (pp. 195–196)

2-1.41   Demonstrate oxygen administration for the infant and child patient. (pp. 195–196)

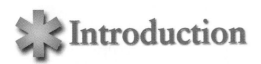 Introduction

Being successful in EMS means understanding priorities. So far you have learned that *your* safety and the safety of *other* EMS professionals at the scene of an emergency is *the* top priority. Now that you have learned how to identify and manage some of the more common hazards at the scene, we will begin discussing issues relating to patient care. We will begin with the single most important priority following personal safety, an open and clear airway for the patient.

Without a clear airway and adequate air exchange, life quickly comes to an end. We can do without many things for an extended amount of time, such as food, water, and shelter, but the human body cannot tolerate even short intervals without oxygen. In this chapter you will learn how to assess the status of a patient's airway as well as differentiate between adequate and inadequate respirations. You will also be introduced to many of the tools available to the EMT for helping maintain an open and clear airway and ensure adequate oxygen.

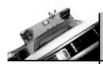

Emergency Dispatch

It is a warm afternoon in late summer and the crew of Unit 281 just lit the well-used barbecue at Post when emergency tones chime from the radio. "281, 2-8-1, start emergency for Baker Lake, on the east side by the boat ramps, for a 23-year-old female who is choking." Mackenzie, an EMT, quickly shuts off the barbecue's propane tank and starts the truck as her partner, Rob, tosses the uncooked chicken back into the refrigerator—for the third time today. A quick drive on Baker Parkway brings them to the park entrance by the boat ramp, where a man is waving at them and pointing toward a woman who is lying on the grass at the edge of the lake.

"We were eating lunch and talking and . . . and then she just started choking," the man gasps as the ambulance rolls to a stop. "I tried those . . . um . . . abdominal thrusts, you know, where you get behind her . . . It didn't seem to work and then she just passed out."

Rob and Mackenzie approach the woman, stepping over the scattered items of a picnic lunch, and find her cyanotic and unresponsive. Mackenzie turns to the man as she is opening the airway kit. "What's her name and how long has it been since she started choking?"

"It's been about . . . I don't know . . . maybe 3 or 4 minutes," he says. "And her name is Shannon."

"Okay, Shannon," Rob says as he performs a head-tilt, chin-lift on the woman. "Hang in there."

2-1.1 Name and label the major structures of the respiratory system on a diagram.

Before going any further with this chapter, it will be helpful to review the anatomy and physiology of the respiratory system found back in Chapter 4. You must be able to identify the following anatomical structures on an anatomical chart of the respiratory system (Figure 7-1A and B):

✳ Nose and mouth

✳ Pharynx

✳ Oropharynx

✳ Nasopharynx

✳ Epiglottis

✳ Trachea

✳ Cricoid cartilage

✳ Larynx

✳ Bronchi and bronchioles

✳ Lungs

✳ Diaphragm

It will also be helpful to review the physiology of the respiratory system including the process of respiration and how oxygen and carbon dioxide are exchanged at the alveoli and cellular levels. Also review the differences in anatomy between the adult and pediatric patient.

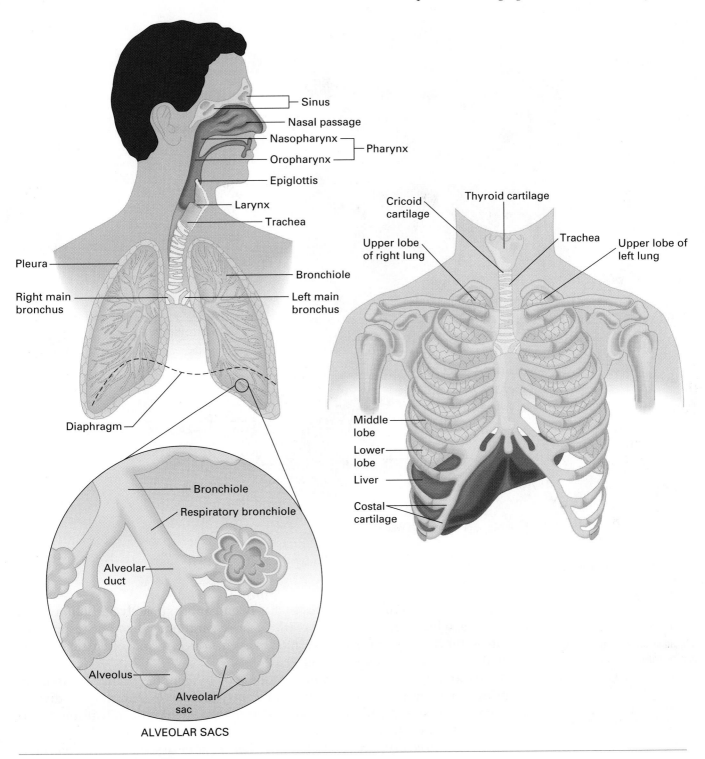

Sinus

Nasal passage

Nasopharynx ⎤
⎥ Pharynx
Oropharynx ⎦

Epiglottis

Larynx

Trachea

Pleura

Bronchiole

Right main bronchus

Left main bronchus

Diaphragm

Cricoid cartilage

Thyroid cartilage

Upper lobe of right lung

Trachea

Upper lobe of left lung

Middle lobe

Lower lobe

Liver

Costal cartilage

Bronchiole

Respiratory bronchiole

Alveolar duct

Alveolus

Alveolar sac

ALVEOLAR SACS

FIGURE 7-1A   The respiratory system.

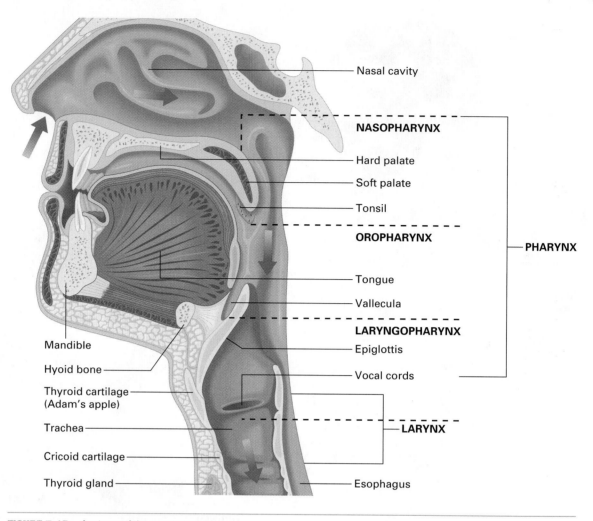

Nasal cavity

NASOPHARYNX

Hard palate

Soft palate

Tonsil

OROPHARYNX

PHARYNX

Tongue

Vallecula

LARYNGOPHARYNX

Mandible

Epiglottis

Hyoid bone

Vocal cords

Thyroid cartilage
(Adam's apple)

Trachea

LARYNX

Cricoid cartilage

Thyroid gland

Esophagus

FIGURE 7-1B Anatomy of the upper airway.

2-1.2 List the signs of adequate breathing.

✳ **respiration**

inhalation and exhalation. May also be called *ventilation.*

When Breathing Is Adequate

It happens nearly 20 thousand times each day and approximately 58 billion times in an average lifetime. It is called breathing or **respiration.** When our respiratory system is functioning normally we hardly even notice it and often take it for granted until something goes wrong.

When we are receiving an adequate supply of oxygen, the primary muscle responsible for respiration is the diaphragm. It is a flat muscle that acts as a divider between the chest and abdominal cavities. It moves up and down, causing air to move in and out of the lungs.

There are three primary characteristics that must be assessed when determining adequacy of breathing. They are:

✳ **Rate**—Rate refers to how many times the patient is breathing per minute and is recorded as a number. Each *inspiration + expiration = 1 respiration.* Respiratory rates can be obtained by counting the number of breaths in one minute. Normal rates for adult, child, and infants are as follows:
  • Adult: 12–20/minute
  • Child: 15–30/minute
  • Infant: 25–50/minute
Depending on the standard practice in your area, there are at least two common methods for counting respirations. One requires counting the respira-

tions for 30 seconds and multiplying by 2 and the second requires counting for 15 seconds and multiplying by 4. You must understand that the shorter your sample the less accurate the total rate. For patients with an irregular breathing pattern, it may be best to count for a full minute to get the most accurate rate.

* **Depth**—The depth of respirations is sometimes referred to as **tidal volume** and is an assessment of the amount of air the patient is moving in and out with each breath. When a patient is breathing adequately, the tidal volume is approximately 400 to 600 ml of air and can be seen as moderate chest or abdominal rise and fall. Depth is commonly recorded as deep, shallow, or normal, depending on how the patient is breathing. In some areas the term "good tidal volume" is used to describe depth that is normal. A low or inadequate tidal volume may result in an inadequate supply of oxygen and/or the build up of dangerous levels of carbon dioxide (CO_2).

* **Ease**—Ease refers to a patient's work of breathing. Normal respirations require little to no effort on the part of the patient. Ease can be recorded as unlabored or labored depending on the situation.

    In addition to rate, depth, and ease, other characteristics that should be assessed with all patients are rhythm and sound. Normal respirations should be steady and regular, much like waves gently crashing on the beach. Irregular respirations are not normal and can be caused by both illness and injury.

    Breath sounds should be assessed on all patients as well. The EMT should use a stethoscope to listen to both lungs in several places. Normal lung sounds are described as equal and clear bilaterally (on both sides). More about assessing lung sounds will be discussed in Chapter 19.

margin note:
* **tidal volume**
the depth of respirations.

When Breathing Is Inadequate

margin note:
2-1.3 List the signs of inadequate breathing.

Inadequate breathing is often the result of inadequate gas exchange (oxygen for carbon dioxide) and can result in the development of at least two problems for the patient, an inadequate supply of oxygen and an excessive buildup of carbon dioxide (CO_2). Regardless of the cause, some of the first responses the body makes to inadequate gas exchange are changes in the way that we breathe and a change in mental status. Signs of inadequate gas exchange can appear anywhere on a sliding scale from very mild, to moderate, to severe. In some instances, the buildup of CO_2 can occur even with an adequate supply of oxygen.

    Signs of inadequate breathing are not always immediately obvious. They can be very subtle, perhaps only mild shortness of breath. In these instances, the only way you would know is by asking the patient, "Do you feel short of breath?" Sometimes if the patient has been short of breath for awhile, he may also appear pale. It is good practice to ask any patient who appears pale if he is having any trouble breathing or if he feels short of breath.

RESPIRATORY DISTRESS

Often the first sign that the patient is not receiving an adequate supply of oxygen is an increased respiratory rate. This is the body's way of saying, "If I can't get enough oxygen at the normal rate, I had better increase the rate to try and make up the difference." If the body is unable to compensate simply by increasing the rate, other mechanisms begin to kick in, making the respiratory distress more obvious (Table 7-1 on page 168).

TABLE 7-1	SIGNS OF AN INADEQUATE GAS EXCHANGE (RESPIRATORY DISTRESS)

∗ Increased respiratory rate (early sign)

∗ Increased work of breathing (labored)

∗ Decreased tidal volume

∗ Increased use of accessory muscles (neck, chest, and abdominal)

∗ Nasal flaring (most common in pediatric patients)

∗ Retractions (above the clavicles, between the ribs, below the ribs) Mostly seen in pediatric patients

∗ Pale skin that may be moist

∗ Decreasing mental status

∗ **respiratory distress**
the body's attempts to compensate for an inadequate supply of oxygen.

Respiratory distress is the body's way of attempting to compensate for an inadequate supply of oxygen (Figure 7-2A and B). In most cases the body does a good job of compensating and, with the assistance of the EMT, some oxygen, and appropriate medications, the patient's respiratory status may return to normal.

RESPIRATORY FAILURE

∗ **respiratory failure**
the reduction of breathing to the point where oxygen intake is not sufficient to support life.

When the body's normal compensatory mechanisms are not able to provide for adequate gas exchange, the patient is in danger of progressing from respiratory distress to **respiratory failure** (Figure 7-3). Respiratory failure occurs when the brain and vital organs have gone too long without an adequate supply of oxygen and can no longer compensate. Some of the first signs of respiratory failure are a decreased mental status and a decreased respiratory rate (Table 7-2).

Respiratory failure is an extreme emergency, and the EMT must begin providing assisted ventilations as soon as possible (Figure 7-4 on page 170). This will be discussed in more detail later in this chapter.

TABLE 7-2	SIGNS OF RESPIRATORY FAILURE

∗ Decreased mental status

∗ Decreased respiratory rate (below normal)

∗ Change in breathing rhythm (irregular)

∗ Breath sounds that become diminished (less obvious)

∗ Decreased chest rise and fall (poor tidal volume)

∗ Skin that may be pale or cyanotic (blue) and cool and clammy

∗ In infants, possible "seesaw" breathing where the abdomen and chest move in opposite directions

∗ Agonal respirations (occasional gasping breaths) that may be seen just before death

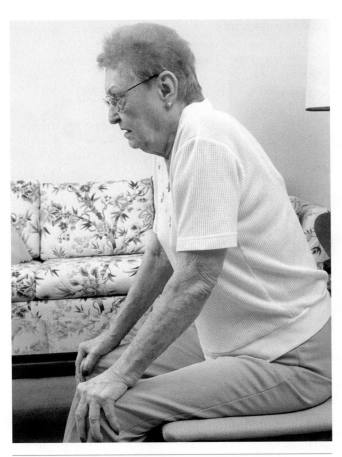

FIGURE 7-2A   Patient displaying signs of respiratory distress.

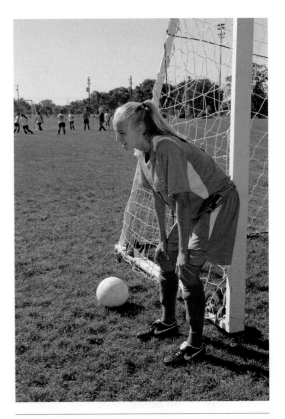

FIGURE 7-2B   A patient in respiratory distress may assume the tripod position.

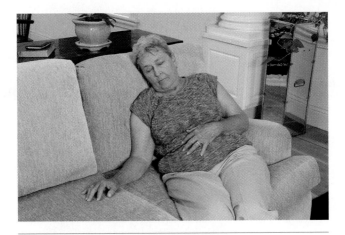

FIGURE 7-3   An unresponsive patient in respiratory failure.

PEDIATRIC DIFFERENCES

As discussed in Chapter 4, there are several differences in anatomy between adult and pediatric patients. Some of these differences may change the way that you care for the patient.

In general, all of the structures of the pediatric respiratory system are smaller and therefore more easily blocked by swelling or foreign material. The tongue

| **PATIENT'S CONDITION** | **WHEN AND HOW TO INTERVENE** |

Adequate breathing:
Speaks full sentences;
alert and calm

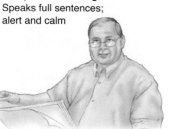

Nonrebreather mask or nasal cannula

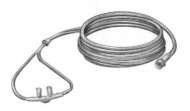

Increasing respiratory distress:
Visibly short of breath;
Speaking 3–4 word sentences;
Increasing anxiety

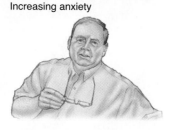

Nonrebreather mask

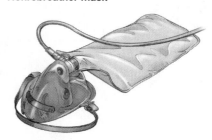

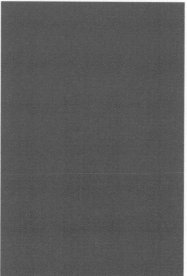

Key decision-making point:

Recognize inadequate breathing before respiratory arrest develops.

Assist ventilations before they stop altogether!

Severe respiratory distress:
Speaking only 1–2 word sentences;
Very diaphoretic (sweaty);
Severe anxiety

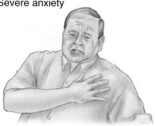

Assisted ventilations
Pocket face mask (PFM),
bag-valve mask (BVM), or
flow-restricted, oxygen-powered
ventilation device (FROPVD)

Assist the patient's own
ventilations, adjusting the
rate for rapid or slow
breathing

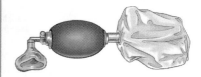

Continues to deteriorate:
Sleepy with head-bobbing;
Becomes unarousable

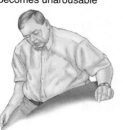

Respiratory arrest:
No breathing

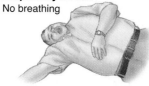

Artificial ventilation
Pocket face mask (PFM),
bag-valve mask (BVM), or
flow-restricted, oxygen-powered
ventilation device (FROPV)

Assisted ventilations at
12/minute for an adult or
20/minute for a child or infant

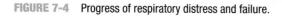

FIGURE 7-4 Progress of respiratory distress and failure.

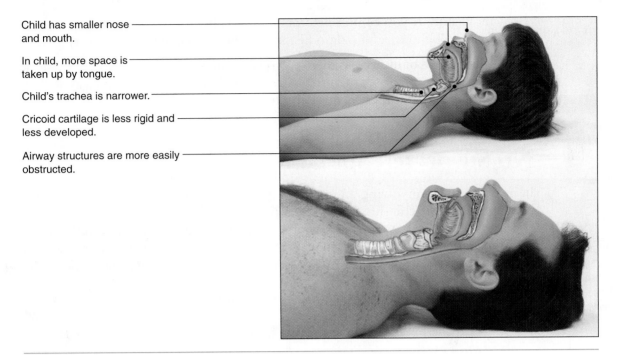

Child has smaller nose and mouth.

In child, more space is taken up by tongue.

Child's trachea is narrower.

Cricoid cartilage is less rigid and less developed.

Airway structures are more easily obstructed.

FIGURE 7-5 Adult and pediatric airways.

takes up proportionately more volume inside the mouth, making it more difficult to visualize the back of the throat. The larynx and trachea are much softer and more susceptible to damage. Being soft, the trachea is also susceptible to collapse if the patient's head is tilted too far back during airway management. While this is not damaging to the child, it will cause a partial airway blockage that will make it more difficult to ventilate the patient. Pediatric patients, especially infants, are abdominal breathers, which means that the abdomen moves more than the chest as they breathe (Figure 7-5).

MANAGING THE AIRWAY

Determining whether or not a patient has a **patent** (open and clear) airway is an essential skill that all successful EMTs must master. In addition, you will need to determine whether a spinal injury is suspected. Your management of that situation is critical and will be among your highest priorities for each patient.

ASSESSING AND OPENING THE AIRWAY

In responsive patients, assessing the airway is achieved quite easily by simply observing the patient and listening to him speak. If he is alert and is able to speak in complete sentences, it can be assumed that he has an open and clear airway. What you must assess at that point is if he is breathing adequately or not.

In the unresponsive patient, determining whether the airway is patent is much more difficult and requires that specific procedures be performed by the EMT, depending on the condition and position of the patient. Factors that must be considered while managing the airway of an unresponsive patient are:

* **Patient position**—If the patient is found face down or on his side and appears to be breathing adequately, there may not be an immediate need to

* **patent**
  in reference to the airway (passage from nose or mouth to lungs), open and clear, without interference to the passage of air into and out of the body.

move him. If you cannot determine if he is breathing adequately, then you must roll him carefully onto his back to begin managing the airway.

* **Mechanism of injury**—Is there reason to believe the patient may have a neck or back injury? If so, the procedure you will use to open the airway will be different than if there is no suspected spinal injury.

No Suspected Spinal Injury

2-1.4 Describe the steps in performing the head-tilt, chin-lift.

* **head-tilt, chin-lift maneuver**

  a means of opening the airway by tilting the head back and lifting the chin. Used when no trauma, or injury, is suspected. See also jaw-thrust maneuver.

In most instances involving an unresponsive patient with no suspected spinal injury, the **head-tilt, chin-lift maneuver** is the most effective means of opening the airway. The tongue is the most common cause of airway obstruction in the unresponsive patient. Because the tongue is attached to the lower jaw, tilting the head back and moving the jaw upward also lifts the tongue, clearing the back of the throat.

To perform the head-tilt, chin-lift (Figure 7-6A–C), follow these steps:

1. With the patient lying supine on a firm flat surface, kneel beside the patient's head.

2. Place the palm of one hand on the patient's forehead and the index and middle fingers of the other hand on the bony part of the jaw just below the chin.

3. Using equal pressure with both hands, tilt the patient's head back as far as it will comfortably go.

4. Once the head is tilted back release pressure on the chin to allow the mouth to open slightly.

5. Place your ear next to the patient's nose and mouth to listen for breathing and observe the chest for adequate rise and fall.

Suspected Spinal Injury

2-1.5 Relate mechanism of injury to opening the airway.

Any patient with an unknown mechanism of injury, or who you believe may have suffered a spinal injury, must be cared for using a slightly different procedure.

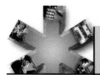

Perspective

Rob—The EMT

"I knew when I heard what happened—that this young lady's boyfriend had tried to perform the Heimlich maneuver on her before she had passed out—that she probably wasn't going to have a head or spine injury. It's not like he's just going to drop his girlfriend to the ground when she becomes unresponsive! So I felt the most effective technique for initially trying to open and look into her airway was the head-tilt, chin-lift. Plus, I knew that we had to get that airway open quick."

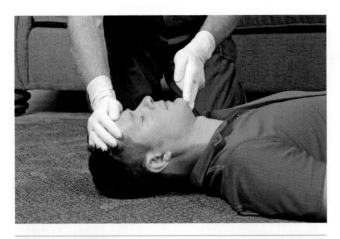

FIGURE 7-6A Place the palm of one hand on the patient's forehead and the index and middle fingers of the other hand on the bony part of the jaw just below the chin.

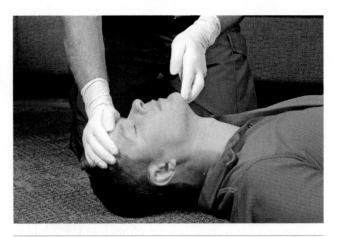

FIGURE 7-6B Using equal pressure with both hands, tilt the patient's head back as far as it will comfortably go.

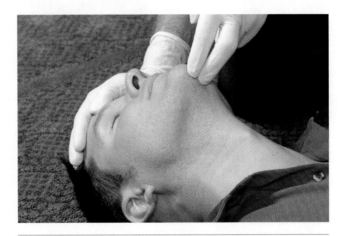

FIGURE 7-6C Correct position for the head-tilt, chin-lift.

Make no mistake; the airway is the top priority with all patients. However, when caring for a patient with suspected spinal injury, we must make every attempt to open the airway without compromising the neck or back. To do this you will use the **jaw-thrust maneuver** (Figure 7-7 on page 174).

To perform the jaw-thrust maneuver, follow these steps:

1. With the patient lying supine on a firm flat surface, kneel at the top of the patient's head.

2. Place your thumbs on the cheekbones on either side of the patients, face.

3. Using the index and middle fingers of each hand at the angles of the patient's jaw, push the jaw upward.

4. Place your ear next to the patient's nose and mouth to listen for breathing and observe the chest for adequate rise and fall.

This procedure is best when at least two rescuers are present. If the patient is not breathing adequately, the first rescuer can maintain an open airway while the second rescuer ventilates the patient. For the single rescuer, a modified jaw-thrust can be performed from the side as well so the rescuer can also ventilate the patient.

2-1.6 Describe the steps in performing the jaw thrust.

* **jaw-thrust maneuver**

a means of correcting blockage of the airway by moving the jaw forward without tilting the head or neck. Used when trauma, or injury, is suspected. See also head-tilt, chin-lift maneuver.

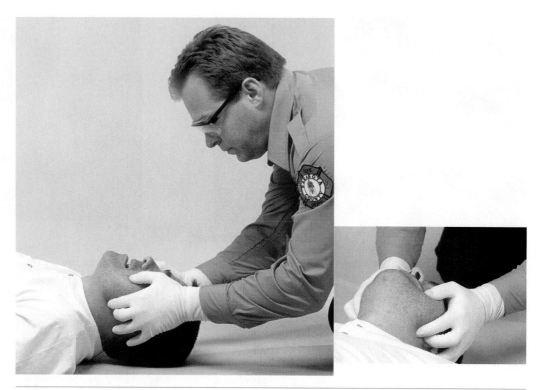

FIGURE 7-7   Jaw-thrust maneuver, side view. Inset shows EMT's finger position at angle of the jaw just below the ears.

COMPLICATIONS

Several factors can make it difficult to establish a patent airway. Trauma to the face will often cause swelling and bleeding that will make it difficult to keep the airway clear. Foreign body airway obstructions (FBAO), such as those caused by food or small objects, are difficult to see and can cause both partial and complete obstructions. The procedure for clearing an FBAO is discussed in detail in Chapter 19. Dental appliances such as crowns, bridges, and dentures can come loose inside the mouth, contributing to the obstruction. Unless they are loose and falling back into the throat, leave these appliances in place. Otherwise remove them with a gloved hand and keep them in a safe place.

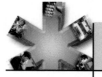

Perspective

The Boyfriend

"That was the scariest thing that I've ever been through! One minute we're having this great picnic by the lake, and the next, Shannon is looking at me with this panic in her eyes and she's grabbing at her throat. Do you know what that's like? I mean, here's this person who you love more than anything in the world and you're looking into her eyes and all you see is fear, just absolute terror. I can't even imagine what it's like to not be able to breathe. I'm so thankful for that ambulance crew. I don't know what I would've done had they not been there."

✳ Stop, Review, Remember!

Multiple Choice

Place a check next to the correct answer.

1. All of the following are signs of inadequate breathing EXCEPT:

   _____ a. use of accessory muscles.

   _____ b. increased respiratory rate.

   _____ c. use of the tripod position.

   _____ d. good chest rise and fall.

2. Adequate respirations are characterized by:

   _____ a. effortless breathing.

   _____ b. poor chest rise.

   _____ c. nasal flaring.

   _____ d. retractions.

3. Which of the following best describes how you should handle a patient you are ventilating who has loose dentures?

   _____ a. Carefully push the dentures back into place.

   _____ b. Remove them with a gloved hand.

   _____ c. Ask a family member to remove them.

   _____ d. Ignore them and keep ventilating.

4. For which of the following patients would the jaw-thrust be most appropriate for opening the airway?

   _____ a. unresponsive 5-year-old from a bicycle accident

   _____ b. 56-year-old with chest pain

   _____ c. unresponsive 27-year-old bee-sting patient

   _____ d. semiresponsive diabetic patient

5. _____ is the most common cause of airway obstruction in the unresponsive patient.

   _____ a. Blood

   _____ b. A foreign body

   _____ c. The tongue

   _____ d. Saliva

Critical Thinking

1. Describe what you would look for when determining if a patient is breathing adequately or not.

   _____

   _____

2. Discuss the difference between respiratory distress and respiratory failure and how each might present.

   _____

   _____

3. Describe how you would manage the airway of a trauma patient whose airway could not be adequately opened using the jaw-thrust maneuver.

   _____

   _____

4. Place an "X" in the appropriate column or columns for each of the signs.

Sign	Distress	Failure
Increased respiratory rate		
Decreased respiratory rate		
Altered mental status		
Use of accessory muscles		
Tripod position		
Nasal flaring		
Decreased heart rate		
Increased heart rate		

2-1.7 State the importance of having a suction unit ready for immediate use when providing emergency care.

The Basics of Suctioning

It is important to take the appropriate BSI precautions whenever you are managing a patient's airway because of the strong likelihood that he may vomit or that you may be exposed to body fluids. Gloves, a mask, and eye protection are the minimum recommended PPE for airway management.

Suction is an important skill that every EMT must learn and practice. The EMT uses suction to assist in maintaining a patent airway that is at risk of becoming blocked by materials such as blood, vomit, and saliva. Noisy respirations are almost always a sign of partial airway obstruction. Gurgling is a strong indication of partial upper airway obstruction caused by fluids. During manual ventilations some of the air enters the stomach and may eventually cause the patient to vomit. You will use suction to minimize the chances that the vomit could enter the lungs. You must have suction ready at all times when caring for unresponsive patients or when manually ventilating a patient.

Most suction units used in the field are adequate for suctioning fluids and small particles of food but are inadequate at picking up or clearing large objects such as chunks of food or teeth. For these objects, a combination of suctioning and finger sweeps may be necessary.

SUCTION DEVICES

Suction devices are quite simple. They consist of a pump, suction tubing, a catheter, and a reservoir to contain the material being suctioned. While there are many brands and styles of suction devices in use today, most field suction units can be divided into three categories: electric, oxygen-powered, and manually operated. (Figure 7-8A–D).

＊ **Electric**—These devices are found permanently mounted in the ambulance for use during transport or can be a battery-powered portable type used on the scene.

＊ **Oxygen-powered**—These typically portable devices function as an accessory to an oxygen regulator. They require an adequate supply of high pressure oxygen to function.

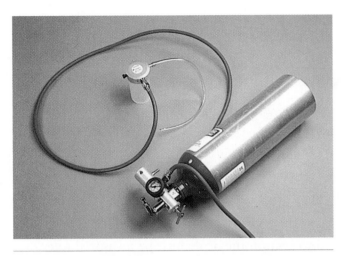

FIGURE 7-8A   An oxygen-powered portable suction unit.

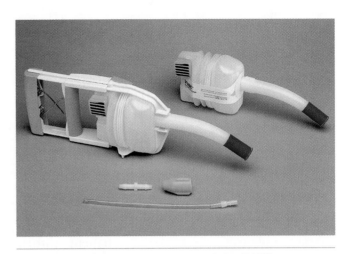

FIGURE 7-8B   Manually operated suction device (V-VAC).

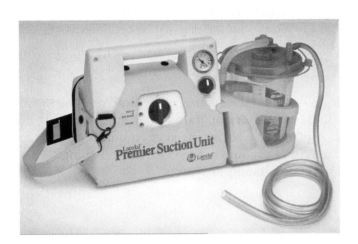

FIGURE 7-8C   A battery-powered portable suctioning unit.

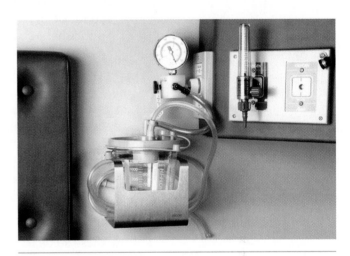

FIGURE 7-8D   A mounted suction unit installed in the ambulance patient compartment.

✳ **Manually Operated**—These devices are generally the most portable and easy-to-use devices. Most are operated by squeezing a handle on the device.

SUCTION CATHETERS

The catheter is the part of the suction unit that is placed into the patient's mouth or nose to assist in removing the material from the airway. Catheters come in a wide variety of styles; however they all fit into one of two basic categories, rigid (hard) or soft (Figure 7-9 on page 178).

✳ **Rigid**—Sometimes called hard or tonsil-tip suction catheters, these catheters are made of nonflexible plastic and can be straight or slightly curved. They are designed primarily for suctioning the mouth (oropharynx) of a semiresponsive or unresponsive patient. In general, catheters used for suctioning the mouth should not be inserted any farther than you can see. It is important when using rigid catheters to avoid touching the center of the back of the throat, as this may stimulate a gag reflex and cause vomiting.

✳ **Soft**—Sometimes referred to as "French" catheters, soft catheters are generally long narrow tubes made of flexible plastic. They are most useful for suctioning through the nose (nasopharynx) of a semiresponsive or unresponsive

FIGURE 7-9 Various types and sizes of suction catheters.

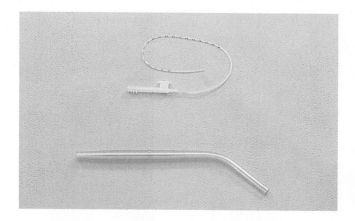

patient. Soft catheters used to suction the nose must be measured to ensure they are not placed too far into the airway. Measure these devices from the tip of the patient's nose to the earlobe prior to insertion. The suction device should be activated only after the catheter is fully inserted into the airway. Soft catheters are also ideal for suctioning the mouths of pediatric patients.

2-1.8 Describe the techniques of suctioning.

Suctioning Techniques

Like all other equipment on an ambulance, the suction unit should be inspected on a daily basis. Because many units are battery operated, they must regularly be charged or the battery replaced. A properly functioning suction unit is capable of developing approximately 300 mmHg of vacuum power. Use the following guidelines when using suction to help clear a patient's airway.

ORAL SUCTIONING

Follow these steps to perform oral suctioning (Scan 7-1):

1. Take appropriate BSI precautions.
2. Attach the appropriate suction catheter to the suction tubing and confirm that the suction tubing is securely attached to the device.
3. Place the tip of the catheter into the mouth as far to one side as possible and only as far as you can see.
4. Activate the suction as you move the tip of the catheter around in small circles on one side of the tongue.
5. Remove the tip and insert it in the same manner on the other side of the patient's mouth. Repeat the procedure.
6. For adult patients suction no more than 15 seconds at a time, child patients 10 seconds, and infants 5 seconds.

NASAL SUCTIONING

Follow these steps to perform nasal suctioning (Scan 7-2 on page 180):

1. Take appropriate BSI precautions.
2. Attach the appropriate suction catheter to the suction tubing and confirm that the suction tubing is securely attached to the device.
3. Measure the device from the tip of the patient's nose to the earlobe.

✳ ✳ ✳ ✳ ✳ ✳ ✳ ✳ ✳ ✳ ✳ ✳ ✳ ✳ ✳ ✳ ✳ ✳ ✳ ✳

SCAN 7-1 | **ORAL SUCTIONING**

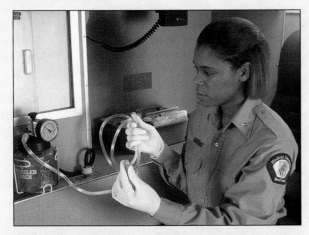

▲ Turn the unit on, attach a catheter, and test for suction at the beginning of your shift.

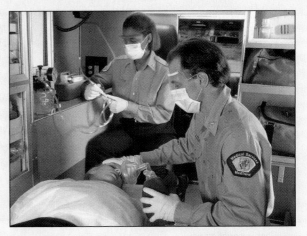

▲ Position yourself at the patient's head and turn the patient's head to the side.

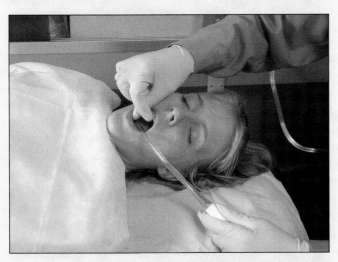

▲ Apply suction only after the rigid tip is in place. Do not lose sight of the tip while suctioning. Suction while withdrawing the tip.

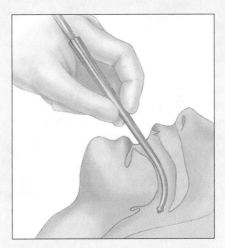

▲ Place the convex side of the rigid tip against the roof of the mouth. Insert just to the base of the tongue.

4. Lubricate the catheter using a water based lubricant.

5. Carefully insert the catheter into one nostril.

6. Once completely inserted, activate the suction and twist the catheter and slowly remove it.

7. Repeat the procedure for the other nostril.

8. For adult patients suction no more than 15 seconds at a time, child patients 10 seconds, and infants 5 seconds.

SCAN 7-2 **NASAL SUCTIONING**

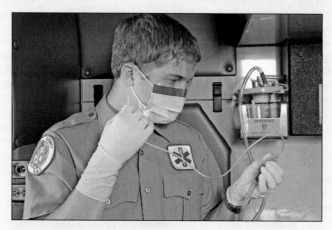

▲ Test the suction unit.

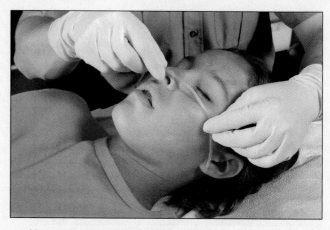

▲ Measure the device against the nose.

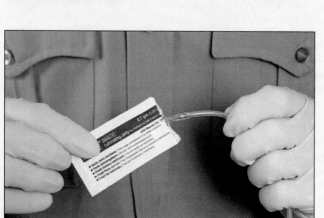

▲ Lubricate the tip.

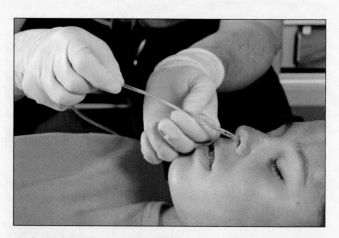

▲ Insert the catheter into the nose.

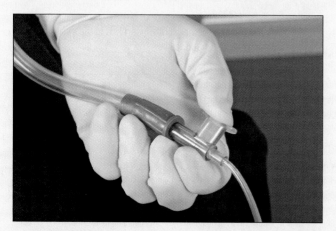

▲ Activate the suction device.

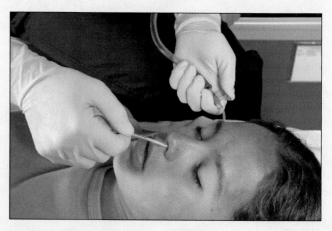

▲ Remove suctioning.

Many suction devices have an adjustment that controls the amount of suction being applied. Consider using lower power settings for pediatric patients. When suctioning newborns and infants, it is best to use a bulb-type suction device.

If your patient is producing secretions as fast as you can suction them, suction as best you can for 15 seconds, then ventilate the patient for 2 minutes, followed by another 15 seconds of suctioning. Repeat this process as necessary during transport.

Suction catheters, tubing, and most reservoirs are disposable and should be handed off to the hospital personnel taking over care of the patient. Otherwise they should be disposed of properly.

THE USE OF AIRWAY ADJUNCTS

EMTs have two mechanical devices (airway adjuncts) they can use to assist in maintaining a patent airway. They are the **oropharyngeal airway,** sometimes referred to as the "oral" airway or OPA, and the **nasopharyngeal airway,** commonly referred to as the "nasal" airway or NPA. It must be clearly understood that both of these devices only *assist* the EMT in maintaining a patent airway. Simply placing either device does not ensure a patent airway. These devices should be used in conjunction with good airway management techniques, such as continuous monitoring for adequate chest rise and fall, head-tilt, chin-lift and jaw-thrust maneuvers, and appropriate suctioning when indicated.

✱ **oropharyngeal airway**
a curved device inserted into the patient's mouth and the pharynx to help maintain an open airway.

✱ **nasopharyngeal airway**
a soft flexible breathing tube inserted through the patient's nose into the pharynx to help maintain an open airway.

2-1.17 Describe how to measure and insert an oropharyngeal (oral) airway.

The Oropharyngeal Airway (OPA)

OPAs are generally made of hard plastic and are designed to minimize the chances that the airway will become blocked by the tongue. They are only used on unresponsive patients who do not have an active gag reflex. Sometimes the only way to determine if an unresponsive patient does not have a gag reflex is to attempt the insertion of an OPA. If the patient begins to gag, you must remove it immediately.

Indications for the use of an OPA:

✱ Unresponsive

✱ No gag reflex

Follow these steps for the proper use of an OPA (Scan 7-3 on pages 182–183):

1. Take appropriate BSI precautions.

2. Manually open the airway using the appropriate method.

3. Select the appropriate size airway by measuring from the corner of the patient's mouth to the earlobe or angle of the jaw.

4. Open the patient's mouth and insert the airway upside down (with the tip facing the roof of the mouth) until it is approximately half way in, then rotate it 180 degrees as you insert it the rest of the way.

5. Allow the flange of the airway to come to rest against the outside of the patient's lips. It is okay to allow the flange to rest no further than the patient's teeth; however if you cannot see the airway, it may have dropped into the mouth and become an obstruction.

SCAN 7-3 INSERTION OF OROPHARYNGEAL AIRWAY

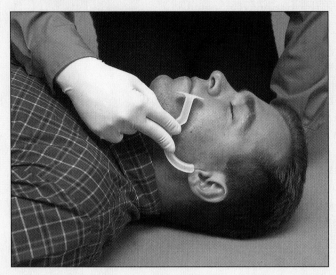

▲ Measure from the corner of the patient's mouth to the tip of the earlobe.

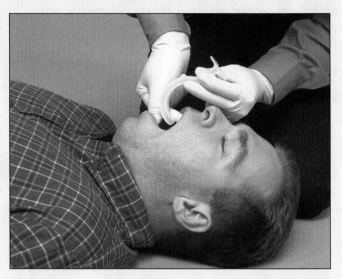

▲ Insert the airway with the tip pointing to the roof of the patient's mouth.

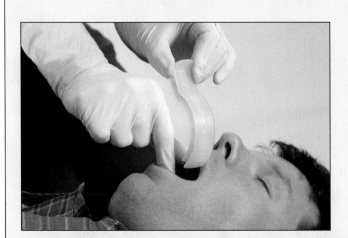

▲ An alternative method is to insert the airway sideways and then rotate it 90°.

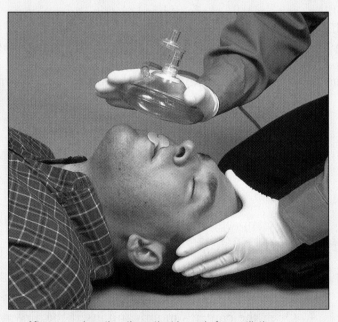

▲ After proper insertion, the patient is ready for ventilation.

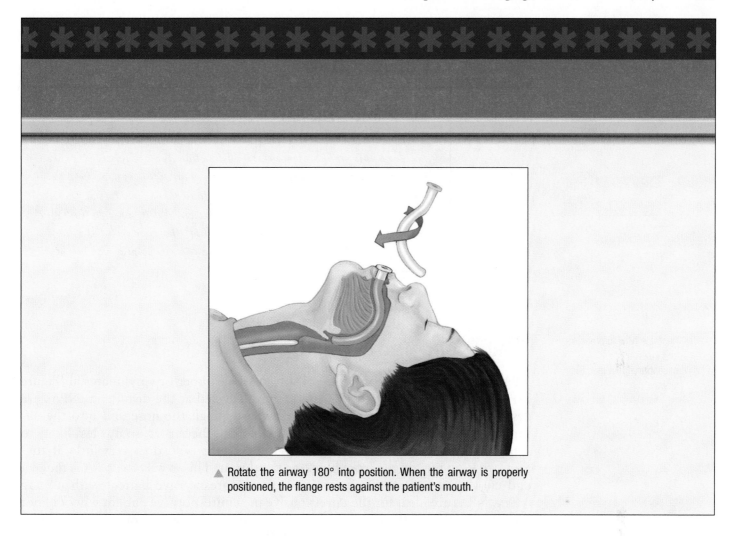

▲ Rotate the airway 180° into position. When the airway is properly positioned, the flange rests against the patient's mouth.

Alternative methods for insertion of an OPA include inserting the airway sideways and rotating it 90 degrees. This is just as effective as long as you ensure that the OPA is resting behind the tongue and not against it, pushing it further back into the airway. The preferred method for inserting an OPA for an infant or small child is to use a tongue blade to press down on the tongue and then insert the OPA right side up directly over the tongue without rotating it (Figure 7-10). Proper insertion of an OPA in an adult is illustrated in Figure 7-11.

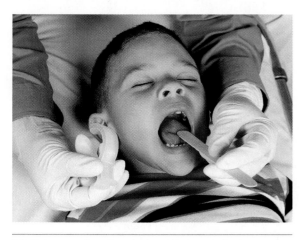

FIGURE 7-10   Insertion of an oropharyngeal airway into a child, using a tongue depressor.

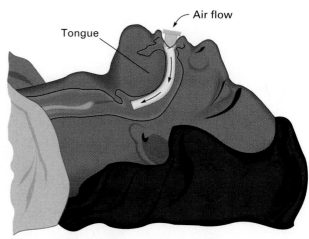

FIGURE 7-11   Oropharyngeal airway that is properly placed. The tongue is kept from falling back to occlude the airway.

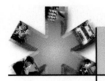

Perspective

Mackenzie—The EMT

"I was actually kind of scared on that call. I had never responded to someone who still had the airway obstruction in place when we arrived. I was ticking through this checklist in my head of things to do for a non-breathing patient, from which adjuncts to use and how to size them to how fast I should squeeze the bag on the BVM if it came to that. And do you know what I kept forgetting? That this poor girl didn't have a patent airway! Luckily Rob remembered the ABCs and went right for the airway."

2-1.18 Describe how to measure and insert a nasopharyngeal (nasal) airway.

The Nasopharyngeal Airway (NPA)

NPAs are short round tubes made of soft flexible rubber or vinyl material (Figure 7-12). They have a flange at the top and are beveled at the distal end. NPAs are designed to help maintain an open pathway through the nose and into the nasopharynx. The NPA should not touch the back of the throat, so it is less likely to stimulate the gag reflex than the OPA. However, the NPA does very little, if anything, to keep the tongue from blocking the throat. This is why the NPA is the second choice between the two airways for an unresponsive patient with no gag reflex. NPAs are ideal for the unresponsive or semiresponsive patient who will not tolerate an OPA or the patient with major trauma to the jaw, or the patient who is convulsing, preventing the use of an OPA.

Follow these steps for the proper use of an NPA (Scan 7-4):

1. Take appropriate BSI precautions.

2. Manually open the airway using the appropriate method.

3. Select the appropriate size airway by first observing the opening of the nostril. Select an airway with a diameter slightly smaller than the opening of the patient's nostril. (*continued on p. 186*)

FIGURE 7-12 Various types of nasopharyngeal airways (NPA).

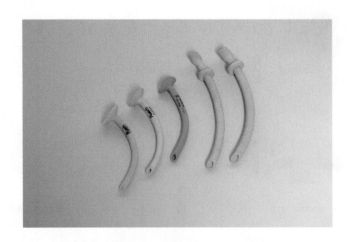

INSERTION OF NASOPHARYNGEAL AIRWAY

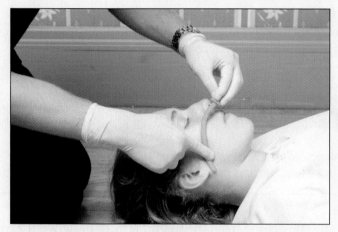

▲ Measure the nasopharyngeal airway from the patient's nostril to the earlobe, or to the angle of the jaw.

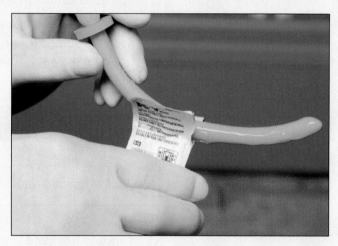

▲ Apply a water-based lubricant before insertion.

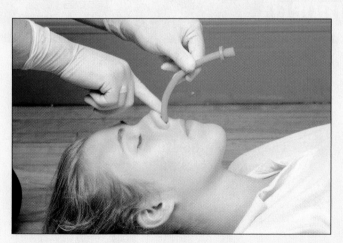

▲ Gently push the tip of the nose upward, and insert the airway with the beveled side toward the base of the nostril or toward the septum (wall that separates the nostrils). Insert the airway, advancing it until the flange rests against the nostril.

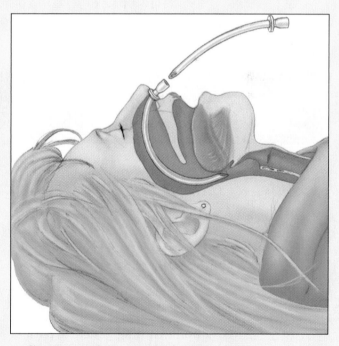

▲ Nasopharnygeal airway properly inserted.

4. Next measure from the tip of the nose to the patient's earlobe. Adjust the flange or cut the airway to the appropriate length.

5. Lubricate the airway using a water-based lubricant.

6. Press gently on the tip of the nose to flare the nostrils, then insert the NPA posteriorly. Make certain that the opening of the bevel is facing inward (toward the septum).

7. Advance the airway until the flange comes to rest against the outside of the nostril.

8. If resistance is felt, try twisting the NPA slightly. If this does not work then remove it and attempt the same procedure on the opposite side.

Clinical Clues: PATIENTS WITH FACIAL TRAUMA

Insertion of an NPA is contraindicated in patients with significant facial trauma. Fractures to the face and skull could allow the airway to pass into a sinus cavity or into the cranium.

It should be noted that all NPAs come from the manufacturer designed for use in the right nostril. This is due to the curvature and the placement of the beveled opening. If the NPA will not easily slide into the right side then you will have to use a pair of scissors to snip the end and change the direction of the beveled opening. This is simple and does not significantly change the length of the NPA.

✳ Stop, Review, Remember!

Multiple Choice

Place a check next to the correct answer.

1. Which of the following patients is most in need of immediate suctioning?

_____ a. an asthma patient with expiratory wheezes

_____ b. a nonbreathing pediatric patient

_____ c. a patient with gurgling sounds while breathing

_____ d. a patient experiencing a severe allergic reaction

2. The most portable and easiest to use of the suction devices is the _____ device.

_____ a. manual

_____ b. battery-operated

_____ c. oxygen-powered

_____ d. ambulance-mounted

3. Which of the following are the indications for inserting an OPA?

_____ a. responsive, active gag reflex

_____ b. unresponsive, no gag reflex

_____ c. responsive, no gag reflex

_____ d. unresponsive, active gag reflex

4. Prior to insertion, an NPA should be measured from the _____ to the _____.

_____ a. middle of the mouth, earlobe

_____ b. angle of the jaw, corner of the mouth

_____ c. tip of the nose, corner of the mouth

_____ d. tip of the nose, earlobe

5. The recommended maximum time allowed for suctioning of an adult patient is _____ seconds.

_____ a. 5

_____ b. 10

_____ c. 15

_____ d. 20

Matching

Match the piece of equipment on the left with the applicable definition on the right.

1. _____ Oxygen-powered suction device

2. _____ Soft suction catheter

3. _____ Bulb syringe

4. _____ OPA

5. _____ NPA

A. This device requires that the patient be unresponsive and have no gag reflex.

B. This is best suited for suctioning an infant's nose and/or mouth.

C. The primary contraindication for this device is face or head trauma.

D. This is most useful for suctioning through the nose of a semiresponsive or unresponsive patient

E. This is typically a portable device that functions as an accessory to an oxygen regulator. It requires an adequate supply of high-pressure oxygen to function.

Critical Thinking

1. Discuss why it is good practice to have a suction device handy whenever you are performing manual ventilations.

_____

_____

_____

2. Discuss why airway adjuncts such as the OPA and NPA cannot be relied upon to maintain a patient's airway by themselves.

_____

_____

_____

3. What are the contraindications for using an NPA and why?

_____

_____

_____

_____

Ventilating Your Patient

Now that you have learned how to assess, establish, and maintain an open and clear airway for your patient, it's time to learn what to do if your patient is not breathing adequately or not breathing at all. Assessing whether an airway is patent is only half of the airway management equation. The other half is assessing the adequacy of the patient's own ventilations and providing the necessary support when needed.

An adult patient who is breathing adequately will have a respiratory rate of between 12 and 20 per minute and show good tidal volume with each breath. This section will focus on the patient who is not breathing adequately (less than 12 times per minute in the case of an adult or too shallowly) and may be in need of ventilatory assistance.

The first thing you will want to assess as you approach a patient is the rise and fall of the chest or abdomen during breathing (Figure 7-13). Is it obvious that he is breathing or is it difficult to tell? If breathing is obvious, then you can assume that tidal volume is adequate and you can move on to assess the adequacy of the rate. If the rate is between 12 and 20 per minute, then the patient is breathing adequately and does not need assisted ventilations, but you may want to consider giving supplemental oxygen. This will be discussed later in this chapter.

If tidal volume is low and you cannot easily see that the patient is breathing, you will have to get more aggressive with your assessment. Kneel beside the patient, establish an open airway using the most appropriate method, and place your ear next to the nose and mouth to listen for breathing while you observe the chest and abdomen for rise and fall. Count the respirations. The chances are that as a patient's respiratory rate gets slower, the respirations will get more shallow as well.

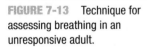
FIGURE 7-13 Technique for assessing breathing in an unresponsive adult.

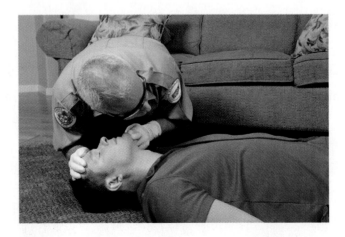

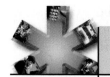

Perspective

Shannon—The Patient

"I woke up with a mask on my face and I was being forced to breathe. It was a totally unnatural feeling . . . and a pretty frightening one! I can remember taking a bite of my sandwich and laughing, and then suddenly I couldn't get a breath. I've never been so scared in my life! I was looking at my boyfriend and trying so hard to breathe. I really thought that I was going to die."

A respiratory rate that is 10 per minute should be a big red flag. You need to compare the rate with the tidal volume, and if the tidal volume is shallow, you may need to assist the patient's ventilations using one of the methods that we will discuss next. A respiratory rate below 10 requires immediate intervention in the way of assisted ventilations.

ASSISTED VENTILATIONS

A patient who is still breathing but who you feel is not breathing adequately either because of rate and/or tidal volume issues needs immediate ventilatory assistance. You can accomplish this by assisting or enhancing the patient's own attempts to breathe with manual ventilations that you provide. The objective is to breathe into the patient as he takes a breath and to make each of his breaths good full breaths by increasing the tidal volume. The exact techniques will vary somewhat, depending on the device that you use. It is preferred to use supplemental oxygen when providing assisted ventilations.

Ventilation Devices

There are several devices available to the EMT to assist with ventilating a patient. They are listed below in the order of preference. While the mouth-to-mouth and mouth-to-stoma techniques are viable options in some situations, they will not be discussed here. These will be covered during your CPR training.

Ventilation devices listed in the order of preference are:

1. Mouth-to-mask with supplemental oxygen

2. Two rescuer bag-valve mask (BVM)

3. Demand valve

4. Single-rescuer BVM

When ventilating a patient, regardless of the device being used, you will want to deliver approximately 12 breaths per minute for an adult, and 20 breaths per minute for pediatric patients. Newborns will require ventilations between 30

2-1.16 List the steps in performing the actions taken when providing mouth-to-mouth and mouth-to-stoma artificial ventilation.

and 50 per minute. The delivery of each breath should be slow and delivered over 1 second. If for any reason you are not able to ventilate using the following techniques, consider a possible foreign body airway obstruction and follow the recommended technique for clearing the obstruction.

Remember to always take appropriate BSI precautions when managing a patient's airway including providing ventilations.

2-1.9 Describe how to artificially ventilate a patient with a pocket mask.

Mouth-to-Mask Technique

In most situations the pocket mask is the easiest barrier device to use and the quickest to deploy. Many EMS professionals and firefighters keep a pocket mask or similar barrier device on their person while on duty (Figure 7-14). This is to ensure they will be ready to provide ventilations without delay should they encounter a nonbreathing patient. For maximum protection against exposure to body fluids a one-way-valve should be used in conjunction with the pocket mask or barrier device.

When used by itself, the pocket mask can allow for the delivery of between 10 and 15 percent oxygen to the patient, because that is how much oxygen remains in each of your exhaled breaths. If possible, use a pocket mask with a supplemental oxygen inlet. This will allow you to deliver much higher concentrations of oxygen when the mask is connected to an oxygen source.

To provide ventilations using a pocket mask, follow these steps (Scan 7-5):

1. Take appropriate BSI precautions.

2. Position yourself at the side or top of the patient's head.

3. Insert an appropriate airway adjunct.

4. Connect the mask to an appropriate oxygen source, if available, at a flow rate of 15 liters per minute (15 lpm).

5. Place the mask over the patient's face, beginning at the top of the nose and walking the mask down so that it rests just below the lower lip.

6. Using both hands, form a tight seal between the mask and the patient's face while maintaining a head tilt or jaw thrust.

7. Take a normal breath and breathe into the one-way valve at the top of the mask. Watch for chest rise and fall.

FIGURE 7-14 A pocket face mask.

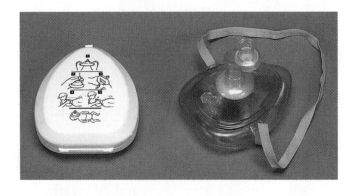

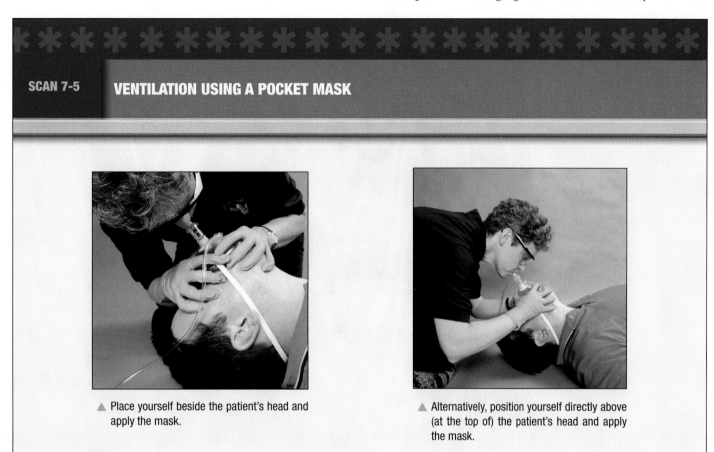

| SCAN 7-5 | **VENTILATION USING A POCKET MASK** |

▲ Place yourself beside the patient's head and apply the mask.

▲ Alternatively, position yourself directly above (at the top of) the patient's head and apply the mask.

Bag-Valve-Mask Technique

A **bag-valve mask (BVM)** consists of a self-inflating bag, a one-way valve, and a face mask. Most BVMs have the capacity to be connected to supplemental oxygen and have an external oxygen reservoir (Figure 7-15 on page 192). Regardless of the configuration, all BVMs are most effective when connected to an oxygen source.

When connected to an oxygen source and used by two rescuers, the BVM is the preferred device for delivering high concentrations of oxygen, up to 100 percent. Used without oxygen, the BVM will deliver room air that is approximately 21 percent oxygen. BVMs come in several sizes, including adult, child, infant, and newborn. The adult-size BVM has a bag capacity or volume of between 1,000 and 1,600 milliliters. If used improperly, the BVM has the potential to deliver smaller volumes than a pocket mask. Be sure to watch the chest and abdomen for adequate rise and fall with each breath. A single rescuer attempting to use a BVM will most likely struggle with trying to maintain an adequate seal while squeezing the bag. For this reason it is a preferred device only when there are two rescuers.

NOTE: *At one time, BVMs were manufactured with "pop-off valves" to prevent overinflation of the patient. It is now known that these valves can release too soon, preventing adequate ventilation of the patient. BVMs with pop-off valves should be taken out of service and replaced.*

2-1.11 List the parts of a bag-valve-mask system.

✳ **bag-valve mask (BVM)**
a hand-held device with a face mask and self-refilling bag that can be squeezed to provide artificial ventilations to a patient. It can deliver air from the atmosphere or oxygen from a supplemental oxygen supply.

2-1.12 Describe the steps in performing the skill of artifically ventilating a patient with a bag-valve mask for one and two rescuers.

FIGURE 7-15   Adult, child, and
infant bag-valve-mask units.

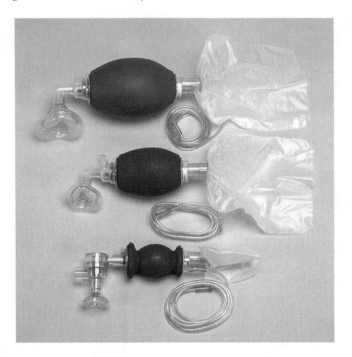

To provide ventilations using a bag-valve mask with a single rescuer, follow these steps (Scan 7-6):

1. Take appropriate BSI precautions.

2. Insert an appropriate airway adjunct.

3. Connect the BVM to an appropriate oxygen source, if available, at 15 lpm.

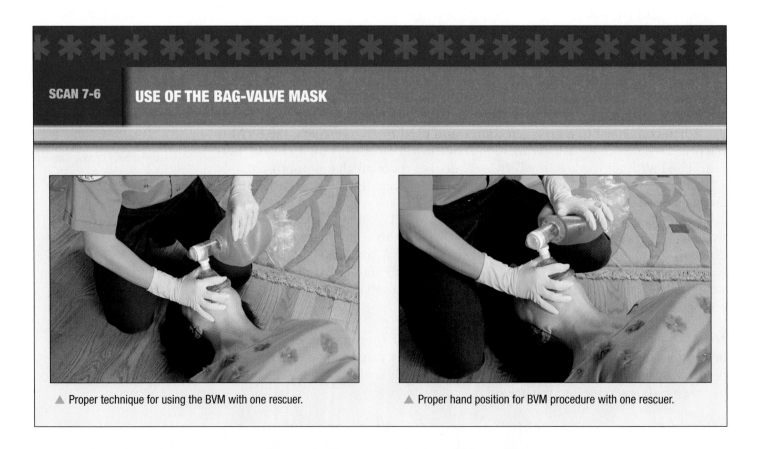

SCAN 7-6   **USE OF THE BAG-VALVE MASK**

▲ Proper technique for using the BVM with one rescuer.

▲ Proper hand position for BVM procedure with one rescuer.

4. Position yourself at the top of the patient's head and place the mask over the patient's face, beginning at the top of the nose and walking the mask down so that it rests just below the lower lip.

5. Using one hand form a "C" around the ventilation port with the thumb and index fingers.

6. Press down firmly on the mask, forming a tight seal between the mask and the patient's face while maintaining a head tilt or jaw thrust. Grasp the mandible with the remaining three fingers.

7. With the other hand, squeeze the bag while watching for chest rise and fall.

To provide ventilations using a bag-valve mask with two rescuers, follow these steps (Scan 7-7):

1. Take appropriate BSI precautions.

2. Insert an appropriate airway adjunct.

3. Rescuer #1 should position himself at the top of the patient's head and place the mask over the patient's face, beginning at the top of the nose and walking the mask down so that it rests just below the lower lip.

4. Using both hands, rescuer #1 forms a tight seal between the mask and the patient's face while maintaining a head tilt or jaw thrust.

5. Rescuer #2 connects the BVM to an appropriate oxygen source, if available, at 15 lpm.

6. Kneeling at the side of the patient's head, rescuer #2 then connects the BVM to the mask and squeezes the bag while watching for chest rise and fall.

2-1.10 Describe the steps in performing the skill of artifically ventilating a patient with a bag-valve mask while using the jaw thrust.

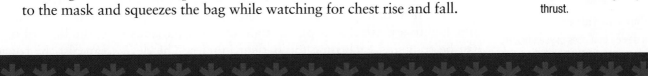

SCAN 7-7   **USE OF BAG-VALVE MASK WITH TWO RESCUERS**

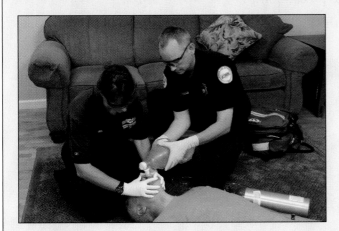

▲ Proper technique for using the BVM with two rescuers.

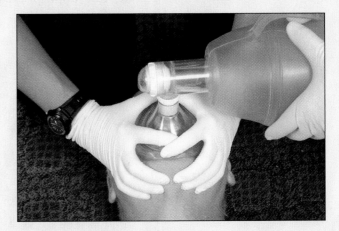

▲ Proper hand placement around the mask.

FIGURE 7-16 Proper technique for performing the jaw-thrust maneuver with two rescuers.

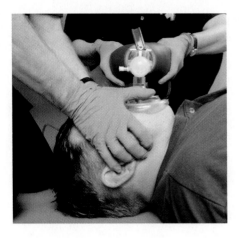

Be sure to use the jaw-thrust maneuver when ventilating a patient with an unknown mechanism of injury or with a suspected spinal injury (Figure 7-16). This can be accomplished by pulling the lower jaw up toward the mask rather than tilting the head back. If the chest does not rise and you are certain there is no airway obstruction, set aside the BVM and attempt to ventilate using the mouth-to-mask technique.

Demand Valve Technique

2-1.15 Describe the steps in artificially ventilating a patient with a flow-restricted, oxygen-powered ventilation device.

✳ **demand valve**

a device that uses oxygen under pressure to deliver artificial ventilations. It has automatic flow restriction to prevent overdelivery of oxygen to the patient. Also called a flow-restricted, oxygen-powered ventilation device (FROPVD).

Sometimes referred to as a flow-restricted, oxygen-powered ventilation device (FROPVD) the **demand valve** is an oxygen-powered ventilation device that provides 100 percent oxygen "on demand" at a peak flow rate of approximately 40 lpm. The flow of oxygen can be triggered by either the patient or the rescuer. When attached to a mask that is placed tight over the patient's face, the flow of oxygen can be triggered each time the patient inhales. The device can also be triggered manually by the rescuer by activating a button or lever on the device itself. Because there is limited control over the pressure delivered by the device, it is recommended that demand valves only be used for adult patients. All demand valves should be configured with an automatic pressure-relief valve and an audible alarm that sounds whenever the relief valve is activated (Figure 7-17).

To provide ventilations using a demand valve, follow these steps (Scan 7-8):

1. Take appropriate BSI precautions.
2. Position yourself at the top of the patient's head.

FIGURE 7-17 A demand valve with activation button.

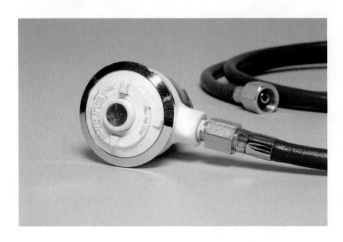

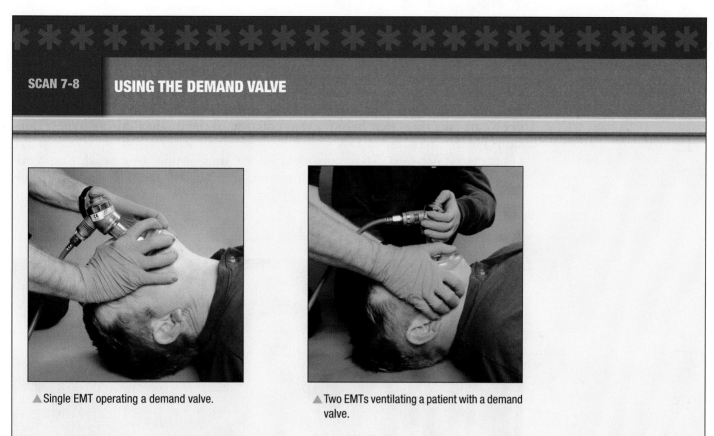

SCAN 7-8   USING THE DEMAND VALVE

▲ Single EMT operating a demand valve.

▲ Two EMTs ventilating a patient with a demand valve.

3. Insert an appropriate airway adjunct.

4. Ensure that the valve of the oxygen tank is open and there is plenty of oxygen.

5. Connect a mask to the demand-valve device.

6. Place the mask over the patient's face, beginning at the top of the nose and walking the mask down so that it rests just below the lower lip.

7. Using both hands, form a tight seal between the mask and the patient's face while maintaining a head tilt or jaw thrust.

8. Activate the device while watching for chest rise and fall.

Be sure to use the jaw-thrust maneuver when ventilating a patient with an unknown mechanism of injury or with a suspected spinal injury. This can be accomplished by pulling the lower jaw up toward the mask rather than tilting the head back. If the chest does not rise and you are certain there is no airway obstruction, set aside the demand valve and attempt to ventilate using the mouth-to-mask technique.

Ventilating Pediatric Patients

The majority of techniques discussed so far apply to all patients, including children and infants. One exception that should be noted pertains to the head-tilt, chin-lift maneuver. While it is best to achieve full extension of the neck in adults, children between the ages of 1 and 8 years generally require only moderate hyperextension of the neck to achieve an adequate airway. Infants require only slight extension, sometimes called the "neutral" or "sniffing" position. The primary reason for avoiding full extension of the neck in pediatric patients is the possibility that the airway could "kink," causing a partial obstruction. This is possible because the tracheas of children and infants do not yet have fully developed cartilage rings that help prevent collapse of the trachea during hyperextension (Figures 7-18 and 7-19).

Pediatric patients also require significantly smaller tidal volumes during ventilation. Care should be taken not to overinflate these patients, as gastric distension occurs more easily in children and infants. Ventilate only until you see adequate chest rise.

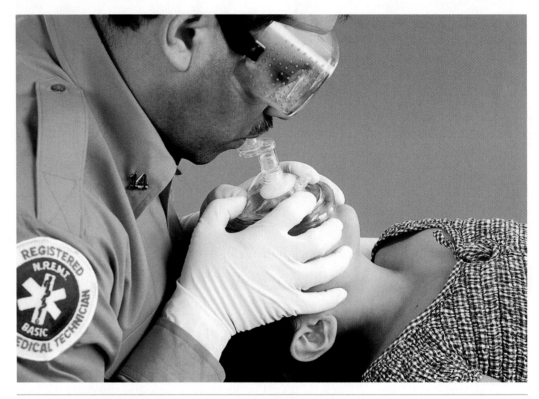

FIGURE 7-18 Ventilation of a child using a pocket face mask.

FIGURE 7-19 One-person ventilation of an infant with a BVM device.

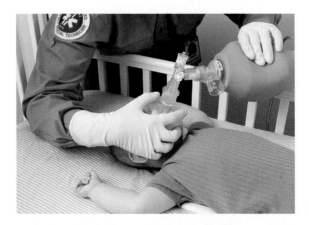

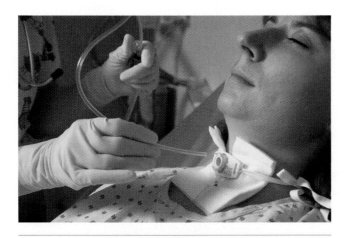

FIGURE 7-20   A stoma with a tracheotomy tube.

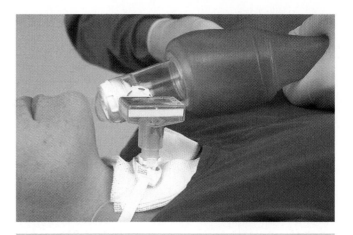

FIGURE 7-21   Artificial ventilation can be accomplished in the patient with a tracheotomy tube by attaching the bag-valve-mask device directly to the tube.

Patients with a Stoma

Some patients may have holes surgically placed in the anterior aspect of the trachea to allow them to breathe. This may have been done secondary to trauma or perhaps the removal of a cancerous tumor. In most instances, there will be an obvious hole (**stoma**) in the front of the neck inferior to the Adam's apple. Sometimes there is a tube inserted into the hole, called a tracheotomy tube (Figure 7-20).

A patient with a tracheotomy or laryngectomy who is having difficulty breathing may have a buildup of secretions at the stoma causing an obstruction. Use a suction device with a soft catheter to help clear the stoma. If necessary, attempt to ventilate the patient using any one of the techniques mentioned above. It may be necessary to seal the stoma with a gloved hand if air is escaping through the stoma during ventilations. If you have no success with conventional ventilations, seal off the mouth and nose and attempt to ventilate through the stoma. Use an infant mask to seal over the stoma as these are typically small and round. A bag-valve-mask device can be connected directly to a tracheotomy tube (Figure 7-21). There is no need to perform a head-tilt, chin-lift or jaw thrust when ventilating through a stoma or tracheotomy tube.

* **stoma**

a permanent surgical opening in the anterior aspect of the trachea through which the patient breathes.

Confirming Adequate Ventilations

Just like being able to assess the adequacy of a patient's own respirations, you must also be able to assess the adequacy of your manual ventilations. The primary sign of adequate ventilations is chest rise and fall. You should observe good chest rise and fall with each ventilation. The rate should be appropriate for the age of the patient. It is also likely that you will see the patient's skin signs and pulse rate improve with adequate ventilations.

When ventilations are inadequate, you will not see good chest rise and fall and the rate will be below or above what is considered acceptable for the age of the patient. It is unlikely that you will see an improvement in the patient's skin signs or pulse rate with inadequate ventilations.

2-1.13 Describe the signs of adequate artificial ventilation using the bag-valve mask.

2-1.14 Describe the signs of inadequate artificial ventilation using the bag-valve mask.

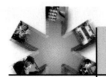

Perspective

Mackenzie—The EMT

"Once Rob cleared the obstruction from Shannon's airway, she was breathing on her own, but it was really shallow and not very effective. So I started assisting her ventilations with a BVM and supplemental oxygen. It was amazing! The color started coming back to her skin and Rob told me that her pulse was returning to normal. The next thing I knew, her eyes opened and she was looking up at me. I remember that look of . . . I don't know . . . confusion, maybe? I guess I'd be pretty confused too if I woke up and someone was ventilating me! I'm so glad that this call turned out good. It was like something out of a textbook or something."

Stop, Review, Remember!

Multiple Choice

Place a check next to the correct answer.

1. What are the two characteristics that must be assessed in order to determine adequacy of respirations?

   _____ a. rate and ease

   _____ b. rate and tidal volume

   _____ c. rate and lung sounds

   _____ d. tidal volume and ease

2. The normal respiratory rate for newborns is between _____ and _____ breaths per minute.

   _____ a. 12, 20

   _____ b. 20, 30

   _____ c. 30, 50

   _____ d. 40, 60

3. The primary mechanism for determining if your ventilations are adequate or not is:

   _____ a. skin color.

   _____ b. lung sounds.

   _____ c. mental status.

   _____ d. chest rise and fall.

4. Because there is limited control over the pressure delivered by this device, it is recommended that the _____ be used only for adult patients.

   _____ a. demand valve

   _____ b. BVM

   _____ c. pocket mask

   _____ d. pressure regulator

5. When attached to supplemental oxygen the BVM can deliver oxygen concentrations as high as _____ percent.

_____ a. 21

_____ b. 44

_____ c. 60

_____ d. 100

Critical Thinking

1. Describe how you would manage an unresponsive adult patient whose respirations are 8 times per minute and shallow.

_____

_____

_____

_____

2. You are caring for a 6-year-old near-drowning patient who is in respiratory arrest. What will be your device of choice for ventilating this patient, and why?

_____

_____

_____

_____

3. List the special factors that must be considered when providing manual ventilations for a pediatric patient.

_____

_____

_____

_____

4. Place an "X" in the box indicating the most appropriate ventilation device for the situation.

Situation	Mouth to Mask	2-Rescuer BVM	Demand Valve	1-Rescuer BVM
You are alone and off duty with an unresponsive nonbreathing infant.				
You, your partner, and a firefighter are ventilating a patient as you carry him down a flight of stairs on a portable stretcher.				
You and a firefighter are ventilating an adult male in the back of an ambulance.				
You are alone in the back of an ambulance and ventilating an 8-year-old near-drowning patient.				
You are ventilating a 20-year-old male who is the third patient from an accidental carbon monoxide poisoning.				

2-1.19 Identify the components of an oxygen delivery system.

Supplemental Oxygen

The Food and Drug Administration has identified medical gases such as oxygen, carbon dioxide, helium, nitrogen, nitrous oxide, medical air, and combinations of these as drugs and requires them to be dispensed by prescription. In its natural state, oxygen is an odorless, colorless, and tasteless gas. Our atmosphere is made up of approximately 21 percent oxygen, 78 percent nitrogen and 1 percent other elements. When our bodies are functioning normally, room air provides an oxygen concentration that is more than adequate to support life.

Good **perfusion** occurs when all cells of the body receive an adequate supply of well oxygenated blood. When a person experiences a serious illness or injury, his body's ability to utilize oxygen is likely to become compromised. This compromise will almost always result in poor perfusion, which can lead to shock and eventually death if not treated properly.

It is safe to say that all victims of illness or injury can benefit from oxygen (Figure 7-22). Some will benefit from larger concentrations while others will respond well to lower concentrations. The point is that oxygen is one of the most important medical interventions the EMT can offer victims of illness and injury.

✳ **perfusion**

the supply of oxygen to and removal of wastes from the cells and tissues of the body as a result of the flow of blood through the capillaries. See also hypoperfusion.

OXYGEN CYLINDERS

Oxygen is stored under pressure in containers known as cylinders, bottles, or tanks. Cylinders can be made of aluminum, steel, or composite materials. Oxygen cylinders come in a variety of sizes with each size designated by a specific letter. Each size also contains a specific amount of oxygen when compressed to approximately 2,015 pounds per square inch (psi). The following list includes the most

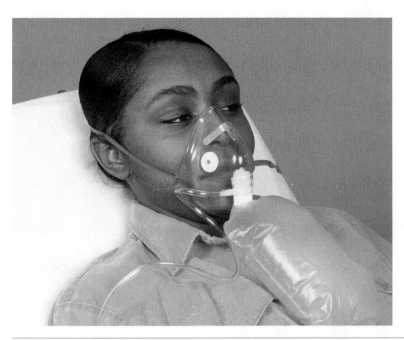
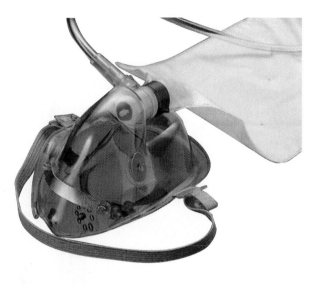

FIGURE 7-22   Patient receiving supplemental oxygen via a nonrebreather mask.

Clinical Clues: OXYGEN USE CRITERIA

The Food and Drug Administration allows oxygen (typically a prescription drug) to be marketed and used as a nonprescription medication under certain criteria:

* That the oxygen unit must deliver a minimum of 6 liters per minute for at least 15 minutes
* That the oxygen unit must be clearly labeled as emergency oxygen
* That the providers be trained in the safe use and storage of oxygen
* That the oxygen unit be packaged with an appropriate delivery device

common cylinder sizes found in EMS along with the approximate volume in liters of oxygen (Figure 7-23 on page 202):

* D cylinder contains up to 425 liters
* Jumbo D cylinder contains up to 640 liters
* E cylinder contains up to 680 liters
* M cylinder contains up to 3,000 liters
* G cylinder contains up to 5,300 liters
* H cylinder contains up to 6,900 liters

Oxygen cylinders are comprised of two main components: the cylinder, which contains the pressurized oxygen, and a valve at the top, which opens and closes the cylinder. The pressure regulator attaches to the cylinder valve when in use.

FIGURE 7-23   Oxygen cylinders.
Left to right: jumbo D cylinder,
D cylinder, and E cylinder.

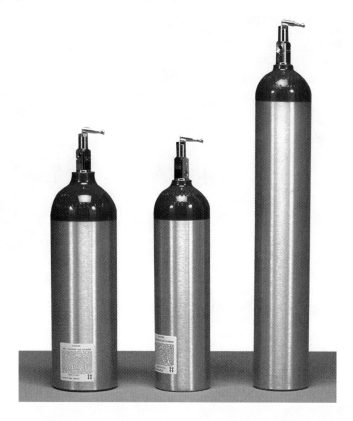

Cylinder Safety

Because oxygen is stored under pressure, care must be used when handling and using oxygen cylinders. The valve of the tank is the most vulnerable part. If damaged it can allow the compressed gas to escape and propel the cylinder at high speed, causing damage to anyone or anything in the way. When not in use, cylinders should be secured so that they cannot fall or roll around (Figure 7-24). When on the scene of an emergency, portable oxygen cylinders should be kept lying down at all times.

Safety features of high-pressure cylinders include:

✳ Hydrostatic testing

✳ Color coding

✳ PIN indexing system

✳ Pressure relief valve

The DOT requires that all compressed-gas cylinders be inspected and pressure tested at specific intervals. The cylinders used in EMS that contain medical grade oxygen must be tested every five years. This test is commonly referred to as a "hydrostatic" test because, following visual inspection, the tank is filled with water and pressurized to 5/3 the service pressure, or approximately 3360 psi, to confirm that no leaks exist. The most recent hydrostatic test date must be stamped into the crown of the cylinder and easily readable (Figure 7-25).

NOTE: *Some oxygen cylinders have met more rigorous inspection and testing standards and are allowed to go up to ten years between test dates. These cylinders have a five-pointed star immediately following the hydrostatic test date stamped into the crown.*

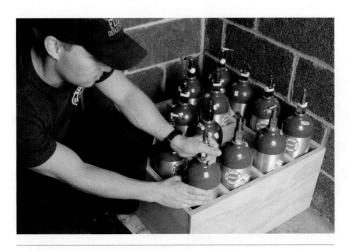

FIGURE 7-24   Portable oxygen cylinders stored properly in a rack. Replace cylinders as necessary.

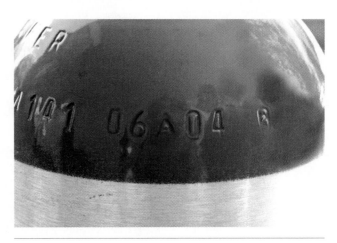

FIGURE 7-25   Standard test stamp.

Clinical Clues: HYDROSTATIC TEST DATE EXPIRATION

A tank that is in service and still contains oxygen when the hydrostatic test date expires does not have to be taken immediately out of service. It can remain in service until such time that it needs to be refilled. At that time it must be removed from service and testing completed before it can be filled and placed back into service.

There are three additional safety features of compressed-gas cylinders used in EMS. The first is color. All medical grade oxygen cylinders are color-coded green to make easy identification of the cylinder contents. The following is a list of common gases and their associated colors:

* Oxygen—green

* Medical air—yellow

* Nitrous oxide—blue

* Carbon dioxide—gray

* Helium—brown

* Nitrogen—black

* Blends of medical gases use a combination of the corresponding color for each component gas. For example, oxygen and carbon dioxide would be green and gray.

Another safety feature is the PIN index system, which is designed to ensure that the proper pressure regulator is used for the appropriate gas. The PIN system consists of two holes strategically placed on the valve of the cylinder. These holes match up with two pins that extend out from the pressure regulator. The pins must line up perfectly or the regulator will not fit properly onto the cylinder valve (Figure 7-26 on page 204).

FIGURE 7-26   The PIN safety system.

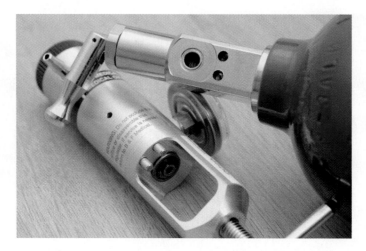

Still another safety feature is the pressure-relief valve. This is located on the cylinder valve and will allow for escape of the gas should the pressure inside the cylinder exceed a predetermined level. The release of pressure will prevent the cylinder from exploding.

PRESSURE REGULATORS

A full oxygen cylinder is pressurized to approximately 2,015 psi. This pressure will vary somewhat depending on the temperature of the environment. For the oxygen to be used by a patient, the pressure must be reduced to allow for a controlled delivery. An appropriate pressure regulator is used for this purpose. A typical pressure regulator will reduce the pressure to between 40 and 60 psi.

Functions of the Pressure Regulator

Pressure regulators can have several functions in addition to simply regulating the pressure inside the cylinder (Figure 7-27). Depending on how they are configured they may be able to provide the following functions:

✳ Pressure gauge

✳ Adjustable-liter-flow outlet

✳ High-pressure port for use with a demand-valve or oxygen-powered suction device

PRESSURE GAUGE

It's probably safe to say that all regulators used in EMS have an integrated pressure gauge (Figure 7-28). Once the regulator is placed onto the cylinder valve and the valve turned on, the pressure gauge will display the amount of pressure inside the cylinder. Gauges are calibrated in pounds per square inch, so the dial will reveal the amount of pressure remaining in the cylinder in psi. For practical purposes a cylinder with 2,000 psi is considered full, 1,000 psi is half full and 500 psi is one quarter full. In many EMS systems, a tank that is less than 500 psi is either refilled or replaced with a full cylinder.

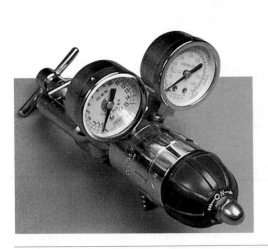
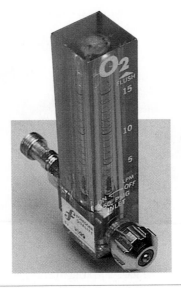
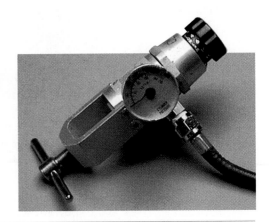

FIGURE 7-27   Different types of pressure regulators: (A) Bourdon gauge flowmeter (pressure gauge), (B) a pressure-compensated flowmeter, and (C) a constant flow selector valve.

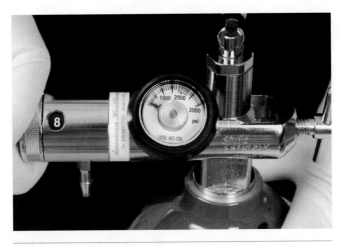

FIGURE 7-28   A pressure gauge.

Clinical Clues: PRESSURE GAUGE SAFETY

Because the gauge utilizes a high-pressure port on the regulator, it is recommended that you NOT look directly at the gauge while turning on the valve. If the gauge was damaged earlier, there is a slight chance that the gauge could burst when the valve is turned on, causing injury to the user.

ADJUSTABLE-LITER-FLOW OUTLET

Most, if not all, regulators have a means of delivering oxygen at a constant flow rate. Medical oxygen is most commonly measured in liters and the flow rate is in liters per minute. Liter-flow valves vary by manufacturer, but a typical regulator will have a liter-flow valve that is adjustable to the following flow rates: 1, 2, 4, 6,

FIGURE 7-29 Liter-flow outlet and dial.

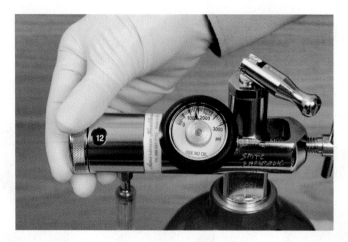

8, 10, 12, 15, 18, 20, 25 (Figure 7-29). The flow rate that you select will be determined by several factors, including which delivery device you are using and how much oxygen you feel the patient needs. In most cases, the higher the flow rate the higher the concentration being delivered to the patient.

REGULATOR ACCESSORIES

Nearly all regulators have additional high-pressure ports that can be used to attach accessories. Two of the most common accessories are the demand-valve and oxygen-powered suction devices. These devices consume a considerable amount of oxygen and will become less effective as the pressure in the cylinder gets low. Be sure to keep a close eye on the pressure in the cylinder and be prepared to change cylinders if necessary.

Attaching a Regulator to the Cylinder

To properly attach a pressure regulator to an oxygen cylinder, follow these steps (Scan 7-9):

1. Remove the protective seal over the cylinder valve.

2. Inspect the valve for cleanliness.

3. Quickly open then shut the cylinder valve to expel any particles of dust or debris.

4. Confirm the presence of an "O" ring and slip the yoke of the pressure regulator over the cylinder valve.

5. Line up the pins on the regulator with the holes on the valve and tighten the thumb screw hand tight.

6. Turn the pressure gauge away from you or others and open the valve one full turn (counterclockwise).

7. Read the pressure gauge and confirm the pressure in the cylinder.

When you are ready to remove the regulator from the cylinder, turn off the valve (clockwise) and bleed all pressure from the regulator by turning on the liter-flow valve until the flow of oxygen stops. It is up to you whether you store the

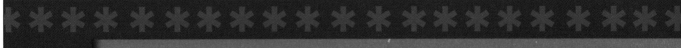

SCAN 7-9   **ATTACHING A PRESSURE REGULATOR TO AN OXYGEN CYLINDER**

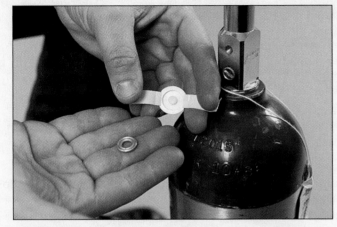

▲ Remove the seal and inspect the valve.

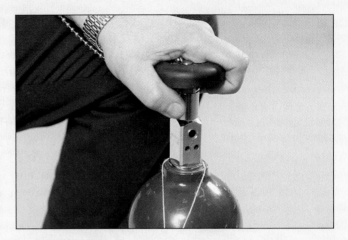

▲ Purge the valve.

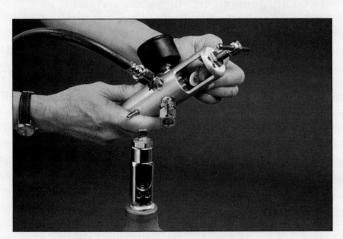

▲ Confirm the presence of an "O" ring on the regulator.

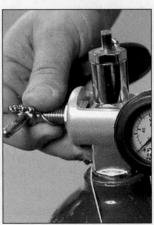

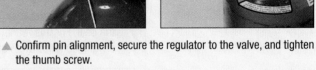

▲ Confirm pin alignment, secure the regulator to the valve, and tighten the thumb screw.

cylinder with the regulator in place on the valve or off the valve. This is often just personal preference. Some agencies have their own policy concerning how portable oxygen cylinders are stored ready for use. Follow your agency's policy.

Oxygen Delivery Devices

To get the oxygen from the cylinder and to the breathing patient in a usable form, an appropriate delivery device is necessary. The two most common delivery devices used in EMS are the nonrebreather mask and the nasal cannula. The device you choose will depend on several factors, including the amount of oxygen you feel the patient needs and the willingness of the patient to accept or tolerate the device.

Regardless of the liter-flow device being used, it is important to determine that the patient is breathing at an adequate rate and volume. Liter-flow devices provide passive oxygen flow, which means that the patient must be breathing adequately on his own to realize any benefit from the oxygen. The purpose of these devices is to increase the concentration of available oxygen to the patient. Liter-flow devices DO NOT provide ventilations for the patient.

Nonrebreather Mask

2-1.20 Identify a nonrebreather face mask and state the oxygen flow requirements needed for its use.

✳ **nonrebreather mask**
a face mask and reservoir bag device that delivers high concentrations of oxygen.

In most situations in the prehospital setting, the nonrebreather mask is the preferred device for delivering a constant flow of oxygen to the breathing patient. It is called a **nonrebreather mask** because the design allows only minimal rebreathing of the patient's exhaled air. It consists of a clear face mask, a one-way valve, an oxygen reservoir, and the supply tubing (Figure 7-30).

Sometimes referred to as a "high-flow" device, the nonrebreather mask works best at a liter-flow rate of 15 lpm. When properly placed, the nonrebreather mask can increase the concentration of available oxygen to 90 percent.

To properly apply a nonrebreather mask to a patient, follow these steps (Scan 7-10):

1. Confirm that the patient is breathing with an adequate rate and tidal volume.

2. Advise the patient that you are going to give him some oxygen.

3. Select the appropriate size mask for the patient.

4. Connect the mask supply tubing to an appropriate oxygen source and adjust the liter flow to 15 lpm.

5. Place your thumb over the one-way valve inside the mask to expedite the filling of the reservoir.

Clinical Clues: NONREBREATHER MASK

Because a nonrebreather mask is not air tight, it will always allow some ambient air in around the seal. For this reason a nonrebreather mask is not capable of providing a breathable oxygen concentration of 100 percent.

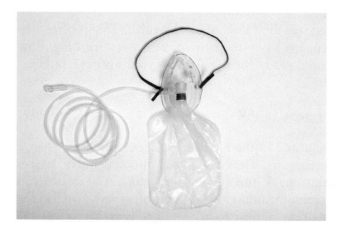

FIGURE 7-30 A nonrebreather mask.

6. Place the mask over the patient's face, starting at the bridge of the nose and walking the mask down the face.

7. Place the elastic band around the patient's head and pull the ends through the mask to ensure a snug fit. Squeeze the aluminum nose strap to help seal the mask across the nose.

Keep a close eye on the reservoir bag as the patient breathes in and out. The bag should NOT completely deflate when the patient breathes in. The bag should also have enough time to completely refill between breaths. If the reservoir becomes deflated or does not refill completely between breaths, increase the liter-flow rate as appropriate.

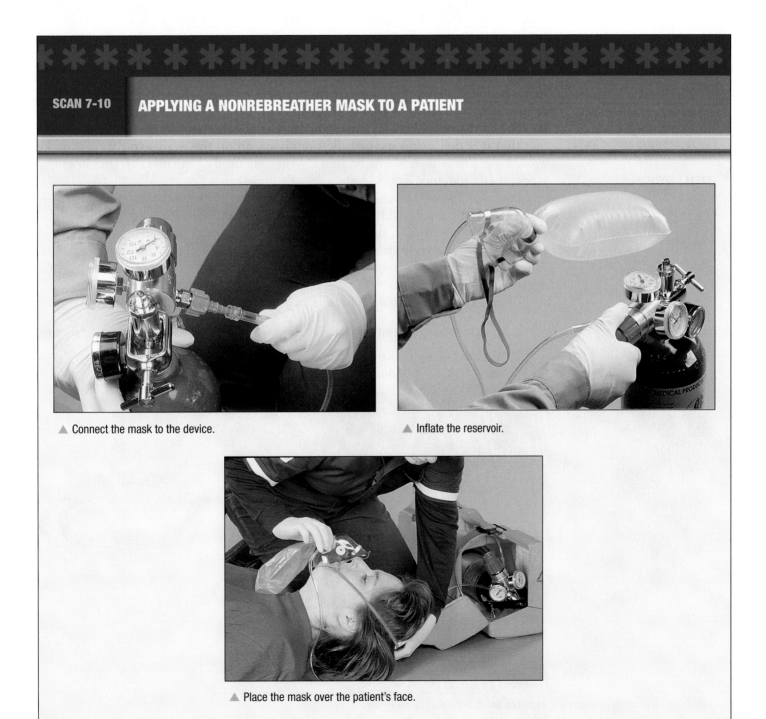

SCAN 7-10   APPLYING A NONREBREATHER MASK TO A PATIENT

▲ Connect the mask to the device.

▲ Inflate the reservoir.

▲ Place the mask over the patient's face.

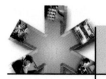

Perspective

Mackenzie—The EMT

"After the patient regained consciousness, I knew that she'd need a good amount of oxygen to help recover from going four or five minutes without any. I chose to put her on a nonrebreather mask with the oxygen set at 15 liters. Because of my nervousness, I forgot to prefill the oxygen reservoir, but Rob was nice enough to remind me."

2-1.21 Describe the indications for using a nasal cannula versus a nonrebreather face mask.

2-1.22 Identify a nasal cannula and state the flow requirements needed for its use.

✳ **nasal cannula**
  a device that delivers low concentrations of oxygen through two prongs that rest in the patient's nostrils.

✳ Nasal Cannula

A **nasal cannula** is used for patients who simply do not tolerate the nonrebreather mask or for patients who are not that critical and may benefit from lower concentrations of oxygen. Patients sometimes feel that their breathing is being restricted by the nonrebreather mask because it covers their entire face, despite the fact that it is delivering oxygen. Before giving up on the mask, you should make every attempt to "coach" the patient into getting used to the mask. If that does not work, many patients will tolerate a nasal cannula just fine.

The nasal cannula consists of a loop of tubing with a pair of prongs (short narrow tubes) that are placed into the patient's nostrils. The loop has an adjustable band and is connected to the supply tubing.

Sometimes referred to as a "low-flow" device, the nasal cannula works best at liter-flow rates between 2 and 6 lpm. When properly placed, the nasal cannula can increase the concentration of available oxygen to approximately 44 percent (Figure 7-31).

To properly apply a nasal cannula to a patient, follow these steps (Scan 7-11):

1. Confirm that the patient is breathing with an adequate rate and tidal volume.

2. Advise the patient that you are going to give him some oxygen.

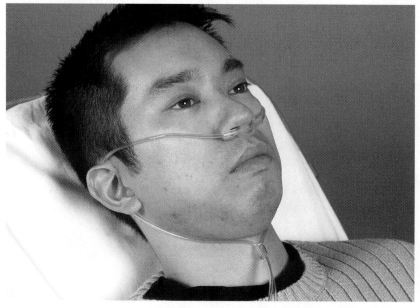

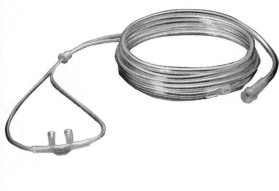

FIGURE 7-31 A nasal cannula properly placed on an adult patient.

✳✳✳✳✳✳✳✳✳✳✳✳✳✳✳✳✳✳✳✳

SCAN 7-11   **APPLYING A NASAL CANNULA**

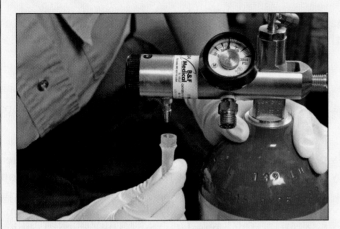

▲ Connect the nasal cannula to the regulator.

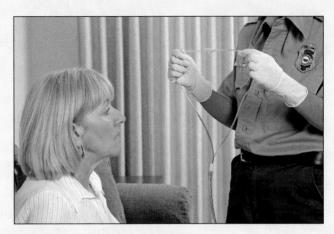

▲ Adjust the nasal cannula to full open.

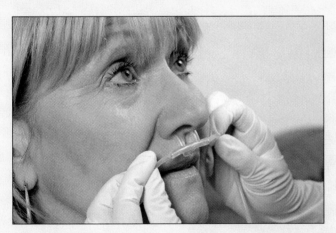

▲ Place the prongs in the patient's nose.

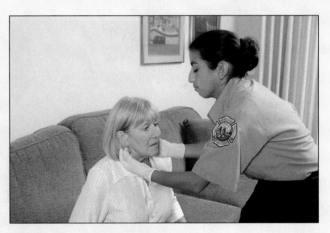

▲ Wrap the tubing around the patient's ears.

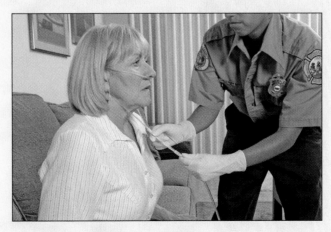

▲ Adjust the slide under the patient's chin.

3. Select the appropriate size cannula for the patient.

4. Connect the cannula supply tubing to an appropriate oxygen source and adjust the liter flow to between 2 and 6 lpm.

5. Slide the adjusting band downward to allow for full expansion of the cannula loop.

6. Grasp the loop with the thumb and index finger of each hand on either side of the prongs.

7. Advise the patient that the prongs will tickle a little bit but will not hurt. Insert the prongs into the patient's nostrils.

8. Slide your fingers along the loop and wrap each side around the patient's ears.

9. Slide the adjusting band up under the chin to take up any slack in the loop. Advise the patient to breathe through his nose.

Some EMS professionals prefer the cannula simply because it makes it easier to hear the patient when they are trying to get a medical history. This is not a good reason to choose the cannula. When a patient is in need of supplemental oxygen, the device of choice should be the nonrebreather mask. Only if the patient will simply not tolerate the mask should you attempt a nasal cannula. The device of choice may also be specified by your local protocols.

FIGURE 7-32 A simple oxygen humidifier.

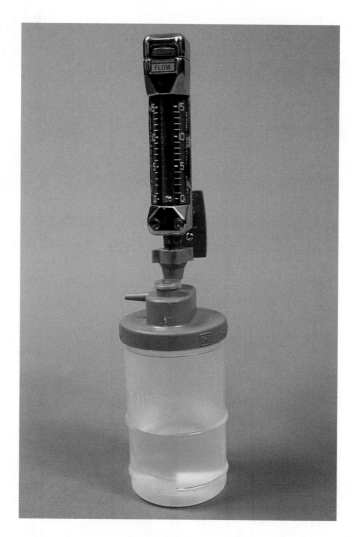

HUMIDIFIED OXYGEN

Compressed oxygen that is stored in cylinders is extremely dry and can cause dryness and irritation to the mucous membranes, especially in the nasal passages (Figure 7-32). If possible, liter-flow oxygen should be run through an oxygen humidifier. An oxygen humidifier is a container of sterile water that is connected to the oxygen supply between the patient and the cylinder. As the oxygen passes through the water, it picks up tiny water molecules. This added moisture minimizes the chances of dryness and irritation that the patient may experience. Humidifiers are found in hospitals and some ambulances and not typically used with portable oxygen cylinders.

✳ Stop, Review, Remember!

Multiple Choice

Place a check next to the correct answer.

1. The oxygen concentration that is normally present in the air we breathe is _____ percent.

   _____ a. 19

   _____ b. 21

   _____ c. 44

   _____ d. 78

2. In round numbers, an oxygen cylinder is considered full if it contains _____ psi of pressure.

   _____ a. 500

   _____ b. 1,500

   _____ c. 2,000

   _____ d. 3,600

3. Which of the following is NOT a safety feature of high-pressure cylinders?

   _____ a. hydrostatic testing

   _____ b. color coding

   _____ c. PIN indexing system

   _____ d. round shape

4. The appropriate liter-flow range for a nasal cannula is between _____ and _____ lpm.

   _____ a. 2, 6

   _____ b. 4, 8

   _____ c. 10, 12

   _____ d. 12, 15

5. A nonrebreather mask that is set at 15 lpm will deliver an oxygen concentration of approximately _____ percent.

   _____ a. 30

   _____ b. 50

   _____ c. 90

   _____ d. 100

Matching

Match the piece of equipment on the left with the applicable definition on the right.

1. _____ Stoma

2. _____ OPA

3. _____ Nonrebreather mask

4. _____ Nasal cannula

5. _____ BVM

A. A low-flow O_2 delivery device that is placed in the nose

B. A device used to provide manual ventilations for a nonbreathing patient

C. A curved plastic device used to keep the tongue from blocking the airway

D. A high-flow oxygen delivery device with an inflatable O_2 reservoir

E. A hole surgically placed in the anterior aspect of the trachea

Critical Thinking

1. What is the difference between medical oxygen and the air that we breathe in the atmosphere?

_____

_____

_____

_____

_____

2. Explain how supplemental oxygen can help improve a patient's perfusion status.

_____

_____

_____

_____

3. Explain why an NRB mask is not capable of providing a breathable oxygen concentration of 100 percent.

_____

_____

_____

_____

_____

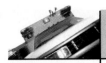

Dispatch Summary

Once Shannon had regained consciousness and started breathing normally with the non-rebreather mask, Mackenzie urged her to be seen by a doctor in the emergency room. At first Shannon declined, citing embarrassment over the whole incident. She soon changed her mind after Rob explained some of the complications that could arise as the result of having choked to the point of unconsciousness.

Rob and Mackenzie then helped Shannon onto their stretcher and into the ambulance where they transported her, still on oxygen and without incident, to Memorial Hospital.

Her boyfriend followed them in his own car.

The Last Word

It cannot be overstated how important a patent airway and adequate ventilations are. Once it has been determined that the scene is safe, these two things become your top priority.

The use of airway adjuncts will assist you in maintaining an open airway, but they must be used in conjunction with close monitoring of the airway.

As an EMT you have several options for ventilating a patient with inadequate or absent respirations. These options are listed here in the order of preference:

1. Mouth-to-Mask
2. Two-rescuer BVM
3. Demand valve
4. Single-rescuer BVM

Whenever possible it is strongly suggested that you use supplemental oxygen when ventilating a patient. Supplemental oxygen increases the concentration available to the patient and helps compensate for inadequate perfusion caused by illness and injury.

Constant-flow delivery devices such as the nonrebreather mask and the nasal cannula are passive devices and require the patient to be moving air adequately on his own in order to benefit from them.

✳ Chapter Review

MULTIPLE CHOICE

Place a check next to the correct answer.

1. During the respiratory assessment of the patient, the EMT must ensure that the patient has an open airway and has adequate:

   _____ a. capillary refill.

   _____ b. skin color.

   _____ c. tidal volume.

   _____ d. pulses.

2. Which of the following are structures of the lower airway?

   _____ a. esophagus, bronchi, larynx

   _____ b. trachea, bronchi, alveoli

   _____ c. nasopharynx, larynx, oropharynx

   _____ d. trachea, pharynx, alveoli

3. The movement of air in and out of the lungs is called:

   _____ a. respiration.

   _____ b. exhalation.

   _____ c. inhalation.

   _____ d. ventilation.

4. Which of the following best describes the most appropriate way to open the airway of a child with no spinal injury?

   _____ a. jaw thrust

   _____ b. head tilt with full extension

   _____ c. the sniffing position

   _____ d. head tilt with slight extension

5. The recommended time allowed for suctioning an infant's airway is _____ seconds.

   _____ a. 5

   _____ b. 10

   _____ c. 15

   _____ d. 20

6. Rigid suction catheters are best suited for suctioning the:

   _____ a. nose of infants.

   _____ b. mouth of an adult patient.

   _____ c. the nose of an adult patient.

   _____ d. the mouth of an infant.

7. Ventilating a patient with a BVM is best if performed:

   _____ a. by a single rescuer.

   _____ b. on responsive patients.

   _____ c. by two rescuers.

   _____ d. in the prone position.

8. Which maneuver is most appropriate for opening the airway of a child with suspected spinal injury?

   _____ a. modified chin lift

   _____ b. head-tilt, chin-lift

   _____ c. jaw thrust

   _____ d. cross-finger technique

9. Which of the following best represents the most appropriate PPE for suctioning a patient?

   _____ a. gloves and face mask

   _____ b. gloves and gown

   _____ c. gloves and eye protection

   _____ d. gloves, mask, and eye protection

10. The appropriate liter-flow rate for a nonrebreather mask is _____ lpm.

   _____ a. 6

   _____ b. 10

   _____ c. 15

   _____ d. 30

CRITICAL THINKING

1. How can you determine if the flow rate on a nonrebreather mask is adequate for the patient's condition?

_____

_____

_____

_____

2. A nonrebreather mask and a cannula are sometimes referred to as "passive" delivery devices. Explain what is meant by "passive" and how these devices differ from the demand-valve or the BVM.

_____

_____

_____

_____

3. Explain why a patient on a nonrebreather mask is not receiving a breathable concentration of 100% oxygen.

_____

_____

_____

_____

CASE STUDIES

Case Study 1

You have responded to a scene where a motorcycle has impacted a guardrail at a high rate of speed. The patient is unresponsive and lying face up. His helmet was removed by firefighters at the scene, and he has an obvious open fracture of the lower left leg. Your initial assessment finds the man's respirations to be 8 and shallow, and you can hear gurgling as he breathes.

1. What is your first priority for this patient?

_____

_____

_____

_____

2. What will you do to address that priority?

_____

_____

_____

3. What device will you use to ventilate this patient?

_____

_____

_____

_____

Case Study 2

You have responded to a possible overdose at a homeless shelter. Upon arrival you find an approximately 30-year-old female lying on the bathroom floor with some vomit near her mouth. She is breathing approximately 10 times per minute and very shallow.

1. What method will you use to open this woman's airway and why?

_____

_____

_____

_____

2. Will you need to provide assisted ventilations for this patient? If so, what device will you use?

_____

_____

_____

_____

3. What position might be the best for this patient as you transport her to the hospital?

_____

_____

_____

_____

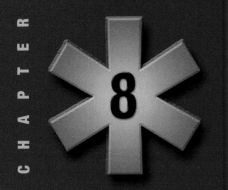

CHAPTER 8

Module Review and Practice Examination

✳ Directions

Assess what you have learned in this module by circling the best answer for each multiple-choice question. When you are done, check your answers against the key provided in Appendix D.

1. After ensuring personal safety, the first priority in patient care is:
   a. checking the patient's pulse.
   b. getting a medical history from the patient.
   c. assessing the patient's airway.
   d. administering oxygen.

2. The structure that prevents food and liquids from entering the trachea is the:
   a. epiglottis.
   b. cricoid cartilage.
   c. epidermis.
   d. carina.

3. The primary muscle(s) used for breathing under normal conditions is/are the:
   a. intercostal muscles between the ribs.
   b. abdominal muscles.
   c. latisimus dorsi muscle of the back.
   d. diaphragm.

4. Which of the following describes a respiratory cycle?
   a. one inspiration + one inhalation
   b. one inspiration
   c. one inhalation + one exhalation
   d. none of the above

5. Your patient is a 6-week-old infant. You should consider her respiratory rate to be normal if it is _____ per minute.
   a. 48
   b. 60
   c. 22
   d. 16

6. Your patient is a 7-year-old male. You should consider his respiratory rate normal if it is _____ per minute.
   a. 60
   b. 48
   c. 28
   d. 12

7. Usually, the earliest sign that someone is not receiving enough oxygen is a/an:
   a. increased tidal volume.
   b. increased respiratory rate.
   c. decreased respiratory rate.
   d. irregular respirations.

8. Which of the following signs is associated with respiratory failure?
   a. flushed skin color
   b. increased tidal volume
   c. increased respiratory rate
   d. decreased mental status

9. If the head of a child is tilted too far back when opening the airway, which of the following may occur?
   a. airway obstruction
   b. a fracture of the cervical vertebrae
   c. damage to the larynx
   d. displacement of the tongue into the pharynx

10. A head-tilt, chin-lift is used to clear the airway from obstruction by:
    a. a foreign body.
    b. the tongue.
    c. swelling due to trauma.
    d. all of the above

11. The best way to open the airway of a patient with a suspected spinal injury is:
    a. placing them in a prone position.
    b. using a head-tilt, chin-lift maneuver.
    c. using a jaw-thrust maneuver.
    d. placing your gloved hand in the patient's mouth to pull the tongue forward.

12. Which of the following PPE is recommended when performing airway management procedures?
    a. gloves
    b. mask
    c. protective eyewear
    d. all of the above

13. Your patient is suspected of taking an overdose of sleeping pills. You note gurgling noises when he attempts to breathe. Which of the following is most likely responsible for this noise?
    a. There is fluid in his lungs.
    b. He has vomited and has fluid in his pharynx.
    c. His tongue is obstructing his airway.
    d. His dentures are obstructing his airway.

14. When suctioning an adult patient's mouth, suction should be applied for no more than _____ seconds.
    a. 5
    b. 10
    c. 15
    d. 20

15. When suctioning the mouth of an infant, suction should be applied for no more than _____ seconds.
    a. 5   c. 15
    b. 10   d. 20

16. Which of the following is the correct sequence for suctioning a patient's mouth?
    1. activate suction
    2. place the tip of the catheter in the mouth
    3. take BSI
    4. remove the suction tip from the mouth
    5. connect the suction catheter to the suction tubing
    a. 3, 5, 1, 2, 4
    b. 3, 5, 2, 1, 4
    c. 5, 3, 1, 2, 4
    d. 5, 3, 2, 4, 1

17. Which of the following steps are required for nasal suctioning of an adult patient, but not for oral suctioning?
    1. BSI
    2. measure the catheter from the tip of the nose to the earlobe
    3. use a water-based lubricant on the suction catheter
    4. suction for no more than 15 seconds
    a. 1, 2, 3, 4
    b. 2, 3, 4
    c. 1, 3, 4
    d. 2, 3

18. The best device for suctioning the nose or mouth of an infant is a/an:
    a. soft (French) suction catheter.
    b. rigid suction tip.
    c. bulb syringe.
    d. large-bore suction tubing.

19. Which of the following statements regarding airway adjuncts is true?
    a. Oropharyngeal airways must not be used in infants.
    b. Oropharyngeal airways eliminate the need for manually opening the airway, but nasopharyngeal airways do not.
    c. Nasopharyngeal airways must never be used in patients with a gag reflex.
    d. Proper manual positioning of the airway is required with the use of oropharyngeal and nasopharyngeal airways.

20. The proper way to measure an oropharyngeal airway is from the _____ to the _____.
    a. tip of the nose; earlobe
    b. nostril; earlobe
    c. corner of the mouth; angle of the jaw
    d. center of the mouth; nostril

21. You are attempting to deliver ventilations to your patient with a bag-valve-mask device, but ventilations are inadequate. How will you know this?
    a. You will not see good chest rise and fall.
    b. The rate is appropriate for the age of the patient.
    c. Skin signs and pulse rate do not improve.
    d. all of the above

22. When delivering ventilations to an adult patient the ideal duration of each ventilation is _____ second(s).
    a. 1
    b. 1 to 1.5
    c. 1.5 to 2
    d. 2 to 2.5

23. For a single rescuer, the preferred technique for ventilating a patient is:
    a. one-rescuer bag-valve mask.
    b. two-rescuer bag-valve mask.
    c. demand-valve device.
    d. mouth-to-mask.

24. Ventilating a patient with a pocket mask delivers _____ percent oxygen in each ventilation.
    a. over 90
    b. 45 to 60
    c. 21
    d. 10 to 15

25. Ventilation with a bag-valve mask device delivers _____ percent oxygen in each ventilation.
    a. over 90
    b. 45 to 60
    c. 21
    d. 10 to 15

26. Another name for a flow-restricted, oxygen-powered ventilation device is:
    a. BVM.
    b. pocket mask.
    c. demand valve.
    d. peak-flow device.

27. Which of the following statements regarding flow-restricted, oxygen-powered ventilation devices is true?
    a. They can only be used on patients who are making respiratory effort on their own.
    b. They can only be used by patients who are not breathing on their own.
    c. They should only be used in adult patients.
    d. They deliver 40 liters per minute of airflow.

28. Which of the following is the most immediate danger associated with using too much volume or delivering each breath too quickly when ventilating a pediatric patient?
    a. filling the stomach with air
    b. creating excessively high oxygen concentrations in the blood
    c. airway obstruction
    d. damage to the trachea

29. Which of the following statements regarding airway management in a patient with a tracheotomy is true?
    a. The EMT must not attempt to suction the stoma; this is a paramedic-level skill.
    b. The best device for ventilating through the stoma is a bag-valve-mask device using an infant mask.
    c. When delivering ventilations through the stoma it is necessary to maintain a head-tilt, chin-lift maneuver.
    d. none of the above

30. Which of the following is used to help identify the contents of a gas cylinder as oxygen?
    a. yellow color coding
    b. a five pointed star on the crown
    c. green color coding
    d. a letter code from A to H, depending on the concentration of oxygen in the tank

31. Once the hydrostatic test date on an oxygen cylinder has passed, which of the following statements is true?
    a. The cylinder may be used until empty but cannot be refilled until the tank is tested.
    b. The oxygen in the cylinder has expired and the tank now contains mostly carbon dioxide.
    c. The cylinder must be immediately removed from service for safety testing.
    d. The cylinder is no longer safe and must be disposed of or recycled.

32. Which of the following serves to ensure that oxygen is delivered to the patient at a safe pressure?
    a. PIN index system
    b. pressure regulator
    c. pressure-relief valve
    d. O ring

33. The best device for delivering oxygen to a breathing patient who needs high-flow oxygen is a/an:
    a. nasal cannula.
    b. bag-valve mask.
    c. nonrebreather mask.
    d. pocket mask.

34. A nonrebreather mask is designed to work best with an oxygen liter flow of _____ liters per minute.
    a. 6
    b. 10
    c. 15
    d. 20

35. The feature of a nonrebreather mask that minimizes the patient's rebreathing of his or her exhaled air is the:
    a. reservoir bag.
    b. supply tubing.
    c. nasal prongs.
    d. one-way valve.

36. A nonrebreather mask, if properly used, can deliver an oxygen concentration of approximately _____ percent.
    a. 16
    b. 21
    c. 50
    d. 90

37. Your 50-year-old female patient has a long history of lung disease. She is having so much difficulty breathing that she cannot speak. Her respirations are 40 per minute, and she is having trouble keeping her eyes open. Which of the following treatments is most appropriate for this patient?
    a. nasal cannula and administering 15 liters per minute of oxygen
    b. nonrebreather mask at 15 liters per minute and administering liters per minute of oxygen
    c. assisting her ventilations with a bag-valve mask and administering supplemental oxygen
    d. assisting her ventilations with a pocket mask and administering 12 liters per minute of oxygen

38. You have applied a nonrebreather mask to a patient who is complaining of difficulty breathing. The patient complains that the mask is "suffocating" her and that she "can't stand it." Which of the following is an appropriate first step?
    a. Automatically switch to a nasal cannula with 6 liters per minute flow of oxygen.
    b. Coach the patient on how to adjust to the nonrebreather mask.
    c. Check to make sure that the reservoir bag is not completely deflating when the patient breathes in.
    d. Remove the mask for 15 seconds every minute to relieve the feeling of suffocation.

39. A nasal cannula, properly used, can deliver an oxygen concentration of up to approximately _____ percent.
    a. 2 to 6
    b. 10 to 15
    c. 40 to 45
    d. 90 to 95

40. A nasal cannula is designed to be used with an oxygen flow rate of _____ liters per minute.
    a. 2 to 6
    b. 2 to 10
    c. 6 to 10
    d. 10 to 15

41. The prongs of a nasal cannula are properly placed when they are:
    a. resting on the upper lip.
    b. inside the nostrils.
    c. resting on the bridge of the nose.
    d. none of the above

42. Which of the following is a drawback to using an oxygen-powered suction device?
    a. It consumes a great quantity of oxygen.
    b. It is not as effective as a manual suction device.
    c. It generates dangerous levels of suction that may injure the patient.
    d. It requires a special regulator that is expensive and typically difficult to find.

43. Before beginning bag-valve-mask ventilations, you must make sure that the patient:
    a. is not making any respiratory effort on his/her own.
    b. has an open airway.
    c. is completely unresponsive.
    d. has adequate tidal volume.

44. Your patient is a 22-year-old male who is having a severe allergic reaction to peanuts. He tells you that his throat feels swollen and he is having trouble breathing. As you attempt to put a nonrebreather mask on the patient, he pushes it away. As you attempt to replace the mask, the patient becomes combative, swatting your hands away. Which of the following should influence how you approach this situation?
    a. You may get in trouble if you bring the patient to the emergency department without a nonrebreather mask in place.
    b. The patient will die immediately without a nonrebreather mask.
    c. The patient may be terrified at the sensation of not being able to breathe.
    d. The patient's fears should not play a role in your decision.

45. Which of the following is required for a BVM to provide adequate ventilation and oxygenation of a patient?
    a. a pop-off valve
    b. an oxygen reservoir
    c. a three-provider ventilation technique
    d. all of the above

46. Which of the following is required for good perfusion?
    a. blood circulation
    b. oxygenation
    c. ventilation
    d. all of the above

47. A full oxygen cylinder is pressurized to approximately _____ pounds per square inch.
    a. 425
    b. 1,000
    c. 2,000
    d. 3,000

48. The most accurate method for obtaining the respiratory rate is to count the respirations for:
    a. 15 seconds.
    b. 30 seconds.
    c. 45 seconds.
    d. 60 seconds.

49. You are the first EMS provider on the scene of a 30-year-old female who is breathing inadequately, possibly due to an overdose of prescription medications. This is the first time you've been put in a situation where there is not a more experienced EMT to help guide you through the call. You can tell that your heart rate is up and you are feeling anxious about the situation. Which of the following should be your primary consideration?
    a. focusing on the priorities of patient care
    b. using your radio to find out how far way additional responders are
    c. finding out exactly what medication the patient took and how much she took
    d. not allowing the patient's family to notice your anxiety

50. Which of the following is NOT one of the three characteristics that must be assessed when checking a patient's breathing?
    a. length of each inspiration
    b. respiratory rate
    c. volume of respirations
    d. regularity of respirations

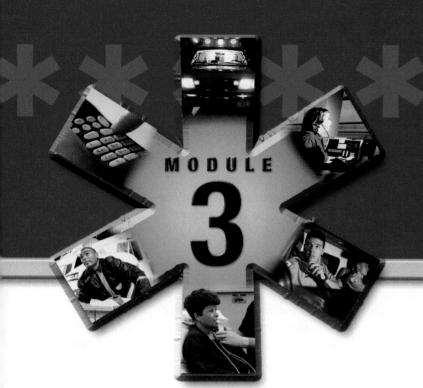

Patient Assessment

> *Listening for Dick's blood pressure was a real challenge on this call. His mother kept talking, Dick kept throwing up or moving his arm to hold onto the garbage can, or I just got the normal junk-noise like the creaking sound of the cuff as it inflated or deflated.*

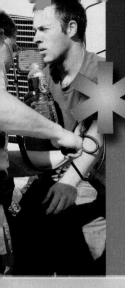

Module Outline

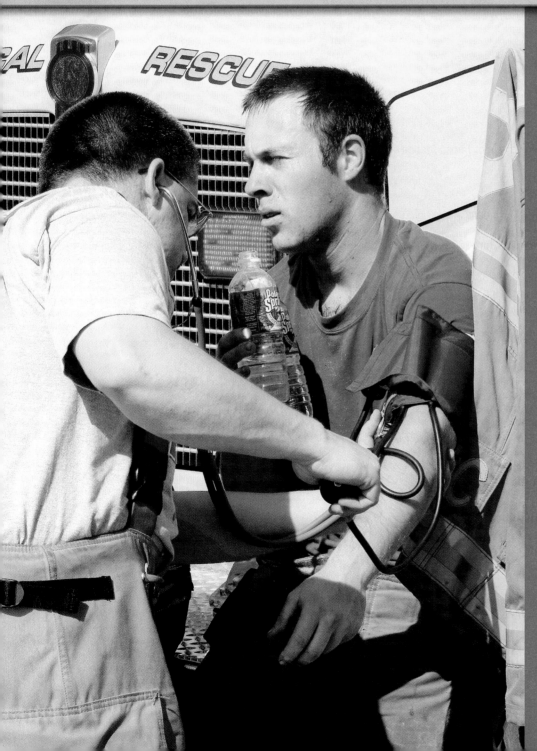

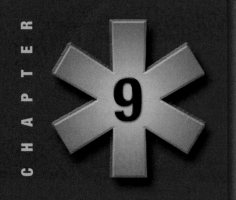
Sizing Up the Scene

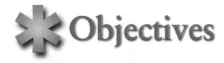

Objectives

Numbered objectives are from the U.S. Department of Transportation 1994 EMT-Basic National Standard Curriculum.

COGNITIVE OBJECTIVES

At the completion of this lesson, the EMT-Basic student will be able to:

3-1.1 Recognize hazards or potential hazards. (pp. 230-233)
3-1.2 Describe common hazards found at the scene of a trauma and a medical patient. (pp. 230-233)
3-1.3 Determine if the scene is safe to enter. (pp. 230–233)
3-1.4 Discuss common mechanisms of injury or nature of illness. (pp. 238–244)

3-1.5 Discuss the reason for identifying the total number of patients at the scene. (pp. 233–234)
3-1.6 Explain the reason for identifying the need for additional help or assistance. (pp. 233–235)

AFFECTIVE OBJECTIVES

At the completion of this lesson, the EMT-Basic student will be able to:

3-1.7 Explain the rationale for crewmembers to evaluate scene safety prior to entering. (pp. 230–231)

3-1.8 Serve as a model for others explaining how patient situations affect your evaluation of mechanism of injury or illness. (pp. 238–244)

PSYCHOMOTOR OBJECTIVES

At the completion of this lesson, the EMT-Basic student will be able to:

3-1.9 Observe various scenarios and identify potential hazards. (pp. 230–231)

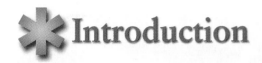

Introduction

The scene size-up is usually considered the most important part of the call. While you will learn many important assessment and treatment skills in the chapters that follow, none of what you learn is likely to be used effectively without a proper scene size-up. In the size-up you will protect yourself, scan the scene for clues about the patient's condition, and call for any additional help you need.

These tasks may seem simple—perhaps even common sense to you. But when you are at the scene of an emergency and you are faced with a sense of urgency, the scene size-up will be the point where you begin a calm, orderly process of assuring your safety and setting the stage for a successful call.

Emergency Dispatch

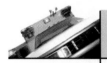

"Hey! We just got a call. I've gotta go!" Mike, an EMT for the county ambulance service, snapped his cell phone shut and grabbed the portable radio. "Go ahead for unit 53."

"Unit 53, please respond to 34472 Rock Canyon Road for a 9-1-1 hang-up. The system shows a history of respiratory distress calls at that address."

"We copy," Mike said as he pulled his seat belt into place and his partner, Erik, pulled the truck onto the road.

The house on Rock Canyon Road was old, poorly tended, and partially obscured by low-hanging tree branches. An old car sat on flat tires in the driveway, rust running across its faded paint, and the windows were blinded by ages of dirt. Neither EMT could see any movement in the house.

"Headquarters, Unit 53," Mike said into the radio. "What's the ETA on the police?"

"They're all tied up with a brawl at the fairground, 53. Sorry."

The two men looked at each other, picked up their equipment, and started toward the house.

The Scene Size-Up

The scene size-up consists of several components: scene safety, body substance isolation, determining if additional resources are necessary (for example, fire department, power company), the number of patients and **mechanism of injury/nature of illness** (Figure 9-1A and B on page 228.)

Each of these components is important in itself. In combination, a foundation is set for the call. You enter a scene knowing that you are protected from disease, that the scene is safe, that any needed help is on the way, and having some sense about your patient even before you talk to or examine him.

Components of the scene size-up are the following:

✳ Body substance isolation precautions

✳ Scene safety

✳ **mechanism of injury**
  a force or forces that may have caused injury.

✳ **nature of illness**
  what is medically wrong with a patient.

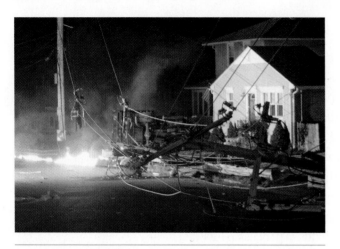

FIGURE 9-1A   An unsafe scene. (© Mark C. Ide.)

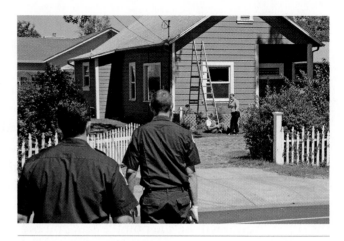

FIGURE 9-1B   A safe scene.

✳ Number of patients

✳ Need for additional resources

✳ Mechanism of injury/nature of illness

BODY SUBSTANCE ISOLATION

You first learned about body substance isolation (BSI) in Chapter 2. It is a concept required on every call. Generally stated, you will take steps to protect yourself from any infectious or potentially infectious substances you encounter. The personal protective equipment (PPE) you must have available at all times includes (Figure 9-2A):

✳ Gloves—to keep your hands from exposure

✳ Face protection—to provide protection of the eyes, nose, and mouth

✳ Respiratory protection—use of N95 masks (Figure 9-2B) or HEPA respirators (Figure 9-2C) to prevent inhalation of microorganisms

✳ Gowns—to protect your clothes from being soiled in circumstances where there are large volumes of blood or fluid or likely splashing of these substances

One vitally important part of infection control is hand washing (Figure 9-3). Because it is done after calls and routinely during the day, we do not always place the value on it we should. Wash your hands after every call—whether or not gloves have been worn. True hand washing involves soap and water with scrubbing to remove any dirt or other materials that may be on your hands, wrists, and exposed distal forearm. The hand washing that some perform, where a small amount of soap is casually spread around and quickly rinsed, is not acceptable or effective in a health care setting.

✳ **alcohol-based waterless hand cleaner**

hand cleaner that can be used in the field when soap and water are not available.

You should also have access to an **alcohol-based waterless hand cleaner** (Figure 9-4 on page 230). This allows you to clean your hands in the field when soap and water aren't available. The Centers for Disease Control and Prevention (CDC) states that this can be as effective as hand washing for hands that are not visibly soiled.

One of the most important concepts in body substance isolation is choosing the correct protection in a given situation. All too often an EMT dons gloves when

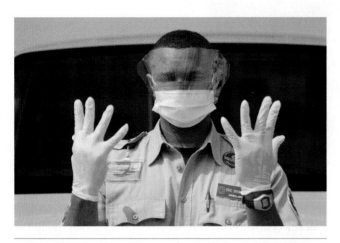

FIGURE 9-2A   Body substance isolation components. (© Ken Kerr.)

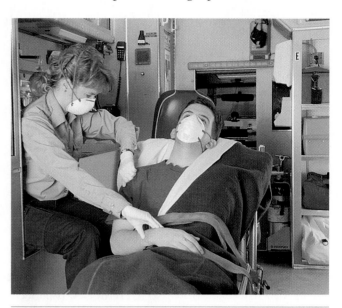

FIGURE 9-2B   Use surgical masks to protect against blood spatters or air-borne disease.

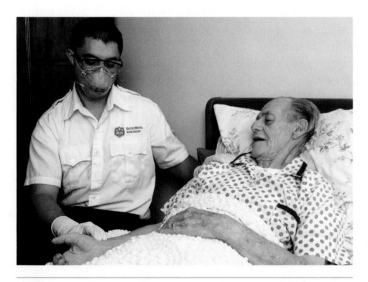

FIGURE 9-2C   Wear a special HEPA respirator to prevent the inhalation of microorganisms.

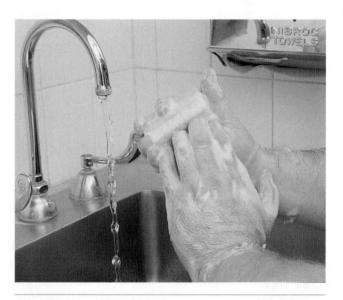

FIGURE 9-3   Hand washing is a vitally important part of infection control.

leaving the ambulance and never thinks of BSI again. This can be dangerous. Consider a situation where you are responding to a fight in the parking lot of a convenience store. The police have made the scene safe and ask you to look at a patient who has facial trauma. He is yelling a bit. Every time he yells, blood sprays from his mouth between the teeth that weren't knocked out. If you are wearing only gloves, you have a high chance of exposure through the mucous membranes of your face—the eyes, nose, and mouth.

In another extreme, some infectious disease experts do not believe gloves are required on each call. If you respond to a patient who complains of abdominal pain and there are no body fluids or substances present (for example, vomitus, urine, feces, blood), gloves are not necessary by definition. Think of the last time you were seen by your personal physician. When the doctor examined you and the nurse took

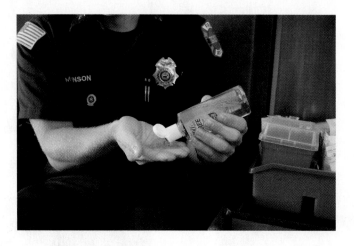

FIGURE 9-4 Alcohol-based waterless hand cleaner.

your blood pressure, pulse, and temperature did either of them wear gloves? Most likely not. Why? Because there was no risk of contact with blood or body fluids.

Think about this: You are called to a nursing home for an elderly woman who is being transported for a feeding tube change. She has chronic diseases that have left her somewhat disoriented. You look but see no blood or body fluids. But you will have to reach under the patient to lift her to the stretcher. You can't see the area under the patient and you can't be sure whether she may have urinated or moved her bowels. In this case, you would wear gloves because you could reasonably expect to find something where you can't see.

The point: BSI precautions are a critical thinking process on each call. You wear precautions against things that are present or can reasonably be expected. Remember also, spreading of infection is a two-way street; you may infect your patient.

Scene Safety

3-1.1 Recognize hazards or potential hazards.

* scene safety

an awareness that you must continually assure the safety of yourself, your crew, and your patient. This is done by teamwork, observation, and communication between members of a crew.

Scene safety is among and perhaps the most important concept you will learn. If you don't remain safe, you will be unable to help your patient, you may become injured and, as a patient, you will now require help that will tax resources and be diverted from your patient. In short, stay safe for both your sake and your patient's.

The safety of your entire crew is also a concern. You will work together with your partner or crew to remain safe. This is done by teamwork, observation, and communication between members of a crew.

Remember that EMS is largely a safe occupation. When you are in the field on calls you will be responding to emergencies. These are dynamic situations that can be unpredictable. This is why they can be dangerous. It is also why we chose to be involved in EMS. Not all calls are the same, and this provides a challenge. It can occasionally pose a danger.

There are a wide variety of hazards, most of which have been covered in chapter 2. These include hazardous materials, violence, danger of injury from unstable vehicles or sharp surfaces in vehicle collisions, and environments and surfaces such as ice, water, or heights. You will learn more about such hazards in chapter 42.

The key to preventing danger is observation. It would be easier if bad things happened only in certain neighborhoods—or only at night. Unfortunately this is not the case. Incidents like domestic violence or a tanker rollover can happen any time, anywhere.

When you approach a scene, do so slowly and carefully. Resist the urge to rush in. Begin your observations long before you arrive on scene. This will give

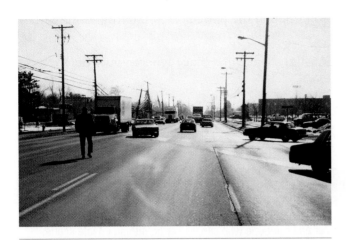

FIGURE 9-5A   Observe the symmetry of telephone poles. (© Daniel Limmer.)

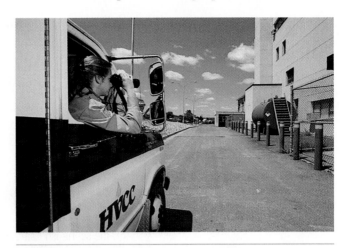

FIGURE 9-5B   Use binoculars to observe a potentially dangerous scene from a distance.

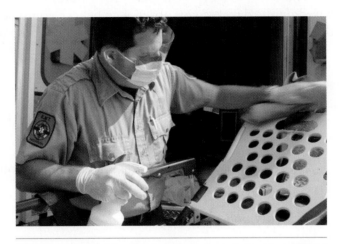

FIGURE 9-5C   Look for objects that may imply the presence of blood or body fluids. (© Ken Kerr.)

you the opportunity to observe and react to the danger before you get in the middle of it.

Examples of observations include (Figure 9-5A–C):

* Observing signs of power lines down, such as a blackout in an area near a scene. You may also observe asymmetry of telephone poles. Poles are relatively evenly spaced. If a pole appears to be missing or at an unusual angle as you approach, this may indicate that wires are down.

* Using binoculars to observe the scene of a highway accident involving a tractor trailer. You will be looking for hazardous material placards, signs of people injured or down, fire, or threat of explosion.

* Observing jagged metal around an area where you will be accessing a patient.

* At the scene of a crime, looking for agitated persons, hostile crowds, or weapons.

* Being alert for potential evidence at crime scenes.

* Look for signs of potential trouble, including evidence of alcohol or drugs on the scene or in use, pets, weapons, violent or agitated persons, unruly

3-1.2   Describe common hazards found at the scene of a trauma and a medical patient.

3-1.3   Determine if the scene is safe to enter.

crowds, and injuries that don't match the patient's explanation of how they occurred, and so on.

✳ Sometimes observing an unusual silence in a place where you would expect panic or activity.

✳ Looking for blood or body fluids or situations where you might expect these substances.

Clinical Clues: SCENE SAFETY

If the scene isn't safe, make it safe or call someone who can. Never go into an unsafe scene.

The scene size-up is the place for careful observation and appropriate action based on the dangers you observe or believe could occur. The actions you take set the stage for your safety as well as the safety of the patient and bystanders at the scene. When you encounter danger, there are actions you can take to remain safe. These include the following:

In cases of violence:

✳ Do not enter a scene until it is safe to do so (Figure 9-6).

✳ Retreat from a scene where there are weapons or violent persons or situations.

✳ Use your equipment as a distraction to aid your retreat from the danger.

✳ Take a position of cover or concealment (Figure 9-7A, B).

✳ Notify police immediately.

In cases of motor vehicle collisions:

✳ Wear appropriate personal protective equipment including turnout gear, gloves, boots, and eye protection (Figure 9-8).

✳ Be alert for unstable vehicles such as those that may roll, move, or tip once you are inside or around them (Figure 9-9).

FIGURE 9-6 Do not enter a scene where there are weapons or violent persons or situations.

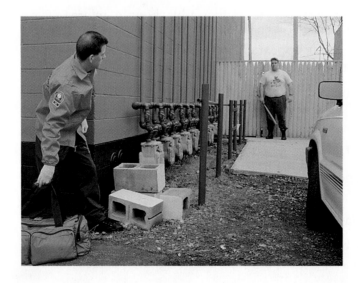

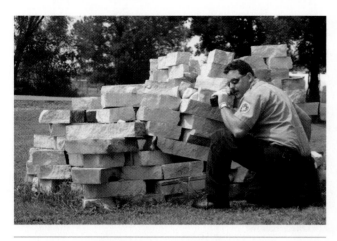

FIGURE 9-7A   Take a position of cover. (© Ken Kerr.)

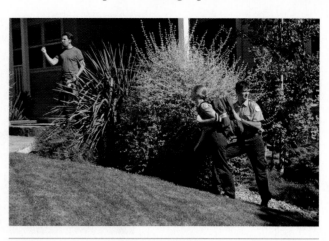

FIGURE 9-7B   Take a position of concealment.

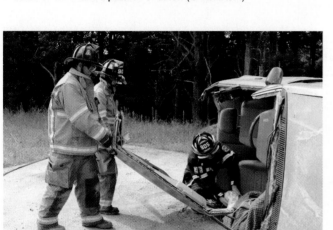

FIGURE 9-8   Wear appropriate personal protective equipment such as, turnout gear, gloves, boots, and eye protection.

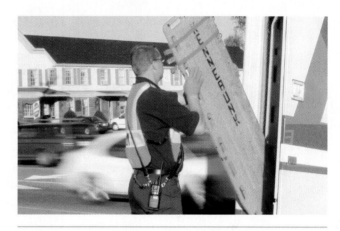

FIGURE 9-9   When providing care on or near the highway, be sure you and your ambulance are safe. (© Daniel Limmer.)

* Be alert for leaking fluid, such as gasoline and hazardous materials.

* Be alert for sharp surfaces, such as jagged metal.

* Notify the fire department and hazardous material units as needed.

In cases of outdoor emergencies:

* Be aware of extremes in weather that may harm you or your patients.

* Do not attempt rescues on or in slopes, heights, confined spaces, or water unless you are trained to do so and have the proper equipment (Figure 9-10 on page 234).

* Notify the appropriate rescue teams for these situations.

Resource Determination and Number of Patients

The experiences of countless EMTs have shown one important fact: If you don't call early for the help you need, you are likely to start caring for patients and for-get. The rule here is simple, call for any help you feel you may need during the

3-1.6 Explain the reason for identifying the need for additional help or assistance.

FIGURE 9-10 Rescues on slopes, from heights, in confined spaces, and in water all require proper training and equipment. (© Ken Kerr.)

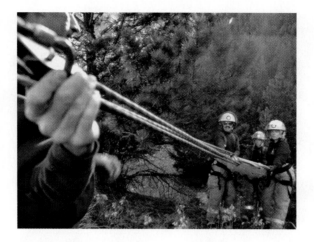

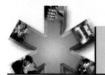

Perspective

Mike—The EMT

"I hate 9-1-1 hang-ups. Most of the time we let the police go in while we wait for the 'all clear,' you know? But sometimes, like this call, we just couldn't wait. There's a history of respiratory calls, the condition of the house and car indicate the possibility of an elderly or disabled person. I just couldn't stand in the driveway and wait when there might be someone right on the other side of the door having a serious medical problem. Wouldn't that be the worst? Lying on the floor, fighting to breathe . . . and you hear the EMTs out in the driveway debating whether or not to approach your house. We just had to check it out."

3-1.5 Discuss the reason for identifying the total number of patients at the scene.

scene size-up. If it turns out that you won't need the help, you can always cancel it. Early is best.

ADDITIONAL AMBULANCES

If you have multiple patients, you will likely need additional ambulances. Even two patients may require different ambulances if they are being transported to different hospitals (Figure 9-11). Consider the intoxicated driver who injured others. It may be unwise to transport him with someone he injured.

If there are many patients you will activate your agency's **multiple casualty incident (MCI)** plan. Some agencies recommend activation of a plan with as few as three patients. Chapters 40 and 41 discuss multiple casualty incidents and triage.

* **multiple casualty incident (MCI)**

any incident involving multiple patients. Most definitions of MCI include a mention of the first in units/resources being overwhelmed.

FIRE DEPARTMENT

While the fire department would obviously be notified for fires, there are many other types of incidents where the fire service is involved. These include hazardous

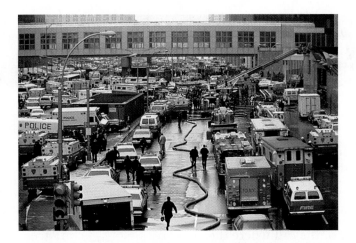

materials, vehicle extrication, and rescue. Some fire departments have special rescue teams (discussed later).

In many areas the fire department can be dispatched for lifting assistance and other situations where additional personnel are necessary.

POLICE ASSISTANCE

While we always consider calling for police when there are immediate threats to our safety, the police may also be of assistance with traffic, patient refusal situations, or situations that aren't yet violent but that you are concerned may erupt while you are there. The police should also be called if, in the course of your time on the scene, you discover drugs, weapons, or a behavioral emergency.

SPECIALIZED TEAMS

There are many different situations you may respond to. Experience, training, and the proper equipment are vital when confronted with situations such as hazardous materials, **weapons of mass destruction, confined spaces,** water rescue and rescue in **high-angle** and **low-angle situations.** Know what teams are available in your area.

UTILITY COMPANIES

You may need the assistance of the utility company to cut power or safely remove wires from the scene.

* **weapons of mass destruction (WMD)**

weapons, devices, or agents intended to cause widespread harm and/or fear among a population.

* **confined spaces**

small, closed-in areas with poor access and egress. Rescues involving confined spaces require specialized training and equipment.

* **high-angle situations**

vertical or above-ground rescue situation requiring specialized training and equipment.

* **low-angle situations**

"off-road" rescue situation requiring specialized training and equipment.

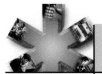

Perspective

Erik—The EMT

"We normally like for the police to go in first on unusual calls or 9-1-1 hang-ups. The way I see it, they got guns and training for that kind of stuff, and I don't. That makes it a real simple choice for me."

Stop, Review, Remember!

Multiple Choice

Place a check next to the correct answer.

1. Which of the following statements best describes the scene size-up?

_____ a. the part of the call where the airway, breathing, and circulation are ensured

_____ b. the part of the call that is completed prior to your arrival on the scene

_____ c. the part of the call that deals with your safety at the scene

_____ d. the part of the call in which important decisions are made that set the stage for the remainder of the call

2. Which of the following may require calling for additional resources at the scene?

_____ a. a motor vehicle collision with two patients

_____ b. a suspected carbon monoxide leak in a house

_____ c. a tanker rollover

_____ d. all of the above

3. Which of the following is not a part of the scene size-up?

_____ a. determining the number of patients

_____ b. determining the nature of the patient's illness

_____ c. determining whether the patient is breathing

_____ d. determining what BSI will be necessary

4. Hand washing is not important if you follow BSI precautions on scene meticulously.

_____ a. true

_____ b. false

5. Never go into an unsafe scene.

_____ a. true

_____ b. false

6. Which of the following statements about a dangerous scene is FALSE?

_____ a. Retreating from the scene is an acceptable tactic.

_____ b. It is acceptable to briefly enter an unsafe scene to remove a patient.

_____ c. Collision scenes frequently have sharp metal and broken glass.

_____ d. Extremes in weather can endanger you and your patient.

Fill in the Blank

For each of the following situations, explain how you may be harmed by potential dangers on the scene and who you would call to handle the situation.

1. A derailed train car with a HazMat placard

   a. Potential dangers: _____

   b. Who would you call? _____

2. A house where you hear an intoxicated person yelling

   a. Potential dangers: _____

   b. Who would you call? _____

3. A motor vehicle collision where there is an occupied vehicle on its side

   a. Potential dangers: _____

   b. Who would you call? _____

4. A hiker has fallen down a steep slope

   a. Potential dangers: _____

   b. Who would you call? _____

Critical Thinking

1. You have responded to a call for an unknown problem. It turns out that it is a domestic violence case, and one of the partners is intoxicated and belligerent. List several things you may have observed while responding to the scene and approaching the apartment that may have warned you about what you found.

   _____

   _____

   _____

   _____

   _____

2. Why is it important to call for additional resources early in a call?

   _____

   _____

   _____

   _____

   _____

Mechanism of Injury and Nature of Illness

After safety has been ensured and it is time to approach the patient, you will shift your focus to the assessment and care you will perform. The few seconds you have as you approach the patient can be very, very important.

3-1.4 Discuss common mechanisms of injury or nature of illness.

Experienced EMTs know that important information can be obtained as you approach. The clues you observe can tell a great deal about your patient.

NATURE OF ILLNESS

You are walking up the stairs into the residence. Things appear calm and safe. The patient's neighbor tells you he saw the patient working in the yard. The patient seemed to stumble and clutch his chest, then fell. The neighbor called 9-1-1 and ran over. He found the neighbor "dazed" but conscious and got him into the house. You approach the patient and notice that he still has his hand clutched in a fist by his chest. He looks pale and sweaty. As you walk by the kitchen counter you observe several medications.

You haven't even begun to talk to your patient, but you have made many observations that are significant to the care you will provide. Can you name them all?

The observations you have made include that the patient is probably very ill (he has his hand to his chest and he is pale and sweaty), that he at one point appears to have had some sort of altered mental status or was stricken (information from the neighbor that the patient was "dazed"), and that he or someone in the residence has a prior medical condition (based on the medications found on the kitchen counter).

This information lets you know that the patient's condition is potentially serious—even before you reach him. This will affect the way you begin care for the patient, call for additional assistance, and set priorities in the initial assessment (chapter 10).

✳ **nature of illness**
what is medically wrong with a patient.

The EMT curriculum explains evaluating **nature of illness** as "determine from the patient, family, or bystanders why EMS was activated." While this description is somewhat limited in comparison to the scenario just presented, the reality is that the scene size-up allows the alert and observant EMT to obtain more than a simple complaint. A significant amount of information that will improve your initial assessment and care can be obtained and processed in a matter of seconds.

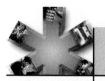

Perspective

Mrs. Roberts—The Patient

"I know I shouldn't have waited so long to call. I had been having trouble breathing for days, and when I finally decided to call, I was really having trouble staying awake. Those guys from the ambulance were really good, though. At first I thought that they must have been psychic! They knew right away that I had COPD and diabetes. They told me later, though, that they had noticed my oxygen stuff next to my television chair and the blood tester on the kitchen table. I think those guys saved my life. Actually, I'm sure of it."

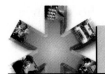

Perspective

Mike—The EMT

"So I got up to the door and knocked—standing off to one side, of course. I listened for a bit to make sure I didn't hear any signs of trouble. I yelled 'Ambulance!' and then listened again. I heard a moan right inside the door, so I looked through the nearest window. I saw an older woman lying on the linoleum . . . man, talk about cyanotic! She looked up at me and I could tell that she was in major panic mode. I noticed a nasal cannula on the kitchen floor and there was an O₂ tank over by a recliner."

Other items to consider in the scene size-up of the medical patient include:

✳ Observation of home oxygen devices, indicating chronic respiratory conditions

✳ Observation of hospital beds in a residence, indicating chronic illness

✳ The condition of the residence in reference to maintenance and cleanliness. Poor living conditions may reflect the overall health of the patient.

✳ Other evidence of illness, for example, in vomiting patients quickly checking the vomitus for evidence of blood.

✳ Odors including those from feces, spoiled foods, or poor hygiene.

MECHANISM OF INJURY

Upon approach to a patient you will first look for hazards to you, your crew, your patient, or bystanders. The **mechanism of injury (MOI)** that hurt the patient may still be capable of hurting you.

Once the scene is safe, you will approach. The observations you make of the scene and the forces that could have caused injury will give you an idea of the patient's potential injuries.

Consider the following situations:

✳ You are called to a motor vehicle collision. You arrive to find a vehicle on its roof. From the damage, it appears it may have rolled over more than once before it came to rest. You look inside the vehicle and see no one. About 20 feet into a ditch on the side of the road, you see a patient lying in an unnatural position.

✳ You are called to a motor vehicle collision. You arrive on a slippery road to find a vehicle into the guardrail. After assuring safety from oncoming traffic, you approach the vehicle. There is very minor damage. The operator of the vehicle is on his cell phone calling a tow truck and says to you. "I'm OK—just slid off the road."

The differences between these extremes are obvious. One patient is potentially very serious and the other appears to be minor or even unhurt. As we begin to

✳ **mechanism of injury (MOI)**

a force or forces that may have caused injury.

discuss mechanism of injury, it is important to note that patients who appear to have experienced a significant mechanism of injury are considered to have a serious injury until proven otherwise—even if they appear fine. The opposite is not true. If the mechanism of injury appears nonsignificant the patient still may be injured—possibly seriously.

In other words, MOI is a one-way sign: If the patient has a significant mechanism of injury they are considered serious, even if they appear without serious injury. If the MOI appears nonsignificant, there is no guarantee that the patient isn't serious.

Another term—used to describe what the mechanism of injury helps you to determine—is **index of suspicion**. This, simply stated, is identifying on the basis of the forces involved that injuries may be possible.

✳ **index of suspicion**

an awareness or suspicion that there may be injuries based on the evaluation of the mechanism of injury.

SIGNIFICANT VERSUS NONSIGNIFICANT MECHANISM OF INJURY

There are many ways a person can be injured. As a result, there is no realistic way to list every possible mechanism of injury that could be considered significant. Some of the commonly accepted factors in assessing significant mechanisms of injury in a motor vehicle collision include:

✳ Position of patient in the vehicle during impact

✳ Use of safety restraints/airbags

✳ Intrusion (crash damage) into the passenger compartment

✳ Approximate speed of vehicle(s)

✳ Object impacted

✳ Damage to inside of vehicle (e.g., bent steering wheel, starred windshield)

✳ Death of other occupant in same vehicle

MOTOR VEHICLE COLLISIONS

In motor vehicle collisions, there are commonly recognized injury patterns based on where the damage is found on the vehicle or the type of collision. Some of these patterns include:

Frontal Impact   In a frontal impact (Figure 9-12), the injuries to the patient depend on many factors. One of the most important is whether or not a patient is wearing a seat

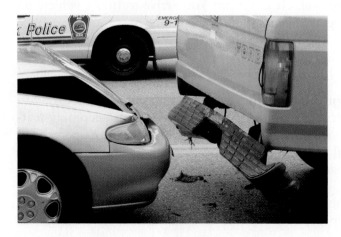

FIGURE 9-12   A collision showing frontal impact. (© Daniel Limmer.)

A.

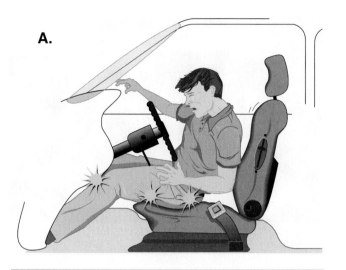

FIGURE 9-13A   In a head-on collision, an unrestrained person may travel in a down-and-under pathway, causing hip, knee, and leg injuries.

B.

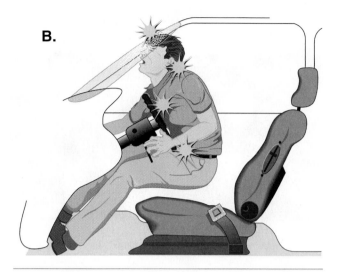

FIGURE 9-13B   In a head-on collision, an unrestrained person may travel in an up-and-over pathway, causing head, neck, chest, and abdominal injuries.

belt—and whether he was wearing it properly. Air bags will also reduce serious injury if deployed—but may even cause injury themselves.

There are two pathways in frontal collisions when patients aren't restrained by seatbelts—down-and-under and up-and-over (Figure 9-13A and B). These describe how the body travels after the collision.

The down-and-under pathway involves the lower body slipping downward in the seat toward the dashboard. Injury is seen in the knees, legs, and hip. There may be injuries to the chest and abdomen from the steering wheel.

The up-and-over pathway involves the body moving upward toward the steering wheel. Injury can be seen in the chest and abdomen from the steering wheel and head injuries from striking the windshield.

In both patterns, the use of seat belts and air bags (Figure 9-14) will offer some protection from these injuries.

Side Impact   In a side impact (Figure 9-15), neck injuries are common and potentially serious because of the significant force from the side causing lateral movement of the cervical spine. Note the amount of intrusion into the passenger compartment. Your

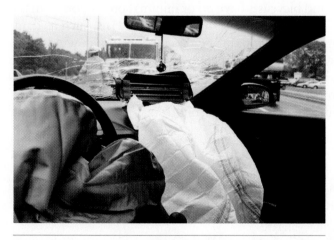

FIGURE 9-14   Air bags offer some protection from injuries. (© Daniel Limmer.)

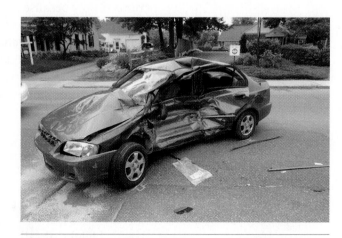

FIGURE 9-15   A collision showing side impact. (© Mark C. Ide.)

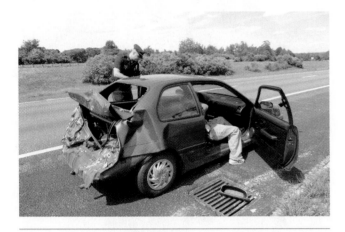

FIGURE 9-16   A rear-end collision. (© Mark C. Ide.)

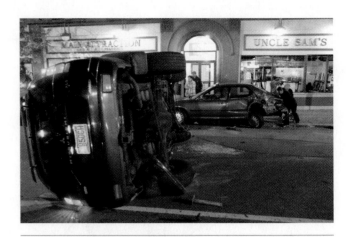

FIGURE 9-17   A rollover. (© Mark C. Ide.)

knowledge of anatomy and physiology may help you in determining possible injuries. Driver's side passengers may receive injury to the spleen, while those on the passenger side may receive liver injuries. Both of these organs can produce significant internal bleeding. Some vehicles now have side-impact air bags that can reduce injury in this type of collision.

Rear-End Collision   Rear-end collisions (Figure 9-16) cause sudden acceleration of the vehicle resulting in the patient initially being thrust backwards in the seat. Known for initially causing "whiplash" injuries to the neck, the patient may also be thrown forward after the initial impact and strike his or her head. Properly positioning the headrest helps reduce whiplash injury.

Rollover   Vehicles that roll over (Figure 9-17) can throw an unrestrained patient around the passenger compartment or partially or completely eject the patient from the vehicle, causing very serious injuries.

Rotational Impact   Vehicles that are struck in one of the quarter panels can be thrown into a spin. As the vehicle spins, the possibility of additional collisions is high. These secondary collisions may be with other vehicles or with stationary objects such as trees or utility poles. Injuries can occur to any part of the body.

Collisions with Pedestrians and Bicyclists   These collisions (Figure 9-18) are potentially serious simply because pedestrians and bicyclists have no or minimal protection from the size and weight of the automobile. You may see certain injury patterns, such as damage to the front of a vehicle from the initial impact or damage to the hood, windshield, or roof where the pedestrian was thrown after being "scooped up" by the vehicle (Figure 9-19). Injury patterns to the pedestrian or bicyclist include lower extremity injury from the initial hood or bumper impact, then injury to the upper body from striking the windshield of the car, and additional injuries from being thrown to the road.

FALLS

Falls are another way patients can be injured. Considerations in the MOI determination of a patient who experienced a fall include:

* Height of fall

* Type of surface landed upon

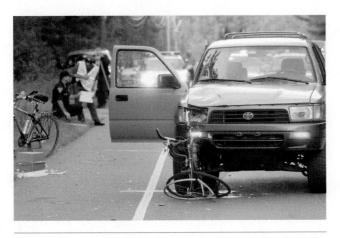

FIGURE 9-18   Collision with a bicyclist. (© Mark C. Ide.)

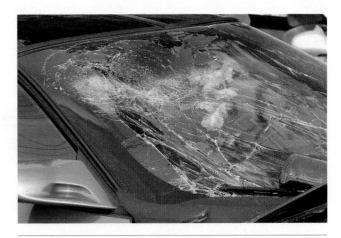

FIGURE 9-19   Damage to the front of the vehicle from the initial impact with a pedestrian. (© Ken Kerr.)

* Part of the body that hit the ground (head, feet, or side first)

* Did he strike anything on the way down? For example, did his head hit a brick ledge?

* Did anything break the fall, such as branches or a window awning?

BLUNT AND PENETRATING TRAUMA

Blunt trauma (Figure 9-20) occurs when an object strikes the body but doesn't physically enter the body. Examples of blunt trauma would be the chest striking the steering wheel or someone being struck by a baseball bat.

Key factors in determining the seriousness of a patient with blunt trauma are the location of the trauma, the item that caused the trauma, how many impacts there were with the blunt object, and the force used. You may observe redness, bruising, or deformity over the area in which the trauma occurred. Internal injuries are possible.

Penetrating trauma is most commonly thought of as knife or gunshot wounds but also includes accidents in which objects are **impaled** (remain in) in the body.

With penetrating trauma, you will see some sort of entry wound but you will not be able to visualize the internal damage caused by the penetration. In a penetrating wound, internal injuries will depend on factors such as the type of object, the length and width of the object, the direction the object was pointed when it entered the body, and the path of the object or bullet within the body.

✳ **blunt trauma**

injury caused by a blow to the body that does not penetrate the skin.

✳ **penetrating trauma**

injury caused by an object that passes through the skin.

✳ **impaled**

penetrating of the body by an object that remains in the body.

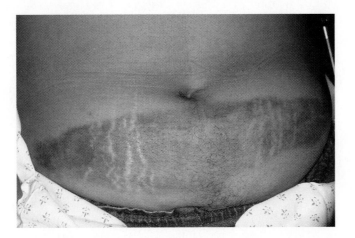

FIGURE 9-20   Blunt trauma occurs when an object strikes the body but doesn't physically enter the body. (Charles Stewart, M.D., and Associates.)

FIGURE 9-21 Cavitation wound.

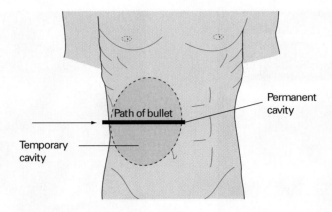

Bullets that enter the body can cause injury in a number of ways. The bullet itself enters the body and destroys any tissue in its path. The energy of the bullet also causes **cavitation** (Figure 9-21), that is, it causes expansion greater than the size of the bullet. It can stretch and tear tissue and may cause damage—or the tissue may simply return to its place without injury.

GUIDELINES FOR SIGNIFICANT MOI

What constitutes a significant MOI is open to interpretation. The following specific situations are generally considered significant mechanisms of injury:

- ✳ Ejection from a moving vehicle
- ✳ Death of a passenger within the same compartment of a vehicle
- ✳ Falls greater than 2–3 times the patient's height
- ✳ Roll-over of a moving vehicle
- ✳ High-speed vehicle collision
- ✳ Vehicle or pedestrian collision
- ✳ Driver or passenger of a motorcycle crash
- ✳ Penetrations of the head, chest, abdomen, or pelvis
- ✳ Significant blunt trauma to the head, chest, abdomen, or pelvis

✳ **cavitation**

expansion of tissue greater than the size of the bullet that penetrated the tissue. The tissue may stretch, tear, or simply return to its place without injury.

Stop, Review, Remember!

Multiple Choice

Place a check next to the correct answer.

1. You approach a motor vehicle collision in which there is a significant amount of impact into the driver's side of the vehicle. Based on your knowledge of anatomy and physiology, which abdominal organ of the driver may most likely be injured?

    _____ a. liver   _____ c. gall bladder

    _____ b. appendix _____ d. spleen

2. Which of the following statements about rear-end accidents is true?

    _____ a. Properly placed head rests can reduce neck injuries.

    _____ b. The down and under pathway is the most common.

    _____ c. Lateral movement of the neck is common in this type of crash.

    _____ d. The first impact often results in contact between the chest and steering wheel.

3. You are riding in the front passenger seat of your ambulance as you approach a collision scene. You notice that the power appears to be out at the houses and businesses near the crash scene. A likely first impression is that:

    _____ a. The power company is doing work in the area.

    _____ b. It is night time but everyone's lights are off.

    _____ c. The collision may have involved a utility pole and wires may be down.

    _____ d. The power company has turned the power off because they were notified that there was an accident at the scene.

4. A significant mechanism of injury tells an EMT that the patient is definitely injured.

    _____ a. true

    _____ b. false

5. Which of the following observations would NOT be significant as part of the nature of illness determination?

    _____ a. observing that the patient has vomited

    _____ b. observing the patient's level of distress

    _____ c. obtaining initial information from a bystander

    _____ d. obtaining a respiratory rate

Identifying

For each patient presentation below write "S" for significant and "N" for nonsignificant mechanism of injury.

1. _____ 3-year-old patient falling 11 feet

2. _____ motor vehicle collision with "starred" windshield

3. _____ man punched in the jaw during a fight

4. _____ woman ejected from a vehicle in a rollover

5. ____ alert child in a car where another passenger was killed

6. ____ a vehicle hit a tree at 75 mph

7. ____ an adult falls 3–4 feet

Critical Thinking

1. Does a significant mechanism of injury guarantee that a patient will be injured? Explain why or why not.

_____

_____

_____

_____

2. List three things that will help determine the damage caused to internal organs by penetrating injuries.

_____

_____

_____

_____

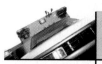 # Dispatch Summary

Once Mike and Erik got to Mrs. Roberts, they found that she was in severe respiratory distress. They began by providing oxygen at 15 liters per minute through a nonrebreather mask and ended up assisting her ventilations with a BVM. Mike also contacted dispatch and requested an immediate ALS intercept at their location.

The patient was transported to Southwest Medical Center where she was diagnosed with pneumonia complicated by other chronic respiratory conditions.

After six days in the ICU, she was released to a skilled nursing facility for ongoing care.

 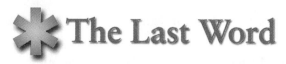 # The Last Word

We have mentioned several times in this chapter that the scene size-up sets the foundation for the entire call. This is true because:

* Safety on every call is critical. You can't help anyone if you are injured. Your BSI determination should prevent exposure while being practical and not going overboard unnecessarily.

* Your determinations about anything else you might need at the scene will get this assistance to you ASAP. Things like the power company, fire department, resources such as lifting assistance, or additional ambulances should be called early.

* And finally, there are clinical implications during the scene size-up. Examining the mechanism of injury will give you an idea of how serious the injuries could possibly be. The steps you take in assessment of the trauma patient are based on your mechanism of injury determination.

The nature of illness is your understanding of the type of complaint for a medical patient. Your observations of the patient, family members, and the scene in general give continued clues about the patient and his condition.

We tend to think of the scene size-up as scene safety and BSI, but you now know there is more. For the alert and interested EMT, the scene size-up sets the entire foundation of the call for safety, for efficiency, and clinically.

 Chapter Review

MULTIPLE CHOICE

Place a check next to the correct answer.

1. Which of the following would indicate a significant mechanism of injury?

   _____ a. an adult falling 5 feet

   _____ b. a motor vehicle collision with a bent steering wheel

   _____ c. a motor vehicle collision in which seat belts were used

   _____ d. a rear seat passenger in a motor vehicle collision

2. Which of the following statements about rotational collisions is false?

   _____ a. Rotational collisions are caused by impact in the front or rear sides of a vehicle.

   _____ b. Rotational collisions may involve multiple subsequent impacts.

   _____ c. Rotational collisions commonly cause "whiplash" injuries.

   _____ d. Rotational collisions can cause multiple or varied injury patterns.

3. Which of the following is NOT a factor in the mechanism of injury determination in a fall?

   _____ a. the height of the fall

   _____ b. the weight of the patient

   _____ c. the surface landed upon

   _____ d. the part of the body that hit the ground

4. When the velocity of a bullet causes expansion of tissue larger than the size of the bullet it is called:

   _____ a. pronation.

   _____ b. cavitation.

   _____ c. velocitation.

   _____ d. expectoration.

5. In a stab wound, the amount of internal damage is very predictable.

   _____ a. true

   _____ b. false

6. The index of suspicion is a numerical scale that rates the probability of serious injury from traumatic injury.

   _____ a. true

   _____ b. false

LISTING

List the components of a scene size-up.

1. _____

2. _____

3. _____

4. _____

5. _____

CRITICAL THINKING

1. You respond to a motor vehicle collision and find the driver in the car. There is significant damage to the front end of the vehicle. How will mechanism of injury determination in this case affect your patient care?

   _____

   _____

   _____

   _____

2. Explain the difference between blunt and penetrating trauma.

   _____

   _____

   _____

   _____

3. List four considerations in determining the mechanism of injury from a fall.

   _____

   _____

   _____

   _____

4. You are caring for a patient who was involved in a motor vehicle collision. His face struck the steering wheel and is bleeding. He may have lost a front tooth. What body substance isolation would be required for this patient? Why?

_____

_____

_____

_____

CASE STUDY

You are contacted by the police for an "intoxicated subject who needs a ride to the hospital or detox or something." You arrive in the early afternoon to find a house in a middle class neighborhood. A police officer meets you at the door. The officer unenthusiastically tells you, "He's upstairs."

You walk upstairs where you observe an obese male patient face down on the floor. You see a small puddle of blood near his forehead. The mattress is half off the bed, tilted down toward where the patient is found. You hear the patient's wife tell a second police officer "No, he is always drunk. He falls like this all the time." You call the patient's name as you approach.

1. What does this scene tell you about the patient's condition?

_____

_____

_____

_____

2. What BSI precautions will you take?

_____

_____

_____

_____

3. Is the patient drunk?

_____

_____

_____

_____

4. What resources, if any, will you need?

_____

_____

_____

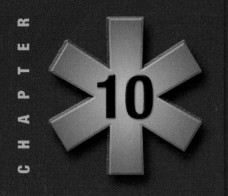

CHAPTER

10 Obtaining Vital Signs and a Medical History

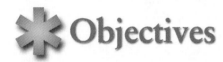
Objectives

Numbered objectives are from the U.S. Department of Transportation 1994 EMT-Basic National Standard Curriculum.

COGNITIVE OBJECTIVES

At the completion of this lesson, the EMT-Basic student will be able to:

1-5.1 Identify the components of vital signs. (pp. 253–254)

1-5.2 Describe the methods used to obtain a breathing rate. (p. 255)

1-5.3 Identify the attributes that should be obtained when assessing breathing. (pp. 255–260)

1-5.4 Differentiate between shallow, labored, and noisy breathing. (pp. 255–258)

1-5.5 Describe the methods to obtain a pulse rate. (pp. 262–264)

1-5.6 Identify the information obtained when assessing a patient's pulse. (pp. 262–264)

1-5.7 Differentiate between a strong, weak, regular, and irregular pulse. (pp. 264–265)

1-5.8 Describe the methods to assess the skin color, temperature, condition (capillary refill in infants and children). (pp. 274–279)

1-5.9 Identify the normal and abnormal skin colors. (pp. 274–275)

1-5.10 Differentiate between pale, blue, red, and yellow skin color. (pp. 274–275)

1-5.11 Identify the normal and abnormal skin temperature. (p. 275)

1-5.12 Differentiate between hot, cool, and cold skin temperature. (p. 275)

1-5.13 Identify normal and abnormal skin conditions. (p. 275)

1-5.14 Describe normal and abnormal capillary refill in infants and children. (pp. 276–277)

1-5.15 Describe the methods to assess the pupils. (pp. 277–279)

1-5.16 Identify normal and abnormal pupil size. (pp. 277–278)

1-5.17 Differentiate between dilated (big) and constricted (small) pupil size. (pp. 277–279)

1-5.18 Differentiate between reactive and nonreactive pupils and equal and unequal pupils. (pp. 277–279)

1-5.19 Describe two methods for assessing blood pressure. (p. 266)

1-5.20 Define systolic pressure. (p. 266)

1-5.21 Define diastolic pressure. (p. 266)

1-5.22 Explain the difference between auscultation and palpation for obtaining a blood pressure. (pp. 266, 269–272)

1-5.23 Identify the components of the SAMPLE history. (pp. 285–287)

1-5.24 Differentiate between a sign and a symptom. (pp. 252–253)

1-5.25 State the importance of accurately reporting and recording the baseline vital signs. (pp. 253–254)

1-5.26 Discuss the need to search for additional medical identification. (p. 289)

AFFECTIVE OBJECTIVES

At the completion of this lesson, the EMT-Basic student will be able to:

1-5.27   Explain the value of performing the baseline vital signs. (p. 251)

1-5.28   Recognize and respond to the feelings patients experience during assessment. (pp. 284–285)

1-5.29   Defend the need for obtaining and recording an accurate set of vital signs. (pp. 253–254)

1-5.30   Explain the rationale of recording additional sets of vital signs. (pp. 254–255, 277)

1-5.31   Explain the importance of obtaining a SAMPLE history. (pp. 285–287)

PSYCHOMOTOR OBJECTIVES

At the completion of this lesson, the EMT-Basic student will be able to:

1-5.32   Demonstrate the skills involved in assessment of breathing. (p. 255)

1-5.33   Demonstrate the skills associated with obtaining a pulse. (pp. 262–264)

1-5.34   Demonstrate the skills associated with assessing the skin color, temperature, condition, and capillary refill in infants and children. (pp. 274–277)

1-5.35   Demonstrate the skills associated with assessing the pupils. (pp. 277–279)

1-5.36   Demonstrate the skills associated with obtaining blood pressure. (pp. 270–272)

1-5.37   Demonstrate the skills that should be used to obtain information from the patient, family, or bystanders at the scene. (pp. 284–288)

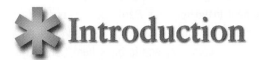 **Introduction**

Taking vital signs and gathering a medical history are not the first things you will do when caring for a patient, and they are not the last things you will do. These tasks always fall somewhere in the middle of your overall patient assessment. We are introducing them here to give you the opportunity to begin practicing these two very important skills. As you will learn later in your training, vital signs and history are taken at specific times during your patient assessment.

Every EMT must eventually master the obtaining and recording of accurate vital signs and the gathering of a detailed patient history. We say "eventually" because it is unrealistic to expect that you will master these skills during your initial EMT training. The objective of this chapter is to help you develop a clear understanding of the purpose and components of these skills. This understanding will be the foundation for hands-on practice during your EMT training. Our hope is that, by the end of your EMT training, you will have the understanding, competency, and confidence to obtain and record accurate vital signs and a medical history on actual patients.

During your initial training, you can take vital signs and gather history information on fellow students and perhaps healthy friends and family members. For the most part, you will be obtaining normal vital sign values and histories. It's a whole new experience when you finally get to take vital signs and obtain a medical history on a real patient in the field or clinical setting.

When caring for actual patients, there is a strong likelihood that the values you obtain will not be within normal limits. This can be challenging at first, and you may question the accuracy of your readings. It will be important to take your time and be patient. Ask your partner to check the signs and compare your results. With enough practice on actual patients, you will quickly gain the same confidence you had in the classroom.

What is important to understand is that developing your vital-sign and history-taking skills can take many months and even years before you become confident in all situations.

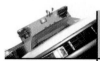

Emergency Dispatch

Derrick and Ray, two EMTs assigned to truck #53 on the south side of town, are just finishing the paperwork on a nonemergent transfer from Filmore Assisted Living to Southwest Hospital when their pagers start vibrating. Ray sighs, pulls the pager from its clip, and reads it.

"They're calling us out for an emergency," he says. Ray replaces the pager on his belt and starts out the door with the stretcher.

"What about 48?" Derrick trails after him with his unfinished paperwork. "I thought 48 was on post and available."

Once in the truck, Ray keys the radio mic and tells dispatch that they're ready for information on the new call.

"Unit 53, please respond to 2305 South Walker Avenue, 2-3-0-5 South Walker, for a priority-two sick person."

Ray pulls the truck out of the Southwest Hospital ambulance parking area, and within minutes they arrive 14 blocks away at the South Walker address.

The small house is set back off of the road with high weeds growing in the front yard, and Derrick and Ray have to fight to get the stretcher, piled with their equipment, to the front door. Derrick knocks on the door and an elderly woman wearing a robe and smoking a cigarette appears. "My son is back here," she says, leading them to a room in the back of the house. "He's been sick for three days. It's just coming out of both ends, you know? He can't keep anything down."

They find the patient, a thin, pale 55-year-old man named Dick, sitting on the edge of his bed with a garbage can containing vomit on the floor in front of him. Ray gets the stethoscope, blood pressure cuff, and a penlight from the jump bag and approaches the man. "Let's see how you're doing, Dick."

1-5.24 Differentiate between a sign and a symptom.

Signs and Symptoms

A lesson on vital signs would not be complete without first discussing the difference between a sign and a symptom. It will also be necessary to understand why certain signs are referred to as "vital" signs while other signs are not. Let's begin our discussion by defining the terms *sign* and *symptom*.

Just like in your daily life, a **sign** is something that you, the EMT, can see or observe or that has a value that can be recorded. For instance, you can see the stop sign at the intersection near your house or the exit sign near the door in the classroom where you are taking your EMT training.

Patients display many signs relating to their current medical condition that we can observe or obtain during assessment, such as skin color, pulse rate, and breath-

✳ **sign**

something that the EMT can see or observe or has a value that can be recorded.

TABLE 10-1	DIFFERENTIATING SIGNS AND SYMPTOMS
EXAMPLES OF SIGNS	**EXAMPLES OF SYMPTOMS**
Skin color, temperature, and moisture	Fatigue
Pulse rate, strength, and regularity	Nausea
Vomiting	Pain
Blood pressure	Headache
Bruise	Double vision
Deformity	Lightheadedness
Swelling	Thirst

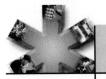

Perspective

Ray—The EMT

"The first thing that I noticed about this guy was that he was obviously sick. He complained of everything from fatigue and lightheadedness to chills and nausea. I could feel that he was running a pretty high fever and, based on the poor turgor of his skin, I'm pretty sure that he was very dehydrated."

ing rate. Some of these signs, such as skin color and breathing rate, we can observe without ever touching the patient. Others, such as pulse rate and blood pressure, require that we touch the patient or use a specialized piece of equipment to obtain a reading or value for the sign.

A **symptom** is very different. We cannot see symptoms; the patient experiences and must describe them to us. The most common symptom that we encounter with our patients is pain. We cannot "see" pain, we can only see signs of it on a patient's face. They must tell us they have pain. Nausea, dizziness, and blurred vision are all symptoms the patient must describe to us. Table 10-1 provides more examples of both signs and symptoms.

∗ **symptom**

something that is experienced and described by the patient as it pertains to his chief complaint.

Vital Signs

Some signs are more important than others—so important in fact that if they are absent it could mean that the patient is clinically dead. The most important of these signs are referred to as "vital" signs because they are vital to life.

1-5.1 Identify the components of vital signs.

1-5.25 State the importance of accurately reporting and recording the baseline vital signs.

Vital Signs

∗ Respirations (presence or absence, rate, depth, and ease)

∗ Pulse (presence or absence, rate, strength, and rhythm)

✳ Blood pressure

✳ Skin signs (color, temperature, and moisture)

✳ Pupils (equality and reactivity to light)

While it can be argued that skin and pupil signs are not exactly vital to life, they are often included in the list of vital signs because they are relatively easy to assess and can tell us a great deal about the patient's current condition.

BASELINE VITAL SIGNS

✳ **baseline vital signs**
the very first set of vital signs obtained on a patient.

Baseline vital signs is a term commonly used that simply refers to the very first set of vital signs obtained on the patient during a call. Baseline vital signs are very important because they establish a standard (baseline) to which all subsequent vital signs will be compared (Figure 10-1).

TRENDING

✳ **trending**
the comparing of multiple sets of vital signs over a period of time in order to reveal a trend in the patient's condition.

A single set of vital signs is an observation. Looking at two sets of vital signs is a comparison. Being able to compare multiple sets of vital signs can reveal a "trend" in the patient's condition. Be careful not to jump too quickly to a conclusion after obtaining your baseline vitals. A single set of vital signs gives us nothing more than a quick "snapshot" of a patient's condition. In fact, it may have very little value unless we can compare it to subsequent sets of vital signs. The taking, recording, and comparing of multiple sets of vital signs over a period of time is called **trending** and is the most accurate method of determining a patient's condition or status.

Taking the vital signs is only half the battle. Being able to accurately record your findings to share with other EMS professionals is just as important. It is impossible to overstate the importance of recording the time vitals were taken and

Clinical Clues: TRENDING

A single set of vital signs is an observation, two sets of vital signs is a comparison, and three sets of vital signs reveal a trend. For stable patients, obtain as many sets of vital signs as practical to reveal any trends in the patient's condition.

FIGURE 10-1 EMT taking vital signs on an adult patient.

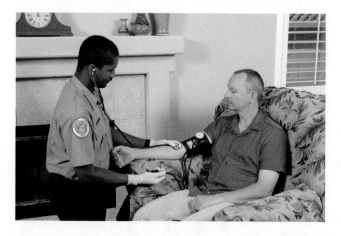

the values. Without a time to reference with each set of vitals, it becomes impossible to know which set came first or how much time elapsed between them, which makes them unusable for purposes of trending. Always record the time with each set of vital signs.

The exact order in which you take and/or record patient vital signs is not all that important. Your instructor will most likely provide a format for recording vital signs that is used in the area or region where you will be working. What is important is that you obtain and record accurate and complete vital signs in a way that will allow for easy comparison. For purposes of consistency while learning this new skill, the following order and format is recommended:

TIME	RESPIRATIONS	PULSE	BP	SKIN	PUPILS

This format allows for easy comparison of multiple sets of vital signs and presents the first three (the most vital of the vital signs) in the order they are most likely going to be obtained while caring for a patient. Again, we don't want you to spend too much time worrying about a format at this point when completeness is the goal. However, like many of the skills you will be learning throughout your training, deciding on a format and sticking to it will minimize the chances that you will skip or forget something important.

Assessing Breathing

Breathing is typically the first vital sign you will be able to assess as you approach your patient. It can reveal a great deal about a patient in less time and with less effort than the other signs. In other words, if your patient is breathing, it is safe to assume he has a pulse and therefore a blood pressure.

In responsive patients, the presence of breathing can often be easily detected from a distance, as you first enter the scene and observe the patient. You will be looking for signs of adequate versus inadequate respirations as you approach (Table 10-2).

For unresponsive patients, the assessment is not so easy from a distance. You may not be able to perform an adequate assessment until you are right next to the patient. In fact, it may be necessary for you to open the airway and place your ear next to the patient's nose and mouth to listen for breathing as you observe the chest for rise and fall.

As you first begin to practice the skill of taking respirations in the classroom, it is easiest to have your patient lying flat in a supine position. Now grasp his wrist, as if you were going to take a pulse, and lay it across his abdomen (Figure 10-2A on page 256). This technique has two benefits. The first is that the patient thinks you are taking his pulse and is less likely to alter his breathing pattern. The second is that you can actually feel the movement of the abdomen as he breathes, and you don't have to stare at his chest, making it obvious that you are counting each breath. Once you have mastered this in the supine-position technique, you can then use the same technique for a patient in the sitting position (Figure 10-2B on page 256).

1-5.2   Describe the methods used to obtain a breathing rate.

1-5.3   Identify the attributes that should be obtained when assessing breathing.

1-5.4   Differentiate between shallow, labored, and noisy breathing.

TABLE 10-2 RESPIRATIONS

NORMAL RESPIRATORY RATES (BREATHS PER MINUTE, AT REST)

Adult	12 to 20
	Above 24: Serious
	Below 10: Serious
Infants and Children	
Adolescent 11–14 years	12 to 20
School age 6–10 years	15 to 30
Preschooler 3–5 years	20 to 30
Toddler 1–3 years	20 to 30
Infant 6–12 months	20 to 30
Infant 0–5 months	25 to 40
Newborn	30 to 50

RESPIRATORY SOUNDS	**POSSIBLE CAUSES/INTERVENTIONS**
Snoring	Airway blocked/Open patient's airway; prompt transport.
Wheezing	Medical problem such as asthma/Assist patient in taking prescribed medications; prompt transport
Gurgling	Fluids in airway/Suction airway; prompt transport
Crowing (harsh sound when inhaling)	Medical problem that cannot be treated on the scene/Prompt transport

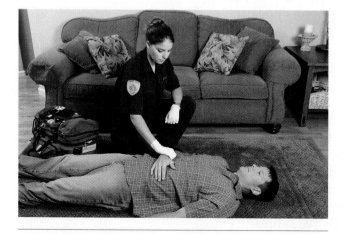

FIGURE 10-2A EMT using the supine-position technique to take respirations.

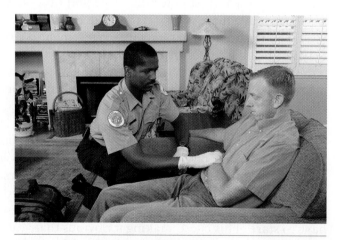

FIGURE 10-2B EMT using the sitting-position technique to take respirations.

CHARACTERISTICS OF RESPIRATIONS

There are four characteristics of respirations that must be assessed and recorded on each patient. They are as follows:

Characteristics of Respirations

✳ Rate

✳ Depth

✳ Ease

✳ Sounds

Some texts group the characteristics of depth, ease, and sounds under the heading "quality." We have broken them out here for ease of understanding.

BREATHING RATE

While it may not be the first thing you will notice about a patient's respirations, you must determine an accurate count of how many times the patient is breathing each minute. All breathing rates are recorded as a per-minute value. To obtain the most accurate value possible, the EMT would have to count respirations for an entire minute. However, this wastes valuable time in the field and may delay important interventions.

Clinical Clues: RESPIRATORY RATE COUNTING

Two common methods for obtaining respiratory rate are as follows:

✳ Count respirations for 30 seconds × 2 = Minute Rate

✳ Count respirations for 15 seconds × 4 = Minute Rate

There are at least two faster methods commonly used for obtaining a breathing rate on patients in the field setting. One method is counting the respirations (1 inhalation plus 1 exhalation = 1 respiration) for 30 seconds and multiplying that value by 2 to get the minute rate. The second method is counting respirations for 15 seconds and multiplying by 4 to get the minute rate. Regardless of which method you use, you should arrive at the same or very similar values. It should be noted that the smaller your sample, the less accurate your value will be. Using samples of less than 15 seconds is not recommended. Also, if your patient has an irregular breathing pattern, you may want to take the time to count the respirations for a full minute to get the most accurate rate.

Every attempt should be made to obtain a respiratory rate without the knowledge of the patient. Once a patient knows you are counting his respirations, he may subconsciously alter his rate. Also, attempting to count respirations while the patient is speaking may result in an inaccurate assessment. You may have to stop asking history questions in order to assess the breathing rate and get an accurate count. Wait for an appropriate time to assess rate.

DEPTH OF BREATHING

Depth of breathing, sometimes referred to as **tidal volume**, is the amount of air moved in and out with each breath. It can be assessed simply by observing the

✳ **tidal volume**

the amount of air moved in and out with each breath.

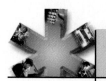

Perspective

Derrick—The EMT

"I let Ray jump right in and get the vitals on this patient. I always have a really hard time with vitals. I think it's mostly the math that gets me, if you know what I mean. You know, what really bothered me about this call, though, is that the other south side truck, number 48, is available, and yet dispatch sent us. That just doesn't make sense, but at least someone is arriving, and we'll do our best.'"

patient's chest for adequate rise and fall. Assessing for adequate tidal volume (depth) can be difficult for the new EMT, because normal tidal volume is often shallow to begin with. It takes time and practice to learn the difference between normal and shallow respirations.

For some patients, the abdomen moves more than the chest during normal breathing. For this reason, you must observe both the chest and abdomen when assessing tidal volume.

Depth of respirations can be characterized as one of the following:

* Normal or good tidal volume (GTV)
* Deep
* Shallow

EASE OF BREATHING

The ease with which a patient is breathing will reveal a lot about his current respiratory status. A patient who is oxygenating well will be breathing easily and will show little if any work of breathing. His respirations can be described as unlabored. On the contrary, a patient in respiratory distress will likely be using accessory muscles and laboring much harder to move air. Labored respirations can be further characterized as mild, moderate, or severe to indicate the patient's level of distress.

You must also observe for the presence of retractions during inspiration. This is the drawing in of the soft tissues, most commonly in the areas above the clavicles and between the ribs. Retractions are most obvious with pediatric patients who are in moderate to severe respiratory distress.

Ease of respirations is described in one of the following ways:

* Unlabored
* Labored (mild, moderate, or severe)

BREATH SOUNDS

Once you are next to the patient, you may be able to hear certain sounds associated with his breathing. Be extra alert when caring for a patient with noisy respirations, as this is almost always a sign of partial airway obstruction! The following are names and descriptions of some of the abnormal sounds that may be heard when a patient breathes. Some sounds may only be heard when using a stethoscope:

∗ **Wheezing**—This is a high-pitched sound that is indicative of lower airway constriction. Wheezing can be heard during both inhalation and exhalation but is more commonly heard during exhalation. Mild wheezes may only be heard with a stethoscope.

∗ **Stridor**—This harsh, high-pitched sound can occur during inhalation or exhalation and is indicative of partial upper airway obstruction. Stridor is heard best in the upper chest or neck area.

∗ **Crackles**—These are fine crackling sounds that can be heard with a stethoscope during inhalation as air is forced through fluid or mucus in the lower airways.

Not all sounds are going to be easily audible. As an EMT you must also assess for the presence or absence of sounds deep within the lungs. To adequately assess lung sounds, you must use an appropriate stethoscope.

You will use the stethoscope to listen over several areas of the chest and back for appropriate or abnormal lung sounds (Figure 10-3). Lung sounds are made by air as it moves in and out of the lungs. When assessing these sounds you are listening for:

∗ the presence of sounds in all lung fields.

∗ equal sounds on both sides of the chest.

∗ clear sounds free of crackles, stridor, or wheezing.

The following are examples of appropriate ways to document respirations:

∗ 16, unlabored with good tidal volume

∗ 24, labored and deep

∗ 8, unlabored and shallow

∗ 32, labored and shallow

∗ **wheezing**

a high-pitched sound that is indicative of lower airway constriction and can be heard during both inspiration and expiration but is more commonly heard during expiration

∗ **stridor**

a harsh high-pitched sound that generally occurs during inhalation but can also occur during exhalation, indicative of partial upper airway obstruction.

∗ **crackles**

a fine-crackling or bubbling sound heard upon inspiration. The sound is caused as air passes through fluid in the alveoli or by the opening of closed alveoli.

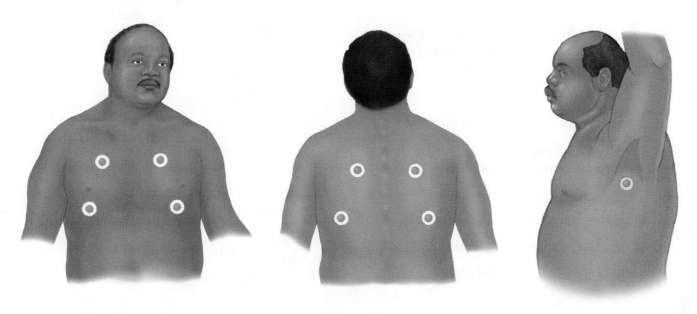

FIGURE 10-3 Auscultate for breath sounds on the upper and lower chest, the upper and lower back, and at the midaxillary line.

To assess a patient's breathing, follow these steps:

1. Take appropriate BSI precautions.
2. Grasp the wrist of the patient as if you were taking his pulse and place his forearm firmly against the upper abdomen.
3. While looking at your watch, feel the movement of each breath against his forearm as you continue to hold it.
4. Count the number of respirations for 15 or 30 seconds and multiply by the appropriate number to get a minute rate.
5. Record the rate along with the characteristics of depth and ease.

* Stop, Review, Remember!

Multiple Choice

Place a check next to the correct answer.

1. Which of the following best describes the difference between a sign and a symptom?

   _____ a. A sign is something the EMT can see or measure; a symptom is something the patient complains about.

   _____ b. A sign is something the patient complains about and a symptom is something the EMT can see or measure.

   _____ c. Assessing signs requires the use of special equipment (blood pressure cuff) while symptoms do not.

   _____ d. Signs and symptoms are essentially the same thing.

2. Which of the following contains the appropriate characteristics of respirations?

   _____ a. rate, depth, and quality

   _____ b. rate, ease, and quality

   _____ c. rate, depth, and ease

   _____ d. rate, depth, and rhythm

3. Which of the following best describes an adult patient who is breathing adequately?

   _____ a. 18, labored, deep

   _____ b. 8, unlabored, shallow

   _____ c. 26, labored, shallow

   _____ d. 12, unlabored, good tidal volume

4. _____ is a high-pitched sound more commonly heard during exhalation than inhalation. It is indicative of lower airway constriction.

   _____ a. stridor

   _____ b. wheezing

   _____ c. crowing

   _____ d. grunting

5. Good tidal volume is a term that most accurately describes which characteristic of breathing?

   _____ a. rate

   _____ b. depth

   _____ c. ease

   _____ d. rhythm

Fill in the Blank

1. A _____ is something that you the EMT can see or observe.

2. A _____ is something the patient describes or complains of.

3. Skin signs and _____ are not exactly vital to life, but they can tell us a great deal about the patient's current condition.

4. The first set of vital signs taken on any patient is referred to as _____ vitals.

5. _____ are recorded as a per-minute value.

Critical Thinking

1. Why is time so important when recording multiple sets of vital signs for the same patient?

   _____

   _____

   _____

   _____

   _____

2. Describe the difference between a sign and a symptom.

   _____

   _____

   _____

   _____

   _____

3. What is meant by the term "baseline" vital signs? Why are baseline vital signs so important?

   _____

   _____

   _____

   _____

   _____

✳ **carotid pulse**

the pulse point located on either side of the anterior neck lateral to the trachea.

✳ **brachial pulse**

pulse point felt in two locations: on the inside of the upper arm and over the medial aspect of the anterior elbow.

✳ **radial pulse**

pulse point located over the lateral aspect of the anterior wrist.

✳ **femoral pulse**

pulse point located deep in the groin between the hip and the inside of the upper thigh.

✳ **popliteal pulse**

pulse point located over the posterior aspect of the knee.

✳ **dorsalis pedis (pedal) pulse**

pulse point located over the anterior foot.

✳ **posterior tibial pulse**

pulse point located over the medial ankle just posterior to the ankle bone.

Assessing the Pulse

A pulse can be thought of as a remote heartbeat. It is the pulsation of the artery as it swells under the pressure of the rushing blood each time the heart pumps. If we could open up the body and see the entire network of arteries, we would see that arteries all pulsate along their entire length. We are only able to feel this pulsing at specific points on the body where the artery lies close to the skin and directly over a firm structure such as a bone. There are several "pulse points" throughout the body, some more easily palpated than others (Figure 10-4). The following is a list of the most common pulse points and their location on the body:

- ✳ **Carotid**—located in the anterior neck
- ✳ **Brachial**—felt in two locations: on the inside of the upper arm and over the medial aspect of the anterior elbow
- ✳ **Radial**—located over the lateral aspect of the anterior wrist
- ✳ **Femoral**—located deep in the groin between the hip and the inside of the upper leg
- ✳ **Popliteal**—located over the posterior aspect of the knee
- ✳ **Dorsalis pedis (pedal)**—located over the anterior (dorsal) foot
- ✳ **Posterior tibial**—located over the medial ankle just posterior to the ankle bone

The most common pulse point used to assess the pulse of a responsive patient is the radial pulse (Figure 10-5). Palpating the radial pulse is less intrusive than pal-

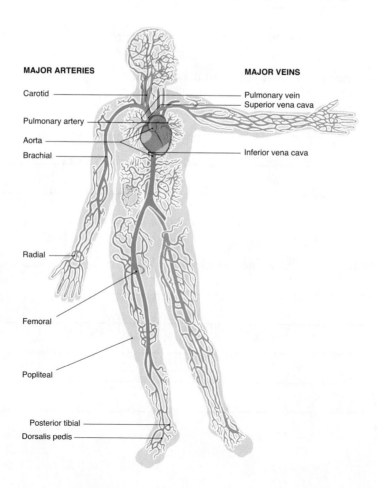

FIGURE 10-4 Pulse points and major arteries throughout the body.

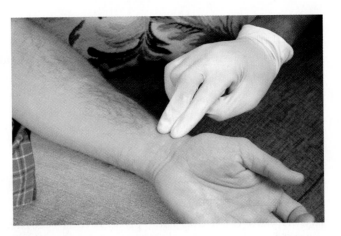

FIGURE 10-5   Proper radial pulse point in the adult patient.

pating the carotid pulse and is as natural as shaking someone's hand as you greet them. The radial pulse is preferred for all responsive patients 1 year and older.

For unresponsive patients older than one year, the carotid pulse is preferred (Figure 10-6), because the carotid is a "central" pulse. It is also one of the last pulses to go away as blood pressure drops and in situations of shock or hypoperfusion. The femoral pulse is also considered a central pulse, because it is located within the core of the body. In contrast, the brachial, radial, and pedal pulse points are called peripheral pulses because they are located in the periphery of the body.

As blood pressure drops, the peripheral pulses become less reliable and can become difficult to palpate. For this reason, the carotid pulse should always be assessed before beginning CPR on any patient over 1 year old and the brachial pulse for patients less than 1 year old (Figure 10-7). Do not assess both carotid pulses at the same time, as this may reduce the blood flow to the brain.

Becoming proficient at palpating pulses requires lots of practice. There are essentially two elements you must master if you want to develop proficiency at taking pulses. The first element is location. You must place your fingers in the correct place or you will not feel the pulse. The second element is pressure. You must learn the correct amount of pressure for each pulse point or you risk not feeling the pulse. Too much pressure and you may cut off the pulse completely. Too little pressure and you will not feel the pulsations. Once you learn these two elements, you will be well on your way to mastering the skill of assessing pulses.

When first learning to assess pulses, you must experiment with different techniques of palpation. Some EMTs have better luck using the tips of the fingers while others prefer the pads of the fingers. Some prefer using two fingers to locate a pulse

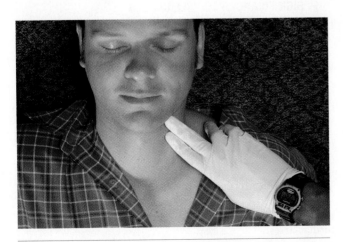

FIGURE 10-6   Proper carotid pulse point in the adult patient.

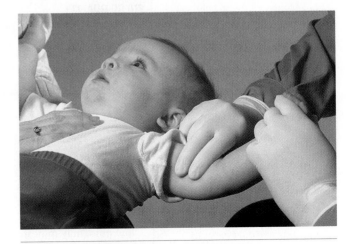

FIGURE 10-7   Brachial pulse point in the infant.

1-5.5 Describe the methods to obtain a pulse rate.

1-5.6 Identify the information obtained when assessing a patient's pulse.

1-5.7 Differentiate between a strong, weak, regular, and irregular pulse.

✳ **bradycardia**

a pulse rate below 60 beats per minute.

✳ **tachycardia**

a pulse rate greater than 100 beats per minute.

while others prefer three fingers. You must try all combinations, and eventually you will find the technique that works best for you.

When assessing a patient's pulse, the EMT should identify the following three characteristics:

✳ Rate

✳ Strength

✳ Rhythm

RATE

Just as with breathing rate, pulse rate is recorded as the number of pulsations (beats) felt in one minute. The same two methods can be used for determining a minute rate for a pulse as are used for breathing. Count the pulse for either 15 seconds and multiply by 4 or 30 seconds and multiply by 2.

The normal range for pulse rates in adults is between 60 and 100 beats per minute. A pulse rate below 60 is referred to as **bradycardia** and a pulse rate greater than 100 is called **tachycardia** (Table 10-3).

TABLE 10-3 PULSE RATES	
NORMAL PULSE RATES (BEATS PER MINUTE, AT REST)	
Adult	60 to 100
Infants and Children	
Adolescent 11–14 years	60 to 105
School age 6–10 years	70 to 110
Preschooler 3–5 years	80 to 120
Toddler 1–3 years	80 to 130
Infant 6–12 months	80 to 140
Infant 0–5 months	90 to 140
Newborn	120 to 160
PULSE QUALITY	**SIGNIFICANCE/POSSIBLE CAUSES**
Rapid and regular	Exertion, fright, fever, high blood pressure, first stage of blood loss
Rapid and regular	Shock, later stages of blood loss
Slow	Head injury, drugs, some poisons, some heart problems, lack of oxygen in children
Irregular	Possible Abnormal Electrical Heart Activity (Arrythmia)
No pulse	Cardiac arrest (clinical death)

Infants and Children: A high pulse in an infant or child is not as great a concern as a low pulse. A low pulse may indicate imminent cardiac arrest.

Clinical Clues: PULSE

Be careful: Sometimes the reason why you may be feeling the pulse as weak is that you are not directly over the pulse point or you are not using the appropriate amount of pressure. The strength of a pulse is simply recorded as either strong or weak.

STRENGTH

Pulses can be anywhere from absent to weak to strong. Many factors contribute to each circumstance. As you learn to assess pulses on fellow classmates, you will find most of them to be strong because all of you are likely young and healthy. You may not ever get to feel a weak pulse until you finally work in the field and encounter patients with real medical problems. The key is to practice taking pulses every chance you get with as many different people as possible. Eventually you will feel pulses that you will describe as weak.

RHYTHM

The rhythm of a pulse is a very important characteristic, because it may reveal a serious heart problem. Normal pulses have a steady, constant, regular rhythm, much like a metronome. Pulses that seem erratic or that skip beats are considered irregular. As an EMT you will record the rhythm of a patient's pulse as either regular or irregular.

To assess the pulse of a patient, follow these steps:

1. Take appropriate BSI precautions.
2. For a responsive patient, grasp the patient's wrist and locate the radial pulse point with the tips of at least two fingers. For an unresponsive patient, locate the carotid artery in the neck.
3. While looking at your watch, count the pulsations of the artery for 15 or 30 seconds and multiply by the appropriate number, 4 or 2 respectively, to get a minute rate.
4. Record the rate along with the characteristics of strength and rhythm.

Assessing Blood Pressure

Blood pressure is the pressure inside the arterial system. It is a very dynamic value and changes constantly as we move about our day. Factors such as blood loss, stress, ambient temperature, and exertion can all influence a patient's blood pressure. In general, the better the blood pressure, the better the perfusion, although this is not universal.

Blood pressure is most often recorded as two separate numbers separated by a horizontal line such as 120/80 (Table 10-4). These two numbers represent two different pressures within the arterial system of the body. Blood pressures are measured in millimeters of mercury (mmHg). Hg is the chemical symbol for mercury on the periodic table of elements. The old style of blood pressure gauges (sphygmomanometers) used the heavy metal mercury much as conventional thermometers do today. Because these were not practical for use in the field,

TABLE 10-4	NORMAL BLOOD PRESSURES IN ADULTS, CHILDREN, AND INFANTS	
PATIENT	**SYSTOLIC**	**DIASTOLIC**
Adult Male	100 + age in years to age 40	60 to 90 mmHg
Adult Female	90 + age in years to age 40	60 to 90 mmHg
Adolescent	90 mmHg (lower limit of normal)	⅔ of systolic pressure
Child 1 to 10 years	90 + (2 × age in years) (upper limit of normal) 70 + (2 × age in years) (lower limit of normal)	⅔ of systolic pressure
Infant 1 to 12 months	70 mmHg (lower limit of normal)	⅔ of systolic pressure

1-5.22 Explain the difference between auscultation and palpation for obtaining a blood pressure.

✳ **auscultation**

the act of listening for sounds made by internal organs such as the lungs and the heart. Also the technique used to listen for pulse sounds when obtaining a blood pressure

✳ **palpation**

the act of examining by feeling with the hands. Also a technique used for obtaining a blood pressure reading.

1-5.20 Define systolic pressure.

✳ **systolic**

the pressure created when the left ventricle contracts and forces blood out into the arteries.

1-5.21 Define diastolic pressure.

✳ **diastolic**

the pressure remaining in the arteries when the left ventricle of the heart is relaxed and refilling.

1-5.19 Describe two methods for assessing blood pressure.

newer fluidless (aneroid) gauges had to be developed. Even though the gauges used in the field today do not contain mercury, they are still calibrated in millimeters of mercury.

There are two methods for obtaining a blood pressure in the field. The **auscultation** (hearing) method requires the use of a blood pressure cuff and a stethoscope, while the **palpation** (feeling) method requires only a blood pressure cuff.

It is recommended that blood pressure be assessed in all patients over the age of 3. Patients under the age of 3 require an especially small blood pressure cuff, and because they move around so much, it is difficult to measure their blood pressure in the field. When assessing young pediatric patients, it is advised that you rely on signs and symptoms other than blood pressure, along with your general impression and other exam findings, to determine the indicated care. These signs and symptoms are often more valuable and take less time to assess.

SYSTOLIC PRESSURE

In a blood pressure reading such as 120/80—which may be spoken as "120 over 80"—the top number is called the **systolic** reading and reflects the pressure inside the artery each time the heart's left ventricle contracts.

DIASTOLIC PRESSURE

The bottom number is called the **diastolic** reading and reflects the pressure inside the artery each time the heart rests between beats.

THE BLOOD PRESSURE (BP) CUFF

The blood pressure cuff is a simple device consisting of a flat bladder (balloon) with two tubes coming off one side. The bladder is contained within a simple fabric cuff or pouch with a Velcro closure. A bulb-and-valve combination is placed on one tube, and the gauge is placed on the other tube (Figure 10-8).

Cuffs come in many sizes, and it is best to use the correct size when taking a blood pressure. A cuff is the correct size if the bladder inside the cuff can cover ap-

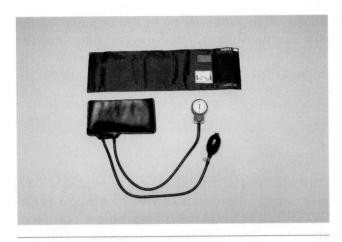

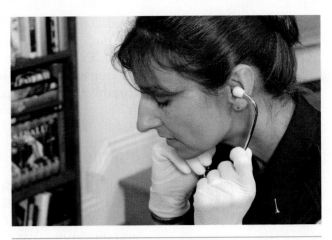

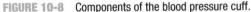

FIGURE 10-8 Components of the blood pressure cuff.

FIGURE 10-9 The proper use of a stethoscope.

proximately 80 percent of the patient's upper arm. For a child under the age of 13, it should cover 100 percent of the arm. A cuff that is too narrow will result in high pressure readings.

To properly place the BP cuff on a patient's arm, pick it up with both hands so that you can feel the top corners of the bladder with the thumb and forefinger of each hand. Now, with the labels facing you, place the center of the bladder directly over the brachial artery located on the inside of the upper arm. The cuff should be placed high enough on the arm to allow access to the brachial pulse point on the anterior aspect of the elbow.

THE STETHOSCOPE

It has been said that the stethoscope is the most important diagnostic tool ever developed. While this may be debatable, what is not debatable is the importance and challenge of learning to use it properly. Like any tool, it must be used often if you ever hope to develop mastery in using it (Figure 10-9).

The typical stethoscope has three main parts:

* Ear pieces
* Tubing
* Diaphragm head

It is important that both the ear pieces and the head be adjusted and placed properly to ensure that you will be able to hear the sounds necessary to record a blood pressure.

THE EAR PIECES

The ear pieces consist of two metal tubes that are curved at one end with plastic or soft rubber ear tips at the end of each tube. The opposite ends are inserted into the rubber tubing. One of the most important aspects of using a stethoscope properly is the placement of the ear pieces. The ear pieces are adjustable and can easily turn in a circular fashion. Pick up the stethoscope and hold the ear pieces, one in each hand. Now adjust them so that they are both pointing slightly forward or outward away from you. This will help ensure that they seat properly inside your ears. Your ear canals are directed forward toward your nose, and by adjusting the ear pieces you can ensure that the openings are pointed directly into your ear canal. Ear pieces that are not adjusted properly may be blocked by the ear itself, making it difficult to hear the sounds of the BP. Once the ear pieces are seated comfortably in your ears, tap gently on the diaphragm to ensure that you can hear well. If not, readjust the ear pieces.

TUBING

Tubing for stethoscopes comes in two basic styles. The most common is "Y" shaped. Each end of the "Y" attaches to an ear piece and the stem of the "Y" connects to the diaphragm. In the other style, a separate tube comes off each ear piece and they connect at the diaphragm. Regardless of which style your instructor recommends, just ensure that the tubing is straight and has no bends or kinks in it.

DIAPHRAGM HEAD

Diaphragm heads also come in two basic styles, the single head and the double head (Figure 10-10). The single head is the most common and the easiest to use when learning to take blood pressures. It consists of a round metallic concave disk that is covered by a plastic diaphragm much like the skin that covers a drum. The diaphragm is held in place over the head by a round threaded ring.

A double head consists of the diaphragm described above on one side and a bell shaped cone on the opposite side. The flat diaphragm is best suited for listening to high-pitched sounds, such as those in the lungs. The bell is used for picking up low-pitched sounds, such as those made by the heart. The diaphragm is the most appropriate side for obtaining a blood pressure, and the bell should not be used to listen for blood pressure.

It is important to realize that the double-headed stethoscope must be adjusted to the side that you want to listen with. When one side is turned on, the other side is closed off so no sound can be heard through it. This is accomplished by holding the tubing right at the head and turning the head. You will feel a click when it is positioned properly. Failing to make this adjustment properly is the single most common reason a new EMT has difficulty hearing when using a double-headed stethoscope. In addition, many stethoscopes have a flat side or marking indicating the "active" side. Please make sure you have the proper side turned on so you will hear the sounds you are listening for.

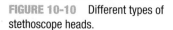

FIGURE 10-10 Different types of stethoscope heads.

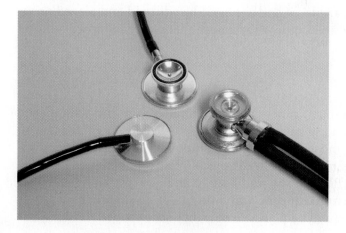

Blood Pressure by Auscultation

Keep in mind that there are two methods of obtaining a blood pressure: auscultation and palpation. Auscultation is the more accurate of the two methods and requires the use of a stethoscope. Learning to take blood pressures using this method can be very cumbersome and frustrating at first, but with enough practice one becomes quite comfortable using this technique. Taking a BP by auscultation requires a relatively quiet environment in order to hear the necessary sounds.

WHAT YOU ARE LISTENING FOR

By far the most challenging part of learning to take blood pressures by auscultation is learning to distinguish blood pressure sounds from the multitude of other sounds caused by movement. Once the BP cuff and stethoscope are in place and the cuff is inflated, you have created a tourniquet and the cuff is restricting all blood flow to the arm. For this reason, do not keep the cuff fully inflated any longer than is absolutely necessary. You must now open the valve near the bulb to release the pressure inside the cuff. At some point as you release the pressure in the cuff, the blood will begin rushing past the cuff with each beat of the heart. This flow of blood past the cuff can be heard through the stethoscope that is placed lower down, over the brachial pulse point. The sound is most often described as a "beat." At the first sound of blood rushing past the cuff or "beat" that you hear, the gauge indicates the systolic blood pressure. You must now continue to listen for the sound of the beats and note when the last sound occurs. This is when the pressure on both sides of the cuff equalizes and the gauge reveals the diastolic pressure.

The exact sounds that you hear will be slightly different with every patient. Sometimes the sounds are loud and distinct and easily heard. Other times they are distant and faint and difficult to hear. Lots of practice on many different people is the only way to develop mastery at taking blood pressures.

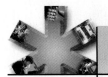

Perspective

Ray—The EMT

"Listening for Dick's blood pressure was a real challenge on this call. His mother kept talking, Dick kept throwing up or moving his arm to hold onto the garbage can, or I just got the normal junk-noise like the creaking sound of the cuff as it inflated or deflated. It can get frustrating. I finally ended up just getting his systolic pressure by palpation—and it was very low. You know, when I was new on the streets and was having trouble getting a pressure, it would make me nervous. That's no lie! I would sit there for a minute with the stethoscope on, looking thoughtful, and then finally succeed in getting a good measurement. I was afraid that if I faked it, I would have a patient die because of that. Even today, I get solid sets of vitals no matter what it takes. There's a reason that they're called vital signs."

When first learning to take blood pressures in class, it is recommended to have your patient lie down on the floor with his arm out to the side. This will allow you to lay the gauge on the floor next to the cuff or on the patient's abdomen where it can be easily seen. It is a good idea to switch arms after every two or three attempts, just to give the arms a break. Once you get comfortable taking blood pressure on a person who is lying down, you can then practice on people in other positions, such as sitting and standing.

To assess a patient's blood pressure by auscultation (Scan 10-1), follow these steps:

1. Take appropriate BSI precautions.

✳ ✳

SCAN 10-1   MEASURING BLOOD PRESSURE BY AUSCULTATION

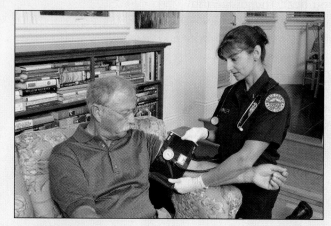

▲ Hold the blood pressure cuff against the inside of the arm and wrap it around the arm.

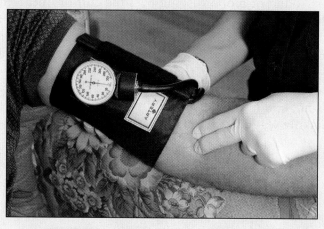

▲ Locate the brachial artery and place the stethoscope over the artery.

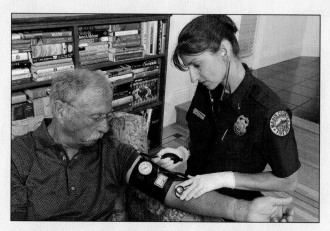

▲ Inflate the cuff, then release the air and watch the guage.

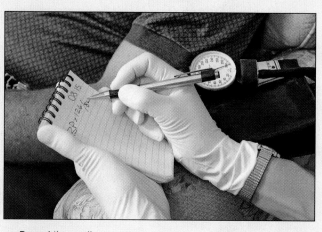

▲ Record the reading.

2. Place the BP cuff appropriately on the upper arm. Ensure that the gauge remains visible.

3. Ask the patient if he knows what his BP is normally.

4. Place the stethoscope in your ears and the diaphragm over the brachial pulse point on the anterior elbow.

5. Ensure that the valve is closed and inflate the cuff to approximately 30 mmHg above where the patient indicated his systolic pressure is normally. If in doubt, inflate to 160 mmHg.

6. Open the valve and deflate the cuff slowly, while listening for the pulse sounds.

7. Note where the needle on the gauge is when you hear the first significant sound (systolic) and the last significant sound (diastolic).

8. Note the time and record your findings.

Blood Pressure by Palpation

An alternative to taking a blood pressure by auscultation is taking it by palpation (feel). This is a great alternative when the environment is too noisy or you want to take vitals on multiple patients as quickly as possible. Blood pressures taken by palpation are not as accurate as those taken with a stethoscope but can still be used to trend a patient if necessary.

Instead of using a stethoscope to "hear" the blood rushing past the cuff, you will use your fingers placed over the radial pulse to "feel" the blood as it causes a pulse. Taking a BP by palpation will only reveal the approximate systolic pressure and does not give the diastolic pressure. You will record a BP taken by palpation as the number over the letter P, such as 120/P.

To assess a patient's blood pressure by palpation (Scan 10-2 on page 272), follow these steps:

1. Take appropriate BSI precautions.

2. Place the BP cuff appropriately on the upper arm. Ensure that the gauge remains visible.

3. Ask the patient if he knows what his BP is normally.

4. Locate the radial pulse in the same arm where you placed the cuff.

5. Ensure that the valve is closed and inflate the cuff to approximately 30 mmHg above where you last feel a radial pulse.

6. Open the valve and deflate the cuff slowly while feeling for the radial pulse to return.

7. Note the location of the needle on the gauge when you feel the first beat return at the radial pulse. This is the approximate systolic blood pressure.

8. Note the time and record your findings.

SCAN 10-2   **MEASURING BLOOD PRESSURE BY PALPATION**

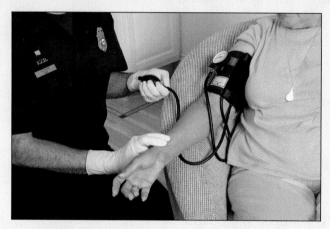

▲ Locate the radial pulse.

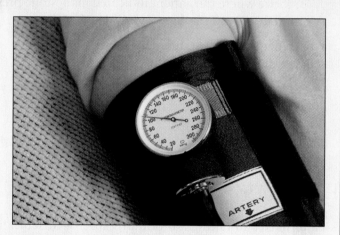

▲ Inflate the cuff and watch the gauge.

Stop, Review, Remember!

Multiple Choice

Place a check next to the correct answer.

1. Which of the following best describes the characteristics you should be looking for when assessing a pulse?

   _____ a. rate, strength, volume

   _____ b. rate, strength, rhythm

   _____ c. rate, regularity, volume

   _____ d. rate, volume, rhythm

2. Which of the following best describes the most common reason(s) you may have difficulty in obtaining a pulse on a healthy patient?

   _____ a. wrong finger placement and too many fingers

   _____ b. using the tips instead of the pads of the fingers

   _____ c. using the pads instead of the tips of the fingers

   _____ d. wrong finger placement and pressure

3. Which of the following is a good question to ask *before* taking a blood pressure on any patient?

   _____ a. Is your blood pressure always low?

   _____ b. Is your blood pressure always high?

   _____ c. What is your blood pressure normally?

   _____ d. When is the last time you had your BP taken?

4. When taking a blood pressure by auscultation, you should continue to inflate the cuff until the gauge reads _____ mmHg higher than the point where the sound of the pulse disappeared.

_____ a. 10

_____ b. 30

_____ c. 50

_____ d. 60

5. Which of the following statements is most accurate about the value of blood pressure in determining a patient's condition?

_____ a. Multiple readings are necessary to reveal a trend.

_____ b. Blood pressure can reveal very little about a patient's condition.

_____ c. Pulses are more revealing than blood pressures.

_____ d. Trending does not pertain to taking blood pressures.

Matching

Match the term on the left with the applicable definition on the right.

1. _____ Auscultation

2. _____ Brachial pulse

3. _____ Bradycardia

4. _____ Diastolic pressure

5. _____ Palpation

6. _____ Pulse

7. _____ Systolic pressure

8. _____ Tachycardia

A. Pressure wave felt over an artery, caused by contraction of the heart
B. The pressure exerted on the walls of the arteries when the heart is at rest
C. Abnormally rapid heart rate (above 100)
D. Pulse point located at the medial aspect of the Upper arm
E. The pressure exerted on the walls of the arteries when the heart is contracting
F. Listening for sounds with a stethoscope
G. Abnormally slow heart rate (below 60)
H. Assessment by touch or feel

Critical Thinking

1. Explain why it is always important to verify the pulse at the carotid artery for patients who are over one year old and do not appear to have a radial pulse.

_____

_____

_____

_____

2. What is the value in asking a patient what his blood pressure is normally prior to taking it yourself?

_____

_____

_____

3. Explain the meaning of the systolic and diastolic readings of a blood pressure.

_____

_____

_____

_____

1-5.8 Describe the methods to assess the skin color, temperature, condition (capillary refill in infants and children).

1-5.9 Identify the normal and abnormal skin colors.

1-5.10 Differentiate between pale, blue, red, and yellow skin color.

1-5.11 Identify the normal and abnormal skin temperature.

1-5.12 Differentiate between hot, cool, and cold skin temperature.

1-5.13 Identify normal and abnormal skin conditions.

✳ **pale**
_____
a whitish skin color indicative of poor perfusion.

✳ **cyanotic**
_____
a bluish skin color indicative of poor oxygenation.

✳ **flushed**
_____
a reddish skin color commonly seen when someone is embarrassed or is suffering a heat-related emergency.

✳ **jaundice**
_____
a yellowish color of the skin and whites of the eyes indicative of poor liver function.

Assessing Skin Signs

The characteristics of a patient's skin can reveal a lot about his current condition. While skin signs are not always accurate and reliable as a single source of information, they can add to the overall picture of the patient. Skin signs are easy to assess and therefore should be included as part of all baseline vital signs.

A patient's skin should be assessed for the following characteristics:

✳ Color

✳ Temperature

✳ Moisture

COLOR

Skin color must be assessed in multiple locations to achieve the best overall assessment. In light-skinned patients, it is easy to identify color changes in the skin of the face. In dark-skinned patients, you must rely on the skin in other areas such as the mucous membranes, conjunctiva, and nail beds for evidence of color change. Skin color can be assessed in the following areas for evidence of good perfusion:

✳ Face

✳ Nail beds

✳ Oral mucosa (inside the lower lip)

✳ Conjunctiva (inside the lower eyelid)

In pediatric patients, the palms of the hands and soles of the feet can also be assessed.

Normal skin color in the locations just listed is pink. Now if you look around and pay close attention, you will notice that while everyone's actual skin color is slightly different, it can still be characterized as pink. Below is a list of abnormal skin colors frequently seen in the field:

✳ **Pale**—a whitish skin color indicative of poor perfusion

✳ **Cyanotic**—a bluish skin color indicative of poor oxygenation

✳ **Flushed**—an unnatural redness seen primarily in the face commonly seen when someone is embarrassed or is suffering a heat-related emergency

✳ **Jaundice**—a yellowish color to the skin and whites of the eyes indicative of poor liver function

TEMPERATURE

A patient's skin temperature is often relative to his immediate environment. Normal skin temperature is warm (Table 10-5). Skin that is hot, cool, or cold may indicate an underlying medical condition. It may also simply be reflecting his environment, so be aware of this when assessing skin temperature.

Use the back of a nongloved hand placed against the patient's forehead to assess skin temperature (Figure 10-11). Skin temperature is characterized as hot, warm, cool, or cold.

MOISTURE

Normal skin is dry to the touch. Skin that is cool and moist or sweaty is called clammy or **diaphoretic.** In either case moisture can be caused by physical exertion and may not have anything to do directly with the patient's current medical condition. Skin moisture is most often characterized as dry, diaphoretic, or clammy (cool and moist).

✳ **diaphoretic**

perspiring, sweaty, moist. A characterization of skin condition.

TABLE 10-5 SKIN TEMPERATURE AND CONDITION	
SKIN TEMPERATURE/CONDITION	**SIGNIFICANCE/POSSIBLE CAUSES**
Cool, clammy	Sign of shock, anxiety
Cold, moist	Body is losing heat
Cold, dry	Exposure to cold
Hot, dry	High fever, heat exposure
Hot, moist	High fever, heat exposure
"Goose pimples" accompanied by shivering, chattering teeth, blue lips, and pale skin	Chills, communicable disease, exposure to cold, pain, or fear

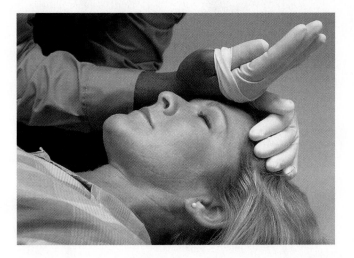

FIGURE 10-11   Use the back of a nongloved hand placed against the patient's forehead to assess skin temperature.

1-5.14 Describe normal and abnormal capillary refill in infants and children.

* **capillary refill test**

a test used to assess perfusion status in the extremities.

CAPILLARY REFILL

The **capillary refill test** is just one tool the EMT can use to assess the perfusion status of a patient. It should be emphasized that the capillary refill test is most reliable in patients younger than 6 years old and is only one element of an overall assessment that should include pulse rate, blood pressure, and skin signs. The capillary refill test is conducted by blanching (pressing until white) a nail bed or the soft tissue of a finger/toe, knee, or upper arm and counting the number of seconds it takes for the capillaries to refill with blood as indicated by the whitened skin turning pink again (Figure 10-12A and B). A capillary refill time of less than 2 seconds is considered normal. A refill time longer than 2 seconds is described as delayed and may be an indication of poor perfusion.

Capillary refill time can also be used to assess the perfusion status of an extremity following an injury. The most common technique for assessing capillary refill time in an adult or child involves pressing a nail bed of the hand or foot and then releasing to observe for refill (Figure 10-12C). This is sometimes difficult, as it requires you to cover the very spot that you are trying to observe for blanching

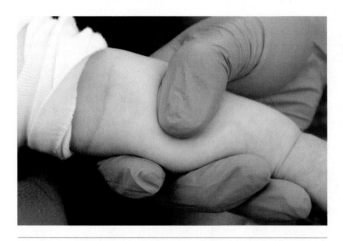

FIGURE 10-12A Press the arm of the infant to assess capillary refill. (© Daniel Limmer.)

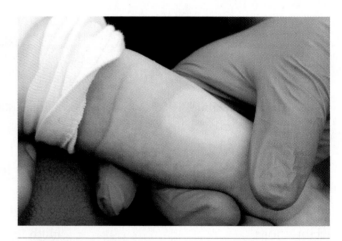

FIGURE 10-12B Release the arm and count the number of seconds it takes for color to return to the skin. (© Daniel Limmer.)

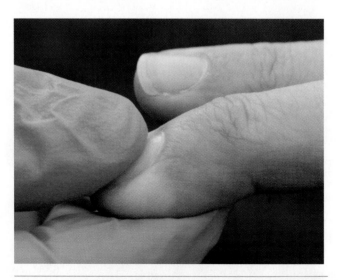

FIGURE 10-12C An alternative method for assessing capillary refill is to squeeze the pad of one finger from both sides. (© Daniel Limmer.)

Clinical Clues: CAPILLARY REFILL

Capillary refill alone should not be used to determine the perfusion status of any patient but should be included in your overall assessment of the patient.

and refill. An alternative method involves squeezing the pad of one finger or toe from both sides (Figure 10-12C). This allows the EMT to observe both the blanching and the refill phase of the test for a more accurate assessment. The capillary refill test requires a well-lit environment in order for you to see the subtle changes in the patient's skin.

Assessing the Eyes

It has been said that the eyes are the windows to the soul. Whether you believe this or not, one thing is certain, the eyes can tell you a lot about a patient's condition. A patient's eyes tell us things we don't even realize we are seeing. That sudden gut feeling we get when we look into someone's eyes and just know that something is very wrong. Some call it intuition, but it is typically triggered by what we see in a patient's eyes.

As an EMT you will want to look each and every patient directly in the eyes as you approach him and introduce yourself. This will help you establish an attitude of caring and compassion for the patient that quickly builds rapport and trust. As you observe a patient's eyes, you will be observing for the following characteristics:

* Pupil size/shape

* Equality of pupil size

* Reactivity to light

PUPIL SIZE AND SHAPE

As you look into a patient's eyes, you will look specifically at the pupil, which is the dark circle in the center of the eye. You will want to assess it for approximate size and see that it is nice and round. To assist in determining approximate pupil size, most EMS-style disposable penlights have a pupil gauge printed on the side. Pupil size can be affected by many things, including medical problems and, of course, ambient light (Figure 10-13 on page 278).

EQUAL PUPIL SIZE

The second characteristic of the eyes that must be assessed is the equality of pupil size between both eyes (bilaterally). This is accomplished by simply observing both pupils and confirming that they are either the same size or not. In some patients you may find that one pupil is larger than the other and this just needs to be noted and documented accordingly. Pupils that are large are referred to as **dilated** (Figure 10-14A on page 278) and pupils that are small are called **constricted** (Figure 10-14B on page 278). Pupils that are not of equal size are documented as unequal (Figure 10-14C on page 278). A simple tool for determining the size of a patient's pupils, the pupil gauge, can be found on the side of most disposable penlights.

1-5.15 Describe the methods used to assess the pupils.

1-5.16 Identify normal and abnormal pupil size.

1-5.17 Differentiate between dilated (big) and constricted (small) pupil size.

* **dilated pupils**
  pupils that are larger than normal.

* **constricted pupils**
  pupils that are smaller than normal.

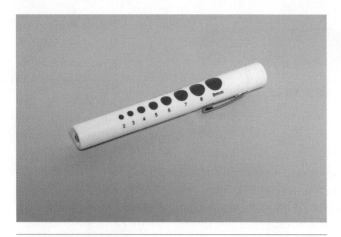

FIGURE 10-13 A gauge tool for determining pupil size can be found on the side of most disposable pen lights.

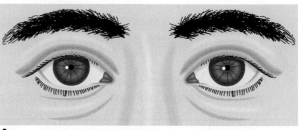

A. Constricted pupils

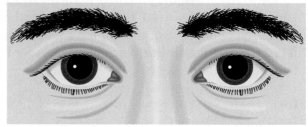

B. Dilated pupils

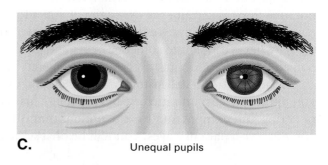

C. Unequal pupils

FIGURE 10-14 (A) Constricted pupils. (B) Dilated pupils. (C) Unequal pupils.

1-5.18 Differentiate between reactive and nonreactive pupils and equal and unequal pupils.

REACTIVITY TO LIGHT

One of the important signs of good perfusion is pupils that respond briskly to the presence or absence of light. Pupils should respond to the sudden introduction of light by constricting and, in contrast, should dilate when light to the pupil is blocked. There are at least two methods that can be used to assess pupil reaction, and each depends on the ambient light at the time.

In a well-lit area such as a bright room or the outdoors on a bright sunny day, it may be of no use attempting to shine a light into someone's eyes. The pupils will likely already be constricted due to the large amount of ambient light. In this situation you will have better results covering each of the patient's eyes, one at a time, with your hand for several seconds, then observing the pupil constrict when you take your hand away. You must learn to be patient when using this method, as it may take some time for the pupil to dilate after you cover the eye. It is a good practice to ask at least 2 or 3 questions pertaining to the patient's medical history while you cover each eye. This will allow enough time for the pupil to dilate and not appear as an awkward silence.

In situations where there is not a lot of ambient light, an artificial light source such as a penlight or flashlight will be necessary. Ask the patient to stare straight ahead as you hold the light just outside his field of vision. With the light turned

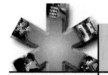

Perspective

Barbara—The Patient's Mother

I didn't understand all of the time that those two EMTs wasted before getting my son to the hospital. Heart pressures and pulses. . . they were even looking at his eyes. I'm from the day when if you were sick, then by God those guys would just load you up and get you to a doctor so he could help you. This poking and prodding in my son's bedroom was an absolute waste of time as far as I'm concerned. It was all just totally unnecessary. . . absolutely unnecessary."

on, quickly move the light from the side directly at his pupil. Watch closely for the pupil to constrict as the light hits it. Then move the light away and watch the pupil dilate slightly and return to its original size.

Both pupils should react to the change in light with the same speed. Pupils that respond slowly to the change in light are documented as sluggish. Pupils that do not respond at all are referred to as fixed. When a person goes into cardiac arrest, the pupils gradually become fixed and dilated.

An acronym that is widely used in EMS to help EMTs remember the characteristics of pupils is **PERRL**. PERRL stands for:

* P – Pupils
* E – Equal
* R – Round
* R – Reactive
* L – Light

✳ **PERRL**

a mnemonic used to evaluate a patient's pupils. The letters stand for Pupils Equal and Round Reactive to Light.

Clinical Clues: PERRL

An earlier version of the PERRL acronym was PERL. The PERRL acronym did not include the "R" for round, which is the shape the pupils should always be. PERRL is now the preferred version.

SYMPATHETIC MOVEMENT

Normally, both eyes move together; when one moves so does the other one. This is called sympathetic movement. When assessing a patient's eyes or just his pupils, you should look for and confirm that both eyes move together.

ORTHOSTATIC VITAL SIGNS

Some EMS systems instruct their EMTs to obtain **orthostatic vital signs** in certain situations. Taking blood pressure and pulse readings with a patient lying or sitting and then again when they are sitting or standing can sometimes reveal that the patient is low on fluid volume. This is typically performed on patients who are not already showing signs of shock but are suspected to be hypovolemic. Chapter 26 discusses hypovolemic shock.

You must first obtain a baseline blood pressure and pulse with the patient lying or sitting. Then have him sit or stand and wait a minute or two for his body to adjust. Retake the blood pressure and pulse. A BP reading that drops more than 20 mmHg, or a pulse that increases more than 20 beats is considered significant and is suggestive of hypovolemia (low fluid volume). Use caution when taking orthostatic vital signs and discontinue if your patient becomes lightheaded or dizzy when he sits or stands up. Do not attempt this on patients with a cardiac history or trauma patients and certainly do not delay transport for this assessment.

REASSESSING VITAL SIGNS

Vital signs are dynamic and ever changing, often with little or no outward signs from the patient. Therefore it is essential that you obtain a thorough and accurate baseline set of vitals as soon as possible and obtain additional sets of vitals as often as appropriate. Each additional set must be immediately compared to the baseline and all previous sets for evidence of a trend.

A patient who you believe may be unstable must have his vitals reassessed every 5 minutes if his condition permits. Do not be concerned about getting additional sets of vitals if the patient requires your immediate care. Patients with a compromised airway or inadequate breathing will need you to perform more important interventions, such as suctioning or assisted ventilations.

A patient who you believe is stable may only need additional vital signs taken every 15 minutes or so. These intervals are recommended guidelines and should be modified to suit the patient's needs and to follow local protocols. It is also recommended that you reassess vital signs following all interventions.

Pulse Oximetry

A tool becoming commonplace in many EMS systems is the pulse oximeter. It is a noninvasive device that can monitor the percentage of hemoglobin that is saturated with oxygen. It consists of a probe that attaches to the patient's finger, toe, or ear lobe and is linked to a computerized unit (Figure 10-15). The unit displays the percentage of hemoglobin saturated with oxygen (SpO_2) together with a digital readout of the patient's pulse rate (Figure 10-16). The device can detect hypoxia before the patient begins to show signs.

Ideally, a patient should be placed on the pulse oximeter prior to receiving supplemental oxygen. Doing so will provide a baseline reading to which later readings with supplemental oxygen can be compared. However, if a patient shows signs of inadequate breathing, do not delay interventions such as supplemental oxygen or manual ventilations for the sake of a baseline pulse oximetry reading. An oxygen saturation (SpO_2) of less than 95 percent is considered ab-

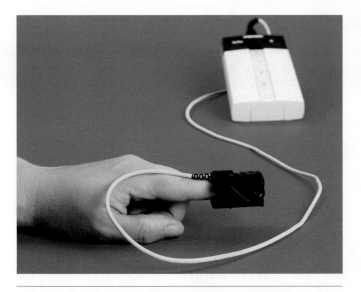

FIGURE 10-15 A pulse oximeter with sensor applied to patient's finger.

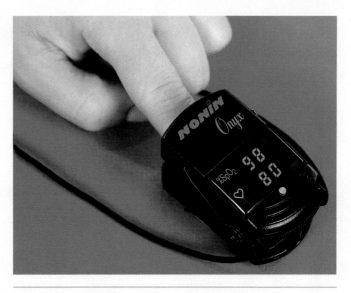

FIGURE 10-16 A mini "finger-size" pulse oximeter with all-in-one sensor and read-out display.

normal and may be indicative of early hypoxia (oxygen deficiency). The pulse oximeter is only one tool in your assessment toolbox. You must continue to use your assessment skills and vital signs to determine the best care for the patient. Just because the pulse oximeter shows a normal saturation of between 95 and 100 percent on room air does not mean the patient should not receive supplemental oxygen.

The effectiveness and accuracy of the pulse oximeter depends on a continuous flow of arterial blood to the tissues. For this reason, there are several situations where the pulse oximeter will not be accurate or effective for determining oxygen saturation. The following is a list of these situations:

* Patients who are in shock or hypothermic

* Cases of carbon monoxide poisoning

* Excessive movement

* Nail polish beneath the probe

Pulse oximetry is most useful in revealing a trend in the patient's oxygen saturation. It will tell you when supplemental oxygen is raising the patient's oxygen saturation, and it will reveal when hypoxia is setting in, because the readings will drop.

Clinical Clues: PULSE OXIMETRY

Do not rely too heavily on the pulse oximeter as the sole indicator of the patient's condition. It is only one piece of the big picture that must include your overall assessment and vital signs.

Stop, Review, Remember!

Multiple Choice

Place a check next to the correct answer.

1. Which of the following is NOT a typical skin sign?

   _____ a. color

   _____ b. sensitivity

   _____ c. temperature

   _____ d. moisture

2. When assessing skin signs, which of the following best describes the term diaphoretic?

   _____ a. hot and red

   _____ b. cool and clammy

   _____ c. hot and moist

   _____ d. cold and moist

3. When assessing a patient's pupils, the two "Rs" in the mnemonic PERRL refers to:

   _____ a. round and reactive to light.

   _____ b. responsive and reactive to pain.

   _____ c. round and refocusing to light.

   _____ d. responsive and reactive to pain.

4. Sympathetic movement of the eyes refers to the ability of the eyes to:

   _____ a. open and close together.

   _____ b. open and close one at a time.

   _____ c. blink.

   _____ d. move together.

5. It is recommended to reassess vital signs every 15 minutes for stable patients and every _____ minutes for unstable patients.

   _____ a. 5

   _____ b. 10

   _____ c. 15

   _____ d. 20

Fill in the Blank

1. Skin signs should be assessed for color, _____, and moisture.

2. The _____ is located on the inside of the mouth and can be used to assess tissue perfusion.

3. The conjunctiva is located _____.

4. A yellowish color to the skin and whites of the eyes, indicative of poor liver function, is called _____.

5. Skin that is moist is often referred to as _____.

Matching

Match the definition on the left with the applicable term on the right.

1. _____ A bluish skin color indicative of poor oxygenation.

2. _____ A reddish skin color commonly seen when someone is embarrassed or is suffering a heat related emergency.

3. _____ Skin color indicative of poor perfusion.

4. _____ A yellowish skin color indicative of poor liver function.

5. _____ Perspiration, skin that is moist.

A. Jaundice
B. Diaphoretic
C. Cyanotic
D. Flushed
E. Pale

Critical Thinking

1. List as many areas on a patient that you can think of for assessing skin color and perfusion status of the patient.

_____

_____

_____

_____

2. List a medical condition that may cause each of the following abnormal skin colors: pale, cyanotic, flushed, and jaundice.

_____

_____

_____

_____

3. Describe the proper method for assessing a patient's skin temperature and moisture and the normal characteristics of each.

_____

_____

_____

_____

Obtaining a Medical History

One of the most important roles that an EMT must learn is that of an investigator. As an investigator your job is to learn as much about the patient's medical history, both past and present, as possible. It is important to obtain a medical history for all patients. However, it is especially important when assessing patients with a medical illness as opposed to an injury.

You will start gathering important history information beginning with the initial dispatch. Dispatches to such common calls as, "difficulty breathing," "chest pain," and "unresponsive person" provide at least some insight into the patient's chief complaint. While the dispatch does not always match up with what you find once on scene, for the most part it is at least close.

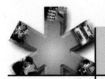

Perspective

Ray—The EMT

"On the surface, Dick's problem seemed like a pretty common intestinal thing. You know, vomiting, diarrhea, chills, and fever. I don't know... stomach flu... or maybe food poisoning? So I was just going to load him up and head out, but then Derrick was wise to start asking him all of these questions about his medical history. Do you know what? Dick is diabetic and undergoing chemo for colon cancer. I behaved very inexperienced for just assuming this was one of those 'middle-aged man living alone with his mom' hypochondria-type cases. This was a very, very sick man and I didn't appreciate that. I guess I'm never going to stop learning out here. Let's hope none of us do."

GENERAL IMPRESSION

✻ **general impression**

an element of the patient assessment that includes assessing approximate age, gender, and level of distress.

Once on scene, your history-taking begins as you approach your patient and begin to form a **general impression** of his condition. The general impression is just one element of your overall patient assessment and includes the following elements:

✻ Approximate age

✻ Gender

✻ Level of distress

As you approach the patient, note his approximate age: Is he elderly, middle-aged, a young adult, or a pediatric patient? Go ahead and estimate his age based on your best guess. Close is good enough for EMS work. You will already know your patient's gender, at least by appearances. The final element of the general impression is the patient's level of distress. Is he in a lot of pain, having difficulty breathing, or simply lying there calm and quiet? Someone with a high level of distress may need immediate attention, so this is an important observation.

Once at the patient's side, introduce yourself and inform him of your level of training and confirm that he has provided permission to care for him. This is typ-

1-5.37 Demonstrate the skills that should be used to obtain information from the patient, family

ically the case if other first responders are already on scene. If you are the first on scene, then you must ask for permission to care for the patient.

CHIEF COMPLAINT

After your introduction, determine the patient's **chief complaint** by asking why you were called. The chief complaint is the primary reason the patient feels he needs assistance, usually described in his own words. The chief complaint for an unresponsive patient may be documented as "unresponsive" or simply "none."

✳ **chief complaint**

the patient's perception of the problem in his own words. It is NOT what the EMT perceives to be the problem.

1-5.23 Identify the components of the SAMPLE history.

SAMPLE HISTORY

There are many tools that EMTs can use to help remember all the questions they must ask while obtaining a patient history. The most common of those tools is a memory device—an acronym that spells the word **SAMPLE**. Each letter of the word represents a specific element of a good patient history. They are as follows:

✳ **SAMPLE**

a mnemonic used in obtaining a patient history. The letters stand for Signs and symptoms, Allergies, Medications, Past pertinent medical history, Last oral intake, and Events leading to the injury or illness.

* ✳ S – Signs and symptoms
* ✳ A – Allergies
* ✳ M – Medications
* ✳ P – Pertinent past medical history
* ✳ L – Last oral intake
* ✳ E – Events leading to the injury or illness

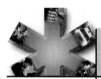

Perspective

Dick—The Patient

"I don't think I've ever been so sick. That was awful. Just vomiting until every muscle in my body ached. I was so tired, I didn't even want to talk. My mother kept trying to call 9-1-1 but I wouldn't let her! I mean, it wasn't until she told me that I was acting just like my father right before he died that I really got concerned. She just lost him two years ago... and... so... how could I argue with her anymore? I may be 55, but she's still my mom. So I let her call for the ambulance and now, I've got to say, I'm glad that she did."

SIGNS AND SYMPTOMS

The *S* in the SAMPLE acronym stands for signs and symptoms and reminds us to assess or reassess any signs and symptoms relating to the chief complaint. One way that you can begin this process is by asking the patient, "Tell me again where you hurt." As he describes where he has pain (a symptom) you must then inspect those areas for any obvious signs of illness or injury. Don't just stop at the most obvious or first place the patient describes as painful. After examining the first painful location, ask if there are any other places that hurt and inspect those as appropriate.

ALLERGIES

All good patient histories include information about known allergies. Known allergies are those things the patient is well aware of that have caused an allergic reaction in the past. This is important for several reasons. For instance, the patient may require medication upon arrival at the hospital, but he may be allergic to a specific medication. Discovering known allergies ahead of time should prevent an unnecessary reaction during his treatment and care. It is good practice to ask about all known allergies including allergies to medications, food, and environmental causes such as bites, stings, and plants.

If the patient advises that he does indeed have a known allergy, then it is a good idea to ask him the last time he had a reaction and what the reaction was like. Was it a minor reaction or was it more severe requiring medical attention? This will provide some insight into how allergic he may be.

MEDICATIONS

Asking a patient what medications he is currently taking can provide important information regarding his medical history. As you become more experienced, you will learn the more common prescription medications and what they are taken for. This can tell you the type of medical conditions for which the patient is being treated, especially if he is unable to describe his own medical history very clearly.

Ask about both prescription and nonprescription medications, including those that don't necessarily pertain to a medical condition, such as birth control pills or patches. Also ask about alternative or holistic medications, dietary supplements, and herbal remedies. Your questioning should include medications from the recent past that the patient may not be currently taking as well as medications he is currently taking (Figure 10-17). Be sure to confirm he has been taking the medications as prescribed.

You are not expected to remember all the names or the purpose of each medication. Ask someone to bring you all the medications the patient is taking and place them in a paper bag for easy reference and transport to the hospital.

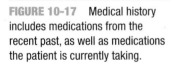 **FIGURE 10-17** Medical history includes medications from the recent past, as well as medications the patient is currently taking.

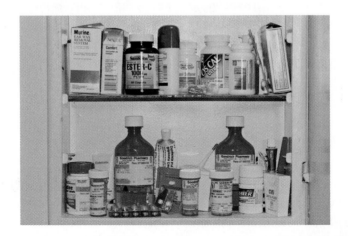

PERTINENT PAST MEDICAL HISTORY

In many situations, the patient's chief complaint relates either directly or indirectly to a past medical complaint or condition. For this reason, a brief assessment of his past medical history is important. Ask about previous or current medical conditions, surgeries, and/or injuries. It is not for you to decide if the previous history is pertinent or not. Let the physician make that decision. You must include as much detail as possible when transferring or documenting your care.

LAST ORAL INTAKE

This question should be asked of all patients but is most important for patients who have suffered a serious injury. Ask the patient when he last had something to eat or drink and an approximate quantity. Should a patient require emergency surgery, it is very important that the surgeons know the time and quantity of food intake, since there is a risk that the stomach contents could be vomited up during surgery.

EVENTS LEADING TO THE INJURY OR ILLNESS

It may be helpful to know what the patient was doing just prior to the event. For instance, if the chief complaint is chest pain it will be important to know if the patient was exerting himself prior to the pain or if he was at rest. It will also reveal something important if the patient has no recollection of events prior to your arrival.

OPQRST Assessment

Another tool used in EMS to help ensure a thorough assessment and medical history related to a medical patient's chief complaint is the mnemonic **OPQRST**. Each of the letters represents a word and each of the words is designed to trigger specific questions that the EMT should ask. The OPQRST mnemonic is especially helpful when the chief complaint is related to pain or shortness of breath:

∗ **OPQRST**
a mnemonic for the questions asked to get a description of the present illness. The letters stand for Onset, Provocation, Quality, Region and Radiate, Severity, and Time.

- ∗ O – Onset
- ∗ P – Provocation
- ∗ Q – Quality
- ∗ R – Region and Radiation
- ∗ S – Severity
- ∗ T – Time

ONSET

The word *onset* is designed to trigger questions pertaining to what the patient was doing when the pain or symptoms began. For example, "What were you doing when the pain began?" or "What were you doing when you first began to feel short of breath?" are questions you might ask related to onset.

PROVOCATION

The word *provocation* is designed to trigger questions pertaining to what might make the pain or symptoms better or worse. For example, "does anything you do make the pain better or worse?", or "does it hurt to take a deep breath or when I push here?" are questions you might ask related to provocation.

QUALITY

The word *quality* is designed to trigger questions pertaining to what the pain or symptom actually feels like. For example, "can you describe how your pain feels?", or "is it sharp or is it dull?" and "is it steady or does it come and go?" are questions you might ask related to quality.

Be careful not to put words in the patient's mouth. Instead provide them with choices and then be patient and allow them to choose. It is also important to use the patient's own words when documenting the call or handing the patient off to the next level of care. If the patient tells you he feels as though an anvil is sitting on his chest, then use his words rather than paraphrasing and stating that he has pressure on his chest.

REGION/RADIATION

The words *region* and *radiation* are designed to trigger questions pertaining to where the pain is originating and to where it may be moving or radiating. For example, "can you point with one finger to where your pain is the most?" or "does your pain move or radiate to any other part of your body?" or "do you feel pain anywhere else besides your chest?" are questions you might ask related to region and radiation.

SEVERITY

The word *severity* is designed to trigger questions pertaining to how severe the pain or discomfort is. A standard 1-to-10 scale is typically used and is presented like this: "On a scale of 1 to 10, with 10 being the worst pain you have ever felt, how would you rate your pain right now?" You can take this a step further by asking the patient to describe the severity of his pain when it first began, using the same scale. Once you have been with the patient awhile and have provided care, you will want to ask the severity question again to see if his pain is getting better or worse.

TIME

The word *time* is designed to trigger questions pertaining to how long the patient may have been experiencing his pain or discomfort. A simple question such as, "when did you first begin having pain today?" or "how long have you had this pain?" will usually suffice.

It is important to point out that there are many different acronyms and mnemonic tools that can be used to assist the EMT in performing a more thorough assessment. We have presented only SAMPLE and OPQRST—two of the more common tools currently used in EMS. Your instructor or EMS system may have different or additional tools. Find the ones that work best for you and that help you do a better job rather than require you to memorize too much.

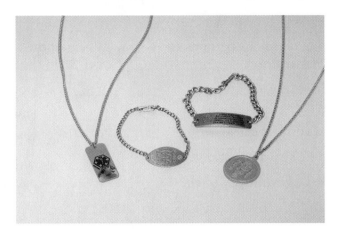

FIGURE 10-18   Various medical ID jewelry and devices.

Medical Identification Jewelry

A valuable resource for medical history is medical identification jewelry (Figure 10-18). These are typically medallions worn around the neck, wrist, or ankle that provide important medical information about the patient. It should be pointed out that the wearing of medical identification jewelry is completely optional, and not all patients with a significant history choose to wear it.

1-5.26 Discuss the need to search for additional medical identification.

 Stop, Review, Remember!

Multiple Choice

1. An appropriate medical history often begins:

   _____ a. with the initial dispatch.

   _____ b. after you arrive on scene.

   _____ c. with the SAMPLE history.

   _____ d. with the detailed assessment.

2. The general impression of the patient consists of the following elements:

   _____ a. approximate age, race, level of consciousness

   _____ b. approximate age, gender, and level of distress

   _____ c. using the pads instead of the tips of the fingers

   _____ d. wrong finger placement and pressure

3. Which of the following best describes the term "chief complaint"?

   _____ a. what the dispatcher tells you over the radio

   _____ b. what the family member tells you about the patient

   _____ c. what the patient states is their problem

   _____ d. any past medical history about the patient

4. Which of the following questions pertains to the "P" in the SAMPLE history?

_____ a. Do you have any allergies to medications?

_____ b. When did you last eat?

_____ c. Do you take any medications?

_____ d. Do you have any history of chest pain?

5. Which of the following questions pertains to the "S" in the SAMPLE history?

_____ a. Do you have pain anywhere?

_____ b. How severe is your pain?

_____ c. Where does your pain originate?

_____ d. What were you doing when the pain began?

Matching

Match up the questions below with the appropriate letter of the OPQRST assessment tool.

1. _____ O
2. _____ P
3. _____ Q
4. _____ R
5. _____ S
6. _____ T

A. What were you doing when the pain/discomfort began?
B. Does anything you do make the pain/discomfort better or worse?
C. Can you describe your pain/discomfort?
D. Is your pain/discomfort sharp or dull?
E. Is your pain/discomfort steady or does it come and go?
F. Where is your pain/discomfort?
G. Does your pain/discomfort radiate anywhere else?
H. How severe is your pain/discomfort now?
I. How long have you had this pain/discomfort?

Critical Thinking

1. Discuss how you might find out if a patient has a previous medical condition without actually asking the question, "Do you have any previous medical history?"

_____

_____

_____

_____

2. List several ways you might ask a patient to describe their pain without leading them to an answer.

_____

_____

_____

_____

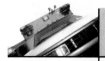

Dispatch Summary

Based on Dick's vital signs, medical history, and apparent dehydration, Derrick and Ray decided to call for an ALS intercept. When the paramedics arrived, they immediately began two IVs of normal saline and, after evaluating Dick with a twelve-lead monitor, began treating him for a cardiac dysrhythmia.

The paramedics complimented the two EMTs on calling for ALS care based on their evaluation of Dick's situation—they had done exactly the right thing.

Dick spent four days in Southwestern's ICU before being released back to his home and has since completed his chemotherapy.

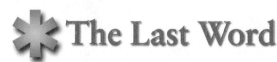

The Last Word

Repeated sets of accurate vital signs help the EMT spot trends in a patient's condition. That trend may be stable, for the better or, in some situations, for the worse. Regardless, vital signs provide valuable information about the patient and should be taken as soon as practical on all patients. Establishing a baseline set of vital signs as early as possible is essential in revealing any trend.

When assessing vital signs be diligent in your effort to obtain information for all characteristics. When assessing breathing, remember to look for:

* Rate
* Depth
* Ease

For pulses you will assess:

* Rate
* Strength
* Rhythm

For skin signs assess for:

* Color
* Temperature
* Moisture

For pupils you will use the PERRL acronym to remind you of the following characteristics:

* Pupils
* Equal
* Round
* Reactive to
* Light

When taking blood pressures, make every attempt to use the auscultation method unless it's just too noisy at the scene, in which case you will use the palpation method.

Reassess vital signs early and often, depending on the condition of your patient. Stable patients should have vitals reassessed approximately every 15 minutes and unstable patients approximately every 5 minutes if their condition allows.

Learning to obtain an excellent medical history is a skill that takes lots of time and experience. Learning to use acronyms such as SAMPLE and OPQRST will help you develop a systematic approach to taking medical histories. Developing a systematic approach will help ensure a complete and thorough history.

✳ Chapter Review

MULTIPLE CHOICE

Place a check next to the correct answer.

1. The five most important vital signs are pulse, respirations, BP, pupils, and:

   _____ a. oxygen saturation.

   _____ b. skin signs.

   _____ c. mental status.

   _____ d. capillary refill.

2. The first set of vital signs obtained on any patient is referred to as the _____ set.

   _____ a. historical

   _____ b. ongoing

   _____ c. baseline

   _____ d. serial

3. _____ can be assessed by watching and feeling the chest and abdomen move during breathing.

   _____ a. Pulse rate

   _____ b. Blood pressure

   _____ c. Skin signs

   _____ d. Respiratory rate

4. Characteristics of respirations include:

   _____ a. rate, depth, and ease.

   _____ b. rate, rhythm, and strength.

   _____ c. rate, depth, and strength.

   _____ d. rate, ease, and quality.

5. The most appropriate location to obtain a pulse for a responsive adult is the _____ artery.

   _____ a. brachial   _____ c. carotid

   _____ b. femoral   _____ d. radial

6. The pulse located at the top of the foot (dorsal aspect) is called the _____ pulse.

   _____ a. tibial

   _____ b. pedal

   _____ c. brachial

   _____ d. dorsal

7. The characteristics of a pulse include:

   _____ a. rate, strength, and rhythm.

   _____ b. rate, ease, and rhythm.

   _____ c. rate, depth, and rhythm.

   _____ d. rate, strength, and quality.

8. Skin that is bluish in color is called:

   _____ a. pale.

   _____ b. flushed.

   _____ c. cyanotic.

   _____ d. jaundice.

9. The term *diaphoretic* refers to:

   _____ a. pupil reaction.

   _____ b. skin temperature.

   _____ c. heart rhythm.

   _____ d. skin moisture.

10. When going from a well-lighted room to a dark room, you would expect the normal pupil to:

_____ a. not react.

_____ b. dilate.

_____ c. constrict.

_____ d. fluctuate.

11. Capillary refill time is most accurate as an assessment tool for perfusion in patients:

_____ a. less than 6 years of age.

_____ b. less than 1 year of age.

_____ c. greater than 8 years of age.

_____ d. greater than 18 years of age.

12. Which of the following is most accurate when describing a palpated blood pressure?

_____ a. It includes only the diastolic pressure.

_____ b. It must be taken on a responsive patient.

_____ c. It can be obtained without a stethoscope.

_____ d. It can be obtained without a BP cuff.

13. A respiratory rate that is less than _____ should be considered inadequate.

_____ a. 4

_____ b. 6

_____ c. 8

_____ d. 10

14. The pressure inside the arteries each time the heart contracts is referred to as the _____ pressure.

_____ a. diastolic

_____ b. pulse

_____ c. systolic

_____ d. mean

15. A _____ is something the EMT can see or measure during the patient assessment.

_____ a. symptom

_____ b. history

_____ c. sign

_____ d. chief complaint

LABELING

Using the illustration, correctly label each of the major pulse points.

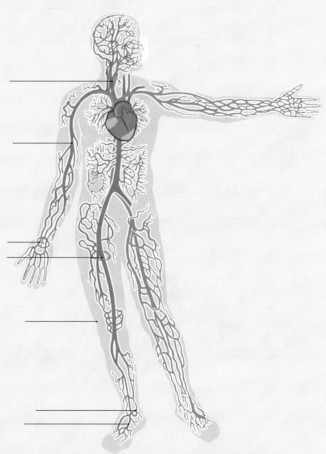

CRITICAL THINKING

1. Describe the importance of recording the time when taking multiple sets of vital signs on an unstable patient.

_____

_____

_____

_____

2. Describe the reasons for not using too small a sample (for example, a 10-second sample versus 15 or 30 seconds) when assessing the pulse rate of a patient.

_____

_____

_____

_____

3. Discuss the differences between an auscultated and palpated blood pressure and when you would use each.

_____

_____

_____

_____

4. Describe how you might assess skin color on dark-skinned patients.

_____

_____

_____

_____

5. Describe how pupils react when perfusion is poor.

_____

_____

_____

_____

CASE STUDIES

Case Study 1

You have been dispatched to the home of an elderly female for abdominal pain. Your SAMPLE history reveals a long history of bleeding ulcers and recent hip replacement surgery. The patient denies any recent history of bloody stools or vomit. Baseline vitals are as follows: Respirations 24 shallow and slightly labored, pulse 96 weak and regular, BP 108/68, skin is pale warm and dry, pupils are PERRL.

1. What conclusions if any can you draw from the patient's baseline vitals?

   _____

   _____

   _____

   _____

2. How often will you want to take vital signs on this patient and why?

   _____

   _____

   _____

   _____

3. How might you determine what this patient's vital signs are normally?

   _____

   _____

   _____

   _____

Case Study 2

You are caring for an approximately 44-year-old male patient who was found on the back porch of his home by his wife. He is alert and oriented upon your arrival but is not sure how he ended up on the ground. He has no obvious signs of trauma and is complaining only of moderate pain to his right elbow and shoulder. His wife states that she had seen him approximately 30 minutes earlier at breakfast before he left to go outside to mow the lawn. His wife tells you he may have been stung by a bee, because he passed out the last time he was stung about a year ago. She shows you an Epi-pen (an epinephrine self-injector) that the doctor gave him the last time he was stung. She also tells you that he has high blood pressure and takes a pill once a day for it.

1. Fill in the appropriate information from the scenario above for each letter of the SAMPLE history.

   _____

   _____

   _____

   _____

2. Would this patient be considered stable or unstable and why?

   _____

   _____

   _____

   _____

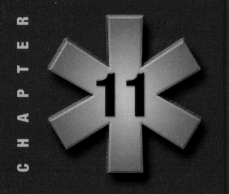
Performing an Initial Assessment

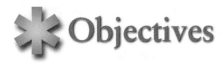 **Objectives**

Numbered objectives are from the U.S. Department of Transportation 1994 EMT-Basic National Standard Curriculum.

COGNITIVE OBJECTIVES

At the completion of this lesson, the EMT-Basic student will be able to:

3-2.1 Summarize the reasons for forming a general impression of the patient. (pp. 299–300)

3-2.2 Discuss methods of assessing altered mental status. (pp. 300–303)

3-2.3 Differentiate between assessing the altered mental status in the adult, child, and infant patient. (p. 303)

3-2.4 Discuss methods of assessing the airway in the adult, child, and infant patient. (p. 303)

3-2.5 State reasons for management of the cervical spine once the patient has been determined to be a trauma patient. (pp. 300–301)

3-2.6 Describe methods used for assessing if a patient is breathing. (pp. 303, 307)

3-2.7 State what care should be provided to the adult, child, and infant patient with adequate breathing. (pp. 303, 307–308)

3-2.8 State what care should be provided to the adult, child, and infant patient without adequate breathing. (pp. 303, 307–308)

3-2.9 Differentiate between a patient with adequate and inadequate breathing. (pp. 303, 307–308)

3-2.10 Distinguish between methods of assessing breathing in the adult, child, and infant patient. (pp. 303, 307)

3-2.11 Compare the methods of providing airway care to the adult, child, and infant patient. (p. 307)

3-2.12 Describe the methods used to obtain a pulse. (pp. 308–309)

3-2.13 Differentiate between obtaining a pulse in an adult, child, and infant patient. (pp. 308–309)

3-2.14 Discuss the need for assessing the patient for external bleeding. (p. 309)

3-2.15 Describe normal and abnormal findings when assessing skin color. (p. 309)

3-2.16 Describe normal and abnormal findings when assessing skin temperature. (p. 309)

3-2.17 Describe normal and abnormal findings when assessing skin condition. (p. 309)

3-2.18 Describe normal and abnormal findings when assessing skin capillary refill in the infant and child patient. (p. 309)

AFFECTIVE OBJECTIVES

At the completion of this lesson, the EMT-Basic student will be able to:

3-2.19 Explain the reason for prioritizing a patient for care and transport. (pp. 299, 300, 310)

3-2.20 Explain the importance of forming a general impression of the patient. (pp. 299, 300)

3-2.21 Explain the value of performing an initial assessment. (p. 299)

PSYCHOMOTOR OBJECTIVES

At the completion of this lesson, the EMT-Basic student will be able to:

3-2.22 Demonstrate the techniques for assessing mental status. (pp. 300–303)

3-2.23 Demonstrate the techniques for assessing the airway. (pp. 303, 306–308)

3-2.24 Demonstrate the techniques for assessing if the patient is breathing. (pp. 303, 306–308)

3-2.25 Demonstrate the techniques for assessing if the patient has a pulse. (pp. 303, 308–309)

3-2.26 Demonstrate the techniques for assessing the patient for external bleeding. (p. 309)

3-2.27 Demonstrate the techniques for assessing the patient's skin color, temperature, condition and capillary refill (infants and children only). (p. 309)

3-2.28 Demonstrate the ability to prioritize patients. (p. 310)

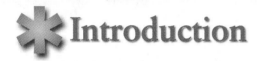 # Introduction

The **initial assessment** is just one component of the skill we refer to as the **patient assessment** and should be performed immediately following the scene size-up. It can easily be argued that the initial assessment is the most important component of the entire patient assessment.

∗ **initial assessment**

a component of the overall patient assessment. The primary objective of the initial assessment is to identify and treat any immediate life threats to the patient.

∗ **patient assessment**

overall evaluation of the patient for life-threatening and non-life-threatening conditions.

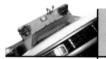 # Emergency Dispatch

"Truck 64, this is headquarters."

"Go ahead," C.J., an EMT, said into the mic after pausing his handheld video game.

"Truck 64, I need you to respond to a code 3 at 377 Grand Avenue for a bleeding victim. The caller states that the patient is a dialysis patient."

"10-4," C.J. dropped the game into the storage bin between the seats and tapped on the truck's siren to alert his partner to the call. Tammy gathered her cash and receipt from the ATM and climbed into the truck.

"There's some sort of bleeding call with a dialysis patient."

"Oh, great," Tammy said as she pulled her latex gloves on. "That probably means a laundry list of other medical problems as well."

Upon arrival at the home, they found a shirtless man waving at them from the porch.

"I don't know what's wrong with her," the man said frantically, as C. J. and Tammy wheeled the cot and equipment toward the front door. "She's diabetic, on dialysis for renal failure, and having a really, really heavy period."

"Could she be pregnant?" Tammy asked.

"Oh, no! No way. I mean, she's having a period. She can't be pregnant."

The man led them to the 32-year-old female patient. She was unresponsive, staring blankly at a wall, and blood was soaking steadily into the couch where she sat.

"How long has she been this way?" Tammy asked, shaking the patient's shoulder.

"About an hour," the man said. "But she always has heavy periods."

"Let's go, C.J.," Tammy slid her hands under the woman's arms. "We need to get her on the cot right now!"

Initial Assessment

The primary objective of the initial assessment is to identify and treat any immediate life threats to the patient. It begins with the formation of a **general impression** and ends with a decision regarding priority for care and transport of the patient.

Components of the initial assessment include:

✳ Formulate a general impression

✳ Determine responsiveness

✳ Determine chief complaint/obvious life threats

✳ Assess airway and breathing

✳ Assess circulation

✳ Determine priority

There are essentially four things from which a patient can die in a short period of time. They are as follows:

✳ Obstructed airway

✳ Absent breathing

✳ Absent pulse

✳ Severe bleeding

The core of the initial assessment consists of assessing the patient for each of these potential problems and providing the indicated care as quickly as possible. You should not feel compelled to always complete an entire patient assessment in each and every situation. In some situations you may be totally occupied with managing a patient's airway on scene and during transport. You will only move on from the initial assessment if all elements are within normal limits and there are no immediate life threats to the patient

> ### Clinical Clues: STEP-BY-STEP ASSESSMENT SKILLS
>
> It is important to point out that you will be learning the patient assessment skills in a step-by-step manner. This will help ensure a structured and thorough approach to your patient assessment. This is somewhat different from the approach you will likely see used in the field on actual patients. A two-person EMS team typically will share the duties of the assessment in an effort to complete it more efficiently.

Forming a General Impression

Once on scene and after completing an appropriate scene size-up, your assessment begins as you approach and form a general impression of the patient's condition (Figure 11-1 on page 300). The general impression is your "first impression" of the patient's immediate condition. Forming a general impression involves using a limited

✳ **general impression**

an element of the patient assessment that includes assessing approximate age, gender, and level of distress.

3-2.1 Summarize the reasons for forming a general impression of the patient.

FIGURE 11-1 As you approach the patient, you will form a general impression of her condition.

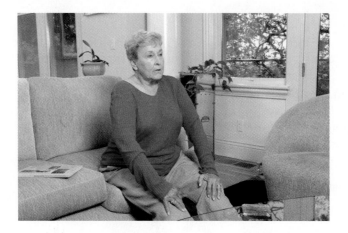

amount of information to make a quick "big sick, little sick" decision. This decision will determine how you begin your care of the patient and his priority for transport.

The specific elements that one uses to form a general impression may vary from person to person and region to region. Below is an example of some elements commonly used to help form a general impression of a patient:

* Approximate age

* Gender

* Level of distress

As you approach the patient note his approximate age: Is he elderly, middle-aged, a young adult, or a pediatric patient. As we advised in chapter 10, go ahead and estimate his age based on your best guess; close is good enough for EMS work. Race and gender will probably be obvious. (Some services include race in the general impression because some medical conditions are more prevalent in certain races. Follow your local guidelines.) The final element of the general impression is level of distress. Does the patient seem to be in a lot of pain, having difficulty breathing, or simply lying there calm and quiet? Someone with a high level of distress may need immediate attention. When verbalized, some typical general impressions might sound something like this, "I observe an approximately 50-year-old male in mild distress." or "I observe an approximately 10-year-old female in severe distress."

While your instructor may ask you to verbalize your general impression as you practice your patient assessment skill in the classroom, it is not typically verbalized during patient care in the field.

Assessing the Patient's Mental Status

3-2.2 Discuss methods of assessing altered mental status.

Up until this point you most likely have not made physical contact with your patient. If you have not, now is the time. You must approach the patient in the most appropriate manner. If he is seated, approach him from straight ahead and kneel to eye level as soon as practical (Figure 11-2). If he is lying down, approach from the side. In either case, make eye contact as soon as possible.

If the patient is in a supine position and you suspect a significant mechanism of injury you may want to gently control his head as you introduce yourself (Figure 11-3). This may prevent him from turning his head in response to your presence and making an existing injury worse. If you are uncertain as to the mechanism of

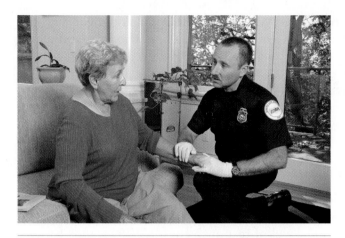

FIGURE 11-2 If the patient is seated, kneel to eye level as soon as practical.

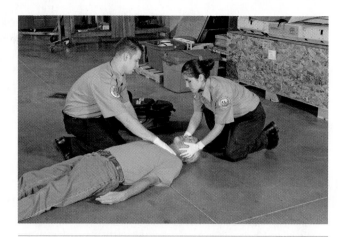

FIGURE 11-3 If the patient is in a supine position and you suspect a significant mechanism of injury, control the head as you introduce yourself.

injury or if you do suspect a spinal injury, direct someone to hold manual cervical stabilization before continuing with the exam.

As you make eye contact, introduce yourself and state your level of training. You may start with something like this, "Hello, my name is Chris and I am an EMT with the ambulance. I'm going to be taking care of you." Pay close attention to his response. Does he make eye contact with you? Is he aware of your presence? Does he engage you verbally by speaking to you or crying out in pain? Does it appear that he is going to allow you to care for him? This is your first assessment of his mental status.

3-2.3 Differentiate between assessing the altered mental status in the adult, child, and infant patient.

3-2.5 State reasons for management of the cervical spine once the patient has been determined to be a trauma patient.

THE RESPONSIVE PATIENT

For patients who are awake, you will want to determine if they are aware of who they are, where they are, what time it is, and what happened. It's not enough just to know that they are responsive; you must attempt to determine if they are alert and oriented. One technique for this is called the A&O assessment. The "A" stands for alert and the "O" stands for oriented. You will want to determine if they are A&O to the following:

* Person (who they are)
* Place (where they are)
* Time (what time it is)
* Event (what happened)

Clinical Clues: TALK TO THE RESPONSIVE PATIENT

One of the best ways of continuously monitoring the airway and breathing status of a responsive patient is to keep him talking. You can attend to other things, such as splinting a suspected fracture or controlling bleeding, while asking him questions. As long as you keep him talking, you know he has an adequate airway.

A patient who is oriented to all four is said to be A&O × 4. A patient who can only tell you his name is A&O × 1. A patient who can tell you who he is and where he is is A&O × 2.

NOTE: In some EMS systems A&O × 3 (person, place, and time) is considered fully aware and is the normal convention for describing a person's mental status. It is important to learn and use the method unique to your system.

THE UNRESPONSIVE PATIENT

Patients are not always fully alert or totally unresponsive. While this is possible, most patients fall somewhere in between. The **AVPU scale** is used to assist in assessing and documenting a patient's level of responsiveness. AVPU stands for:

> ✳ A – Alert
>
> ✳ V – Verbal
>
> ✳ P – Painful
>
> ✳ U – Unresponsive

Alert The alert patient is one who is responsive and alert to his surroundings and is aware of your presence. As just mentioned, the A&O scale can be used to further define the level of awareness for responsive patients.

Verbal The word "verbal" refers to a patient who by all appearances is unresponsive. He is most likely lying down and motionless as you approach him. However, when you speak to him or ask him if he can hear you, he responds in some meaningful way. He may respond to the sound of your voice by opening his eyes or trying to speak. When left alone, he once again appears unresponsive. A patient who responds only to verbal stimulus may have a depressed gag reflex and is at risk for airway compromise. Monitor his airway closely.

Painful When an unresponsive patient does not respond to the sound of your voice, you may attempt to stimulate a response by inflicting an appropriate painful stimulus. The emphasis here is on *appropriate*. Moderate pinches of the skin such as between the finger and thumb or the trapezies, or rubbing the patient's sternum with your knuckles are considered appropriate and not harmful to the patient as long as it's not excessive. An appropriate response to painful stimulus would be movement of the hands toward the point of pain. Sometimes the patient may also moan or groan. A patient who responds only to painful stimulus may have a depressed gag reflex and is at high risk for airway compromise. Monitor his airway closely.

Unresponsive The unresponsive patient offers no response to verbal or painful stimulus and must be considered a high priority for transport. He may have little to no gag reflex, so airway compromise is a major concern. Continue to assess his level of responsiveness throughout your care and transport and document any change in responsiveness. Review Table 11-1.

✳ **AVPU scale**

a method for classifying a patient's level of responsiveness, or mental status. The letters stand for Alert, Verbal, Painful, and Unresponsive.

3-2.4 Discuss methods of assessing the airway in the adult, child, and infant patient.

TABLE 11-1   INITIAL ASSESSMENT OF ADULTS, CHILDREN, AND INFANTS

	ADULTS	CHILDREN 1–5 YEARS	INFANTS TO 1 YEAR
Mental Status	AVPU: Is patient alert? responsive to verbal stimulus? responsive to painful stimulus? unresponsive? If alert, is patient oriented to person, place, and time?	As for adults	If not alert, shout as a verbal stimulus, flick feet as a painful stimulus.(Crying would be infant's response).
Airway	Trauma: jaw-thrust Medical: head-tilt, chin-lift Both: Consider oro- or nasopharyngeal airway, suctioning	As for adults, but see chapter 7 for special child airway techniques. If performing head-tilt, chin lift, do so without hyperextending the neck.	As for children, but see chapters 7 and 36 for special infant airway techniques.
Breathing	If respiratory arrest, perform rescue breathing. If depressed mental status and inadequate breathing (slower than 8 per minute), give positive pressure ventilations with 100% oxygen. If alert and respirations are more than 24 per minute, give 100% oxygen by nonrebreather mask.	As for adults, but normal rates for children are faster than for adults. (See chapter 7 for normal child respiration rates.) Parent may have to hold oxygen mask to reduce child's fear of mask.	As for children, but normal rates for infants are faster than for children and adults. (See chapter 7 for normal infant respiration rates.)
Circulation	Assess skin, radial pulse, bleeding. If cardiac arrest, perform CPR. See chapters 27 and 28 on how to treat for bleeding and shock.	Assess skin, radial pulse, bleeding, capillary refill. See chapter 9 for normal child pulse rates (faster than for adults). If cardiac arrest, perform CPR. See chapters 27 and 28 on how to treat for bleeding and shock.	Assess skin, brachial pulse, bleeding, capillary refill. See chapter 7 for normal infant pulse rates (faster than for children and adults). If cardiac arrest, perform CPR. See chapters 27 and 28 on how to treat for bleeding and shock.

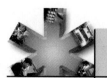

Perspective

Tammy—The EMT

"That poor girl was on her way out. The only thing that she responded to was pain—and then it was only to move her eyes toward me. There was blood everywhere on that couch . . . even some on the carpet. I know that some women have heavy periods, but this poor girl was bleeding out. All I knew was that we needed to get her to the hospital, and fast."

 ## Stop, Review, Remember!

Multiple Choice

Place a check next to the correct answer.

1. The general impression is determined immediately following the:

   _____ a. determination of the chief complaint.

   _____ b. scene size-up.

   _____ c. initial assessment.

   _____ d. SAMPLE history.

2. Which letter in the AVPU responsiveness scale refers to a patient who responds only when you rub his sternum?

   _____ a. A   _____ c. P

   _____ b. V   _____ d. U

3. A patient that is A&O × 3 is oriented to what?

   _____ a. person, place, and event

   _____ b. place, time, and event

   _____ c. person, place, and age

   _____ d. person, place, and time

4. A patient who is apparently asleep but who opens his eyes when spoken to is referred to as _____ on the AVPU scale.

   _____ a. Alert

   _____ b. Verbal

   _____ c. Painful

   _____ d. Unresponsive

5. One of the biggest concerns when caring for a patient who is unresponsive is:

   _____ a. absent breathing.

   _____ b. internal bleeding.

   _____ c. airway compromise.

   _____ d. an absent pulse.

Fill in the Blank

1. The initial assessment should be performed immediately following the _____.

2. The primary objective of the initial assessment is to identify and treat _____.

3. The initial assessment begins with the formation of a _____.

4. The _____ is designed to provide a quick "big sick, little sick" determination.

5. A patient who is A&O × 4 is said to be alert and oriented to person, place, time and _____.

6. A patient who responds to the sound of your voice by opening his eyes or trying to speak is said to be _____ on the AVPU scale.

Critical Thinking

1. Describe why the initial assessment is such an important component of the overall patient assessment.

   _____

   _____

   _____

   _____

2. What elements are you considering when you formulate a general impression of a patient?

   _____

   _____

   _____

   _____

3. A patient who is A&O × 2 can tell you what information?

   _____

   _____

   _____

   _____

Determining the Chief Complaint

✳ **chief complaint**

the patient's perception of the problem in his own words.

Simply stated, the **chief complaint** is the patient's perception of the problem in his own words. It is NOT what you the EMT perceive to be the problem. You may have been dispatched to a call for "chest pain"; however when you arrive your patient states that he is having difficulty breathing. When you ask if he is having any chest pain he states, "Yes, but I can't seem to catch my breath."

There may be times when the patient has several complaints and does not say that one is worse than the other. With these patients, you must do your best to decide which is the most serious of the complaints and provide care accordingly. One suggested approach to determining the patient's chief complaint is to use the following formula when you initiate contact with the patient: "Hello. My name is Dan and I'm with the rescue squad. What seems to be the problem today?" The first thing out of the patient's mouth will likely be his chief complaint.

IDENTIFYING APPARENT LIFE THREATS

As we have stated before, the primary purpose of the initial assessment is to identify and care for all immediate life threats. Some of these threats are more obvious than others. As you approach the patient, you need to look for and identify any obvious threats that may not be directly related to the ABCs. Such things as open chest wounds, impaled objects, or entrapment may need to be addressed before continuing on with the rest of the initial assessment.

> ### Clinical Clues: SAFETY
>
> Sometimes there are obvious life threats even before you begin your initial assessment of the patient. Things such as exposure to flames and unstable vehicles must be addressed prior to beginning your formal assessment.

3-2.11 Compare the methods of providing airway care to the adult, child, and infant patient.

Assessing the Patient's Airway

As you introduce yourself to the patient and assess his mental status, you will simultaneously be assessing the status of his airway. This is easier to accomplish for responsive patients, because it can be deduced that if they are talking they must have a clear airway. If for any reason they do not have a clear airway, such as with a choking patient, you must immediately clear the airway using the appropriate method. Once you are comfortable that they have a clear airway, you will assess for adequacy of breathing. This will be covered a little later.

Assessing for an open airway in an unresponsive patient takes a little more work. If you are not certain the airway is open, you must manually open it using the appropriate method. The specific method you use to open the airway will depend on the patient's age and the mechanism of injury. For a medical patient in whom you do not suspect a spinal injury, you will use the head-tilt, chin-lift maneuver. For a patient with an unknown MOI or one in whom you suspect a spinal injury, you must perform the jaw-thrust maneuver. Refer to chapter 7 for details on both of these maneuvers.

If for any reason you believe the airway is compromised, you must immediately perform the appropriate procedures to clear the airway.

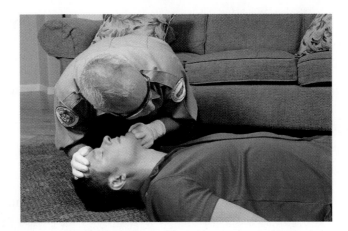

FIGURE 11-4 Perform an initial assessment of the adequacy of breathing by looking, listening, and feeling for breathing.

ASSESSING FOR ADEQUACY OF BREATHING

It is not enough to know the patient has a clear airway. You must confirm that he is breathing at an appropriate rate and moving an adequate amount of air (tidal volume) with each breath. The method for initially assessing the adequacy of breathing is the same for all patients. You must assess rate, depth, and ease by observing the chest for rise and fall and assess for signs of difficulty breathing, such as increased rate and use of accessory muscles (Figure 11-4). Even if breathing appears adequate, consider the need for supplemental oxygen.

A respiratory rate that is greater than 24 is considered inadequate, and the patient should receive oxygen by nonrebreather mask at 15 lpm. A rate less than 10 is also inadequate and may require assisted ventilations by bag-valve mask or similar device. Regardless of the device, the use of supplemental oxygen is recommended. For unresponsive patients, consider the need for an appropriate airway adjunct.

OXYGEN THERAPY

It is during the initial assessment that you will make your first determination of whether the patient would benefit from supplemental oxygen. While it is probably safe to say that all patients will benefit from supplemental oxygen, this does not mean that all patients MUST receive supplemental oxygen. That decision is up to the EMT and is based on many factors, including but not limited to mechanism of

3-2.6 Describe methods used for assessing if a patient is breathing.

3-2.7 State what care should be provided to the adult, child, and infant patient with adequate breathing.

3-2.10 Distinguish between methods of assessing breathing in the adult, child, and infant patient.

3-2.8 State what care should be provided to the adult, child, and infant patient without adequate breathing.

3-2.9 Differentiate between a patient with adequate and inadequate breathing.

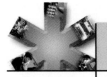

Perspective

C.J.—The EMT

"That lady's airway was fine; I could hear her breathing and grunting as we moved her, but her respiratory rate was a little slow and shallow. When we moved her to our cot, I put a nonrebreather on her with 15 liters of oxygen. I figured between her poor breathing and the major blood loss, a bunch of oxygen would be her best bet. Even with the oxygen, I knew we needed to keep an eye on her breathing rate and volume during the transport."

injury (MOI) or nature of illness (NOI), level of distress, and signs and symptoms. If you decide initially to not provide oxygen, this does not mean that you cannot change your mind later. Perhaps you will want to initiate oxygen once you have the majority of the history from the patient. The point is, you must constantly reassess the need for appropriate interventions, and oxygen can be initiated at any time.

3-2.12 Describe the methods used to obtain a pulse.

3-2.13 Differentiate between obtaining a pulse in an adult, child, and infant patient.

Assessing for Adequacy of Circulation

Once you have determined that the airway is clear and the patient is breathing adequately, you must assess for adequacy of circulation. This is accomplished by locating an appropriate pulse point. For responsive patients greater than 1 year of age, use the radial pulse (Figure 11-5A). For responsive pediatric patients less than 1 year old, use the brachial pulse in the upper arm (Figure 11-5B).

For unresponsive patients greater than 1 year of age use the carotid pulse (Figure 11-6). For unresponsive patients under 1 year of age, use the brachial pulse. If a pulse cannot be located, immediately begin CPR. If the patient is greater than 1 year of age, attach an automated external defibrillator if available (follow local protocol).

In pediatric patients under the age of 6, you can use the capillary refill test to help determine the adequacy of perfusion. A capillary refill time of less than 2 seconds is

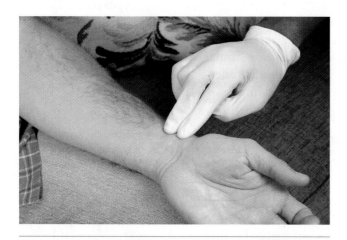

FIGURE 11-5A   Assess the radial pulse in the adult patient.

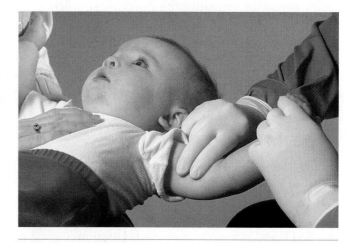

FIGURE 11-5B   Assess the brachial pulse in the infant.

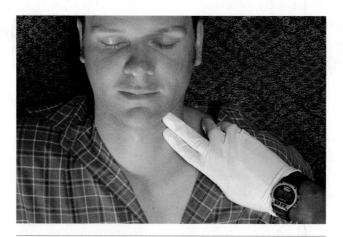

FIGURE 11-6   For unresponsive patients over the age of 1, assess the carotid pulse.

considered normal. Remember that the capillary refill test is only one component in the overall patient assessment and should not be used as the sole determination of adequate or inadequate perfusion.

Assessing for Serious Bleeding

Quickly assess the patient for evidence of serious external bleeding. Look for obvious blood pooling beneath the patient or blood stained clothing. Cut away clothing or carefully roll the patient to control obvious bleeding.

3-2.14 Discuss the need for assessing the patient for external bleeding.

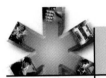

Perspective

Tammy—The EMT

"I'd never seen vaginal bleeding like that, except maybe post delivery. It was just running out. As soon as we got her on the cot, I grabbed a trauma dressing and tried to control the bleeding as best I could, but I knew that the hospital was the only place where this girl was going to have a chance."

Assessing Skin Signs

Assess the patient's skin color, temperature, and moisture. Begin by looking at and feeling the skin of the face, lips, and conjunctiva. Observe for and document any abnormal findings. Normal skin signs are pink, warm, and dry. Abnormal skin signs include skin that is pale, flushed, or a color other than pink. Skin that is sweaty, extremely hot, or cool to the touch may also be a sign of underlying injury or illness.

In addition to the skin signs just mentioned, capillary refill time should be assessed in all pediatric patients. A capillary refill time of less than 2 seconds is considered normal in most patients. See also chapter 10 regarding capillary refill.

3-2.15 Describe normal and abnormal findings when assessing skin color.

3-2.16 Describe normal and abnormal findings when assessing skin temperature.

3-2.17 Describe normal and abnormal findings when assessing skin condition.

3-2.18 Describe normal and abnormal findings when assessing skin capillary refill in the infant and child patient.

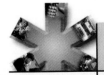

Perspective

The Husband

"I've been with her through a lot of medical stuff, you know? Diabetic problems, dialysis. . . you name it. But I've never seen her so pale and cold. It scared me enough to call 9-1-1! She's just never been that bad before."

Determining Patient Priority

You will use all of the information that you have gathered during your initial assessment to determine the treatment and transport priority for your patient. Depending on his condition, a patient can be placed into a high, medium, or low priority. This priority will determine such things as how quickly he should receive care and how quickly you must get him to the hospital. The following is a list of factors that might place a patient in a high priority category:

* Poor general impression
* Unresponsive
* Altered mental status
* Difficulty breathing
* Signs of shock
* Complicated childbirth
* Chest pain with BP <100 systolic
* Uncontrolled bleeding
* Severe pain anywhere

Patient condition will determine his priority and priority will determine how quickly he receives care and transport. In some cases, his priority will also determine whether or not an ALS intercept is indicated.

CONTINUING YOUR ASSESSMENT

Once you have completed the initial assessment and have identified and cared for all immediate life threats to the patient, you may move on to the next component of the patient assessment. You may not, however, move on if any of the critical components of the initial assessment still need attention. For instance, if the patient is not breathing adequately, you must assist him accordingly. If there is severe external bleeding, you must perform the appropriate techniques to control the bleeding before doing anything else.

In some situations, you may spend all of your time dealing with issues related to the initial assessment and never complete a full assessment. Do not delay transport simply to complete a full assessment. If the patient is a high or medium priority, consider loading him into the ambulance and continuing care while en route to an appropriate receiving facility.

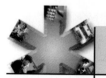

Perspective

Tammy—The EMT

"What priority was she? You're kidding, right? Just look at the initial assessment. One, she had a tremendously poor general appearance. Two, she was all but unresponsive. And three . . . she was losing blood fast and I couldn't stop it. It just doesn't get more serious than all that."

Stop, Review, Remember!

Multiple Choice

Place a check next to the correct answer.

1. The best maneuver for opening the airway of an unresponsive medical patient is the _____ maneuver.

   _____ a. jaw-thrust

   _____ b. head-thrust

   _____ c. head-tilt, chin-lift

   _____ d. jaw-tilt

2. The assessment for adequacy of breathing includes:

   _____ a. rate, depth, and ease.

   _____ b. rate, strength, and rhythm.

   _____ c. rate, depth, and volume.

   _____ d. rate, ease, and volume.

3. Assessment of circulation should occur immediately following assessment of:

   _____ a. pulse.

   _____ b. mental status.

   _____ c. airway.

   _____ d. breathing.

4. When performing an initial assessment, the control of serious bleeding should occur:

   _____ a. before airway and breathing.

   _____ b. after circulation assessment.

   _____ c. at the end.

   _____ d. immediately.

5. The decision to administer supplemental oxygen occurs during which step of the initial assessment?

   _____ a. determining chief complaint

   _____ b. assessing mental status

   _____ c. assessing breathing

   _____ d. determining priority

Matching

Match the definition on the left with the applicable term on the right.

1. _____ A patient's perception of his problem stated in his own words

2. _____ The primary objective of the initial assessment

3. _____ Preferred method for opening the airway of a patient with an unknown MOI

4. _____ Preferred pulse for assessing circulation in an unresponsive adult

5. _____ Preferred pulse for assessing circulation in an unresponsive infant

A. Identify life threats
B. Chief Complaint
C. Carotid
D. Brachial
E. Jaw-thrust

Critical Thinking

1. Describe how you would assess the airway of a responsive patient versus an unresponsive patient.

_____

_____

_____

_____

2. How would you determine the adequacy of an unresponsive patient's breathing?

_____

_____

_____

_____

3. How will you determine if a patient would benefit from supplemental oxygen?

_____

_____

_____

_____

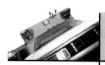

Dispatch Summary

The patient was placed gently on the cot in the Trendelenburg position, covered with a blanket, given oxygen via nonrebreather mask at 15 lpm, and rushed to the nearest hospital.

The patient was immediately admitted into surgery where her bleeding—determined to have been caused by a miscarriage—was successfully controlled. She was released from the hospital several days later.

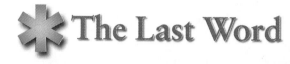 **The Last Word**

An initial assessment must be performed on each and every patient with the primary goal being to identify and care for all immediate life threats. You must ensure that all elements of the initial assessment are addressed properly before moving on with the rest of the patient assessment:

✳ As you approach the patient, form a general impression to begin to make the "big sick, little sick" determination. The general impression can include:
  - Approximate age
  - Gender
  - Level of distress

✳ Determine level of responsiveness using the A&O and/or the AVPU scales.

✳ Determine the chief complaint and mitigate any immediate life threats.

✳ Confirm that the patient has a clear airway.

✳ Confirm that the patient is breathing with an adequate rate and tidal volume.

✳ Consider the need for supplemental oxygen.

✳ Confirm the presence of adequate circulation.

✳ Identify and care for any obvious external bleeding.

✳ Make an informed determination regarding priority for care and transport.

 Chapter Review

MULTIPLE CHOICE

Place a check next to the correct answer.

1. Which of the following is NOT a component of the initial assessment?

　_____ a. general impression

　_____ b. chief complaint

　_____ c. vital signs

　_____ d. priority

2. The general impression includes such elements as the patient's age, gender, and:

　_____ a. level of distress.

　_____ b. chief complaint.

　_____ c. mechanism of injury.

　_____ d. level of responsiveness.

3. Which of the following is the most appropriate reason for forming a general impression?

　_____ a. Determine level of responsiveness.

　_____ b. Determine the patient's chief complaint.

　_____ c. Identify any immediate life threats.

　_____ d. Establish a first impression of patient's condition.

4. A patient who is awake and able to respond appropriately is said to be _____ on the AVPU scale.

　_____ a. alert　　　　_____ c. painful

　_____ b. verbal　　　_____ d. unresponsive

5. Confirming that a patient is alert and oriented includes establishing that he is aware of person, _____, time, and event.

　_____ a. complaint　　_____ c. surroundings

　_____ b. place　　　　_____ d. age

CRITICAL THINKING

1. We mentioned four things from which a person can die in a short period of time. Discuss each of them and how they would lead to the death of the patient.

_____

_____

_____

_____

2. Can you think of any other conditions not included in the above list that can cause the death of a patient?

_____

_____

_____

_____

3. What is the purpose of forming a general impression of each and every patient?

_____

_____

_____

_____

4. Why is it important to use the patient's own words when relaying or documenting the patient's chief complaint?

_____

_____

_____

_____

CASE STUDIES

Case Study 1

You have responded to a single-vehicle rollover. Upon arrival, you are told by bystanders that the car is over the side of the road and against a tree. You safely make your way to the vehicle but are unable to gain access to the patient. You have called for the extrication team and have established verbal contact with the patient.

1. How might you conduct an initial assessment from your position outside the vehicle?

_____

_____

_____

2. What elements of the initial assessment will be most difficult to assess without making patient contact?

_____

_____

_____

_____

Case Study 2

You have been dispatched to a convalescent hospital for an unknown medical problem. Upon arrival, you are escorted back to one of the patient rooms where you find an unresponsive female patient lying on the floor of the bathroom. One of the nursing staff tells you she has a history of falling all the time, and they were unable to get her back into bed due to the patient being in too much pain.

1. Describe how you will perform your initial assessment on this patient.

_____

_____

_____

_____

2. She remains unresponsive and you are unable to determine if she is breathing adequately. What will you do next?

_____

_____

_____

_____

3. She now appears to be breathing adequately but you are unable to palpate a radial pulse. What will you do next?

_____

_____

_____

_____

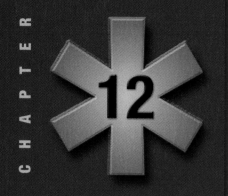

CHAPTER 12

Assessing the Trauma Patient

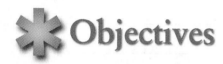

Objectives

Numbered objectives are from the U.S. Department of Transportation 1994 EMT-Basic National Standard Curriculum.

COGNITIVE OBJECTIVES

At the completion of this lesson, the EMT-Basic student will be able to:

3-3.1   Discuss the reasons for reconsideration concerning the mechanism of injury. (pp. 319–322)

3-3.2   State the reasons for performing a rapid trauma assessment. (pp. 324–325)

3-3.3   Recite examples and explain why patients should receive a rapid trauma assessment. (p. 324)

3-3.4   Describe the areas included in the rapid trauma assessment and discuss what should be evaluated. (p. 325)

3-3.5   Differentiate when the rapid assessment may be altered in order to provide patient care. (p. 329)

3-3.6   Discuss the reason for performing a focused history and physical exam. (pp. 330–331)

3-5.1   Discuss the components of the detailed physical exam. (pp. 331–332)

3-5.2   State the areas of the body that are evaluated during the detailed physical exam. (pp. 332–334)

3-5.3   Explain what additional care should be provided while performing the detailed physical exam. (p. 335)

3-5.4   Distinguish between the detailed physical exam that is performed on a trauma patient and that of the medical patient. (pp. 326–329, 331–332)

AFFECTIVE OBJECTIVES

At the completion of this lesson, the EMT-Basic student will be able to:

3-3.7   Recognize and respect the feelings that patients might experience during assessment. (p. 326)

3-5.5   Explain the rationale for the feelings that these patients might be experiencing. (p. 326)

PSYCHOMOTOR OBJECTIVES

At the completion of this lesson, the EMT-Basic student will be able to:

3-3.8   Demonstrate the rapid trauma assessment that should be used to assess a patient based on mechanism of injury. (pp. 326–329)

3-5.6   Demonstrate the skills involved in performing the detailed physical exam. (pp. 331–332)

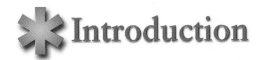 **Introduction**

Good patient care is directly related to a good patient assessment. In other words, if your assessment is thorough, it is likely that the associated care will be appropriate as well. If the assessment is poor, it stands to reason that the care provided will be less than optimal. This chapter will focus specifically on the assessment of the trauma patient. The next chapter will discuss the assessment of the medical patient.

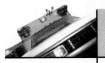 ## Emergency Dispatch

"**U**nit 44: 44, I need you to respond to an emergency at Joy's Truck Stop on I-40 and Morgan." The dispatcher's voice, normally monotone and emotionless, was coming in rapid bursts from the radio. "You've got a 53-year old-male trapped between two trailers. Extrication is also en route."

Several minutes later, when Preston and Michelle, the EMTs on truck 44, arrived at Joy's, the scene was in chaos. A woman was crying hysterically behind the steering wheel of a pickup truck with a fifth-wheel trailer trapped and the male patient—whose swollen right arm seemed to blend into the metal folds of the damaged trailers—was arguing with a trucker who was trying to apply some sort of tourniquet. Blood was running freely down the jagged metal before falling into pools on the concrete.

"Oh, boy," Preston took a deep breath and grabbed his equipment pack. "Let's hope that the extrication crew gets here quick."

The Trauma versus the Medical Patient

While it can be argued that all patients have medical problems, the medical profession, including EMS, divides all patients into one of two fundamental categories. This categorization is based on whether the chief complaint is related to an illness or injury.

Patients whose chief complaint is related to an illness such as difficulty breathing, chest pain, or headache are categorized as "medical" patients. Patients whose chief complaint is related to an injury are categorized as "trauma" patients. Simply stated, injury equals trauma and illness equals medical. This differentiation is important, because the specific assessment path you will follow will be different for each category.

The flow chart in Figure 12-1 on page 318 shows all of the components of a patient assessment for both medical and trauma patients. This chapter will focus specifically on the trauma assessment path that is shown on the left-hand side of the flowchart.

PATIENT ASSESSMENT

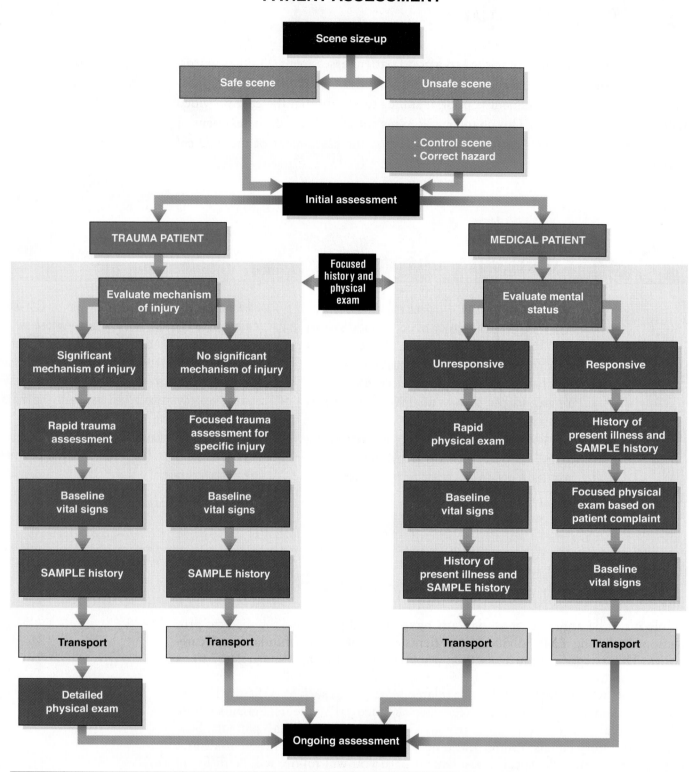

FIGURE 12-1 Components of patient assessment for both medical and trauma patients.

As you will notice, both the trauma and the medical assessments begin with common elements performed in the same order each time. These components are as follows:

* BSI precautions

* Scene size-up

* Initial assessment

Other elements, such as vital signs, SAMPLE history, and ongoing assessments are common to both but will be performed in a different order.

It cannot be overstated how important each of the beginning components—BSI precautions, scene size-up, and initial assessment—is to the well being of both the EMT and the patient. Only after ensuring that you are protected, the scene is safe, and all aspects of the initial assessment are addressed will you move on to complete your patient assessment of the trauma or medical patient.

Management of the Trauma Patient

Trauma patients are managed differently than most medical patients in the pre-hospital setting. Trauma to the body results in injury to soft tissues, organ systems, and/or bones and can result in significant blood loss. For this reason, time is a critical factor in the survival of the trauma patient. As a general rule, it is recommended to limit on-scene time to 10 minutes or less when caring for trauma patients, especially those with serious injuries from a significant mechanism of injury. For many of these patients, the sooner they can get to surgery the more likely they will survive. The 10-minute rule serves as a guideline only and may not be possible with patients who need significant extrication.

REEVALUATING THE MECHANISM OF INJURY

Evaluation of the mechanism of injury (MOI) is critical when caring for the trauma patient. You made your first assessment of the MOI during the scene size-up and identified to the best of your ability any major MOI, such as a fall, motor vehicle collision, or blunt trauma (Figure 12-2). Now you must take a closer look at the specific factors involved in the MOI and make predictions about potential injury based on those factors.

3-3.1 Discuss the reasons for reconsideration concerning the mechanism of injury.

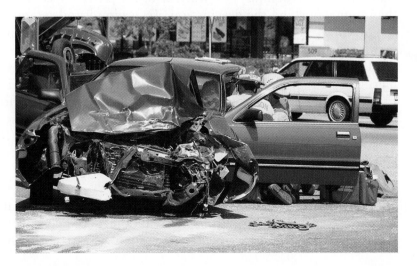

FIGURE 12-2   The significant MOI at this scene is a frontal impact motor vehicle collision. (© Eddie M. Sperling.)

Factors that should be assessed during the reevaluation of the MOI following a vehicle collision are as follows:

* Ejection from a vehicle

* Position of patient in the vehicle during impact

* Use of safety restraints/airbags

* Intrusion into the vehicle

* Approximate speed of vehicle(s) at the time of the collision

* Object impacted

* Damage to inside of vehicle

* Death of other occupant in same vehicle

* Loss of consciousness or altered mental status

Factors that should be assessed during the reevaluation of the MOI following a fall from height are as follows:

* Height of fall

* Surface landed on

* Position when hitting the ground (head, feet, or side first)

* Anything struck on the way down

* Loss of consciousness

As you will notice when you study the trauma side of the patient assessment flow chart (review Figure 12-1), you will find two parallel assessment paths for the trauma patient. The path that you will follow for a specific trauma patient will depend on the evaluation of one critical piece of information, the mechanism of injury. If the MOI is considered to be "significant" you will follow the path on the left, and if it is "not significant" you will follow the path on the right.

SIGNIFICANT MECHANISM OF INJURY

There is much debate regarding the difference between significant and not significant mechanisms of injury. We will attempt to provide specific examples of each and the rationale behind the designation. To begin to understand what is meant by a "significant" MOI, you need to have at least a fundamental understanding of human anatomy. The majority of the body's vital organs are contained within the skull, chest, abdomen, and pelvis. Therefore, when these areas sustain injury the vital organs that lie within them are at serious risk for damage. The most immediate risk is the loss of blood from tissue and vessel damage. In addition to physical damage to these vital organs, their function can become compromised. When one organ begins to fail, it creates a domino affect, and other vital organs begin to fail as well.

✻ **multi-system trauma**

term referring to the multiple organ systems that are generally affected by significant mechanisms of injury.

A term often associated with victims of significant MOI is **multi-system trauma.** The term *multi-system* refers to the multiple organ systems that are generally affected by significant MOIs.

For a patient who has sustained a mechanism of injury that you suspect could have caused damage to the skull, chest, abdomen, or pelvis, you must consider this a significant MOI and follow the appropriate assessment path (Figure 12-3). The

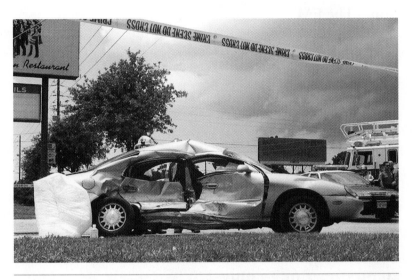

FIGURE 12-3 A motor vehicle collision with significant intrusion into the passenger compartment is considered a significant MOI. (© Eddie M. Sperling.)

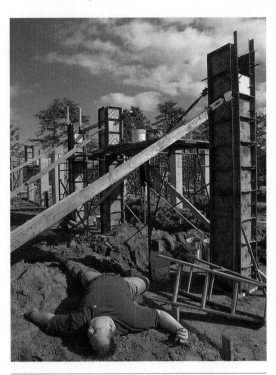

FIGURE 12-4 The MOI is a fall from a significant height.

following are examples of mechanisms of injury that are commonly considered significant:

* Ejection from a moving vehicle

* Death of a passenger within the same compartment of a vehicle

* Falls greater than 20 feet (Figure 12-4)

* Rollover of a moving vehicle

* High-speed vehicle collision

* Vehicle versus pedestrian collision

* Driver or passenger of a motorcycle crash

* Trauma resulting in a loss of consciousness or altered mental status

* Penetrations of the head, chest, abdomen, or pelvis

* Significant blunt trauma to the head, chest, abdomen, or pelvis

Less force is needed to cause significant injury with pediatric patients. Falls greater than 10 feet should be considered significant MOIs with these patients.

It should be understood by the EMT that, while safety devices such as seat belts and airbags do save lives, they may also cause injury. Seat belts, even when properly worn, can cause bone and soft-tissue injury to the pelvis, lower abdomen, and shoulder.

It should also be understood that airbags may not deploy at low speeds, thus allowing the occupant to strike the steering column, dash board, or windshield. Significant injury is still possible with an airbag if the occupant is not wearing a seatbelt. Lift the deployed airbag when possible and assess the dash or steering column for damage that may suggest a serious MOI.

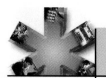

Perspective

Preston—The EMT

"I've got to be honest! I've never seen a mechanism like that before! I mean, it seemed like it was just his arm that was involved, but was anything else injured? Could his torso have been smashed in the initial collision? Was I going to focus so much on this nasty, essentially amputated arm that I was going to miss some really life-threatening injury that wasn't so obvious? As I was approaching the patient I just kept wondering things like 'Am I supposed to c-spine this guy?' You know how you go over and over what you learned in class, trying to see if you can remember anything that applies to your current situation? That was truly an amazing call. It kind of encompassed everything about trauma."

NO SIGNIFICANT MECHANISM OF INJURY

As already noted, significant mechanisms of injury typically involve injury to the head, chest, abdomen, or pelvis, resulting in damage to multiple body systems. Mechanisms of injury that are not significant, while they may be painful and destructive, typically do not cause life-threatening injuries. Most isolated injuries to the extremities are considered not significant.

 Stop, Review, Remember!

Multiple Choice

Place a check next to the correct answer.

1. Which of the following best defines the term *multi-system trauma*?

   _____ a. obvious injuries to multiple bones

   _____ b. suspected injury to multiple body systems

   _____ c. multiple mechanisms of injury

   _____ d. multiple patients

2. Which of the following elements of the patient assessment is NOT common to all assessments?

   _____ a. focused trauma assessment

   _____ b. initial assessment

   _____ c. scene size-up

   _____ d. BSI precautions

3. Which of the following most represents a significant MOI?

_____ a. a right foot that was run over by a forklift

_____ b. a 20-foot fall onto concrete

_____ c. an 8-foot fall from a ladder onto asphalt

_____ d. crush injury to both lower legs

4. Falls greater than _____ feet should be considered as significant mechanisms of injury for pediatric patients.

_____ a. 2   _____ c. 5

_____ b. 3   _____ d. 10

5. The first time that MOI is assessed is during the:

_____ a. scene size-up.

_____ b. initial assessment.

_____ c. rapid trauma assessment.

_____ d. detailed physical exam.

Critical Thinking

1. Provide two examples each of what would be considered a "medical" patient and a "trauma" patient.

_____

_____

_____

_____

2. If you knew you were responding to a fall victim, what questions would you like to have answered before you arrive on scene?

_____

_____

_____

_____

3. For each of the patients below, determine whether the MOI is significant or not significant:

1. 57-year-old male who was found unresponsive beneath a ladder in his garage _____

2. 13-year-old female whose hand was run over by a car _____

3. 22-year-old female who was struck by a car while crossing the street _____

4. 32–year-old female who was struck by a car while riding a motorcycle _____

5. 7- year-old male who fell while running and has deformity to his right wrist _____

Determining the Appropriate Assessment Path

3-3.3 Recite examples and explain why patients should receive a rapid trauma assessment.

Deciding whether or not the mechanism of injury is significant will determine which specific assessment path you will follow. When caring for a patient who you believe has sustained a significant MOI, you will perform a rapid trauma assessment. When caring for a patient who you believe has NOT sustained a significant MOI, you will perform a focused trauma assessment based on the chief complaint. The chart in Figure 12-5 shows these two assessment paths side by side.

RAPID VERSUS FOCUSED ASSESSMENT

The first major decision point in the patient assessment comes immediately following the initial assessment. At this point you will decide between the rapid trauma assessment and the focused trauma assessment. That decision is made based on the mechanism of injury. The rapid assessment is for more critical patients while the focused assessment is for less critical patients.

FIGURE 12-5 Components of patient assessment for a trauma patient.

ASSESSMENT OF TRAUMA PATIENT

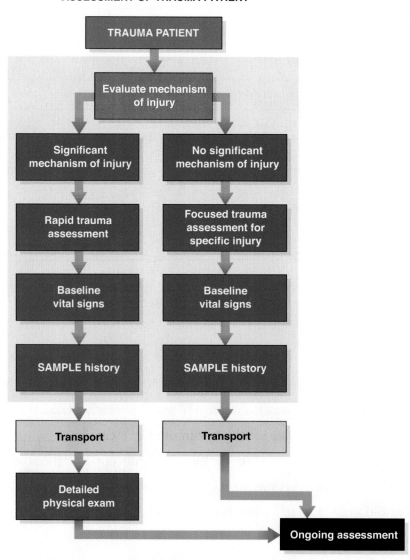

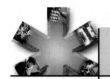

Perspective

Michelle—The EMT

"We didn't have much time with this poor guy. I could tell right away that his arm was done for, if you know what I mean. There was just enough tissue still attached to keep him trapped, which is unfortunate because the initial crush and the sharp metal edges were keeping his veins open and bleeding. I just kept thinking, 'Move fast, move fast, move fast'. I don't know but I might have even been saying it out loud!"

RAPID TRAUMA ASSESSMENT

The primary purpose of the rapid trauma assessment is to quickly identify all areas of injury or suspected injury not already addressed by the initial assessment. It involves a rapid head-to-toe physical examination of the patient, looking for obvious signs of injury.

The following areas are assessed during the rapid trauma assessment:

* Head
* Neck
* Chest
* Abdomen
* Pelvis
* Back
* Extremities

Remember to maintain appropriate spinal precautions with all trauma patients. In most cases, trauma patients will be a high priority for transport. Consider the need for ALS backup or an ALS intercept if appropriate.

As you perform the rapid trauma assessment, you will be looking for signs of obvious or suspected injury. The mnemonic **DCAP-BTLS** is a tool that can be used by the EMT to assist in remembering the most obvious signs of injury.

* **D—Deformities**—A deformity is a deviation from the normal shape or size of a body part. These are typically caused by broken bones or soft-tissue swelling. You must inspect and palpate all areas of the body, looking for signs of deformity.

* **C—Contusions**—Contusions are areas of soft tissue that have been damaged although the skin remains intact. They are characterized by discoloration and swelling. Another name for the discoloration is bruising.

* **A—Abrasions**—Abrasions are the wearing down or rubbing away of the superficial layers of skin. One of the most common forms of abrasion is known as road rash and is caused when a person slides along the pavement at a high rate of speed.

3-3.2 State the reasons for performing a rapid trauma assessment.

3-3.4 Describe the areas included in the rapid trauma assessment and discuss what should be evaluated.

* **DCAP-BTLS**

a mnemonic used to identify the obvious signs of injury. The letters stand for Deformities, Contusions, Abrasions, Punctures/Penetrations, Burns, Tenderness, Lacerations, and Swelling.

✳ **P—Punctures/Penetrations**—Punctures are often difficult-to-see small holes in the skin caused by sharp objects. Punctures are evidence of potentially serious injuries, depending on how deeply the objected penetrated the skin. All penetrations should be noted, whether puncture-size or larger.

✳ **B—Burns**—Burns occur when the skin is damaged by thermal, chemical, or electrical contact. Assess burned areas for the amount of body surface affected and the depth of the burns. See chapter 30 for more specific information on the assessment and care of burns.

✳ **T—Tenderness**—Tenderness is the pain caused when an area of the body is being palpated. Pay particular attention to tenderness in the chest, abdomen, and pelvic areas, as this could be a sign of serious internal injury.

✳ **L—Lacerations**—Lacerations can be caused by either sharp or blunt objects and are often characterized by a jagged open wound or cut. Bleeding from lacerations can be anywhere from minimal to severe, depending on the extent of soft-tissue and vessel damage. You must control all serious bleeding before moving on with your exam.

✳ **S—Swelling**—Swelling is a localized enlargement of soft tissue typically caused by an accumulation of blood and other fluids. In most cases, where you find swelling you will also find tenderness. Gently palpate the area of swelling and note if you can leave an indentation with your finger. *Edema* is another word for swelling.

To find these signs, you will need to expose the patient. This means removing or cutting away clothing in order to see and palpate the area or areas of the body you are assessing. Be sure to tell the patient what you are doing and offer reassurance as necessary. Protect the patient's privacy and take steps to prevent unnecessarily long exposure to cold. Document all appropriate information.

PERFORMING THE RAPID TRAUMA ASSESSMENT

Using appropriate BSI precautions, inspect and palpate the following areas of the patient's body, looking for any sign of possible injury. When an injury is discov-

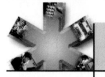

Perspective

Jim—The Patient

"It's all a little hazy, actually. I remember the fifth-wheel lurching toward another truck and I think I tried to stop it. How stupid is that? I can remember this big, bright flash and I think I couldn't breathe for a second. And then my arm . . . oh man. I definitely remember my arm! I actually felt the bone crumble and the pain . . . it was like nothing I've . . . I've never felt anything like that before. It hurt so bad that I couldn't even feel the rest of my body! When they asked if I hurt anywhere else I remember yelling, 'Look at my arm! Do something about my arm!'"

ered, you must decide if it is life threatening or not. For those injuries that you suspect could be life threatening, you must stop your exam and provide the indicated care. For non-life-threatening injuries, you may proceed with your exam and provide the indicated care when appropriate.

HEAD

Palpate and inspect the head for DCAP-BTLS, including **crepitation** (grating sound or feeling as bones rub together) of the cranial bones. Run your fingers through the hair, noting any evidence of blood (Figure 12-6). You must maintain stabilization of the cervical spine as you palpate and inspect.

NECK

Palpate and inspect the neck for DCAP-BTLS, including **jugular vein distention (JVD), tracheal deviation,** and crepitation (Figure 12-7). Immediately following assessment of the neck, apply an appropriate cervical collar.

CHEST

Palpate and inspect the chest for DCAP-BTLS, including **paradoxical movement** of the chest wall, **subcutaneous emphysema,** and crepitation (Figure 12-8 on page 328). Assessment of the chest should also include bilateral auscultation of breath sounds.

ABDOMEN

Palpate and inspect the abdomen for DCAP-BTLS (Figure 12-9 on page 328). Note any **tenderness, rigidity, distention,** or **guarding,** and watch the patient's face for signs of pain.

PELVIS

Palpate and inspect the pelvis for DCAP-BTLS, including evidence of wetness that may be caused by blood or loss of bladder control. If there is no major complaint of pain to the pelvis, place one hand on each hip bone and gently compress the pelvis down and inward (Figure 12-10 on page 328). Note any tenderness or instability.

✳ **crepitation**

the grating sound or feeling of broken bones rubbing together. Also called crepitus.

✳ **jugular vein distention (JVD)**

bulging of the neck veins.

✳ **tracheal deviation**

displacement of the trachea laterally from the midline.

✳ **paradoxical movement**

movement of a part of the chest in the opposite direction to the rest of the chest during inhalation and exhalation.

✳ **subcutaneous emphysema**

crackling sensation caused by air just underneath the skin.

✳ **tenderness**

pain that is elicited through palpation.

✳ **rigidity**

tenseness, immovability, stiffness, an inability to bend or be bent.

✳ **distention**

a condition of being stretched, inflated, or larger than normal.

✳ **guarding**

body defense mechanism, to prevent the movement of an injured part.

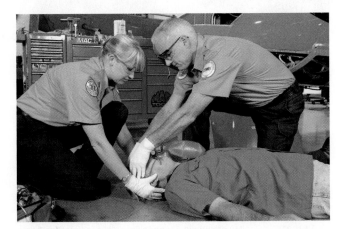

FIGURE 12-6   Use both hands to palpate and inspect the head.

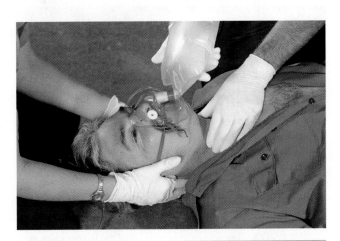

FIGURE 12-7   Palpate the neck for tracheal deviation.

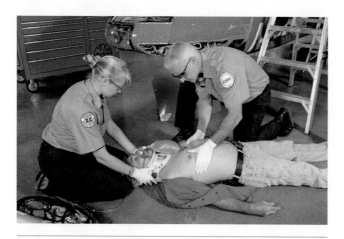

FIGURE 12-8   Use both hands to palpate and inspect the chest.

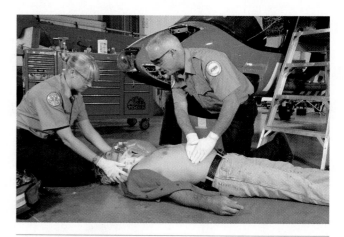

FIGURE 12-9   Use both hands to palpate and inspect the abdomen.

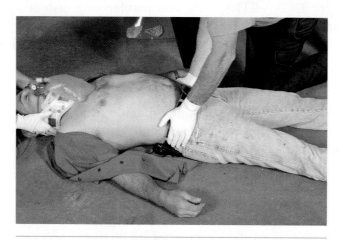

FIGURE 12-10   Use both hands to examine the pelvis for injury.

BACK

Palpate and inspect the back for DCAP-BTLS including paradoxical movement, subcutaneous emphysema, and crepitation (Figure 12-11A). Do your best to palpate as much of the back without rolling the patient or compromising the spine. If necessary, maintain spinal immobilization and roll the patient to perform a complete assessment of the back (Figure 12-11B).

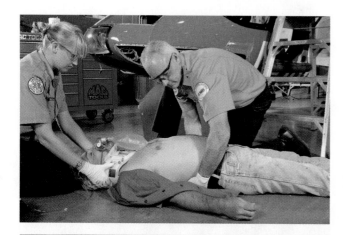

FIGURE 12-11A   Use one hand to slide under the lrumbar spine to palpate the back.

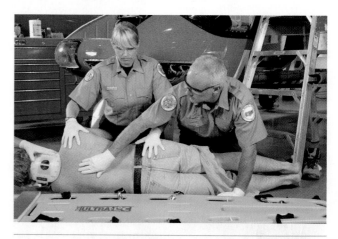

FIGURE 12-11B   Maintain spinal immobilization to inspect the back prior to rolling onto a backboard.

EXTREMITIES

Palpate and inspect each extremity for DCAP-BTLS (Figures 12-12 and 12-13). Assess the hands and feet for circulation, sensation, and motor function (CSM). When evaluating motor function, do so with both extremities simultaneously (Figure 12-14A and B). This will allow you to detect slight differences in strength from one side to the other.

If at any point during the rapid trauma assessment you discover what could be a life-threatening injury not found during the initial assessment, you must stop the exam and provide care for the problem immediately. It is important to remember that all potential life threats must be addressed as they are found. Examples of immediate life threats that need immediate intervention include:

3-3.5 Differentiate when the rapid assessment may be altered in order to provide patient care.

* Facial injuries that compromise the airway—have suction ready to help clear the airway of blood and other fluids.

* Chest wall injuries that result in inadequate breathing—be prepared to provide manual ventilations with a BVM if necessary.

* Open wounds with serious uncontrolled bleeding—be prepared to stop and use the appropriate bleeding control steps.

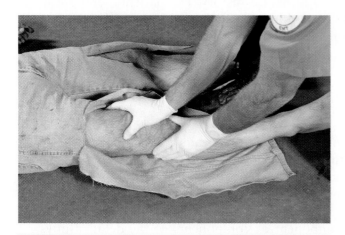

FIGURE 12-12 Use both hands to palpate and inspect the leg.

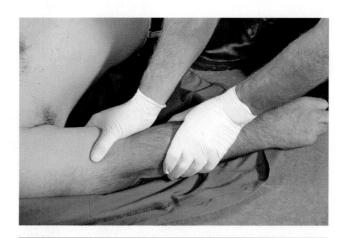

FIGURE 12-13 Use both hands to palpate and inspect the arm.

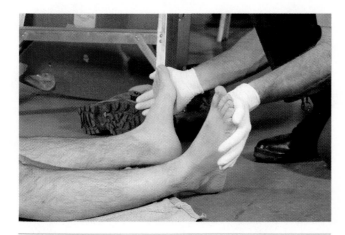

FIGURE 12-14A Use both hands to assess motor function bilaterally in the feet.

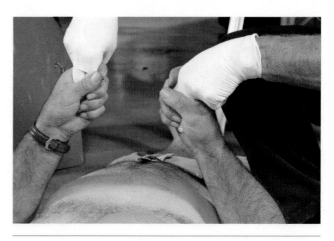

FIGURE 12-14B Use both hands to assess motor function bilaterally in the hands.

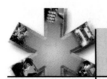

Perspective

Annette—The Wife

"Oh my God I feel so bad about what I did to my husband. It was all my fault. Just . . . just totally my fault. But I couldn't believe that they left him there for as long as they did. And this lady from the ambulance is asking me things like, 'Is he diabetic?' and 'Does he have any heart problems or anything?' and . . . I'm like, 'Look at him! His arm is stuck! What good is it to know if he's taking (expletive) high blood pressure medicine?' Really!"

Baseline Vital Signs and SAMPLE History

Following the rapid trauma assessment you must obtain a baseline set of vital signs (Figure 12-15) and gather a SAMPLE history. For patients who are unresponsive or unable to provide a good history, look to witnesses, bystanders, or family members for this information. Remember to reassess vital signs at least every 5 minutes for the critical patients and compare the results to the baseline set.

Focused Trauma Assessment

When caring for trauma patients who have not sustained a significant MOI, you will perform a focused assessment based on his chief complaint. For instance, if your patient had a lacerated leg or had his foot crushed you would focus your assessment on the injured extremity and not waste time completing an exam of his entire body (Figure 12-16).

3-3.6 Discuss the reason for performing a focused history and physical exam.

You can use the specific component or components of the detailed physical exam that relate to the patient's chief complaint to serve as your focused trauma assessment. The detailed physical exam will be discussed in the next section.

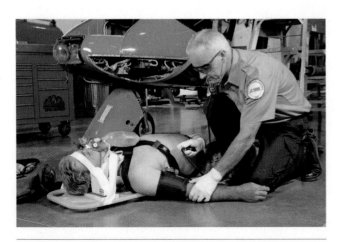

FIGURE 12-15 Take a baseline set of vital signs.

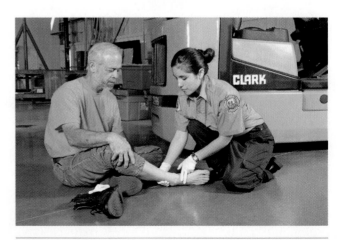

FIGURE 12-16 Perform a focused assessment based on the patient's chief complaint.

Following the focused trauma assessment, you will obtain a baseline set of vital signs and gather as much of the SAMPLE history as possible. Remember to reassess vital signs every 15 minutes for the noncritical patient.

The Detailed Physical Exam

The detailed physical exam (Scan 12-1) is a more thorough version of the rapid trauma assessment and involves closer inspection and palpation of all body regions. In order to expedite transport of the patient, the detailed physical exam is

3-5.1   Discuss the components of the detailed physical exam.

3-5.4   Distinguish between the detailed physical exam that is performed on a trauma patient and that of the medical patient.

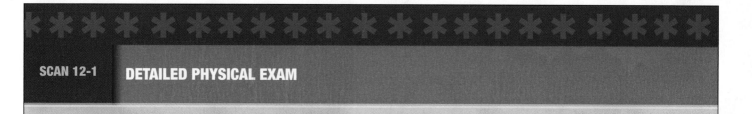

| SCAN 12-1 | **DETAILED PHYSICAL EXAM** |

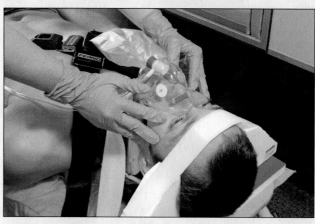

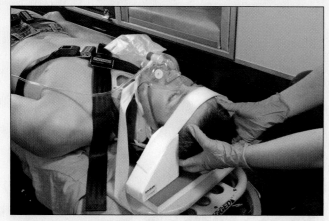

▲ Run your gloved hands over the scalp and through the hair. Note any blood on your gloves.

▲ Palpate the face, forehead, and jaw, and ask the patient to smile. Look for equality of facial expression.

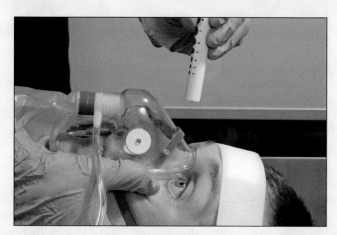

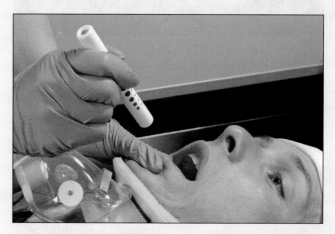

▲ Observe the pupils using an appropriate light source. Expose the conjunctiva by pulling down the lower eyelid.

▲ Observe for drainage of blood or cerebrospinal fluid, flaring of nostrils, and damage to teeth. Look behind the ears for bruising (Battle's sign).

(continued on the next page)

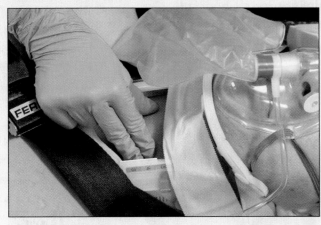

▲ Observe for JVD and run thumb and forefinger along both sides of the trachea to confirm proper alignment. Note any retractions above the clavicles.

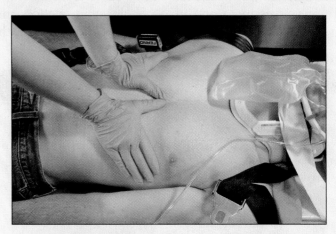

▲ Palpate the chest with both hands, feeling for soft spots and crepitation (subcutaneous emphysema), listen for equal breath sounds and observe for paradoxical movement of the ribs.

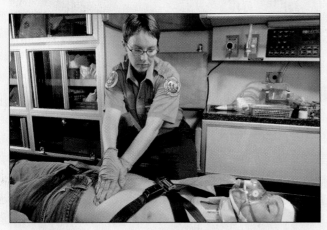

▲ Palpate each quadrant of the abdomen with both hands. Observe the patient's face for signs of grimacing, and note body language for evidence of guarding.

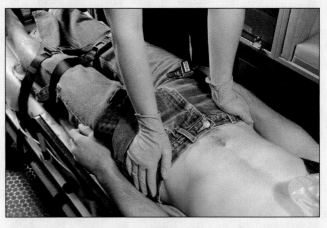

▲ Palpate both sides of the pelvis gently with both hands. Press downward and inward gently. Observe for signs of wetness that may be blood or urine.

(continued on the next page)

3-5.2 State the areas of the body that are evaluated during the detailed physical exam.

typically performed in the back of the ambulance while en route to the receiving hospital. Whether or not a patient receives a detailed physical will depend on his overall condition. Stable patients without a life-threatening condition will typically receive a detailed physical while more critical patients will not. This is because, for critical patients, most of your time will be spent managing immediate life threats while en route to the hospital.

DETAILED PHYSICAL EXAM *(continued)*

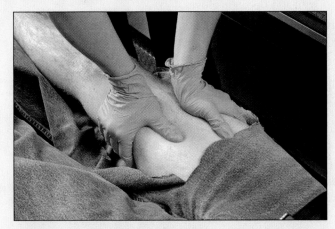

▲ Palpate each leg with both hands and assess distal pulses, sensation, and the push/pull of both feet simultaneously.

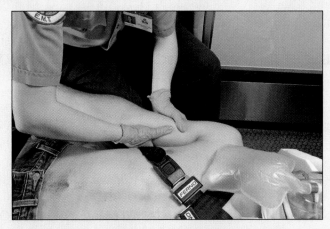

▲ Palpate each arm with both hands, and assess distal pulses, sensation, and the squeeze of both hands simultaneously.

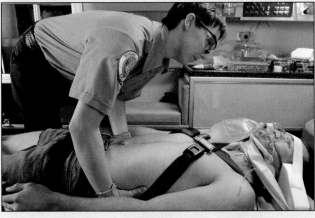

▲ Palpate as much of the back as you can with both hands, feeling for soft spots (paradoxical movement) and crepitation (subcutaneous emphysema).

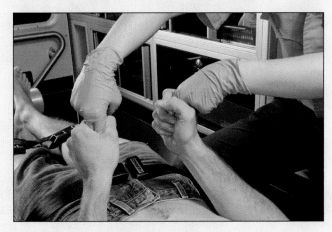

▲ Use both hands to perform the grip test.

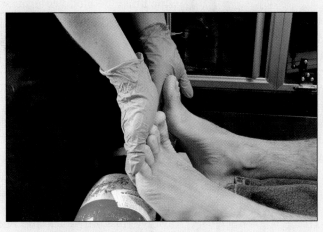

▲ Perform the foot-flex test against both feet.

Table 12-1 is a breakdown of the elements of the detailed physical exam:

TABLE 12-1	ELEMENTS OF A DETAILED PHYSICAL EXAM FOR A TRAUMA PATIENT	
AREA/REGION	**WHAT**	**HOW**
Head (cranium and scalp)	Pain, DCAP-BTLS, crepitation, blood	Run your gloved hands over the scalp and through the hair. Note any blood on your gloves.
Face	Pain, DCAP-BTLS, crepitation, equality of facial muscles	Palpate the face, forehead, and jaw and ask the patient to smile. Look for equality of facial expression.
Eyes	Pain, DCAP-BTLS, equality, reactivity and size of pupils, pink moist conjunctiva (good perfusion)	Observe the pupils using an appropriate light source. Expose the conjunctiva by pulling down the lower eyelid.
Ears	Pain, DCAP-BTLS, drainage, bruising	Observe for drainage of blood or cerebrospinal fluid. Look behind the ears for bruising (Battle's sign)
Nose	Pain, DCAP-BTLS, drainage, singed nostrils, nasal flaring, foreign body	Observe for drainage or evidence of smoke inhalation or burning. Flaring of the nostrils may be a sign of respiratory distress.
Mouth	Pain, DCAP-BTLS, loose/broken teeth (dentures), foreign material, pink moist tissue	Observe for damage to the teeth. Remove anything that may cause an obstruction such as blood or foreign material. Observe for pink moist tissue.
Neck	Pain, DCAP-BTLS, jugular vein distention, tracheal deviation, accessory muscle use, medical alert jewelry, stoma, scars	Observe for JVD, run thumb and forefinger along both sides of trachea to confirm proper alignment. Note any retractions above the clavicles.
Chest	Pain, DCAP-BTLS, chest rise and fall, subcutaneous emphysema, paradoxical movement, breath sounds, scars	Palpate the chest with both hands feeling for soft spots (paradoxical movement) and crepitation (subcutaneous emphysema), listen for equal breath sounds.
Abdomen	Pain, DCAP-BTLS, distention, rigidity, guarding, and scars	Palpate each quadrant of the abdomen with both hands. Observe the patient's face for signs of grimacing and note body language for evidence of guarding.
Pelvis	Pain, DCAP-BTLS, crepitation, and wetness	Palpate both sides of the pelvis gently with both hands. Press downward and inward gently. Observe for signs of wetness which may be blood or urine.
Legs	Pain, DCAP-BTLS, distal circulation, sensation and motor function, scars, track marks, medical jewelry	Palpate each leg with both hands, assess distal pulses, sensation, and push/pull of both feet simultaneously.
Arms	Pain, DCAP-BTLS, distal circulation, sensation and motor function, scars, track marks, medical jewelry	Palpate each arm with both hands, assess distal pulses, sensation, and squeeze both hands simultaneously to perform the grip test.
Back	Pain, DCAP-BTLS, crepitation, paradoxical movement, scars	Palpate as much of the back as you can with both hands, feeling for soft spots (paradoxical movement) and crepitation (subcutaneous emphysema). If appropriate, roll the patient maintaining c-spine precautions and palpate and observe the entire back and buttocks.

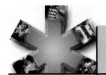

Perspective

Preston—The EMT

"So his arm was gone. Unfortunately, the extrication process completed the amputation, but at least it allowed us to assess the injury, stop the bleeding, and get him on the way to the hospital. It was then that I found crepitation in his ribs on the right side and some tenderness in his abdomen. I think that the guy did get pretty smashed after all, but the trailers came to rest where only his arm was trapped. I actually ended up being a lot more concerned about his chest and potential abdominal bleeding than the damage to his arm."

Management of Secondary Injuries

During the detailed physical exam you will have identified as many signs and symptoms of injury as possible. Once you have completed the detailed exam, you must provide the indicated care for as many of the secondary injuries as appropriate. Small wounds should be covered with dressings and extremity injuries should be immobilized as well as possible. For patients with a significant MOI, extremity injuries are a low priority and can easily be managed by packaging the patient on a long backboard.

For patients with a less significant MOI, suspected fractures can be managed utilizing appropriate splinting techniques. More on splinting will be covered in chapter 31.

3-5.3 Explain what additional care should be provided while performing the detailed physical exam.

ONGOING ASSESSMENT

Once all immediate life threats and secondary injuries have been managed, it is important to complete periodic ongoing assessments of the ABCs, interventions, and vital signs. Stable patients should be reevaluated approximately every 15 minutes and unstable patients approximately every 5 minutes. The specifics of the ongoing assessment will be discussed in more detail in chapter 14.

Stop, Review, Remember!

Multiple Choice

Place a check next to the correct answer.

1. A patient who has sustained a significant MOI should receive which type of assessment?

   _____ a. focused trauma

   _____ b. focused medical

   _____ c. rapid trauma

   _____ d. rapid medical

2. Which of the following represents the correct assessment path for a patient who has sustained a nonsignificant MOI?

   _____ a. focused trauma assessment, baseline vitals, SAMPLE history

   _____ b. rapid trauma assessment, baseline vitals, SAMPLE history

   _____ c. focused trauma assessment, SAMPLE history, baseline vitals

   _____ d. rapid trauma assessment, SAMPLE history, baseline vitals

3. Subcutaneous emphysema is typically found during the assessment of the:

   _____ a. extremities.

   _____ b. skull.

   _____ c. chest and back.

   _____ d. pelvis.

4. Falls greater than _____ feet should be considered significant mechanisms of injury for pediatric patients.

   _____ a. 2   _____ c. 5

   _____ b. 3   _____ d. 10

5. An ongoing assessment should be conducted approximately every _____ minutes for unstable patients.

   _____ a. 5   _____ c. 15

   _____ b. 10   _____ d. 20

Matching

Match the term on the left with the applicable definition on the right.

1. _____ The grating sound or feeling of broken bones rubbing together.

2. _____ Displacement of the trachea laterally from the midline.

3. _____ Bulging of the neck veins.

4. _____ Movement of a part of the chest in the opposite direction to the rest of the chest during inhalation and exhalation.

5. _____ Air trapped beneath the skin.

A. Paradoxical movement
B. Subcutaneous emphysema
C. Tracheal deviation
D. Jugular vein distention
E. Crepitation

Critical Thinking

1. List the differences between a rapid trauma assessment and a focused trauma assessment.

   _____

   _____

   _____

   _____

2. Explain the reasons for performing both the rapid trauma assessment and the focused trauma assessment.

   _____

   _____

   _____

   _____

3. During a rapid trauma assessment you discover a pool of blood beneath the patient. What should you do?

   _____

   _____

   _____

   _____

4. Describe your assessment of a patient who has suffered an injury to his lower right leg when a large crate fell against it, causing deformity.

   _____

   _____

   _____

   _____

5. For each of the patients below, select the most appropriate assessment path:

   a. 66-year-old male who was found unresponsive on the couch at home _____

   b. 13-year-old female whose hand was run over by a car _____

   c. 22-year-old female with sudden onset of severe abdominal pain _____

   d. 31-year-old male who was struck by a car while riding a motorcycle _____

   e. 8-year-old female who was pulled unresponsive from a hot tub _____

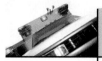

Dispatch Summary

Jim had been covered with blankets and placed on 15 liters of oxygen via nonrebreather mask and Preston had started a large bore IV line prior to the arrival of the extrication crew. Once he was freed, a tourniquet was needed to stop Jim's bleeding and he was subsequently transported to the Four Corners Trauma Center in the Trendelenburg position due to the onset of shock.

The hospital found that Jim had six fractured ribs, a hemopneumothorax, and a dislocated hip in addition to the arm injury. He ultimately survived and is in good health, but his arm was too badly damaged to be reattached. In a few weeks he will receive his new prosthetic arm.

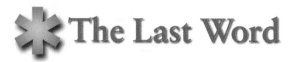

The Last Word

Good patient care depends on a good thorough assessment of each and every patient. The focused history and physical exam is a systematic approach to the assessment of both the trauma and the medical patient.

Trauma and medical patients require slightly different approaches to assessment.

The specific assessment path for the trauma patient is determined by the significance of the mechanism of injury. A rapid trauma assessment is used for the patient who has suffered a significant MOI affecting multiple body systems.

The focused trauma assessment is used for patients with an injury that is isolated to a noncritical area of the body, such as an extremity.

Once one of the above assessments is completed and all immediate life threats are being managed appropriately, the EMT should complete a detailed physical exam. In most situations, the detailed physical is completed while en route to the hospital.

Ongoing assessment of the ABCs, vital signs, and interventions must be conducted at frequent intervals until the patient can be delivered to an appropriate receiving hospital.

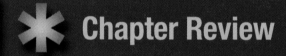

Chapter Review

MULTIPLE CHOICE

Place a check next to the correct answer.

1. Which of the following patients best meets the criteria for a rapid trauma assessment?

    _____ a. 16-year-old female who fell 20 feet

    _____ b. 23-year-old male who twisted an ankle

    _____ c. 41-year-old male with severe chest pain

    _____ d. 77-year-old female who fainted during a meal

2. After performing a rapid trauma assessment and taking vital signs you should obtain a _____ history.

    _____ a. brief

    _____ b. detailed

    _____ c. SAMPLE

    _____ d. focused

3. Which component of the patient assessment is most often performed during transport to the hospital?

   _____ a. initial assessment

   _____ b. baseline vitals

   _____ c. focused assessment

   _____ d. detailed assessment

4. Which of the following would not be a routine component of the chest assessment?

   _____ a. paradoxical movement

   _____ b. distention

   _____ c. crepitation

   _____ d. tenderness

5. The purpose of the ongoing assessment is to:

   _____ a. identify any injuries missed during other assessments.

   _____ b. detect any changes in the patient's condition.

   _____ c. determine effectiveness of interventions.

   _____ d. all of the above

6. All of the following are factors that should be evaluated when assessing the MOI of a fall victim EXCEPT:

   _____ a. height of fall.

   _____ b. speed of fall.

   _____ c. the position in which he landed.

   _____ d. whether he lost consciousness.

7. Falls greater than _____ feet are considered significant mechanisms of injury for adult patients.

   _____ a. 5

   _____ b. 10

   _____ c. 15

   _____ d. 20

8. A _____ is a deviation from the normal shape or size of a body part.

   _____ a. deformity

   _____ b. contusion

   _____ c. puncture

   _____ d. abrasion

9. Tenderness, rigidity, distention, and guarding are characteristics that must be assessed when examining the:

   _____ a. head.

   _____ b. chest.

   _____ c. abdomen.

   _____ d. pelvis.

10. When caring for trauma patients who have not sustained a significant MOI, you will perform a focused assessment based on his:

    _____ a. MOI.

    _____ b. chief complaint.

    _____ c. mental status.

    _____ d. age.

CRITICAL THINKING

1. Discuss how and why trauma patients are cared for differently than medical patients.

   _____

   _____

   _____

2. What is the purpose of reevaluating the mechanism of injury when caring for trauma patients?

   _____

   _____

   _____

3. Compare and contrast the objectives of the rapid trauma and focused trauma assessment.

_____

_____

_____

_____

4. What is the purpose of the detailed physical exam?

_____

_____

_____

_____

CASE STUDIES

Case Study 1

You have been dispatched to a vehicle collision on a two-lane highway leading out of the city. En route, you are advised by law enforcement at the scene that there is one fatality and two others with injuries. Once on scene, you are directed over to a two-door sedan with what appears to be an adult female lying across the front seat.

1. What factors can you quickly evaluate that will help you determine the mechanism of injury for this patient?

_____

_____

_____

_____

_____

_____

_____

2. What will be the most appropriate assessment path for this patient?

_____

_____

_____

_____

_____

_____

_____

3. What immediate life threats can you expect?

_____

_____

_____

_____

_____

_____

Case Study 2

You have been called to a multi-story condominium complex for a fall victim. On arrival, you are led over to an adult female seated on the ground at the base of some stairs. She is alert and in obvious pain. She states that she was carrying some boxes down the stairs and just missed the last step. She has pain and deformity to her right wrist and pain in her right ankle with significant swelling.

1. What questions will you want to ask regarding the mechanism of injury to rule out possible neck or spine injury?

_____

_____

_____

_____

_____

_____

2. What assessment path is most appropriate for this patient?

_____

_____

_____

_____

_____

_____

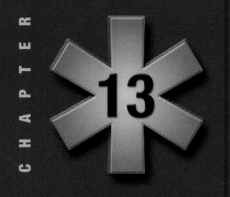

CHAPTER 13

Assessing the Medical Patient

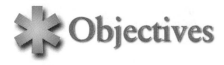

Objectives

Numbered objectives are from the U.S. Department of Transportation 1994 EMT-Basic National Standard Curriculum.

COGNITIVE OBJECTIVES

At the completion of this lesson, the EMT-Basic student will be able to:

3-4.1   Describe the unique needs for assessing an individual with a specific chief complaint with no known prior history. (p. 345)

3-4.2   Differentiate between the history and physical exam that are performed for responsive patients with no known prior history and responsive patients with a known prior history. (p. 358)

3-4.3   Describe the needs for assessing an individual who is unresponsive. (pp. 344, 346–347)

3-4.4   Differentiate between the assessment that is performed for a patient who is unresponsive or has an altered mental status and other medical patients requiring assessment. (pp. 345–346)

AFFECTIVE OBJECTIVES

At the completion of this lesson, the EMT-Basic student will be able to:

3-4.5   Attend to the feelings that these patients might be experiencing. (p. 345)

PSYCHOMOTOR OBJECTIVES

At the completion of this lesson, the EMT-Basic student will be able to:

3-4.6   Demonstrate the patient assessment skills that should be used to assist a patient who is responsive with no known history. (pp. 351–357)

3-4.7   Demonstrate the patient assessment skills that should be used to assist a patient who is unresponsive or has an altered mental status. (pp. 346–350)

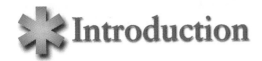# Introduction

As we stated in the last chapter on trauma assessment, good patient care is directly related to a good patient assessment. In general, a good patient assessment will almost always result in the patient receiving the most appropriate care. This is especially true when caring for the patient with a medical complaint. This chapter is similar to the previous chapter but will introduce the skill of patient assessment specifically for the medical patient. If you have not already done so, we strongly encourage you to read the previous chapter before continuing here.

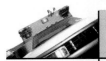

Emergency Dispatch

"He isn't normally like this," the elderly woman explained to Mike, an EMT for the city fire department. "He usually talks all of the time and is, you know, active."

They were standing over the bed of 78-year-old Al Hernandez, who was watching them quietly with a pleasant look on his face.

"Mr. Hernandez, can you talk to me?" Mike said to him loudly. "Can you say something?"

The man simply stared up at Mike with the hint of a smile on his lips.

"So he normally responds when you ask him a question?"

"Oh, heavens, yes. Sometimes you can't shut him up!"

"Can he get out of bed?"

"Before this started he could. He played golf three times a week. Now he just lies in bed and doesn't say anything."

"How long has it been since he stopped talking?"

"Oh . . . about four days."

"Four days seems a long time to wait to call 9-1-1."

"Well," the old woman shrugged her shoulders. "I thought he would just get better."

The Trauma versus the Medical Patient

As you will remember from the last chapter, the medical profession, including EMS, divides all patients into one of two fundamental categories. This categorization is based on whether the patient's chief complaint is related to an illness or injury.

Patients whose chief complaint is related to an illness, such as difficulty breathing, chest pain, or headache, are categorized as "medical" patients. Patients whose chief complaint is related to an injury are categorized as "trauma" patients. Simply stated, injury equals trauma and illness equals medical. This differentiation is important, because the specific assessment path you will follow will be different for each category.

Figure 13-1 on page 344 is a flow chart showing all of the components of a patient assessment for both medical and trauma patients. This chapter will focus specifically on the medical assessment path that is shown on the right-hand side of the flowchart.

PATIENT ASSESSMENT

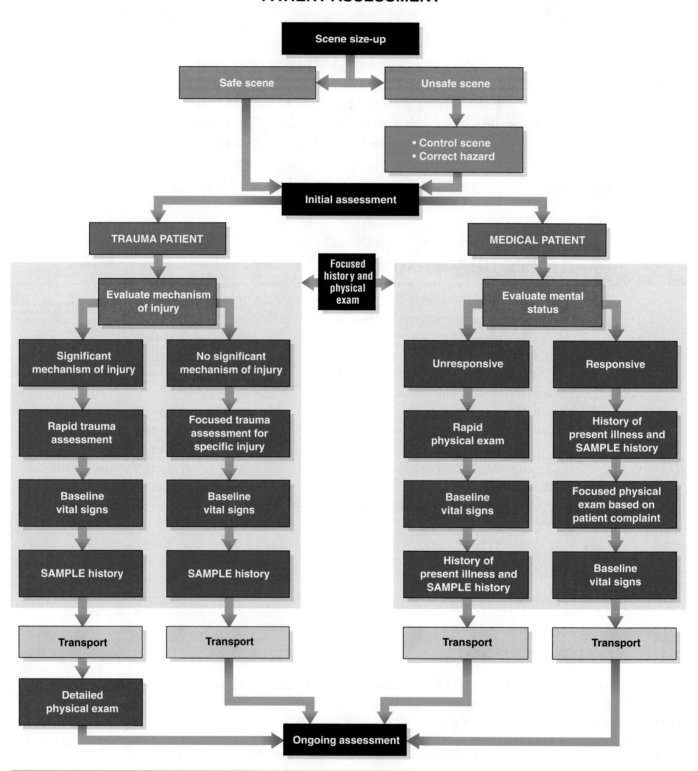

FIGURE 13-1 Components of patient assessment for both medical and trauma patients.

As you will notice, several elements of the patient assessment are common to both medical and trauma patients. The common components are as follows:

* BSI precautions

* Scene size-up

* Initial assessment

It cannot be overstated how important each of these components is to the well-being of both the EMT and the patient. Only after ensuring that you are protected, the scene is safe, and all aspects of the initial assessment are addressed will you move on to complete your patient assessment.

3-4.1 Describe the unique needs for assessing an individual with a specific chief complaint with no known prior history.

Management of the Medical Patient

Medical patients are managed differently than most trauma patients in the pre-hospital setting. For trauma patients with a significant mechanism of injury, time on scene must be limited so the patient can reach the hospital quickly for surgery. For most medical patients—especially those who are responsive—a more thorough assessment at the scene is usually appropriate. You will also need to attend to the feelings of the responsive patients as you progress through the assessment.

As already noted, in most situations involving medical patients transport time to an appropriate receiving hospital is not the most critical factor. Instead, a thorough investigation into the patient's present and past medical history is the focus of the assessment. However, there are some medical conditions, such as an acute stroke, that require time-sensitive drug therapies that must also be considered when deciding the priority of the patient. This will be discussed in more detail in chapter 21.

REEVALUATING THE PATIENT'S MENTAL STATUS

Evaluation of the patient's mental status is critical when caring for a medical patient and will be the criterion used to decide which assessment path to follow. When you study the medical side of the patient assessment flow chart you will find two parallel assessment paths: the rapid medical assessment and the focused medical assessment (Figure 13-2 on page 346). The specific path that you will follow for your medical patient will depend upon your evaluation of the patient's level of responsiveness.

If your patient is unresponsive or unable to provide any meaningful information about his condition, you will follow the rapid medical assessment path. If the

3-4.3 Describe the needs for assessing an individual who is unresponsive.

3-4.4 Differentiate between the assessment that is performed for a patient who is unresponsive or has an altered mental status and other medical patients requiring assessment.

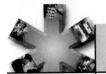

Perspective

Mike—The EMT

"How are you supposed to do a mental status evaluation, or gather a good history . . . or even determine a chief complaint . . . if the patient can't communicate at all? And the way that he just smiled at me, I honestly thought that he was just being difficult! At first, that actually made me kind of angry until I realized that this all might just be a serious problem."

ASSESSMENT OF MEDICAL PATIENT

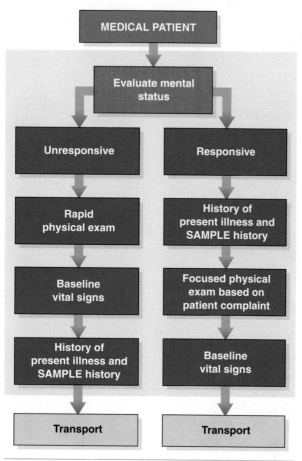

FIGURE 13-2 Components of patient assessment for medical patients.

ASSESSMENT OF UNRESPONSIVE PATIENT

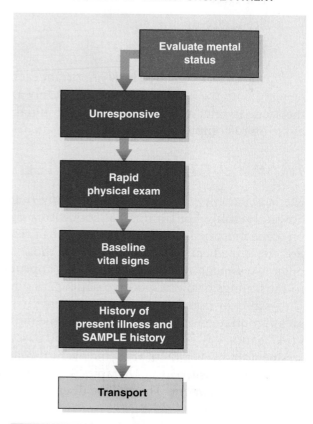

FIGURE 13-3 Patient assessment of the unresponsive medical patient.

patient is responsive enough to provide meaningful information about his condition, then you will follow the focused medical assessment path.

You made your first assessment of mental status during the initial assessment, using the AVPU scale. Now you must take a closer look and evaluate mental status a little further.

RAPID VERSUS FOCUSED ASSESSMENT

The first major decision point in the patient assessment comes immediately following the initial assessment. At this point you will decide between a rapid medical assessment and a focused medical assessment. The medical assessment is not as simple as the trauma assessment. That decision is made based on your evaluation of the patient's history, chief complaint, and mental status (Figure 13-3).

Rapid Medical Assessment of the Unresponsive Patient

The primary purpose of the rapid medical assessment is to quickly identify any important signs and symptoms not already addressed by the initial assessment. It involves a rapid head-to-toe physical examination of the patient, looking for obvious signs and symptoms of illness.

The following areas are assessed during the rapid medical assessment:

* Head

* Neck

* Chest

* Abdomen

* Pelvis

* Back

* Extremities

If you are caring for what appears to be a medical patient, but you cannot positively rule out an injury to the head, neck, or spine, you must maintain appropriate spinal precautions. The typical call for the "possible overdose" or "drunk" in the alley is one that you must be careful with. It is very possible that this person was assaulted and may have an injury. In almost all cases, unresponsive patients will be a high priority for transport. Consider the need for ALS backup or an ALS intercept if appropriate.

 Stop, Review, Remember!

Multiple Choice

Place a check next to the correct answer.

1. The "A" in the AVPU mental status assessment scale stands for:

   _____ a. annoying.

   _____ b. alert.

   _____ c. ability to move.

   _____ d. ability to speak.

2. Which of the following elements of the patient assessment is NOT common to all assessments?

   _____ a. focused medical assessment

   _____ b. initial assessment

   _____ c. scene size-up

   _____ d. BSI precautions

3. The first time that mental status is assessed is during the:

   _____ a. scene size-up.

   _____ b. initial assessment.

   _____ c. rapid trauma assessment.

   _____ d. detailed physical exam.

Ordering

Put the following elements of the rapid medical assessment in the correct order.

∗ SAMPLE history

∗ Baseline vitals

∗ Rapid medical assessment

∗ Transport

Critical Thinking

1. Compare and contrast the focus of the medical and trauma assessments.

_____

_____

_____

2. Describe how you would manage a suspected overdose patient who was found unresponsive behind the local homeless shelter.

_____

_____

_____

3. Would you need to consider spinal precautions for the above patient? If so, why?

_____

_____

_____

Performing the Rapid Medical Assessment

Using appropriate BSI precautions, inspect and palpate the areas of the patient's body discussed in the following section, looking for any sign of possible illness (Scan 13-1). When something is discovered, you must decide if it is life threatening or not. For those signs that you suspect could be life threatening, you must stop your exam and provide the indicated care. For non-life-threatening signs, you may proceed with your exam and provide the indicated care when appropriate.

Keep in mind that the airway of an unresponsive patient is at risk of becoming compromised at any time. Continue to monitor the patient's airway and breathing status throughout your exam.

HEAD

Palpate and inspect the head for symmetry and scars. Remember to maintain stabilization of the cervical spine if you suspect any possibility of trauma.

✳ ✳

SCAN 13-1   RAPID MEDICAL ASSESSMENT, VITAL SIGNS, AND HISTORY

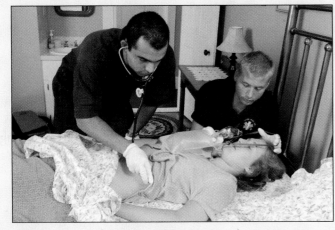

▲ Perform a rapid assessment of the entire body.

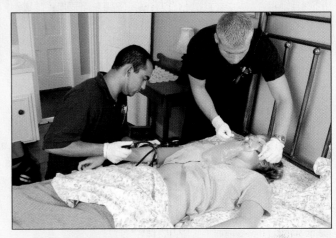

▲ Assess the patient's baseline vital signs.

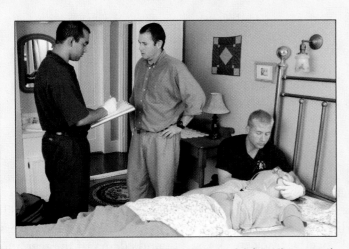

▲ Interview family and bystanders to get as much information as possible about the patient's problem.

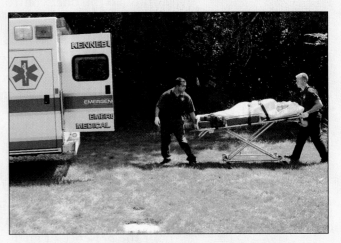

▲ Perform interventions as needed and transport the patient.

NECK

Palpate and inspect the neck for a **stoma, jugular vein distention (JVD), tracheal deviation,** medical jewelry, scars, and accessory muscle use.

CHEST

Palpate and inspect the chest for equal rise and fall, subcutaneous emphysema, retractions, and scars. Assessment of the chest should also include bilateral auscultation of breath sounds (Figure 13-4 on page 350).

✳ **stoma**

opening in the anterior neck that connects to the trachea.

✳ **jugular vein distention (JVD)**

bulging of the neck veins.

✳ **tracheal deviation**

displacement of the trachea laterally from the midline.

FIGURE 13-4 Listening to lung sounds of an unresponsive patient.

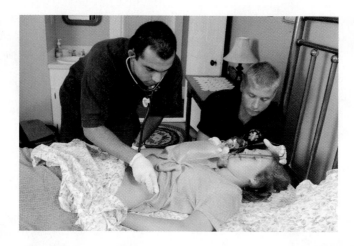

ABDOMEN

✳ **distention**

a condition of being stretched, inflated, or larger than normal.

✳ **rigidity**

abnormal sense of firmness in the abdomen on palpation indication disease or trauma within.

✳ **guarding**

body defense mechanism to further prevent pain during abdominal examination.

Palpate and inspect the abdomen for **distention**, tenderness, **rigidity**, **guarding**, scars, or pulsating masses. Guarding, grimacing, and moaning are indications that the patient is experiencing pain.

PELVIS

Palpate and inspect the pelvis for evidence of wetness that may be caused by blood or loss of bladder control.

BACK

Palpate and inspect the back for subcutaneous emphysema and scars. If necessary, roll the patient to perform a complete assessment of the back.

EXTREMITIES

Palpate and inspect each extremity as appropriate. Assess each for circulation, sensation, and motor function (CSM). When evaluating motor function, do so with both upper extremities and both lower extremities simultaneously. This will allow you to detect slight differences in strength from one side to the other. Assess for the presence of medical jewelry, track marks, scars, and edema of the feet and ankles.

If at any point during the rapid medical assessment you discover what could be a life-threatening injury or condition, you must stop the exam and care for the problem immediately. It is important to remember that all potential life threats must be addressed as they are found.

Baseline Vital Signs and Medical History

Following the rapid medical assessment, you must obtain a baseline set of vital signs and gather an appropriate medical history. For patients who are unresponsive or unable to provide a good history, look to witnesses, bystanders, or family members for this information. For the unresponsive patient, remember to reassess vital signs at least every 5 minutes and compare the results to the baseline set.

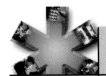

Perspective

Al's Wife

"Now, that fireman was a nice enough boy, but he was somewhat annoying. He kept asking about Al's blood pressure history and if he had ever had a stroke or anything like that. He was just all over the map! And what was his little tiff about me waiting 4 days to call? It doesn't matter if it's 4 minutes or 4 years ... my Al was perfectly comfortable. He just had some trouble talking. That kind of stuff happens when you get as old as we are."

Focused Medical Assessment of the Responsive Patient

When caring for medical patients who are responsive you will perform a focused medical assessment based on his chief complaint (Figure 13-5). For instance, if your patient has difficulty breathing or chest pain, you would focus your assessment on the chief complaint and not waste time completing an exam of his entire body (Figure 13-6).

MEDICAL ASSESSMENT OF RESPONSIVE PATIENT

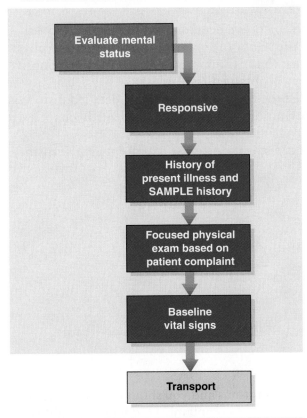

FIGURE 13-5   Patient assessment of the responsive medical patient.

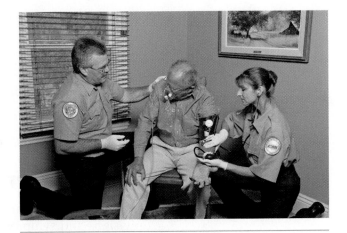

FIGURE 13-6   If the patient's chief complaint is chest pain, focus your assessment in that area.

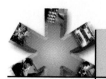

Perspective

Mike—The EMT

"So, here was my conundrum. Al was conscious . . . his eyes moved. I would consider him more or less responsive. But he couldn't communicate with me at all. So was I supposed to do a rapid assessment . . . or a focused one? You read about these things, and act them out in class . . . but when you're there . . . looking down at an actual patient, you realize that in the real world you have to actually think about and apply the knowledge that you got in school. Does that make any sense? I just keep finding these patients that don't fit neatly into one category or another."

You will use specific components of the detailed physical exam that are related to your patient's chief complaint to guide your focused medical assessment. The detailed physical exam will be discussed a little later in this chapter.

During the focused medical assessment you will first obtain a detailed history from the patient. This history will include information about the current problem as well as any previous medical issues that may be pertinent.

The SAMPLE History

The core of the focused medical assessment is a detailed medical history. Note that for the responsive medical patient, the history is obtained first, before the physical exam and vitals. This is in contrast to the trauma patient and the unresponsive medical patient for whom the history is obtained last.

One commonly used tool to assist the EMT in completing a detailed history is the acronym SAMPLE. The SAMPLE acronym was introduced back in chapter 10 but we will present it again here for your review.

Each letter of the word represents a specific element of a good patient history. They are as follows:

∗ S – Signs and symptoms

∗ A – Allergies

∗ M – Medications

∗ P – Pertinent past medical history

∗ L – Last oral intake

∗ E – Events leading to the injury or illness

SIGNS AND SYMPTOMS

The *S* in SAMPLE stands for signs and symptoms and you should assess or reassess any signs and symptoms relating to the chief complaint. One way to begin is by asking, "Can you tell me where you hurt." Inspect the areas the patient mentions (his symptoms) for any obvious signs of illness or injury. After examining the first painful location, ask if there are any others and inspect those as appropriate. Ask about **referred pain.**

ALLERGIES

All good patient histories include information about known allergies. Known allergies are things the patient has had an allergic reaction to in the past. This is important for several reasons. It may be the cause of the patient's chief complaint or he may be allergic to a medication he might be given at the hospital. Ask about all known allergies, including allergies to the following:

* Medications

* Food

* Environmental allergies (bites, stings, plants)

If the patient has a known allergy, ask the last time he had a reaction and what the reaction was like. Was it a minor reaction or was it more severe, requiring medical attention?

MEDICATIONS

Ask the patient what medications he is currently taking. As you become familiar with the more common prescription medications and what they are taken for, this can tell you the type of medical conditions the patient is being treated for.

Ask about both prescription and nonprescription medications including those that don't necessarily pertain to a medical condition such as birth control pills or nicotine patches. Also ask about medications from the recent past that he may not be currently taking as well as medications he is currently taking (Figure 13-7). Confirm he is taking the medications as prescribed.

Ask someone to bring you all the medications the patient is taking and place them in a paper bag for easy reference and transport to the hospital.

PERTINENT PAST MEDICAL HISTORY

In many situations, the patient's chief complaint may relate directly or indirectly to a past medical complaint or condition. Ask about previous or current medical conditions, surgeries, and/or injuries. Inform the physician at the hospital if this information is pertinent. Include as much detail as possible when transferring or documenting your care.

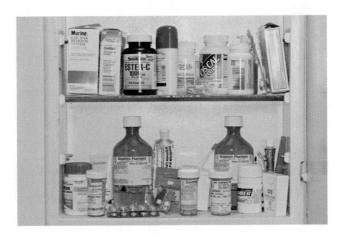

FIGURE 13-7   Part of the SAMPLE history includes questioning the patient about medications he is currently taking as well as those he has taken in the recent past.

LAST ORAL INTAKE

Ask the patient what he last ate or drank. Should a patient require emergency surgery, the surgeons need to know the time and quantity of food intake, because stomach contents could be vomited during surgery.

EVENTS LEADING TO THE INJURY OR ILLNESS

What was the patient doing just prior to the event? For instance, if the chief complaint is chest pain, was the patient exerting himself prior to the pain or was he at rest? Or does the patient, perhaps, have no recollection of events prior to your arrival?

The OPQRST Mnemonic

Another mnemonic that was introduced in chapter 10 is OPQRST, which can help trigger questions about a patient's pain or discomfort.

- ✳ O – Onset
- ✳ P – Provocation
- ✳ Q – Quality
- ✳ R – Region/Radiation
- ✳ S – Severity
- ✳ T – Time

ONSET

"What were you doing when the pain began?" or "What were you doing when you first began to feel short of breath?" are questions you might ask related to onset.

PROVOCATION

"Does anything you do make the pain better or worse?" or "Does it hurt to take a deep breath or when I push here?" are questions you might ask related to provocation.

QUALITY

"Can you describe how your pain feels?" or "Is it sharp or is it dull?" and "Is it steady or does it come and go?" are questions you might ask related to quality.

Be careful not to put words in the patient's mouth. Instead provide them with choices and allow them to choose. Use the patient's own words when documenting the call or handing the patient off to the next level of care.

REGION/RADIATION

"Can you point to your worst pain?" or "Does your pain move or radiate to another part of your body?" and "Do you feel pain anywhere else?" are questions you might ask related to region and radiation.

SEVERITY

A standard 1 to 10 scale is typically used to evaluate the severity of pain or discomfort. You might ask, "On a scale of 1 to 10 with 10 being the worst pain you have ever felt, how would you rate your pain right now?" You can also ask the patient to describe the severity of his pain when it first began, using the same scale. Later, ask the severity question again to see if the pain is getting better or worse.

TIME

You will want to know how long the patient has been experiencing his pain or discomfort. A question such as, "When did you first begin having pain today?" or "How long have you had this pain?" will usually suffice.

Your instructor or EMS system may have different acronyms, mnemonics, or additional tools such as these. Find the ones that work best for you.

Additional Medical Assessments

Scan 13-2 shows additional medical assessments to be performed in response to the history obtained from the patient, family, and bystanders. To expedite transport, as with the detailed exam for a trauma patient, these assessments for a medical patient are typically performed in the back of the ambulance while en route to the receiving hospital. Performing these assessments will depend on the patient's overall condition. Stable patients without a life-threatening condition will typically receive a more detailed exam while more critical patients will not because most of your time will be spent managing immediate life threats.

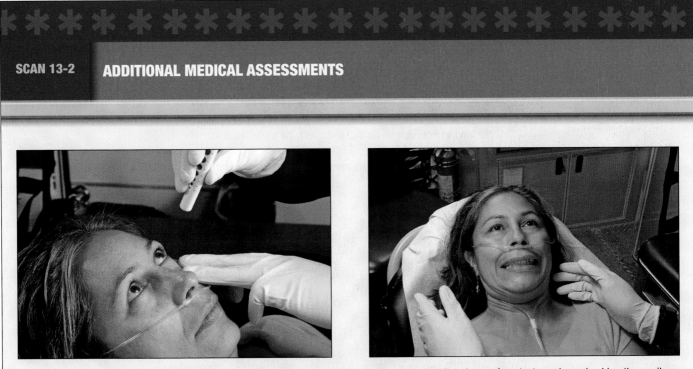

SCAN 13-2   ADDITIONAL MEDICAL ASSESSMENTS

▲ For patients with altered mental status or signs of neurological problems, such as suspected stroke, perform tests such as checking the pupils as well as strength in the extremeties. As part of a prehospital stroke scale, observe for facial symmetry.

(continued on the next page)

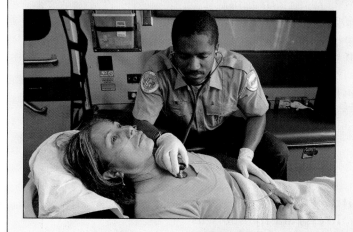

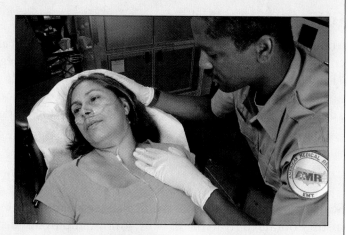

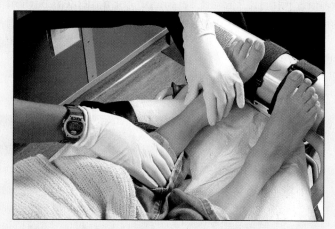

▲ For patients with suspected cardiac or respiratory problems, listen for lung sounds, observe for JVD and check the ankles for fluid.

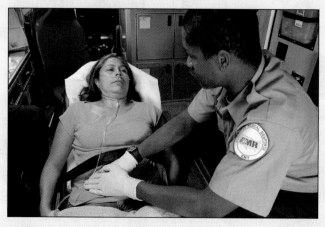

▲ For patients with abdominal pain, nausea or vomiting, palpate the abdomen.

Please also refer to chapter 12, Assessing the Trauma Patient, The Detailed Physical Exam, and note the difference in the detailed physical exams for the trauma and the medical patient.

Table 13-1 is a breakdown of assessment elements for the medical patient. Assessments are based on the history as obtained from the patient, family or bystanders.

TABLE 13-1	ADDITIONAL MEDICAL ASSESSMENTS	
AREA/REGION	**WHAT**	**HOW**
Head (cranium and scalp)	Pain, symmetry, and scars	Run your gloved hands over the scalp and through the hair. See also chapter 33.
Face	Pain, equality of facial muscles	Palpate the face, forehead, and jaw and ask the patient to smile. Look for equality of facial expression. See also chapter 21.
Eyes	Pain, equality, reactivity and size of pupils, pink moist conjunctiva, yellow discoloration sclera (jaundice)	Observe the pupils using an appropriate light source. Expose the conjunctiva by pulling down the lower eyelid. See also chapter 21.
Ears	Pain, drainage	Observe for drainage of blood or cerebrospinal fluid.
Nose	Pain, drainage, singed nostrils, nasal flaring, foreign body	Observe for drainage or evidence of smoke inhalation or burning. Flaring of the nostrils may be a sign of respiratory distress.
Mouth	Pain, loose/broken teeth (dentures), foreign material, pink moist tissue	Observe for damage to the teeth. Remove anything that may cause an obstruction such as blood or foreign material. Observe for pink moist tissue.
Neck	Pain, jugular vein distention, tracheal deviation, accessory muscle use, medical alert jewelry, stoma, scars	Observe for JVD, run thumb and forefinger along both sides of trachea to confirm proper alignment. Note any retractions above the clavicles.
Chest	Pain, chest rise and fall, subcutaneous emphysema, breath sounds, scars	Palpate the chest with both hands feeling for equal rise and fall, subcutaneous emphysema, listen for equal breath sounds. See also chapters 19 and 20.
Abdomen	Pain, distention, rigidity, guarding, and scars	Palpate each quadrant of the abdomen with both hands. Observe the patient's face for signs of grimacing and note body language for evidence of guarding. See also chapters 25 and 31.
Pelvis	Pain and wetness	Palpate both sides of the pelvis gently with both hands. Press downward and inward gently. Observe for signs of wetness that may be blood or urine.
Legs	Pain, distal circulation, sensation and motor function, scars, track marks, medical jewelry	Palpate each leg with both hands, assess distal pulses, sensation, and push/pull of both feet simultaneously. See also chapters 32 and 34.
Arms	Pain, distal circulation, sensation and motor function, scars, track marks, medical jewelry	Palpate each arm with both hands, assess distal pulses, sensation, and squeeze both hands simultaneously to perform the grip test.
Back	Pain, subcutaneous emphysema, sacral edema, scars	Palpate as much of the back as you can with both hands feeling for subcutaneous emphysema. If appropriate, roll the patient and palpate and observe the entire back and buttocks. See also chapter 34.

BASELINE VITAL SIGNS

Following the SAMPLE history and the focused medical assessment for the responsive medical patient, you must obtain a baseline set of vital signs. Remember to reassess vital signs every 15 minutes if the patient is stable or every 5 minutes if the patient is unstable, and compare the results to the baseline set.

Management of Signs and Symptoms

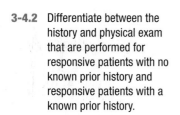

3-4.2 Differentiate between the history and physical exam that are performed for responsive patients with no known prior history and responsive patients with a known prior history.

During the history and physical exam, you will have identified as many signs and symptoms relating to the chief complaint as possible. At this point you must provide the indicated care for as many of the secondary signs and symptoms as appropriate.

As you have already seen, your assessment and care of the medical patient will be driven by several factors, including level of responsiveness, chief complaint, and prior medical history. One of the most important pieces of information you can gather is whether the patient has a history of problems relating to his chief complaint. If the chief complaint is associated with a prior medical history, you will focus your attention on what the patient may be doing to care for the problem and how it has been cared for in the past. Many times the patient has medication at hand, such as a metered dose inhaler or nitroglycerin, that can be used to help the problem.

A patient with no prior medical history is much more of a challenge to the EMT. The importance of a thorough SAMPLE and OPQRST history is critical in determining the most appropriate care for the patient. While it is not always important to know exactly what is causing the patient's problems, a thorough history can reveal clues to the indicated care.

ONGOING ASSESSMENT

Once all immediate life threats have been managed, it is important to complete periodic ongoing assessments of the ABCs, interventions, and vital signs. Stable patients should be reevaluated approximately every 15 minutes and unstable patients at least every 5 minutes. The specifics of the ongoing assessment will be discussed in more detail in chapter 14.

 Stop, Review, Remember!

Multiple Choice

Place a check next to the correct answer.

1. A patient who is alert and oriented should receive which type of assessment?

   _____ a. focused medical

   _____ b. focused trauma

   _____ c. rapid medical

   _____ d. rapid trauma

2. Which of the following represents the correct assessment path for a patient who is unresponsive?

_____ a. focused medical assessment, baseline vitals, SAMPLE history

_____ b. rapid medical assessment, baseline vitals, SAMPLE history

_____ c. focused medical assessment, SAMPLE history, baseline vitals

_____ d. rapid medical assessment, SAMPLE history, baseline vitals

3. Distention is typically found during the assessment of the:

_____ a. extremities.

_____ b. abdomen.

_____ c. chest and back.

_____ d. pelvis.

4. Which of the following assessments is typically performed in the ambulance while on the way to the receiving facility?

_____ a. detailed physical

_____ b. rapid medical

_____ c. focused medical

_____ d. rapid trauma

5. An ongoing assessment should be conducted every _____ minutes for stable patients.

_____ a. 5

_____ b. 10

_____ c. 15

_____ d. 20

Matching

Match the term on the left with the applicable definition on the right.

1. _____ Stoma

2. _____ Jugular vein distention (JVD)

3. _____ Tracheal deviation

4. _____ Distention

5. _____ Guarding

6. _____ Referred pain

A. Bulging of the neck veins

B. Pain that is felt in a location other than where the pain originates

C. Opening in the anterior neck that connects to the trachea

D. A condition of being stretched, inflated, or larger than normal

E. Displacement of the trachea, lateral from the midline

F. Body defense mechanism, to prevent movement of an injured part

Critical Thinking

1. What are the indications for performing a rapid medical assessment? Provide a description of a patient who would fit the criteria for this assessment.

_____

_____

_____

_____

2. List at least three findings you might observe when assessing the neck of a medical patient.

_____

_____

_____

_____

3. List at least three findings you might observe when assessing the abdomen of a medical patient.

_____

_____

_____

_____

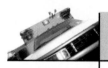

Dispatch Summary

Al Hernandez was transported without incident to Saint Anthony Hospital on Broadway and 23rd. Subsequent tests showed that Mr. Hernandez had suffered a major stroke, but with the extended time before help was sought, he was not considered a candidate for fibrinolytic therapy.

He has since been placed into the Spring County Advanced Care Facility for follow-up care, but has so far showed no signs of regaining either his ability to speak or move successfully.

The Last Word

Good patient care depends on a thorough assessment of each and every patient. The focused history and physical exam is a systematic approach to the assessment of both the trauma and the medical patient.

Trauma and medical patients require slightly different approaches to assessment.

The specific assessment path for the medical patient is determined by the level of responsiveness. A rapid medical assessment is used for the patient who is unresponsive or unable to provide any meaningful history pertaining to his condition or chief complaint.

The focused medical assessment is used for the patient who is responsive and able to provide a meaningful history of his problem.

Once one of the above assessments is completed and all immediate life threats are being managed appropriately, the EMT should complete a detailed physical exam. In most situations, the detailed physical is completed while en route to the hospital.

Ongoing assessment of the ABCs, vital signs, and interventions must be conducted at frequent intervals until the patient can be delivered to an appropriate receiving hospital—every 15 minutes for a stable patient, every 5 minutes for an unstable patient.

 # Chapter Review

MULTIPLE CHOICE

Place a check next to the correct answer.

1. The vital signs of a stable patient should be reassessed at least every _____ minutes.

   _____ a. 5

   _____ b. 10

   _____ c. 15

   _____ d. 20

2. The criterion for determining the most appropriate assessment path for a medical patient is the:

   _____ a. chief complaint.

   _____ b. level of responsiveness.

   _____ c. level of pain.

   _____ d. mechanism of injury.

3. Which of the following is the most appropriate assessment tool for evaluating the chief complaint for a medical patient?

   _____ a. SAMPLE

   _____ b. OPQRST

   _____ c. AVPU

   _____ d. DCAP-BTLS

4. The _____ is a quick head-to-toe examination of an unresponsive medical patient.

   _____ a. rapid medical assessment

   _____ b. focused medical assessment

   _____ c. detailed physical exam

   _____ d. ongoing assessment

5. An appropriate focused history should include both _____ and OPQRST assessments.

   _____ a. AVPU

   _____ b. DCAP-BTLS

   _____ c. SAMPLE

   _____ d. ongoing

6. The detailed physical exam should be performed:

   _____ a. after obtaining vital signs.

   _____ b. after the ongoing assessment.

   _____ c. immediately prior to the initial assessment.

   _____ d. immediately following the initial assessment.

7. The *E* in the SAMPLE assessment acronym stands for:

   _____ a. events leading to the problem.

   _____ b. events following the problem.

   _____ c. exercise induced problem.

   _____ d. evaluation of the problem.

8. The vital signs of an unstable patient should be reassessed at least every _____ minutes.

   _____ a. 5

   _____ b. 10

   _____ c. 15

   _____ d. 20

9. Swelling that is found in the ankles and lower back of some medical patients is called:

_____ a. distention.

_____ b. edema.

_____ c. deformity.

_____ d. ascites.

10. In the unresponsive medical patient, vital signs should be obtained:

_____ a. before the rapid assessment.

_____ b. following the rapid assessment.

_____ c. as often as possible.

_____ d. every 15 minutes.

ORDERING

List the steps in the correct order of the assessment paths for both a responsive and an unresponsive medical patient.

Responsive:

Focused history

Focused physical exam

Baseline vitals

Transport

Unresponsive:

Rapid medical assessment

Baseline vitals

Focused history

Transport

CRITICAL THINKING

1. Provide at least three examples each of patient that would be categorized as trauma and medical.

_____

_____

_____

2. Discuss how and why medical patients are cared for differently than trauma patients.

_____

_____

_____

_____

3. What is the purpose of reevaluating the mental status when caring for medical patients?

_____

_____

_____

_____

4. What is the purpose of the ongoing assessment?

_____

_____

_____

CASE STUDIES

Case Study 1

You have completed an initial assessment, physical exam, vitals, and SAMPLE history on a 66-year-old female with an altered mental status. You are now loaded in the ambulance and en route to the hospital. While conducting a detailed physical exam on the patient you begin to hear gurgling upon inspiration.

1. What might the presence of gurgling say about this patient?

   _____

   _____

   _____

   _____

2. How will you alter your assessment to address this new development?

   _____

   _____

   _____

   _____

Case Study 2

You have responded to an office building for a man having chest pain. On your arrival, you are escorted to a third-floor office where you find an approximately 50-year-old male in moderate distress. The man states that he is experiencing a "tightness" in his chest, which started approximately 30 minutes ago and came on while he was walking up the stairs to his office. He also states that he is having difficulty breathing.

1. Which assessment path is most appropriate for this patient and why?

   _____

   _____

   _____

   _____

2. List at least two questions for each of the elements of the OPQRST assessment mnemonic.

   _____

   _____

   _____

   _____

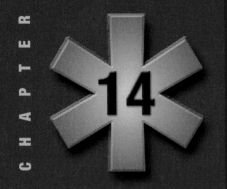

14

Performing an Ongoing Assessment

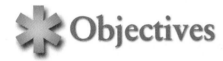

Objectives

Numbered objectives are from the U.S. Department of Transportation 1994 EMT-Basic National Standard Curriculum.

COGNITIVE OBJECTIVES

At the completion of this lesson, the EMT-Basic student will be able to:

3-6.1 Discuss the reasons for repeating the initial assessment as part of the ongoing assessment. (pp. 365–367)

3-6.2 Describe the components of the ongoing assessment. (pp. 366–367)

3-6.3 Describe trending of assessment components. (p. 366)

AFFECTIVE OBJECTIVES

At the completion of this lesson, the EMT-Basic student will be able to:

3-6.4 Explain the value of performing an ongoing assessment. (pp. 365–366)

3-6.5 Recognize and respect the feelings that patients might experience during assessment. (p. 367)

3-6.6 Explain the value of trending assessment components to other health professionals who assume care of the patient. (p. 365)

PSYCHOMOTOR OBJECTIVES

At the completion of this lesson, the EMT-Basic student will be able to:

3-6.7 Demonstrate the skills involved in performing the ongoing assessment. (pp. 369–373)

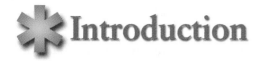 **Introduction**

It can be argued that, of all the elements of the patient assessment, the **ongoing assessment** is second only to the initial assessment in terms of importance and priority. As you will remember from chapters 12 and 13, the purpose of the initial assessment is to identify and care for all immediate life threats to the patient. The ongoing assessment is a continuous rechecking of the patient's condition to ensure that everything checked previously is still okay (Figure 14-1).

Just because the patient appeared stable when you first arrived on scene does not mean this will remain the case. A patient's condition can change at any time, and it is critical that you continuously reassess specific elements of the patient assessment, regardless of his injuries or chief complaint.

3-6.1 Discuss the reasons for repeating the initial assessment as part of the ongoing assessment.

* **ongoing assessment**
  a continuous recheck of the patient's condition to ensure that everything checked previously is still okay.

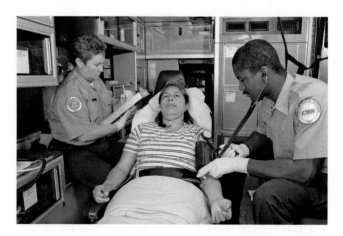

FIGURE 14-1   Ongoing assessment in the ambulance.

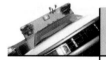

Emergency Dispatch

"Unit 1-9, unit 1-9," the dispatcher's voice came over the radio, bringing Conrad and his partner, Stephanie, to attention. "Please respond to an assault at the 'Los Rios' Bar at 13963 Bockwelder Avenue. Meet with P.D. on scene."

"Copy," Stephanie mumbled into the mic and stretched her arms wide in the cab of the truck.

"I just knew we were gonna get a call," said Conrad.

The patient was a Hispanic man who spoke no English and had been beaten severely. One eye was swollen shut, his avulsed nose dangled just above his top lip, and several teeth were missing. His nose and mouth were bleeding steadily, and his shirt was soaked with blood.

Although the patient looked bad, Conrad found that his vitals were actually pretty normal. They loaded him up and proceeded, low priority, to the local hospital.

About 5 minutes into the transport, Stephanie decided to recheck the man's vital signs. She found that his blood pressure had dropped and his pulse rate was increasing.

"Let's move it, Conrad!" Stephanie yelled up to the cab of the truck. "There's something definitely going wrong with this guy!"

Trending and the Ongoing Assessment

3-6.3 Describe trending of
assessment components.

✳ **trending**

the comparing of multiple sets
of vital signs over a period of
time in order to reveal a trend in
the patient's condition.

✳ **interventions**

actions taken to correct or
improve a patient's condition.

You learned about **trending** in chapter 10. Patients who are struck suddenly by an
injury or illness are at risk of getting much worse in a rather short period of time.
For this reason, we must closely watch several key elements over time in order to
spot any life-threatening trends. As we assess a component at any point in time,
such as breathing rate or mental status, we are simply taking a "snapshot" of that
component.

With several of these snapshots, we can begin to compare them and spot
changes from one snapshot to the next. Sometimes these changes show us that the
patient is getting better. In other instances they reveal that the patient is getting
worse, and you may need to alter or initiate specific **interventions.**

ELEMENTS OF AN ONGOING ASSESSMENT

3-6.2 Describe the components
of the ongoing assessment.

An ongoing assessment (Scan 14-1) is not a repeat of an entire patient assessment. Instead, it is a reassessment of those elements most critical to the well-
being of the patient. The following are the key components of the ongoing
assessment:

* ✳ Repeat the initial assessment
* ✳ Recheck vital signs
* ✳ Repeat assessment of chief complaint or injuries
* ✳ Check effectiveness of interventions
* ✳ Confirm priority

A CONTINUOUS PROCESS

Ongoing assessments are a continuous process. You do not, however—and *should
not*—wait until the end of your assessments to begin performing ongoing assessments. Elements of the more formal ongoing assessment should be checked all

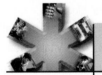

Perspective

Stephanie—The EMT

*"Holy cow, that was close! Here I am just bopping along, thinking that
it's just more physical exam and find that the poor guy's got like five or
six stab wounds to the side of his abdomen! Just like that . . . it goes from
a low priority to a critical patient. It threw me, because he was wearing
dark sweat pants, which soaked up much of the blood, and it appeared
that all of the blood on his shirt was from his nose and mouth. I don't
even want to think about what would have happened if I hadn't done the
ongoing assessment."*

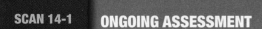

SCAN 14-1   **ONGOING ASSESSMENT**

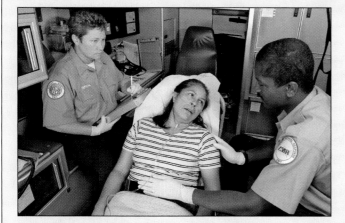

▲ Reassess ABCs of the responsive patient.

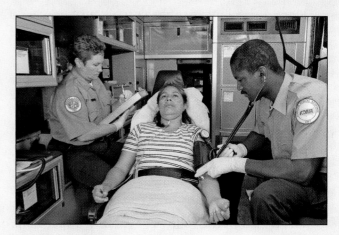

▲ Recheck vitals.

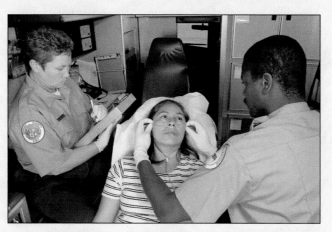

▲ Check effectiveness of interventions, such as oxygen, as necessary.

along the way. For example, when you first arrive at the patient's side, you will assess mental status by asking the patient some simple questions. Based on his response to your questions you will make an initial evaluation of his mental status, but it does not stop there. As you go on with your assessment, you should be continually asking questions and evaluating his responses. A patient who is talking and responding appropriately is in good shape at that moment. As soon as he begins to get quiet or respond inappropriately, his condition may be changing. By continuously interacting with your patient and asking him questions, you will become immediately aware if his condition changes.

Stop, Review, Remember!

Multiple Choice

Place a check next to the correct answer.

1. What is the term used to describe the comparison of multiple sets of vital signs over time?

   _____ a. trending

   _____ b. tasking

   _____ c. continuation

   _____ d. approximation

2. Which of the following is NOT an element of the ongoing assessment?

   _____ a. vital signs

   _____ b. initial assessment

   _____ c. interventions

   _____ d. scene size-up

3. Asking a patient the status of his pain is related to which element of the ongoing assessment?

   _____ a. vital signs

   _____ b. initial assessment

   _____ c. focused assessment

   _____ d. assess interventions

4. Which of the following statements most accurately describes when to perform an ongoing assessment?

   _____ a. once at the end of the detailed physical exam

   _____ b. continuously throughout your assessment

   _____ c. once at the beginning and once at the end

   _____ d. once at the beginning of the exam

5. An informal way to conduct an ongoing assessment of your patient is to:

   _____ a. keep the blood pressure cuff on and pumped up during transport.

   _____ b. have your partner keep the head tilted at all times.

   _____ c. continuously interact with your patient by talking to him.

   _____ d. use painful stimuli to keep him awake.

Fill in the Blank

1. The ongoing assessment should be performed at least every 15 minutes for stable patients and every _____ minutes for unstable patients.

2. The elements of the ongoing assessment include a recheck of the _____ assessment, a recheck of _____ signs, a repeat assessment of the chief _____, a check of the effectiveness of _____, and a confirmation of care and _____ priority.

3. _____ is the term used to describe the comparison of multiple sets of vital signs over time.

Critical Thinking

1. What is the importance of reevaluating the elements of the initial assessment during the ongoing assessment?

   _____

   _____

   _____

   _____

2. List the components of the ongoing assessment and what you will be looking for with each component.

   _____

   _____

   _____

   _____

3. Describe the concept of "trending" and how it applies to patient care.

   _____

   _____

   _____

   _____

Looking for Changes

Once you have completed the majority of your patient assessment, you must look back and reassess specific elements to ensure that the patient's needs are being met. Reassessing these elements will help identify changes in the patient's condition that may require changes in the care you provide.

RECHECK OF THE INITIAL ASSESSMENT

As you will remember from chapter 11, the core components of the initial assessment include mental status, airway, breathing, and circulation or pulse and the control of severe bleeding. Your reassessment during the ongoing assessment will include evaluation of the patient's mental status, ensuring that the patient is breathing at an acceptable rate and tidal volume, and ensuring that he has an adequate pulse (Figure 14-2 on page 370). It may be necessary to perform such interventions as suctioning, insertion of an airway adjunct, administration of oxygen, or perhaps performing CPR, depending on the patient's condition.

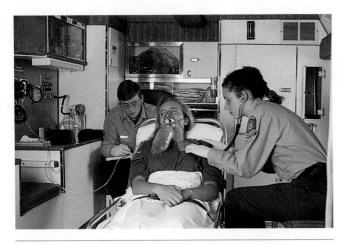

FIGURE 14-2   Ongoing assessment of a responsive patient.

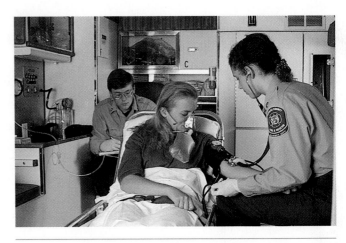

FIGURE 14-3   Recheck vitals on a responsive patient.

You will also need to assess all open wounds for evidence of bleeding and control any bleeding that has not already been managed.

RECHECK VITAL SIGNS

Now is the time to obtain another set of vital signs (Figure 14-3). It will be important to compare this set to the baseline set and any additional vital signs measurements obtained earlier. Comparing vital signs helps you identify a trend in the patient's condition and adjust your care as necessary. Remember to document all findings clearly and accurately, including the time at which the signs were obtained.

As you talk to the patient, pay close attention to his skin signs. Oftentimes you will see a change in color or moisture that may tip you off that the patient is getting worse.

REASSESS CHIEF COMPLAINT/INJURIES

One thing is certain, a patient's condition is dynamic and may change at any time, including his chief complaint. As you provide reassurance and care, some of the original symptoms may go away or new and different ones may appear (Figure 14-4). For instance, upon your arrival, a patient may have a chief com-

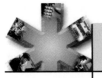

Perspective

Conrad—The EMT

"Although I missed the stab wounds when I did the initial assessment, at least I got a good set of baseline vitals! Hey, without those, Steph never would have been able to 'trend' that guy and see the change in his condition—and she may not have seen the red flag during the ongoing assessment."

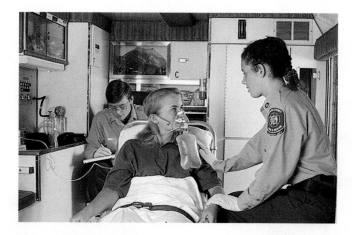

FIGURE 14-4   Reassess the chief complaint of a responsive patient.

plaint of chest pain, but after several minutes of oxygen his pain is nearly gone and he is now complaining of only shortness of breath. It is important to stay aware of how the patient is feeling and what his complaints are throughout your time with him.

CHECK EFFECTIVENESS OF INTERVENTIONS

It is your goal as an EMT to provide the most appropriate care for the patient based on the patient's condition. For that reason you must constantly evaluate the care you provide (Figure 14-5). Is the oxygen set at the right flow rate? Am I using the most appropriate delivery device? Is the bleeding still controlled or has it started to flow again? Is the traction splint still holding traction? These are just some of the things you must constantly be asking yourself relative to the care you are providing. One of the best ways to assess the effectiveness of our interventions is to simply ask the patient how he is feeling.

CONFIRM CARE AND TRANSPORT PRIORITY

As a patient's condition changes, for the better or for the worse, we must change his priority for both care and transport (Figure 14-6A and B on page 372). If you are caring for only one patient, then he should receive your undivided attention, and the only thing you might change is the urgency with which you get him to the hospital. If you are caring for multiple patients, you may have to adjust both who gets cared for first and who gets transported first, second, or third, based on their condition.

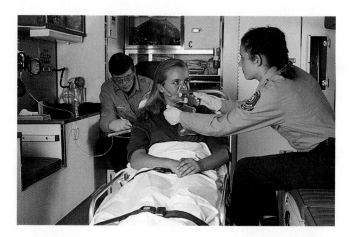

FIGURE 14-5   Adjust interventions in a responsive patient, if necessary.

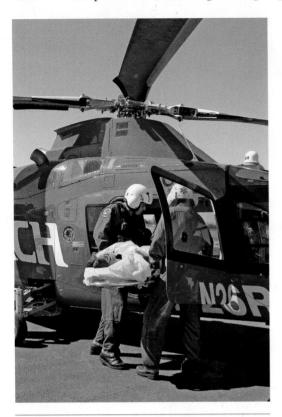

FIGURE 14-6A As a patient's condition changes, the priority for transport should be reassessed.

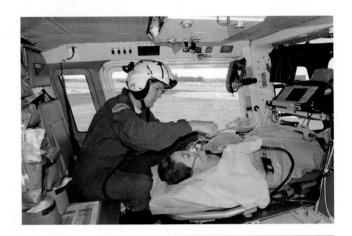

FIGURE 14-6B Ongoing assessment should continue during transport.

When to Reassess

UNSTABLE PATIENTS

As a rule of thumb, and once you have completed a thorough ongoing assessment, it is advised to reassess at least the initial assessment every 5 minutes for unresponsive patients and those patients you feel are unstable or whose condition is likely to deteriorate quickly. Examples of unstable patients include but are not limited to patients with:

* An altered mental status
* Respiratory distress
* Chest pain
* Multi-system trauma
* Signs and symptoms consistent with shock

The idea here is that unstable patients may deteriorate quickly, but if something goes wrong, you will be able to identify it quickly and provide the appropriate care. More frequent vital signs also mean that you are more likely to spot a trend in the patient's condition sooner and therefore anticipate the care he will need before his condition gets too bad.

STABLE PATIENTS

Stable patients are those whose condition is not likely to change any time soon. They are typically patients with a non-life-threatening injury or chief complaint

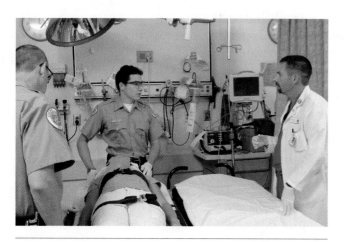

FIGURE 14-7A   The EMT hands off the care of the patient to the next level.

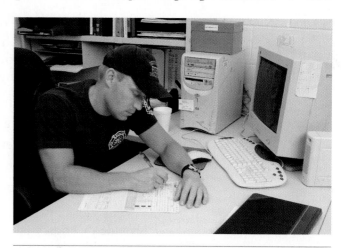

FIGURE 14-7B   After handing off the patient, complete the Patient Care Report form.

but who still need the attention of a higher level of care. Of course vital signs are always important, but more formal ongoing assessments are not typically needed as often for stable patients. It is generally recommended that stable patients be re-assessed at least every 15 minutes to observe for and note any significant changes in condition.

Documentation

It is especially important to document the patient's condition when you arrive on the scene, including the care that you provide and the response of the patient to your care (Figure 14-7A and B). The ongoing assessment will reveal if the signs and symptoms are getting better, worse, or remaining the same. Document as best you can any and all changes that the patient experiences in your care.

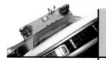

Dispatch Summary

Stephanie initiated oxygen therapy at 15 lpm via nonrebreather mask. The patient was then rushed to Baptist Tower Hospital, the city's Level One trauma center, and taken directly into surgery. He was found to have multiple intestinal punctures and a small liver laceration.

The patient survived the surgery but spent several weeks in ICU battling an infection and a bout with septic shock.

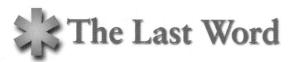 **The Last Word**

It is your continuous assessment of the patient that is likely to reveal any changes in his condition and is called the ongoing assessment.

Ongoing assessments are, just as the name implies, ongoing throughout the entire time you are with your patient.

One of the easiest ways to constantly assess the responsive patient is by talking to him and asking him questions. The appropriateness of his responses should be consistent throughout the patient assessment.

A complete ongoing assessment should include the following elements:

* ✳ Recheck the initial assessment
* ✳ Recheck vital signs
* ✳ Repeat assessment of chief complaint or injuries
* ✳ Check effectiveness of interventions
* ✳ Confirm care and transport priority

Pay close attention to any changes seen during the ongoing assessment, and provide the indicated care as appropriate. Reassess unstable patients every 5 minutes; stable patients every 15 minutes.

Document all changes in the patient's condition following the call.

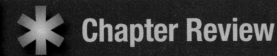

Chapter Review

MULTIPLE CHOICE

Place a check next to the correct answer.

1. Ensuring that all bleeding from open wounds is controlled is part of what element of the ongoing assessment?

   _____ a. vital signs

   _____ b. initial assessment

   _____ c. focused assessment

   _____ d. interventions

2. Which of the following is NOT an example of an unstable patient?

   _____ a. a patient with an altered mental status

   _____ b. a patient with an open fractured ankle

   _____ c. a patient with a history of asthma and in severe respiratory distress

   _____ d. a patient with a chest injury who was ejected from a vehicle rollover

3. A patient whose condition is not likely to get worse in the very near future can be described as:

   _____ a. a medical patient.

   _____ b. unstable.

   _____ c. stable.

   _____ d. a trauma patient.

4. Which of the following patients would be considered unstable?

   _____ a. 33-year-old male with an altered mental status

   _____ b. 6-year-old female with a bleeding cut on the hand

   _____ c. 66-year-old female with emphysema

   _____ d. 26-year-old male with a history of seizures

5. Which of the following ongoing assessment findings is least important during the assessment of a trauma patient?

   _____ a. the abdomen has become distended.

   _____ b. bandages have become blood soaked.

   _____ c. oxygen is still flowing through the nonrebreather mask.

   _____ d. the patient's bladder is full.

CRITICAL THINKING

1. Describe the concept of "trending."

_____

_____

_____

_____

2. Which element of the ongoing assessment do you feel is the most important and why?

_____

_____

_____

_____

CASE STUDIES

Case Study 1

You are caring for a 12-year-old female who began having difficulty breathing during a soccer practice. She has a history of asthma and her mother, who was at the practice, had her take several puffs of her inhaler. Initially the girl seemed to be getting better, but during transport to the hospital her breathing became more labored with audible wheezes.

1. What factors will you want to focus on during your ongoing assessment of this patient?

_____

_____

_____

_____

2. How will you adjust your care to accommodate this girl's worsening trend?

_____

_____

_____

_____

Case Study 2

You have responded to a residence for an unknown medical problem. Upon arrival you are presented with an approximately 70-year-old male who is sitting in a recliner in front of the television. He appears alert but seems to be fixated on the television, which is not even on. You step into his line of sight and introduce yourself. He shifts his gaze to look at you but does not respond in any other way. His wife tells you that he has a history of strokes and acted this way the last time he had one a year ago.

1. What are your initial concerns for this patient and what will they be as you transport?

   _____

   _____

   _____

   _____

2. How often will you want to provide ongoing assessments for this patient?

   _____

   _____

   _____

   _____

3. What will be the most appropriate position for this patient during transport?

   _____

   _____

   _____

   _____

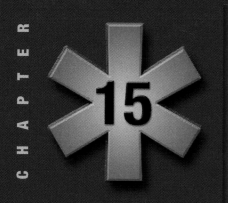

Communications in EMS

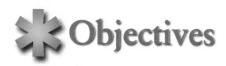

Objectives

Numbered objectives are from the U.S. Department of Transportation 1994 EMT-Basic National Standard Curriculum.

COGNITIVE OBJECTIVES

At the completion of this lesson, the EMT-Basic student will be able to:

3-7.1 List the proper methods of initiating and terminating a radio call. (pp. 384–385)

3-7.2 State the proper sequence for delivery of patient information. (pp. 387–388)

3-7.3 Explain the importance of effective communication of patient information in the verbal report. (pp. 388–390)

3-7.4 Identify the essential components of the verbal report. (pp. 391–392)

3-7.5 Describe the attributes for increasing effectiveness and efficiency of verbal communications. (pp. 380–381)

3-7.6 State legal aspects to consider in verbal communication. (pp. 379–380)

3-7.7 Discuss the communication skills that should be used to interact with the patient. (p. 380)

3-7.8 Discuss the communication skills that should be used to interact with the family, bystanders, and individuals from other agencies while providing patient care and the difference between skills used to interact with the patient and those used to interact with others. (pp. 380–381)

3-7.9 List the correct radio procedures in the following phases of a typical call: (p. 385)
- To the scene
- At the scene
- To the facility
- At the facility
- To the station
- At the station

AFFECTIVE OBJECTIVES

At the completion of this lesson, the EMT-Basic student will be able to:

3-7.10 Explain the rationale for providing efficient and effective radio communications and patient reports. (pp. 378–380)

PSYCHOMOTOR OBJECTIVES

At the completion of this lesson, the EMT-Basic student will be able to:

3-7.11 Perform a simulated, organized, concise radio transmission. (p. 385)

3-7.12 Perform an organized, concise patient report that would be given to the staff at a receiving facility. (p. 392)

3-7.13 Perform a brief, organized report that would be given to an ALS provider arriving at an incident scene at which the EMT-Basic was already providing care. (pp. 386, 388, 389, 391–392)

✳ Introduction

The best patient care available would suffer if we were unable to communicate properly. Our assessment and care would have no meaning to the patient if we didn't talk to them—in fact it would cause emotions ranging between fear and annoyance. And imagine if you performed that excellent care and treatment but didn't communicate your findings to the doctors and nurses at the hospital. The patient's assessment and care would start again from scratch.

Consider one other important point: What if *you* were this patient? How would you feel if no one listened to you? If no one talked to you? If one medical professional didn't talk to the other?

Communication is more than efficiency; it lets people know we are taking care of them and respect them as patients and as *people*.

✳ **communication**
the exchange of common symbols—written, spoken, or other kinds, such as signing and body language.

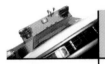

Emergency Dispatch

"So, what do we have here?" Dr. Orwell had come into the room right after EMTs Jared and Melanie finished transferring their patient to the hospital bed.

"This here is Mr. Thompson . . . " Melanie began.

"Tamblyn," the patient winced. "My last name is Tamblyn."

"Okay," Melanie smiled and moved on. "Mr. Tamblyn called because he was having pain on his right."

"Left."

" . . . left side . . . and it's gone on for most of the day."

"Most of the week. I told you a week."

"Does he have any allergies?" Dr. Orwell looked over her glasses at Melanie, frowning. Melanie stretched her exam glove between her fingers.

"Uh . . . yes, I think so," Melanie said, sounding unsure.

"Yes!" the patient roared. "What's wrong with you? I told you that I'm allergic to morphine! Back at my house you asked me, 'Are you allergic to anything?' and I very clearly said, 'Yes, I'm allergic to morphine'!"

The doctor looked from one EMT to the other and opened the exam room door. "Thanks for bringing Mr. Tamblyn in. I think I can take it from here."

The Role of Communications

Communication is a vital part of being an EMT. While much of your time in class will be dedicated to medical knowledge and skills, the role of communication must not be underestimated. Consider the following scenarios:

✳ You are called to a patient who is hyperventilating. The patient is anxious, breathing rapidly, and getting dizzier and dizzier. You apply oxygen to the patient. You get yourself at a level slightly lower than the patient and use a soft voice to get the patient's attention and then calm her down. You coach her to take slower, deeper breaths. The patient improves.

* You are called to a patient with chest pain. You find a man in his 50s with his wife looking on anxiously. As the man describes his chest pain, you apply some oxygen and reassure him. You note that the man is so worried he is trembling. You stop briefly and explain that you are taking care of him and are going to bring him to the hospital. Your calm demeanor provides reassurance throughout treatment and transport. He relaxes somewhat. His pulse comes down a little and his pain diminishes.

* You find a woman who was involved in a motor vehicle collision with relatively minor front-end damage to her vehicle. She has a minor head injury. She was not wearing a seat belt, and there was no air bag in her vehicle. She is anxious and her pulse is a bit rapid. You recognize this as a sign of possible shock—but also one of anxiety. You get the patient out of the car with a long board and into the ambulance. The entire time you are reassuring and talking with the patient. She actually has made a few jokes so you joke appropriately with her. In the ambulance she seems relaxed and calmer. Her pulse has dropped to within normal limits and has stayed stable.

In each of the foregoing cases, communication was a key component of your patient care (Figure 15-1). In the first case, calming the hyperventilating patient is an established clinical treatment. In the second case, the man with chest pains felt better after he was given oxygen and reassured. Anxiety causes an increased pulse; an increased pulse causes the heart to work harder and use more oxygen, which causes chest pain. Reassurance is a valuable clinical tool that likely reduced this man's chest pain. In the final case, you were unsure if the woman was simply nervous from the crash or had hidden injuries and shock. Your calming, reassuring manner and checking vital signs frequently led you to answer your question properly: Her nervousness and rapid pulse were caused by anxiety.

While in each case you gave oxygen, which also helped, the role of compassionate interpersonal communication can't be given too much importance.

If you work or volunteer at an ambulance or fire department—or have even been a patient—you will find that one of the things that patients remember most is the way they were treated. Letters of thanks that come to ambulance squads do not talk primarily of the clinical care. They say things such as, "You took good care of me," or "Thank you for taking such good care of my mother." People remember how they were treated. Something as simple as talking kindly to the patient can make a huge difference.

3-7.6 State legal aspects to consider in verbal communication.

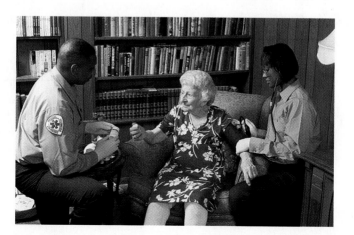

FIGURE 15-1 Communication is a critical component of patient care.

3-7.7 Discuss the communication skills that should be used to interact with the patient.

Proper communication and a caring attitude can also reduce legal liability. It is believed that patients are less likely to file a lawsuit if they feel that they were treated well. Good communication will also help you obtain the maximum amount of information from your patient, helping you make better care decisions.

3-7.5 Describe the attributes for increasing effectiveness and efficiency of verbal communications.

3-7.8 Discuss the communication skills that should be used to interact with the family, bystanders, and individuals from other agencies while providing patient care and the difference between skills used to interact with the patient and those used to interact with others.

INTERPERSONAL COMMUNICATION

Effective interpersonal communication includes:

* **Listening**—You can't communicate without listening. Recall how annoyed you get at the drive-through window when your order isn't right. Now place this annoyance in the context of a life-and-death situation. If you don't listen, you will not appear to care, regardless of how reassuring you sound. Plus, listening will help you obtain vital history information. Listening will also help you detect things that are important but not said out loud.

* **Speaking in a calm, reassuring tone**—Your demeanor, as noted in the small scenarios that opened this chapter, has a tremendous influence on the patient in both a personal and a clinical sense. It may well be the thing that the patient remembers most about the call.

* **Speaking slowly and clearly**—Patients will be nervous and confused and may even have an altered mental status. You should always talk slowly and clearly so the patient can understand. Avoid the unnecessary use of medical abbreviations, jargon, or big words.

* **Using body language and position**—Your body language and position tell the patient something. If you are standing above a sitting patient with your arms crossed, you are in a position of authority, appearing disinterested. When it is safe and appropriate to do so, get down to the patient's level—particularly with children. Make eye contact (Figure 15-2). Looking constantly at the clipboard or elsewhere also establishes poor relations.

* **Touching, when appropriate**—There are times when a hand on a shoulder or arm establishes a level of warmth and concern. A handshake shows respect. If a patient refuses transport but promises to call his personal physician, the handshake may "seal the deal."

* **Honesty**—Honesty is critical in patient care. Believe it or not, even the youngest patients are able to sense dishonesty. And patients often know the answer to questions like "Could it be serious?" or "Are you taking me to the psychiatric center?" before they ask. If you don't know, you can always

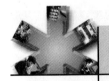

Perspective

Mr. Tamblyn—The Patient

"Good lord! How do they let people like that work on an ambulance? She asks questions and then doesn't listen to the answers. I mean, why bother? What if someone was dying? What if she was trying to give someone something that he is allergic to? That's just unbelievable to me."

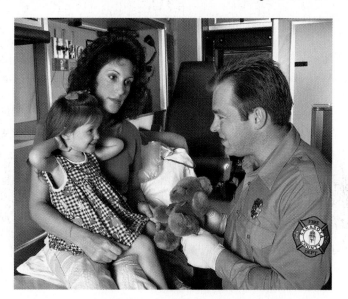

FIGURE 15-2 You should place yourself slightly lower than the patient with no barriers between you, and make eye contact as you speak with the patient.

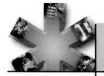

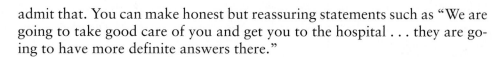

Perspective

Jared—The EMT

"I just started working with Melanie last week, and what happened today is unfortunately not uncommon. It's like . . . like she's so intent on getting through all of the 'official' assessment questions that, instead of listening to the answers, she's thinking of the next question. I've tried to talk to her about it—that we ask the questions to get an accurate picture of the patient's overall situation—but she keeps telling me that I'm just new and that she's in paramedic school. At least I can remember my patient's name!"

admit that. You can make honest but reassuring statements such as "We are going to take good care of you and get you to the hospital . . . they are going to have more definite answers there."

Your communication will make a difference in the patient's prehospital experience and can even help the patient's clinical condition. One other way to say this is *treat every patient the way you would want to be treated. You won't go wrong.*

BARRIERS TO EFFECTIVE COMMUNICATION

Many of your patients will speak to you and hear what you have to say. Others may not hear or understand what you say. Likewise your ability to hear and understand some patients will be an issue or a challenge in providing effective care. There are many barriers to communication, including patients who are hard of hearing, deaf, blind, speak a different language, or have a different culture than you. These barriers occur across all groups of people and can occur anywhere.

Patients who are hearing impaired may have some hearing or they may not be able to hear at all. These patients may know sign language or be able to read lips.

Face your patient when speaking. If the patient does lip read, speak slowly and clearly but do not speak in an unusually slow or exaggerated manner. Family members or acquaintances may know sign language and translate for you. In other cases, you may be able to communicate by writing notes back and forth with the patient.

Some patients, especially in the geriatric population, have some hearing loss (also known as being "hard of hearing") but do still have some ability to hear. By speaking up slightly and facing the patient when you speak, you will be able to communicate effectively.

Patients who are blind or have limited eyesight will require extra care and explanation of what you are doing. This will help reduce anxiety. If you are going to have contact with the patient (for example, palpating a part of the body or applying a nonrebreather mask), you must tell the patient before you touch him. Explain things and procedures (for example, stretcher movement or splinting) you may take for granted as self-explanatory.

Patients who speak a language other than your own will also pose a communication challenge. Use a friend or relative to translate if possible. Some pocket guides that have medical translations are available. Some EMS agencies and many hospitals subscribe to translation services available over the phone. Know the languages spoken in your community and have resources available if you encounter a patient and require a translator.

Often these same patients may have certain cultural beliefs that can affect the care to which they are receptive. Family members and acquaintances again may be able to help you understand these cultural factors and also help you communicate more effectively.

The patients we have just discussed pose challenges for communication. The level of compassion and clinical care for these patients should equal that given to patients with full ability to communicate. These patients usually possess normal intelligence. So be careful not to shout, talk down to, or assume that the patient has reduced mental capacity when this is not true.

Communication Systems

* **9-1-1 system**
  a system for telephone access to report emergencies.

* **base station radio**
  a two-way radio at a fixed site such as a hospital or dispatch center.

* **mobile radio**
  a two-way radio that is used or affixed in a vehicle.

* **portable radio**
  a handheld two-way radio.

* **mobile data terminals (MDTs)**
  computers that are mounted in a vehicle and connected to the base station by radio modem. In addition to full functionality as a computer, the MDT will display dispatch information for calls and may provide the ability to enter information for prehospital care reports.

Communication systems link patients to dispatchers, to ambulances, and to hospitals and are a vital part of what we do. Communication systems improve efficiency, reduce response times, and allow us to contact the hospital with vital patient information before we arrive. Yes, communications systems are involved in almost everything we do.

You will recall that lay people activate the EMS system in most areas by calling 9-1-1. In an enhanced **9-1-1 system** the location (address) is displayed on the computer screen.

At the dispatch center is a **base station radio.** This is a radio or radio system located at a stationary site. Hospital radios are also base stations (Figure 15-3).

In the field, **mobile radios** are radios that are mounted in vehicles. These transmit at a lower power than base station radios (but more than many portable radios described next) (Figure 15-4).

Portable or handheld **radios** are carried with an EMT or worn in a belt case so the radio may be used anywhere the EMT is (Figure 15-5). This is very important in the event additional help is required. With a portable radio, the EMT will not have to return to the ambulance to call for assistance.

Many ambulances and fire apparatus are equipped with **mobile data terminals (MDTs).** These computers are mounted in the vehicle and connected to the base station by radio modem. In addition to full functionality as a computer, the MDT

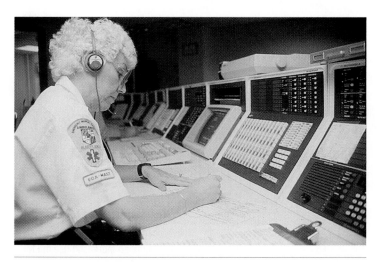

FIGURE 15-3   The dispatcher determines the appropriate level of response according to the established guidelines.

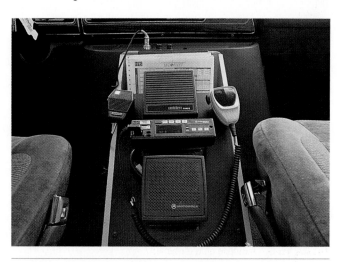

FIGURE 15-4   A mobile (vehicle-mounted) radio.

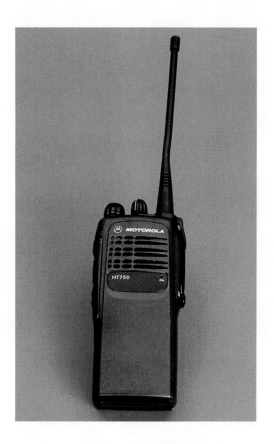

FIGURE 15-5   A handheld portable radio.

will display dispatch information for calls and may provide the ability to enter information for prehospital care reports (Figure 15-6 on page 384).

Some systems use repeaters when radio frequencies must span large distances or difficult terrain. A **repeater** receives transmissions from a low-powered radio (e.g., a portable radio) and rebroadcasts it at greater power on a different frequency (Figure 15-7 on page 384). Radio frequencies are assigned by the Federal Communications Commission (FCC).

Cellular phones have found an increased use in EMS recently (Figure 15-8 on page 384). They may be used in systems where radio signals are unavailable or expensive to create. The walkie-talkie-type features on some cell phones are very similar to two-way portable radios.

* **repeater**

a device that picks up signals from lower-power radio units, such as mobile and portable radios, and retransmits them at a higher power. It allows low-power radio signals to be transmitted over longer distances.

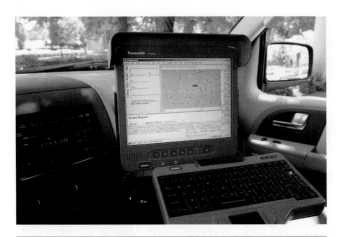

FIGURE 15-6   A mobile data terminal.

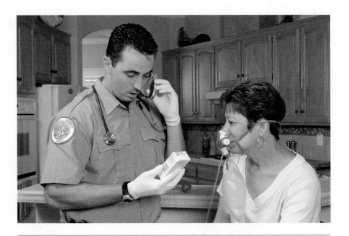

FIGURE 15-7   Cellular phones have found an increased use in EMS.

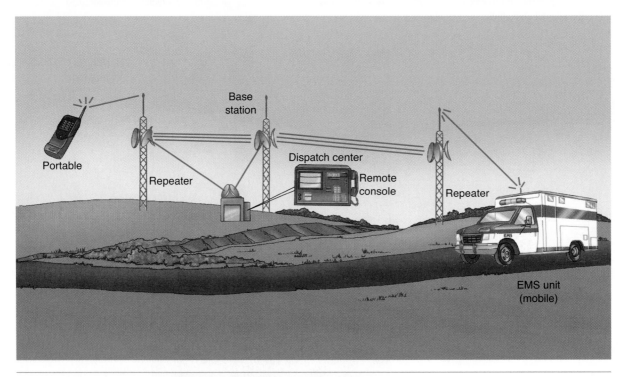

FIGURE 15-8   An example of an EMS communication system using repeaters.

3-7.1 List the proper methods of initiating and terminating a radio call.

RADIO COMMUNICATION

When working as an EMT, you will use the radio many times each day. When you use a radio, whether it be a portable or a mobile radio, the following guidelines will be helpful in making your radio communications clear:

* Make sure the radio is on and the volume is properly adjusted.

* Listen before transmitting. Do not transmit over someone who is already speaking.

* Press the "push to talk" or "PTT" button for 1 second before beginning to speak.

* Speak with your mouth about 2–3 inches from the microphone.

* Address the unit you are calling by its name or radio identifier (for example, number).

∗ The unit being called will acknowledge by saying "Go ahead" or another approved code meaning the same thing.

∗ Speak clearly and slowly.

∗ Keep transmissions brief.

∗ Avoid unnecessary or confusing codes. Use only those that are approved, meaningless phrases such as "be advised," and things like "please" and "thank you," since courtesy is assumed.

∗ Do not use patient names on the air. People with scanners will be able to hear this information. Do not put judgments or negative comments over the air for that same reason.

The transmissions procedures required on an EMS call vary from agency to agency. Some of the more common transmissions required during a call include:

∗ Dispatch information

∗ En route

∗ On scene

∗ En route to the hospital

∗ Arriving at the hospital

∗ In service

∗ Back in quarters

Table 15-1 shows examples of these radio transmissions on a typical call.

3-7.9 List the correct radio procedures in the following phases of a typical call:
- To the scene
- At the scene
- To the facility
- At the facility
- To the station
- At the station

TABLE 15-1 TYPICAL RADIO TRANSMISSIONS	
TRANSMISSION	**TIME**
Dispatcher: Rescue 29, respond to 1422 Clinton Avenue for a report of a male patient with chest pain.	1123 hours
Rescue 29: Responding to 1422 Clinton.	1123 hours
Dispatcher: Rescue 29, I am still on the phone with the patient.	1125 hours
He reports chest pain and some dizziness.	
Rescue 29: 10-4.	
Rescue 29: On scene.	1128 hours
Rescue 29: Rescue 29, Dispatch. Can we get ALS response here?	1130 hours
Dispatcher: Rescue 29, Medic 2 is en route.	1131 hours
Rescue 29: Dispatch, Rescue 29 is en route to Mercy Hospital. Medic 2 is on board.	1144 hours
Rescue 29: Rescue 29 is out at Mercy.	1202 hours
Rescue 29: Rescue 29 is in service returning Medic 2 to her vehicle.	

✳ Stop, Review, Remember!

Multiple Choice

Place a check next to the correct answer.

1. The time you were given the call via the radio is called the:

_____ a. en route time.

_____ b. dispatch time.

_____ c. on-scene time.

_____ d. in-service time.

2. The radio mounted in the ambulance is called a _____ radio.

_____ a. portable

_____ b. mobile

_____ c. base

_____ d. walkie-talkie

3. Which of the following statements in reference to repeaters is true?

_____ a. Repeaters reduce the signal from radio to radio to reduce interference.

_____ b. Repeaters are installed only on base station radios.

_____ c. Repeaters retransmit and boost signals on the same frequency.

_____ d. Repeaters retransmit and boost signals on a different frequency.

4. The _____ is responsible for allocating EMS radio frequencies.

_____ a. Department of Homeland Security

_____ b. Department of Transportation

_____ c. Federal Communication Commission

_____ d. Federal Emergency Management Agency (FEMA)

5. Touching a patient can be used as an effective tool for communicating with your patient.

_____ a. true

_____ b. false

6. Calming a patient may help his medical condition.

_____ a. true

_____ b. false

Matching

Match the communication activity described on the left with the type of radio listed on the right.

1. _____ Two EMTs acknowledge and call en route to a call via radio from their ambulance

2. _____ The hospital receives a call-in report from EMTs in the field via radio

3. _____ The dispatcher transmits a call to an ambulance

4. _____ An EMT calls for ALS assistance via radio from the patient's living room

A. Base station
B. Mobile radio
C. Portable radio
D. Cell phone

Critical Thinking

1. You are called to a scene and find a deaf adult patient. How will you communicate with the patient? Give two methods you may try.

_____

_____

_____

_____

2. Differentiate between a portable, a mobile, and a base station radio.

_____

_____

_____

_____

Medical Communication

Not only will you communicate with your patients, for each patient you care for and transport you will also communicate with other medical professionals. You may call a physician for medical direction, request an advanced life support (ALS) provider, call the hospital on the radio to give a report, and also provide a verbal report to the hospital staff on your arrival.

These reports are important because they transfer medical information between health care providers. The reports should be pertinent and concise while containing all of the appropriate information. Contacting a busy emergency department by radio or when dropping off a patient, you will provide an accurate, clinically relevant report.

What does clinically relevant mean? It means that the report contains information on the patient's present complaint and condition, any pertinent medical history, physical exam findings and vital signs, any interventions you have provided, and changes (improvement or worsening) you have seen in the patient's condition.

COMMUNICATING WITH THE HOSPITAL VIA PHONE OR RADIO

You will contact the hospital for advice or to advise them that you are coming in with a patient so they can be prepared. This communication is done from a phone or radio (not in person).

It is important that you paint a picture of your patient so the physician can provide any orders or advice accurately. These reports contain the following information:

* Identify your unit (ambulance identifier) and your level of certification—in this case EMT (Figure 15-9 on page 388).

* Your estimated time of arrival (ETA)

3-7.2 State the proper sequence for delivery of patient information.

3-7.4 Identify the essential components of the verbal report.

FIGURE 15-9 Give a radio report to the hospital prior to your arrival with the patient.

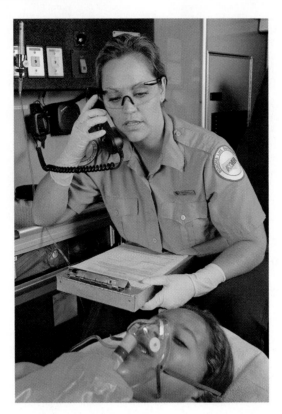

* The patient's age and gender

* The patient's chief complaint

* A brief, pertinent history of the present illness or injury

* Relevant past medical history

* Vital signs including mental status

* Pertinent findings of your examination

* The care you have provided

* The patient's response to your care

A sample call-in report is as follows:

Mercy Hospital, this is Ambulance 21. How do you copy?

Mercy here, 21. Loud and clear. Go ahead.

Mercy, Ambulance 21 is 10 minutes from your location at the EMT level with a 47-year-old male patient who complains of leg pain after a fall from a ladder. The fall was from about 4 feet. We noted deformity to the left tib/fib. The patient denies other injury. The patient has no past medical history or meds. He is alert and oriented, and never lost consciousness. His pulse is 94 strong and regular, respirations 16, BP 124/86, pupils equal and reactive, skin warm and dry. We have splinted the leg and have good circulation and neuro distal to the injury. We've applied ice. He is in quite a bit of pain but seems stable.

3-7.3 Explain the importance of effective communication of patient information in the verbal report.

Mercy to Ambulance 21, we'll be expecting you. You'll be going to the cast room.

Ambulance 21 10-4 and clear.

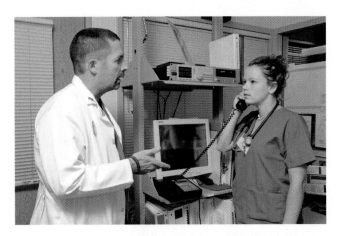

FIGURE 15-10   A nurse or physician at the hospital will take your report prior to arrival.

This is a significant amount of information. Each bit is pertinent and relevant. Read the report above while timing yourself on a watch with a second hand. Your author read this in 30–40 seconds. (You can hear this and the next reports on the CD that accompanies this text.)

What does the nurse or physician at the other end of the radio get from this (Figure 15-10)? They know that a 47-year-old, otherwise healthy man fell a relatively short distance from a ladder and may have broken his leg. He denies further injury, didn't lose consciousness, and his vital signs seem good. You've splinted the leg and he doesn't seem to have nerve or circulatory problems.

That is what is meant by concise and relevant. There are some things that may be in his medical history and are not important for the radio report. For example, if the patient had hernia surgery 7 years ago (and it has been fine since then), it doesn't go in the radio report. The fact that he has bunions, occasional indigestion, or broke his arm once as a child has no significance to this condition and would only serve to clog an otherwise excellent report with unnecessary facts.

Let's look at a report with a more complicated problem:

Mercy, Ambulance 21. How do you copy?

Mercy to Ambulance 21. Loud and clear. Go ahead.

Mercy, we are en route to your location at the basic level with a 15 minute ETA. We are treating a 64-year-old female patient who complains of difficulty breathing. The difficulty began suddenly and awoke her from sleep. She is able to speak 5-to-6-word sentences before catching her breath. She reports having a heart attack last year and has high blood pressure. She takes furosemide and atenolol. She is alert and oriented. Slightly anxious. Pulse 104 and regular, respirations 24, BP 146/92, skin warm and dry, pupils equal and reactive. We have found that she sleeps on several pillows and has some edema in her ankles. We put her in the Fowler's position and are giving oxygen by NRB mask at 15 liters which brought her oxygen saturation from 95% to 98% and reduced her anxiety. Over.

OK, Ambulance 21. Sounds good. We'll be awaiting your arrival in 15. Mercy out.

In this case the patient was having difficulty breathing. You were able to add some additional physical findings such as the edema and sleeping elevated on pillows. You also provided pulse oximetry readings and your positioning of the patient. The hospital now knows that this is a potentially serious situation based on her cardiac history, medications, and complaint.

REQUESTING ADVICE FROM A PHYSICIAN

There are times you will call a medical direction physician or medical director for advice. There are many reasons this will occur. Some of the most common include when protocols require this contact (for example, to assist a patient with medication administration), patient refusal situations, and any time you feel you would benefit from speaking to a physician.

The format for your report to the physician is similar to the call-in radio report except that you will be asking a question at the end of a report. The question may be specific: "May I assist this patient with the use of her inhaler?" or looking for input or advice: "Do you think it is appropriate for this patient to refuse transportation?" or "Do you think that this patient should receive nitroglycerin?"

When requesting permission to assist patients with their own medications—or to administer medications you may carry on the ambulance—there are additional facts a physician will require. You must be very specific. These include:

* Do the patient's signs and symptoms match the condition the drug is intended for?

* Does the patient have any allergies to medications?

* Has the patient taken any of the medication already? If so has the patient had any response?

* Vital signs take on increased importance when considering medication orders.

When you speak to a physician and obtain an order to assist with or administer a medication, you should always repeat the order back to the physician for confirmation. If the physician gives an order that doesn't make sense to you or indicates a misunderstanding of the information you presented, ask for clarification or explanation before carrying out any order.

This is an example of a radio report in which the EMT requests an order to administer a medication:

Mercy Hospital, this is Ambulance 21.

Mercy is on, 21. Go ahead.

Ambulance 21 requesting a physician for medical direction request.

Stand by, 21.

Ambulance 21 this is Dr. Perkins. Go ahead with your report.

Dr. Perkins, we are en route to your location, 20-minute ETA, with a 32-year-old female patient who complains of shortness of breath after exercising. She reports a history of asthma for which she has an albuterol inhaler. No other health problems or allergies. She is alert, oriented, and anxious. Vitals are pulse 110 strong and regular, respirations 28 and labored. We can hear wheezing without a stethoscope. BP 138/88. Skin is warm but slightly moist. As we said, we have wheezing and also mild accessory muscle use. She is speaking about 4-word sentences. Her oxygen sats were 92 when we arrived. Oxygen at 15 lpm via nonrebreather brought that up to 95. She has an albuterol inhaler prescribed to her and is not expired. She used it for "two or three puffs," which caused slight improvement. We'd like to coach her and make sure it is being done properly and administer two more puffs of the albuterol. Over.

OK, 21. Get her to take two more puffs of the albuterol inhaler—timed well and with deep breaths. You said that you were 20 minutes out, so give it 5 minutes, and if her vitals remain OK you can administer two more puffs of the albuterol. Let me know if there are any changes. Monitor her breathing carefully. If I don't hear back, I'll see you in 20 minutes.

Confirming 2 puffs of albuterol now. Timed well with deep breaths. Two more in 5 minutes if vitals remain OK.

These orders are confirmed. Please advise of any significant changes in the patient's condition. Mercy out.

Ambulance 21 out.

There may be times when your medical direction physician may not be at the hospital to which you are taking the patient. In this case, you will also need to notify the receiving hospital with a radio report.

VERBAL REPORTS AT THE HOSPITAL

3-7.4 Identify the essential components of the verbal report.

When you arrive at the hospital, the nurse or physician meeting you at the hospital should already know the information you called in via the radio (Figure 15-11). In this case you will be able to provide a verbal report that summarizes and updates the information given over the radio. If the information hasn't been relayed to the person you are dealing with, or if partial information was relayed, you will need to provide a full report.

Information contained in the verbal report includes:

* Restating the chief complaint

* Significant changes in the patient's condition since the radio report

* History information not previously presented (may include medications)

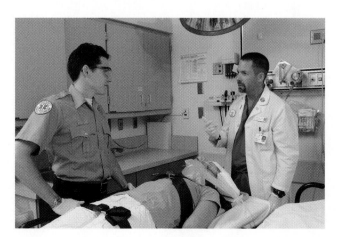

FIGURE 15-11   Once you arrive at the hospital, you will give a verbal report that summarizes all of the information on the patient.

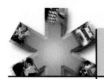

Perspective

Dr. Orwell—The Physician

"Most of the ambulance crews are great at communicating with both the patient and us at the ED. But sometimes a mistake is made. What if the patient is unresponsive when he is brought in and I need to make decisions based on the medical information that an EMT gathered at the scene? I could decide on a course of action that kills my patient just because an EMT wasn't actually listening when a family member was talking. And let me tell you . . . I cannot trust that EMT and will address the mistakes."

* Treatments that were administered en route

* Subsequent vital signs taken en route

* Additional pertinent information not presented in the radio report

An example of a verbal report follows. This report pertains to the patient for whom you requested orders from medical direction to administer her inhaler.

Hi. This is our patient, Sally Farnsworth. We called in. Did you get the info?

Yes, I heard it on the radio.

OK. She has a history of asthma and developed shortness of breath after exercising. She says it is similar to previous attacks. She used her albuterol inhaler twice. We did four more puffs en route spaced five minutes apart as ordered. She has felt considerable relief. Her pulse and respirations have come down a bit. Her sats are up to 98%. Doing better.

OK. Very good. Sally, I'm Hal Chapman, the nurse who is going to take care of you today. Let's get you moved over to our stretcher.

Stop, Review, Remember!

Multiple Choice

Place a check next to the correct answer.

1. Which of the following is NOT a part of the hospital radio report?

    _____ a. the chief complaint

    _____ b. the patient's sex

    _____ c. a complete medical history

    _____ d. vital signs

2. Which of the following items would not be appropriate in the radio report to the hospital?

    _____ a. the patient's blood pressure

    _____ b. the fact that you splinted a suspected leg fracture

    _____ c. the patient's complete medication list

    _____ d. the patient has had prior heart attacks

3. Which of the following statements best describes the content of a radio report?

    _____ a. fair and balanced

    _____ b. concise and relevant

    _____ c. lengthy and complete

    _____ d. short and fast

4. How does a "request for order" from a physician differ from a basic call-in report?

    _____ a. Less medication information is required for physician advice when compared to a call-in.

    _____ b. You frequently ask questions at the end of a call-in report.

    _____ c. Requests for physician advice may include more than one set of vital signs.

    _____ d. Call-in reports are generally longer than requests for advice or orders.

5. Which statement reflects the differences between the call-in radio report and the in-person hand-off report at the hospital?

    _____ a. The hand-off report states all information from the radio report plus any new information you have obtained.

    _____ b. If the person receiving the report at the hospital heard the radio report, no further report is necessary.

    _____ c. The verbal report at the hospital is given by the patient; the radio report is given by the EMT.

    _____ d. The hand-off report highlights core information, medications, treatments, and changes in the patient's condition.

Critical Thinking

1. List the components of the call-in radio report to the hospital.

   _____

   _____

   _____

   _____

2. List two things that are different between the call-in report (radio) and the hand-off report (in person at the hospital).

   _____

   _____

   _____

   _____

3. How would a physician or nurse at the hospital view you upon arrival at the hospital when your radio report was hurried and incomplete?

   _____

   _____

   _____

   _____

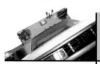

Dispatch Summary

Mr. Tamblyn was released later the same day with a diagnosis of a pulled abdominal muscle. He has since recovered fully. Dr. Orwell contacted the Field Supervisor for the ambulance company and made a formal complaint about Melanie's poor communication skills—a third such complaint. Melanie was placed into a remedial training program and is showing marked improvement in her listening and other communication abilities.

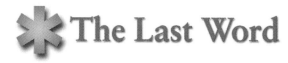

The Last Word

Communication in EMS is more than talking. The communication you have with patients is important—sometimes therapeutic. It is likely the part of the call the patient will remember most.

Your communication with other health care professionals has a direct relation to the care you give and the care the patient will receive at the hospital. Your communications must be accurate, yet concise.

The radio systems used in your area are vital for communication. Radios, whether they are base stations, mobiles, portables, cell phones, or computers, are used for communicating calls and other vital information. Radios must be treated well and maintained so they will be ready when you need them.

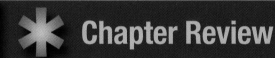

Chapter Review

MULTIPLE CHOICE

Place a check next to the correct answer.

1. You are helping another new EMT with his issued radio. Which piece of advice would not be appropriate?

   _____ a. Listen before transmitting.

   _____ b. Speak with your mouth as close as possible to the microphone for best sound transmission.

   _____ c. Don't use patients' names or other specific identifying information on the air.

   _____ d. Push the "PTT" button for one second before you speak.

2. Patients who are unable to hear at all would likely be benefited by your:

   _____ a. shouting.

   _____ b. speaking quickly to avoid frustration.

   _____ c. writing down questions.

   _____ d. placing a stethoscope in his ears and speaking into the diaphragm or bell.

3. In order to obtain an order from a physician to administer medications, you will need to present additional information. Which of the following considerations is NOT correct?

   _____ a. Do the patient's signs and symptoms match the condition the drug is intended for?

   _____ b. Does the patient have any allergies to medications?

   _____ c. Has the patient taken any of the medication already? If so, has the patient had any response?

   _____ d. Vital signs take on decreased importance when considering medication orders.

4. A repeater boosts signal transmission from a base station to mobile or portable radios in the field.

   _____ a. true

   _____ b. false

5. Shouting at patients who have communication difficulties shows that you are taking extra effort and is usually appreciated.

   _____ a. true

   _____ b. false

CRITICAL THINKING

1. You are called to a 75-year-old patient who is complaining of chest pain. She is extremely anxious and seems fearful of going to the hospital. Describe several things you have learned in this section that you will use to calm the patient and help get her to accept transport.

_____

_____

_____

_____

2. Why is it important to notify the dispatcher of key events such as en route, at scene, en route to the hospital, and so on?

_____

_____

_____

3. Imagine you are a patient who is being cared for by an EMT. How would you react if the EMT wasn't listening or making eye contact but stood above you and talked to another person (e.g., spouse, parent) to obtain your medical history and history of the present illness?

_____

_____

_____

_____

4. You receive an order from a physician to assist the patient with one sublingual nitroglycerin spray and to have the patient chew 4 baby aspirins (total 324 mg). How would you confirm this with the physician? Write down your response.

_____

_____

_____

_____

5. What four additional things (over and above the call-in radio report) will you need to tell the physician when asking for permission to assist a patient with his medication?

_____

_____

_____

_____

6. Why is it important to limit the amount of information given in the radio report to the most pertinent information?

_____

_____

_____

_____

7. Your grandmother has fallen and is being cared for by EMTs. What would you expect from the EMTs in reference to the way they treat your grandmother?

_____

_____

_____

_____

RECONSTRUCT THE RADIO REPORT

The following radio reports have been taken apart and placed in individual sentences. Reassemble the reports by numbering the sentences in the correct order of presentation.

Radio Report 1

_____ We have splinted the extremity and applied cold. She has good circulation and sensation distal to the injury.

_____ A 27-year-old female patient.

_____ Her pulse is 86 strong and regular, respirations 16, BP 106/74, pupils equal and reactive, skin warm and dry.

_____ Patient is alert and oriented. She never lost consciousness.

_____ Complains of an ankle injury sustained while hiking. She slipped from a rock and twisted the ankle.

_____ En route to your facility with a 17-minute ETA.

_____ Patient has a history of asthma but has no complaint of difficulty breathing.

_____ She is resting comfortably with minor pain in the ankle.

_____ There is swelling and deformity of the left ankle. Patient did not fall and denies further injury.

Radio Report 2

_____ Vital signs are pulse 104 regular and weak, respirations 26, BP 152/94, skin pale and moist, pupils equal and reactive.

_____ He developed the shortness of breath after having an increased cough and sputum production for a week.

_____ We administered oxygen and placed the patient in a position of comfort.

_____ He is alert and oriented.

_____ 86-year-old male patient.

_____ He is speaking 5-to-6-word sentences. He has produced some brown sputum. Initial oxygen saturation was 88%.

_____ We are en route to your location with a 5-minute ETA.

_____ Complaining of shortness of breath.

_____ His sats came up to 94% with oxygen and he is breathing a little easier.

_____ He has a history of emphysema and MI.

CASE STUDY

You are called to a residence for an unknown medical problem. The dispatcher says she is unable to understand the caller. The police are also dispatched.

You arrive on the scene and find the police talking to a teenage male in the doorway. Once you are waved in by the police, you find that the patient doesn't speak English. The patient, a 50-year-old Hispanic man, was cleaning windows when he fell from the ladder. His wife, who speaks broken English, called for help.

You find the son does speak fluent English and will translate.

1. Can you use the son as a translator? Why or why not?

_____

_____

_____

_____

2. Would the information you receive from the son/interpreter be accurate? How can you assure accuracy?

_____

_____

_____

_____

3. Will you be able to perform an assessment at a normal pace? If not, will it be faster or slower? Why?

_____

_____

_____

_____

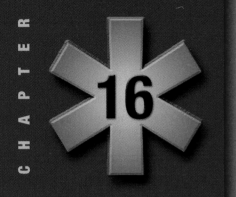

CHAPTER 16

Documenting Your Assessment and Care

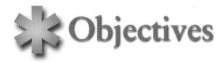 **Objectives**

Numbered objectives are from the U.S. Department of Transportation 1994 EMT-Basic National Standard Curriculum.

COGNITIVE OBJECTIVES

At the completion of this lesson, the EMT-Basic student will be able to:

3-8.1 Explain the components of the written report and list the information that should be included in the written report. (pp. 405–406)

3-8.2 Identify the various sections of the written report. (pp. 405–406)

3-8.3 Describe what information is required in each section of the prehospital care report and how it should be entered. (pp. 405–407)

3-8.4 Define the special considerations concerning patient refusal. (pp. 412–413)

3-8.5 Describe the legal implications associated with the written report. (p. 401)

3-8.6 Discuss all state and/or local record and reporting requirements. (pp. 414–415)

AFFECTIVE OBJECTIVES

At the completion of this lesson, the EMT-Basic student will be able to:

3-8.7 Explain the rationale for patient care documentation. (p. 401)

3-8.8 Explain the rationale for the EMS system gathering data. (p. 401)

3-8.9 Explain the rationale for using medical terminology correctly. (p. 405)

3-8.10 Explain the rationale for using an accurate and synchronous clock so that information can be used in trending. (p. 405)

PSYCHOMOTOR OBJECTIVES

At the completion of this lesson, the EMT-Basic student will be able to:

3-8.11 Complete a prehospital care report. (pp. 401–404)

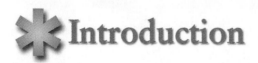

Introduction

Documenting your assessment and care is a vitally important part of your role as an EMT. Your written reports—known as run reports or prehospital care reports (PCRs)—will follow a patient through the health care system as the only lasting representation of your work.

Of course documentation has many other uses. It is used in the short term by emergency department personnel to reference your assessment findings and determine what care was given in the field.

Good documentation also plays an important role in minimizing your liability. If someone questioned the care you gave, would you want thorough documentation of your quality care—or would a quick and shoddy attempt at writing down a few things be enough? There is no doubt you would want to develop a reputation for thorough documentation. Good documentation is more than legal protection. Good documentation should also be a matter of pride in what you do.

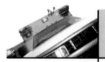

Emergency Dispatch

"**M**r. Devlin," the attorney said, rolling his pencil on the table and looking at the tiled ceiling for a moment before continuing. "Take us back to that night. Just explain what happened, in your own words, and try to be as detailed as possible. Keep in mind that a deposition is just like a trial, and you've sworn to tell the truth."

EMT Joe Devlin looked around the conference table at the others present but dropped his gaze when he encountered the face of the woman who was suing his employer, the North County Ambulance Service.

"Yeah, sure," he said. What did he remember about that call? He had been searching his memory ever since the guys showed up with the subpoena at work. He glanced at his copy of the PCR, but the narrative wasn't very helpful—just a couple of hastily written sentences that made this incident sound like every other call that he had ever been on. "Well . . . we arrived to find the patient . . . um . . . that lady's husband . . .

in some distress. I guess . . . um . . . according to my narrative . . . we transported him to Midway Hospital."

"Actually, Mr. Devlin," the attorney sat up straight and pointed his pencil at Joe. "You transported Mr. O'Neil to Riverside Community Hospital . . . not Midway. As a matter of fact, our contention is that had you taken the patient to Midway he might still be alive today. But please, continue. I might suggest that you don't use that PCR, though. We found that it's full of errors. Just tell us from memory, if you can."

Joe glanced at the patient's address on the PCR. Portland Drive. Why *wouldn't* he have taken that patient to Midway? Going to Riverside would have added 20 minutes to the transport time. There *must* have been a reason.

"I'm sorry," Joe shook his head. "I don't remember what happened . . . it was over a year ago. I just . . . I . . . don't know."

"Thanks, Mr. Devlin." The attorney smiled and set his pencil down on a blank legal pad. "We don't have any other questions for you."

Prehospital Care Reports

Reporting and documentation is a very important skill. In spite of this you may still hear some EMTs after a call dreading the documentation or complaining about having to do the **run report.**

The documentation you provide is a direct extension of the care you perform. When you perform excellent, patient-centered prehospital care, your patient will be grateful and you will feel proud of the care you gave. Poor documentation performed after this great care will tarnish the record of what you have done by anyone reviewing the documentation later.

The reporting done in EMS can take on many names, depending on your region or service. Some call the reports simply run reports, others **PCRs—prehospital care reports** or patient care reports (Figures 16-1A and B on pages 402–403). Some reports are now done totally on computers (Figure 16-2 on page 404). Regardless of how the reports are completed, there are many reasons for accurate and complete documentation. These include:

* **Continuity of care**—Your report may be referenced at any time during the hospital care of the patient. After you leave the hospital, the report may be referenced for the vital signs you obtained early in the call, medications or treatments you administered, or your observations at the scene.

* **Education**—Your written report may be used as an example for others of proper documentation. If you responded to an unusual or challenging call, it may be used as a basis for training other providers who may encounter similar patients or situations.

* **Administrative**—The report will be used for the documentation of billing information and can be used to do statistical analysis on issues that affect your agency, such as response times and staffing.

* **Quality**—Reports created by you and others in your agency will be reviewed as part of a Continuous Quality Improvement (CQI) or Total Quality Management (TQM) process.

* **Research**—Reports are often used to research important clinical issues in EMS, such as specific treatments for patients with airway problems or shock.

* **Legally**—The report you created is a legal document. It may be called into court for a number of reasons:
    * As evidence in a legal action where your patient is suing someone who caused the injuries
    * As evidence in a criminal action where your patient was the victim of a crime
    * As documentation when you or another member of the team that treated the patient is accused of improper medical care or treatment of the patient

When your report is called to attention in a legal matter, you may be required to go to court to testify. You may be asked to testify about your observations on the call, what others may have said, the care you provided, that you created the report, and that it accurately depicts the events of the call.

Documentation plays a large role in minimizing the exposure to liability for you and your agency. The old saying "If you didn't document it, you didn't do it" is true when it comes to liability. For example, someone may look at your written report and observe that you didn't give oxygen to a patient with chest pain. You, of course, recognize that it is a vitally important part of the care for chest pain and are sure you did. However, if it wasn't documented, the only conclusion a person reading your report could reach is that it wasn't done.

* **run report**
    written documentation of the call and patient encounter. Also called a prehospital care report.

* **prehospital care report (PCR)**
    written documentation of the call and patient encounter. Also called a patient care report or a run report.

3-8.5 Describe the legal implications associated with the written report.

MAINE **✻EMS**   **PRESS DOWN, YOU ARE MAKING THREE COPIES.**

RUN REPORT #	Mo.	Day	Year	M T W Th	F S Sun	SERVICE NAME		SERVICE NO.	VEHICLE NO.	ALS ☐ Performed ☐ Back-up called	SERVICE RUN NO.
746118											

NAME	BILLING INFORMATION

STREET OR R.F.D.

CITY/TOWN	STATE	ZIP

AGE/DATE OF BIRTH	☐ Male ☐ Female	PHONE

INCIDENT LOCATION:	ADDRESS	CITY/TOWN

TRANSPORTED TO:	TREATING/FAMILY PHYSICIAN	CREW LICENSE NUMBERS

TRANSPORTATION/COMMUNICATIONS PROBLEMS

☐ Medical
  ☐ Cardiac
  ☐ Poisoning/OD
    ☐ Respiratory
  ☐ Behavioral
    ☐ Diabetic
  ☐ Seizure
    ☐ CVA
  ☐ OB/Gyn
    ☐ Other _____

☐ Trauma
  ☐ Multi-Systems Trauma
  ☐ Head
    ☐ Spinal
  ☐ Burn
    ☐ Soft Tissue Injury
  ☐ Fractures
    ☐ Other _____

☐ Code 99

☐ MEDICATIONS   ☐ ALLERGIES

CHIEF COMPLAINT:

R	L	LUNG SOUNDS
☐	☐	CLEAR
☐	☐	ABSENT
☐	☐	DECREASED
☐	☐	RALES
☐	☐	WHEEZE
☐	☐	STRIDOR

TYPE OF RUN
☐ Emergency Transport
☐ Routine Transfer
☐ Emergency Transfer
☐ No Transport
☐ Refused Transport

TIME	CODE	ODOMETER	
			Call Received
			Enroute
			At Scene
			From Scene
			At Destination
			In Service

TIME	PULSE	RESP	BP	PUPILLARY RESPONSE	SKIN	VERBAL RESPONSE	MOTOR RESPONSE	EYE-OPENING RESPONSE	CAPILLARY REFILL
						5 4 3 2 1	6 5 4 3 2 1	4 3 2 1	☐ Normal ☐ None ☐ Delayed
						5 4 3 2 1	6 5 4 3 2 1	4 3 2 1	☐ Normal ☐ None ☐ Delayed
						5 4 3 2 1	6 5 4 3 2 1	4 3 2 1	☐ Normal ☐ None ☐ Delayed

☐ MVA   ☐ Concern AOB/ETOH   SEAT BELTS: ☐ Used   ☐ Not Used   ☐ N/A   ☐ Helmet Used

MUTUAL AID: Assisted/Assisted by Service # _____   Time Called: _____

PATIENT'S SUSPECTED PROBLEM:	**746118**	

☐ Medication Administered   ☐ Defib Lic.# _____

☐ Monitor   ☐ Chest Decomp

☐ Pacing   ☐ Caricothyrotomy

MEDICAL CONTROL	☐ Written Order/Protocol ☐ Verbal Order/Protocol

IV ☐ SUC LIC.# _____   Total Attempts
    ☐ UNSUC LIC.# _____

Cleared Airway	Extrication			
Artificial Respiration/BVM	Cervical Immobilization			
Oropharyngeal Airway	KED/Short Board			
Nasopharyngeal Airway	Long Board			
CPR–Time:	Restraints			
Bystander CPR	Traction Splinting			
AED	General Splinting			
Suction	Cold Application			
Oxygen–LPMin ___ ☐ Nasal ☐ Mask	MAST Inflated			
Pulse Oximetry				
Autovent				

EOA ☐ SUC LIC.# _____ Total Attempts
     ☐ UNSUC LIC.# _____

ET ☐ SUC LIC.# _____ Total Attempts
    ☐ UNSUC LIC.# _____

LIC #	EKG RHYTHM	TIME	MEDS/DEFIB/C-VERT	DOSE W/S	ROUTE

NAME OF E.D. TREATING PHYSICIAN	SIGNATURE OF CREW MEMBER IN CHARGE	COPY 1 HOSPITAL

FIGURE 16-1A   A prehospital care report.

TRIP #			
MEDIC #			
BEGIN MILES			
END MILES			
CODE___/___	PAGE___/___		
UNITS ON SCENE			

Rural/Metro
Ambulance
50 Years of Serving Others

EMERGENCY TRIP SHEET – CONDITION CODES 1 THROUGH 71

BILLING USE ONLY			
DAY			
DATE			
RECEIVED			
DISPATCHED			
EN-ROUTE			
ON SCENE			
TO HOSPITAL			
AT HOSPITAL			
IN-SERVICE			

NAME	SEX M F DOB ___/___/___
ADDRESS	RACE
CITY STATE ZIP	
PHONE ( ) - PCP DR.	
RESPONDED FROM CITY	
TAKEN FROM ZIP	
DESTINATION REASON	
SSN - - MEDICARE # MEDICAID #	
INSURANCE CO INSURANCE # GROUP #	
RESPONSIBLE PARTY ADDRESS	
CITY STATE ZIP PHONE ( ) -	
EMPLOYER	

CREW	CERT	STATE #

TIME	ON SCENE (1)	ON SCENE (2)	ON SCENE (3)	EN-ROUTE (1)	EN-ROUTE (2)	AT DESTINATION
BP						
PULSE						
RESP						
EKG						

IV THERAPY
SUCCESSFUL Y N # OF ATTEMPTS _____
ANGIO SIZE _____ ga.
SITE _____
TOTAL FLUID INFUSED _____ cc
BLOOD DRAW Y N INITIALS _____

INTUBATION INFORMATION
SUCCESSFUL Y N # OF ATTEMPTS _____
TUBE SIZE _____ mm
TIME _____ INITIALS _____

MEDICAL HISTORY	CONDITION CODES				
	TREATMENTS				

MEDICATIONS	TIME	TREATMENT	DOSE	ROUTE	INIT
ALLERGIES					
C/C					
EVENTS LEADING TO C/C					
PERTINENT FINDINGS					
ASSESSMENT					

TREATMENT	GCS E___V___M___TOTAL =
	GCS E___V___M___TOTAL =
	HOSPITAL CONTACTED
	CPR BEGUN BY B P TIME BEGUN
EMS SIGNATURE	AED USED Y N BY:
LIFETIME SIGNATURE AUTHORIZATION	RESUSCITATION TERMINATED - TIME

I request that payment of authorized Medicare benefits be made on my behalf to Rural/Metro Ambulance for any ambulance service or supplies provided to me by Rural/Metro Ambulance. I authorize any holder of medical information or documentation about me to release to the Health Care Financing Administration and its agents and carriers, as well as to Rural/Metro Ambulance any information or documentation needed to determine these benefits payable for related services or any services provided to me by Rural/Metro Ambulance now or in the future.

Signature _____ Date _____ ( ) OSHA REGULATIONS FOLLOWED

FIGURE 16-1B A prehospital care report. (Rural/Metro Ambulance Service, Youngstown, Ohio.)

FIGURE 16-2 A computerized form for run documentation. (Westech, Inc.)

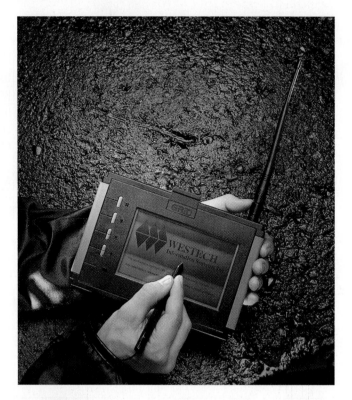

Perspective

Joe Devlin—The EMT

"Oh man, that couldn't have gone worse. I mean, I'm a good EMT. I really am, and I know for a fact that I just wouldn't have taken a critical patient to a particular hospital if one was closer. Maybe Midway diverted us . . . or the patient requested Riverside. I don't know. But now I look like the bad guy just because I don't remember and my PCR was a piece of junk."

Good documentation alone won't protect you from liability. One of the most significant ways we can minimize liability is to treat people compassionately and provide quality care. Documenting shoddy, incomplete, or inaccurate care of people you haven't treated well will not help prevent lawsuits at all.

Clinical Clues: COMPASSIONATE CARE

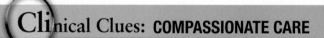

High quality, compassionate care supported by good documentation can greatly minimize your exposure to liability.

COMPONENTS OF THE PREHOSPITAL CARE REPORT

There are two ways prehospital care reports can be completed: on paper and via computer. Computer-based reports are becoming increasingly common in EMS. Regardless of how the reports are completed, the data that goes into each is the same.

Each report has several sections. Each of the sections provides specific, important information. These sections include:

Run Data—This section includes information about the call itself, such as the unit and crew members responding, the date and time of the call, the name of the ambulance service, and certification levels of those providing care. Times recorded must be accurate and synchronous (by clocks or watches that show the same time). Be sure to use the time given to you by the dispatcher when noting times on your report, and then make sure the time your watch shows does not differ from the dispatch center's official time. This time synchronization is important, especially in determining how long a patient has been in cardiac arrest, documenting trends in the patient's condition, and measurement of system efficiency such as response times.

Patient Data—This section includes all the information about the patient such as:

* name, address, date of birth, sex
* nature of the call
* insurance information
* detailed information on the patient's complaint
* mechanism of injury, assessment
* care administered before (by bystanders) and after the arrival of the EMT
* vital signs
* SAMPLE history
* changes in condition throughout the call

The information in each of the sections of the report can be entered in various ways (review Figure 16-1). These include:

* **Fill-in**—You would write the patient's name, address, date of birth, insurance information, and vital signs in spaces labeled for this use.
* **Check boxes**—Some care reports have boxes that can be checked for information such as patient history, nature of illness, and care provided.
* **Narrative**—Space is provided for you to write narrative information—your objective "story" documenting the patient's history, assessment, or care information that does not otherwise fit in check boxes or that requires expansion on the details.

Narrative portions of the prehospital care report are usually the most challenging to write. When writing the narrative, do not use radio codes or slang. Abbreviations are acceptable if they are standard and understood by hospital and other EMS personnel. Be sure to use proper spelling in your report, even if you must use a medical dictionary. Knowledge of medical terminology and proper spelling of terms will make your reports clearer and more accurate.

The information you write in the narrative should be **objective** rather than **subjective**. Objective information is that which you have personally observed and can attest to. Subjective information is that which is not first hand or is subject to interpretation. The statement "The patient has a one-inch laceration on his forehead" is objective. Statements that begin or could begin with "I think . . ." or "It seems . . ." usually contain subjective information. Examples of subjective statements include "I don't believe this patient is telling the truth" or "His car was

3-8.1 Explain the components of the written report and list the information that should be included in the written report.

3-8.2 Identify the various sections of the written report.

3-8.3 Describe what information is required in each section of the prehospital care report and how it should be entered.

* **run data**

  information about the call itself, such as the unit and crew members responding, the date and time of the call, and the name of the ambulance service

* **patient data**

  all the information about the patient (name, address, date of birth), insurance information, and detailed information on the patient's complaint, assessment, care, and vital signs.

* **objective**

  information that you have personally observed, can measure, or can attest to.

* **subjective**

  information that is not first hand or that is subject to interpretation.

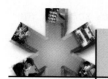

Perspective

Thomas Powell, Esq.—The Plaintiff's Attorney

"As soon as I saw that PCR I knew that we had a slam dunk! Come on . . . it's been a year since the tragic loss of Mr. O'Neil and that narrative gave no reason whatsoever for the extended transport. In fact . . . it even named the wrong hospital. This EMT may be good at his job, but I knew that he wasn't going to remember anything about this call . . . and his documentation 'skills' made my job that much easier!"

probably going 90 miles an hour when it hit the tree." In short, avoid writing conclusions that are not fact based.

One way to put pertinent items into your report that you may not have witnessed yourself is to put the words of the patient or family member/bystander between quotation marks. For example: "Patient states that he took '40 or 50 sleeping pills.'" You weren't there when he allegedly took the pills. The information comes from what the patient said, and your report reflects this. Another example might be information from a bystander. You could report: "An associate of the patient stated that the patient had '10 or 12 beers' before he fell."

Your narrative should also include observations of the scene, such as mechanism of injury, suicide notes, approximate blood loss observed at the scene, living conditions, and care given by bystanders.

NARRATIVE DOCUMENTATION

There are several ways to document information in the narrative section of your report. The most important consideration is that the narrative section is legible, accurate, and contains appropriate information. Some agencies and regions have preferred methods of narrative documentation.

* **timeline or sequential**
  method of narration that tells the story of the call as it happened in a step by step, chronological narrative.

* **SOAP**
  acronym for Subjective, Objective, Assessment, and Plan. A method of documentation in which each letter stands for a specific portion of the narrative.

Timeline or Sequential—This method of narration tells the story of the call as it happened in a step-by-step, chronological narrative.

SOAP—An acronym for Subjective, Objective, Assessment, and Plan, each letter stands for a specific portion of the narrative:

* Subjective—This includes what the patient says in response to your questions, such as the history of the present illness (including OPQRST). It also includes the patient's medical history as well as information from family and bystanders.

* Objective—This is the information you obtain from the physical examination. You may observe a wound or observe the patient in a posture indicating pain or distress. Vital signs and other physical assessments (e.g., lung sounds, palpation) are also included here.

* Assessment—The assessment section is where you consider the subjective and objective information and make an assessment of the patient's overall

condition. Examples might be that a patient who developed substernal chest discomfort with nausea and diaphoresis after exertion may have cardiac-related chest pain or that a patient who fell and has pain and deformity in the lower leg has a suspected fracture.

* Plan—This is the plan you create for the care of the patient. In the case of the patient with chest discomfort, you will administer oxygen, prevent exertion, and assist him with prescribed nitroglycerin if he has it. In the event of the suspected leg fracture, you would plan on immobilizing the leg, applying ice for pain, and so on.

CHART—This is another helpful acronym and stands for Chief complaint, History, Assessment, Rx (or treatment), and Transport.

Examples of narratives written in the SOAP and CHART formats are shown in Figure 16-3 and Figure 16-4 on page 408.

* **CHART**
acronym for Chief complaint, History, Assessment, Rx (or treatment), and Transport. A method of documentation in which each letter stands for a specific portion of the narrative.

S: Patient complains of difficulty breathing. She reports that it came on while jogging and was accompanied by a "tightness like I can't breathe." She reports a history of asthma for which she takes an albuterol inhaler. This episode seems to the patient to be exactly like asthma attacks she has had in the past. She reports that she is usually able to breathe easier with an inhaler. She states that she took two puffs from her inhaler without significant relief.

O: Patient appears obviously short of breath and is using accessory muscles to breathe. She is in the tripod position. Wheezes are audible without a stethoscope. Lung sounds and wheezing are present in all fields of the chest by auscultation. Vital signs P: 102 strong and regular, R: 28 and adequate, BP 118/84, skin pink, warm and moist. Pupils equal/react. SaO2 93% before oxygen.

A: Patient has signs and symptoms which are identical to asthma attacks she has had in the past. They also match a clinical picture of asthma.

P: Oxygen administration was begun immediately and medical control was contacted to assist the patient with additional doses of her albuterol inhaler. Dr. Cook from County General approved two puffs, reevaluation and two more puffs. The patient experienced some relief from our first two. After reassessment and stable vital signs (noted above) a second set of puffs was administered with greater relief. SaO2 increased to 98% and the patient was no longer using accessory muscles.

FIGURE 16-3 The SOAP format.

C: "I'm having an asthma attack."

H: Patient reports difficulty breathing which developed while jogging about 10 minutes ago. It is accompanied by a tightness in her chest when she tried to breathe. Patient has a history of asthma for which she takes an albuterol inhaler. She has taken two puffs with minimal relief. She denies allergies, other medications or additional medical history. She had a light breakfast this AM.

A: Patient exam reveals patient seated on a bench in tripod position using accessory muscles to breathe. Patient is breathing with an adequate tidal volume. She is able to speak 4–5 word sentences. Wheezes are audible without a stethoscope. Lung sounds are equal bilaterally with wheezes in all lobes of the lungs. Initial vital signs P: 102 strong/regular, R: 28 shallow and slightly labored, but adequate, BP 118/84, skin warm and moist. Pupils equal and react. SaO2 93%
R: Oxygen provided via NRB mask at 15 lpm. Dr. Cook at County General contacted via radio who approved 2 puffs of her albuterol inhaler spaced 5 mins apart with reevaluation. The first two puffs were administered with some relief. Vitals stable (noted above) so two additional puffs gave more relief. Patient no longer used accessory muscles, could speak full sentences and SaO2 increased to 98%.

T: Patient transported to County General code 1 with the patient's difficulty breathing improved. Report given to RN in room 4—rails up.

FIGURE 16-4   The CHART format.

Stop, Review, Remember!

Multiple Choice

Place a check next to the correct answer.

1. Prehospital care reports may be used for all of the following EXCEPT:

   _____   a. part of the Quality Improvement process.

   _____   b. research.

   _____   c. as evidence in court.

   _____   d. for dissemination to the media.

2. You cannot be sued if you have documented your call properly and accurately.

   _____ a. true

   _____ b. false

3. Insurance information would be included in which section of the prehospital care report?

   _____ a. run data

   _____ b. patient data

   _____ c. check boxes

   _____ d. assessment data

4. Which of the following is considered part of the run data?

   _____ a. patient's name

   _____ b. date and time of the call

   _____ c. vital signs

   _____ d. the name of the medical control physician

5. The patient's blood pressure would be recorded in which type of space on the report?

   _____ a. fill-in   _____ c. narrative

   _____ b. check boxes _____ d. subjective

6. Which of the following statements correctly describes subjective and objective information?

   _____ a. Objective information is what you hear from others; subjective information is what you see.

   _____ b. Objective information is what you see; subjective information is information that can be definitively proved by other sources.

   _____ c. Objective information is what you reasonably believe to be true; subjective information is false.

   _____ d. Objective information is something you observe; subjective information is that which is not first hand or that requires interpretation.

Labeling

Label each of the following statements as either objective (O) or subjective (S).

1. _____ Based on his injuries, the patient must have jumped from the upper floors.

2. _____ The patient has a bone protruding from his mid-shaft lower leg.

3. _____ The patient has wheezes audible without a stethoscope.

4. _____ Due to his high level of intoxication, he obviously had a lot to drink.

5. _____ The patient states she has chest discomfort that radiates to her neck and jaw.

6. _____ The patient has an area of bruising over the fifth to ninth ribs on the left side.

Fill in the Blank

Fill the following vital signs into the report in the appropriate spaces:

	TIME	RESP	PULSE	B.P.	LEVEL OF CONSCIOUSNESS	R PUPILS L	SKIN
V I T A L S I G N S		Rate: ☐ Regular ☐ Shallow ☐ Labored	Rate: ☐ Regular ☐ Irregular		☐ Alert ☐ Voice ☐ Pain ☐ Unresp.	☐ Normal ☐ ☐ Dilated ☐ ☐ Constricted ☐ ☐ Sluggish ☐ ☐ No-Reaction ☐	☐ Unremarkable ☐ Cool ☐ Pale ☐ Warm ☐ Cyanotic ☐ Moist ☐ Flushed ☐ Dry ☐ Jaundiced
		Rate: ☐ Regular ☐ Shallow ☐ Labored	Rate: ☐ Regular ☐ Irregular		☐ Alert ☐ Voice ☐ Pain ☐ Unresp.	☐ Normal ☐ ☐ Dilated ☐ ☐ Constricted ☐ ☐ Sluggish ☐ ☐ No-Reaction ☐	☐ Unremarkable ☐ Cool ☐ Pale ☐ Warm ☐ Cyanotic ☐ Moist ☐ Flushed ☐ Dry ☐ Jaundiced
		Rate: ☐ Regular ☐ Shallow ☐ Labored	Rate: ☐ Regular ☐ Irregular		☐ Alert ☐ Voice ☐ Pain ☐ Unresp.	☐ Normal ☐ ☐ Dilated ☐ ☐ Constricted ☐ ☐ Sluggish ☐ ☐ No-Reaction ☐	☐ Unremarkable ☐ Cool ☐ Pale ☐ Warm ☐ Cyanotic ☐ Moist ☐ Flushed ☐ Dry ☐ Jaundiced

11:17 hours Pulse 94 strong and regular, respirations 22 and labored, BP 112/74 Pupils equal and react to light. Skin cool and moist.

11:22 hours Pulse 88 strong and regular, respirations 20 and labored, BP 108/70 Pupils equal and react to light. Skin cool and dry.

Critical Thinking

1. Some say "Documentation is the best way to minimize liability." Defend or disagree with that statement and give your reasons.

_____

_____

_____

_____

CONFIDENTIALITY

Your prehospital care reports contain confidential information. This confidentiality is governed by many laws, including the Health Insurance Portability and Accountability Act (HIPAA) that was discussed in chapter 3.

The information in your report can only be distributed to those individuals allowed by law to see the report or whom the patient has given written authorization to see the report. Generally the hospital will receive a copy of the report, the EMS agency will keep a copy of the report, and often an additional copy goes to a regional or state EMS agency for data collection and research.

EMS reports may be used within an agency or region for Quality Improvement review. Patients are often asked to sign a form that allows your agency to share information with insurance companies and billing agencies.

CORRECTIONS AND FALSIFICATION

When you are writing a report, there will be times when you write something inadvertently or incorrectly. An example might be writing that the pulse was 87 instead of 78. In this case you would cross out the incorrect item with a single line, initial it, and write the correct number beside or above it (Figure 16-5).

This would also work in the narrative where you wrote, "The patient has no medical history," and then you realize that she did take a medicine for diabetes. This could be corrected by crossing out the entire sentence or just the "no medical history" portion and writing the correct information beside or above it.

You use a single line instead of completely covering the wrong information, because making the entry completely unreadable would look like an attempt to hide something.

If an error is discovered after a report has been submitted, make the correction just described, but note the time and date the correction was made. If the change has significance to patient care, billing, or research, amended copies should be sent to those affected.

Falsification of a report is very serious. Honesty and integrity are essential traits of an EMT. Never write false information in a prehospital care report. Likewise, never leave out any information from a report—even about something that was done in error.

There are two types of errors—**omission** and **commission**. Errors of omission are those where something wasn't done that should have been. Examples include not giving oxygen when you should have or not asking a patient if he had allergies before giving a medication.

Errors of commission are actions done that shouldn't have been done, especially actions that cause harm to a patient. Assisting a patient with a medication that wasn't his own or using a stretcher in a manner that caused injury to a patient are examples of errors of commission.

* **falsification**

   documentation of false information in a prehospital care report.

* **omission**

   errors of omission are those where something wasn't done that should have been.

* **commission**

   errors of commission are actions done that shouldn't have been done, especially actions that cause harm to a patient.

COMMENTS   PATIENT COMPLAINS OF PAIN IN HIS ~~RIGHT~~ ^{DL} LEFT SHOULDER THAT RADIATES TO THE LEFT ARM.

FIGURE 16-5   The proper way to make a correction.

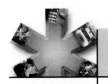

Perspective

Joe—The EMT

"I've been trying to figure out why I wrote the wrong hospital on that PCR—I never do that. The only thing I can think is . . . we must have gotten diverted en route . . . and I hate the paperwork so much that I always zip through it as soon as I can. I bet I had that sorry excuse for a PCR done before we ever got diverted."

Other times you may find yourself tempted to document things that didn't happen but would make you and your report look better—in other words, as noted earlier, falsification. One example is vital signs. It is always recommended that you take two or more sets of vital signs, even on short transports. Remember that a change in vital signs over time provides the most significant clinical information.

But what if you only did one set of vitals and your squad required that you obtain a minimum of two sets on every patient? Maybe you were checking splints and oxygen or even comforting the patient and lost track of time. Never write down a set of vitals you did not take. If you were busy performing other important patient care tasks, document this information in the narrative.

There are other times you may have forgotten to give oxygen to the patient, or perhaps he was so anxious he wouldn't tolerate the mask or cannula on his face. Never write down that you gave a medication or treatment that wasn't actually given. This could negatively affect patient care decisions later at the hospital.

The run report should not cover up any of these types of errors. If an error happens, it should be documented along with when you identified the error and what was done to correct the situation. The hospital and your supervisor should also be notified of the error.

As said earlier, it is important to give clinically competent, people-oriented care at all times. As a human being there is always a possibility that you will make an error. Work diligently to prevent errors and document them honestly if they do occur.

Special Issues in Documentation

There are times, such as patient refusal of care, that documentation has special importance. There are also times when the documentation procedures and requirements may change or are different than usual. An example of this is a call where there are multiple patients (also known as a multiple casualty incident or MCI—see chapters 40 and 41) and there isn't time to document each patient in detail at the scene. The following sections will discuss some of these special issues.

3-8.4 Define the special considerations concerning patient refusal.

PATIENT REFUSAL

In most instances, patients who call for help need to go to the hospital. Occasionally you will find patients who do not want to accept your care and/or transportation. Chapter 3 discussed methods to convince the patient to go to the hospital. It also stated that documentation of your attempts at convincing the patient were very important, since refusal situations are a significant source of risk and liability for EMTs.

You should take your time when trying to talk your patient into accepting your care and transportation. You may be able to break down barriers or the patient's fears and change his mind. Be prepared to take the time necessary with each patient. Even if your documentation of the patient refusal is meticulous, if the times recorded by the dispatcher show you were only on scene for 5 minutes your efforts will appear minimal, regardless of what you document.

In a patient refusal situation, you should document the following information:

✳ Any assessment and care you performed for the patient

✳ That the patient is competent and is of legal age to refuse and has the ability to make an informed decision (not intoxicated or otherwise incompetent)

✳ That the patient was told the risks of refusing care; this includes worsening of the current problem up to and including death

✳ That efforts were made to convince the patient to accept care; document these efforts that may include (but not be limited to) reassurance, involving family members or friends, offering to call a relative or personal physician, helping arrange care for a pet.

✳ Any efforts made to protect the patient if he does refuse, including contacting a family member or friend to stay with him, scheduling a visit that day with a personal physician, or providing phone stickers with EMS access numbers and advising the patient that he can call back at any time

Some systems recommend or require that you contact medical direction in refusal situations. The physician may offer suggestions, offer to talk to the patient, or in some cases agree with the refusal if follow-up care is arranged through a personal physician. Document this conversation in your prehospital care report.

In most areas or systems, you will ask your patient to sign a "refusal form." This form asks the patient to acknowledge that care and transportation were offered by EMS and refused by the patient. It may indicate some of the items above, including the fact that harm may come to the patient. It is sometimes called a "waiver" or "release," because it may have legal language releasing the crew and agency from liability if harm comes to the patient.

This will not prevent a lawsuit, but it may help to show that the patient was aware of the risks and that you acted appropriately.

Some EMS systems have refusal checklists (Figure 16-6 on page 414) that help EMTs remember and perform all of the necessary steps both to properly care for the patient and to reduce the potential for liability.

MULTIPLE CASUALTY INCIDENTS

Patients should always receive the best possible care followed by thorough documentation of the care provided. In the case of multiple casualty incidents (MCIs), this documentation may have to be done later because patient care is a priority.

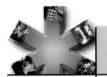

Perspective

Mrs. O'Neil—The Wife

"I actually felt kind of bad for that EMT. I know that there are things about Artie's death that even I don't remember now. It seemed that my whole case ended up turning on that hospital issue though, you know? But that could've been Artie's fault. He swore to me that he'd never go to Midway again after the problem with his colonoscopy results there . . . and I'm the one who told them to take him there. For all I know he asked to go to Riverside once they were driving. Well, I guess the point is, my husband of 35 years died and now my life is a wreck. After my attorney said that it may have been the ambulance's fault, I had no choice but to sue. Right?"

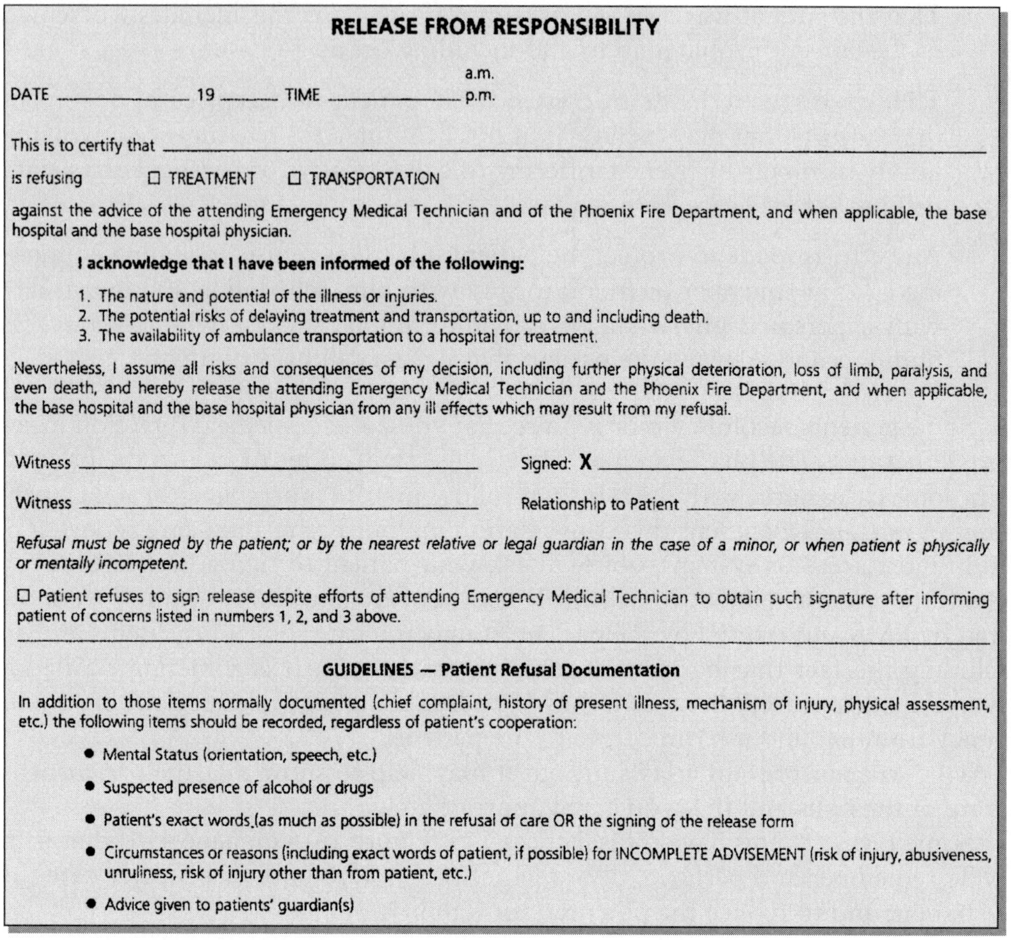

RELEASE FROM RESPONSIBILITY

DATE _____ 19 ____ TIME _____ a.m. / p.m.

This is to certify that _____

is refusing ☐ TREATMENT ☐ TRANSPORTATION

against the advice of the attending Emergency Medical Technician and of the Phoenix Fire Department, and when applicable, the base hospital and the base hospital physician.

I acknowledge that I have been informed of the following:

1. The nature and potential of the illness or injuries.
2. The potential risks of delaying treatment and transportation, up to and including death.
3. The availability of ambulance transportation to a hospital for treatment.

Nevertheless, I assume all risks and consequences of my decision, including further physical deterioration, loss of limb, paralysis, and even death, and hereby release the attending Emergency Medical Technician and the Phoenix Fire Department, and when applicable, the base hospital and the base hospital physician from any ill effects which may result from my refusal.

Witness _____   Signed: **X** _____

Witness _____   Relationship to Patient _____

Refusal must be signed by the patient; or by the nearest relative or legal guardian in the case of a minor, or when patient is physically or mentally incompetent.

☐ Patient refuses to sign release despite efforts of attending Emergency Medical Technician to obtain such signature after informing patient of concerns listed in numbers 1, 2, and 3 above.

GUIDELINES — Patient Refusal Documentation

In addition to those items normally documented (chief complaint, history of present illness, mechanism of injury, physical assessment, etc.) the following items should be recorded, regardless of patient's cooperation:

● Mental Status (orientation, speech, etc.)

● Suspected presence of alcohol or drugs

● Patient's exact words (as much as possible) in the refusal of care OR the signing of the release form

● Circumstances or reasons (including exact words of patient, if possible) for INCOMPLETE ADVISEMENT (risk of injury, abusiveness, unruliness, risk of injury other than from patient, etc.)

● Advice given to patients' guardian(s)

FIGURE 16-6 A refusal checklist. (Phoenix Fire Department Emergency Medical Services, City of Phoenix, Arizona.)

The proper transfer of information from the field to the hospital is still important. Hospital staff would still like to know what the patient's complaint and condition was in the field and to determine if there have been any changes during transport.

The need for concise but accurate information at MCIs is met by specialized forms such as the triage tag (Figure 16-7). This allows notation of injuries, care, and vital signs on a compact form that stays with the patient. Multiple copies allow one copy to remain at the scene and another to accompany the patient to the hospital.

3-8.6 Discuss all state and/or local record and reporting requirements.

SPECIALIZED REPORTS

Most calls you go on will require some form of a prehospital care report. There are special situations where you will be required to document specific information on your report or complete a second report with this information.

Mandated reporting of certain crimes is an example of where additional report forms may be needed. When reporting child or elder abuse, your local social service agencies may have a special form to use. These forms will have questions specific to the needs of their agency and investigation of the matter.

Supplemental reports may be used for calls that were of a very long duration or where there was a significant use of resources. Documentation of these events will be too long to fit in a standard prehospital care report.

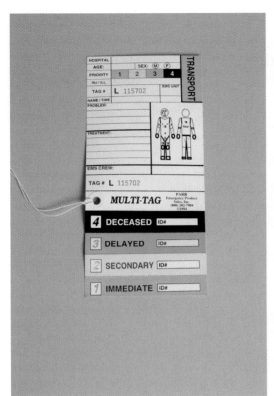

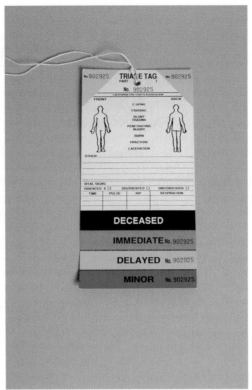

FIGURE 16-7 Examples of triage tags.

Other times, special documentation is needed because of a motor vehicle collision involving an EMS vehicle or when there is a conflict between emergency personnel at a scene.

✳ Stop, Review, Remember!

Multiple Choice

Place a check next to the correct answer.

1. HIPAA stands for the:

   _____ a. Health Insurance Privacy Amendment Act.

   _____ b. Health Information Purpose and Accountability.

   _____ c. Health Insurance Portability and Accountability Act.

   _____ d. Health Industry Perspective and Accountability Access.

2. EMS reports can be used for all of the following EXCEPT:

   _____ a. sharing information on patients with dangerous, communicable diseases.

   _____ b. billing purposes.

   _____ c. Quality Improvement.

   _____ d. research.

3. An error in a run report should be corrected by:

   _____ a. crossing out all indications of the error.

   _____ b. leaving the error as is and noting it at the end of the report.

   _____ c. crossing the error out with a single line and writing the correct information in.

   _____ d. covering the error with a thick black marker on all copies and writing the corrected information in at the end of the report.

4. Which of the following statements regarding documentation of patient refusal is NOT correct?

   _____ a. The patient's age and mental state should be documented.

   _____ b. A patient's prior knowledge of the risks of refusing treatment releases an EMT from explaining and documenting them again.

   _____ c. For some conditions it is appropriate to tell the patient that serious harm or even death could come from refusing care.

   _____ d. You should document any care you did give the patient before he refused transportation.

5. Giving a patient a medication to which he is allergic is an example of an error of omission.

   _____ a. true

   _____ b. false

6. If you do not have the time to do a second set of vital signs, it is acceptable to duplicate the earlier vital signs if the patient's condition is unchanged.

   _____ a. true

   _____ b. false

7. When documenting a patient refusal, you should document all attempts you made to convince your patient to go to the hospital.

   _____ a. true

   _____ b. false

8. Patients are required to sign a waiver or "refusal form" if they do not wish to accept your care or transportation.

   _____ a. true

   _____ b. false

9. If you document accurately, you will not get sued.

   _____ a. true

   _____ b. false

10. It is acceptable to document in less detail when treating patients at a multiple casualty incident.

    _____ a. true

    _____ b. false

Critical Thinking

1. Your EMS Chief read a report you wrote two days ago and in it found the following statement: "The patient was unconscious and oriented × 3." She was sure you meant "conscious" and brought it to your attention. How should this report be amended 2 days after it was written?

   _____

   _____

2. **Make It Right.**   Correct the error in each statement using proper documentation procedure.

   a. The patient weighs approximately 190 kg. (You meant to write 90 kg.)

   _____

   b. The patient has no allergies to medications. (Actually, the patient is allergic to penicillin.)

   _____

   c. The blood pressure increased when the patient stood up. (It really decreased.)

   _____

   d. Pulse 88 strong and regular, respirations 18, blood pressure 88/126, pupils equal and react to light. (Blood pressure is really 126/88.)

   _____

   e. The respirations are 16 and deep, there are equal sounds bilaterally. (You meant to say that there were equal _breath_ sounds bilaterally.)

   _____

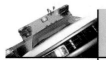

Dispatch Summary

Mrs. Arthur O'Neil won a settlement against the North County Ambulance Service for $1.3 million. The case is on appeal.

Joe Devlin has since become a paramedic for North County and is now well known for his clear, concise, and accurate PCRs.

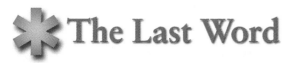

The Last Word

Documentation is a critical skill. It is the only record of the care you provide long after you have dropped the patient off at the hospital. This report, when accurate and complete, will provide a lasting record of quality care. When shoddy, incomplete, or inaccurate, the record kept by your report is not one you would be proud of.

Your documentation is used in court in many different situations. The trial may be one in which you and your report are a witness—or a defendant. Accurate and thorough documentation will help you in both situations. The other practice that is vital to your work as an EMT and one that will help in liability prevention is treating each patient carefully and compassionately.

Your documentation will also be important in specific situations like patient refusals, one of the leading causes of lawsuits against EMS. Your documentation of the time and effort you spend with your patients who refuse care will be of great value.

Although not the glamorous part of EMS you see on television and in the newspapers, documentation is clearly an extremely important part of what you do as an EMT.

✳ Chapter Review

MULTIPLE CHOICE

Place a check next to the correct answer.

1. Which of the following would NOT be legally able to receive a copy of your patient care report?

_____ a. the patient's clergy

_____ b. the state EMS agency

_____ c. the Quality Improvement committee

_____ d. the ambulance service headquarters

2. Signing a refusal-of-care or transportation form prevents the patient from suing you or your EMS agency in the future.

_____ a. true

_____ b. false

3. You are writing your patient's history on your pre-hospital care report at the hospital and inadvertently write down a medication not taken by the patient. You should:

_____ a. leave it as is since you did not give the medication.

_____ b. cross out the wrong information with a single line.

_____ c. totally cross out the area where the medication was listed so no one could ever see it.

_____ d. shred the report you are writing, due to confidentiality issues, and begin again.

4. "The patient states he was going 75 miles per hour when he hit the tree" is a/an _____ statement.

_____ a. sworn

_____ b. attestable

_____ c. objective

_____ d. subjective

5. Giving aspirin to a patient who is allergic to aspirin is an error of _____.

_____ a. omission.

_____ b. operation.

_____ c. commission.

_____ d. neglect.

CRITICAL THINKING

1. List three ways you can envision your prehospital care report being used after you complete it.

_____

_____

_____

2. You are completing your report at the hospital and realize that you only took one set of vital signs on your patient. He had vomited during the short trip to the hospital and you just didn't have time. Your partner says, "Just write down a set that is close to the first. It'll keep the boss off our backs. You know he was stable, and they didn't change anyway." What should you do?

_____

_____

_____

3. How is documentation at a multiple casualty incident (MCI) different than on a call with a single patient?

_____

_____

_____

_____

4. **Name That Error.** While we always try to prevent errors—determine if the errors below are errors of omission (O) or commission (C).

a. _____ You don't administer oxygen to a patient with chest pain.

b. _____ You fail to identify inadequate breathing in an unresponsive patient.

c. _____ You assist a patient with his prescribed nitroglycerin even though he took Viagra yesterday (a contraindication).

d. _____ You don't immobilize the spine of a person involved in a motor vehicle collision even though he complains of neck pain.

e. _____ You hit the release mechanism on the stretcher prematurely. The stretcher drops from the elevated position to the lowered position in a freefall and injures the patient.

CASE STUDY

Imagine you are a patient who was transported in an ambulance. You are in a coffee shop 3 days later and hear two EMTs talking about your care. Others in the coffee shop can also hear what is going on.

1. How would you feel about this? What would you do?

_____

_____

_____

_____

2. If you complained about this to the supervisor of the EMTs or a local official, what would happen to the EMTs?

_____

_____

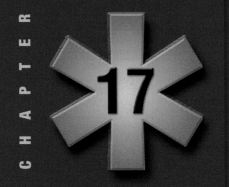

CHAPTER 17 — Module Review and Practice Examination

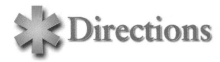

Directions

Assess what you have learned in this module by circling the best answer for each multiple-choice question. When you are done, check your answers against the key provided in Appendix D.

1. Which of the following is part of the scene size-up?
   _____ a. determining the number of patients
   _____ b. checking the patient's airway
   _____ c. determining the patient's chief complaint
   _____ d. performing an initial assessment

2. Determining the need for BSI is part of the:
   _____ a. dispatch information.
   _____ b. initial assessment.
   _____ c. scene size-up.
   _____ d. general impression.

3. The best way to protect yourself and your crew from hazards at a scene is:
   _____ a. relying on dispatch information.
   _____ b. always responding with a crew of at least 3 EMS providers.
   _____ c. wearing body armor.
   _____ d. observation

4. You are approaching the porch of a house to which you have been dispatched for an "injured person." Suddenly, the door swings open and you are confronted by a male in his 60s who is armed with a shotgun. He yells, "Get out of here before I blow your heads off!" Which of the following is the best course of action?
   _____ a. Immediately call for law enforcement.
   _____ b. Retreat immediately to a safe distance from the house.
   _____ c. Explain that you were called here to help someone who is injured.
   _____ d. Throw your oxygen cylinder at the man to try to disarm him.

5. The time to call for additional resources to assist you at the scene is:
   _____ a. after you receive the dispatch information.
   _____ b. when you are performing the scene size-up.
   _____ c. after you have triaged your patients.
   _____ d. during the initial assessment.

6. In addition to looking for signs of danger, the scene size-up can also give clues about:
   _____ a. whether the patient is chronically ill.
   _____ b. the patient's past medical history.
   _____ c. how the patient was injured.
   _____ d. all of the above.

7. Which of the following is a patient symptom?
   _____ a. hot, dry skin
   _____ b. headache
   _____ c. irregular pulse
   _____ d. a bruise

8. Which of the following is a patient sign?
   _____ a. depth of respiration
   _____ b. nausea
   _____ c. pain
   _____ d. itching

9. Which of the following is NOT a vital sign?
   _____ a. pupil response
   _____ b. blood pressure
   _____ c. skin temperature
   _____ d. reaction to painful stimulus

10. The first set of vital signs obtained from a patient is known as the _____ vital signs.
    _____ a. trending
    _____ b. size-up
    _____ c. baseline
    _____ d. normal

11. When assessing respirations, all of the following are assessed EXCEPT:
    _____ a. strength.
    _____ b. rate.
    _____ c. depth.
    _____ d. sounds.

12. A patient who breathes 4 times in a 15-second period has a respiratory rate of:
    _____ a. 4.
    _____ b. 8.
    _____ c. 16.
    _____ d. 20.

13. The most accurate method for counting respirations is to count them for a period of:
    _____ a. 10 seconds.
    _____ b. 15 seconds.
    _____ c. 30 seconds.
    _____ d. 1 minute.

14. The amount of air that moves in and out of the lungs with each respiration is the _____ volume.
    _____ a. tidal
    _____ b. minute
    _____ c. resting
    _____ d. lung

15. In respect to assessing respirations, the term *retraction* refers to:
    _____ a. an abnormal sound heard during inspiration.
    _____ b. shallow respirations.
    _____ c. drawing in of the soft tissues between the ribs.
    _____ d. prolonged inspiration with short expiration.

16. The presence of wheezing is an indication of:
    _____ a. upper airway obstruction.
    _____ b. partial upper airway obstruction.
    _____ c. fluid in the airway.
    _____ d. lower airway obstruction.

17. When assessing the pulse of a responsive adult, the preferred site of assessment is the _____ artery, located in/on the _____.
    _____ a. carotid, anterior neck
    _____ b. femoral, wrist
    _____ c. radial, wrist
    _____ d. radial, elbow

18. When assessing the pulse of an unresponsive adult, the preferred site is the _____ artery, located in/on the _____.
    _____ a. brachial, neck
    _____ b. radial, wrist
    _____ c. femoral, groin
    _____ d. carotid, neck

19. All of the following are peripheral pulses EXCEPT:
    _____ a. femoral.
    _____ b. popliteal.
    _____ c. dorsalis pedis.
    _____ d. radial.

20. All of the following are assessed when checking the pulse EXCEPT:
    _____ a. rate.
    _____ b. rhythm.
    _____ c. duration.
    _____ d. strength.

21. Blood pressure should be assessed in all patients _____ old or older.
    _____ a. 6 months
    _____ b. 1 year
    _____ c. 3 years
    _____ d. 5 years

22. When recording a blood pressure reading, the _____ pressure is recorded on top.
    _____ a. pulse
    _____ b. diastolic
    _____ c. venous
    _____ d. systolic

23. The use of a stethoscope to listen to the sounds of the blood pressure is called:
    _____ a. palpation.
    _____ b. auscultation.
    _____ c. insufflation.
    _____ d. perpetuation.

24. Cyanosis is an indication of:
    _____ a. poor perfusion.
    _____ b. liver disease.
    _____ c. poor oxygenation.
    _____ d. fever.

25. You are assessing a patient whose skin and whites of his eyes have a yellowish color. This would be documented as:
    _____ a. pallor.
    _____ b. cyanosis.
    _____ c. jaundice.
    _____ d. turgor.

26. Pupils that do not respond at all to changes in light are described as:
    _____ a. fixed.
    _____ b. dilated.
    _____ c. constricted.
    _____ d. PERRL.

27. The _____ is the primary reason why the patient summoned EMS, described in his or her own words.
    _____ a. general impression
    _____ b. initial assessment
    _____ c. chief complaint
    _____ d. pertinent history

28. To determine *provocation*, the "P" in OPQRST, which of the following questions should be asked?
    _____ a. What were you doing when your pain started?
    _____ b. Does anything make the pain worse or better?
    _____ c. Can you describe what your pain feels like?
    _____ d. Does the pain go anywhere else other than your chest?

29. Which of the following is NOT used to determine a patient's level of orientation?
    _____ a. awareness of who they are and who other people are
    _____ b. recall of what led to the EMS call
    _____ c. ability to calculate a simple addition or subtraction problem
    _____ d. awareness of the day and date

30. The purpose of the initial assessment is to:
    _____ a. determine immediate threats to life.
    _____ b. get a baseline set of vital signs.
    _____ c. form a general impression.
    _____ d. detect any possible hazards at the scene.

31. When caring for a patient with significant trauma, the scene time should be kept to a maximum of _____ minutes.
    _____ a. 5
    _____ b. 10
    _____ c. 15
    _____ d. 30

32. Which of the following is considered a significant mechanism of injury?
    _____ a. a wound to the pelvis
    _____ b. death of an occupant of the other vehicle
    _____ c. a fall from greater than 8 feet
    _____ d. being a backseat passenger of an automobile

33. Your patient is a 32-year-old mechanic who dropped an engine block on his right foot. When you arrive, the engine block has been lifted off the patient's foot. He is cursing and yelling at you to "hurry up and give me something for the pain." The most appropriate assessment for this patient is a(n):
    _____ a. initial assessment followed by a rapid trauma assessment.
    _____ b. initial assessment only.
    _____ c. initial assessment followed by a focused trauma assessment.
    _____ d. rapid trauma assessment followed by a focused trauma assessment.

34. The rapid trauma assessment includes:
    _____ a. vital signs.
    _____ b. checking the chest for deformities.
    _____ c. checking the reaction of the pupils.
    _____ d. formulating a general impression.

35. Your patient is a 50-year-old male who was burned when he poured gasoline into a smoldering pile of leaves to try to "get the fire burning." While your partner and the first-responding EMTs assess the patient, you are trying to get a medical history from his wife. She is impatient with your questions and tells you she doesn't understand why you need to know all these things. Which of the following is the best response?
    _____ a. "I'm just trying to do my job."
    _____ b. "Please, ma'am, could you just answer the questions?"
    _____ c. "Some medical problems and medications can complicate injuries. The more we know, the better we can help your husband."
    _____ d. "I know this all seems unnecessary. Please, just trust me on this."

36. A trauma patient who is unstable should be reevaluated every _____ minutes.
    _____ a. 1 to 2
    _____ b. 5
    _____ c. 10
    _____ d. 15

37. Which of the following statements is true regarding the assessment of a responsive medical patient?
    _____ a. A rapid physical examination is performed before the history is obtained.
    _____ b. A thorough, head-to-toe examination is performed.
    _____ c. An initial assessment is not necessary.
    _____ d. The history is obtained before performing a focused physical examination.

38. When asking about a patient's allergies, you should ask about:
    _____ a. only allergies to medications.
    _____ b. allergies to medications and environmental factors, such as bees or wasps.
    _____ c. allergies to medications and foods.
    _____ d. allergies to food, medications, and environmental factors, such as bees or wasps.

39. When assessing the severity of pain, you should ask the patient to rate how bad his or her pain is on a scale from 1 (least severe) to:
    _____ a. 5.
    _____ b. 10.
    _____ c. 25.
    _____ d. 100.

40. The process of obtaining and comparing vital signs over time is called:
    _____ a. trending.
    _____ b. profiling.
    _____ c. follow-up.
    _____ d. verifying.

41. Which of the following is a component of good communication with your patients?
    _____ a. touch
    _____ b. listening
    _____ c. tone of voice
    _____ d. all of the above

42. The radio that is mounted in a vehicle is a:
    _____ a. base station.
    _____ b. portable radio.
    _____ c. mobile radio.
    _____ d. repeater.

43. The piece of equipment that amplifies and rebroadcasts weaker radio signals is called a/an:
    _____ a. cell.
    _____ b. PTT.
    _____ c. MDT.
    _____ d. repeater.

44. In terms of documenting patient care, which of the following is a subjective statement?
    _____ a. The patient was found sitting at the kitchen table.
    _____ b. The patient stated he developed abdominal pain after eating.
    _____ c. Oxygen was administered at 15 liters per minute with a nonrebreather mask.
    _____ d. Bystanders were performing CPR when we arrived on the scene.

45. Which of the following best describes a chronological method of documentation?

_____ a. writing things down in the order they occurred

_____ b. first describing the patient's complaint, then what you observed, your overall impression, and finally, the care you gave the patient

_____ c. stating the chief complaint, history, assessment, treatment, and transport information

_____ d. documenting the assessment in a head-to-toe order

46. HIPAA regulations apply to:

_____ a. what radio frequencies are assigned to EMS systems.

_____ b. decisions about where patients are to be transported.

_____ c. the confidentiality and privacy of medical information.

_____ d. standard codes that can be used in radio transmissions.

47. In completing your documentation, you inadvertently write that the patient complained of pain to his left leg, when in fact it was his right. Which of the following is the best way to correct this situation?

_____ a. Discard the PCR and start a new one.

_____ b. Use correction fluid and write over the mistake.

_____ c. Black out the mistake with a marker, make the correction, and initial it.

_____ d. Draw a single line through the mistake, make the correction, and initial it.

48. Mrs. Jemenez is suing your employer and has named you in the suit. When you review your PCR, you recall that Mrs. Jemenez was an especially difficult patient. She was rude and demanding. Finally, after loading Mrs. Jemenez into the ambulance, you remember losing your patience and telling her if she didn't have anything nice to stay that she needed to be quiet. Your care of Mrs. Jemenez is well documented. She is a diabetic who had lost circulation to her left foot. Although you at first documented that it was her right foot, you corrected the mistake. Her foot was amputated in the hospital. Mrs. Jemenez claims that if you had treated her properly, she would not have lost her foot. What is the most likely reason why Mrs. Jemenez is suing?

_____ a. a breakdown in communications

_____ b. poor prehospital medical care

_____ c. poor medical care in the hospital

_____ d. initial documentation that it was the right foot

49. It has been a tough day for Mark. He forgot to get a second set of vital signs on his last patient, Mr. Bridlove. He knows if he leaves the space for the second set of vitals blank, he'll be reprimanded by his supervisor. Mark decides to write in a set of vital signs to avoid yet more paperwork. Mark's actions are best described as:

_____ a. negligence.

_____ b. fraud.

_____ c. falsification.

_____ d. error of commission.

50. Which of the following should be included in documentation of patient refusals?

_____ a. that the patient was informed of the risks of refusing care

_____ b. that you attempted to convince the patient to accept care

_____ c. any care you performed

_____ d. all of the above

51. Tidal volume refers to the _____ of breathing.

_____ a. rate

_____ b. rhythm

_____ c. ease

_____ d. depth

52. Hearing crackles when listening to the lungs with a stethoscope is an indication of:
    _____ a. poor technique of listening to breath sounds.
    _____ b. lower airway constriction.
    _____ c. partial upper airway obstruction.
    _____ d. fluid in the alveoli.

53. In dark skinned individuals skin color changes can best be detected by observing the:
    _____ a. inside of the lower eyelid.
    _____ b. back of the hand.
    _____ c. nape of the neck.
    _____ d. medial (inside aspect) of the arm.

54. Taking orthostatic vital signs is recommended when:
    _____ a. a patient's chief complaint is dizziness.
    _____ b. caring for a trauma patient with possible internal bleeding.
    _____ c. a patient may have low blood volume but does not have signs of shock.
    _____ d. caring for a cardiac patient.

55. Which of the following best depicts a patient whose level of consciousness is described as verbal?
    _____ a. The patient is able to speak, even though the words may or may not make sense.
    _____ b. The patient is able to speak and the words spoken are appropriate.
    _____ c. The patient appears unresponsive but responds in some manner to your voice.
    _____ d. The patient cries out in response to painful stimulus.

56. Which of the following does NOT necessarily place a patient into a high-priority category for treatment and transport?
    _____ a. vomiting
    _____ b. pale, cool skin with a weak, rapid pulse
    _____ c. unresponsiveness
    _____ d. difficulty breathing

57. Which of the following is the correct sequence of assessment steps for a trauma patient with NO significant mechanism of injury?
    _____ a. rapid trauma assessment, baseline vital signs, SAMPLE history, detailed physical exam
    _____ b. SAMPLE history, baseline vital signs, rapid trauma assessment
    _____ c. focused trauma assessment, baseline vital signs, SAMPLE history
    _____ d. baseline vital signs, SAMPLE history, focused trauma assessment, detailed physical exam

58. For a responsive medical patient, which of the following assessment components comes first?
    _____ a. baseline vital signs
    _____ b. history
    _____ c. focused physical exam
    _____ d. detailed physical exam

59. When palpating a patient's abdomen you note that the patient tenses up his abdominal muscles. This finding is known as:
    _____ a. tenderness.
    _____ b. rigidity.
    _____ c. guarding.
    _____ d. distention.

60. Upon greeting your 65-year-old female patient, you realize she has a hearing impairment. Which of the following should you do first to improve communication?
    _____ a. Face the patient and speak clearly.
    _____ b. Get the history from a family member.
    _____ c. Talk as loudly as you can without shouting.
    _____ d. Speak loudly, slowly, and with exaggerated emphasis on words.

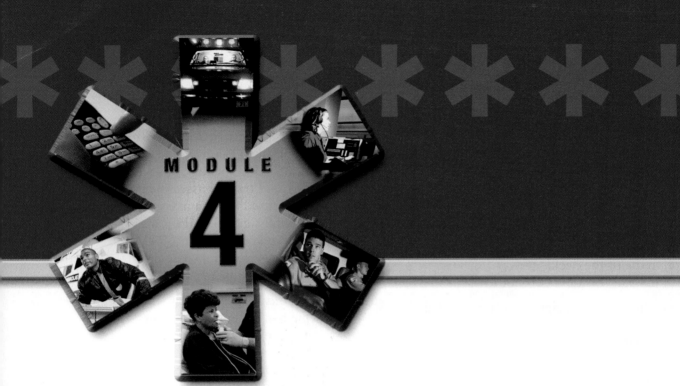

Medical Emergencies

" *I honestly thought I was going to die . . . At first I can remember being frustrated with the ambulance people . . . All that aside, I probably wouldn't be here right now without them.* "

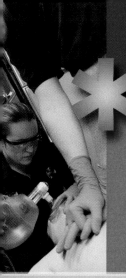

Module Outline

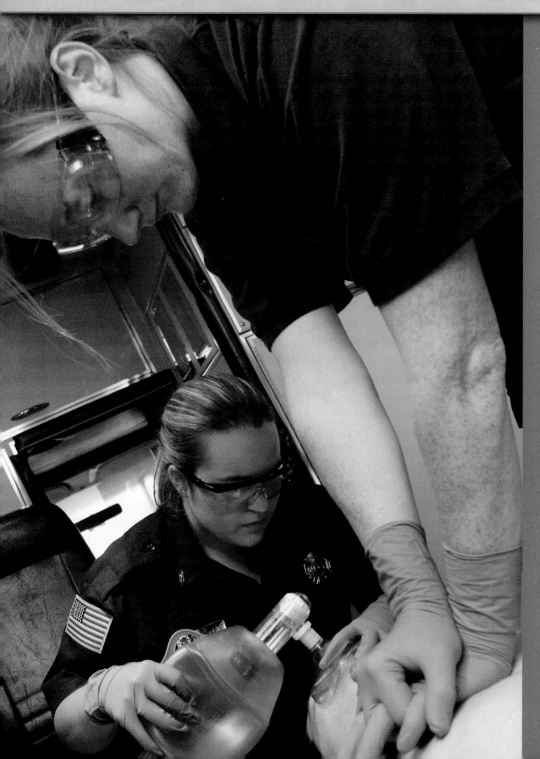

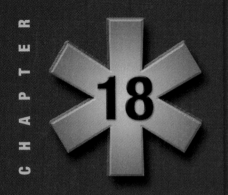

CHAPTER 18

Understanding Pharmacology

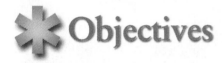

Objectives

Numbered objectives are from the U.S. Department of Transportation 1994 EMT-Basic National Standard Curriculum.

COGNITIVE OBJECTIVES

At the completion of this lesson, the EMT-Basic student will be able to:

4-1.1 Identify which medications will be carried on the unit. (pp. 436–440)

4-1.2 State the medications carried on the unit by the generic name. (pp. 436–440)

4-1.3 Identify the medications with which the EMT-Basic may assist the patient with administering. (pp. 436–440)

4-1.4 State the medications the EMT-Basic can assist the patient with by the generic name. (pp. 436–440)

4-1.5 Discuss the forms in which the medications may be found. (pp. 430–431)

AFFECTIVE OBJECTIVES

At the completion of this lesson, the EMT-Basic student will be able to:

4-1.6 Explain the rationale for the administration of medications. (pp. 429, 434)

PSYCHOMOTOR OBJECTIVES

At the completion of this lesson, the EMT-Basic student will be able to:

4-1.7 Demonstrate general steps for assisting patient with self-administration of medications. (pp. 436–437)

4-1.8 Read the labels and inspect each type of medication. (pp. 434–435)

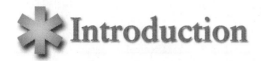# Introduction

Pharmacology is an important concept for EMTs—or any health care provider. Administering medications can help relieve breathing difficulty or chest pain and make a tremendous difference in the life of your patient. Administering a medication is also a tremendous responsibility for the EMT. This chapter will introduce you to principles of pharmacology and the drugs you may have available to you as an EMT.

Pharmacology can be simply defined as the study of medications. At some point you will be asked to administer a medication to a patient or assist a patient with a medication. To do this you must know details about the medication and how it will affect your patient—in both good and bad ways. This includes everything from the medications appearance to its actions.

Consider the following situations where the same medication was administered to three different patients:

* You assist a patient who is experiencing chest pain to take his own prescribed medication (nitroglycerin). The medication relieves the pain.

* You assist another patient with his own prescribed medication who does not experience any relief from the pain.

* You administer the same medication to a third patient and it causes a dangerous drop in blood pressure.

Medications can relieve pain or help a patient with a serious medical condition such as diabetes, chest pain, or breathing difficulty. In each case, the same medication can also have negative effects. This is why the study of pharmacology is important and why we say the ability to administer medications is a significant responsibility to be taken seriously.

This chapter will talk about how medications are named, provided, and administered, how they act, and why one medication can act differently in different patients.

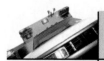# Emergency Dispatch

EMT Rory Ellis squinted at his watch in the dim light of the convenience store parking lot and whistled softly. 0402 hours.

"Looks like we made it without another late call," he said to his partner, who immediately shot him a horrified look.

"Aw man! You just jinxed us!" Brett, also an EMT, closed his eyes and slumped into the seat.

"Oh, come on, you don't really believe . . . " Rory was interrupted by the emergency tones on the radio.

"Sorry, 2-12, but I've got a call at your post and there's nobody closer," the dispatcher said. "It's a priority-one chest pain in the south parking lot of the K&W Supermarket on Fourth Street. You're looking for a delivery driver sitting by a semi."

(continued on next page)

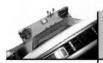

Emergency Dispatch

(continued)

"I told you," Brett smiled at Rory as he picked up the microphone and keyed it. "Ok, 2-12 copies. We're on our way."

The patient was Kenny, a 53-year-old male who was pale, cool, diaphoretic, and complaining of "a real heaviness" in his chest, accompanied by shortness of breath.

"Do you have a history of heart problems?" Rory asked as Brett positioned the blood pressure cuff.

"I had a heart attack about three years ago," the man grimaced.

"Can you take aspirin and do you carry nitro?" Brett was now pumping the blood pressure cuff up.

"I already took two baby aspirin, but I don't have my . . . no wait," The man looked toward his delivery truck. "I'm driving number three today. I carry a little spray bottle . . . nitroglycerin . . . in the glove box. I totally forgot."

Rory climbed up into the cab, fished the small red bottle from the truck's glove box, and confirmed the information on the prescription label. He was just preparing to spray a dose under the man's tongue when Brett pulled the stethoscope from his ears.

Brett quickly grabbed Rory's arm. "Don't give him any nitroglycerin! His BP is too low. Let's load him and go."

✳ **inhaler**

a spray device with a mouthpiece that contains an aerosol form of a medication that a patient can spray into his airway.

✳ **generic**

the medication name found in the U.S. Pharmacopoeia.

✳ **United States Pharmacopoeia (USP)**

government listing of all medications

✳ **albuterol**

a medication used to dilate bronchioles in patients with respiratory disorders.

✳ **trade name**

the medication name a pharmaceutical company gives to a drug. It could also be referred to as a brand name.

✳ **chemical name**

the medication name that reflects the chemical structure of the medication.

Medications

Each medication has several names. Each refers to the same medication but is described differently.

We will use a common medication found in **inhalers** as an example.

The **generic** name is the one listed in the **United States Pharmacopoeia (USP)**, a government listing of all medications.

In this case, the generic name is **albuterol** (albuterol, USP).

The **trade name** is the name a pharmaceutical company gives to a drug. It could also be referred to as a brand name.

The trade names for albuterol include Proventil, Ventolin, and others. Each manufacturer of albuterol will have a different trade name for it.

The **chemical name** is the name that reflects the chemical structure of the medication. You won't commonly see this as you practice as an EMT.

The chemical name for albuterol is albuterol sulfate.

Medications come in several forms. The forms are specifically designed to allow the medication to be absorbed at the appropriate rate and achieve its designated effect at the proper time and location.

Medications that are *injected* act very quickly. Medications that are taken *orally* (by mouth) reach the intended area much more slowly because they require digestion and absorption. *Inhaled* medications reach the lungs quickly. Others are *absorbed* by the mucus membranes in the mouth. The forms of medications you may see are as follows:

* Liquids for **injection** (epinephrine)
* **Gels** (oral glucose)
* **Tablets** (nitroglycerin)
* **Suspensions** (activated charcoal)
* Fine powder for inhalation (metered-dose inhaler)
* **Sublingual** spray (nitroglycerin)
* Gas (oxygen)
* **Nebulized** (vaporized) (respiratory medication)
* **Transdermal** (nicotine patch or nitroglycerin patch)

4-1.5 Discuss the forms in which the medications may be found.

* **injection**
  placement of medication in or under the skin with a needle and syringe.

* **gels**
  jelly-like form of medication.

* **tablets**
  small disk-like compressed form of medication.

* **suspensions**
  solid medication mixed in a fluid. Must be shaken before giving.

* **sublingual**
  beneath the tongue.

* **nebulized**
  process of mixing air and medication to produce a mist, which is inhaled.

* **transdermal**
  through or by way of the skin.

 # Stop, Review, Remember!

Multiple Choice

Place a check next to the correct answer.

1. A medication's generic name is:
   _____ a. its chemical structure.
   _____ b. its "brand name."
   _____ c. the name listed in the USP.
   _____ d. a name based on the brand name of the medication.

2. A medication found in gel form is:
   _____ a. epinephrine.
   _____ b. oxygen.
   _____ c. nitroglycerin.
   _____ d. glucose.

3. The device that dispenses medication in fine-powder form is the:
   _____ a. nonrebreather oxygen mask.
   _____ b. nebulizer.
   _____ c. metered-dose inhaler.
   _____ d. oxylizer.

4. A medication given to one person may have a different reaction when given to another person.
   _____ a. true
   _____ b. false

5. Sublingual medications are given:

_____ a. under the tongue.

_____ b. by injection under the skin.

_____ c. as an ointment on the skin.

_____ d. by inhalation or vapor.

Matching

Match the definition on the left with the applicable term on the right.

1. _____ The medication name found in the U.S. Pharmacopoeia

2. _____ The medication name that reflects the chemical structure of the medication

3. _____ Solid medication mixed in a fluid. Must be shaken before giving

4. _____ The medication name a pharmaceutical company gives to a drug. It could also be referred to as a brand name

5. _____ Process of mixing air and medication to produce a mist

A. Chemical name
B. Generic name
C. Nebulized
D. Trade name
E. Suspension

Critical Thinking

1. What is the difference between a metered-dose inhaler and a nebulizer?

_____

_____

_____

_____

2. A member of your family has gone to the cardiologist and received a prescription for nitroglycerin. The prescription was filled at your local pharmacy. Since you are an EMT, he stops by to ask you about his medication. Upon opening the pharmacy bag you notice the medication container says "Nitrostat." Is there a difference between nitroglycerin and Nitrostat? Use chapter 20 of this text or a drug reference to answer this question.

_____

_____

_____

_____

_____

3. You are in a discussion with another EMT who tells you, "It doesn't matter if you put the nitroglycerin pill under the patient's tongue or he chews it or swallows it. It all goes to the same place." Do you agree or disagree with this? Why?

   _____

   _____

   _____

   _____

   _____

4. Using this text or a drug reference source for each of the following medication names, list whether it is a trade name, chemical name, or generic name.

   Nitrostat _____

   Albuterol sulfate _____

   Activated charcoal _____

   Nitroglycerin _____

   Proventil _____

   Glucose _____

   Actidose _____

   Epinephrine _____

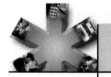

Perspective

Kenny—The Patient

"Okay, God, you win. I really don't want to die! I was so good after my heart attack, you know? I exercised and watched my diet and, I just did everything that my doctor said. But then after awhile, little by little, I sort of . . . stopped. Now here, almost three years later, I'm back to coffee and donuts, fast food, and cigarettes. But I'm done now. I'm definitely not as indestructible as I thought. Man oh man was I lucky today! Okay, I'll admit, I'm scared now."

Administering Medications

It is worth repeating that administering a medication is a significant responsibility. There are rules for administering medications. These rules set the reason the medication is administered, how the medication is administered, and how much of the medication is administered. We also expect the medication to cause certain responses in the body and recognize that negative or unexpected effects may occur. And there are situations where you wouldn't administer the medication because it may do more harm than good.

There are actually formal names for each of the rules and expectations described in the previous paragraph. These concepts will apply each and every time you administer, or consider administering, a medication. The formal terms are:

✳ **indication**

   reason a medication is administered.

✳ **route**

   how the medication is administered.

✳ **dose**

   how much of the medication is administered.

✳ **actions**

   desired responses in the body a medication may cause. Also called the desired effect.

✳ **side effects**

   any action of a drug other than the desired action.

✳ **contraindications**

   situations where a medication should not be administered because it may do more harm than good.

✳ **Indication**—the reason the medication is administered (for example, chest pain or poisoning)

✳ **Route**—how the medication is administered (for example, sublingual, injection, or inhalation)

✳ **Dose**—how much of the medication is administered

✳ **Actions**—certain responses expected in the body, also called the desired effect

✳ **Side effects**—negative effects or actions other than the desired actions

✳ **Contraindications**—situations where you wouldn't administer the medication because it may do more harm than good

When you administer a medication, it will often be after consulting a physician (medical director) by radio or phone. After presenting your patient and his condition to the physician, you may receive an order to administer a medication.

When receiving a medication order, it is important to acknowledge the order, then repeat it back to the physician for verification. Once it is confirmed, write down the medication, dose, route, and any other specific information. You may be told to administer one sublingual nitroglycerin now and another one in 5 minutes if the patient's blood pressure remains over 120 mmHg systolic. It is important to remember the order exactly. Writing it down will help assure that it is done correctly.

After receiving the order and writing it down, you should select the medication from your kit (if it is one that is carried on the ambulance) or obtain it from your patient (if it is one prescribed to the patient). Verify the medication name on the container and the expiration date and all of the "six rights." (Figure 18-1). En-

FIGURE 18-1 Examine the patient's medication with the patient present. Confirm the expiration date.

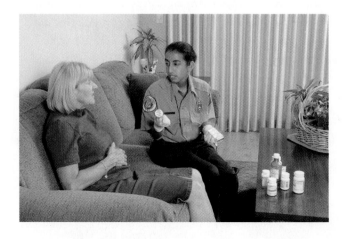

sure that the medication is uncontaminated. For example, if it is a liquid, ensure that it is normal (usually clear) and free of particles or impurities. Be sure the patient is not allergic to the medication you wish to administer.

After a medication is given it is important to reassess the patient. This will include determining the effect the patient felt from receiving the medication (better, worse, or no change) and reassessing vital signs. This reassessment is often performed as part of an ongoing assessment en route to the hospital.

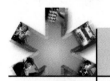

Clinical Clues: COMMUNICATING WITH MEDICAL DIRECTION

If an order from a physician does not seem to make sense to you, ask the physician for clarification. Remember that the physician can't see the patient. His information is based on your radio report. If part of your transmission is distorted or if there is a misunderstanding on either end, an order could be incorrect. It is always better to ask for clarification and express concerns you have than to administer a medication in error.

The **six rights** are often cited as a way to remember all things you must check when administering a medication to the patient. These include:

* **Right medication**—Is this the right medication for the patient's condition? Is the medication I am about to administer the medication I believe it is? Have I checked and rechecked the label to verify this? Is the medication current (not expired)?

* **Right dose**—Am I giving the correct amount of medication?

* **Right route**—Am I giving the medication through the correct route (the way it is intended to be administered)?

* **Right patient**—Does this medication belong to the patient I am about to give it to?

* **Right time**—Is it the right time to give the medication? Will the medication treat the patient's condition? Are there any reasons not to give the medication, such as contraindications or allergies?

* **Right documentation**—Have I documented the patient's condition before administration as well as documenting the patient's response to the medication? Have I rechecked and recorded vital signs after administering the medication?

* **six rights**

  memory aid to remember all things you must check when administering a medication to the patient. These include: right medication, right dose, right route, right patient, right time, and right documentation.

Perspective

Rory—The EMT

"I'm glad that Brett was thinking. I apparently wasn't. In my brain I was jumping through the chest-pain protocol at a million miles per hour, you know? Aspirin . . . nitro . . . the whole thing. But I forgot one of the most important 'rights' when administering medication. It definitely was not the right time. I never thought to ask Brett for the guy's BP before readying the nitro. I was about to risk this guy's life by skipping over an entire junction of the cardiac protocols. I've got to learn to slow down, I really do. Also I learned again how important my partner is."

4-1.1 Identify which medications will be carried on the unit.

4-1.2 State the medications carried on the unit by the generic name.

4-1.3 Identify the medications with which the EMT-Basic may assist the patient with administering.

4-1.4 State the medications the EMT-Basic can assist the patient with by the generic name.

Prehospital Medications

The following section provides an introduction to the most common prehospital medications. Each medication will be covered in greater detail in the chapter in which it applies (for example, nitroglycerin in the cardiac chapter, inhalers in the respiratory emergencies chapter).

Medicine is an ever-changing science. As research and experience dictate, some medications are added or deleted from the medications EMTs use. In most cases, the number of medications and ways they are administered have increased over the past 10 years.

For example, aspirin has been shown to reduce the risk of death for patients who are in the midst of a heart attack (myocardial infarction). Therefore, many EMS systems now allow their EMTs to carry and administer aspirin as part of their chest pain protocols.

Another example is the epinephrine auto-injector used to treat severe allergic reactions. EMTs have been allowed to assist patients in using their auto-injector for many years. But because these allergic reactions can be deadly and patients don't always have their auto-injector with them, many ambulances now carry epinephrine auto-injectors as part of their equipment.

Your instructor and system protocols will tell you what medications are allowed in your area.

Epinephrine is used to treat serious allergic reactions called anaphylaxis (chapter 22). It is supplied in an auto-injector that injects the medication into the muscle or soft tissue of the lateral aspect of the mid-thigh (Figure 18-2). It can be injected through most pants. The medication reverses the most serious effects of these allergic reactions: low blood pressure and constricted bronchioles in the lungs.

Nitroglycerin is a **smooth-muscle relaxant** that is used to treat chest pain. It is supplied as tablets (Figure 18-3) that are placed under the tongue to dissolve or spray that is sprayed directly under the tongue (Figure 18-4). The smooth-muscle-relaxant properties of nitroglycerin dilate blood vessels and help reduce the workload of the heart—which helps to relieve chest pain. A dangerous side effect associated with nitroglycerin is that it may reduce blood pressure too much. You will need to check the patient's blood pressure before and after administration. Nitroglycerin tablets also remain potent for only about 6 months after the bottle has been opened. They must also be protected from light. Nitroglycerin is contraindicated for a patient whose systolic blood pressure is less than 100 mmHg and/or

* **epinephrine**

  a medication used to treat serious allergic reactions called anaphylaxis.

* **nitroglycerin**

  a medication used to treat chest pain.

* **smooth-muscle relaxant**

  a medication that relaxes smooth muscles, for example, as nitroglycerin relaxes the muscle in blood vessels and permits an increased blood flow.

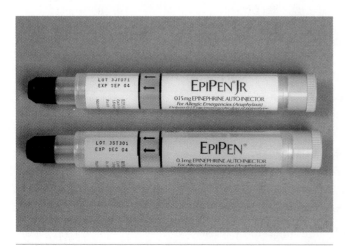

FIGURE 18-2 Adult and child-size EpiPens.

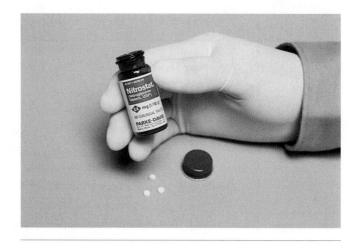

FIGURE 18-3 Nitroglycerin tablets.

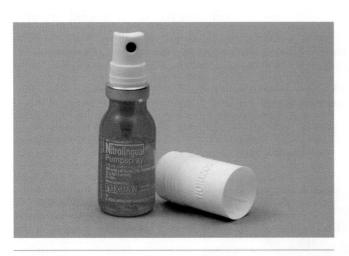

FIGURE 18-4   Nitroglycerin spray.

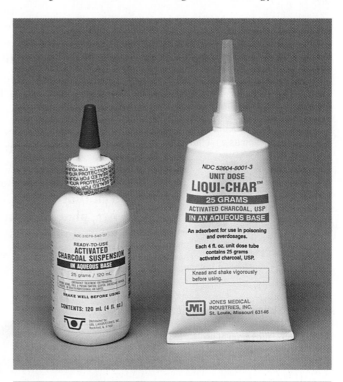

FIGURE 18-5   Activated charcoal may be used in poisoning cases.

who is taking medication to treat erectile dysfunction. Some EMS system's protocols contraindicate nitroglycerin at 110 or 120 mmHg. Follow your local protocol.

Activated charcoal is used to treat certain cases of poisoning or overdose (Figure 18-5). It is a substance that is made specifically to have a large surface area for maximum absorption (binding the poison). Once the poison binds to the charcoal, it is prevented from being absorbed into the body. Since activated charcoal is not recommended for all poisonings, follow the advice of medical direction or the poison control center in the use of this medication.

Oral glucose is a **carbohydrate** used to treat patients with suspected low blood sugar. If a patient has a history of diabetes and an altered mental status but retains a gag reflex, glucose can cause an amazing improvement in the patient's condition.

∗ **activated charcoal**

a medication used to treat certain cases of poisoning or overdose.

∗ **oral glucose**

a medication used to treat patients with suspected low blood sugar.

∗ **carbohydrate**

source of fuel for the body.

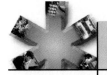

Perspective

Brett—The EMT

"82 over 56! In what universe is it okay to give nitroglycerin to a patient with a BP like that? And what if he took Viagra or another one of those drugs that you can't give nitro with? This is a big responsibility. I just shudder when I think what could have happened if I wasn't right there, taking the patient's pressure. Now what do I do? This kind of thing has happened once too often with Rory. I guess I should go to the supervisor, right? I don't know. I hate being in this position."

✳ **inhaled bronchodilators**

> medication used to open up bronchioles that are constricted due to a respiratory disease such as asthma.

✳ **aspirin**

> medication used both during a heart attack and as a method to prevent heart attacks.

✳ **blood clotting**

> clumping together of blood cells.

✳ **platelets**

> components of the blood; membrane-enclosed fragments of specialized cells.

✳ **oxygen**

> a medication used to increase the amount of circulating oxygen in the blood stream.

Oral glucose is squeezed onto a tongue depressor and placed between the patient's cheek and gum (Figure 18-6). It is rapidly absorbed through the oral mucosa.

Inhaled bronchodilators as the name implies, open up bronchioles that are constricted due to a respiratory disease such as asthma. These may be administered in two ways: via fine powder through a metered-dose inhaler (Figure 18-7) or through a nebulizer that creates a continuous vapor inhaled by the patient (Scan 18-1).

Aspirin, the common household pain reliever that has been around for over 100 years, has now been recommended both during a heart attack and as a method to prevent heart attacks (Figure 18-8). It is the ability of this medication to prevent **blood clotting** that causes the benefit to the heart. When a blood vessel in the heart narrows, **platelets** form and can block the artery. Aspirin prevents this from happening. You must be sure to ask the patient if he has an allergy to aspirin.

Oxygen is a gas and is often not even considered a drug—but it is. As a matter of fact, in some states you can't get oxygen without a prescription (Figure 18-9 on

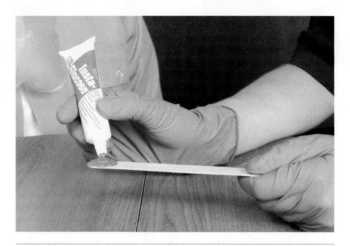

FIGURE 18-6 Oral glucose may be administered by squeezing it on a tongue depressor and placing it between the cheek and gum.

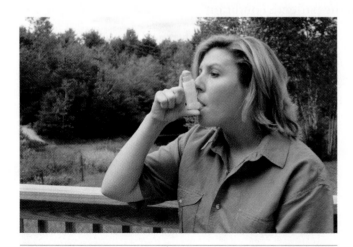

FIGURE 18-7 A prescribed inhaler may help a patient who has respiratory problems.

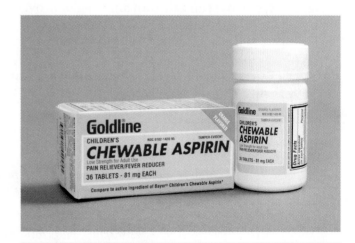

FIGURE 18-8 Aspirin may be administered to patients with suspected cardiac conditions.

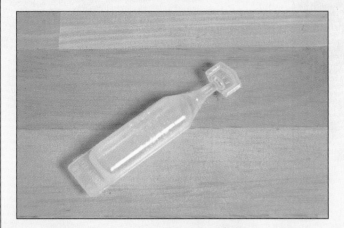

▲ Individual dose of albuterol for use on a nebulizer.

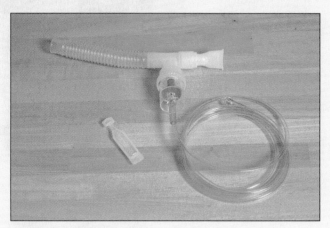

▲ Nebulizer administration set.

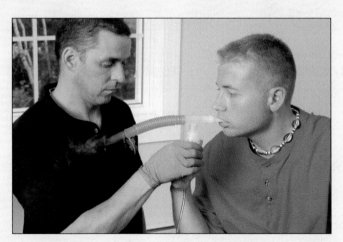

▲ Have the patient seal his lips around the nebulizer mouthpiece and breathe deeply. Instruct the patient to hold his breath for 2 to 3 seconds if possible. Continue until medication is gone from the chamber.

page 440). Many if not most of your patients will receive oxygen as part of your prehospital care. Oxygen administration was discussed in depth in chapter 7. Check your local protocols.

The medications used in your EMS system may differ slightly from the medications listed in Table 18-1 on page 440. Ask your instructor or refer to your local protocols to learn about the medications you may administer.

FIGURE 18-9 A patient receiving oxygen with assistance.

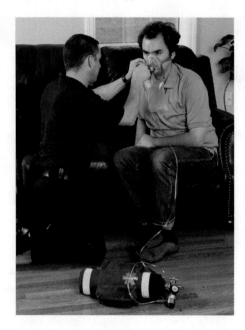

TABLE 18-1	PREHOSPITAL MEDICATIONS		
MEDICATION	CARRIED ON THE AMBULANCE OR PATIENT'S OWN	FORM	INDICATION (USE)
Epinephrine	Patient's own. Carried on the ambulance in many areas	Auto-injector	Severe allergic reactions (anaphylaxis)
Nitroglycerin	Patient's own	Tablet or spray administered under the tongue (sublingually)	Cardiac-related chest pain
Oral glucose	Carried on the ambulance	Gel (oral)	Diabetic patients with suspected low blood sugar
Activated charcoal	Carried on the ambulance	Suspension	Some poisoning and overdose patients
Albuterol/prescribed inhaler	Patient's own. Some areas now carry these for EMTs	Fine powder for inhalation	Asthma, chronic lung conditions
Albuterol (nebulized)	Patient's own. Some areas carry on ambulance for EMTs	Nebulized (aerosolized)	Severe asthma and chronic lung conditions
Aspirin	Patient's own or carried on the ambulance	Tablet (chewable)	Chest pain
Oxygen	Carried on the ambulance Patients may be on home oxygen	Gas	Various including respiratory distress, chest pain, shock, many others

✳ Stop, Review, Remember!

Multiple Choice

Place a check next to the correct answer.

1. Which of the following medications is supplied as a suspension?

   _____ a. glucose

   _____ b. epinephrine

   _____ c. activated charcoal

   _____ d. aspirin

2. Which of the following medications is supplied as a tablet?

   _____ a. nitroglycerin

   _____ b. albuterol

   _____ c. activated charcoal

   _____ d. proventil

3. You assist a patient with his inhaler. Almost immediately the patient feels shaky and like his heart has sped up. These sensations would be called:

   _____ a. contraindications.

   _____ b. actions.

   _____ c. indications.

   _____ d. side effects.

4. The medication that is designed to adsorb poisons and prevent them from entering the body is:

   _____ a. nitroglycerin.

   _____ b. activated charcoal.

   _____ c. aspirin.

   _____ d. albuterol.

5. Oxygen is a drug.

   _____ a. true

   _____ b. false

Matching

Match each medication form on the left with the medication on the right that comes in that form.

1. _____ Liquids for injection

2. _____ Gels

3. _____ Tablets

4. _____ Suspensions

5. _____ Fine powder for inhalation

6. _____ Sublingual spray

7. _____ Gas

8. _____ Nebulized (vaporized)

A. Oxygen
B. Nitroglycerin
C. Epinephrine
D. Oral glucose
E. Activated charcoal
F. Albuterol

Critical Thinking

1. Is nitroglycerin carried on your ambulance? Describe your local protocols regarding administering or assisting in the administration of nitroglycerin.

   _____

   _____

   _____

   _____

2. You call medical direction because you are treating a patient experiencing a severe allergic reaction and request an order for epinephrine. The doctor approves the order and says, "OK, go ahead and put the epinephrine in the IV line." What should you do?

   _____

   _____

   _____

   _____

3. Your patient uses an inhaler. What form of medication is in the inhaler? How does the inhaler work?

   _____

   _____

   _____

   _____

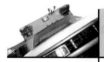

Dispatch Summary

The patient was placed on high-flow oxygen via a nonrebreather mask and transported with lights and siren to the Midwest Heart Hospital. He was stabilized there and underwent tests that indicated he had suffered his second mild heart attack. The patient was released several days later with a new determination to improve his health.

Based on Brett's report to the supervisor, Rory was interviewed and placed in remedial training with a Field Training Officer. He has since improved greatly as an EMT and is now very careful to think through each situation prior to taking action. Brett and Rory plan to become partners again during the next shift-bid.

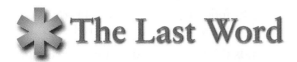

The Last Word

As has been said throughout this chapter, medication administration is a serious responsibility. It is important to understand the concepts presented in the chapter.

Medications have different names, including the generic name, trade name, and chemical name. These medications come in many forms ranging from gels (glucose) to gas (oxygen). Each medication is given for a specific reason or indication. A contraindication is a situation when a medication shouldn't be given. Each drug has fairly predictable side effects.

A drug has expected actions. For example, a nitroglycerin tablet or spray will often relieve chest pain. It also may have side effects, or negative effects, such as lowering the patient's blood pressure. And each medication is given by a specific route. Some are oral, others are injected, and some are breathed in through inhalers. Always use the proper route when administering medications.

There are many medications that EMS providers can administer or assist with. These change over time as research reveals additional benefits and/or risks of a medication. Prehospital medications include oxygen, oral glucose, activated charcoal, epinephrine auto-injector, prescribed inhalers, nitroglycerin, and sometimes aspirin. Each medication and its administration will be discussed in subsequent chapters. Always consider the "six rights" when administering medications.

Chapter Review

MULTIPLE CHOICE

Place a check next to the correct answer.

1. When receiving an order from medical direction, you should:

   _____ a. write down the order, then administer the medication.

   _____ b. repeat the order as confirmation, write down the order, administer the medication.

   _____ c. write down and repeat the order, confirm it with the patient, then administer the medication.

   _____ d. confirm the order with a second physician, write down the order, administer the medication.

2. Which of the following is NOT one of the "rights" of medication administration?

   _____ a. medication

   _____ b. dose

   _____ c. patient

   _____ d. action

3. Aspirin, when carried on the ambulance, is administered when _____ is suspected.

   _____ a. pain

   _____ b. fever

   _____ c. heart attack

   _____ d. infection

4. Reassessment of a patient after administering a medication is often done as part of the:

_____ a. initial assessment.

_____ b. scene size-up.

_____ c. focused history.

_____ d. ongoing assessment.

5. Which of the following questions would you ask to determine "right patient" in the six "rights?"

_____ a. Is this the correct drug for this patient?

_____ b. Is this the right amount of the drug for this patient?

_____ c. Is this patient allergic to this drug?

_____ d. Is this medication prescribed to the patient?

MATCHING

Match the term on the left with the definition on the right.

1. _____ Indication

2. _____ Route

3. _____ Dose

4. _____ Actions

5. _____ Side effects

6. _____ Contraindications

A. What we expect the medication to do within the body
B. The reason the medications are administered
C. Situations when you wouldn't administer a medication
D. Negative effects that may occur
E. How much of the medications are administered
F. How the medications are administered

CRITICAL THINKING

1. What is the difference between a side effect and a contraindication?

_____

_____

_____

_____

2. You have just administered nitroglycerin for chest pain and begin to reassess the patient. For what will you reassess?

_____

_____

_____

_____

3. You are at a high school football game where a student is having breathing difficulty. The patient says he has asthma, but his inhaler is inside the locked school. Another student has an inhaler for asthma. Can you use the other student's inhaler? Why or why not?

_____

_____

_____

_____

4. List the "six rights" of medication administration and one question you can ask to verify each.

_____

_____

_____

_____

CASE STUDY

This case study will require you to integrate information from chapter 16 and this chapter.

You are called to a patient with chest pain. John Gillis is 67 years old. The patient reports that he was mowing the lawn when the pain started. This was about 10 minutes ago. He came in and sat down in the air conditioning. You find him pale, cool, and sweaty. He reports that although his chest pain has subsided, it is still significant. He describes it as "5" on a 0–10 scale. Previously it was "8."

His vital signs are: pulse 96 strong and regular, respirations 20 and slightly labored, blood pressure 124/86, pupils equal and reactive. Skin as noted above.

The patient has taken one of his nitroglycerin tablets that he received after his first and only other bout of chest pain "4 or 5 months ago." Otherwise the patient is healthy. He takes an aspirin a day for prevention of heart attacks and Lipitor for high cholesterol.

Assuming (until you study cardiac emergencies in chapter 20) that this patient would benefit from nitroglycerin:

1. Compose a radio report to your medical direction physician requesting an order for administration of sublingual nitroglycerin.

_____

_____

_____

_____

2. What side effect(s) might you see from the administration of nitroglycerin?

_____

_____

_____

_____

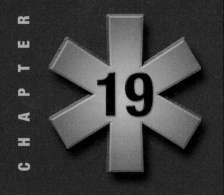

CHAPTER 19

Patients with Respiratory Distress

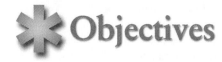 Objectives

Numbered objectives are from the U.S. Department of Transportation 1994 EMT-Basic National Standard Curriculum.

COGNITIVE OBJECTIVES

At the completion of this lesson, the EMT-Basic student will be able to:

4-2.1 List the structure and function of the respiratory system. (pp. 447–449)

4-2.2 State the signs and symptoms of a patient with breathing difficulty. (pp. 451–453)

4-2.3 Describe the emergency medical care of the patient with breathing difficulty. (pp. 461–462)

4-2.4 Recognize the need for medical direction to assist in the emergency medical care of the patient with breathing difficulty. (pp. 464–465)

4-2.5 Describe the emergency medical care of the patient with breathing distress. (pp. 461–462)

4-2.6 Establish the relationship between airway management and the patient with breathing difficulty. (pp. 451–457)

4-2.7 List signs of adequate air exchange. (pp. 451–457)

4-2.8 State the generic name, medication forms, dose, administration, action, indications, and contraindications for the prescribed inhaler. (pp. 464–470)

4-2.9 Distinguish between the emergency medical care of the infant, child, and adult patient with breathing difficulty. (pp. 462–463)

4-2.10 Differentiate between upper airway obstruction and lower airway disease in the infant and child patient. (pp. 462–463)

AFFECTIVE OBJECTIVES

At the completion of this lesson, the EMT-Basic student will be able to:

4-2.11 Defend EMT-Basic treatment regimens for various respiratory emergencies. (pp. 463–470)

4-2.12 Explain the rationale for administering an inhaler. (pp. 463–466)

PSYCHOMOTOR OBJECTIVES

At the completion of this lesson, the EMT-Basic student will be able to:

4-2.13 Demonstrate the emergency medical care for breathing difficulty. (pp. 461–462)

4-2.14 Perform the steps in facilitating the use of an inhaler. (pp. 465–467)

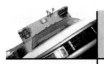 # Introduction

Patients with respiratory distress will require your clinical as well as your emotional care. Respiratory distress can be the presenting problem in a variety of serious conditions, such as heart attack, fluid in the lungs (congestive heart failure), and worsening of long-term lung conditions such as emphysema. The patient experiencing shortness of breath may literally feel he is going to die. The feeling is one of the most frightening sensations there is—for both the patient and loved ones who worry about the patient.

This chapter discusses the patient who experiences respiratory distress or has "shortness of breath," some of the conditions that can cause this feeling, and the treatment you will provide to these patients.

Emergency Dispatch

The light drizzle that had been falling on the ambulance windshield for an hour had just progressed to a steady downpour when the radio broke the silence.

"Unit 2, respond to 1163 Courtside Avenue for an adult male in respiratory distress."

"Unit 2, 10-4." Brent, a new EMT, switched on the windshield wipers and looked up and down the deserted street before pulling out and activating the emergency lights.

Brent and his partner, Joanne, first saw the patient as they rolled to a stop in front of the address. The man was sitting in the tripod position on the front steps of his home, drenched by the rain and waving his arm feebly.

"You . . . gotta . . . help . . . me." The man struggled with each word as they approached. The rain poured down onto them, soaking everything, including the stretcher.

"Quick, let's get him in the truck!" Joanne shouted, her words almost silenced by overhead thunder.

Thomas, the patient, was pale and struggling frantically to breathe. His eyes were wide with fear, and with each attempted breath he pounded on the plastic cabinet doors in the back of the ambulance.

"I'll get a nonrebreather," Brent said, sliding one of the compartment doors aside with a trembling hand.

"Forget that," Joanne said through a tangle of wet hair. "We're gonna have to bag him."

Respiratory Anatomy and Physiology Review

A sound knowledge of respiratory anatomy and physiology will allow you to understand the signs and symptoms presented by your patient. This knowledge will also help you understand some of the basic **pathophysiology** (disease processes) you will find when you obtain a patient history and find that the patient has had respiratory conditions in the past. See chapter 4, for further review of the respiratory system.

4-2.1 List the structure and function of the respiratory system.

✳ **pathophysiology**
the study of how disease affects normal body processes.

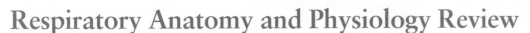

Moving oxygen into the bloodstream and to the tissues and the removal of waste products generated by the body is essential to life. This is the primary function of the respiratory system.

Air enters the body through the mouth and nose. The area behind the mouth is known as the oropharynx. The area behind the nose is the nasopharynx. Then the air moves into the larynx. The larynx contains the vocal cords and the entrance to the trachea. This opening is protected by the epiglottis (Figure 19-1). The epiglottis folds down during swallowing to prevent solids and liquids from entering the lungs. When foreign substances enter the lungs, it is referred to as **aspiration.**

The trachea splits into two mainstem bronchi. Each bronchus continues to split into smaller bronchioles, eventually ending at the alveoli (Figure 19-1). The alveoli are sacs whose appearance is often referred to as grape-like clusters. This is where the transfer of oxygen into the bloodstream and the removal of carbon dioxide from the blood stream are performed. The alveoli are very small. One blood cell at a time approaches one alveolus, and the exchange of oxygen and carbon dioxide takes place through their very thin walls. Of course there are millions of alveoli, enough to supply the body with oxygen even during times of exertion, such as running.

The lungs, positioned in the chest cavity, are covered by pleura. The **parietal pleura** is attached to the chest wall while the **visceral pleura** is attached to the surface of the lung. There is a "potential space" between these two layers, which is called the pleural cavity. In cases of chest injury, air or blood could enter this space and cause the partial or total collapse of a lung. Chapter 31 will discuss this type of injury in greater detail.

Dead space (Figure 19-2) in the lung is any place where oxygen is *not* exchanged—anywhere other than the alveoli. When air enters the body, it must travel through the mouth and nose, through the oropharynx and nasopharynx, into the larynx, the trachea, bronchi, and through bronchioles before the air reaches the alveoli. This means that about 150 mL of air you breathe in doesn't even reach the alveoli where the gas exchange—oxygen for carbon dioxide—takes place.

✳ **aspiration**

when foreign substances enter the lungs.

✳ **parietal pleura**

membrane that is attached to the chest wall.

✳ **visceral pleura**

membrane that is attached to the lung surface.

✳ **dead space**

areas of the lungs outside the alveoli where gas exchange with the blood does not take place.

FIGURE 19-1 Overview of the upper and lower airways.

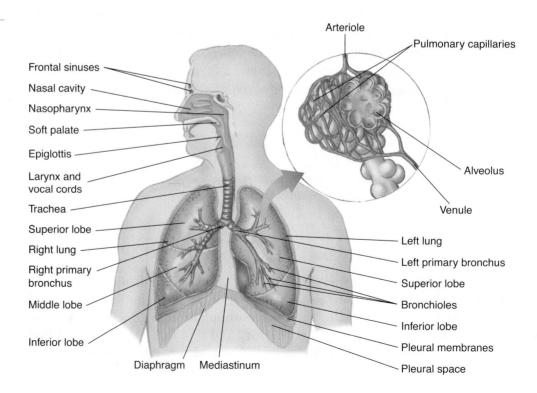

Frontal sinuses
Nasal cavity
Nasopharynx
Soft palate
Epiglottis
Larynx and vocal cords
Trachea
Superior lobe
Right lung
Right primary bronchus
Middle lobe
Inferior lobe
Diaphragm
Mediastinum

Arteriole
Pulmonary capillaries
Alveolus
Venule
Left lung
Left primary bronchus
Superior lobe
Bronchioles
Inferior lobe
Pleural membranes
Pleural space

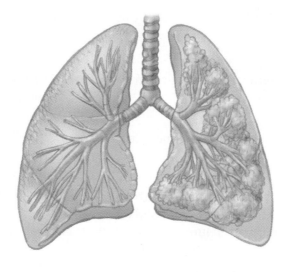

FIGURE 19-2 Dead space in the lung.

☐ Lung tissue

☐ Dead space (bronchi and bronchioles)

☐ Alveoli/gas exchange areas

The average inhalation by an adult is about 500 mL. Of this 500 ml, only about 350 ml actually reach the alveoli. This is normal. A problem develops when the patient begins to breathe shallowly. If only 200–250 ml of air is breathed in, very little gets to the alveoli for gas exchange. This is one cause of **hypoxia** as well as a cause of the build up of carbon dioxide, **hypercarbia.**

✳ **hypoxia**

an insufficiency of oxygen in the body's tissues.

✳ **hypercarbia**

excessive carbon dioxide in the blood.

 Stop, Review, Remember!

Multiple Choice

Place a check next to the correct answer.

1. Foreign substances entering the lungs is referred to as:

   _____ a. reflux.

   _____ b. pneumothorax.

   _____ c. inhalation.

   _____ d. aspiration.

2. Alveoli are often described as:

   _____ a. multi-cellular.

   _____ b. grape-like clusters.

   _____ c. pressure-filled vesicles.

   _____ d. venous-pressure driven.

3. Hypoxia is a reduced level of:

   _____ a. blood volume.

   _____ b. carbon dioxide in the blood.

   _____ c. oxygen in the blood.

   _____ d. hemoglobin.

Fill in the Blank

1. The area that is posterior to the mouth and above the larynx is called the _____.

2. Oxygen is transferred to the blood and waste products are removed in the _____.

3. The _____ is the tissue that folds over the tracheal opening to prevent solids and liquids from entering the lungs.

4. The lung has two pleura. The _____ pleura is attached to the chest wall; the _____ pleura is attached to the surface of the lungs.

5. Areas where no transfer of oxygen takes place in the lungs are called _____ .

Critical Thinking

1. Describe the structures air passes through from the point it enters the mouth/nose until it gets to the alveoli.

_____

_____

_____

_____

2. What is the main purpose of the respiratory system?

_____

_____

_____

_____

Assessment of the Respiratory Distress Patient

Respiratory distress, also called difficulty breathing or shortness of breath, is a common complaint seen by EMS providers. It is an extremely frightening feeling for your patient and one that almost always indicates some sort of serious underlying condition.

There are many levels of respiratory distress, ranging from very mild to those that involve inadequate breathing or pending respiratory arrest.

Unlike a broken bone, where you can look and see a deformity, breathing difficulties may not be as obvious. The patient's ability to speak, his body position and muscles used to breathe, the patient's history, and what he tells you will help form your assessment and treatment plan.

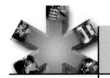

Perspective

Joanne—The EMT

"I tell you, sometimes the assessment is quick and simple. Like that guy in the rain. Was he breathing adequately? No. Did he need assistance right away? Definitely! Was I able to determine why he wasn't breathing right? No. Did I need to know the reason before I could help him? Obviously not."

PATIENT ASSESSMENT

The assessment of the respiratory distress patient includes assessments that must be done immediately (for example, Is the patient breathing? Is the breathing adequate?) and others that may be performed later in your assessment for example, history (Figures 19-3A and B).

Remember that you will assess breathing adequacy and apply oxygen during the initial assessment.

Scene Size-Up   The scene size-up can give you important information in reference to the patient with respiratory distress. As you approach the patient do you see home oxygen devices or medications? What position is the patient in? Positions such as the **tripod position** (Figure 19-4 on page 452) or the appearance of anxiety, restlessness, or altered mental status indicates a patient in serious condition.

Initial Assessment   During the initial assessment note the adequacy of breathing. Look for an adequate rate and depth of breathing. Note the work of breathing and look for use of **accessory muscles.** You may also listen with a stethoscope to determine if you hear air moving in and out of each lung and that it is equal on both sides. You may also note cyanosis or other poor skin colors (pale or grey) with diaphoresis.

4-2.2   State the signs and symptoms of a patient with breathing difficulty.

4-2.6   Establish the relationship between airway management and the patient with breathing difficulty.

4-2.7   List signs of adequate air exchange.

* **tripod position**

   position that may be assumed during respiratory distress to facilitate breathing. The patient usually sits or may stand or crouch, leaning forward with hands placed on the bed, chair, table, or knees.

* **accessory muscles**

   muscles in the neck, chest, back, and abdomen used to assist ventilations in respiratory distress.

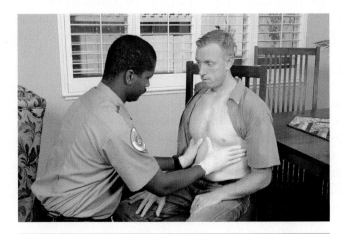

FIGURE 19-3A   Assess the adequacy of breathing. Assess both rate and depth.

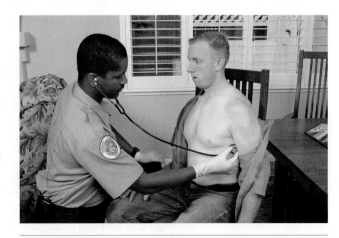

FIGURE 19-3B   Auscultate for adequate movement of air in and out of the lungs.

FIGURE 19-4   A patient in the tripod position.

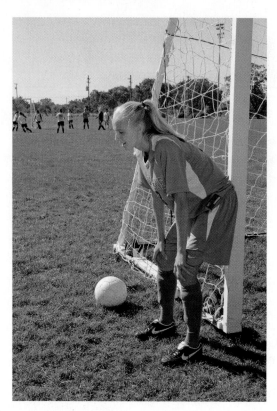

FIGURE 19-4   A patient in the tripod position.

If the patient with respiratory distress is breathing adequately, administer oxygen by nonrebreather mask. If the patient is breathing inadequately, or not at all, provide ventilations with a pocket face mask or BVM.

The patient's general appearance will also provide important clues about the level of respiratory distress. As already noted, poor skin signs such as pale, moist skin may indicate a patient in severe distress. Altered mental status is an early indicator of hypoxia or hypercarbia. This may range from anxiety to combativeness to a sleepy, head-bobbing appearance.

At the conclusion of the initial assessment, you will make a priority determination. High-priority patients include all patients with respiratory distress, but remember that patients with altered mental status, elevated pulse rates, poor skin color and diaphoresis, accessory muscle use, and inability to speak more than a few words at a time are very sick patients who may require ventilation with a BVM or pocket face mask and could be in imminent danger. See the next Clinical Clues box for additional signs of significant distress.

History   The history is important in any medical patient. Obtain a SAMPLE history. Use the OPQRST mnemonic to obtain information in reference to the signs and symptoms (See Table 19-1 on page 454).

The history is important because past conditions may provide clues to current problems. Medications taken by the patient will also be relevant to the patient's condition. You may be able to assist the patient with medications to help his distress. In medical patients, the history is often a greater source of information than the physical examination.

Respiratory problems are often a sign of underlying cardiac problems. Some patients having a heart attack may not have traditional signs and symptoms (e.g., chest pain or discomfort), and the only symptom is respiratory distress. In some

Clinical Clues: SIGNIFICANT RESPIRATORY DISTRESS

Clues your patient is in *significant* distress include:

* Altered mental status including unresponsiveness, sleepiness, head-bobbing, agitation, or anxiety
* Severe difficulty breathing including ability to speak only a few words per sentence or the inability to speak
* Poor skin color including pale, grey, or cyanotic (blue). Cool, moist skin
* Use of accessory muscles
* Abnormally slow or fast respiratory rates
* Increased pulse rate (pulse rate will decrease in pediatric patients)
* Shallow respirations with any respiratory rate
* Noisy breathing (usually audible even without a stethoscope) including **wheezing, gurgling, snoring,** and **stridor**

NOTE: All patients who present with respiratory distress are potentially a high priority. This list describes the patients who are in serious condition and unstable. Patients with *any* of these signs are serious—all signs do not have to be present.

* **wheezing**
  high-pitched, musical lung sounds created by air moving through constricted air passages.

* **gurgling**
  intermittent low-pitched sounds. Indicative of fluids in the upper airway.

* **snoring**
  intermittent low-pitched sounds heard during inhalation. Often indicative of partial upper airway obstruction caused by the tongue and associated soft tissue.

* **stridor**
  a harsh high-pitched sound that generally occurs during inhalation but can also occur during exhalation, indicative of partial upper airway obstruction.

cases the respiratory distress is what the patient notices most, but upon being asked, he may indicate that he has pain or discomfort in the chest, neck, jaw, or arm.

Vital Signs   You will assess vital signs every 5 minutes for the unstable patient and every 15 minutes for the stable patient. Many of your respiratory distress patients will be unstable and require the more frequent vital sign checks. Specific things to look for in vital signs include:

* Abnormal pulse rate—In response to hypoxia the heart rate will increase. In adult patients who are near death, and in pediatric patients as an earlier response to hypoxia, the pulse rate may be abnormally slow.

* Abnormal respiratory rate or depth—The respiratory rate will usually rise in the presence of respiratory distress. But be aware that abnormally high or low rates and low respiratory volumes may require ventilation.

* Skin color changes—The skin may become pale, cyanotic, cool, and moist.

Remember that it is a trend in vital signs over time that provides the most information.

Physical Examination   Your physical assessment of the patient continues what you started in the initial assessment. Patients in respiratory distress should be carefully and frequently monitored to detect inadequate breathing as soon as it begins. Observe the following:

* The patient's overall appearance—considered in the initial assessment and throughout the call. Look for anxiety, uneasiness, increased **work of breathing,** and positioning (for example, tripod).

* How many words the patient can speak before having to catch his breath. The fewer words spoken, the more serious the distress.

* **work of breathing**
  effort needed for adequate ventilation.

TABLE 19-1	**MEDICAL HISTORY—RESPIRATORY**

SAMPLE HISTORY

* S—Signs and Symptoms—Use the OPQRST mnemonic (below) to obtain this information.
* A—Allergies—Does the patient have any allergies? Anaphylaxis (allergic reactions) may cause respiratory distress.
* M—Medications—Ask the patient if he takes any medications. Find out when he last took his medications. Remember that you may be able to assist some patients with a prescribed inhaler.
* P—Past History—Does the patient have any medical problems? Any respiratory or cardiac problems? Ever experienced anything like this before? Has he been told he has asthma, emphysema, or chronic bronchitis?
* L—Last oral intake—When did the patient last eat or drink?
* E—Events—What was the patient doing when this came on?

OPQRST

* O—Onset—What were you doing when the distress began?
* P—Provocation—Does anything make the distress better or worse?
* Q—Quality—Can you describe the feeling you have?
* R—Radiation—Does the feeling seem to spread to any other part of your body? Do you have pain anywhere else?
* S—Severity—On a 1–10 scale (where 1 is best and 10 is worst) how would you rate your distress?
* T—Time—How long have you had this feeling? How long have you been in distress?

OTHER IMPORTANT QUESTIONS/PERTINENT NEGATIVES

* Do you have chest pain or discomfort?
* Do you have pain or discomfort in your neck, jaw, or arms?
* Have you ever had a heart problem?
* Have you noticed swollen ankles or weight gain recently?
* Have you had to sleep on more pillows recently?

✳ **pertinent negatives**

  questions that are important to know the answers to—even if the answer is no.

* Use of accessory muscles in the chest and neck.
* Listen to the patient's chest with a stethoscope. Listen for air entry in both sides of the chest. You should be able to hear air moving in and out on both sides. The sound should be equal between the two lungs. Some systems train EMTs to listen for and document abnormal sounds (for example, crackles or wheezes). These are described later in the chapter.

✳ **pulse oximetry**

  use of an electronic device, a pulse oximeter, to determine the amount of oxygen carried by the hemoglobin in the blood, known as the oxygen saturation or SpO_2.

* **Pulse oximetry** (Figure 19-5)—Many systems now have a pulse oximeter available on the ambulance. This device will determine the percent of hemoglobin in the blood that is saturated by oxygen. However, never withhold oxygen from a patient who appears to have respiratory distress, even

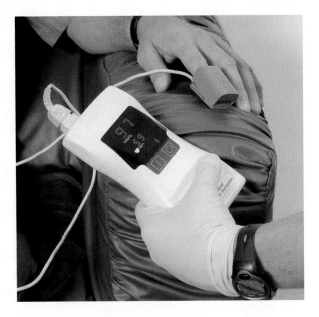

FIGURE 19-5   Pulse oximetry.

when his pulse oximeter readings are normal. The device is useful to show improvement or decline in the patient's condition (for example, increased "sats" after administration of oxygen). Generally readings below 95 percent indicate hypoxia. Readings below 90% indicating more severe hypoxia. As with any equipment: *Treat the patient, not the device.*

ABNORMAL BREATHING PATTERNS

There are several specific and identifiable abnormal breathing patterns that indicate serious underlying conditions. These patterns and the conditions that cause them are:

* ∗ **Cheyne-Stokes respirations**—Deep respirations alternating with very shallow respirations. There may also be periods of **apnea** in the cycles. Cheyne-Stokes are seen in patients who have brain injury or end-stage brain tumors (Figure 19-6A).

* ∗ **Central neurogenic hyperventilation**—Seen in head injuries or strokes that involve the brainstem. As the name implies there are very rapid, deep ventilations (Figure 19-6B).

* ∗ **Kussmaul's respirations**—Another presentation of rapid, deep ventilations, but this is usually caused by very acidic blood as in some diabetic conditions and aspirin overdose (Figure 19-6C).

∗ **Cheyne-Stokes respirations**
deep respirations alternating with very shallow respirations. There may also be a period of apnea in the cycles. Seen in patients who have brain injury or end-stage brain tumors.

∗ **apnea**
absence of any breathing or respiratory effort.

∗ **hyperventilation**
breathing that is abnormally rapid and deep.

∗ **central neurogenic hyperventilation**
very rapid, deep respirations usually caused by head injuries or strokes that involve the brainstem.

∗ **Kussmaul's respirations**
rapid, deep ventilations usually caused by very acidic blood such as some diabetic conditions and aspirin overdose.

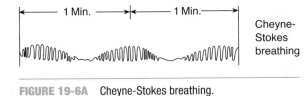

Cheyne-Stokes breathing

FIGURE 19-6A   Cheyne-Stokes breathing.

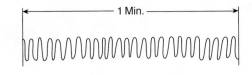

Central neurogenic hyperventilation

FIGURE 19-6B   Central neurogenic hyperventilation.

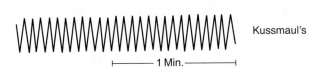

Kussmaul's

FIGURE 19-6C   Kussmaul's respirations.

✳ **asthma**

a disease that has attacks involving bronchoconstriction and mucus production with significant difficulty breathing.

✳ **bronchoconstriction**

constriction of the bronchioles in the lungs, caused by allergies, respiratory infections, exercise, or emotion.

✳ **triggers**

allergies, respiratory infections, exercise, or emotion that may cause bronchoconstriction.

✳ **mucus**

slippery secretion that lubricates and protects airway surfaces.

✳ **status asthmaticus**

prolonged, life-threatening asthma attack, often not responding to the patient's own medications.

✳ **chronic bronchitis**

condition where the lining of the bronchiole is inflamed. Excess mucus is formed and remains in the airway. The accumulations become severe as the body is unable to clear the mucus from the airway.

✳ **emphysema**

condition where the walls of the alveoli break down and lose surface area.

✳ **stale air**

air that remains in the alveoli increasing carbon dioxide levels in the lungs.

✳ **drive to breathe**

stimulation to breathe. Usually related to the level of carbon dioxide in the blood.

RESPIRATORY DISEASES AND CONDITIONS

There are some common respiratory diseases that you will encounter as an EMT. While it is not necessary to diagnose these conditions as you care for your patient, knowing about the diseases will help you communicate with the patient and health care providers about the patient's history and condition.

Asthma (Figure 19-7A) is a chronic lung disease that is characterized by periodic episodes of shortness of breath. That is, it doesn't affect the patient every day—just when there are attacks. Attacks are episodes of **bronchoconstriction** caused by **triggers** such as allergies, respiratory infections, exercise, or emotion. In cases of prolonged constriction **mucus** can develop and plug small airways, severely restricting air flow. Asthma attacks can be life threatening. **Status asthmaticus** is a prolonged, life-threatening asthma attack, that often does not respond to the patient's own medications.

Chronic bronchitis (Figure 19-7B) is a condition where the lining of the bronchiole is inflamed. Excess mucus is formed and remains in the airway. The accumulations become severe, because the body is unable to clear the mucus from the airway.

Emphysema (Figure 19-7C) is a condition where the walls of the alveoli break down and lose surface area. This significantly limits the ability to exchange gases in the alveoli and permits **stale air** to remain in the alveoli, increasing carbon dioxide levels in the lungs. Chronic bronchitis and emphysema are considered chronic obstructive pulmonary diseases (COPD).

Hypoxic Drive Normally, the **drive to breathe** is controlled by carbon dioxide levels in the blood. The body is stimulated to breathe when there is an excess of carbon dioxide and to *stop* breathing when carbon dioxide levels fall. In some

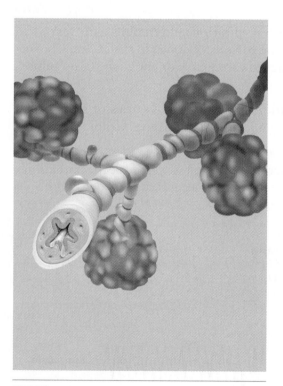

FIGURE 19-7A Asthma.

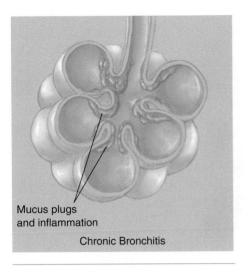

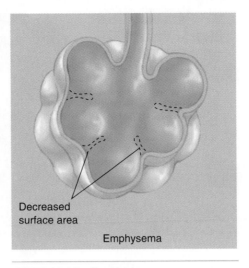

FIGURE 19-7B   Chronic bronchitis.

FIGURE 19-7C   Emphysema.

patients with COPDs such as emphysema, a **hypoxic drive** develops in which the body is stimulated to breathe by below-normal oxygen levels rather than by elevated carbon dioxide levels. In theory, patients with hypoxic drive may stop breathing with higher than normal oxygen levels in the blood. The concern is that when oxygen is administered to these patients, it may cause them to stop breathing.

Hypoxic drive is rare. The rule in EMS is to never withhold oxygen from a patient who needs it. This includes patients in respiratory distress with a COPD history. When patients with these conditions have difficulty breathing, they need oxygen. These patients can also have heart attacks and trauma—both of which require oxygen and aren't related to a respiratory problem.

In short, never withhold oxygen from a patient who needs it.

LUNG AUSCULTATION

Listening to the lungs with a stethoscope, called **auscultation,** can be done for two reasons: to listen for air movement in and out and to listen for abnormal sounds.

When listening for air movement, note whether the sound of air moving in and out is present as well as equal between both sides. This can be done by listening at the **midaxillary** line over both lungs.

Listening for abnormal sounds is more difficult. There are many sounds that can be heard in different areas of the chest. Locating and identifying a specific sound is challenging—especially in a moving ambulance. Auscultating lung sounds must be done in several areas of the lungs. Figures 19-8A and B on page 458 shows these areas. The left lung has two lobes while the right lung has three. You should listen over each area in the front and back. The bases of the lung are only effectively auscultated from the back. The specific abnormal lung sounds you may hear include:

✳ **Wheezing**—High pitched musical sounds created by air moving through constricted air passages. It is heard in asthma, emphysema, and chronic bronchitis. It can also be heard in some cases of **pulmonary edema.**

✳ **hypoxic drive**

when the stimulus to breathe is the amount of oxygen in the blood rather than the normal drive to breathe that is related to the amount of carbon dioxide in the blood.

✳ **auscultation**

assessment technique of listening, usually with a stethoscope.

✳ **midaxillary**

a line drawn vertically from the middle of the armpit to the ankle.

✳ **pulmonary edema**

a condition of fluid in the lungs.

FIGURE 19-8A Auscultate for breath sounds.

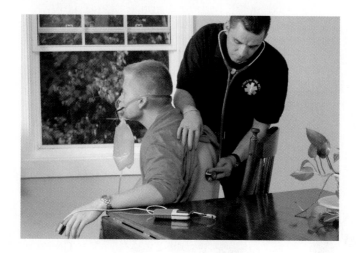

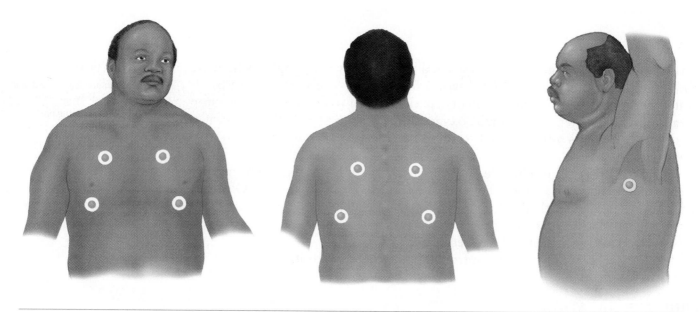

FIGURE 19-8B Auscultate for breath sounds on the upper and lower chest, the upper and lower back, and at the midaxillary line.

✳ **crackles**

lung sounds created in pulmonary edema when alveoli, closed because of fluid, open. They are usually heard on inspiration as fine crackling sounds.

✳ **rhonchi**

low-pitched snoring or rattling sounds caused by secretions in the larger airways. These may be seen in chronic lung diseases and possibly pneumonia.

✳ **Crackles**—These are the sounds created in pulmonary edema when alveoli, closed because of fluid, open. They are usually heard on inspiration as fine crackling sounds (as the name implies).

✳ **Rhonchi**—Lower-pitched snoring or rattling sounds caused by secretions in the larger airways. These may be seen in chronic lung diseases and possibly pneumonia.

✳ **Stridor**—A high pitched sound that is heard on inspiration. It indicates some sort of obstruction or narrowing of the upper airway (trachea or larynx).

Clinical Clues: LUNG SOUNDS

Listening to and evaluating lung sounds is challenging. Lung sounds should be evaluated in a quiet area (e.g., the patient's residence or in the ambulance—before leaving the scene, without the additional road noise). If you are going to evaluate lung sounds, realize, as with other vital signs, that it is how the sounds change over time that is important—especially when administering a medication. Listen before and after assisting or administering any medication and note changes.

One pitfall when listening to lung sounds is the "quiet chest." You may have a patient who had wheezes early in the call. Later in the call you note there are no more wheezes. This could be for one of two reasons: The patient has improved (as a result of a medication) or *the patient's respirations have become so shallow that there is not enough air moving in and out to make the wheezing noise any more.* This means that the patient's respirations are inadequate. If you simply thought "great, no more wheezing," you would falsely assume that the patient was better when he was actually developing inadequate breathing.

✳ Stop, Review, Remember!

Multiple Choice

Place a check next to the correct answer.

1. Which of the following is an indication of severe respiratory distress in adults?

   _____ a. warm, dry skin

   _____ b. speaking 6 or 8 words per breath

   _____ c. pulse rate of 128

   _____ d. respiratory rate of 10/minute

2. You are called to an agitated patient with a respiratory rate of 40/minute and shallow. You note poor skin color. His wife tells you he complained of difficulty breathing about an hour ago and has worsened. What device would you use to treat this patient's condition?

   _____ a. nasal cannula

   _____ b. simple face mask

   _____ c. nonrebreather mask

   _____ d. bag-valve mask

3. Cyanosis is a _____ color of the skin and/or mucous membranes.

   _____ a. black

   _____ b. pink

   _____ c. pale

   _____ d. blue

4. Hypoxic drive is best described as the body:

   _____ a. liking carbon dioxide more than oxygen.

   _____ b. using increased levels of oxygen as a drive to breathe.

   _____ c. using low oxygen levels as the drive to breathe.

   _____ d. using low carbon monoxide levels as the drive to breathe.

5. Emphysema is a chronic obstructive pulmonary disease (COPD).

_____ a. true

_____ b. false

6. Chronic bronchitis is a condition where the lining of the bronchiole is inflamed.

_____ a. true

_____ b. false

Fill in the Blank

1. OPQRST stands for O_____, P_____, Q_____, R_____, S_____, T_____.

2. A question that would be appropriate for the "Q" in OPQRST is: Can you _____ the distress?

3. A patient who is sitting up and leaning forward with his hands on his knees is said to be in the _____ position.

4. When determining whether the breathing is adequate or not, it is important to check both _____ and _____.

5. A patient in respiratory distress who is breathing adequately would be given oxygen via _____.

Critical Thinking

1. Why are a patient's medical history and current medications important?

_____

_____

_____

_____

_____

2. What generally provides more information for a responsive medical patient: history or physical examination? Why?

_____

_____

_____

_____

_____

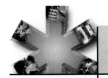

Perspective

Thomas—The Patient

"I honestly thought that I was going to die. It was what I imagine trying to take deep breaths underwater would be like. Just a struggle, you know? At first I can remember being frustrated with the ambulance people . . . then I was just angry. It seemed like it took forever for them to get to my house, and then they started asking me all of these questions. It was no use, though. I just couldn't talk. I know that they were just doing their jobs and all, but while they're going through their checklist steps and hooking up whatever little things that they hook up, I'm losing my life. I had a lot more at stake than they did. All that aside, though, I probably wouldn't be here right now without them. I guess I can't overlook that."

Care of the Respiratory Distress Patient

Your care of the respiratory distress patient is vital and begins with your actions in the initial assessment. During the initial assessment, you will ensure a patent airway and adequate breathing—efforts that must be continued through the entire call. You will apply oxygen or administer ventilations as necessary and will suction the patient if excess fluids or solids make him unable to maintain his own airway.

4-2.3 Describe the emergency medical care of the patient with breathing difficulty.

The final step in the initial assessment is determining a patient priority. For patients with a high priority for transport, prompt transportation is part of a treatment plan. This should be done concurrently with the focused history and vitals when possible.

Take the following steps:

* Complete an initial assessment. Ventilate and suction the patient if necessary. A patient who is adequately breathing with a patent airway will receive oxygen by nonrebreather mask. A patient with minor distress or severe anxiety when a mask is placed on his face may receive oxygen by nasal cannula. Follow local protocols.

4-2.5 Describe the emergency medical care of the patient with breathing distress.

* Realize that difficulty breathing is very scary to the patient. Patients who are hypoxic may also be anxious and argumentative. Reassure the patient and provide emotional care and patience as you meet and care for him.

* Determine a patient priority. If the patient is a high priority for transport, begin preparation for transport while completing the next steps.

* Patients who are breathing adequately should be allowed to assume a position of comfort. When on the stretcher, this is often a sitting position or on a stretcher with the head elevated. Once a patient's breathing becomes inadequate, you will choose the correct patient position to provide ventilations for him.

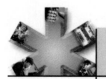

Perspective

Brent—The EMT

"That was a scary call for me. I had never seen someone that bad off. Any second I expected him to just die. Right there in front of me. I know that you can only struggle to breathe for so long before your body just gives up. And if he wasn't at that point, he was right on the line. I was trying to be calm, though, but that kind of backfired. I was moving too slow and I could tell that the patient knew it. And every time that I told him to calm down and try to inhale as I squeezed the BVM, he looked up at me like . . . like if he had the energy he'd kick my butt or something! I definitely learned a lot on that call. All in all, though, even though I feel I didn't do everything perfectly, I know that we made a difference for that guy."

✳ Perform a focused history and physical examination. Obtain a SAMPLE history from the patient or family members/bystanders.

✳ Assist the patient with his prescribed inhaler if the patient meets the indications in protocols and medical direction approves. (See the information on administering a prescribed inhaler later in the chapter.) Many patients now have home **nebulizers** with which you may also be able to assist. Check with your instructor and consult local protocol.

✳ Perform ongoing assessments frequently en route to the hospital.

✳ **nebulizers**

devices that continuously administer a vaporized medication, as opposed to the inhaler that provides a one-time dose.

4-2.9 Distinguish between the emergency medical care of the infant, child, and adult patient with breathing difficulty.

4-2.10 Differentiate between upper airway obstruction and lower airway disease in the infant and child patient.

✳ **croup**

viral illness characterized by inspiratory and expiratory stridor and a seal-barklike cough.

Respiratory Distress in Infants and Children

You may be called to help infants and children who experience respiratory distress. There are some significant differences between the adult and child patient. Often the lungs of an adult have undergone years of abuse from smoking and/or occupational or environmental exposure to substances that harm the lungs. Adults will have more chronic respiratory diseases, such as emphysema and chronic bronchitis. Also, normal breathing rates for infants and children are faster than an adult's.

You will see certain diseases more often in children. Children experience infectious diseases of the upper airway such as **croup** and infections of the lower airways such as pneumonia. Asthma often begins at an early age. You must also be aware of the potential for foreign body airway obstruction in small children, especially toddlers.

Clinical Clues: INFANTS AND CHILDREN

Remember that an abnormally low pulse rate in an infant or child with respiratory distress is a sign of inadequate oxygen (hypoxia) that requires immediate intervention.

Your care for the infant or child patient will be similar to an adult's in that you will provide oxygen, reassurance, and transport. There will, of course, be differences in the way you would comfort an infant or child patient. Many times, a younger patient will not tolerate an oxygen mask or understand why it is on his face. Dosages for assisted medications will be less for pediatric patients, or inhalers will dispense a specific pediatric dose.

Chapter 36 covers pediatric respiratory assessment and care in detail.

Transportation of the Patient with Respiratory Distress

Patient positioning is a key part of patient care for the respiratory distress patient. Attempting to have a patient in this condition lie down may cause considerable anxiety and worsen his condition. Because of this, the choice of an appropriate transportation device is critical.

In many cases your wheeled stretcher will not fit through some doorways and around corners. There are two basic choices for transporting a patient to the stretcher: sitting up or lying down. The stair chair is the device of choice for patients who are breathing adequately and would be made worse by lying down (Figure 19-9). Patients who require ventilation are often transported on a Reeves stretcher or backboard to the stretcher. Remember: *It is inappropriate to have respiratory patients walk to the stretcher.* Any unnecessary exertion will make the condition worse.

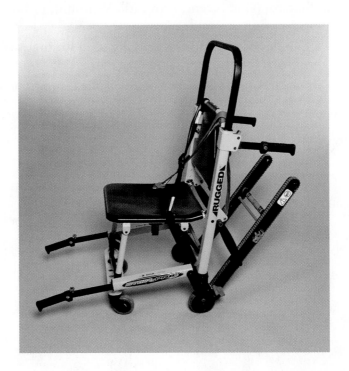

FIGURE 19-9   A stair chair.

4-2.8 State the generic name, medication forms, dose, administration, action, indications, and contraindications for the prescribed inhaler.

Respiratory Medications and Administration Devices

Respiratory medications generally take two forms: medications to help improve breathing immediately by dilating the bronchioles and medications that help over a long time by preventing attacks (for example, steroids). It is important to be sure that you administer the correct type of medication to a patient who is having difficulty breathing. Medications of each type are listed in Table 19-2. The most common medication used in inhalers and nebulizers is albuterol.

Medications may be administered by inhaler (Figure 19-10) or by small-volume nebulizer (SVN) (Figure 19-11). Both work effectively in administering medications. Patients with more severe or chronic (long-term) conditions are more likely to have a nebulizer. The medications used in the different devices are the same but can differ in dosage.

4-2.4 Recognize the need for medical direction to assist in the emergency medical care of the patient with breathing difficulty.

ADMINISTERING OR ASSISTING WITH RESPIRATORY MEDICATIONS

As an EMT, your ability to administer or assist patients with administering medications is based on protocols and approval of medical direction. These vary widely from region to region. Your instructor will explain the protocols and reg-

TABLE 19-2 RESPIRATORY MEDICATIONS
Examples of medications used in emergencies to improve breathing: albuterol (Combivent, Proventil, Ventolin), pirbuterol acetate (Maxair), ipratroprium bromide (Atrovent) **Examples of medications that are used for long-term prevention of breathing problems** (not to be used in acute attacks): flunisolide (AeroBid), beclomethasone dipropionate (Vanceril), fluticasone and salmeterol (Advair)

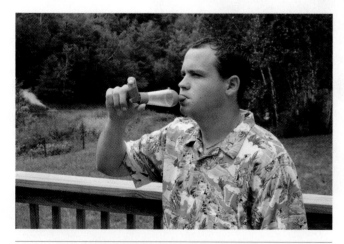

FIGURE 19-10 A prescribed inhaler with an attached spacer may help a patient who has respiratory problems.

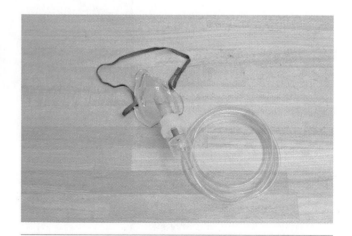

FIGURE 19-11 A small-volume nebulizer with a mask attached.

ulations in your area and will explain the use of the two devices already mentioned: the prescribed inhaler and the small-volume nebulizer (SVN).

Before considering or beginning the administration of any medication you must consider the six "rights": right medication, right dose, right route, right patient, right time, right documentation. Don't forget that sixth right: The patient's condition both before and after the medication administration must be documented.

Administering medications also involves indications and contraindications. Indications for administration of respiratory medications include:

✳ The patient is exhibiting signs of a respiratory emergency (for example, short of breath or wheezing)

✳ The patient has a medication prescribed to him for this respiratory condition

✳ Medical direction (either on-line or by protocol) has approved the use of this medication.

General contraindications include:

✳ Inability of the patient to use the device (for example, patient is unresponsive or breathing inadequately)

✳ Device or medication is not prescribed to the patient

✳ Medical direction does not approve of the administration

✳ The patient has already exceeded the maximum dose

✳ The medication is inappropriate for the treatment of acute breathing difficulty, such as an inhaled corticosteroid.

PRESCRIBED INHALER

The prescribed inhaler, also known as a **metered-dose inhaler,** is a device that patients use to breathe in medication (Figure 19-12). The medication is very effective because it is breathed into the lungs directly and acts immediately—much better and faster than a pill that would take time to be digested and absorbed.

The prescribed inhaler contains a fine powder that is inhaled directly into the lungs. Because this is a fine powder—not a gas—that is inhaled, it is *critical* that the inhaler be used properly. If the inhaler spray isn't timed properly with breathing (that is, activating the inhaler after beginning a deep breath), the

✳ **metered-dose inhaler**
device that patients use to breathe in medication.

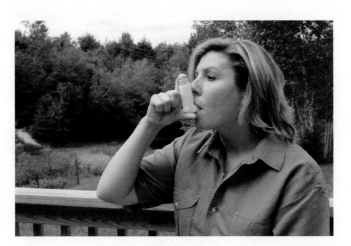

FIGURE 19-12 A metered-dose inhaler.

FIGURE 19-13 A spacer device attached to a metered-dose inhaler.

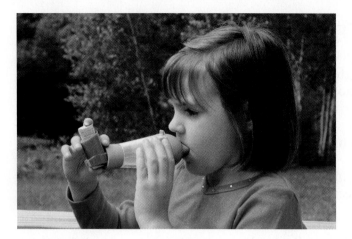

FIGURE 19-13 A spacer device attached to a metered-dose inhaler.

powder will deposit on the moist membranes of the mouth and tongue and not enter the lungs. A device called a spacer helps eliminate the need for such exact timing (Figure 19-13).

Inhalers can have side effects. Since the medication works on the **sympathetic nervous system,** it is possible that the patient's pulse will increase and the patient may feel anxious or jittery after taking the medication.

To use a prescribed inhaler (Scan 19-1):

* Obtain an order from medical direction or assure the patient and medication meet the criteria of your standing orders.

* Verify the six "rights."

* Check the inhaler for the expiration date.

* Verify that the patient has not exceeded the maximum dosage.

* Ensure that the inhaler is at room temperature or warmer.

* Shake the inhaler several times.

* Remove any oxygen mask or device from the patient and have him exhale deeply.

* Have the patient put his lips around the inhaler and begin to inhale deeply.

* Have the patient depress the handheld inhaler as he continues to inhale deeply.

* Instruct the patient to hold his breath for as long as he comfortably can, which allows the medication to be absorbed.

* Replace the nonrebreather mask or other oxygen device.

* Wait for several breaths and administer a second dose if approved by medical direction or protocol.

After administering a prescribed inhaler, or any medication, reassess the patient. Assess the patient's respiratory distress. Observe the patient for any changes in signs such as work of breathing, accessory muscle use, and ability to speak. Observe for changes in vital signs. Document any changes you observe (the sixth "right").

* **sympathetic nervous system**

part of the nervous system that activates the "fight or flight" response.

USING A PRESCRIBED INHALER

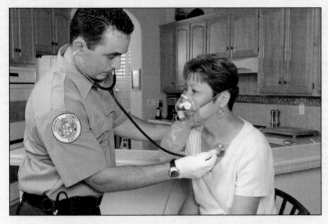

▲ Assess the patient's breathing and obtain a patient history.

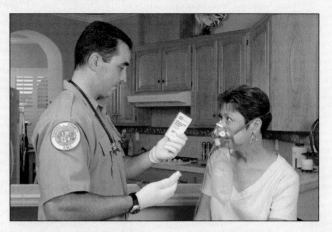

▲ Check the patient's medication to verify the "six rights."

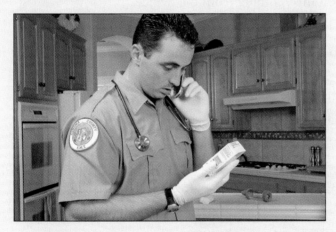

▲ Contact medical direction before administering the medication.

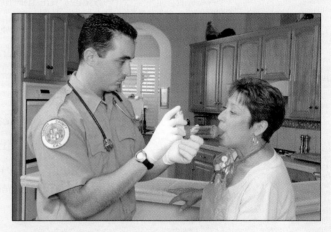

▲ Assist the patient in using the inhaler properly.

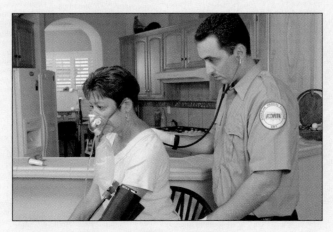

▲ Reassess the patient's breathing and vital signs.

SMALL-VOLUME NEBULIZER

✳ **small-volume nebulizer (SVN)**

method of continuously administering a vaporized medication, as opposed to the inhaler that provides a one-time dose.

The **small-volume nebulizer (SVN)** (Figures 19-14A and B) is a method of continuously administering a medication—as opposed to the inhaler that provides a one-time dose. The nebulizer works by having the patient inhale oxygen (or sometimes air) that has been run through a liquid medication. This creates a vapor containing the medication. SVNs are commonly found in the homes of patients with chronic respiratory conditions and those who have frequent attacks.

You may be allowed to assist the patient in the set-up and use of the SVN. In some regions, EMTs have begun carrying medications like albuterol on the ambulance to administer to patients via SVN after contacting medical direction.

The medications given via SVN are often the same medications contained in inhalers—just given in different form. The indications, contraindications, and side effects are similar.

To administer a medication via SVN (Scan 19-2):

✳ Obtain an order from medical direction to administer the medication.

✳ Assure the six "rights."

✳ Be sure there are no contraindications to administering the medication.

✳ Put the liquid medication in the chamber.

✳ Attach oxygen tubing to the chamber and set the flow rate at 6–8 lpm.

✳ Observe the medication mist coming from the device.

✳ Have the patient seal his lips around the mouthpiece and breathe deeply.

✳ Instruct the patient to hold his breath for a few seconds after breathing if possible.

✳ Continue until the medication is gone from the chamber.

✳ Reassess the patient's level of distress and vital signs.

✳ Document the patient's response to the medication (the sixth "right").

✳ Additional doses may be ordered by medical direction if the patient is still in distress and there have been no adverse effects from the medication.

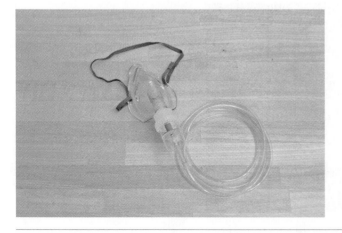

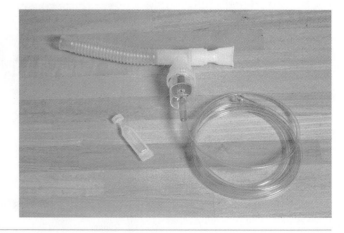

FIGURE 19-14   (A) A small-volume nebulizer (SVN) with an attached mask.   (B) A small-volume nebulizer with mouthpiece.

SCAN 19-2 USING A SMALL-VOLUME NEBULIZER (SVN)

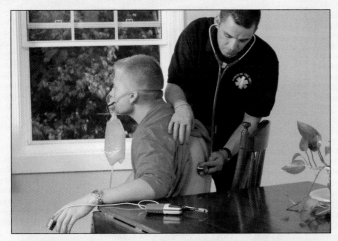

▲ Identify the patient as a candidate for nebulized medication per protocol (for example, history of asthma with respiratory distress). Administer oxygen and assess vital signs. Be sure the patient is not allergic to the medication.

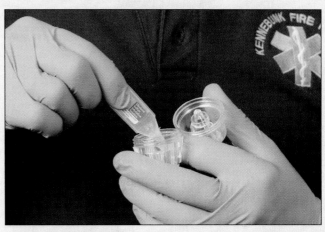

▲ Ensure the six "rights" (right medication, right dose, right route, right patient, right time, right documentation). Prepare the nebulizer. Put the liquid medication in the chamber. Attach the oxygen flow for 6–8 liters per minute (or according to the manufacturer's recommendations).

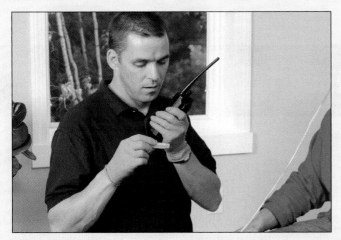

▲ Obtain permission from medical direction to administer or assist with the medication.

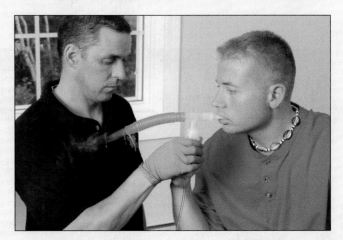

▲ Have the patient seal his lips around the mouthpiece and breathe deeply. Instruct the patient to hold his breath for 2 to 3 seconds if possible. Continue until medication is gone from the chamber.

(continued on the next page)

✳✳✳✳✳✳✳✳✳✳✳✳✳✳✳✳✳✳✳✳

SCAN 19-2 | **USING A SMALL-VOLUME NEBULIZER (SVN)—(continued)**

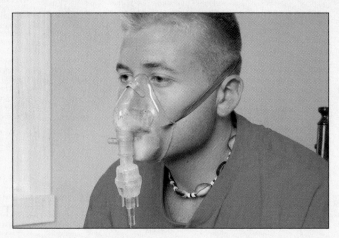

▲ Alternative device; A mask delivers the medication.

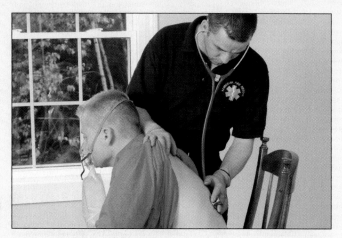

▲ Reassess the patient's level of distress and vital signs. Additional doses may be authorized by medical direction if the patient continues to be in distress and the patient is not having adverse effects from the medication.

✳ Stop, Review, Remember!

Multiple Choice

Place a check next to the correct answer.

1. Which of the following is not a common side effect of a prescribed inhaler?

    _____ a. tremors

    _____ b. decreased pulse

    _____ c. jittery feeling

    _____ d. anxiety

2. Why is timing breathing important when using an inhaler?

    _____ a. The medication is a fine powder and must get to the lungs.

    _____ b. The medication is a gas, but since it is lighter than air it must be forcefully inhaled.

    _____ c. The medication has a short half-life once out of the inhaler.

    _____ d. none of the above

3. Which of the following is NOT a sign of hypoxia?

   _____   a. elevated pulse rate

   _____   b. pink skin color

   _____   c. elevated respiratory rate

   _____   d. anxiety

Fill in the Blank

1. SVN stands for _____ _____ _____.

2. You may assist a patient with his inhaler with approval from _____ _____.

3. A _____ may be attached to an inhaler to improve the inhalation of medication.

4. Adequately breathing patients with respiratory distress generally prefer being transported in a _____ position.

5. You can only assist patients with medication that is _____ to them.

Critical Thinking

1. List the six "rights" of medication administration.

   _____

   _____

   _____

   _____

   _____

   _____

2. You are caring for a patient with emphysema who is having significant respiratory distress. You begin to administer oxygen, but your partner says, "No, he may have a hypoxic drive." Should you administer oxygen? Why or why not?

   _____

   _____

   _____

   _____

   _____

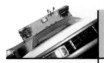

Dispatch Summary

The patient was loaded into the ambulance and a BVM with supplemental O_2 was used to assist his ventilations until an ALS unit could arrive and provide more advanced care.

The patient remained in the hospital for several days before being released back home with two inhalers—one to use in an emergency and another (a steroid) to prevent future attacks.

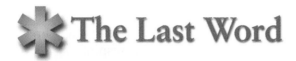

The Last Word

Patients experiencing respiratory distress should be considered to be in a serious condition—not only because of the medical problems that cause difficulty breathing but also because patients with difficulty breathing sincerely believe that they will die unless they are able to breathe easily again. The feeling of not being able to breathe is terrifying.

In chapter 7, and again in this chapter, you learned about adequate versus inadequate breathing. This is one of the most important determinations you will make as an EMT. You will see patients in various levels of respiratory distress. Remember that anxiety, poor skin color, and an elevated pulse are all signs of significant hypoxia.

Oxygen is the universal treatment for patients with respiratory distress. Provide high-concentration oxygen via nonrebreather mask for patients with respiratory distress. If you use a pulse oximeter, never withhold oxygen because of a high oxygen saturation reading. You may be allowed to assist a patient with his inhaler or, in some areas, to provide nebulized albuterol as a pharmacological treatment for respiratory distress.

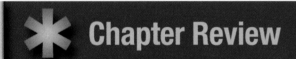

Chapter Review

MULTIPLE CHOICE

Place a check next to the correct answer.

1. The respiratory disease that results in constriction of the bronchioles as a result of allergies, exercise, or emotional stress is called:

   _____ a. emphysema.

   _____ b. chronic bronchitis.

   _____ c. hyperventilation.

   _____ d. asthma.

2. Which of the following is NOT part of the initial assessment of the respiratory patient?

   _____ a. checking for bleeding

   _____ b. administering oxygen

   _____ c. obtaining a pulse rate

   _____ d. determining adequacy of breathing

3. Inhaled medications that open up constricted bronchioles are called:

_____ a. bronchospastics.

_____ b. broncholytic.

_____ c. bronchodilators.

_____ d. bronchocompliant.

4. The grape-like clusters of sacs where gas is exchanged in the lungs are called:

_____ a. alveoli.

_____ b. bronchioles.

_____ c. capillaries.

_____ d. pulmonary venules.

5. You are called to a "sick person" at 4224 Malaprop Circle. You arrive to find an older man in a chair. His chin is on his chest. He is pale and sweaty. He only groans when you loudly ask him what is wrong. To begin care you should:

_____ a. open his airway in the chair.

_____ b. apply oxygen by nonrebreather mask.

_____ c. move the patient to the floor.

_____ d. determine a history from a family member.

6. Which of the following is one of the six "rights"?

_____ a. Right preparation

_____ b. Right patient

_____ c. Right location

_____ d. Right form of medication

7. A patient is complaining of difficulty breathing. He awoke short of breath. He reports that he has been sleeping on more pillows recently and has noticed weight gain and "puffy" ankles. You suspect his condition is:

_____ a. asthma.

_____ b. chronic bronchitis.

_____ c. congestive heart failure.

_____ d. emphysema.

8. You are called to a 68-year-old male who is complaining of shortness of breath. It began after he ran to the mailbox and back in the rain, and it hasn't subsided for 15 minutes. He is breathing 24 times per minute. You hear air moving in and out of both lungs. The patient is able to speak about 6 or 7 words before having to catch his breath. He looks a bit anxious. This patient should receive oxygen by:

_____ a. nasal cannula at 2 lpm.

_____ b. nasal cannula at 6 lpm.

_____ c. nonrebreather mask at 15 lpm.

_____ d. bag-valve mask with supplemental oxygen and reservoir.

9. You are assisting a patient with her prescribed inhaler. You should instruct the patient to do which of the following before activating the inhaler?

_____ a. Inhale half way, then stop and activate the inhaler.

_____ b. Exhale fully, then activate the inhaler.

_____ c. Activate the inhaler, then breathe in deeply.

_____ d. Begin to breathe in deeply, then activate the inhaler.

10. Which of the following questions or examinations would be most appropriate in the assessment of a patient with difficulty breathing?

_____ a. "Can you wiggle your fingers and toes?"

_____ b. checking pupillary reaction

_____ c. "Do you have any chest tightness or discomfort?"

_____ d. palpating abdominal quadrants

MATCHING

Match the respiratory physical exam finding on the left with the definition on the right.

1. _____ Stridor

2. _____ Wheezes

3. _____ Rhonchi

4. _____ Crackles

5. _____ Pedal edema

6. _____ Jugular venous distention

A. Distention of veins in the neck
B. Fluid accumulation in the ankles
C. Sound caused by alveoli opening
D. High-pitched upper airway sound
E. High-pitched, musical sound
F. Rattling sound

Match the patient presentation with the appropriate oxygen administration device.

1. _____ A 17-year-old male patient who fell from a moving truck and appears to have multiple fractures.

2. _____ A 78-year-old man who complains of chest pain and has a history of emphysema.

3. _____ A 42-year-old male patient who is believed to have overdosed on a pain reliever. He is sleepy and has respirations of 6/minute and shallow.

4. _____ An extremely anxious 66-year-old female patient with a history of severe congestive heart failure who is breathing 44 times per minute.

5. _____ An 82-year-old male patient who was complaining of chest pain and has now stopped breathing.

6. _____ A 32-year-old male with a history of panic attacks who complains of difficulty breathing.

7. _____ A 27-year-old man who was hit in the chest with a baseball bat. He is conscious, alert, and breathing deeply at 20/minute.

8. _____ A 13-year-old female having an asthma attack. The patient is breathing at 24/minute. You hear lung sounds bilaterally.

9. _____ A 69-year-old woman complaining of fatigue and difficulty breathing. Her respirations are 16 and a bit shallow.

10. _____ A 59-year-old male in an automobile collision with significant MOI. He complains of slight pain to his neck and nothing else. Pulse 104, respirations 20 and deep.

A. Nonrebreather mask at 15 lpm
B. BVM with supplemental oxygen
C. No oxygen required

CRITICAL THINKING

1. Why might a patient who is conscious and breathing require ventilation with a BVM or pocket face mask?

_____

_____

_____

_____

2. Can you really tell that a patient with respiratory distress is in serious condition (sick) as you approach the patient and before you examine him?

_____

_____

_____

_____

3. Why are pulse and skin color so important as signs of respiratory distress?

_____

_____

_____

_____

CASE STUDIES

Case Study 1

Your ambulance is dispatched to a call for a patient experiencing respiratory distress at a local assisted-living facility. You arrive at a safe scene and find the female patient sitting in a wheelchair just inside the door. Her husband is sitting on the couch with his walker nearby.

You introduce yourself to the patient, who seems only slightly short of breath. Her name is Marie. She holds a handful of tissues she has been bringing up phlegm into. "I haven't been feeling that well," she says. "I've had a cough and some breathing problems." She brings up a sizeable wad of phlegm and spits it into the tissues. It is off-white with yellow streaks. "See." Her skin is pink, warm, and dry. She is talking in full sentences, and her pulse at the wrist feels slightly rapid.

A short distance away, her husband, Frank, is trying to get off the sofa and is reaching for his walker. He is a big man and doesn't seem very steady on his feet. As you note this, Janice, one of the health aides, comes in with copies of some paperwork for the hospital. She is talking with a patient in the next room. "OK, Mr. Henry. I'll be right there. Just let me check on Marie."

1. Is Marie breathing adequately? Why?

_____

_____

_____

_____

2. How much oxygen would you place Marie on and by which device?

_____

_____

_____

_____

3. Do you have any responsibility to help her husband? What help does he need?

_____

_____

_____

_____

4. If the health aide tells you Marie has an inhaler, would you use it? Why or why not?

_____

_____

_____

_____

Case Study 2

You are called to a college running track for a patient with difficulty breathing. You find a 19-year-old female standing but leaning forward with her hands on her knees. The phys ed teacher tells you that she has asthma. The patient is able to speak to you and confirms the history of asthma.

1. Which of the following would indicate severe respiratory distress in this asthma patient?
   a. pulse of 128/min
   b. ability to speak only 6 or 7 words without catching her breath
   c. oxygen saturation of 97 percent
   d. wheezes with adequate air exchange

2. All of the following are indications for assisting with a prescribed inhaler EXCEPT:
   a. patient experiencing respiratory difficulty.
   b. patient with inadequate breathing.
   c. inhaler prescribed to the patient.
   d. medical direction approves of its use.

Case Study 3

You are called to a patient with respiratory distress. You arrive to find a patient sitting in a chair, slumped slightly to the side. You note that the patient is an 80-year-old male who responds only by slight groaning to very loud stimulus. He is limp and his skin is pale, cool, and moist.

1. To assess the airway of the patient above you should:
   a. open the airway and evaluate breathing in the chair.
   b. open the airway, listen for breathing, and auscultate lung sounds in the chair before moving the patient.
   c. move the patient to the floor, open the airway, and evaluate breathing.
   d. move the patient to the stretcher and perform the airway and breathing assessments en route to the hospital. This is a critical patient.

2. In this patient you are likely to find:
   a. adequate breathing.
   b. inadequate breathing.
   c. central neurogenic hyperventilation.
   d. normal breathing.

3. This patient would receive an ongoing assessment at least every _____ minutes.
   a. 5
   b. 10
   c. 15
   d. 20

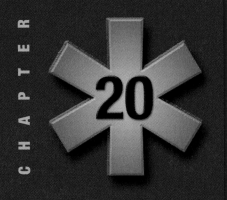

CHAPTER 20

Patients with Cardiac Problems

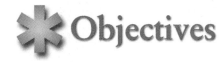

Objectives

Numbered objectives are from the U.S. Department of Transportation 1994 EMT-Basic National Standard Curriculum.

COGNITIVE OBJECTIVES

At the completion of this lesson, the EMT-Basic student will be able to:

4-3.1   Describe the structure and function of the cardiovascular system. (pp. 481–485)

4-3.2   Describe the emergency medical care of the patient experiencing chest pain or discomfort. (pp. 501–506)

4-3.3   List the indications for automated external defibrillation. (p. 509)

4-3.4   List the contraindications for automated external defibrillation. (p. 510)

4-3.5   Define the role of EMT-B in the emergency cardiac care system. (pp. 485–486)

4-3.6   Explain the impact of age and weight on defibrillation. (p. 509)

4-3.7   Discuss the position of comfort for patients with various cardiac emergencies. (p. 496)

4-3.8   Establish the relationship between airway management and the patient with cardiovascular compromise. (p. 494)

4-3.9   Predict the relationship between the patient experiencing cardiovascular compromise and basic life support. (pp. 486–487)

4-3.10   Discuss the fundamentals of early defibrillation. (pp. 508–509)

4-3.11   Explain the rationale for early defibrillation. (p. 508)

4-3.12   Explain that not all chest pain patients result in cardiac arrest and do not need to be attached to an automated external defibrillator. (p. 508)

4-3.13   Explain the importance of prehospital ACLS intervention if it is available. (p. 487)

4-3.14   Explain the importance of urgent transport to a facility with advanced cardiac life support if it is not available in the prehospital setting. (p. 487)

4-3.15   Discuss the various types of automated external defibrillators. (p. 512)

4-3.16   Differentiate between the fully automated and the semiautomated defibrillator. (p. 512)

4-3.17   Discuss the procedures that must be taken into consideration for standard operations of the various types of automated external defibrillators. (p. 514)

4-3.18   State the reasons for assuring that the patient is pulseless and apneic when using the automated external defibrillator. (p. 509)

4-3.19   Discuss the circumstances which may result in inappropriate shocks. (p. 510)

4-3.20   Explain the considerations for interruption of CPR when using the automated external defibrillator. (p. 516)

4-3.21   Discuss the advantages and disadvantages of automated external defibrillators. (p. 509)

4-3.22   Summarize the speed of operation of automated external defibrillation. (p. 508)

4-3.23   Discuss the use of remote defibrillation through adhesive pads. (p. 509)

4-3.24   Discuss the special considerations for rhythm monitoring. (p. 509)

4-3.25   List the steps in the operation of the automated external defibrillator. (p. 514)

4-3.26   Discuss the standard of care that should be used to provide care to a patient with persistent ventricular fibrillation and no available ACLS. (p. 514)

4-3.27 Discuss the standard of care that should be used to provide care to a patient with recurrent ventricular fibrillation and no available ACLS. (p. 514)

4-3.28 Differentiate between the single rescuer and multi-rescuer care with an automated external defibrillator. (p. 514)

4-3.29 Explain the reason for pulses not being checked between shocks with an automated external defibrillator. (p. 512)

4-3.30 Discuss the importance of coordinating ACLS trained providers with personnel using automated external defibrillators. (p. 514)

4-3.31 Discuss the importance of post-resuscitation care. (p. 516)

4-3.32 List the components of post-resuscitation care. (p. 516)

4-3.33 Explain the importance of frequent practice with the automated external defibrillator. (pp. 519–520)

4-3.34 Discuss the need to complete the Automated Defibrillator: Operator's Shift Checklist. (pp. 517–518)

4-3.35 Discuss the role of the American Heart Association (AHA) in the use of automated external defibrillation. (pp. 485, 519)

4-3.36 Explain the role medical direction plays in the use of automated external defibrillation. (p. 519)

4-3.37 State the reasons why a case review should be completed following the use of the automated external defibrillator. (p. 519)

4-3.38 Discuss the components that should be included in a case review. (p. 519)

4-3.39 Discuss the goal of quality improvement in automated external defibrillation. (p. 519)

4-3.40 Recognize the need for medical direction of protocols to assist in the emergency medical care of the patient with chest pain. (p. 503)

4-3.41 List the indications for the use of nitroglycerin. (p. 503)

4-3.42 State the contraindications and side effects for the use of nitroglycerin. (p. 505)

4-3.43 Define the function of all controls on an automated external defibrillator, and describe event documentation and battery defibrillator maintenance. (pp. 512–519)

AFFECTIVE OBJECTIVES

At the completion of this lesson, the EMT-Basic student will be able to:

4-3.44 Defend the reasons for obtaining initial training in automated external defibrillation and the importance of continuing education. (p. 519)

4-3.45 Defend the reason for maintenance of automated external defibrillators. (p. 517)

4-3.46 Explain the rationale for administering nitroglycerin to a patient with chest pain or discomfort. (p. 503)

PSYCHOMOTOR OBJECTIVES

At the completion of this lesson, the EMT-Basic student will be able to:

4-3.47 Demonstrate the assessment and emergency medical care of a patient experiencing chest pain/discomfort. (p. 502)

4-3.48 Demonstrate the application and operation of the automated external defibrillator. (p. 515)

4-3.49 Demonstrate the maintenance of an automated external defibrillator. (pp. 517–519)

4-3.50 Demonstrate the assessment and documentation of patient response to the automated external defibrillator. (p. 519)

4-3.51 Demonstrate the skills necessary to complete the Automated Defibrillator: Operator's Shift Checklist. (p. 518)

4-3.52 Perform the steps in facilitating the use of nitroglycerin for chest pain or discomfort. (pp. 504–505)

4-3.53 Demonstrate the assessment and documentation of patient response to nitroglycerin. (pp. 504–505)

4-3.54 Practice completing a prehospital care report for patients with cardiac emergencies. (p. 519)

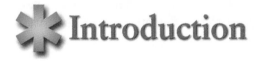 **Introduction**

According to American Heart Association (AHA) statistics, coronary heart disease (CHD) is the single leading cause of death in America today. One of every five deaths in the United States is caused by CHD. Coronary heart disease causes both angina (chest pain) and heart attacks. There are approximately 1.2 million new or

FIGURE 20-1 A patient showing a classic sign of chest pain.

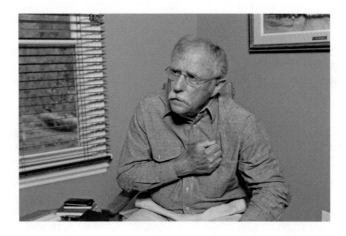

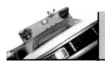

* **cardiac arrest**

the stopping of the heart, resulting in a loss of effective circulation.

* **automated external defibrillator (AED)**

electrical device that automatically analyzes the heart rhythm and, if appropriate, provides a measured dose of electricity through the heart in an attempt to defibrillate or convert the heart into a normal rhythm.

recurrent cases of cardiac-related chest pain and heart attack each year. The AHA estimates that approximately 13.5 million people (6.9 percent of the population) in the United States alone suffer from some form or degree of CHD.

These statistics tell us that, as an EMT, you will see plenty of patients whose chief complaint is chest pain (Figure 20-1). For many of these patients, prompt recognition and transport to an appropriate receiving hospital may mean the difference between life and death. For patients suffering **cardiac arrest,** the key to survival may be the prompt application of an **automated external defibrillator (AED).**

Emergency Dispatch

"Unit 77, Unit 7-7," the dispatcher's voice crackled from D'juan's portable radio, interrupting the relative quiet of the emergency room. "We are at level zero with calls holding. I need you to go 10-8 for an unresponsive patient."

"Copy." D'juan sighed and shrugged his shoulders at the nurse he had been talking to. "What's the address?"

Eight minutes later, D'juan and Tom pulled up to the home in a residential neighborhood. It was one of several housing developments in this city of more than 200,000 people.

As they maneuvered the stretcher through the front door, they found a fire crew performing CPR on the patient—a 63-year-old woman.

"Her husband says that she was having trouble breathing," a sweating fireman said, wiping his forehead with the back of a gloved hand. "Then she just screamed and fell down. We got here about 2 minutes after that and our AED shocked her once. Everytime we reanalyzed, no shock was advised. So we've been doing CPR for about 9 or 10 minutes."

Tom quickly looked around the room, assessing the scene, and his eyes stopped on the helpless gaze of the patient's husband. "Help her," his eyes begged. "She's all I've got."

"Headquarters, this is 7-7," D'juan said into his portable radio. "Confirming cardiac arrest. We are going to prepare for transport; what is the ETA of the ALS unit?"

Review of Circulatory System

Before continuing with this chapter, it will be helpful to review some of the basic anatomy and physiology of the **circulatory system**. Also known as the cardiovascular system, the circulatory system is comprised of three main components: the heart, the blood, and the vessels that carry the blood throughout the body. Certain illnesses as well as injuries can affect one or all of these vital components, thereby reducing the effectiveness of the circulatory system.

PERFUSION

The concept of **perfusion** is the adequate supply of well-oxygenated blood throughout the entire body, including the vital organs and other tissues. When the circulatory system is functioning properly, a patient is said to be perfusing well.

Signs of good perfusion include:

∗ Normal skin signs

∗ Normal mental status

∗ Normal vital signs

When a person is not perfusing well, it is most often due to a malfunction of one or more of the components of the circulatory system.

Signs and symptoms of poor perfusion include:

∗ Abnormal skin signs (pale color, cool temperature)

∗ Altered mental status (sluggishness, confusion, or decreased responsiveness)

∗ Abnormal vital signs (increased pulse and respiratory rate, decreased blood pressure)

A properly functioning circulatory system along with an adequate blood pressure is essential for good perfusion.

THE HEART

The heart serves as the pump in the system and is responsible for the continuous flow of blood throughout the body (Figure 20-2 on page 482). The heart is made up of four interconnected chambers; the top two chambers are the **atria** and the bottom two chambers are the **ventricles**. Deoxygenated blood enters the heart at the right atrium and then flows down into the right ventricle. The right ventricle then pumps the blood into the lungs so it can pick up valuable oxygen and rid itself of waste products such as carbon dioxide. Upon leaving the lungs, the blood reenters the heart at the left atrium, then flows down into the left ventricle. The left ventricle is the largest and most muscular chamber of the heart because it must then pump blood out to the entire body.

CONDUCTION SYSTEM

One of the unique properties of the heart is **automaticity**. This is the ability of each and every heart muscle cell to generate an electrical impulse. When the heart is functioning normally, electrical impulses begin and end along the **conduction pathway** (Figure 20-3 on page 482). This pathway begins at the **sinoatrial node** at

4-3.1 Describe the structure and function of the cardiovascular system.

∗ **circulatory system**

the system made up of the heart, the blood vessels, and the blood. Also called the cardiovascular system (*cardio* referring to the heart; *vascular* referring to the blood vessels).

∗ **perfusion**

the adequate supply of well-oxygenated blood to body tissues, especially the vital organs. (*Hypoperfusion* is inadequate perfusion.)

∗ **atria**

the two upper chambers of the heart. There is a right atrium (which receives unoxygenated blood returning from the body) and a left atrium (which receives oxygenated blood returning from the lungs).

∗ **ventricles**

the two lower chambers of the heart. There is a right ventricle (which sends oxygen-poor blood to the lungs) and a left ventricle (which sends oxygen-rich blood to the body).

∗ **automaticity**

the ability of all heart muscle cells to generate an electrical impulse.

∗ **conduction pathway**

the pathway of electrical impulses through the heart, which causes the heart to beat. The cardiac conduction pathway begins at the sinoatrial node and flows down the center of the heart eventually branching across both ventricles.

∗ **sinoatrial node**

beginning of the cardiac conduction pathway, located at the top of the heart near the right atrium.

FIGURE 20-2 Cross-section of the heart.

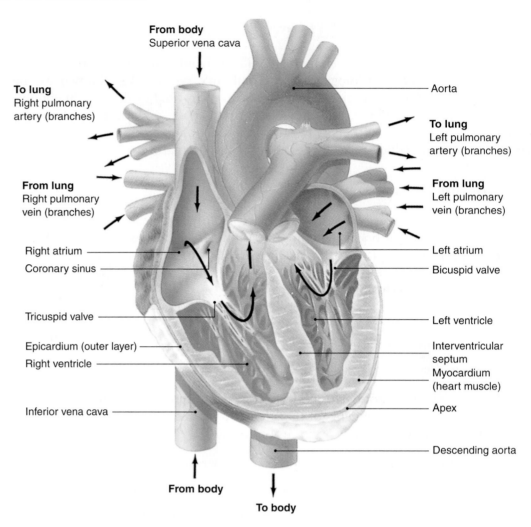

FIGURE 20-2 Cross-section of the heart.

From body
Superior vena cava

To lung
Right pulmonary
artery (branches)

Aorta

To lung
Left pulmonary
artery (branches)

From lung
Right pulmonary
vein (branches)

From lung
Left pulmonary
vein (branches)

Right atrium

Coronary sinus

Left atrium

Bicuspid valve

Tricuspid valve

Left ventricle

Epicardium (outer layer)

Interventricular septum

Right ventricle

Myocardium (heart muscle)

Inferior vena cava

Apex

Descending aorta

From body

To body

FIGURE 20-3 The cardiac conduction pathway, highlighted in green.

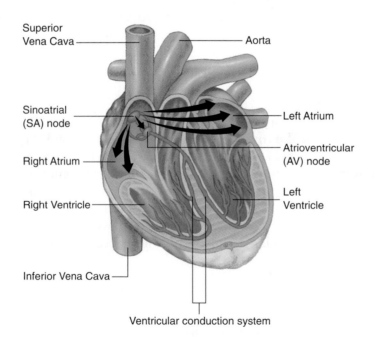

FIGURE 20-3 The cardiac conduction pathway, highlighted in green.

Superior
Vena Cava

Aorta

Sinoatrial
(SA) node

Left Atrium

Atrioventricular
(AV) node

Right Atrium

Left
Ventricle

Right Ventricle

Inferior Vena Cava

Ventricular conduction system

the top of the heart near the right atrium and flows down the center of the heart, eventually branching across both ventricles. Certain medical conditions, such as a heart attack, can cause damage to this electrical pathway, resulting in dangerous heart rhythms and even cardiac arrest.

THE VESSELS

The vessels are the plumbing of the circulatory system. They are often described by their function, location, and whether they carry blood to or from the heart. All vessels that carry blood away from the heart are called **arteries,** while vessels that carry blood to the heart are called **veins.**

Arteries begin as larger vessels and eventually terminate in tiny vessels called **arterioles.** On the contrary, veins begin as tiny **venules** that empty into larger vessels before entering the heart. The tiny vessels that join arterioles and venules and where oxygen and nutrients are exchanged for waste products are called **capillaries** (Figure 20-4).

The following is a list of just some of the major vessels of the body, along with their location and function (Figure 20-5 on page 484):

* **Aorta**—The largest artery in the body, it is attached directly to the left ventricle. It is responsible for carrying oxygenated blood directly from the heart to the major areas of the body.

* **Venae cavae**—They are the largest veins of the body and deliver deoxygenated blood from the body directly into the heart through the right atrium.

* **arteries**
  any blood vessels carrying blood away from the heart.

* **veins**
  any blood vessel returning blood to the heart.

* **arterioles**
  the smallest kind of artery.

* **venules**
  the smallest kind of vein.

* **capillaries**
  tiny vessels that connect arterioles and venules.

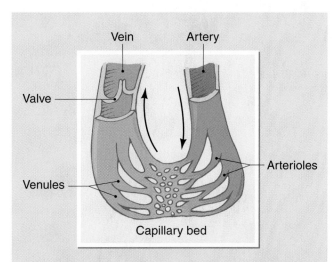

FIGURE 20-4 Arteries, capillaries, and veins.

From the heart, oxygen-rich blood is carried out into the body by arteries. The arteries gradually branch into smaller arteries called arterioles. The arterioles gradually branch into tiny vessels called capillaries.

In the capillaries, the blood gives up oxygen and nutrients, which move through the thin walls of the capillaries into the body's cells. At the same time, carbon dioxide and other wastes move in the opposite direction, from the cells and through the capillary walls, to be picked up by the blood.

On its return journey to the heart, the oxygen-poor blood, now carrying carbon dioxide and other wastes, flows from the capillaries into small veins called venules which gradually merge into larger veins.

MAJOR ARTERIES

MAJOR VEINS

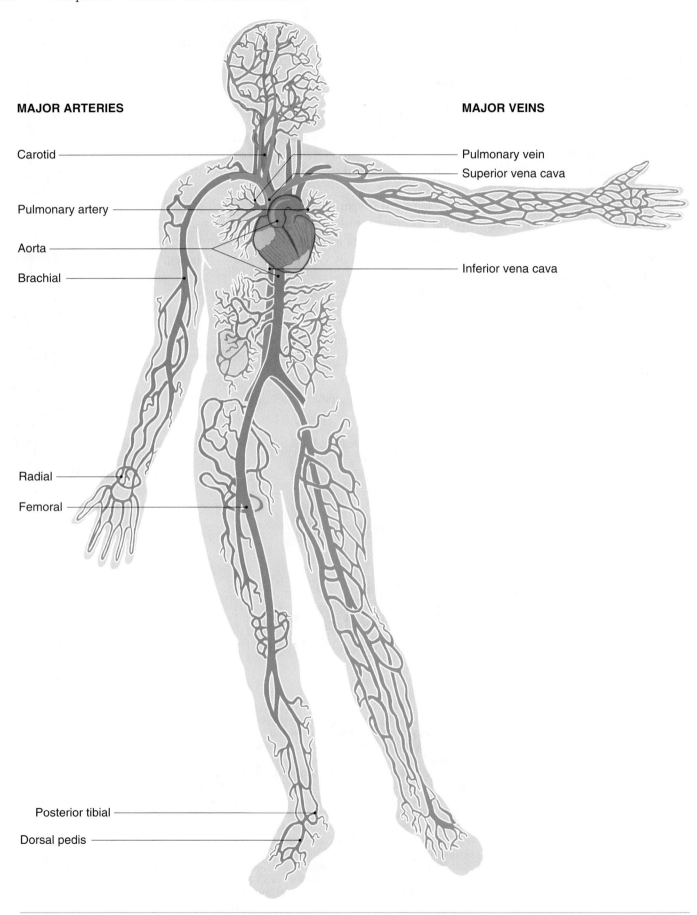

Carotid

Pulmonary artery

Aorta

Brachial

Radial

Femoral

Posterior tibial

Dorsal pedis

Pulmonary vein

Superior vena cava

Inferior vena cava

FIGURE 20-5 The circulatory system.

* **Coronary arteries**—They are the small arteries that carry oxygenated blood to the heart muscle itself. A disruption in flow through these arteries can cause pain and damage to the heart muscle.

* **Pulmonary arteries**—These are the only arteries in the body that carry de-oxygenated blood. They carry blood from the heart and into the lungs to be oxygenated.

* **Pulmonary veins**—The only veins in the body that carry oxygenated blood, they bring freshly oxygenated blood from the lungs into the left atrium.

* **Carotid arteries**—Found in the neck along both sides of the trachea, these arteries carry blood to the head.

* **Brachial arteries**—Located on the inside of each arm between the armpit and the elbow, these arteries carry blood to each arm.

* **Radial arteries**—Located on the thumb side of the anterior wrist, these arteries carry blood to the hands.

* **Femoral arteries**—Located in the anterior groin area, these arteries supply blood to the lower extremities.

THE FUNCTION OF THE BLOOD

Blood serves many essential functions as it is carried by the circulatory system and flows throughout the body. Its most fundamental duty is to carry oxygen and nutrients to the cells and remove waste products generated by cell metabolism.

Blood is made up of several components, each with a specialized function or functions. The major components of blood are as follows:

* **Plasma**—This is the clear, yellowish fluid in which the other components of blood are suspended.

* **Red blood cells**—These are disc-shaped cells responsible for transporting oxygen and carbon dioxide to and from the tissues.

* **White blood cells**—These are any of the colorless or white cells in the blood that help protect the body from infection and disease.

* **Platelets**—These are irregularly shaped cell fragments that are responsible for promoting rapid blood clotting.

To perform these very important functions and sustain life, blood must be present in a sufficient amount. There is a direct connection between the volume of blood within the circulatory system, blood pressure, and perfusion. When a patient loses blood from within the circulatory system, blood pressure will eventually fall and perfusion will become inadequate to keep the patient alive.

The Chain of Survival

You may remember, from your CPR training, learning about the "Chain of Survival." Developed by the American Heart Association and recognized by most, if not all, of the national organizations supporting CPR training, the Chain of

4-3.5 Define the role of EMT-B in the emergency cardiac care system.

Chain of Survival

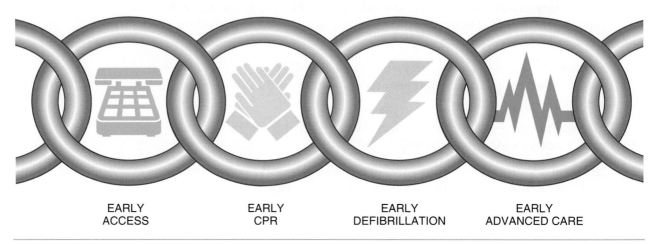

EARLY
ACCESS

EARLY
CPR

EARLY
DEFIBRILLATION

EARLY
ADVANCED CARE

FIGURE 20-6   The chain of survival. (American Heart Association.)

Survival consists of four essential components or "links" necessary for the successful care of out-of-hospital cardiac arrest victims (Figure 20-6). The four links are:

✳ early access to EMS

✳ early CPR

✳ early defibrillation

✳ early access to advanced life support

4-3.9 Predict the relationship between the patient experiencing cardiovascular compromise and basic life support.

When any one of the four links is weak or missing, the likelihood of a successful patient outcome is greatly diminished. As an EMT in your community, you will likely be involved in some manner with all four of these links. At the very least, as an EMT working within an EMS system, you will be directly involved in the first three.

EARLY ACCESS TO EMS

In most emergencies, EMS must rely on willing and informed bystanders to access the EMS system in the most efficient way possible. Thanks to technology, there are more ways to access the EMS system than ever before. You must understand how the system works and when one method is better than another for accessing the system. You must do your part to educate the public on how the system works and encourage them to activate EMS when appropriate.

EARLY CPR

Basic life support (BLS) care and CPR are the foundation of any good EMS system. Without these basic skills, many more victims of cardiac arrest would die unnecessarily. As an EMT, you have a duty to keep your skills sharp as you may have to initiate or take over for bystander CPR at the scene of a cardiac arrest. As a member of the EMS system, you should also become and advocate for CPR training and encourage laypersons to become trained.

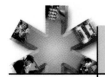

Perspective

Jordan—The Fire Major

"Man, it went like clockwork at first. We got there, determined that she was in full arrest, and slapped the AED on. It shocked the first time, but then it said "no shock advised" the rest of the time. She was still in full arrest, so I guess we shocked her into asystole or something. That happens. Most of the time, though, the AED works like a charm. I've even had people go from full arrest to sitting up and talking before the ambulance even gets there."

EARLY DEFIBRILLATION

It is important to minimize the time between cardiac arrest and defibrillation. As automated external defibrillators (AEDs) become more common and are used by more and more laypersons, the likelihood that you will have a viable patient when you arrive at the scene of a cardiac arrest is greatly increased.

EARLY ADVANCED CARE

The fourth and final link in the chain is early advanced care. In most EMS systems this refers to early access to advanced life support (ALS) EMTs and paramedics. These individuals possess the advanced skills and equipment necessary to help stabilize a cardiac patient in the field. In most areas of the country, the patient no longer must wait until arrival at the hospital to begin receiving lifesaving advanced care. Research has shown that the sooner a patient receives advanced-level care, the better his chances for a positive outcome.

You must know the system you are working in and all the available resources. In some systems, the fastest way to access advanced life support is to simply call dispatch for an ALS back-up and have them respond directly to the scene. In more rural systems, it may save valuable time to request an ALS intercept, load the patient, begin transporting toward the hospital, and meet the ALS crew along the way. In other systems, it may be that ALS is still not available in the field, and you must initiate rapid transport to the most appropriate facility. Regardless of the type of system you may be working in, ALS care is a vital link in the chain of survival.

Cardiac Compromise

The term cardiac compromise (also called Acute Coronary Syndrome) is used to describe patients who present with specific signs and symptoms that may indicate some type of emergency relating to their heart. Medical conditions such as **myocardial infarction (MI)** (heart attack), **angina** (chest pain), and **congestive heart failure (CHF)** are some of the most common types of cardiac compromise. The following is a list of some of the more common signs and symptoms of cardiac compromise:

1. Chest discomfort—typically described as pain or a dull pressure, tightness or squeezing sensation in the chest. It may also radiate to the arms, shoulders, back, or jaw.

4-3.13 Explain the importance of prehospital ACLS intervention if it is available.

4-3.14 Explain the importance of urgent transport to a facility with advanced cardiac life support if it is not available in the prehospital setting.

* **myocardial infarction (MI)**

occlusion or blockage of one or more of the coronary arteries resulting in damage to the heart muscle. Also called a heart attack.

* **angina**

literally a pain in the chest. Occurs when one or more of the coronary arteries are unable to provide an adequate supply of oxygenated blood to the heart muscle. Also called angina pectoris.

* **congestive heart failure (CHF)**

an overload of fluid in the body's tissues that results when the heart is unable to pump an adequate volume of blood.

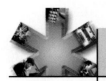

Perspective

Ted—The Husband

"Joanie has CHF. We've known that for awhile. And she's diabetic. But we're very careful about her medications—we really take all of that stuff very seriously. When Joanie was complaining about her breathing, I thought immediately of the CHF, because that happens sometimes. But when she screamed and fell down . . . I felt . . . I don't know . . . like I was a little kid again or something. Just helpless."

2. Sudden onset of sweating (diaphoresis)

3. Shortness of breath (dyspnea)

4. Nausea/vomiting

5. Anxiety, irritability

6. Feeling of impending doom

7. Abnormal pulse rate (may be rapid and/or irregular)

8. Abnormal blood pressure (may be high or low)

9. Epigastric pain (upper abdomen)

Cardiac compromise can have many causes and can present with any or all of the above signs and symptoms. The point is, not all patients experience the same signs and symptoms in the same order and therefore will present differently. As an EMT, you must use your assessment skills to quickly perform an appropriate history and physical exam to identify the potential for cardiac involvement. When in doubt, treat for the worst possible scenario and initiate immediate transport and ALS backup if available.

MYOCARDIAL INFARCTION (HEART ATTACK)

The medical term for heart attack is *myocardial infarction (MI)*. *Myo-* means muscle, *cardial-* means heart, and *infarction* means death of tissue due to a loss of adequate blood supply. It is important to understand that an MI and cardiac arrest are not one and the same. In its simplest definition, a cardiac arrest is the sudden stopping of the heart, resulting in a loss of effective circulation. Patients suffering a cardiac arrest are unresponsive, nonbreathing, and have no palpable pulses. These patients should receive immediate CPR and the application of an AED. While it is true that many cardiac arrests are the result of an MI, most MIs do not result in a cardiac arrest.

The heart is a living organ that must have an adequate supply of well-oxygenated blood to continue to function properly. The heart receives its blood supply through vessels known as **coronary arteries** (Figure 20-7). When these arteries become excessively narrow or blocked from disease and can no longer supply the heart with enough oxygenated blood, the tissue of the heart begins to die.

⁎ **coronary arteries**

small arteries that carry oxygenated blood to the heart muscle itself. A disruption in flow through these arteries can cause pain and damage to the heart muscle.

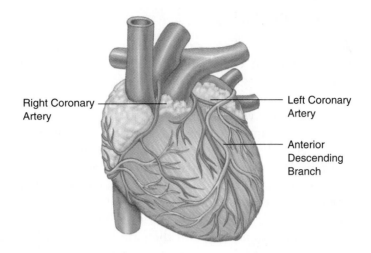

Right Coronary
Artery

Left Coronary
Artery

Anterior
Descending
Branch

FIGURE 20-7   The coronary arteries.

There are many factors that will ultimately determine whether or not an MI will result in a cardiac arrest, but the most common factors are where the damage occurs on the heart and how extensive an area actually dies. Damage that occurs to a large area, over an important electrical pathway, or to the left ventricle is more likely to cause a cardiac arrest than an MI that is very small or occurs to a less critical area of the heart.

SIGNS AND SYMPTOMS OF AN MI

The signs and symptoms of an MI can occur suddenly—as often portrayed in movies and on television. However, in real life their onset is often more gradual and subtle. It is not unusual for a patient to awaken in the morning with mild chest, back, or arm pain and some shortness of breath. He will often experience nausea, which makes him think it may be the flu. This gradual onset is not consistent with what the patient understands a heart attack is, and therefore he may delay seeking care until symptoms worsen. This delay can be detrimental and may lead to cardiac arrest before he seeks medical care. Chest pain from an MI typically lasts more than a few minutes and is not relieved by rest.

Some studies suggest that nearly half of patients who experience a heart attack do not have chest pain as the primary symptom. Common yet atypical symptoms of an MI include the following:

* Shortness of breath

* Nausea

* Dizziness, weakness, and fainting

* Abdominal pain

* Fatigue.

Patients most likely to have atypical symptoms are women, diabetics, and the very elderly (although they can certainly have classic heart attack symptoms as well). During an acute MI, these populations more often experience nausea and vomiting, indigestion, back, neck, or jaw pain, and less often experience the chest pain that is so common in middle-aged men.

As an EMT, you must be very aware of all the possible presentations of cardiac compromise and not just the typical "Hollywood" presentation of the man who suddenly grasps his chest and falls to the ground. You must be very suspicious of the elderly, female, or diabetic patients who may be insisting it's just indigestion and will be just fine. You must provide care presuming the worst possible scenario.

ANGINA PECTORIS

A slightly less dangerous type of cardiac compromise is angina pectoris or, as it is more commonly called, angina. Literally translated *angina pectoris* means "pain in the chest." Angina occurs when one or more of the coronary arteries are unable to provide an adequate supply of oxygenated blood to the heart muscle. While this may sound like what happens in an MI, the similarity ends here. With angina there is no actual damage to the heart muscle. The supply of oxygenated blood is never cut off entirely, and the pain is caused by the muscles starving for more blood and oxygen. Angina is often triggered by exertion. Exertion such as physical activity creates a demand on the heart muscle that the coronary arteries, which have been narrowed by disease or spasm, are unable to meet. The pain increases until the patient must stop the activity and rest. Within a few minutes, the demand on the heart returns to normal and the pain begins to subside and eventually goes away. Some patients are prone to angina attacks and must take medication such as nitroglycerin to help increase circulation to the heart. Nitroglycerin will be discussed in more detail later in this chapter.

SIGNS AND SYMPTOMS OF ANGINA

The signs and symptoms of angina are nearly identical to those of an MI. For that reason, it is important to treat all patients who you feel are experiencing cardiac-related pain as though they were having an MI and seek immediate advanced medical care. Do not try to distinguish between an MI and angina; this must be left up to the doctors and other specialists at the hospital.

✳ Stop, Review, Remember!

Multiple Choice

Place a check next to the correct answer.

1. Which vessels supply blood to the heart muscle?

    _____ a. pulmonary veins

    _____ b. pulmonary arteries

    _____ c. coronary arteries

    _____ d. coronary veins

2. Which chamber of the heart pumps blood to the body?

    _____ a. left atrium

    _____ b. left ventricle

    _____ c. right atrium

    _____ d. right ventricle

3. One out of every _____ deaths in the U.S. is attributed to coronary heart disease.

    _____ a. 2

    _____ b. 5

    _____ c. 10

    _____ d. 25

4. Most cardiac arrests are due to:

    _____ a. a myocardial infarction.

    _____ b. angina.

    _____ c. diabetes.

    _____ d. trauma.

5. Chest pain from angina will typically be of a
   _____ duration than/to that of an MI.

   _____   a. slightly longer

   _____   b. similar

   _____   c. much longer

   _____   d. shorter

Fill in the Blank

1. _____ is the flow of well-oxygenated blood throughout the entire body including the vital organs and other tissues.

2. The top two chambers of the heart are called the _____ and the bottom two chambers are the ventricles.

3. _____ is the ability of all muscle cells in the heart to stimulate an electrical impulse.

4. All vessels that carry blood away from the heart are called _____ while vessels that carry blood to the heart are called _____.

5. The four links in the "Chain of Survival" are early access to EMS, early _____, early access to defibrillation, and early _____.

6. Conditions such as _____, are some of the most common causes of cardiac compromise.

Critical Thinking

1. Describe what you might look for to determine a patient's perfusion status.

   _____

   _____

   _____

2. Describe how a myocardial infarction can lead to cardiac compromise.

   _____

   _____

   _____

3. Describe the difference between an MI and angina.

   _____

   _____

   _____

CONGESTIVE HEART FAILURE

Congestive heart failure (CHF) is a term used to describe an overload of fluid in the body's tissues that results when the heart is unable to pump an adequate volume of blood. Because the heart is unable to manage the normal amount of fluid volume, fluid begins to back up within the circulatory system. If left untreated, this backup of fluids can result in excessive fluid buildup in the lower extremities, sacrum, and lungs. Patients with CHF usually present with difficulty breathing as a chief complaint, due to the accumulation of fluids in the lungs. CHF can be both a **chronic** problem and an **acute** one as well. Some of the causes of chronic CHF include diseased heart valves and hypertension. A patient can also experience an acute episode of CHF secondary to an MI.

SIGNS AND SYMPTOMS OF CHF

Unlike angina and MI, which typically present with a chief complaint of chest pain or discomfort, the acute CHF patient will typically have difficulty breathing. However, patients with CHF can also develop MIs and angina, and they may present with chest pain or discomfort in addition to shortness of breath. These patients often have a history of cardiac problems and, for that reason, will likely have a long list of prescribed medications.

If the patient is standing or seated, you will usually see obvious swelling of the feet and ankles (pedal edema), as gravity will pull the excess fluids to these areas. If he is confined to a bed, you may see edema in the sacral area (sacral edema), since this will usually be the lowest part of the body and, once again, gravity pulls the excess fluid downward. Depending on the amount of fluid in the lungs, the patient may experience increased shortness of breath while lying down. Be alert for this and be prepared to place the patient in a position of most comfort. You may also see some **jugular vein distention** (**JVD**) when the patient is in the sitting position as a result of the increased pressure inside the circulatory system (Figure 20-8).

CARDIAC ARREST

The ultimate cardiac compromise is *cardiac arrest*. The heart has failed completely as a pump and circulation is no longer adequate to support life. While there may still be some electrical activity and movement within the heart, it is not able to circulate blood. The victim of cardiac arrest will be unresponsive, pulseless, and non-breathing and will require immediate CPR and the placement of an AED. AEDs are now being recommended for patients as young as 1 year of age. Be sure to consult your local protocols concerning the use of AEDs.

✳ **chronic**

slow-onset or long-term. Opposite of acute.

✳ **acute**

sudden-onset. Opposite of chronic.

✳ **jugular vein distention (JVD)**

bulging of the neck veins.

FIGURE 20-8 A patient with jugular vein distention. (Edward T. Dickinson, M.D.)

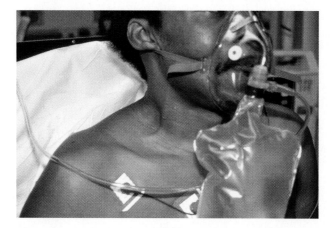

Assessment of the Cardiac Patient

As with all patients, good care depends on a good assessment. We will now discuss the elements of a good assessment when you are caring for a patient with suspected cardiac compromise.

You should begin thinking about your assessment and care even as you respond to the call. In most cases, it will be a call for chest pain. What personal protective equipment will you want to wear? Who will perform the history and physical exam, you or your partner? What equipment will you want to bring into the scene with you? How will you get a history if the patient is unable to provide one? These are just some of the things you can be thinking about as you safely drive to the scene.

SCENE SIZE-UP AND INITIAL ASSESSMENT

Once you have completed an appropriate scene size-up and determined that the scene is safe for you and your partner, you will need to perform an initial assessment. As you enter the scene and approach the patient, pay particular attention to the patient's body language. Is the patient sitting comfortably talking to others (Figure 20-9A) or is the patient showing signs of distress—sitting upright, leaning forward with hands on knees (tripod position) (Figure 20-9B), perhaps holding a clenched fist to his chest (Figure 20-9C on page 494) with a troubled or painful facial expression? What is his color like, and does he appear to be diaphoretic or having difficulty breathing? Many of these signs will be obvious as you approach your

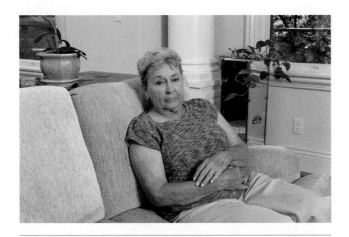

FIGURE 20-9A A patient who does not appear to be in distress.

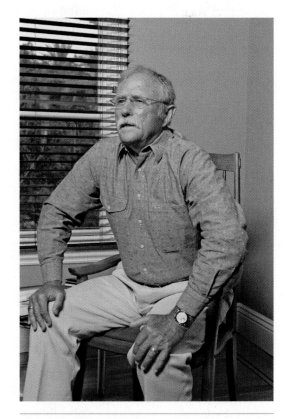

FIGURE 20-9B A patient in the tripod position to ease breathing difficulty.

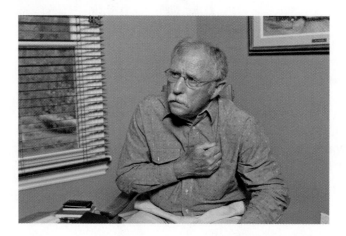

FIGURE 20-9C A patient with a clenched fist over chest as a sign of chest pain or discomfort.

patient. Trust your gut. If the patient looks bad and you don't like what you see, consider this patient as a high priority for transport. Confirm the patient's chief complaint (nature of illness). Are his signs and symptoms consistent with what he is telling you?

Look at the patient's immediate environment. Do you see anything, such as a home oxygen supply source or medication bottles on the table or night stand, that may give you clues to his current medical history?

Based on your general impression and your assessment of the ABCs you must make an initial decision regarding transport priority. If ALS is available in your area, you may want to consider calling it to the scene or setting up an intercept en route to the hospital if it has not already been dispatched.

4-3.8 Establish the relationship between airway management and the patient with cardiovascular compromise.

Depending on the level of responsiveness of the patient, airway management may play an important role. If the patient is responsive, it will be easy to determine the status of his airway because he will be talking and relaying information about his history. For patients with a decreased level of responsiveness, you must pay close attention to the status of the airway and adequacy of breathing. Most protocols for patients with cardiac compromise mandate the administration of supplemental oxygen. *Do not move past the initial assessment without considering the need for supplemental oxygen.*

SAMPLE HISTORY

Based on the chief complaint of chest pain or discomfort you will want to move directly into your SAMPLE history and focus your questions on the chief complaint.

Your line of questioning here will be directed at the chief complaint of chest pain or discomfort. The mnemonic OPQRST is a common tool used to assess chest pain or discomfort. Be sure to look the patient in the eyes as you ask questions and be very clear that he understands your questions. Remember that he is likely very frightened and distracted by what is happening with his body. Below is a review of OPQRST and some sample questions for each component:

✳ **Onset**—What were you doing when the pain/discomfort began?

With this question, you are trying to determine if the patient was at rest or may have been involved in some physical activity when the pain began. While it may not change how you treat the patient, this information will be valuable to the physician who will be treating the patient at the hospital.

* **Provocation**—Does anything you do make the pain/discomfort better or worse?

This question helps to determine if anything the patient does in terms of movement or positioning makes the pain get better or worse. Cardiac-related chest pain is typically a constant pain that will not change with palpation or position. While the patient may feel as though he can breathe easier in one position over another, the pain/discomfort will not usually change. Exertion or strenuous activity may also provoke pain or discomfort.

* **Quality**—Can you describe how your pain/discomfort feels?

Try to get the patient to describe his pain/discomfort in his own words. Be careful with this one, because it is easy to accidentally lead the patient by your line of questioning. For instance, if the patient is having difficulty finding words to describe what he is experiencing, he may agree with the first suggestion you offer. A better way to explore what he is feeling is to offer contrasting choices and allow him to select the most appropriate word. For example you might ask, "Is your pain/discomfort sharp or dull?" or "Is your pain/discomfort steady, or does it come and go?" You must remember that his mind may be very distracted by what is happening to him so be patient and allow the patient enough time to process the question and provide an appropriate response. Pay attention and notice any use of the clenched fist to describe his pain.

* **Region/radiate**—Can you point with one finger where the pain/discomfort is the most? Does your pain/discomfort move or radiate anywhere else?

The focus of this question is to determine where the pain/discomfort is located and if it appears to be moving or radiating anywhere else. Watch the patient carefully after you ask this question. Is he able to pinpoint the pain or does he motion with an open hand over his chest or other area suggesting the pain is spread out and perhaps radiating.

* **Severity**—On a scale of 1 to 10, how would you rate your pain/discomfort?

This question will help you determine just how much pain/discomfort the patient is experiencing from the event. It will be important to ask this question three different times. The first time you ask, you are trying to determine the level of discomfort at that moment. You must then ask, "What level was the pain when it first began?" This will provide insight into whether or not the pain has gotten better, worse, or stayed the same from the time of onset until your arrival. You will want to ask the question again after you have provided some care and comfort or nitroglycerin to the patient—perhaps 5 or 10 minutes after your arrival and the patient having been on oxygen for most of that time. The purpose here is to determine if your calming demeanor, and the oxygen or medication are having any affect on the patient's condition.

* **Time**—When did you first begin feeling this pain/discomfort?

In many cases of cardiac compromise, time plays an important factor. While it will not and should not affect the way you care for your patient, it is a very important part of the history that can affect intervention at the hospital. You will want to ask when the pain/discomfort first began, but you will also want to know

Clinical Clues: CARDIAC COMPROMISE

Clues your patient is in significant distress, unstable, or serious and is a high priority for transport include:

✳ Altered mental status, including unresponsiveness, sleepiness, head-bobbing, agitation, or anxiety

✳ Chief complaint of chest, neck, back, or jaw pain/discomfort

✳ Severe difficulty breathing, including inability to speak or ability to speak only a few words per sentence

✳ Poor skin color, including pale, grey, or cyanotic (blue); Cool, moist skin

✳ Abnormally slow or fast respiratory rates

✳ Increased pulse rate (greater than 100)

✳ Decreased pulse rate (less than 60)

✳ Irregular rhythm of the pulse

✳ Shallow respirations with any respiratory rate

✳ Noisy breathing (usually audible even without a stethoscope) including wheezing, gurgling, snoring, stridor

NOTE: All patients who present with suspected cardiac compromise are a high priority. This list describes the patients who are in serious condition and unstable. Patients with any of these signs are serious—all do not have to be present.

---

if the patient felt bad or had any other symptoms prior to the onset of the pain/ discomfort. As we mentioned earlier in this chapter, many patients begin feeling nausea, lightheadedness, shortness of breath, and fatigue long before the pain or discomfort begins.

If you have not already done so, consider the use of supplemental oxygen at this time. There are many differing opinions as to whether to use a nasal cannula or a nonrebreather mask for these patients. Which device is not as important as getting the patient on some level of oxygen flow. Follow local protocols.

If the patient is currently taking any medications such as nitroglycerin or a respiratory inhaler, you will want to determine if he has taken any of that medication prior to your arrival and what the results were. You will also need to consider assisting the patient with additional doses if indicated and allowed by local protocol.

4-3.7 Discuss the position of comfort for patients with various cardiac emergencies.

Also, consider the position of the patient if you have not already done so. In most cases, the patient will be in the position of most comfort when you arrive. However, some patients are less able to move on their own, so you must ask if the patient would feel better in a different position. For the majority of patients experiencing chest pain, sitting upright (Fowler's) or slightly reclined (semi-Fowler's) is the position of most comfort (Figure 20-10). If you find a patient lying down, ask if he would like to try sitting up and assist him into this position if he feels it will help. Do not decide for a patient which position is best.

If he is responsive, always make a suggestion first and allow the patient to decide. Once he decides on a position of comfort, then assist him in getting into that position. If your patient is unresponsive or simply unable to remain safely in a seated position, then lay him down and place him in the recovery position as appropriate.

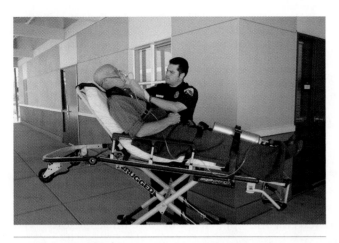

FIGURE 20-10   Cardiac patient in the semi-Fowler's position being prepared for transport.

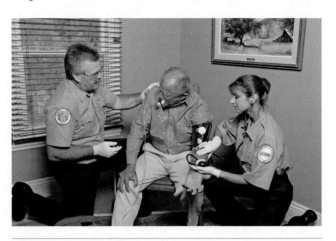

FIGURE 20-11   In a team of two, one EMT should take vital signs while the other completes the SAMPLE history.

VITAL SIGNS

In a typical team of two, one EMT will be getting baseline vital signs while the other completes the SAMPLE history (Figure 20-11). Don't forget to ask the patient what his blood pressure is normally *before* you take your reading. This will help you know what to expect and be able to determine if it is normal for the patient. Get a complete baseline as soon as possible and take subsequent sets approximately every 5 minutes. Be sure to document all vitals carefully and compare them for evidence of a trend.

FOCUSED PHYSICAL EXAM

Assuming your patient is responsive, you will now perform a physical exam focusing on the chief complaint.

As you perform your exam, you will be looking and palpating for signs and symptoms of cardiac compromise. Table 20-1 on page 498 will provide specific examples of what to look for when performing your exam as well as what the finding may mean.

Continue to question the patient about his signs and symptoms throughout your examination and during transport. Keep a close eye on whether he appears to be getting better or worse. Consider increasing the oxygen liter flow if his symptoms do not subside at least a little within the first 5 or 10 minutes.

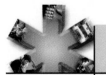

Perspective

D'juan—The EMT

"The fire-rescue guys were doing a great job with CPR when we arrived. In fact I could feel a great carotid pulse with each compression. As soon as they stopped compressions in order to ventilate, the pulse just stopped. That was kind of eerie, if you ask me. Just goes to show you that CPR really does circulate blood."

TABLE 20-1	SIGNS AND SYMPTOMS OF CARDIAC COMPROMISE	
BODY AREA	**ASSESSMENT FINDINGS**	**POSSIBLE CAUSE**
Head	Observe for abnormal skin signs.	Skin that is pale may be an indication of poor perfusion.
Neck	Observe for jugular vein distention, accessory muscle use, and medical alert necklace.	JVD may be a sign that fluid is backing up in the circulatory system. This is often seen in CHF patients. Use of accessory muscles is frequently an indication of respiratory difficulty. Medical alert jewelry may provide valuable information about the patient's history.
Chest	Observe for adequate chest rise and fall, auscultate breath sounds. Palpate the chest where the patient states it hurts.	Good chest rise and fall is important for all patients. This is an important part of adequate respirations. Listen carefully for lung sounds in all fields. Noisy breath sounds may be an indication of fluid in the lungs which is often caused by CHF. Palpate any areas of pain as appropriate to identify if palpation causes more pain or not.
Abdomen	Palpate for pain and pulsating mass.	Be thorough and palpate all four quadrants of the abdomen. Be patient and hold your hands over each area for a few seconds feeling for a pulsating mass. This may be an indication of problems with the abdominal aorta (aneurysm).
Legs and Arms	Assess for distal circulation-sensation-motor function as well as evidence of pedal edema and medical alert jewelry.	Some of the first areas to show evidence of poor circulation are the extremities. Carefully assess for circulation, sensation, and motor function in all four extremities. Look especially for evidence of swelling in the feet and ankles. This can be an important finding in CHF patients who spend much of their time sitting or standing. The fluid that backs up from the circulatory system is drawn to the lowest part of the body by gravity. Medical alert jewelry can provide valuable information about the patient's medical history.

Stop, Review, Remember!

Multiple Choice

Place a check next to the correct answer.

1. Asking a patient to describe what his pain/discomfort feels like is associated with which part of the OPQRST assessment mnemonic?

   _____ a. provocation

   _____ b. quality

   _____ c. onset

   _____ d. severity

2. During which phase of your patient assessment should you first be considering the need for supplemental oxygen?

   _____ a. scene size-up

   _____ b. initial assessment

   _____ c. SAMPLE history

   _____ d. focused physical exam

3. Pedal and JVD are most often seen with which medical condition?

   _____ a. myocardial infarction

   _____ b. angina

   _____ c. congestive heart failure

   _____ d. cardiac arrest

4. Which of the following questions is most appropriate for the "Q" of the OPQRST assessment mnemonic?

   _____ a. Can you describe for me what your pain/discomfort feels like?

   _____ b. How long have you had this pain?

   _____ c. What were you doing when the pain began?

   _____ d. Does anything you do make the pain better or worse?

5. The position of comfort is decided by the:

   _____ a. EMT.

   _____ b. family members.

   _____ c. medical director.

   _____ d. patient.

Signs and Symptoms

List as many signs and symptoms as you can for the following medical conditions and the treatment(s) that would be appropriate for the EMT to provide:

Condition	Signs	Symptoms	Treatment
CHF			
MI			
Angina			

Critical Thinking

1. Describe why edema is often found in the ankles and sacral area of patients experiencing CHF.

_____

_____

_____

_____

_____

2. Describe the difference between cardiac arrest and myocardial infarction (heart attack).

_____

_____

_____

_____

_____

3. Provide an example of at least one appropriate question to ask a possible cardiac-compromise patient for each letter of the SAMPLE history acronym.

_____

_____

_____

_____

_____

Caring for the Patient with Cardiac Compromise

One of the most important aspects of caring for a suspected cardiac patient is a calm professional demeanor and plenty of comfort and reassurance. The following steps can be used to provide care for most patients presenting with the signs and symptoms of cardiac compromise (Scan 20-1 on page 502). Remember, it is not important that you determine the patient's specific problem, such as MI, angina, or CHF; the treatment should be based on the patient's presentation and should be the same regardless.

1. Take appropriate BSI precautions.

2. Perform an appropriate initial assessment and administer supplemental oxygen.

3. Obtain a thorough SAMPLE history, utilizing the OPQRST assessment mnemonic.

4. Obtain a baseline set of vital signs.

5. Perform an appropriate focused physical exam.

6. Assist with the administration of the patient's prescribed nitroglycerin (follow local protocol).

7. Perform regular ongoing assessments and adjust your care as appropriate.

8. Transport as soon as practical and consider the need for an ALS backup or intercept.

4-3.2 Describe the emergency medical care of the patient experiencing chest pain or discomfort.

Clinical Clues: CHEWABLE BABY ASPIRIN

Some EMS systems are allowing EMTs to administer chewable baby aspirin for patients with suspected cardiac pain. This should be included in your treatment plan if allowed by local protocol.

SCAN 20-1 | CARING FOR THE PATIENT WITH SIGNS AND SYMPTOMS OF CARDIAC COMPROMISE

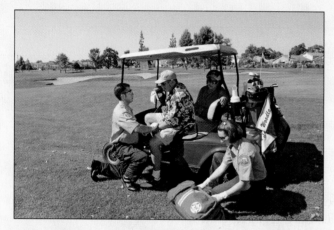

▲ Use appropriate BSI while performing initial assessment.

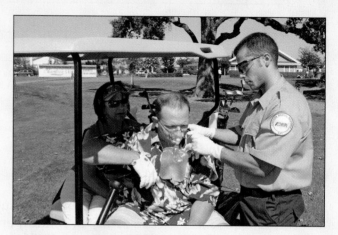

▲ Administer supplemental oxygen.

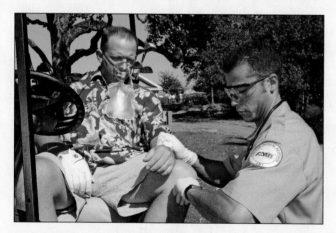

▲ Obtain a set of baseline vital signs.

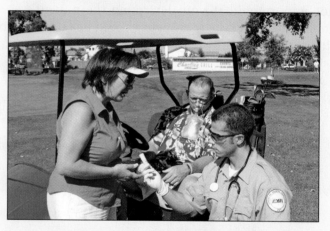

▲ Obtain a history including any medications taken by the patient.

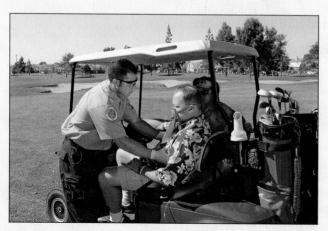

▲ Perform the appropriate focused physical exam.

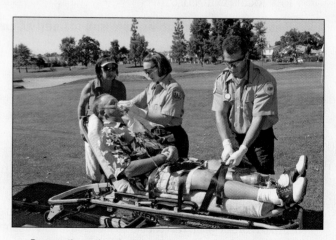

▲ Prepare the patient for transport.

Medical direction plays an important role in every EMS system across the country. This is especially true when you are caring for patients with cardiac emergencies. It has been by the advisement of qualified physician medical directors and through the development of specific treatment guidelines and protocols that we have been able to improve upon the care that these patients receive. As you learn to function as an EMT, make sure you learn the specific protocols that direct the care you will provide.

4-3.40 Recognize the need for medical direction of protocols to assist in the emergency medical care of the patient with chest pain.

ASSISTING WITH NITROGLYCERIN

During your SAMPLE history, you will have determined if the patient had been prescribed any medications for his condition. One of the most common medications prescribed to patients with a cardiac history is nitroglycerin (Figure 20-12A and B). A derivative of the infamous explosive, medical nitroglycerin is used to dilate blood vessels in an effort to help improve circulation to the heart muscle.

4-3.41 List the indications for the use of nitroglycerin.

Once you have determined that the patient is experiencing what is suspected to be cardiac-related chest pain, the following criteria must be met before you can assist the patient in taking his own nitroglycerin (Scan 20-2 on page 504):

1. *The patient has his own prescription with him.* Be sure to confirm the "six rights" and that the prescription has been issued in the name of the patient and not another family member.

2. *The prescription is current and not expired.* In some cases the expiration date on the bottle may be missing or difficult to read; do not administer medication that you cannot confirm is current.

3. *The patient has not taken Viagra or a similar medication (Cialis, Levitra) for erectile dysfunction within the past 24 hours.* Be advised that, in some EMS systems, the requirement may be that the patient has not taken these medications within the past 48 or 72 hours. In other systems, the protocol is to contact medical direction prior to the administration of nitroglycerin for patients who take erectile dysfunction medications at all.

4. *The patient has a systolic blood pressure of at least 100.* This requirement also varies from region to region and may range from 90 mmHg to 120 mmHg. Nitroglycerin may also be contraindicated in patients with very rapid or slow pulses. Always check your local protocols.

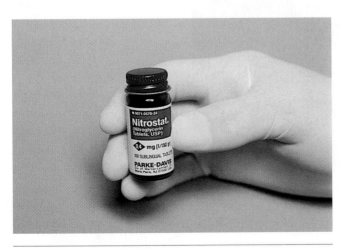

FIGURE 20-12A   Nitroglycerin tablets.

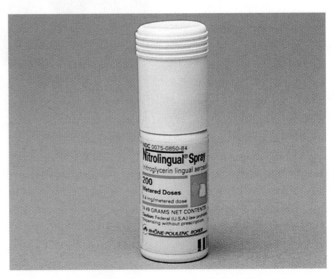

FIGURE 20-12B   Nitroglycerin spray.

SCAN 20-2 **ASSISTING WITH THE ADMINISTRATION OF NITROGLYCERIN**

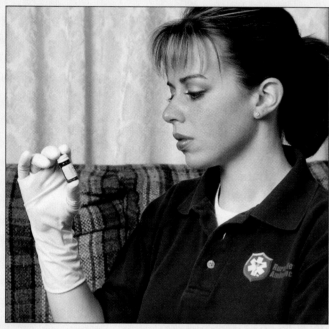

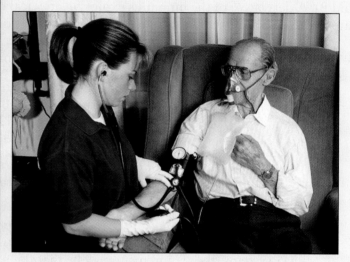

▲ Inspect medication container and confirm indications and "six rights" of administration.

▲ Confirm blood pressure.

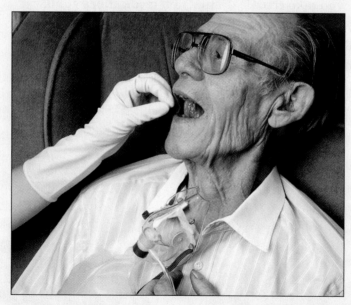

▲ Place pill under tongue.

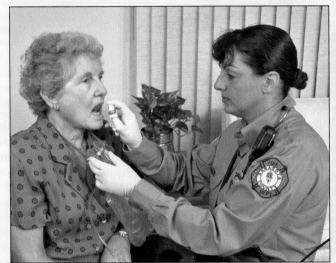

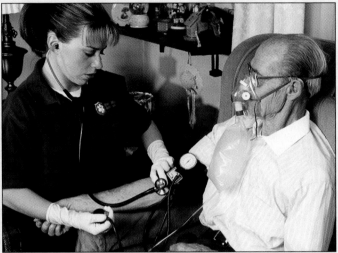

▲ Alternatively, when using a spray, spray nitroglycerin under the tongue.

▲ Reassess blood pressure with oxygen back on within 2 minutes of administering nitroglycerin.

Typical instructions for the administration of nitroglycerin are to place one tablet (or one spray) beneath the tongue (sublingually) and allow it to dissolve completely. If the medication is in pill form, instruct the patient not to swallow it. If the patient does not experience an improvement in symptoms within 3 to 5 minutes, repeat the dose every 5 minutes up to a maximum of three doses in a 15-minute period of time. *Follow local protocols.*

Following each dose, you must reassess vital signs and confirm that the patient's systolic blood pressure remains above 100 mmHg. Because nitroglycerin has the potential to cause a significant drop in blood pressure, resulting in the patient becoming light-headed and possibly unresponsive, allow the administration of this medication only with the patient securely seated or lying down.

If at any point the patient's systolic blood pressure drops below 100 mmHg, or if a significant increase in pulse or decrease in responsiveness occurs, initiate transport to an appropriate receiving facility while continuing the history and physical exam and providing the indicated care en route.

4-3.42 State the contraindications and side effects for the use of nitroglycerin.

Clinical Clues: GLOVES AND NITROGLYCERIN

Always wear gloves when handling or assisting with the administration of nitroglycerin. Do not allow the tablets or spray to come in contact with your skin, as doing so may allow the medication to be absorbed into your bloodstream.

FIGURE 20-13   Aspirin.

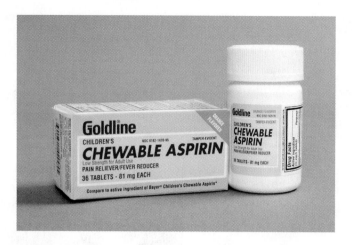

THE USE OF ASPIRIN

In addition to nitroglycerin, aspirin has proven to be highly beneficial for the treatment of patients suspected of having a cardiac event. Aspirin minimizes the formation of blood clots within the circulatory system and reduces that chance of serious heart damage due to clotting (Figure 20-13).

Many EMS systems are adding the administration of aspirin to the list of EMT skills. *Follow local protocols.*

✳ Stop, Review, Remember!

Multiple Choice

Place a check next to the correct answer.

1. Supplemental oxygen helps the cardiac patient by:

   _____ a. acting as a pain reliever.

   _____ b. increasing circulation to the heart.

   _____ c. increasing the concentration of oxygen in the blood.

   _____ d. dilating the coronary arteries.

2. Which of the following is NOT a link in the "Chain of Survival"?

   _____ a. Early access

   _____ b. Early CPR

   _____ c. Early diagnosis

   _____ d. Early advanced care

3. A common side effect of nitroglycerin is:

   _____ a. decreased pulse rate.

   _____ b. increased blood pressure.

   _____ c. dry mouth.

   _____ d. headache.

4. The patient's blood pressure must be at least _____ systolic prior to the administration of nitroglycerin.

   _____ a. 80

   _____ b. 100

   _____ c. 110

   _____ d. 120

5. Which of the following actions should be performed following each administered dose of nitroglycerin?

_____   a. Repeat vital signs.

_____   b. Increase oxygen flow.

_____   c. Lay the patient down.

_____   d. Contact medical direction.

Fill in the Blank

The following criteria must be met before you may assist a patient with administering nitroglycerin:

1. Confirm that the patient has a _____ for nitroglycerin.

2. Confirm that the medication has not _____.

3. Confirm that the patient has not taken any medication for erectile dysfunction in the past _____ hours.

4. Confirm that the patient has a _____ blood pressure of at least _____.

Critical Thinking

1. Describe how nitroglycerin helps the patient who is experiencing cardiac-related chest pain.

_____

_____

_____

_____

2. What are the contraindications to allowing a patient to take his own nitroglycerin?

_____

_____

_____

_____

3. How does supplemental oxygen help the patient experiencing cardiac compromise?

_____

_____

_____

Fundamentals of Early Defibrillation

❋ **dysrhythmias**

  any variations from the normal rate or rhythm of the heart. Also called arrhythmias.

❋ **arrhythmias**

  see dysrhythmias.

❋ **ventricular fibrillation (VF or v-fib)**

  one of the most common electrical rhythms associated with sudden cardiac arrest in which the ventricles of the heart contract spontaneously and in an uncoordinated manner, thus preventing the heart from circulating any meaningful amount of blood.

Depending on what source you read, anywhere from 300,000 to 450,000 people die each year in the United States from sudden cardiac arrest. It is believed that many of these people could be saved with the strengthening of the "Chain of Survival." Research has shown that with strong links in the chain we can reduce the incidence of death from cardiac arrest.

For many years the weak link in the "Chain of Survival" has been early defibrillation. While many ambulances and fire departments carry and use these defibrillators, there is often a significant delay in delivering the first shock due to long response times. Research has shown that the sooner a victim of sudden cardiac arrest can receive a shock, the better the likelihood of a positive outcome. Because AEDs require so little training to operate, they are being placed in more and more public places, allowing for quicker delivery of shocks following collapse.

HOW AEDS SAVE LIVES

Not all patients experiencing a heart attack (MI) go into cardiac arrest. In fact, the majority of MI patients actually remain responsive and survive the event. A number of procedures performed at the hospital can help these patients lead normal lives following a heart attack.

AEDs are designed specifically to help convert the heart rhythm of victims of sudden cardiac arrest (Figure 20-14). While the term cardiac arrest does imply that the heart has stopped pumping blood, it often times remains "electrically active." This electrical activity that remains in the heart can be any one of a number of uncoordinated electrical rhythms called **dysrhythmias** or **arrhythmias.** One of the most common electrical rhythms associated with sudden cardiac arrest is **ventricular fibrillation** or simply **VF** or **v-fib** (Figure 20-15). VF causes the ventricles of the heart to contract spontaneously and in an uncoordinated manner, thus preventing the heart from circulating any meaningful amount of blood. A patient

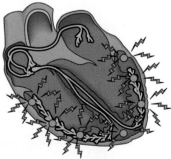

Chaotic electrical discharge as seen on an ECG tracing.

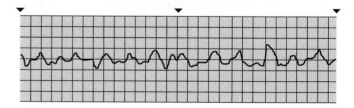

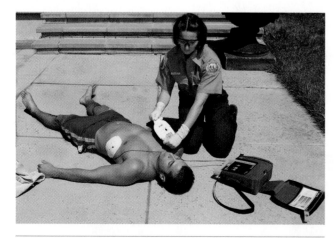

FIGURE 20-14   AEDs are designed specifically to help convert heart rhythms of victims of sudden cardiac arrest.

FIGURE 20-15   Ventricular fibrillation is associated with chaotic electrical discharge in the ventricles.

in VF will not have any palpable pulses and is rendered unresponsive, pulseless and nonbreathing within seconds following the onset of VF.

The job of the AED is to automatically analyze the heart rhythm and "reboot" the heart, not unlike rebooting a computer that has locked up. The AED provides a measured dose of electricity through the heart in an attempt to defibrillate or convert the heart into a normal rhythm.

ADVANTAGES OF AEDS

AEDs offer many advantages over the traditional manual defibrillator used by both hospital and EMS personnel.

* **Ease of operation**—It is easier to learn to operate an AED than it is to learn CPR. The newest machines provide extremely detailed instructions for the operator, which minimizes confusion and costly delays in care.

* **Speed of operation**—The ease of operation and layperson access allow for the opportunity to deliver a shock to the patient sooner than having to wait for EMS to arrive.

* **Safer operation**—An AED uses adhesive electrode pads to both analyze and deliver a shock, making a "hands-off" operation that is safer for both the patient and the operator. Once placed, the large electrode pads also allow for more consistent shocks over a larger area than most manual defibrillator paddles.

* **Continuous monitoring**—Once the AED pads are in place and the device is turned on, it will continually analyze the patient's rhythm at regular intervals and advise if a shock is necessary, making the job of the rescuer easier. Some devices also have an LCD screen that shows a real-time moving image of the patient's heart rhythm.

INDICATIONS FOR THE USE OF AN AED

As we mentioned earlier, not all patients will benefit from the use of an AED. A responsive patient complaining of chest pain is clearly not in VF; therefore the AED will not help him. A patient must meet the following criteria before it is recommended that you place an AED:

* The patient must be unresponsive.

* The patient must be pulseless.

* The patient must be nonbreathing.

* The patient must have a clear airway.

* The patient must be 1 year of age or older.*

In 2004 the American Heart Association released a document recommending the use of AEDs on patients as young as 1 year of age. While not required, it is preferred that special pediatric pads be used for pediatric patients. The AHA does not recommend for or against the use of AEDs on patients younger than 1 year of age. Check with your local protocols.

It is important to confirm that the patient does indeed have a clear airway before attaching the AED. Even if the patient is in VF, he cannot be successfully

4-3.21 Discuss the advantages and disadvantages of automated external defibrillators.

4-3.23 Discuss the use of remote defibrillation through adhesive pads.

4-3.24 Discuss the special considerations for rhythm monitoring.

4-3.3 List the indications for automated external defibrillation.

4-3.6 Explain the impact of age and weight on defibrillation.

4-3.18 State the reasons for assuring that the patient is pulseless and apneic when using the automated external defibrillator.

resuscitated until the airway is open and you are able to provide adequate ventilations during CPR.

4-3.4 List the contraindications for automated external defibrillation.

CONTRAINDICATIONS

Now that AED use is recommended for pediatric patients, there are essentially no contraindications for its use in unresponsive, pulseless, and nonbreathing patients. While not contraindicated, the use of AEDs for the treatment of cardiac arrest due to trauma or hypothermia has proven less effective and may not be included in treatment protocols for these specific patients. You will need to verify any contraindications for AED use with your local EMS agency.

4-3.19 Discuss the circumstances which may result in inappropriate shocks.

  While it is possible that an AED could deliver an inappropriate shock, it is extremely unlikely. A couple of ways to minimize the likelihood of inappropriate shocks is to place an AED only on a patient who meets all the appropriate criteria and to keep the AED in good working order by performing regularly scheduled maintenance checks.

 # Stop, Review, Remember!

Multiple Choice

Place a check next to the correct answer.

1. Abnormal electrical rhythms of the heart are called:

  _____ a. anomalies or dysrhythmias.

  _____ b. aberrancies or anomalies.

  _____ c. anginas.

  _____ d. dysrhythmias.

2. Early defibrillation is the _____ link in the "Chain of Survival."

  _____ a. first _____ c. third

  _____ b. second _____ d. fourth

3. The primary cause of cardiac arrest in adult patients is:

  _____ a. ventricular fibrillation.

  _____ b. trauma.

  _____ c. vehicle accidents.

  _____ d. respiratory arrest.

4. Which of the following is NOT a criterion for the placement of an AED? The patient must:

  _____ a. be unresponsive.

  _____ b. be pulseless.

  _____ c. be nonbreathing.

  _____ d. be lying on a metal surface.

5. The use of AEDs is now being encouraged for patients as young as _____ year(s) of age.

  _____ a. 1

  _____ b. 3

  _____ c. 5

  _____ d. 8

Fill in the Blank

1. When given to suspected MI and angina patients, aspirin acts as a _____ and minimizes the formation of blood clots.

2. Early application of an AED is the _____ link in the chain of survival.

3. One of the most common electrical rhythms associated with sudden cardiac arrest is _____.

4. The use of AEDs for the treatment of cardiac arrest due to _____ and hypothermia has proven less effective and may not be included in treatment protocols for these specific patients.

Critical Thinking

1. What makes AEDs today so easy to operate?

_____

_____

_____

_____

_____

2. Discuss the role that time plays in the successful resuscitation of a cardiac arrest patient.

_____

_____

_____

_____

3. Discuss at least two advantages that AEDs have over the more traditional manual defibrillators.

_____

_____

_____

_____

_____

Types of AEDS

While there are many manufacturers and models of AED on the market today, defibrillators all operate using the same principles: they analyze the heart rhythm of a patient without a pulse and based on that analysis will decide whether a shock is appropriate (Figures 20-16A-B).

Initially there were two types of defibrillators, fully automated and semi-automated. The fully automated defibrillator is turned on and attached to the patient and as the name implies, requires minimal or no input from the EMT. Semi-automated defibrillators require constant interaction with the device including pressing the "analyze" and shock buttons when prompted to do so.

Most defibrillators in use today are semi-automated defibrillators. Another distinction between defibrillators is **monophasic** vs. **biphasic**. Monophasic defibrillators deliver shocks at set energy levels to all patients. Biphasic defibrillators are newer and more technologically advanced. These devices measure the resistance of the chest and deliver more effective shocks at lower energy levels and patterns.

The American Heart Association sets specific guidelines for the energy levels delivered by monophasic defibrillators. Biphasic defibrillators deliver shocks based on manufacturer's recommendations and measurements of the patient obtained by the defibrillator. Since AEDs are pre-programmed you will not have to choose or specify an energy level before defibrillating a patient.

RHYTHM ANALYSIS

One of the design features that make AEDs so simple to use is the sophisticated rhythm analysis software. The electrode pads capture the patient's heart rhythm and send it to a microprocessor in the main unit for interpretation (Figure 20-17). The rhythm is then quickly analyzed for several criteria to ensure that it is indeed a shockable rhythm. Because of the sophistication of the analysis software, there is little chance of an inappropriate shock being delivered. The software is specifically designed to identify both shockable and nonshockable rhythms. The safety of the device is further enhanced by the activation of the shock button ONLY if the software detects a shockable rhythm. This prevents the operator from inadvertently delivering an inappropriate shock.

There are two rhythms that an AED would consider shockable. The first is ventricular fibrillation (V-fib), which we explained earlier. The second is a rhythm

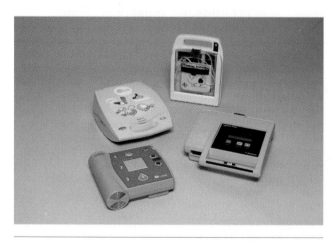

FIGURE 20-16A Automated and semi-automated AEDs.

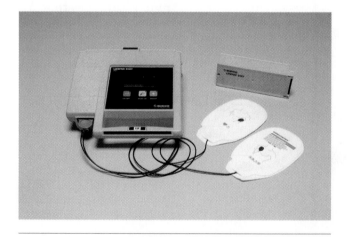

FIGURE 20-16B An AED and its components.

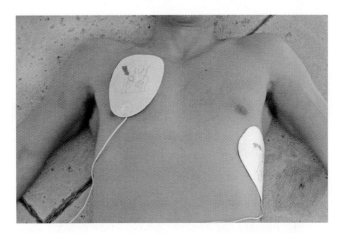

FIGURE 20-17   Pediatric patient with properly placed AED pads.

called rapid ventricular tachycardia (V-tach). It is not important that you know what each of these rhythms looks like, because that is the job of the AED.

The energy delivered by an AED is measured in units called joules. A joule is the amount of energy delivered by one watt of power in one second. For instance a 100-watt light bulb uses 100 joules every second. Depending on the age and model of the AED, it may deliver anywhere from 150 to 360 joules each time it delivers a shock. Some models provide shocks with increasing energy levels, while others use the same energy level for all shocks. Newer models are able to utilize lower energy settings due to biphasic technology.

ANALYZE/SHOCK SEQUENCE

Once the AED is turned on, it will begin a set of preprogrammed voice commands designed to assist the rescuer in following the correct sequence of steps. After the electrode pads are properly placed on the patient, it will follow a preset sequence of analyze and shock phases.

If, after the first analyze phase, the AED recognizes a shockable rhythm, the voice prompt will state that a shock is advised and prompt the rescuer to press the shock button. Following delivery of each shock, the AED will advise the rescuer to perform CPR for 2 minutes before analyzing the heart rhythm again. This sequence of analyze, delivery of a single shock, and 2 minutes of CPR will repeat as appropriate.

Analyze/Shock Sequence

* Single shock

* 2 minutes of CPR

* Single shock

* 2 minutes of CPR

* Single shock

New resuscitation guidelines are allowing local Medical Directors to recommend 2 minutes of CPR (5 cycles) before attempting defibrillation when the response time is greater than 4 to 5 minutes. This will help ensure that the heart is adequately perfused before the first shock. Always know and follow your local protocols.

If there is no return of spontaneous pulses, begin CPR.

OPERATING AN AED

The AED should be applied and used immediately in any witnessed arrest, but in cases of unwitnessed arrest, defibrillation should not occur until about 2 minutes of CPR have been done. Follow your local protocols. Once you have confirmed that the scene is safe and your initial assessment has confirmed that your patient meets all the criteria for the application of an AED, perform the following steps (Scan 20-3):

1. Turn on the AED.
2. Place electrode pads (you may have to stop CPR if already in progress).
3. Confirm that no one is touching the patient.
4. Initiate the analyze phase (may require that you press the analyze button depending on the type of AED).
5. If a shock is advised, confirm everyone is clear of the patient and press the shock button if required. Then provide CPR for two minutes.
6. If no shock is advised, perform CPR for 2 minutes.
7. Follow the voice prompt of your AED. About every 2 minutes, you will be directed to clear the patient while the AED analyzes the rhythm. You may also be prompted to recheck the pulse.
8. Transport as soon as practical.

Continue to follow the voice prompts from the AED until ALS takes over or you arrive at an appropriate receiving facility.

Should you find yourself transporting a responsive patient who suddenly goes into cardiac arrest, initiate CPR while your partner stops the ambulance and climbs into the back of the ambulance to assist. You must continue CPR until your partner can properly place the AED on the patient.

Regardless of whether you are alone or working with another rescuer, the steps for using an AED are essentially the same. If you are alone, you must turn on the AED and then perform your assessment of the patient. With two rescuers, one of you will perform the assessment while the other prepares the AED for use.

CPR and the use of an AED are only two of the four links in the "Chain of Survival." Whenever possible, integrate your care with advanced life support care to maximize the likelihood of patient survival. ALS care will provide more advanced airway care as well as the necessary medications to help the patient regain a normal heart rhythm.

RECURRENT VENTRICULAR FIBRILLATION

Once you have regained a pulse during resuscitation, continually monitor the patient's carotid pulse during transport. A patient in cardiac arrest may regain and lose a pulse several times during a resuscitation attempt. If you are unable to palpate a carotid pulse, initiate the analyze phase of the AED.

Once you have begun transport of a cardiac arrest patient, it may be necessary to come to a complete stop in the ambulance in order to allow the AED to properly analyze the patient's rhythm. Motion can cause the electrodes to pick up inappropriate electrical activity and the machine may advise *"Check Electrodes."* If this occurs while in motion, stop the ambulance and press the analyze button to reinitiate the analyze phase.

SCAN 20-3   OPERATING AN AED

The AED should be applied and used immediately in any witnessed arrest, but in cases of unwitnessed arrest, defibrillation should not occur until about 2 minutes of CPR have been done. Follow your local protocols.

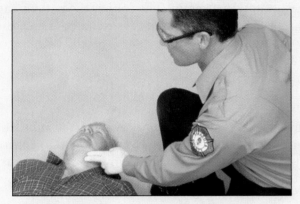

▲ Confirm the patient is in cardiac arrest by assessing for a pulse.

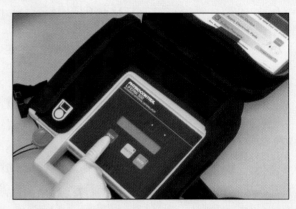

▲ If no pulse, initiate CPR and turn on the AED. Some systems may require you to perform 2 minutes of CPR before activating the AED. Follow local protocols.

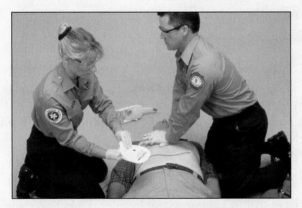

▲ Place electrode pads on the patient's bare chest.

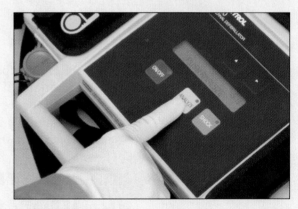

▲ Confirm that no one is touching the patient and initiate the analyze phase.

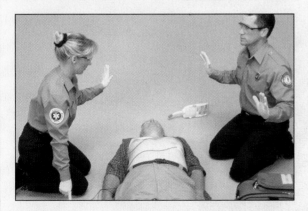

▲ If a shock is indicated, again confirm that no one is touching the patient and press the shock button.

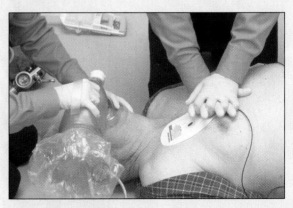

▲ After the shock or if shock is not indicated, perform 2 minutes of CPR. Follow further prompts of the AED.

4-3.20 Explain the considerations for interruption of CPR when using the automated external defibrillator.

INTERRUPTION OF CPR

Interrupt CPR for the following reasons when using an AED:

NOTE: Interrupting compressions severely reduces circulation of blood throughout the body. Interruptions in CPR during AED use must be limited to analysis of the rhythm and delivering shocks to the patient.

✳ During the analyze phase

✳ During the shock phase

It is important to keep CPR going as long as possible and minimize the times that CPR is interrupted during a resuscitation attempt. The sooner the patient can receive a shock, the better his chances of being successfully resuscitated. Once the AED is on the scene, do not delay the application of the device. Stop CPR, if necessary, to apply the pads and initiate the analyze phase.

4-3.31 Discuss the importance of post-resuscitation care.

4-3.32 List the components of post-resuscitation care.

POST-RESUSCITATION CARE

Should the patient be fortunate enough to regain a pulse following CPR and defibrillation, there is still much you must do during transport to the hospital to ensure a successful outcome. Post-resuscitation care consists of the following components:

✳ Rapid transport to an appropriate receiving facility

✳ Continuous monitoring of patient's airway, breathing, and circulatory status

✳ Consideration of ALS intercept for advanced care

✳ Use of supplemental oxygen

✳ Completion of focused history and physical exam

Monitor your patient continuously and carefully during transport and be prepared to initiate CPR and the AED as appropriate (Figure 20-18). Consider taking an additional rescuer such as a firefighter or other Emergency Responder with you in the ambulance. The extra hands will become very helpful should the patient go back into cardiac arrest during transport.

SAFETY CONSIDERATIONS

Use of AEDs have proven to be successful in saving many lives and have an excellent safety record. However, they are not invulnerable. They must be respected and

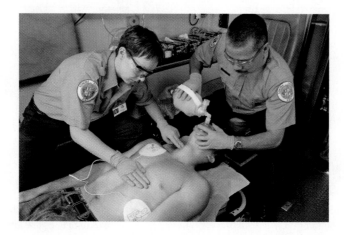

FIGURE 20-18   Continue to provide ventilations and monitor the pulse of a post-arrest patient with AED pads still in place.

handled with care. The following safety tip regarding moisture must be followed to ensure a safe environment for everyone working with or around an AED:

Ensure that the patient's chest is completely dry before placing the electrode pads. Moisture on the chest from sweat, rain, or other sources can cause the electrical energy to travel (arc) across the chest rather than through the chest. This may cause burning of the skin and will not provide proper defibrillation. It is also important to make certain the patient is not lying in a puddle of water prior to defibrillation. While simply lying on wet ground is not a problem, lying in a puddle of standing water may cause arcing and places other rescuers at risk of being shocked. Carefully move the patient out of the standing water before defibrillation. Remove the medication patch and wipe any remaining medication from the skin before placing the defibrillator pad.

Defibrillator Maintenance

Like any piece of equipment used for the care and transport of a patient, the AED has specific maintenance requirements that must be followed to ensure proper function of the device.

Self-Diagnostic Checks

* Most if not all AEDs have built-in sophisticated diagnostic software that performs automated self checks at regular intervals. These self checks ensure that all internal circuitry is operating normally and require little if any work on the part of the operator. A visible indicator and/or audible tone will alert the operator should one of these self checks find a malfunction in the device (Figure 20-19).

* Defibrillator malfunction is frequently due to a battery failure. It is important to inspect the batteries on a regular basis and confirm they are not leaking and have not expired. Batteries have a limited life and must be changed once expired. Expiration dates are clearly marked on all batteries.

ROUTINE INSPECTIONS

In addition to the self checks, each AED manufacturer provides a detailed maintenance checklist for each device (Figure 20-20 on page 518). Depending on where the AED is being used the inspection may be performed daily, weekly, or monthly. At a minimum, all AEDs must be checked every 30 days to ensure they are ready for service.

4-3.34 Discuss the need to complete the Automated Defibrillator: Operator's Shift Checklist.

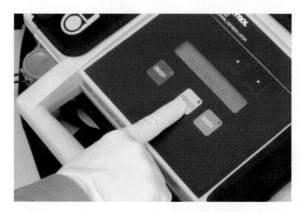

FIGURE 20-19   Visual indicator (display) of an AED device.

AUTOMATED DEFIBRILLATORS: OPERATOR'S SHIFT CHECKLIST

Date: _____ Shift: _____ Location: _____

Mfr/Model No.: _____ Serial No. or Facility ID No.: _____

At the beginning of each shift, inspect the unit. Indicate whether all requirements have been met. Note any corrective actions taken. Sign the form.

	Okay as found	Corrective Action/Remarks
1. Defibrillator Unit Clean, no spills, clear of objects on top, casing intact		

2. Cables/Connectors
 	
  a. Inspect for cracks, broken wire, or damage
  b. Connectors engage securely		

3. Supplies
 	
  a. Two sets of pads in sealed packages, within expiration date   *g. Spare charged battery
  b. Hand towel   *h. Adequate ECG paper
  c. Scissors   *i. Manual override module, key or card
  d. Razor   *j. Cassette tape, memory module, and/or event card plus spares
  * e. Alcohol wipes
  * f. Monitoring electrodes		

4. Power Supply
 	
  a. Battery-powered units
    (1) Verify fully charged battery in place
    (2) Spare charged battery available
    (3) Follow appropriate battery rotation schedule per manufacturer's recommendations
  b. AC/Battery backup units
    (1) Plugged into live outlet to maintain battery charge
    (2) Test on battery power and reconnect to line power		

5. Indicators/*ECG Display
 	
  * a. Remove cassette tape, memory module, and/or event card   *e. "Service" message display off
  b. Power on display   *f. Battery charging; low battery light off
  c. Self-test ok   g. Correct time displayed — set with dispatch center
  * d. Monitor display functional		

6. ECG Recorder a. Adequate ECG paper b. Recorder prints		

7. Charge/Display Cycle
 	
  * a. Disconnect AC plug — battery backup units   *e. Manual override functional
  b. Attach to simulator   f. Detach from simulator
  c. Detects, charges, and delivers shock for "VF"   *g. Replace cassette tape, module, and/or memory card
  d. Responds correctly to non-shockable rhythms		

8. *Pacemaker
 	
  a. Pacer output cable intact   c. Inspect per manufacturer's operational guidelines
  b. Pacer pads present (set of two)		

☐ **Major problem(s) identified** **(OUT OF SERVICE)**		

Applicable only if the unit has this supply or capability

Signature: _____

FIGURE 20-20 A typical AED maintenance check list. (Laerdal.)

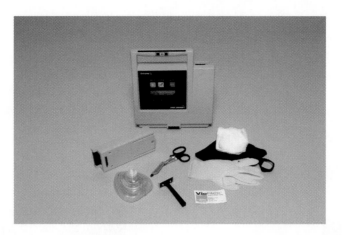

FIGURE 20-21 Supplies should be stored with the AED and inspected at regular intervals.

In addition to ensuring that the device is in working order, the operator must see that the necessary supplies are stored with the AED (Figure 20-21). The following list of supplies should be stored with the AED and inspected at regular intervals:

* Extra set of electrode pads

* Extra battery

* Shaver for removal of chest hair

* Scissors for cutting away clothing

* Supply of 4 × 4 gauze pads for wiping away moisture

* Protective gloves and barrier mask

Medical Direction

In most states, AED programs must have medical oversight. This is most often provided by the EMS system's Medical Director. Medical directors provide oversight of the deployment of AEDs and training requirements of personnel who will be using the devices. They must also review each incident where an AED was used. Following the use of an AED, a written report must be submitted to the Medical Director along with the data downloaded from the device. The Medical Director will review all details concerning the event and provide feedback for program quality improvement.

In addition, most AEDs require the prescription of a physician before they can be purchased. One AED manufacturer has received Federal Food and Drug Administration (FDA) approval for the sale of one specific model of AED designed for home use.

Whether as part of an EMS system or in the private sector, one of a Medical Director's primary goals is to ensure the continuous quality improvement (CQI) of the AED program. The goal of CQI is to ensure that local EMS systems are providing the best possible care at all times to victims of cardiac arrest. By reviewing each incident where an AED was used, important statistical information can be gathered that will assist in making improvements to the AHA guidelines and protocols that direct how AEDs are used.

Like any skill that you might use as an EMT, make sure you review procedures and practice using the AED as often as necessary to maintain proficiency. Cardiac arrest is a time-sensitive emergency, and maintaining proficiency with the AED will minimize unnecessary delays in providing care for the patient.

4-3.36 Explain the role medical direction plays in the use of automated external defibrillation.

4-3.37 State the reasons why a case review should be completed following the use of the automated external defibrillator.

4-3.38 Discuss the components that should be included in a case review.

4-3.39 Discuss the goal of quality improvement in automated external defibrillation.

4-3.33 Explain the importance of frequent practice with the automated external defibrillator.

4-3.35 Discuss the role of the American Heart Association (AHA) in the use of automated external defibrillation.

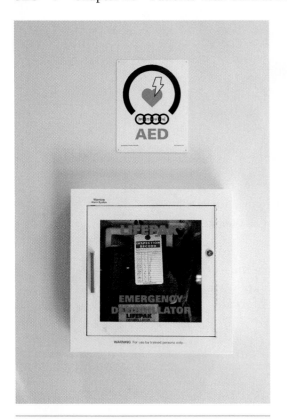

FIGURE 20-22A AEDs are available in many public places in a special identifying cabinet.

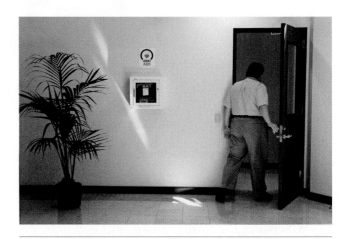

FIGURE 20-22B The lobby of a building is a logical place for housing an AED.

Public Access Defibrillation

It is only a matter of time before you respond to the scene of a cardiac arrest and find an AED in use by someone from a private company or organization. Amusement parks, airports, shopping malls, and even some cities and towns are developing what are known as public access defibrillation programs, making AEDs available in public places (Figures 20-22A and B).

The American Heart Association and similar organizations have developed specific training and implementation programs for the public use of AEDs. These organizations are promoting public access defibrillation programs in an effort to decrease the time to shock following collapse from a cardiac arrest.

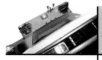

Dispatch Summary

Once on scene, the paramedics intubated the patient, started a jugular IV, and implemented the cardiac drug protocols. Incredibly, the patient regained a pulse and a low but steady blood pressure. She was then quickly transported to the city's heart hospital where she was transferred to their care in the same precarious condition.

Whether she lived or not is unknown. Sometimes EMS personnel just do what they can and never have the opportunity to follow up or learn whether they ultimately made a difference.

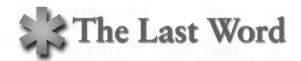 # The Last Word

Patients with the signs and symptoms of cardiac compromise make up a large percentage of the calls you will see as an EMT. Your understanding of the cardiovascular system and the signs and symptoms that appear when it begins to malfunction is essential to the well-being of your patients.

While the causes of cardiac compromise can be many and varied, the presentation is often very similar. The following are just some of the more common signs and symptoms of cardiac compromise:

* Chest discomfort—typically described as a dull pressure, tightness, or squeezing sensation in the chest. It may also radiate to the arms, shoulders, back, or jaw.
* Sudden onset of sweating (diaphoresis)
* Shortness of breath (dyspnea)
* Nausea/vomiting
* Anxiety, irritability
* Feeling of impending doom
* Abnormal pulse rate (may be rapid, slow, and/or irregular)
* Abnormal blood pressure (may be high or low)
* Epigastric pain (upper abdomen)

When in doubt, provide care for the worst possible scenario and initiate transport and access to ALS care as soon as possible.

Stay up on the basics of CPR and the use of an AED, as these skills are the foundation of all EMS systems.

AEDs are an essential link in the chain of survival and are becoming more and more common as organizations such as the American Heart Association are promoting public access defibrillation programs.

AEDs are designed to be placed on unresponsive, pulseless, and nonbreathing patients who are 1 year of age or greater. They can convert a deadly heart rhythm into a normal one with electrical shocks.

Sophisticated software will analyze the patient's rhythm and determine if a shock is indicated. Depending on the type of AED being used, it will either prompt the operator to push a button to deliver the shock or will deliver it automatically.

AEDs can be easily integrated into single- or multiple-rescuer CPR scenarios. Whenever possible, call for ALS backup or request an ALS intercept.

Chapter Review

MULTIPLE CHOICE

Place a check next to the correct answer.

1. The primary vessels responsible for supplying the heart muscle with blood are the:

   _____ a. cardiac veins.

   _____ b. pulmonary arteries.

   _____ c. coronary arteries.

   _____ d. pulmonary veins.

2. Nitroglycerin is indicated for the treatment of:

   _____ a. angina.

   _____ b. pectoris.

   _____ c. anxiety.

   _____ d. shortness of breath.

3. Which of the following is NOT a side effect of nitroglycerin?

   _____ a. drop in blood pressure

   _____ b. headache

   _____ c. pulse rate changes

   _____ d. shortness of breath

4. _____ is caused by a backup of fluids from the circulatory system when the heart can no longer pump blood efficiently.

   _____ a. Angina

   _____ b. CHF

   _____ c. An MI

   _____ d. SOB

5. Which of the following is NOT a typical sign or symptom of cardiac compromise?

   _____ a. chest discomfort

   _____ b. low back pain

   _____ c. nausea and vomiting

   _____ d. shortness of breath

6. It is recommended that the AED inspection checklist be completed at least every _____ to ensure readiness for an emergency.

   _____ a. day

   _____ b. week

   _____ c. 30 days

   _____ d. year

7. You are operating an AED on an adult victim of cardiac arrest. The AED has just delivered a shock. What should happen next?

   _____ a. The AED will analyze again and deliver a shock if indicated.

   _____ b. The AED will advise to check pulse and to begin CPR if no pulse.

   _____ c. You should begin CPR immediately; a pulse check is not required.

   _____ d. You should assess for pulse and breathing and transport. The AED will not deliver any more shocks.

8. Which of the following is NOT considered a component of post-resuscitation care?

   _____ a. rapid trauma assessment

   _____ b. rapid transport

   _____ c. monitoring of ABCs

   _____ d. administration of supplemental oxygen

9. When using an AED, CPR is commonly interrupted for all of the following reasons EXCEPT during:

   _____ a. rhythm analysis.

   _____ b. delivery of shocks.

   _____ c. placement of electrode pads.

   _____ d. warm-up of the device.

10. You are on the scene of a cardiac arrest and the AED has given a "no shock advised" prompt. What should you do next?

   _____ a. Initiate another analyze phase.

   _____ b. Remove the electrode pads.

   _____ c. Assess for pulse and breathing.

   _____ d. Perform CPR for 2 minutes.

CRITICAL THINKING

1. Discuss the difference between a heart attack and a cardiac arrest.

   _____

   _____

   _____

   _____

2. Discuss the role of the EMT in the "Chain of Survival."

   _____

   _____

   _____

   _____

3. Discuss the differences between fully automatic and semiautomatic AEDs.

   _____

   _____

   _____

   _____

4. What are the two rhythms that an AED will recognize as shockable?

   _____

   _____

   _____

   _____

5. Discuss the role of the Medical Director in an AED program.

   _____

   _____

   _____

   _____

CASE STUDIES

Case Study 1

You have been dispatched to a local gym for a man down. Upon arrival, you find an approximately 60-year-old male unresponsive on the floor. A gym employee is performing CPR and advises that the patient collapsed about 10 minutes ago and that the employee started CPR almost immediately. You direct the employee to stop CPR while you check for a carotid pulse. You feel a pulse. The man, however, is still not breathing.

1. How will you proceed with caring for this man?

   _____

   _____

   _____

   _____

2. After a few minutes of rescue breathing, you discover that the patient no longer has a pulse. What will you do next?

   _____

   _____

   _____

   _____

3. The AED has delivered 1 shock. What will you do next?

   _____

   _____

   _____

   _____

Case Study 2

While working the first aid station at the local county fair, an approximately 45-year-old man is brought to the station by some family members. The family states that he is having trouble breathing and needs some assistance. You sit the man down in the station and begin to assess him. He reveals that his primary complaint is a pressure on his chest, which seems to be causing the difficulty breathing. He states that he had a similar episode about 6 months ago and had a stent inserted into one of his coronary arteries. He denies any other history other than high cholesterol, for which he takes Lipitor. His BP is 106/68, pulse 88 strong and regular. He appears a little pale and sweaty.

1. How will you begin your care for this patient?

   _____

   _____

   _____

   _____

2. The man states that he has some nitroglycerin in his wife's purse and asks if he should take one. What will you want to know before you assist him in taking a nitro pill?

   _____

   _____

   _____

   _____

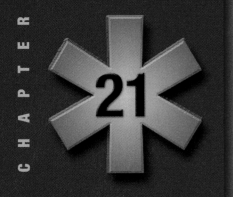

CHAPTER

21

Patients with Altered Mental Status

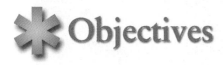
Objectives

Numbered objectives are from the U.S. Department of Transportation 1994 EMT-Basic National Standard Curriculum.

COGNITIVE OBJECTIVES

At the completion of this lesson, the EMT-Basic student will be able to:

4-4.1 Identify the patient taking diabetic medications with altered mental status and the implications of a diabetes history. (pp. 535–537, 538)
- List the signs and symptoms of hyperglycemia.
- List the signs and symptoms of hypoglycemia.
- List at least 3 history questions specific to the patient with a known diabetic history.

4-4.2 State the steps in the emergency medical care of the patient taking diabetic medicine with an altered mental status and a history of diabetes. (pp. 537–539)

4-4.3 Establish the relationship between airway management and the patient with altered mental status. (pp. 527, 528)

4-4.4 State the generic and trade names, medication forms, dose, administration, action, and contraindications for oral glucose. (pp. 539–540)

4-4.5 Evaluate the need for medical direction in the emergency medical care of the diabetic patient. (p. 538)

AFFECTIVE OBJECTIVES

At the completion of this lesson, the EMT-Basic student will be able to:

4-4.6 Explain the rationale for administering oral glucose. (p. 539)

PSYCHOMOTOR OBJECTIVES

At the completion of this lesson, the EMT-Basic student will be able to:

4-4.7 Demonstrate the steps in the emergency medical care for the patient taking diabetic medicine with an altered mental status and a history of diabetes. (pp. 538–539)

4-4.8 Demonstrate the steps in the administration of oral glucose. (p. 540)

4-4.9 Demonstrate the assessment and documentation of patient response to oral glucose. (p. 542)

4-4.10 Demonstrate how to complete a prehospital care report for patients with diabetic emergencies. (pp. 541, 542)

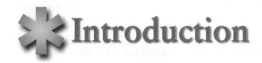

Introduction

Patients who experience a sudden illness or suffer a significant mechanism of injury will often become confused, violent, or slow to respond to your questions or events around them. These patients are said to have an **altered mental status** (**AMS**). A patient can be described as having an AMS anytime he is not acting normally or appears abnormally sleepy, confused, violent, or even completely unresponsive (Figure 21-1). A patient with an AMS becomes particularly serious when the patient's level of responsiveness decreases to a point at which he may not be able to maintain his own airway.

A patient who presents with an AMS should be considered unstable and a high priority for transport.

4-4.3 Establish the relationship between airway management and the patient with altered mental status.

* **altered mental status (AMS)**

appearing abnormally sleepy, confused, violent, or even completely unresponsive.

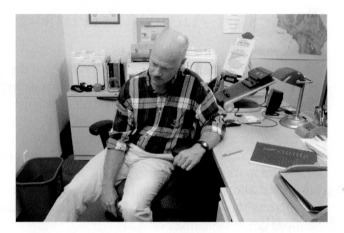

FIGURE 21-1 A patient exhibiting possible signs of an altered mental state.

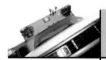

Emergency Dispatch

EMTs Ray and Jason pulled into the small, desolate parking lot just before the police arrived, their headlights illuminating a tow truck with the driver's door hanging open and a man lying motionless on the pavement not far from it.

"I drove by about ten minutes ago," one of the officers told them, adjusting his duty belt after climbing from the police cruiser. "He was hooking that car up and he waved at me. He seemed fine."

Ray surveyed the scene and then cautiously approached the patient—a man approximately 35–40 years old, wearing a tow-company uniform, with a messy tangle of long hair obscuring his face. The first thing that Ray noticed was blood oozing thickly from the man's scalp. A quick inspection with his gloved fin-

gers exposed a 3-centimeter laceration just above the man's right ear. The man groaned.

"We're from the ambulance," Ray said. "We're here to help you. What happened?"

The man groaned louder and said something unintelligible. He was trying to sit up.

"Relax . . . hold on," Ray said, trying to keep the man from moving his head or neck.

"What . . . what . . . help me!" The man began to shout, pulling away from Ray and trying to get to his knees.

"We are trying to help." Jason knelt next to Ray and tried to gently restrain the man.

"You . . . uh . . . you . . . why are . . . I mean . . . oh God . . . " The man stammered as he began pushing

(continued on p. 528)

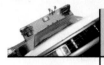

Emergency Dispatch

(continued)

the EMTs' hands away. "There's a green . . . a green . . . oh . . . what am I saying? Were we talking? Just now? Get the hell away from me!"

"We gotta get this guy boarded," Ray said to Jason, and then he turned to the police officers. "Can you guys help hold him? We can't let him move around like this!"

✳ **hypoglycemia**

abnormally low blood glucose level.

✳ **hyperglycemia**

abnormally high blood glucose level.

✳ **seizures**

interruptions of normal brain function caused by bursts of abnormal electrical signals in the brain.

✳ **stroke**

condition that occurs when the blood supply to an area of the brain is interrupted.

FIGURE 21-2 Common causes of an altered mental status.

Causes of Altered Mental Status

There are many causes of an AMS including both illnesses and injuries. For many of these patients the underlying cause is often a decrease in perfusion to the brain. Patients experiencing such medical conditions as **hypoglycemia** (low blood sugar), **hyperglycemia** (high blood sugar), **seizures**, **strokes** (brain attack), and poisonings will almost always have some degree of AMS. Patients experiencing a traumatic event such as a head injury or significant blood loss will also commonly present with an AMS. While it is not the responsibility of the EMT to always know the cause of a patient's AMS, becoming familiar with some of the more common causes will allow you to provide the most appropriate care. In every case, be sure to gather as thorough a medical history as possible. See Figure 21-2 for some of the more common causes of AMS.

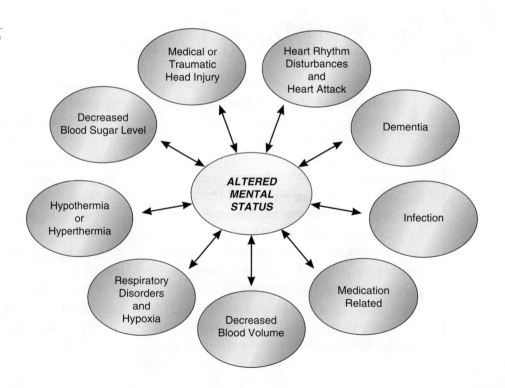

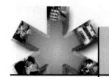

Perspective

Ray—The EMT

"I'm still not sure what happened. One minute this guy is just doing his job and the next he's got a head laceration and is obviously altered. The cops thought that he might have been mugged or something. We never found his wallet. But it was obvious that he didn't know what was going on. If you take a patient with a head wound who starts off unresponsive and then wakes up but is talking gibberish and starts resisting help, it sends up all sorts of red flags."

SIGNS AND SYMPTOMS OF AN AMS

Determining if a patient is actually presenting with an altered mental status is not always easy. In some patients with psychiatric disorders, mental retardation, or certain chronic medical conditions, such as **dementia,** an AMS may be their normal presentation. It is always important to refer to family or caregivers to determine the patient's baseline mental status before forming any conclusions on your own.

The following is a list of some of the more common signs and symptoms of an altered mental status:

* Decreased level of responsiveness

* Confusion

* Sluggish to respond

* Disorientation

* Asking repeated questions

* Abnormal pupils

* Loss of bowel or bladder control (incontinence)

* Obvious signs of injury to the head

* Agitation or unusually violent behavior

Remember that an AMS can range from slight confusion to complete unresponsiveness and may get better or worse during your care. Pay close attention to your patient and continually monitor his mental status for changes. For most patients, the best way to monitor the mental status is to maintain constant verbal communication with them. Continually ask questions and monitor their responses.

> * **dementia**
> condition involving gradual development of memory impairment and cognitive disturbance.

Emergency Medical Care

It is worth repeating: It is not essential that you determine the exact cause of a patient's AMS in order to care for him. In most cases your care will center on maintaining an open airway, ensuring adequate breathing, and monitoring circulatory status as well as the patient's safety and yours (Figure 21-3A on page 530).

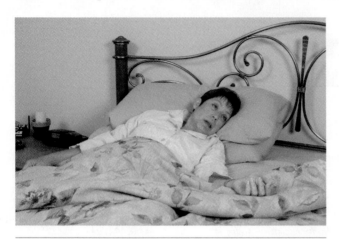

FIGURE 21-3A This patient's altered mental status is likely caused by a medical condition.

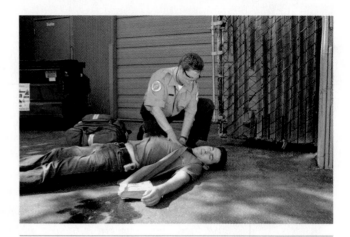

FIGURE 21-3B Some cases of altered mental status can be caused by traumatic injury.

Maintain a high index of suspicion for possible spinal injury with any patient presenting with an AMS and an unknown history (Figure 21-3B). This may not be the case with the 87-year-old male found unresponsive in bed, but it is required for the 50-year-old patient found out behind the grocery store or in the alley. Bottom line: When you can't rule out a serious mechanism of injury, provide appropriate spinal precautions.

INITIAL ASSESSMENT

As you approach your patient, note how you find him. Is he in a seated position with eyes open or is he lying motionless on the ground? In what kind of an environment did you find him? Is there any chance he could have been injured? Regardless of how he is found, your initial assessment will center on the patency of his airway and the adequacy of his respirations. Maintain spinal precautions as appropriate.

You can use the AVPU scale to make an initial assessment of his mental status. AVPU stands for:

✳ A – Alert

✳ V – Responds to verbal stimulus

✳ P – Responds to painful stimulus

✳ U – Completely unresponsive

If the airway is not clear, position the patient's head, provide suction as necessary, and attempt to insert an airway adjunct. Once you have established a clear airway, confirm that respiratory rate and tidal volume are adequate. For patients who are not breathing adequately, provide assisted ventilations as necessary. For patients who have adequate respirations, provide supplemental oxygen using a nonrebreather mask at 15 lpm.

Assess the adequacy of circulation by confirming the presence of an adequate pulse and noting skin signs (color, temperature and condition). Most patients with an AMS should be considered unstable and, therefore, require rapid transport to an appropriate receiving facility.

FOCUSED HISTORY

For medical patients the history often provides the most valuable information. Obtain a SAMPLE history and talk to family members, friends, bystanders, or other caregivers regarding how the patient may have been feeling prior to the onset of an AMS. Do your best to determine his baseline mental status and to be able to describe how his current condition differs from his normal state of mind.

PHYSICAL EXAM

The physical exam is performed after the initial assessment when the patient appears to have a traumatic injury or if a patient believed to have a medical condition is unresponsive. The physical exam may help find hidden injuries or medical alert devices that give clues to why the patient has an altered mental status.

Perform examinations specific to the patient's condition if appropriate, such as blood glucose monitoring.

GLASGOW COMA SCALE

Once the initial assessment is completed and immediate life threats managed, a common and useful additional tool for determining mental status and patient response is the Glasgow Coma Scale (GCS) (Figure 21-4 on page 532). It utilizes 3 specific assessment findings to arrive at a score that can be shared with other care providers and used in your documentation. The best possible score is 15 and the lowest possible score is 3. A score of 3 indicates the absence of any response to the following three GCS assessment areas:

* Eye opening

* Verbal response

* Motor response

The Glasgow Coma Scale provides a more detailed and thorough assessment than the preliminary AVPU scale.

VITAL SIGNS

Obtain a complete set of baseline vital signs as soon as possible and record them with the correct time. Remember that an AMS is a strong indicator of some other underlying problem. Repeat the vital signs at frequent intervals and always compare to the baseline set. Note any changes that might indicate a trend in the patient's condition for better or worse. Because hypoxia is a frequent cause of AMS, include pulse oximetry as part of your initial and ongoing vital sign assessment.

POSITION FOR TRANSPORT

How you position the patient for transport will depend on whether you suspect a spinal injury or not. If you are unable to rule out the possibility of trauma, you must take appropriate spinal precautions and transport the patient supine on a long board. If injury is not suspected, then it may be best to place the patient in the recovery (lateral recumbent) position for transport unless the patient requires constant airway management or ventilation. Place the patient in a supine position. Be sure to position the patient so he is facing you during transport. It is much easier to monitor and manage a patient's airway if you can see the airway at all times. Keep suction ready in case the patient vomits.

FIGURE 21-4 The Glasgow Coma Scale.

Glasgow Coma Scale

Eye opening	Spontaneous	4	
	To Voice	3	
	To Pain	2	
	None	1	
Verbal response	Oriented	5	
	Confused	4	
	Inappropriate Words	3	
	Incomprehensible Sounds	2	
	None	1	
Motor response	Obeys Command	6	
	Localizes Pain	5	
	Withdraw (pain)	4	
	Flexion (pain)	3	
	Extension (pain)	2	
	None	1	
Glasgow coma score total			

ONGOING ASSESSMENT

The elements of the ongoing assessment are the same regardless of what kind of patient for whom you are caring.

* Recheck the initial assessment.
* Recheck vital signs.
* Repeat assessment of chief complaint or injuries.
* Obtain additional history if possible.
* Consider ALS intercepts.
* Check effectiveness of interventions.
* Confirm care and transport priority.

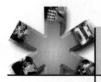

Perspective

Jason—The EMT

"Boarding that guy was a no-brainer. I mean, a head injury with altered mentation and no clue about the mechanism? There just simply was no other way to handle this patient."

Stop, Review, Remember!

Multiple Choice

Place a check next to the correct answer.

1. The preliminary assessment of a patient's mental status should be conducted during which segment of the patient assessment?

    _____ a. scene size-up

    _____ b. initial assessment

    _____ c. SAMPLE history

    _____ d. detailed physical exam

2. Which of the following is NOT one of the characteristics of the Glasgow Coma Scale?

    _____ a. eye opening

    _____ b. verbal response

    _____ c. motor response

    _____ d. grip strength

3. In most cases, the appropriate position for transport for patients with an altered mental status is the _____ position.

    _____ a. supine

    _____ b. prone

    _____ c. recovery

    _____ d. Fowler's

4. A patient who opens his eyes only when you speak to him, provides confused responses, and withdraws from pain, would have a GCS score of:

    _____ a. 11.

    _____ b. 9.

    _____ c. 7.

    _____ d. 5.

5. Which of the following best describes how often vital signs should be repeated on an unresponsive patient?

    _____ a. only once

    _____ b. every 15 minutes

    _____ c. every 5 minutes

    _____ d. twice

Glasgow Coma Scale Activity

For each of the following patient descriptions, identify the appropriate GCS score:

1. 22-year-old male who is awake and his eyes are open. He is confused and is only able to tell you where he hurts. _____

2. 45-year-old female who responds only to pain by opening her eyes, is moaning and withdraws from your painful stimulus.

    _____

3. 76-year-old female who appears unconscious and does not open her eyes. She offers no verbal response to your questions and offers no motor response. _____

Critical Thinking

1. Describe at least six common causes of altered mental status.

   _____

   _____

   _____

   _____

2. Discuss why a patient with an altered mental status would or would not be considered a high-priority patient.

   _____

   _____

   _____

   _____

3. Discuss why the position of the patient with an altered mental status is so important during transport.

   _____

   _____

   _____

   _____

The Diabetic Patient

* **diabetes**

  medical condition that results when a person's pancreas will no longer produce an adequate supply of insulin or when the body loses the ability to utilize insulin properly.

* **insulin**

  hormone required for the transfer of glucose (sugar) from the blood to the tissues and cells where it can be used for fuel.

* **glucose**

  blood sugar.

Diabetes is a medical condition that results when a person's pancreas will no longer produce an adequate supply of **insulin** or when the body loses the ability to utilize insulin properly.

Insulin is required to facilitate the transfer of **glucose** (sugar) from the blood to the tissues and cells where it can be used for fuel. One of the biggest users of glucose is the brain, and when the brain does not receive an adequate supply it begins to shut down, causing an altered mental status. Without insulin, glucose levels in the blood can continue to rise to dangerous levels. Similarly, glucose levels will rise in the blood if the cells lose their ability to take the sugar from the bloodstream.

A diabetic patient must carefully monitor the level of glucose in his blood stream (Figure 21-5). Diabetics can manage their glucose levels in several ways. Some are able to control glucose levels simply by eating properly and minimizing the intake of sugar and starchy foods that the body converts to sugar. Others must take oral medications to help stimulate the cells to better utilize what insulin the pancreas does produce. Many diabetics must take daily injections of insulin in or-

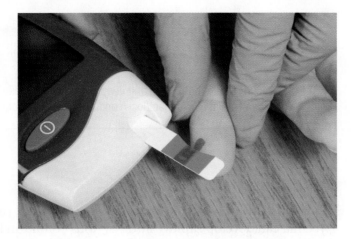

FIGURE 21-5   Blood glucose monitoring is performed by analyzing a small drop of blood from a patient's finger.

der to control the level of glucose in the blood. Regardless of the method, diabetics are constantly walking a fine line between too much and too little sugar in the blood.

There are essentially two types of diabetic emergencies you will encounter in the field:

* Hyperglycemia (abnormally high blood glucose levels)

* Hypoglycemia (abnormally low blood glucose levels)

If left untreated, both of these conditions will result in an altered mental status.

HYPERGLYCEMIA

When glucose levels get too high, hyperglycemia (diabetic coma) will result. If left untreated, hyperglycemia can develop into a severe condition called **diabetic ketoacidosis** (DKA), also known as **diabetic coma.** Hyperglycemia can take many hours (24 to 72) to develop to a point where the patient begins showing obvious signs and symptoms. In general, hyperglycemia occurs when the patient does not take his medication as prescribed and continues to eat, or increases the amount of food intake without adjusting his insulin intake. In some cases, especially those involving children, profound hyperglycemia with an altered mental status may be the initial presentation that ultimately results in the diagnosis of diabetes. Signs and symptoms of hyperglycemia include:

* Altered mental status

* Frequent urination

* Extreme thirst

* Abdominal cramping

* Nausea and vomiting

* Headache

* Fruity odor to breath

* Hot dry skin

* Unresponsiveness

* Rapid, deep respirations

4-4.1 Identify the patient taking diabetic medications with altered mental status and the implications of a diabetes history.

* **diabetic ketoacidosis**

a hyperglycemic condition in which an absence of insulin causes the body to metabolize other sources of energy such as fat. The blood becomes acidic and the condition may result in a fruity breath odor and AMS.

* **diabetic coma**

altered mental status resulting from untreated hyperglycemia.

Clinical Clues: KUSSMAUL'S RESPIRATIONS

Respirations that are both rapid and deep are frequently seen in patients with extreme hyperglycemia (diabetic ketoacidosis) and are called Kussmaul's respirations.

HYPOGLYCEMIA

✳ **insulin shock**

condition resulting from untreated hypoglycemia.

When glucose levels get too low, hypoglycemia will result. If left untreated, hypoglycemia can develop rapidly into a serious condition known as **insulin shock.** The signs and symptoms of hypoglycemia can develop quickly (30 minutes to 2 hours) and most often are caused by the patient taking a routine dose of insulin without balancing it with a proper meal. Hypoglycemia can also develop in the patient who does everything right but burns off the calories too quickly through exercise. A diabetic who is sick with certain illnesses can sometimes become hypoglycemic when he takes his normal dose of insulin but is unable to eat or keep the food down. Signs and symptoms of hypoglycemia include:

* Rapid onset of altered mental status
* Hunger
* Slurred speech
* Appearing intoxicated
* Confusion
* Dizziness
* Headache
* Blurred vision
* Irritability
* Cool, clammy skin

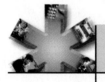

Perspective

Ray—The EMT

"I totally forgot to check our guy's blood sugar. It turns out that the ED nurses did . . . it was a normal 108 . . . so it wouldn't have made a difference in this case. It could have, though. I just tunneled in and figured it was either an assault or some sort of accident while hooking that car up. Thinking about it now, though, that whole incident could very well have been caused by hypoglycemia. Believe me, I won't overlook that again!"

* Elevated heart rate (tachycardia)

* Seizures

* Unresponsiveness

EMERGENCY CARE: THE DIABETIC PATIENT

When caring for a patient who presents with an altered mental status you must complete a thorough history, including asking if the patient has a history of diabetes. In some instances the patient, family members, or other caregivers can provide you with this information. When no one is available to provide this information, look for medical alert jewelry on the patient's neck, wrists, and ankles. You should also inspect the scene for evidence of diabetes medications. Insulin comes in a liquid form and must be kept refrigerated. Be sure to look in the refrigerator, if there is one at the scene, for insulin vials.

Common diabetes medications (Figure 21-6 and 21-7) include:

* Insulin (for injection)

* Diabinese (pill form)

* Orinase (pill form)

* Micronase (pill form)

* Glucophage (pill form)

* Oral glucose (paste or tablet form)

* Glucagon (for injection)

4-4.2 State the steps in the emergency medical care of the patient taking diabetic medicine with an altered mental status and a history of diabetes.

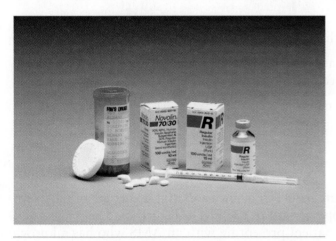

FIGURE 21-6   Common diabetic medications.

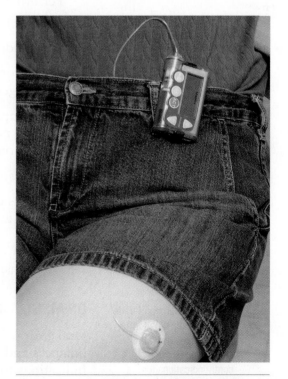

FIGURE 21-7   A typical insulin pump and injection site.

When gathering a SAMPLE history on a known diabetic patient, in addition to the normal questions you will want to determine the answers to the following:

* **When did you last eat?**—— You will want to know when and what the patient had last to eat.

* **Do you take diabetes medications?**—— This will help determine the type of diabetic he is. Type I diabetics require insulin injections, often for life. Type II diabetics' glucose levels are often controlled by diet or oral medications or a combination of the two.

* **Have you taken your medication today as prescribed?**—— This will help the hospital staff determine the cause of the patient's problem and provide the most appropriate care.

4-4.5 Evaluate the need for medical direction in the emergency medical care of the diabetic patient.

Again, it is not essential that you know for certain which it may be, hyperglycemia or hypoglycemia. The focus of your care will be to manage the patient's ABCs and obtain a thorough history. When you are uncertain as to which it may be, it is appropriate to treat the problem as hypoglycemia and provide oral glucose if indicated and allowed by protocol and/or medical direction. Providing glucose to the hypoglycemic patient is likely to improve his condition within a few minutes. If he happens to be hyperglycemic already, the small dose provided by you will not make a significant difference in his condition. When in doubt, and depending on the system in which you are working, contact medical direction before administering oral glucose to any patient. *Follow local protocols.*

Management of the airway and breathing status are of the utmost importance with patients presenting with an AMS. If the use of oral glucose is indicated and your local treatment protocols allow for its use, you must be very certain the patient is capable of protecting his own airway. One way to determine this is by asking the patient to swallow. If he can follow your directions and is able to swallow easily, he is likely to be responsive enough for you to administer oral glucose safely.

Perform the following steps when caring for a patient presenting with an AMS and a history of diabetes:

1. Conduct an appropriate scene size-up and take the necessary BSI precautions.

2. Perform an initial assessment and consider the need for supplemental oxygen.

3. Complete a focused history (SAMPLE) and physical examination and confirm prior history of diabetes, last oral intake, and last time and dose of medication taken.

4. If responsive, confirm that the patient can swallow without difficulty.

5. Consider the administration of oral glucose in accordance with local protocols and/or medical direction.

6. Perform ongoing assessments as necessary.

7. Transport in the recovery position.

4-4.4 State the generic and trade names, medication forms, dose, administration, action, and contraindications for oral glucose.

ORAL GLUCOSE

Oral glucose is an over-the-counter (OTC) medication that is carried on most ambulances and is within the scope of care of the EMT (Figure 21-8 on page 540). Indications for its use are any patient presenting with an AMS who has a known history of diabetes that is controlled by medication.

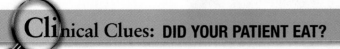

Clinical Clues: DID YOUR PATIENT EAT?

* If a patient has eaten but has not taken his medication, there is a strong possibility they may be experiencing an episode of hyperglycemia.

* If the patient has not eaten and has taken his medications, the probability of hypoglycemia is high.

Once you have administered the oral glucose to a patient (Figures 21-9A and B on page 540), you may see an improvement in his condition within a few minutes. Continue to monitor his mental status and ABCs throughout transport. If the patient becomes unresponsive, remove any material from his mouth, if possible, place him in the recovery position, and provide the indicated care.

BLOOD GLUCOSE MONITORING

The diabetic patient must manage the delicate balance between hyper- and hypoglycemia every day of his life. The ability to maintain this balance requires that he take his medications appropriately, eat a balanced diet, and monitor his blood glucose level. Thanks to modern technology there is a quick and easy tool for

---

Medication: Oral Glucose

- **Generic Name:**—Oral Glucose

- **Trade Names:**—Glutose, Insta-Glucose

- **Contraindications:**—An unresponsive patient or responsive patient who is unable to swallow adequately.

- **Medication Form:**—Gel or tablets (Gel is the most common form used in EMS)

- **Dosage:**—Tubes come in dosages between 15 and 45 mg. Most often, one tube represents one dose.

- **Administration:**—
  1. Confirm signs and symptoms and history of diabetes.
  2. Obtain an order from medical direction or follow local protocols.
  3. Confirm that patient is responsive enough and can swallow adequately.
  4. Have the patient squeeze the tube into his mouth in small quantities and have him swallow it immediately until tube is empty.
  5. Alternative method is to squeeze a small amount of glucose onto a tongue depressor and place it in the patient's mouth between cheek and gums.
  6. Monitor airway patency and perform ongoing assessments as necessary.
  7. Transport in the recovery position.

- **Actions:**—Oral glucose is a fast-acting concentration of glucose rapidly absorbed into the bloodstream, increasing the blood glucose level.

- **Side Effects:**—None when administered properly. May be aspirated into the upper or lower airway if the patient is not capable of managing his own airway.

FIGURE 21-8   Tubes of oral glucose.

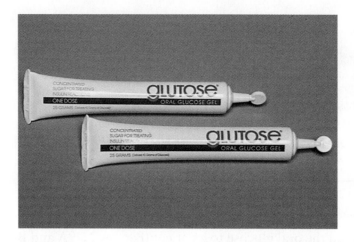

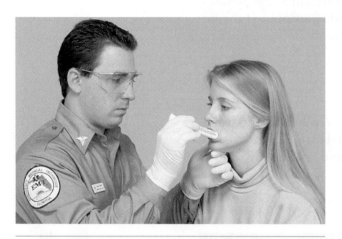

FIGURE 21-9A   One method of administering oral glucose is to squeeze the tube of oral glucose between the patient's cheek and gum.

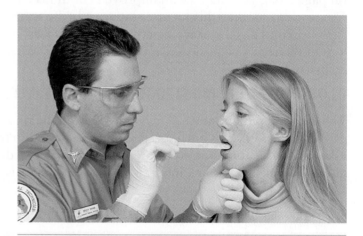

FIGURE 21-9B   Another method of administering oral glucose is to squeeze the glucose onto the end of a tongue depressor, which can then be placed between the patient's cheek and gum.

measuring the level of glucose in the blood and it is called a glucose meter or sometimes simply a glucometer (Figure 21-10).

Blood glucose levels are measured in milligrams per 100 milliliters of blood (deciliters) and are expressed as mg/dl. For most patients, the normal values for blood glucose range between 80 and 120 mg/dl. A patient who is symptomatic

FIGURE 21-10   A glucometer helps the diabetic patient monitor blood sugar levels.

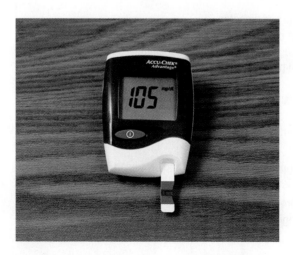

with a value less than 80 mg/dl is consistent with hypoglycemia. Typically, symptoms of hypoglycemia are not evident until 50 mg/dl. A symptomatic patient with a value greater than 120 mg/dl is consistent with hyperglycemia.

Blood glucometers are small, simple to use, and provide accurate results. For that reason, most diabetic patients use them to monitor their blood glucose levels anywhere from once to several times each day. Knowing the results helps them determine how much to eat or how much medication they may need at any given time. By keeping their glucose levels stable, they will experience fewer complications, both short and long term.

Because glucometers are so common and easy to use, you are likely to encounter them in the field while caring for a diabetic patient. Some EMS systems are now allowing EMTs to carry and use glucometers as a matter of normal protocol for managing the diabetic patient. They provide definitive results when the patient cannot provide an appropriate history or is unresponsive.

Not all glucometers are created equal. While similar, each has specific instructions for use and requires calibration with compatible test strips. For these reasons, it is not advised that you use the patient's own glucometer if you are going to obtain a glucose reading. If your system does not allow EMTs to obtain glucose readings, have the patient or appropriate caregiver obtain a reading using the patient's own device. If you are allowed by protocol to obtain glucose readings, only do so with the device provided by your agency. Follow these steps when using a glucometer to obtain blood glucose readings (Scan 21-1 on page 542):

Using A Blood Glucose Meter

1. Utilize proper BSI precautions.

2. Pull out the device, a test strip, a lancet, and some small gauze pads.

3. Confirm that the test strips have been calibrated to the device and, if appropriate, place the strip in the device.

4. Prepare the patient by cleaning the tip of one finger with an alcohol wipe.

5. Once the alcohol has dried, stick the finger using the lancet. Wipe away the first drop of blood that appears. It may be necessary to squeeze the finger to produce a second drop.

6. Apply one drop of blood to the test strip.

7. Read and record the value given by the device. This may take 15 to 60 seconds.

8. Assess the puncture site and provide pressure to control bleeding if necessary.

Clinical Clues: GLUCOMETERS

Specific directions for obtaining a blood glucose sample may differ, depending on the device being used. Always follow the manufacturer's directions for the specific device you are using.

And remember: Glucometers provide just one small piece of the total patient assessment puzzle. Do not neglect the initial assessment of the ABCs, thinking you need to know the glucose level of your patient. Focus on basic assessment skills first, and utilize the glucometer to confirm your assessment findings. Some EMS systems using glucometers recommend that glucose levels be checked during transport to the hospital only.

✳✳✳✳✳✳✳✳✳✳✳✳✳✳✳✳✳✳✳✳

SCAN 21-1 **USING A BLOOD GLUCOSE METER**

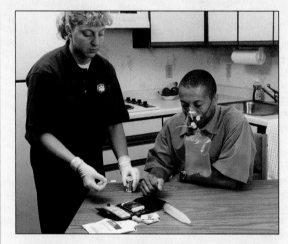

▲ Prepare the glucometer.

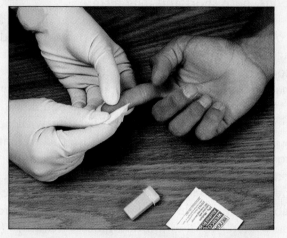

▲ Clean the site.

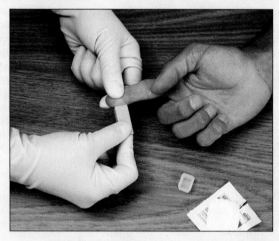

▲ Perform the finger stick.

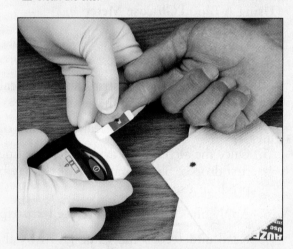

▲ Waste the first drop of blood onto a dressing. Drop the second blood drop onto the test strip.

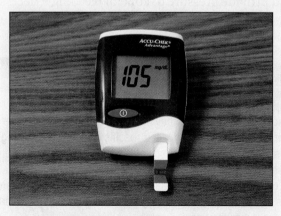

▲ Read and record the blood glucose value displayed on the glucometer.

Stop, Review, Remember!

Multiple Choice

Place a check next to the correct answer.

1. Hypoglycemia, if left untreated, will result in:

   _____ a. insulin shock.

   _____ b. insulin coma.

   _____ c. diabetic shock.

   _____ d. diabetic coma.

2. Hyperglycemia, if left untreated, will result in:

   _____ a. insulin shock.

   _____ b. insulin coma.

   _____ c. diabetic shock.

   _____ d. diabetic coma.

3. A diabetic patient who has eaten regular meals over the past several hours but has not taken his medication will most likely develop:

   _____ a. hypoglycemia.

   _____ b. insulin shock.

   _____ c. hyperglycemia.

   _____ d. diabetic shock.

4. Which of the following is a contraindication for administering oral glucose to a known diabetic patient?

   _____ a. low blood glucose readings

   _____ b. unresponsive patient

   _____ c. The patient is able to swallow easily.

   _____ d. The patient has taken insulin recently.

5. A typical dose of oral glucose would be:

   _____ a. 5 mg.

   _____ b. 10 mg.

   _____ c. one tube.

   _____ d. two tubes.

Matching

Match the definition on the left with the applicable term on the right.

1. _____ A medical condition that results when a person's pancreas will no longer produce an adequate supply of insulin.

2. _____ It is required to facilitate the transfer of glucose (sugar) from the blood to the tissues and cells where it can be used for fuel.

3. _____ If left untreated this condition can develop into what is referred to as diabetic coma.

4. _____ If left untreated this condition can develop into what is referred to as insulin shock.

5. _____ A device used to measure the blood glucose level in patients.

A. Hypoglycemia
B. Hyperglycemia
C. Glucometer
D. Diabetes
E. Insulin

Critical Thinking

1. Describe the relationship between blood glucose and insulin.

_____

_____

_____

_____

2. Describe the medical conditions that can occur when hypoglycemia and hyperglycemia go untreated.

_____

_____

_____

_____

3. List some of the questions you might ask a known or suspected diabetic patient.

_____

_____

_____

_____

* **seizures**

    interruptions of normal brain function caused by bursts of abnormal electrical signals in the brain.

* **convulsions**

    full-body muscle contractions lasting up to several minutes.

* **epilepsy**

    a neurological disorder characterized by sudden recurring attacks of motor, sensory, or psychic malfunction with or without loss of consciousness or convulsive seizures.

* **febrile seizures**

    seizures caused by a sudden increase in fever. Most common in children.

Management of the Seizure Patient

Seizures are another common cause of altered mental status. They occur when an area or areas of the brain receive a burst of abnormal electrical signals that temporarily interrupts normal electrical brain function. Depending on the location and severity of the seizure, the patient may experience anything from a brief lapse in awareness or uncontrolled spasm of an extremity to a total loss of consciousness accompanied by full-body muscle contractions (**convulsions**) lasting up to several minutes (Figure 21-11).

Seizures are not a disease but a sign of some underlying problem possibly caused by an injury, disease, or other abnormal condition. One of the most common causes of seizures in adults is a medical condition called **epilepsy**. Epilepsy is a neurological disorder characterized by sudden recurring attacks of motor, sensory, or psychic malfunction with or without loss of consciousness or convulsive seizures. The most common cause of seizures in children is a high fever; these are referred to as **febrile seizures**. Febrile seizures should be considered a true emergency and attempts should be made to cool the child during transport to the hospital. Cool by removing clothing to the underwear, sponging with tepid water, and fanning. Don't use alcohol, ice or cold water, which can cause hypothermia.

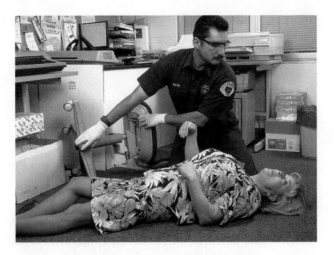

FIGURE 21-11 Care of the seizure patient should center on protecting her from harm.

There are many other common causes of seizures (Figure 21-12):

* *Alcohol withdrawal*—Patients who are chronic alcoholics who abruptly stop drinking alcohol go through withdrawal and will often experience seizures due to the changes their body goes through during the withdrawal process.

* *Traumatic Injury*—Patients who sustain an injury to the head will often experience seizures following the injury.

* *Brain Tumors*—As a tumor grows inside or around the brain, pressure on the brain can cause seizure activity.

* *Infection*—Generalized infections within the body and localized infections within the brain are also capable of causing seizure activity.

FIGURE 21-12 Common causes of seizures.

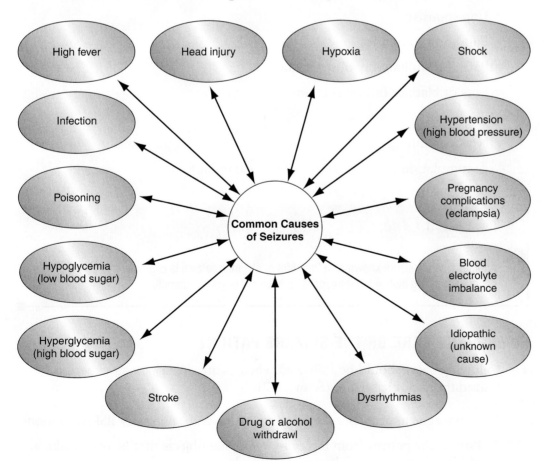

✳ *Metabolic*—Changes or imbalances in the body's chemistry are frequently the cause of seizures.

✳ *Hypoxia*—Insufficient oxygen to the brain may lead to seizure activity.

Clinical Clues: COMMON CAUSE OF SEIZURES

In adult patients, the most common cause of seizures you may see is the failure to properly take their prescribed anti-seizure medications.

✳ **generalized tonic-clonic seizure**

seizure characterized by a loss of consciousness, convulsions. Also called a grand mal seizure.

One of the most obvious and dramatic type of seizures is called a **generalized tonic-clonic seizure.** Generalized tonic-clonic seizures are characterized by a loss of consciousness and convulsions (full-body muscle contractions). These can be very dramatic and frightening to watch for the first time but are usually not life threatening. It is very possible for a person experiencing a generalized tonic-clonic seizure to lose consciousness while standing and injure himself during a fall to the ground. You must carefully consider the need for spinal precautions when caring for a generalized tonic-clonic seizure patient.

During a generalized tonic-clonic seizure the patient may also experience anywhere from a partial to a complete airway obstruction. This is normal and expected and no attempt should be made to insert anything into the mouth of a convulsing patient. Due to the short duration of most seizures, it is appropriate to wait until the seizure has stopped before providing airway care.

Signs and Symptoms of a Generalized Tonic-Clonic Seizure include:

✳ Unresponsive

✳ Full-body convulsions

✳ Partial-to-full airway obstruction

✳ Loss of bladder or bowel control

✳ Fixed gaze on one side

✳ Noisy breathing

✳ Accumulation of fluids in the airway (foaming)

Clinical Clues: PETIT MAL SEIZURE

Another type of seizure known as a Petit Mal or absence seizure is characterized by the patient appearing awake but unresponsive to verbal or painful stimuli.

EMERGENCY CARE OF THE SEIZURE PATIENT

The following steps should be followed when caring for a person experiencing a generalized tonic-clonic seizure (Scan 21-2):

1. Conduct an appropriate scene size-up and take the necessary BSI precautions.

2. Protect the patient from injury by removing objects that he may strike and placing something soft beneath his head.

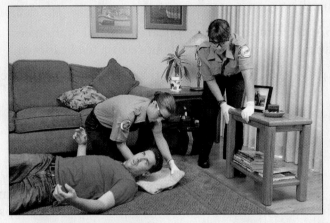

▲ Protect the patient from injury by removing objects that he may strike and by placing something soft beneath his head.

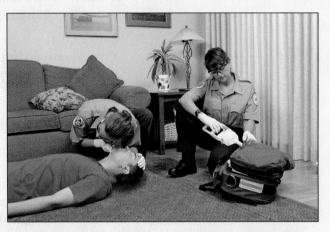

▲ Once the convulsions have stopped, assess the airway. Suction if necessary.

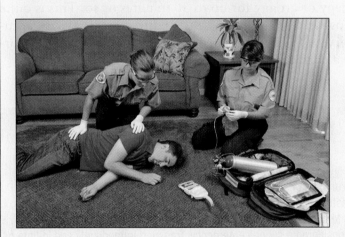

▲ Roll the patient onto his side to allow drainage of secretions.

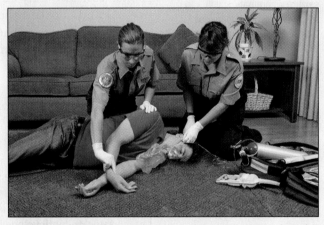

▲ Provide oxygen to the patient.

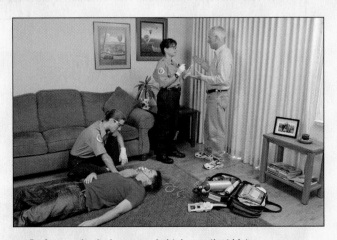

▲ Perform a physical exam and obtain a patient history.

3. Consider the use of supplemental oxygen by nonrebreather mask while he is still convulsing.

4. Get suction ready.

Once the convulsions have stopped continue your care by completing the following steps:

1. Perform an initial assessment and consider the need for supplemental oxygen if not already started. Suction as necessary.

2. Complete a focused SAMPLE history and physical examination. Remember to determine if the patient has been prescribed antiseizure medications.

3. Consider placing the patient in the recovery position if there is no suspected spinal injury (Figure 21-13).

4. Perform ongoing assessments as necessary.

5. Transport the patient in the recovery position.

A seizure patient experiencing convulsions should not be forcibly restrained. The emphasis of your care should be on protecting the patient from hurting himself as his body shakes and thrashes about. Move any obstacles away from the patient and place something soft beneath the patient's head.

Following a generalized tonic-clonic seizure, the patient will remain unresponsive or also may be sleepy or groggy for up to 30 minutes or so. This is quite normal and is called the **postictal** phase. Because the patient may have an accumulation of fluids in the airway following the convulsion, it is especially important to immediately ensure a clear airway and adequate breathing.

✳ **postictal**

period following a generalized seizure where patient will remain unresponsive or also may be sleepy or groggy for up to 30 minutes or so.

✳ **status epilepticus**

multiple seizures without a period of consciousness between them, or one continuous seizure lasting 10 minutes or more.

Clinical Clues: STATUS EPILEPTICUS

In general, seizures are rarely life threatening. They can however become life threatening if the patient has multiple seizures in a row. Repeated seizures without regaining consciousness or one continuous seizure lasting 10 minutes or more can result in the brain becoming hypoxic and eventually lead to brain damage and even death. This is a condition known as **status epilepticus** and is considered a serious emergency. Transport immediately and initiate an ALS intercept if available. This condition is life-threatening.

FIGURE 21-13 Following a seizure, place the patient in the recovery position.

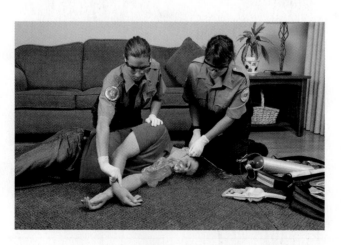

As you gather a history of the incident, be sure to ask witnesses if they saw the patient fall, how he landed, how the patient was moving during the convulsion, and how long the convulsion lasted.

Management of the Stroke Patient

Another patient who is seen fairly regularly in the prehospital setting and who presents with an altered mental status is the patient who has suffered a **stroke.**

A stroke occurs when the blood supply to an area of the brain is interrupted. The interruption can be the result of a blocked artery (ischemic stroke) or a ruptured artery (hemorrhagic stroke) (Figures 21-14A and B). Blood flow can also be interrupted from pressure on the surface of the brain caused by bleeding in the skull or from the formation of a tumor. Because of the way nerve paths from the brain cross, a stroke affecting one side of the brain will cause symptoms, such as weakness, on the opposite side of the body.

Strokes most often occur suddenly and with little warning. They can produce a range of affects from mild symptoms that last only minutes or hours to severe symptoms such as unresponsiveness and respiratory arrest. The severity of the stroke depends on many factors, including the cause (ischemic or hemorrhagic), the location within the brain, the size of the artery affected, and the age of the patient. Generally speaking, hemorrhagic strokes tend to produce the most severe symptoms and have the poorest outcomes for the patient.

SIGNS AND SYMPTOMS OF A STROKE

Patients who have suffered a stroke may present with some or all of the following signs and symptoms:

* Altered mental status up to and including unresponsiveness

* Numbness, weakness, or paralysis of one side of the body (hemiparesis)

* Slurred or garbled speech

* **stroke**

condition that occurs when the blood supply to an area of the brain is interrupted.

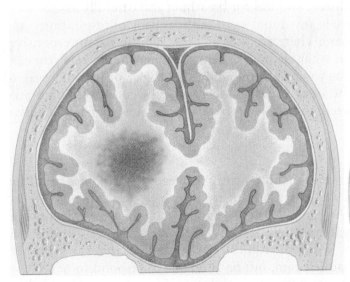

FIGURE 21-14A   Hemorrhagic stroke: intracerebral.

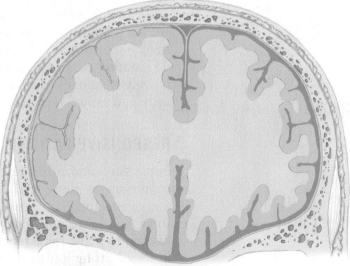

FIGURE 21-14B   Hemorrhagic stroke: subarachnoid.

* Facial droop

* Abnormal pupils, unequal or sluggish to respond

* Abnormal vision, blurred or double vision

* Severe headache

* Nausea and/or vomiting

* Dizziness

* Loss of bladder/bowel control

* Seizures

* **transient ischemic attack (TIA)**

also called mini-stroke, this condition presents as a stroke but signs and symptoms resolve usually within 24 hours.

You may have also heard of a condition called **transient ischemic attack (TIA)**. TIA presents with signs and symptoms similar to a stroke which go away usually within 24 hours. Recently, stroke experts have discovered that certain TIA patients whose neurological symptoms seem to have resolved within hours have in fact suffered permanent brain injuries. This discovery reinforces your training that it is not your responsiblity to distinguish between a stroke and a TIA in the field. Treat all patients with any stroke-like symptoms as a high-priority patient.

ASSESSMENT OF THE STROKE PATIENT

Your assessment of the suspected stroke patient will differ slightly, depending on the patient's level of responsiveness. Obtain a history. If the patient is unable to communicate, obtain the history from a family member or bystander. Be sure to ask exactly when the symptoms began. As you will remember from the chapter on patient assessment, you must perform a rapid medical assessment if the patient is unresponsive and a focused medical assessment if he is responsive.

UNRESPONSIVE PATIENT

Many unresponsive patients will be found in a lying position; if not, then lay him down. Be sure to rule out any possibility of spinal injury before moving the patient. If he is lying face down, carefully roll him over and begin your initial assessment.

As with any patient, focus on the adequacy of the airway and respirations. Take your time as you look, listen, and feel for breathing and carefully assess both rate and tidal volume. If there is any doubt as to the adequacy of respirations, assist his respirations as necessary. There are typically few signs in the unresponsive stroke patient that will reveal what is going on. For this reason, the best you can do is gather as much history as you can from family, caregivers, or bystanders. Do not waste valuable time at the scene. These patients must be considered high priority and should be transported immediately to an appropriate receiving facility.

RESPONSIVE PATIENT

Strokes are sudden and quiet events that often are unnoticed or are blamed on other conditions by those around the patient. In many instances, the patient remains awake and apparently alert. An example is the husband and wife who are enjoying some quiet time together watching television. The wife decides to go into the kitchen to make some lunch. When she returns a few minutes later, she finds her husband sitting just as she had left him, but he is unable to respond to her. He is able to look at her and makes attempts to speak but can only produce garbled or slurred words that don't make sense.

Upon arrival, you will likely find an apparently alert patient with a worried or frightened look on his face. Once you are certain that the ABCs are intact, focus your attention on your history and physical assessment. Perform an examination for stroke such as the Cincinnati Prehospital Stroke Scale. Note any difference in these assessments from one side to the other. A new-onset weakness may be an indication of a stroke on the opposite side of the brain. Look closely at the pupils and note any differences between them. In some victims of stroke, the affected pupil will become sluggish, unresponsive, or dilated.

It is important to understand the fear and frustration that responsive stroke patients are experiencing. They know something is terribly wrong but are unable to communicate well or ask questions about what is going on. For this reason be sure to communicate continuously with your patient and explain everything that is happening. Provide lots of reassurance to both the patient and the family members who are present.

CINCINNATI PREHOSPITAL STROKE SCALE

There are several assessment tools that can be helpful when assessing a responsive patient suspected of having a stroke. One of the most common of these tools is the Cincinnati Prehospital Stroke Scale (CPSS). The CPSS uses three assessment characteristics to evaluate for the likelihood of a stroke.

* **Facial droop**—Have the patient look directly at you and smile or show his teeth. Observe if the facial muscles do not move symmetrically or if there is facial droop on one side or the other (Figure 21-15).

* **Arm drift**—Have the patient hold both arms straight out in front of them and close his eyes. Observe for arm drift, one arm that drops down while the other remains up. It is also significant if the patient cannot bring both arms up together (Figure 21-16 on page 552).

* **Abnormal speech**—Observe for slurred speech, inappropriate words, or an inability to respond verbally.

Presence of an abnormality in any one of the three areas of the CPSS indicates a strong likelihood of a stroke.

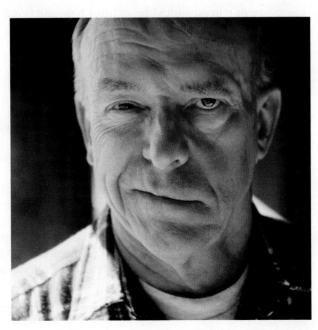

FIGURE 21-15 Assess for facial droop. The face of a stroke patient often has an abnormal drooped appearance on one side. (Michal Heron Photography.)

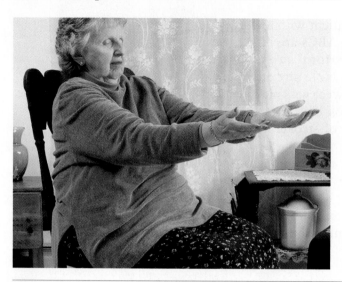 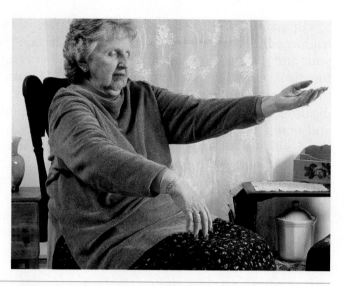

FIGURE 21-16A and B Assess for arm drift by asking the patient to close her eyes and extend her arms for 10 seconds. (A) A patient who has not suffered a stroke can usually hold arms in an extended position with eyes closed. (B) A stroke patient will often display arm drift. That is, one arm will remain extended but the arm on the affected side will drift downward.

EMERGENCY CARE OF THE STROKE PATIENT

The following steps should be followed when caring for a person with a suspected stroke (Scan 21-3):

1. Perform an appropriate scene size-up and take the necessary BSI precautions.

2. Perform an appropriate initial assessment and provide the necessary airway and breathing support.

3. Provide supplemental oxygen as appropriate.

4. Perform an appropriate focused history and physical exam based on the chief complaint.

5. Consider placing the patient in the recovery position. Avoid elevating the patient's head unless he cannot tolerate lying flat.

6. Perform ongoing assessments as necessary and focus on adequacy of airway and breathing.

Clinical Clues: FIBRINOLYTICS

Recent advances in stroke care include the development of clot-busting drugs called "fibrinolytics." These are drugs that can break up the clot that is causing the disruption of blood flow in the brain. Not all stroke patients are candidates for these drugs, but one thing is certain: The sooner a suspected stroke patient gets to the hospital the sooner he can be evaluated for the use of fibrinolytics. The general rule is that patients must receive these drugs within 3 hours following the initial onset of symptoms. However, patients must be evaluated with a head CT scan.

SCAN 21-3   **CARE OF THE STROKE PATIENT**

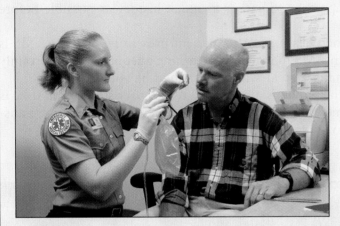

▲ Apply oxygen.

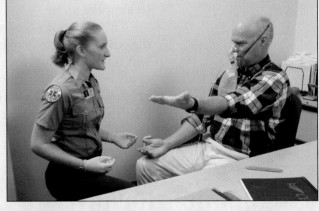

▲ Perform a focused exam including a Cincinnati Stroke Scale.

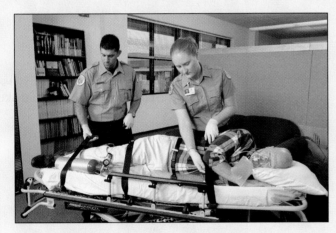

▲ Place the patient in the recovery position as appropriate.

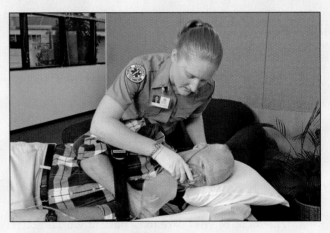

▲ Reassess the patient's ABCs.

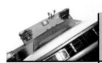

Dispatch Summary

The patient was secured to a spine board, given high-flow O₂ and transported with lights and siren to the University Trauma Center downtown. There, he was found to have a skull fracture with some intracranial bleeding.

He has since made a full recovery but still has no recollection about the events of that night.

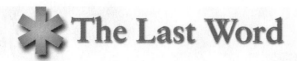

The Last Word

There are, perhaps, almost as many causes of an altered mental status as there are patients. However, several common causes are seen in EMS, including diabetic emergencies, seizures, and strokes.

While it is not essential for you to identify the specific cause of a patient's altered mental status, it is important to gather as much history as possible before leaving the scene.

The focus of all care when dealing with a patient presenting with an AMS is the ABCs. A patients with an AMS may not be breathing adequately and certainly will be less able to maintain his own airway, especially if he vomits.

Continuously monitor the patient's airway and respiratory status even if he is responsive. Provide supplemental oxygen as soon as practical, and initiate transport to an appropriate receiving facility.

✳ Chapter Review

MULTIPLE CHOICE

Place a check next to the correct answer.

1. Which of the following is NOT a typical cause of stroke?

    _____ a. blocked artery

    _____ b. ruptured artery

    _____ c. dilated artery

    _____ d. pressure on an artery

2. The focus of your care for a patient who is actively convulsing should center on:

    _____ a. keeping the patient from injuring himself.

    _____ b. keeping the patient from injuring others.

    _____ c. keeping the patient's mouth open.

    _____ d. getting a good history.

3. The most common cause of seizures in children under the age of 2 is:

    _____ a. injury.

    _____ b. hypoxia.

    _____ c. infection.

    _____ d. high fever.

4. Which of the following is NOT one of the assessment findings in the Cincinnati Prehospital Stroke Scale?

    _____ a. facial droop

    _____ b. headache

    _____ c. arm drift

    _____ d. abnormal speech

5. Clot-busting drugs (fibrinolytics) are most effective when they can be administered within _____ hours following the onset of stroke symptoms.

    _____ a. 3

    _____ b. 6

    _____ c. 9

    _____ d. 12

6. Without _____, a patient's blood sugar levels can become dangerously elevated.

    _____ a. potassium

    _____ b. sodium

    _____ c. insulin

    _____ d. glucose

7. All of the following are potential causes of hypo-glycemia EXCEPT:

_____ a. excessive blood sugar.

_____ b. excessive exercise.

_____ c. skipping meals.

_____ d. excess insulin.

8. The condition in which a patient experiences pro-longed or multiple seizures without regaining con-sciousness is known as:

_____ a. status asthmaticus.

_____ b. grand mal.

_____ c. tonic-clonic.

_____ d. status epilepticus.

9. The condition caused by interruption of blood flow to the brain by a blocked artery or hemorrhage is:

_____ a. seizure.

_____ b. stroke.

_____ c. syncopal episode.

_____ d. status epilepticus.

10. One of the most common causes of seizures in the adult patient is:

_____ a. trauma.

_____ b. taking too much prescribed medication.

_____ c. a high fever.

_____ d. not taking prescribed medications.

CRITICAL THINKING

1. Discuss the causes and types of seizures.

_____

_____

_____

_____

2. Discuss a situation when a seizure may become life threatening and what you would do for the patient in that situation.

_____

_____

_____

_____

3. Describe the difference between an ischemic and a hemorrhagic stroke.

_____

_____

_____

_____

CASE STUDIES

Case Study 1

You have been dispatched to the second floor of an office building for an unknown medical problem. Upon arrival, you are led over to an approximately 60-year-old male who is seated at his desk and appears awake but is staring straight ahead. One of his coworkers tells you that he came by his friend's desk to go to lunch and found him acting strangely and difficult to understand. You discover a medical bracelet that states the man is an insulin-dependent diabetic. As you begin to ask the man questions, he responds by looking at you and speaking; however his words are difficult to understand. He has a rapid pulse and his skin appears pale and moist.

1. What information will you attempt to gather from the patient or his friend?

_____

_____

_____

_____

_____

_____

_____

2. You are able to determine that the man did indeed take his normal dose of morning insulin but has had nothing to eat since. What is most likely this man's problem?

_____

_____

_____

_____

_____

_____

_____

3. How will you care for this patient?

_____

_____

_____

_____

_____

_____

_____

Case Study 2

You have responded to an assisted-living facility for a possible stroke and arrive to find an approximately 80-year-old female sitting at a table in the recreation room. The facility manager states that one minute she was playing bridge with her friends at the table and the next she couldn't talk. The patient is awake and appears alert; however she is only able to make garbled sounds as she attempts to speak. You notice that the right side of her mouth has a slight droop and she is moving her left hand but not her right.

1. You decide to assess this woman using the Cincinnati Prehospital Stroke Scale. What factors of this patient's presentation will you be assessing?

_____

_____

_____

_____

_____

_____

_____

2. Based on her presentation, which side of the brain has the stroke likely occurred?

_____

_____

_____

_____

_____

_____

3. How will you care for this patient?

_____

_____

_____

_____

_____

_____

_____

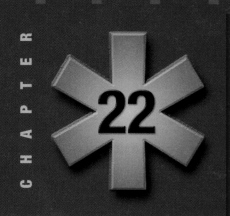

CHAPTER

22

Patients with Allergies

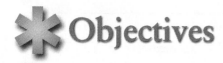

Objectives

Numbered objectives are from the U.S. Department of Transportation 1994 EMT-Basic National Standard Curriculum.

COGNITIVE OBJECTIVES

At the completion of this lesson, the EMT-Basic student will be able to:

4-5.1 Recognize the patient experiencing an allergic reaction. (p. 562)

4-5.2 Describe the emergency medical care of the patient with an allergic reaction. (p. 565)

4-5.3 Establish the relationship between the patient with an allergic reaction and airway management. (p. 565)

4-5.4 Describe the mechanisms of allergic response and the implications for airway management. (pp. 562–563)

4-5.5 State the generic and trade names, medication forms, dose, administration, action, and contraindications for the epinephrine auto-injector. (pp. 569–572)

4-5.6 Evaluate the need for medical direction in the emergency medical care of the patient with an allergic reaction. (p. 565)

4-5.7 Differentiate between the general category of those patients having an allergic reaction and those patients having an allergic reaction and requiring immediate medical care, including immediate use of epinephrine auto-injector. (pp. 561–562)

AFFECTIVE OBJECTIVES

At the completion of this lesson, the EMT-Basic student will be able to:

4-5.8 Explain the rationale for administering epinephrine using an auto-injector. (pp. 565–567)

PSYCHOMOTOR OBJECTIVES

At the completion of this lesson, the EMT-Basic student will be able to:

4-5.9 Demonstrate the emergency medical care of the patient experiencing an allergic reaction. (pp. 565–568)

4-5.10 Demonstrate the use of epinephrine auto-injector. (pp. 567–568)

4-5.11 Demonstrate the assessment and documentation of patient response to an epinephrine injection. (pp. 571, 572, 573)

4-5.12 Demonstrate proper disposal of equipment. (p. 568)

4-5.13 Demonstrate completing a prehospital care report for patients with allergic emergencies. (p. 572)

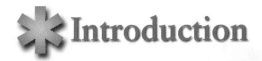 **Introduction**

Nearly everyone experiences some type of allergic reaction during his lifetime. While most allergic reactions are mild, some reactions can be very severe and become life threatening if not treated promptly. In this chapter we will discuss what happens to the body during an allergic reaction and how to distinguish between a mild and a severe reaction capable of causing death.

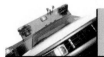

Emergency Dispatch

Harold and his wife Shannon, EMT partners for the city ambulance service, pulled into the parking lot of The Ice Cream Station and stopped near a frantically waving woman.

"Quick! He's on the floor!" The woman shouted as the pair quickly stacked their equipment on the cot and followed her. "The after-school crowd came in a little while ago, and this one boy just started acting really . . . really . . . I don't know. He's just really sick!"

The patient, a 13-year-old male, was unresponsive, cyanotic, and obviously swollen around his face and neck. The shop employees were trying to keep the area clear as a sea of faces jostled for better views and talked in forced whispers.

"He's not breathing," Shannon knelt next to the boy. "Give me an OPA and call for ALS."

A young girl stepped from the crowd and burst into loud sobs, holding her shaking hands over her mouth. "Oh my God . . . I'm so sorry! This is all my fault."

"What do you mean, honey?" Shannon was struggling to get the adjunct into the boy's airway—and losing the battle. She finally tossed it aside, and Harold attempted to ventilate the boy with the BVM. No luck.

"He kept making this big deal about him and . . . and peanuts." The girl was sobbing harder now. "And we didn't believe it . . . and we . . . I . . . tricked him into eating them."

"O, crap." Harold looked from the crying girl to the crowd of students. "Does he have an auto-injector? Have you ever seen him with a thing that looks like a really fat pen . . . maybe with a plastic cap on one end?"

Their blank stares answered his question.

"Let's just go Harold! We can't wait for the ALS unit to get here . . . we're gonna have to meet up with them on the road somewhere. This isn't looking good."

An Immune Response

Allergic reactions are caused when the body becomes exposed to specific substances for which it has sensitivities (Figure 22-1 on page 560). Substances that cause sensitivities are called **allergens** and can be just about anything. Common allergens include:

* **Insect bites/stings**—Bees and wasps are the most common.

* **Food**—Just about any food can become an allergen, but nuts and shellfish seem to be common.

* **allergic reactions**

the body's exaggerated response when exposed to specific substances to which it has sensitivities.

* **allergens**

substance that causes sensitivity.

FIGURE 22-1 Common substances that may cause allergic reactions.

Insect stings

Plants

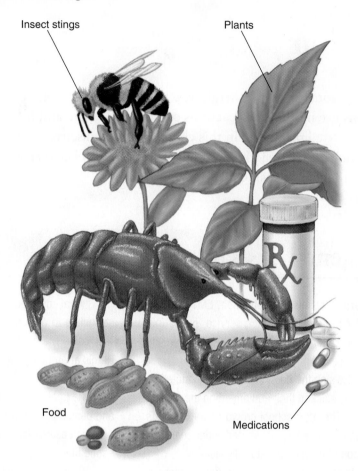

Food

Medications

✳ **Plants**—Poison oak, poison ivy, and pollen are common plant allergens.

✳ **Medications**—Like food, any medication has the potential to become an allergen. Penicillin is an allergen for some people.

✳ **Others**—Latex, mold, dust, chemicals, and animal dander are also common allergens.

Allergens can enter the body through several paths, such as contact with the skin (absorption), inhalation into the lungs, ingestion into the digestive tract, and injection through the skin as in the case of an insect sting. The exposure to an allergen causes an exaggerated response by the immune system as it attempts to attack and fight off the allergen. Most reactions occur soon after exposure to the allergen and occur more frequently in people with a family history of allergies.

While a first-time exposure may produce only a mild reaction, repeated exposures may lead to more serious reactions. Once a person has had a previous sensitization, even a very small amount of allergen can trigger a severe reaction.

Allergic reactions can vary from very mild localized reactions confined to a small area of the body to severe and life-threatening systemic reactions that affect the entire body. These severe reactions are called **anaphylaxis.**

Most reactions occur within seconds or minutes after exposure to the allergen, but some can occur after several hours, particularly if the allergen causes a reaction only after it is partially digested. In very rare cases, reactions develop after 24 hours.

✳ **anaphylaxis**

sudden, severe allergic reaction.

MILD AND MODERATE ALLERGIC REACTIONS

Mild allergic reactions are often confined to a specific area of the body, such as the swelling around the area of a bee sting or the localized reaction from exposure to poison oak (Figures 22-2A and B). Moderate allergic reactions can also involve a more generalized body response such as **hives,** itching or wheezing.

Common signs and symptoms of a mild or moderate allergic reaction include:

✳ Itching on the skin, especially at or near the point of contact.

✳ Hives (Figure 22-3)

✳ Reddish skin (flushing)

4-5.7 Differentiate between the general category of those patients having an allergic reaction and those patients having an allergic reaction and requiring immediate medical care, including immediate use of epinephrine auto-injector.

✳ **hives**

red, itchy, possibly raised blotches on the skin, possibly from insect bites or food allergy.

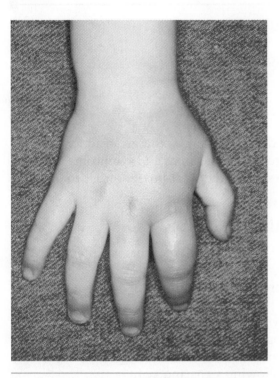

FIGURE 22-2A   Localized reaction from a bee sting. (Photo Researchers, Inc.)

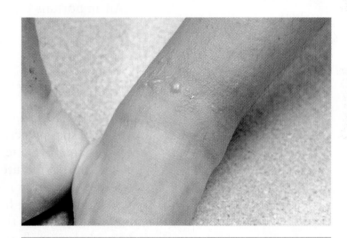

FIGURE 22-2B   Localized reaction from exposure to poison oak.

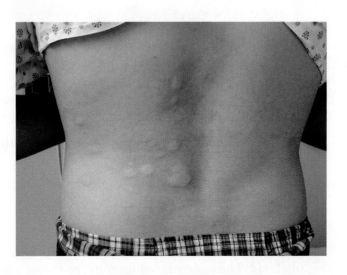

FIGURE 22-3   Hives are a common response to an allergic reaction. (Charles Stewart, M.D. & Associates.)

Clinical Clues: LATEX ALLERGY

Allergies to latex are becoming more common in the EMS profession. It is now known that frequent exposure to latex, such as when an EMT wears latex gloves while providing patient care, can cause a latex sensitivity. If you now use latex gloves and have noticed your hands becoming dry, red, swollen, and itchy following glove use, you may be developing a sensitivity to latex. Try switching to a nonlatex-style glove and see if your symptoms go away. It is important to know that some patients you will be caring for may also have an allergy to latex. Caring for a patient who is sensitive to latex while wearing latex gloves can cause a reaction in the patient. It is becoming common practice to include this question as part of the history gathering.

✳ Minor wheezing

✳ Swelling at or near the point of contact

✳ Swollen, watery, itchy eyes

✳ Increased heart rate

An important characteristic of mild and moderate allergic reactions is that they reach a point and do not continue to get worse. Signs and symptoms may persist for several hours but are not progressive and do not pose a threat to life.

SEVERE ALLERGIC REACTIONS (ANAPHYLAXIS)

4-5.1 Recognize the patient experiencing an allergic reaction.

✳ **anaphylactic shock**
progression of a severe allergic reaction. May result in death.

Anaphylaxis is a sudden and severe allergic reaction that occurs within minutes of exposure. Anaphylactic reactions progress rapidly and can lead to a condition known as **anaphylactic shock.** If left untreated or if treatment is delayed, death can occur within 15 minutes.

A severe reaction is characterized by many of the same signs and symptoms as a moderate reaction; however, they progressively worsen and become life threatening. In addition to those of mild and moderate reactions, the patient experiencing anaphylaxis will present with the following signs and symptoms:

✳ Swelling to the face, neck, throat, tongue, hands and/or feet

✳ Tightness in the chest

✳ Rapid, labored, or noisy breathing

✳ Severe wheezing

✳ Cough

✳ Hoarseness (losing the voice)

✳ Stridor (a high-pitched sound heard on inhalation or exhalation)

✳ Increased heart rate

✳ Decreased blood pressure

4-5.4 Describe the mechanisms of allergic response and the implications for airway management.

✳ Altered mental status

There are two primary mechanisms at work in the patient experiencing severe anaphylaxis. The exaggerated immune response causes the blood vessels to dilate

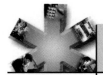

Perspective

Shannon—The EMT

"That was just a bad call. It was the worst allergic reaction that I've ever seen; we couldn't get an airway and . . . and what kid with such a severe peanut allergy doesn't have an auto-injector? We even searched his backpack. If only he had an epinephrine auto-injector, we would have at least had a shot at slowing down his reaction."

Clinical Clues: ANAPHYLAXIS

Assessment findings indicate the presence of anaphylaxis in a person with allergic reactions and signs of shock (hypoperfusion) OR respiratory distress.

while causing the airway passages to constrict. Blood vessel dilation causes the blood pressure to drop, which decreases the perfusion to the brain and other vital organs. As if this weren't enough, the body is struggling to bring in an adequate supply of oxygen because the air passages are progressively getting smaller.

For these reasons, the allergic patient who presents with signs of shock (hypoperfusion) OR respiratory distress must be considered to be experiencing anaphylaxis and MUST receive the appropriate care *immediately!*

* Stop, Review, Remember!

Multiple Choice

Place a check next to the correct answer.

1. _____ are/is caused when the body becomes exposed to specific substances for which it has sensitivities.

   _____ a. Allergens

   _____ b. Allergic reactions

   _____ c. Anaphylaxis

   _____ d. AMS

2. Which of the following is NOT a common allergen?

   _____ a. bee stings

   _____ b. shellfish

   _____ c. vinyl gloves

   _____ d. medications

3. All of the following are common signs and symptoms of an allergic reaction EXCEPT:

_____ a. decreased pulse rate.

_____ b. difficulty breathing.

_____ c. hives.

_____ d. itchy watery eyes.

4. The two clinical findings that indicate the presence of a severe reaction (anaphylaxis) are:

_____ a. difficulty breathing and altered mental status.

_____ b. altered mental status and hypoperfusion.

_____ c. increased heart rate and decreased blood pressure.

_____ d. difficulty breathing and hypoperfusion.

5. Signs and symptoms of this reaction may last for several hours but typically do not progressively get worse.

_____ a. mild

_____ b. severe

_____ c. anaphylaxis

_____ d. allergen

Fill in the Blank

1. _____ are caused when the body becomes exposed to specific substances for which it has sensitivities.

2. Substances that cause sensitivities are called _____ and can be just about anything.

3. _____ are often confined to a specific area of the body, such as the swelling around the area of a bee sting.

4. A sudden and severe allergic reaction that occurs within minutes of exposure is called _____.

5. If left untreated or if treatment is delayed, a severe reaction will develop into _____ and death can occur within 15 minutes.

Critical Thinking

1. Describe the role that allergens play in an allergic reaction.

_____

_____

_____

_____

2. Describe the differences between a mild and a severe allergic reaction.

_____

_____

_____

_____

3. Describe how the body responds during a severe allergic reaction.

_____

_____

_____

_____

Emergency Care: Allergic Reactions

CARING FOR MILD OR MODERATE REACTIONS

Most mild or moderate reactions will take care of themselves with time, but there are some things you should do regardless of the reaction. Perform a focused medical assessment and gather as much history as you can pertaining to what may have caused the reaction, if there have been any past reactions, and how the patient responded. Pay close attention to the respiratory and mental status as you perform your assessment. If the reaction was caused by an insect bite or sting, placing a cool gauze or washcloth over the sting site may help with the pain, swelling, and itching. If the patient refuses to be transported, be sure to inform him of the signs and symptoms of anaphylaxis and instruct him to call EMS should his condition worsen. If the patient refuses transport, be sure to stay with him long enough to determine that the signs and symptoms are not getting worse. Patients presenting with signs and symptoms of a mild or moderate reaction are not candidates for **epinephrine.**

CARING FOR A SEVERE REACTION

Scene Size-Up   Be sure to know what you are walking into. A person who was stung by a swarm of bees may create a hazard for the EMTs who could enter the scene and become stung themselves. If possible, move the patient to a safe place, such as indoors or the back of the ambulance, before initiating care.

Initial Assessment   Determine the chief complaint and focus your attention on the adequacy of the airway and breathing. Some patients may present with a chief complaint of dizziness or lightheadedness due to dropping blood pressure. Others may have a chief complaint of breathing difficulty because of the constriction of the air passages. Administer supplemental oxygen by nonrebreather mask. Airway compromise is likely to occur, so be prepared to provide manual ventilations if either the rate or the tidal volume falls below acceptable minimums. Proper airway management is critical.

Focused History and Physical Exam   Assuming your patient is responsive, you will perform a focused medical exam. For unresponsive patients, perform a rapid medical exam. In addition to the typical SAMPLE history you will want to obtain the answers to the following questions:

* Any previous history of allergies or similar reactions?

* What was the patient exposed to?

4-5.2 Describe the emergency medical care of the patient with an allergic reaction.

* **epinephrine**
  a hormone produced by the body. As a medication, it constricts blood vessels and dilates respiratory passages and is used to relieve severe allergic reactions.

4-5.3 Establish the relationship between the patient with an allergic reaction and airway management.

4-5.6 Evaluate the need for medical direction in the emergency medical care of the patients with an allergic reaction.

✳ How was he exposed?

✳ When did the signs and symptoms begin?

✳ How have the signs and symptoms progressed?

✳ What interventions have been used so far?

✳ Does the patient have a prescription for and carry epinephrine?

✳ Has he used the epinephrine yet?

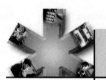

Perspective

Harold—The EMT

"There are those cases—and luckily they seem to be few and far between—where we just don't really have a chance. I think this was one. This kid had no airway, and as anyone who's been in an EMT course for 2 minutes knows, no 'A' makes 'B' and 'C' pretty insignificant. On that entire call, we never moved beyond step 'A'; forget about the medical exam and history."

Obtain a set of baseline vitals as soon as practical. Your partner can be doing this while you complete the history and physical.

If the patient has a prescription for an epinephrine auto-injector and has the medication with him, instruct him to self-administer or assist him in doing so. Follow local protocols. Contact medical direction as appropriate.

It will be important to watch your patient closely for signs of improvement and reassess vitals shortly after administration of the medication. Document the patient response to the medication. If the patient does not have an epinephrine auto-injector available, transport immediately.

Ongoing Assessment   Constant monitoring of the anaphylaxis patient is essential, as his condition is progressive, and you may need to assist his breathing at any moment. In addition to the typical elements of the ongoing assessment, you will want to assess and document any changes in the patient's condition following the administration of the epinephrine.

Follow these steps when caring for the patient with anaphylaxis (Scan 22-1):

1. Conduct a careful scene size-up and use the appropriate BSI precautions.

2. Perform an initial assessment and initiate high-flow oxygen by nonrebreather mask.

3. Perform a focused medical history and physical exam.

4. Assist with the administration of the patient's own epinephrine auto-injector, if available. Follow local protocols and contact medical direction as appropriate.

5. Transport to the closest appropriate facility and/or initiate an ALS intercept, if available.

6. Perform ongoing assessments as appropriate.

7. Document all assessment findings, care provided, and any responses to care by the patient.

If at any time your patient becomes unresponsive or you determine that respirations are not adequate, begin providing assisted ventilations with a bag-valve mask with supplemental oxygen. Do not wait for the patient to stop breathing

SCAN 22-1   **TREATING A PATIENT WITH ANAPHYLAXIS**

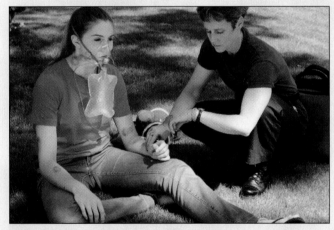

▲ Perform an initial assessment. Provide high-concentration oxygen by nonrebreather mask.

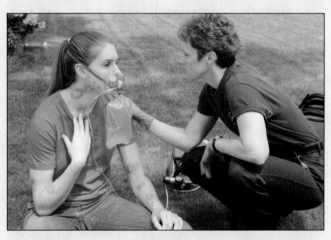

▲ Perform a focused history and physical exam. Obtain a SAMPLE history.

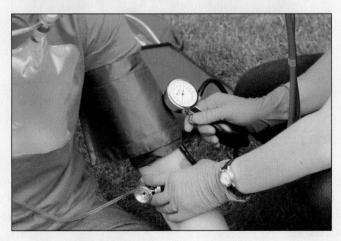

▲ Take the patient's vital signs.

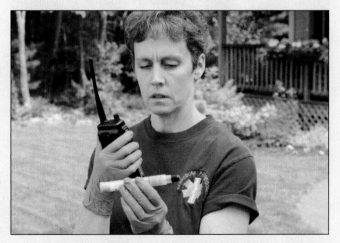

▲ Find out if the patient has a prescribed epinephrine auto-injector and if it is prescribed for this patient. Then check the expiration date and for cloudiness or discoloration if liquid is visible. Contact medical direction.

(continued on the next page)

✳✳✳✳✳✳✳✳✳✳✳✳✳✳✳✳✳✳✳✳✳

SCAN 22-1 | **TREATING A PATIENT WITH ANAPHYLAXIS** *(continued)*

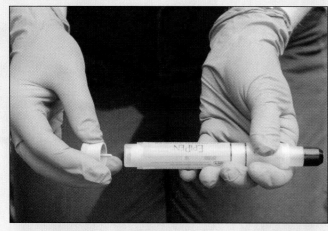

▲ If medical direction orders the use of the epinephrine auto-injector, prepare it for use by removing the safety cap.

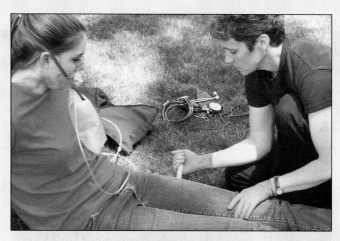

▲ Then press the injector against the patient's thigh to trigger release of the spring-loaded needle and inject the dose of epinephrine into the patient.

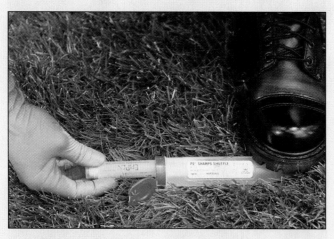

▲ Dispose of the used injector in a portable biohazard container.

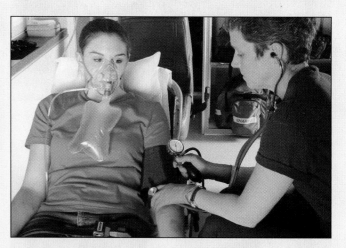

▲ Perform an ongoing assessment, paying special attention to the patient's ABCs and vital signs en route to the hospital.

completely before assisting his respirations. Place the patient in a supine position, attempt to insert an airway adjunct, and provide assisted ventilations as necessary. Have suction at the ready should the patient vomit. Transport immediately and request an ALS intercept if available.

EPINEPHRINE: A TREATMENT FOR SEVERE ANAPHYLAXIS

✳ **adrenaline**
see epinephrine.

Epinephrine has already been mentioned several times. Also known as **adrenaline**, epinephrine is a hormone produced by the adrenal glands, which are located above

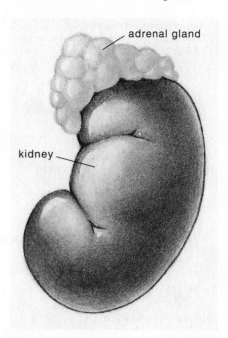

FIGURE 22-4   The adrenal gland is located on the top of each kidney. It is responsible for the production of adrenaline. (Dorling Kindersley)

the kidneys (Figure 22-4). It is a very potent stimulant that primarily affects the sympathetic nervous system. When epinephrine is released into the bloodstream, it quickly causes an increase in heart rate, constriction of the blood vessels and dilation of the air passages. For these reasons, epinephrine is the ideal medication for the patient experiencing anaphylaxis, who has constricted air passages and dilated blood vessels (Figure 22-5 on page 570). On the down side, the body's supply of epinephrine is limited and its effects last for only a few minutes. Because the symptoms of anaphylaxis progress beyond the effects of the body's own supply of epinephrine, another source of epinephrine is needed to control the life-threatening reaction.

Epinephrine can be manufactured in the laboratory and has been for many years. It has also been available as a treatment for anaphylaxis for decades in the form of ANA-Kits and Epi-Kits, which sometimes required the manual drawing up of the solution and injection into the patient. Today, a tool called an epinephrine auto-injector or Epi-Pen makes the delivery of the medication much simpler (Figure 22-6 on page 571).

Medication Name

> **Generic**—Epinephrine
>
> **Trade**—Adrenalin
>
> **Delivery system**—Auto-injection pen designed for self-administration (Figure 22-7 on page 571)

Indications   A patient must meet the following three criteria before administration:

1. Patient must exhibit signs and symptoms of anaphylaxis, including respiratory distress and/or hypoperfusion (shock).

2. Patient has a prescription for the medication.

3. Medical direction or local protocols authorizes the use for this patient.

Contraindications   There are no contraindications when used for severe anaphylaxis.

Medication Form   Liquid form of a 1:1000 concentration

4-5.5   State the generic and trade names, medication forms, dose, administration, action, and contraindications for the epinephrine auto-injector.

A grave medical emergency
Severe allergic reaction to an injected, inhaled, or ingested foreign protein can occur within minutes, even seconds.

Early signs and symptoms
• Flushing, itching. Skin rash.
• Sneezing. Watery eyes and nose.
• Airway swelling.
• Cough. "Tickle" or "lump" in the throat that cannot be cleared.
• Gastrointestinal complaints.

The signs and symptoms of an allergic reaction may swiftly lead to:

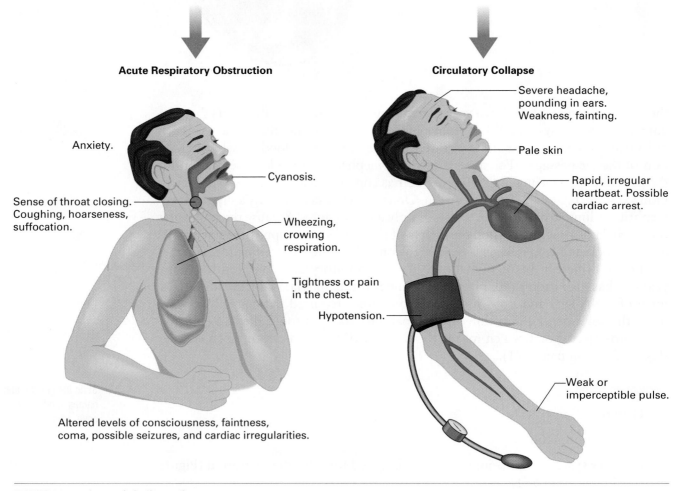

FIGURE 22-5   An anaphylactic reaction.

Dosage   Auto-injectors are available in both adult and pediatric dosages. Adult has a yellow label and the pediatric has a white label.

Adult—one adult auto-injector 0.3 mg

Pediatric—one infant/child auto-injector 0.15 mg

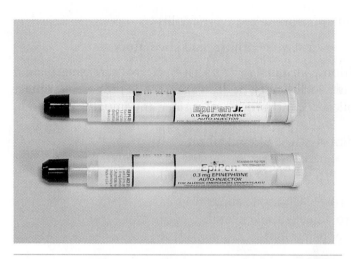

FIGURE 22-6   Pediatric and adult epinephrine auto-injectors (Epi-Pens).

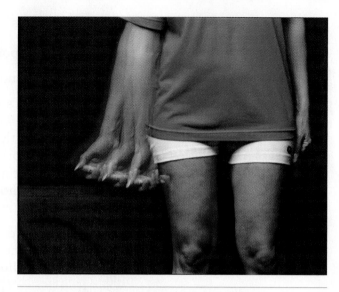

FIGURE 22-7   Patient self-administering an auto-injector.

Actions

Dilates the airway passages (bronchioles).

Constricts blood vessels.

Side Effects

* Increases heart rate
* Pale skin (pallor)
* Dizziness
* Chest pain
* Headache
* Nausea and vomiting
* Excitability, anxiousness

Administration

1. Follow local protocols and contact medical direction as appropriate.

2. Obtain the patient's prescribed medication and confirm:
   a. Medication presented to you is indeed prescribed for the patient.
   b. Medication has not expired. Most auto-injectors have a 2-year shelf life. Medication will discolor (yellowish) when expired.

3. Remove the safety cap from the auto-injector.

4. Place the tip of the auto-injector against the lateral portion of the patient's thigh midway between the waist and the knee. You may inject through clothing if necessary.

5. Push the injector firmly against the thigh until the injector activates. Hold the injector in place for at least 10 seconds.

6. Document the time and any response to the medication.

7. Dispose of the injector in an appropriate biohazard sharps container.

Reassessment Strategies

1. Initiate transport to an appropriate receiving facility as soon as practical.

2. Continually monitor the airway, breathing, and circulatory status.

3. If the patient's condition continues to worsen—such as decreasing mental status, increasing breathing difficulty, or decreasing blood pressure—contact medical direction. Follow local protocols. Consider and initiate the following as appropriate:
   • Administer an additional dose of epinephrine.
   • Treat for shock (hypoperfusion).
   • Prepare to initiate CPR and AED use if indicated.

4. Patient condition improves. Continue supportive care.
   • Evaluate the need to adjust supplemental oxygen.
   • Treat for shock (hypoperfusion).

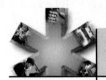

Perspective

The Patient's Mother

"Eric should have had his Epi-Pen, but this was the one day he forgot it at home. He usually keeps it in his backpack. But he was running late today and couldn't find one of his shoes. And, you know, he hadn't had an attack in a couple of years. You know the worst part? When I came home from the hospital, I put Eric's stuff up in his room, and his Epi-Pen was just sitting there on his dresser. I picked it up and haven't been able to put it down since."

Epinephrine auto-injectors come in two single-use dosages, adult and pediatric. The adult dose is 0.3 mg, recommended for patients greater than 66 pounds and carries a bright yellow label. The pediatric dose is 0.15 mg and carries a white label. It is recommended for children weighing between 33 and 66 pounds. Sometimes a single dose of epinephrine may not be enough to completely reverse the effects of an anaphylactic reaction. For that reason, the patient's physician may have prescribed more than one auto-injector.

The beneficial effects of epinephrine occur within minutes following administration. However, the effects of the epinephrine may only last between 10 and 20

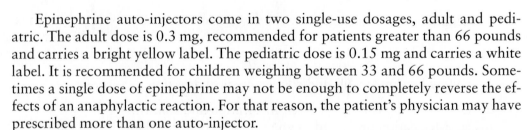

Clinical Clues: PATIENT COMMUNICATION AND EPINEPHRINE

To minimize patient anxiety, prepare the patient for how he is going to feel after administration of the epinephrine. Tell him that he will feel his heart rate begin to increase; he may feel jittery and get a headache. If the patient is prepared for what is about to happen, he is less likely to be surprised and scared, which will only make things worse.

minutes. It is important that you initiate transport and/or an ALS interface as soon as possible. Continue to seek more advanced medical care even if the patient states that he feels better. Complete all necessary documentation.

Bring the used auto-injector with you to the hospital. Handle the auto-injector carefully following the injection. The needle will remain exposed from the end of the device and you must prevent yourself or anyone else from getting stuck. The manufacturer recommends pressing the exposed needle against a hard surface and bending it over. Then place the injector *needle first* into the plastic storage tube. A small amount of fluid will remain in the device following injection. DO NOT attempt to use the same device a second time.

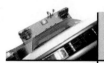

Dispatch Summary

The boy never regained consciousness and was pronounced dead in the emergency department of the Palm Harbor Regional Hospital. The medical director has since authorized the city's EMS system to stock all of the ambulances with epi-nephrine auto-injectors and train the crews in their use. The next time that Harold, Shannon, or any of their EMT coworkers are confronted with an anaphylactic patient, they will have the tools available to help avoid a similarly tragic result.

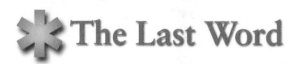

The Last Word

Nearly everyone experiences at least a mild allergic reaction at sometime in his life.

While most reactions do not represent a threat to life, severe reactions known as anaphylaxis progress rapidly and can be deadly.

Anaphylaxis is differentiated from mild and moderate reactions by the fact that it causes difficulty breathing and/or signs and symptoms of shock (hypoperfusion).

Rapid assessment, care, and transport are essential for the survival of victims of anaphylaxis.

Epinephrine can be life saving if given in time. It may only be administered to patients with a prescription who happen to be carrying their own medication. Follow local protocols when administering or assisting with the administration of epinephrine and consult medical direction as appropriate.

Epinephrine slows or reverses the effects of anaphylaxis by constricting blood vessels and dilating the airways.

Chapter Review

MULTIPLE CHOICE

Place a check next to the correct answer.

1. The care for anaphylaxis should focus on:

   _____ a. maintaining responsiveness.

   _____ b. patient comfort.

   _____ c. obtaining a thorough history.

   _____ d. airway and breathing adequacy.

2. Which of the following would NOT be an appropriate history question for the patient experiencing an allergic reaction?

   _____ a. When did your symptoms begin?

   _____ b. What did you last have to eat? Is there a family history of allergies?

   _____ c. Do you have a prescription for epinephrine?

   _____ d. Have you had similar reactions in the past?

3. When should supplemental oxygen be initiated when caring for a patient with an allergic reaction?

   _____ a. immediately

   _____ b. after the scene size-up

   _____ c. during the initial assessment

   _____ d. after the focused history and physical

4. The adult dose of epinephrine is:

   _____ a. 0.15 mg.

   _____ b. 1.5 mg.

   _____ c. 3.0 mg.

   _____ d. 0.3 mg.

5. The effect of epinephrine lasts as little as _____ minutes:

   _____ a. 10 to 20

   _____ b. 5 to 10

   _____ c. 20 to 30

   _____ d. 30 to 60

6. Anaphylaxis is commonly associated with _____ compromise.

   _____ a. neurogenic

   _____ b. airway

   _____ c. mental status

   _____ d. cerebrovascular

7. Which of the following is NOT a sign or symptom of anaphylaxis?

   _____ a. itching

   _____ b. difficulty breathing

   _____ c. decreased pulse rate

   _____ d. swelling of the throat

8. A pediatric Epi-pen contains the following dose of epinephrine:

   _____ a. 1.5 mg

   _____ b. 0.15 mg

   _____ c. 3.0 mg

   _____ d. 0.30 mg

9. A common cause of allergic reaction in an increasing number of EMS professionals is:

   _____ a. latex gloves.

   _____ b. vinyl gloves.

   _____ c. paper face masks.

   _____ d. cleaning solution.

10. A severe allergic reaction will cause the blood vessels to _____ while at the same time causing the airways to _____.

    _____ a. constrict, dilate

    _____ b. dilate, constrict

    _____ c. contrict, constrict

    _____ d. dilate, dilate

CRITICAL THINKING

1. Describe how the emergency care might differ between a patient with a mild allergic reaction and one with a severe allergic reaction.

   _____

   _____

   _____

   _____

2. Describe how epinephrine affects the body when given to a victim of anaphylaxis.

   _____

   _____

   _____

   _____

3. Discuss the critical elements of your patient reassessment following the administration of epinephrine.

   _____

   _____

   _____

   _____

CASE STUDIES

Case Study 1

You have been dispatched to a campground for a person with difficulty breathing. Upon your arrival, a park aid escorts you to a campsite where several people are surrounding what appears to be an approximately 40-year-old female lying on a picnic table. A man who identifies himself as the woman's husband tells you that they were just breaking down the tent when his wife suddenly screamed and shouted that she had just been bitten by something under her right arm near the armpit. As you attempt to get a history from the woman, she appears sleepy and confused and is unable to provide any valuable history.

1. What will be your first priority for this patient in terms of assessment and care?

   _____

   _____

   _____

   _____

2. Your initial assessment reveals that she has an open airway with a respiratory rate of 10 and shallow. Her pulse is rapid and weak. Does this patient require further care pertaining to her respiratory status? If so, what care will you provide?

_____

_____

_____

_____

3. What questions will you want to ask the husband regarding her medical history?

_____

_____

_____

_____

Case Study 2

You have responded to a local park for a possible allergic reaction and are met in the parking lot by a pair of frantic parents holding what appears to be an approximately 3-year-old boy. The father states that his son was stung two times by bees and is concerned that he may be having an allergic reaction to the stings. You begin to assess the child while he is being held by his father and see one sting mark on his hand and another on his shoulder. Both are small red dots similar to mosquito bites. The child appears calm, considering the circumstances. His mother states that he was stung about 15 minutes ago.

1. What will you look for to determine the extent of this boy's reaction to the bee stings?

_____

_____

_____

2. The boy appears to be breathing adequately and his level of alertness seems appropriate for his age. His hand appears to be getting more swollen just in the 10 minutes that you have been on scene. What type of reaction is this boy likely experiencing?

_____

_____

_____

3. The parents are insisting that you get the boy to the hospital before he has a severe reaction. How will you handle this request? What care will you provide for the child?

_____

_____

_____

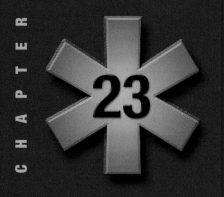

CHAPTER 23

Patients with Environmental Emergencies

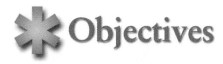

Objectives

Numbered objectives are from the U.S. Department of Transportation 1994 EMT-Basic National Standard Curriculum.

COGNITIVE OBJECTIVES

At the completion of this lesson, the EMT-Basic student will be able to:

4-7.1 Describe the various ways that the body loses heat. (pp. 579–580)

4-7.2 List the signs and symptoms of exposure to cold. (pp. 583–584)

4-7.3 Explain the steps in providing emergency medical care to a patient exposed to cold. (pp. 585–588)

4-7.4 List the signs and symptoms of exposure to heat. (pp. 591–592)

4-7.5 Explain the steps in providing emergency care to a patient exposed to heat. (pp. 592–593)

4-7.6 Recognize the signs and symptoms of water-related emergencies. (pp. 596–597)

4-7.7 Describe the complications of near-drowning. (pp. 597–598)

4-7.8 Discuss the emergency medical care of bites and stings. (pp. 601–602)

AFFECTIVE OBJECTIVES

No affective objectives identified.

PSYCHOMOTOR OBJECTIVES

At the completion of this lesson, the EMT-Basic student will be able to:

4-7.9 Demonstrate the assessment and emergency medical care of a patient with exposure to cold. (pp. 586–588)

4-7.10 Demonstrate the assessment and emergency medical care of a patient with exposure to heat. (pp. 590–593)

4-7.11 Demonstrate the assessment and emergency medical care of a near-drowning patient. (pp. 596–598, 600)

4-7.12 Demonstrate completing a prehospital care report for patients with environmental emergencies. (p. 604)

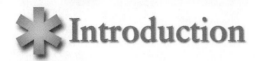

Introduction

Environmental emergencies involve exposure to heat and cold. Exposure to heat and cold is inevitable, even common, but when it becomes excessive true emergencies can develop. Interestingly, the amount of heat or cold necessary to cause problems varies considerably from person to person. This chapter will provide the information to identify and treat emergencies resulting from excesses in heat and cold.

Water emergencies are environmental emergencies involving drowning and near-drowning. Many people participate in water sports today (Figure 23-1). If you have recreational areas—or even swimming pools—in your area, you will be called to respond to submersion incidents.

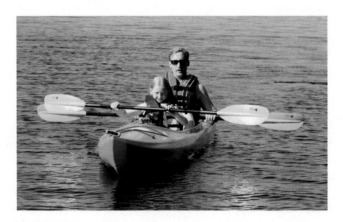

FIGURE 23-1 Today, many people enjoy water sports. (©Daniel Limmer.)

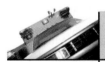

Emergency Dispatch

"You're headed to an oilfield out on County Road 23," Heather, the midday dispatcher, said. "You're supposed to look for a small white sign on the south side of the road that says . . . um . . . 'Rig number 119.' "

"Okay, and do we have a nature yet?" EMT Jay Collins asked, turning the ambulance's air conditioner up to high. He was still sweating.

"They think it's the heat," Heather responded. "And now they're telling us that they'll have someone on the county road to wave you in."

"Ten-four," Jay responded and turned to his partner, Al Brackin. "A heat call? Imagine that. Heck, it's only 108 degrees."

The patient, a middle-aged man clad in a fire-retardant jumpsuit, was sitting in a shady spot at the foot of a towering oil derrick. One of his coworkers was fanning him with a rag.

"How are you feeling, sir?" Al approached the patient and peeled his exam glove from the back of his hand in order to touch the man's skin. Hot and dry.

"There's a . . . um . . . I'm not . . . " The man blinked his eyes several times and shook his head as if to clear it. "I'm kind of sick, I think."

"Let's get this guy in the ambulance now." Al said to Jay as he slid his hands under the man's arms to lift him.

The Environment

Environmental emergencies can happen in a wide range of situations. Hunting, skiing, hiking, and ice fishing are common ways people experience emergencies relating to cold. Those outside for prolonged times in the summer, those working in hot industrial settings, and firefighters are among those who experience heat emergencies.

Of course each person handles extremes of temperature differently. A geriatric patient who has fallen and remains on a cool tile floor for a relatively short time may experience the same level of **hypothermia** that a teenager may experience after many hours outside in very cold weather. Likewise, an infant outside in August for a short time may experience **hyperthermia** at the levels an adult may experience after strenuous exertion or many hours in the same environment.

Some patients who are younger, older, or have significant circulatory problems may develop hypothermia even at or near room temperature. Pay careful attention to factors such as the temperature where the patient is found, clothing worn, age and condition of the patient prior to the exposure, and contact with any surfaces that may worsen the condition.

* **hypothermia**
  abnormally low core body temperature.

* **hyperthermia**
  abnormally elevated core body temperature.

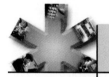

Perspective

Al—The EMT

"Man, what a classic case of hyperthermia! The guy's out working in temperatures over a hundred degrees, in a jumpsuit. He starts getting faint, his skin is hot and dry, and it was pretty obvious that he was having trouble thinking straight. That was just an absolute textbook example of heat stroke. Sometimes you have to stop and think if the surrounding temperature might be an issue on a call, but other times it's just obvious."

Temperature and the Body

The body closely and carefully regulates its temperature. The process of maintaining proper body temperature is called **temperature regulation** and is performed by the brain through various processes, including hormonal regulation.

Hypothermia and hyperthermia occur when the body isn't able to regulate temperature any longer. Another way to describe the balance of hot versus cold is that hypothermia is when heat loss exceeds heat produced by the body's metabolism. Hyperthermia is when heat gained (from metabolism and environment) exceeds heat lost.

Heat is lost through a number of means (Figure 23-2 on page 580). These include:

* **Radiation**—Body heat is emitted into the environment.

* **Conduction**—Body heat is transferred to an object with which the body is in contact.

* **temperature regulation**
  the body's ability to maintain a stable core temperature.

4-7.1 Describe the various ways that the body loses heat.

∗ **Convection**—Body heat is lost to surrounding air that becomes warmer, rises, and is replaced with cooler air.

∗ **Evaporation**—Body heat is lost when perspiration is changed from liquid to vapor.

∗ **Respiration**—Heat leaves the body with each breath.

Consider these methods of heat loss when you are treating patients with emergencies related to heat or cold.

If you have a patient with hypothermia, care will be geared toward preventing heat loss. You will prevent each of the mechanisms of heat loss just described from taking heat from your patient. This will be accomplished by covering the patient with blankets to prevent losses through radiation and convection and placing blankets under the patient to prevent conductive loss. We also add heat to the patient by placing hot packs in his armpits and groin (adds heat through conduction).

With hyperthermia, the principles apply in reverse. We remove clothes and fan the patient (allows conduction, convection, and evaporation of perspiration) and use cold packs and sometimes water to cool the patient's skin (conduction).

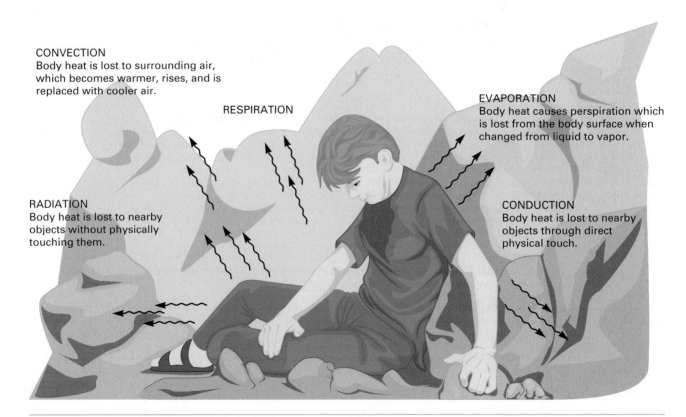

CONVECTION
Body heat is lost to surrounding air, which becomes warmer, rises, and is replaced with cooler air.

RESPIRATION

EVAPORATION
Body heat causes perspiration which is lost from the body surface when changed from liquid to vapor.

RADIATION
Body heat is lost to nearby objects without physically touching them.

CONDUCTION
Body heat is lost to nearby objects through direct physical touch.

FIGURE 23-2 Mechanisms of heat loss.

Stop, Review, Remember!

Multiple Choice

Place a check next to the correct answer.

1. Hypothermia is best explained as:

_____ a. low heart rate.

_____ b. the body loses more heat than it generates.

_____ c. the body generates more heat than it loses.

_____ d. the body is unable to moderate temperature.

2. Applying cold packs to a patient's armpits is an example of temperature regulation by:

_____ a. conduction.

_____ b. convection.

_____ c. radiation.

_____ d. evaporation.

3. When evaluating a patient for hyperthermia, which of the following is least important?

_____ a. the patient's age

_____ b. the environmental temperature

_____ c. the patient's clothing

_____ d. the patient's blood pressure

4. The process by which the body retains or releases heat in normal situations is called:

_____ a. hypothermia.

_____ b. hyperthermia.

_____ c. temperature regulation.

_____ d. convection/conduction reaction (CCR).

5. Hypothermia can occur at a normal room temperature.

_____ a. true

_____ b. false

Matching

Match the situations on the left with the method of heat loss or gain on the right.

1. _____ A patient is lying on the floor of his patio in the winter.

2. _____ A patient has cold packs placed in his armpits and groin.

3. _____ The patient breathes rapidly.

4. _____ You cover the top of a patient with blankets.

5. _____ You remove a patient's wet clothing.

6. _____ You administer warm, humidified oxygen.

A. Radiation
B. Conduction
C. Convection
D. Evaporation
E. Respiration

Critical Thinking

1. Explain the difference between hyperthermia and hypothermia.

_____

_____

_____

_____

2. You are called to a patient who is experiencing hyperthermia. He is outside on baseball bleachers. Using what you know about heat loss methods, how could you cool this patient?

_____

_____

_____

_____

Local Cold Emergencies and Hypothermia

Cold emergencies can be divided into two general categories: generalized and localized. Hypothermia is a generalized emergency; that is, it affects the whole body. A localized cold emergency, for example frostbite, affects one local area.

GENERALIZED HYPOTHERMIA

As already noted, hypothermia is caused when the body loses more heat than it creates. This can occur in a number of ways. For example, if a person is out in a cold environment without adequate clothing, hypothermia will eventually develop. There are factors that can make hypothermia more severe and rapid in onset. These include:

* Wind-chill (Figure 23-3) is caused by the convection of moving air.

* Submersion in cold water increases the rate of heat loss.

* Geriatric patients are more susceptible to heat loss due to reduced circulation and compensatory mechanisms.

* Very young children have large surface areas, less insulating body fat, and less muscle mass (which results in less shivering to generate heat).

* Medical and traumatic conditions such as shock, burns, diabetic conditions, head injury, or infection.

* Drugs (both legal and illicit) and alcohol.

WIND-CHILL INDEX

FIGURE 23-3   Wind chill index.

WIND SPEED (MPH)	WHAT THE THERMOMETER READS (degrees °F.)											
	50	40	30	20	10	0	–10	–20	–30	–40	–50	–60
	WHAT IT EQUALS IN ITS EFFECT ON EXPOSED FLESH											
CALM	50	40	30	20	10	0	–10	–20	–30	–40	–50	–60
5	48	37	27	16	6	–5	–15	–26	–36	–47	–57	–68
10	40	28	16	4	–9	–21	–33	–46	–58	–70	–83	–95
15	36	22	9	–5	–18	–36	–45	–58	–72	–85	–99	–112
20	32	18	4	–10	–25	–39	–53	–67	–82	–96	–110	–121
25	30	16	0	–15	–29	–44	–59	–74	–88	–104	–118	–133
30	28	13	–2	–18	–33	–48	–63	–79	–94	–109	–125	–140
35	27	11	–4	–20	–35	–49	–67	–82	–98	–113	–129	–145
40	26	10	–6	–21	–37	–53	–69	–85	–100	–116	–132	–148

Little danger if properly clothed	Danger of freezing exposed flesh	Great danger of freezing exposed flesh

Source: U.S. Army

SIGNS AND SYMPTOMS OF GENERALIZED HYPOTHERMIA

When called to an emergency involving exposure to cold, begin with identifying situations that could have led to exposure as well as any of the factors just listed that could have accelerated hypothermia. During your initial and focused assessments you will note the exterior skin temperature. Be sure to feel an area beneath the patient's clothing (rather than an exposed surface) to get a better idea of the patient's skin temperature. Use the back of your hand to get the most accurate reading of the patient's temperature without interference from your own. If possible, feel the skin over the abdomen to make this determination.

4-7.2   List the signs and symptoms of exposure to cold.

Other signs and symptoms of generalized hypothermia include:

∗ Altered mental status, including confusion, mood changes, and speech difficulty. The patient's judgment may be affected, causing him to remove clothing

∗ Decreased motor function including poor coordination

∗ Diminished sense of cold sensation

∗ Pupils that respond slowly or sluggishly.

There are also a series of signs and symptoms that can vary based on the severity of the hypothermia (how low the body temperature has dropped). It is critical to identify symptoms early before they become more severe (Figure 23-4 on page 584). Early determinations will also include evaluating risk factors (age, alcohol or drug use and submersion).

Signs and symptoms of hypothermia that vary with severity include:

∗ **Shivering**

Early – present

Late – absent

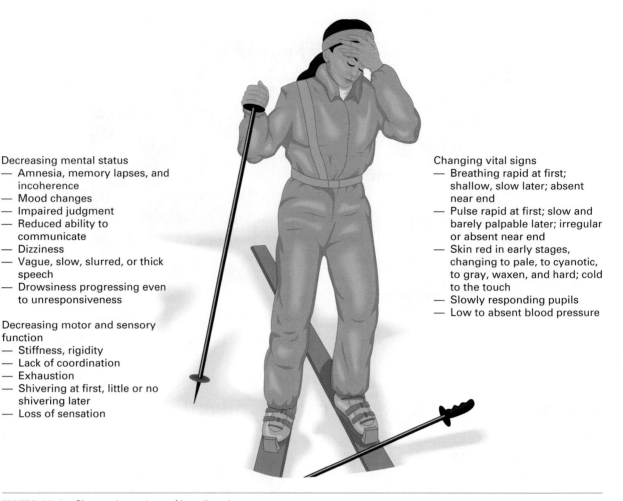

Decreasing mental status
— Amnesia, memory lapses, and incoherence
— Mood changes
— Impaired judgment
— Reduced ability to communicate
— Dizziness
— Vague, slow, slurred, or thick speech
— Drowsiness progressing even to unresponsiveness

Decreasing motor and sensory function
— Stiffness, rigidity
— Lack of coordination
— Exhaustion
— Shivering at first, little or no shivering later
— Loss of sensation

Changing vital signs
— Breathing rapid at first; shallow, slow later; absent near end
— Pulse rapid at first; slow and barely palpable later; irregular or absent near end
— Skin red in early stages, changing to pale, to cyanotic, to gray, waxen, and hard; cold to the touch
— Slowly responding pupils
— Low to absent blood pressure

FIGURE 23-4 Signs and symptoms of hypothermia.

✳ **Breathing**

Early – rapid

Late – slow, shallow eventually absent

✳ **Pulse/Circulatory**

Early – rapid

Late – slow, becoming difficult to palpate, may be irregular. Eventually absent. Low to absent blood pressure.

✳ **Skin**

Early – red

Late – pale, becoming cyanotic (blue and/or gray) then hard

✳ **Musculoskeletal**

Early – shivering, loss of coordination as hypothermia progresses

Late – muscular rigidity, joint and muscle stiffness

Emergency care for patients with generalized hypothermia is centered around removing the patient from the cold environment and preventing further heat loss.

4-7.3 Explain the steps in providing emergency medical care to a patient exposed to cold.

* Protect yourself and ensure your safety from hazards, including hypothermia.

* Remove any wet clothing and cover the patient with blankets.

* Handle the patient gently. Avoid rough movements or jarring, as this could cause abnormal and dangerous heart rhythms.

* Do not allow the patient to walk or exert himself.

* Administer oxygen. If available, warm, humidified oxygen is best.

* Do not allow the patient to eat or drink substances containing stimulants, such as caffeine.

Some care steps depend on the patient's mental status. A decreased mental status indicates a more severe condition that is handled differently.

If the patient has a normal mental status (is alert and acting appropriately), he may be given **active rewarming.** This includes covering the patient with blankets, turning the heat in the ambulance on high, and placing hot packs in the patient's **axillae** (armpits), groin, and neck (Figure 23-5).

If the patient has an altered mental status (ranging from confusion to unresponsiveness), use **passive rewarming** techniques (Figure 23-6). This technique includes covering the patient with blankets and raising the temperature in the ambulance, but hot packs *will not* be used.

When you find an unresponsive patient who is apparently hypothermic, be sure to spend 30 to 45 seconds checking for a pulse before starting CPR. In some cases, a pulse may be present but very slow and difficult to palpate.

An old adage you may hear, "A patient isn't dead until he is warm and dead," favors resuscitation of patients submerged in cold water and others found pulseless in the cold. Research in this area is ongoing. Current beliefs are that patients found within a short time after submersion may in fact be resuscitated past the 5 to 10 minutes that is often fatal in **normothermic** patients. When the patient has been submerged for a longer period of time (more than 30 minutes) or when the patient's body has undergone significant freezing, resuscitation attempts are

* **active rewarming**
  application of an external heat source to rewarm the body of a hypothermic patient. See also passive rewarming.

* **axillae**
  armpits.

* **passive rewarming**
  covering a hypothermic patient and taking other steps to prevent further heat loss and help the body rewarm itself. See also active rewarming.

* **normothermic**
  normal body temperature.

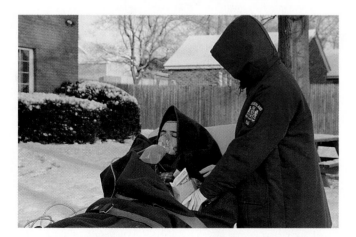

FIGURE 23-5   One way to actively warm the patient is to place heat packs in the groin, armpits, and neck. Insulate the packs to prevent burns.

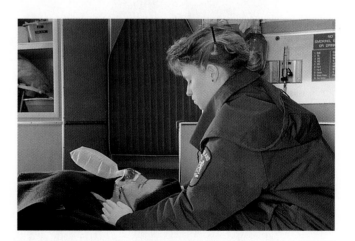

FIGURE 23-6   Passive rewarming includes wrapping the patient in blankets and turning up the heat in the patient compartment.

likely to be futile. Follow your local protocols in reference to performing CPR on hypothermic patients.

LOCAL COLD INJURY

Local cold injuries involve damage to local tissues of one or more parts of the body but do not involve a generalized lowering of the body temperature as seen in hypothermia—although hypothermia may also be present in the patient who has a local cold injury. Local cold injuries are commonly referred to as **frostbite** or **frostnip**.

✳ **frostbite**

Local cold injury. Damage to local tissues from exposure to cold temperatures. See also frostnip.

✳ **frostnip**

early or superficial frostbite.

Many of the same risk factors of hypothermia apply to local cold injury. Additionally the extremities and exposed areas of the head (especially the nose and ears) are susceptible to local cold injury. The two stages of local cold injury are known as early or superficial cold injury and late or deep cold injury (Figure 23-7).

Signs and symptoms of early or superficial local cold injury include:

✳ Loss of normal skin color. Skin may be pale or appear "blanched."

✳ Loss of feeling and sensation in the area.

✳ A tingling sensation when rewarmed

✳ Skin that is soft to the touch (not frozen)

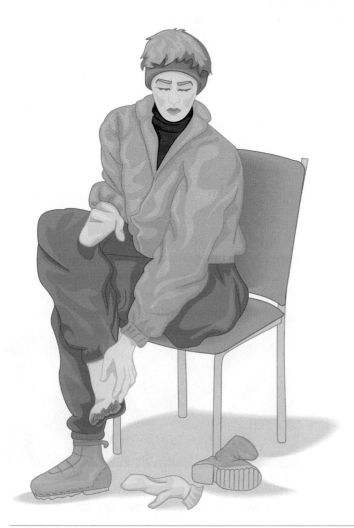

EARLY OR SUPERFICIAL COLD INJURY usually involves the tips of the ears, the nose, the cheek bones, the tips of the toes or fingers, and the chin. The patient is usually unaware of the injury. As exposure time lengthens or temperature drops, the patient will lose feeling and sensation in the affected area. The skin remains soft but cold to the touch, and normal skin color does not return after palpation. As the area rewarms, the patient may report a tingling sensation.

LATE OR DEEP COLD INJURY involves both the skin and tissue beneath it. The skin itself is white and waxy with a firm to completely solid, frozen feeling. Swelling and blisters filled with clear or straw-colored fluid may be present. As the area thaws, it may become blotchy or mottled, with colors from white to purple to grayish-blue. Deep cold injury is an extreme emergency and can result in permanent tissue loss.

FIGURE 23-7   Stages of local cold injury.

Late or deep cold injuries are those that develop after prolonged exposure or that affect deeper tissues (Figures 23-8A and B). Signs and symptoms of late, deep cold injury include:

* White, waxy skin

* Firm or frozen-feeling skin

* Swelling

* Blisters

* Upon thawing, the skin may appear mottled, flushed, or cyanotic

Emergency care for local cold injuries involves some core components and some differences based on the depth of the injury.

All patients with local cold injuries should be removed from the cold environment, have wet or restrictive clothing removed, and receive oxygen.

If the injury appears early or superficial:

* Splint the extremity

* Cover the extremity to preserve warmth

* Avoid rubbing or massaging the area

* Do not reexpose the injury to the cold

If the injury appears to be deep or as a result of prolonged exposure to the cold, follow the steps above for early or superficial cold injury **and:**

* Remove jewelry

Do not:

* Rewarm or apply heat

* Rub or massage the part

* Break blisters

* Allow the patient to walk on the affected extremity

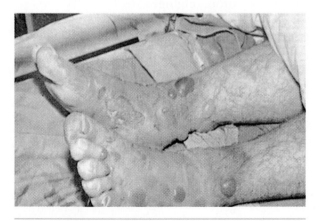

FIGURE 23-8A   In late or deep cold injury, the skin may appear white and waxy and feel firm to solidly frozen. Swelling and blisters may be present.

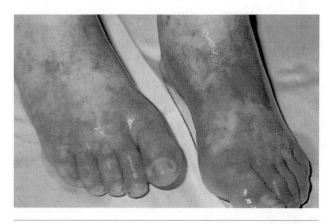

FIGURE 23-8B   As a late or deep cold injury thaws, it may become blotchy or mottled and colored from white to purple to grayish-blue.

Cold injuries often occur in remote locations resulting in delays accessing and transporting the patient to the hospital. If a delay in transport or a long transport time is anticipated, rewarming may be performed.

To rewarm a local cold injury, place the affected part in warm (not hot) water. Water should be slightly warmer than normal body temperature but should not exceed 105 to 108 degrees Fahrenheit. Since the body part will be anywhere from cold to frozen, stir the water to ensure that warm water remains in contact with the body. You may need to add additional warm water or to change the water, depending on the amount of time it takes to thaw the body part.

Thaw until color and sensation return and the body part is soft. This process may cause significant pain for the patient as sensation returns. Once thawed, it is critical to dry the part and maintain warmth for the patient and the affected part to prevent refreezing or hypothermia. Only rewarm the part if you can be sure that the limb will not refreeze.

 Stop, Review, Remember!

Multiple Choice

Place a check next to the correct answer.

1. Which of the following is NOT a factor contributing to hypothermia?

   _____ a. alcohol

   _____ b. geriatric patients

   _____ c. pediatric patients

   _____ d. shivering

2. Water used to rewarm a local cold injury should be:

   _____ a. 50 degrees.

   _____ b. 90 degrees.

   _____ c. 105 degrees.

   _____ d. 125 degrees.

3. Shivering begins late in hypothermia.

   _____ a. true

   _____ b. false

4. Signs and symptoms of generalized hypothermia include all of the following EXCEPT:

   _____ a. mood changes.

   _____ b. decreased motor function.

   _____ c. sluggish pupil response.

   _____ d. increased sensation in the extremities.

5. Which statement about determining body temperature is most correct?

   _____ a. You should check the patient's forehead, because the head receives an increased blood supply.

   _____ b. You should check the patient's feet, because this is the most distal part of the patient's circulation.

   _____ c. You should check the abdomen or another area under the patient's clothes to get an area less affected by external temperature.

   _____ d. You should avoid determining body temperature, because this may cause cardiac arrest.

6. You should spend an increased time checking the pulse of a hypothermic patient, sometimes as long as 30 to 45 seconds.

   _____ a. true

   _____ b. false

Fill in the Blank

1. There are two categories of local cold injury: _____ and _____.

2. Freezing of tissue (for example, fingers or toes) is called _____.

3. Hypothermia occurs when the body _____ more heat than it _____.

4. Loss of heat through an object in contact with the body is called _____.

Critical Thinking

1. Explain the difference between hypothermia and local cold injury.

   _____

   _____

   _____

2. What is the difference between active and passive rewarming?

   _____

   _____

   _____

3. For each of the following list the early and late signs of hypothermia: shivering, breathing, pulse, and skin.

   _____

   _____

   _____

Heat Exposure and Hyperthermia

As discussed at the beginning of this chapter, body temperature is the sum of heat given off and the heat generated by the body's metabolism. This section will discuss conditions that occur when the body temperature becomes too high.

Serious increases in body temperature usually occur when the environmental temperature is so high that it prevents the body from losing heat by radiation. High humidity reduces the ability of the body to lose heat through sweating and evaporation. The presence of one or both of these conditions often sets the stage for a heat emergency (Figure 23-9).

CONTRIBUTING FACTORS

Factors in heat emergencies—other than environmental temperature and humidity—vary from person to person. The elderly often experience heat emergencies as a result of poor temperature-control mechanisms in the body. Medications may also reduce the elderly patient's ability to regulate temperature. In those who are bedridden or have limited mobility, it may not be possible to leave a hot environment. You may recall hearing news reports of elderly people in cities who died as a result of living on an upper floor in a non-air-conditioned apartment during a heat wave.

Newborns and infants (those in the first year of life) also have heat regulation problems. In these patients, the ability to regulate heat has not been fully developed. Making things worse is the fact that infants are not able to remove clothes.

Preexisting problems and medical conditions can predispose any patient to heat emergencies. Some of these include:

* Psychiatric disorders (both because of the medications taken and the patient's poor judgment)
* Heart disease
* Diabetes
* Fever
* Fatigue
* Obesity
* Dehydration

Dehydration can be caused by reduced fluid intake or from perspiration. It is estimated that exercise or hard labor can cause a loss of up to 1 liter of loss in an hour. This also causes a loss of important **electrolytes,** such as sodium. Electrolyte balance is critical to many body functions.

❋ **electrolyte**

a substance that, in water, separates into electrically charged particles.

ASSESSMENT OF THE PATIENT WITH A HEAT EMERGENCY

4-7.4 List the signs and symptoms of exposure to heat.

Your assessment of the heat-emergency patient will consider conditions such as environment, patient age, and preexisting conditions in addition to the signs and symptoms you observe.

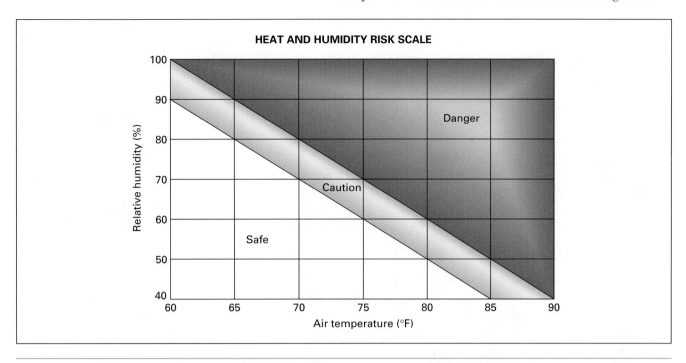

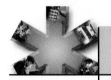

Perspective

The Oil Rig Supervisor

"Sometimes it's so hard to prevent heat emergencies out here on the job. It's tough, physical work and on days like today . . . it's not like we can just shut down so everyone can take a break. I try to make them drink water, but as the old saying goes . . . ."

Signs and symptoms seen in the patient experiencing a heat emergency include (Figure 23-10 on page 592):

✳ Weakness or exhaustion

✳ Dizziness

✳ Fainting or feeling faint

✳ Rapid heart rate

✳ Muscular cramps

✳ Altered mental status

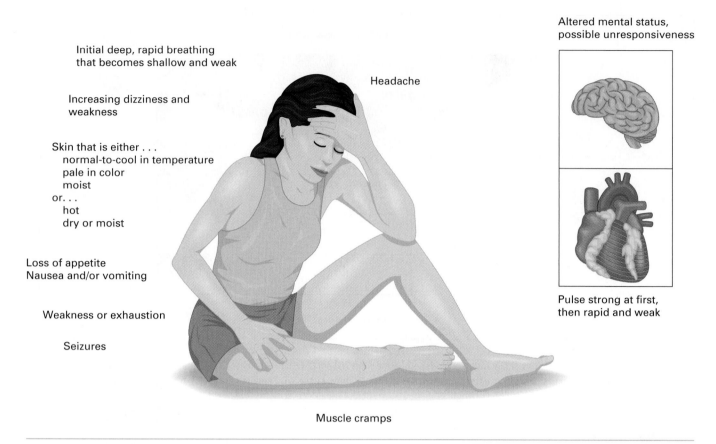

Initial deep, rapid breathing
that becomes shallow and weak

Increasing dizziness and
weakness

Skin that is either . . .
    normal-to-cool in temperature
    pale in color
    moist
or. . .
    hot
    dry or moist

Loss of appetite
Nausea and/or vomiting

Weakness or exhaustion

Seizures

Headache

Muscle cramps

Altered mental status,
possible unresponsiveness

Pulse strong at first,
then rapid and weak

FIGURE 23-10 Signs and symptoms of heat emergency.

The signs and symptoms just listed can occur in all heat-emergency patients. Among the most significant features, in combination with these signs and symptoms, are the color, temperature, and condition of the patient's skin.

＊ Skin that is moist and pale with normal-to-cool temperature usually indicates a less serious heat condition.

＊ Skin that is hot and dry or moist indicates a serious heat emergency.

EMERGENCY CARE FOR HEAT EMERGENCIES

4-7.5 Explain the steps in providing emergency care to a patient exposed to heat.

Care for heat emergencies is based on patient presentation. Patients who have cool skin are cared for differently than those with hot skin.

All patients will benefit from being removed from the hot environment. The most practical location for this is the back of the ambulance. Not only can you begin transport but you can use the air conditioning as a means of cooling the patient. If you know you are responding to a heat emergency, turn the air conditioner in the back of the ambulance on before you go to the patient's side so it will be cool when you return.

For patients with cool skin (may be dry or moist) (Figure 23-11):

＊ Administer oxygen

＊ Loosen or remove clothing

＊ Fan the patient to provide extra cooling

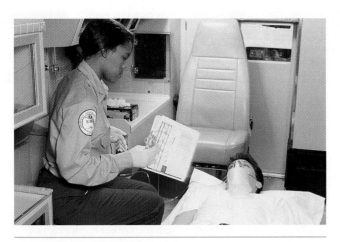

FIGURE 23-11   If the skin is moist, pale, and normal-to-cool, place the patient in a cool environment and fan to promote cooling.

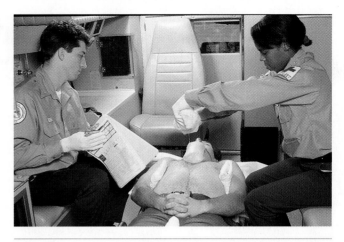

FIGURE 23-12   If the skin is hot and dry or moist, promote cooling by applying cool packs, fanning, and pouring cool water over the patient's body.

* Place the patient supine with legs elevated

* If the patient is unresponsive, place the patient on his left side and monitor the airway for vomiting

* Water may be given to patients who are responsive, have a gag reflex, and are not nauseated. (Follow local protocols.)

For patients with hot skin (may be dry or moist) (Figure 23-12):

* Administer oxygen

* Remove clothing

* Apply cold packs to the neck, armpits, and groin

* Wet the skin and fan the patient aggressively to promote cooling

* Transport immediately

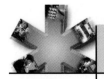

Perspective

Jay—The EMT

"I can't even guess that guy's temperature, but he was way overheated. So we got him in the truck, turned the A/C on high, cut off his jumpsuit, and packed him with ice packs. And our service just bought us these cool little fans . . . the kind with the squirt bottles attached to them. Have you seen those? They work great on patients like these. Some of us . . . not mentioning any names . . . but some of us have been known to use them between calls on hot afternoons. Not me, of course."

Stop, Review, Remember!

Multiple Choice

Place a check next to the correct answer.

1. Patients experiencing a more serious heat emergency will have which skin characteristics?

   _____ a. cool, moist

   _____ b. pale, moist

   _____ c. hot, moist

   _____ d. cool, pale

2. Which of the following treatments would NOT be appropriate for a patient with hot, moist skin?

   _____ a. remove clothing

   _____ b. offer cool water to drink

   _____ c. place ice packs in the groin

   _____ d. place an unresponsive, breathing patient on his side

3. Rewarming of a local cold injury should occur in which of the following scenarios?

   _____ a. a patient in severe pain 10 minutes from the hospital

   _____ b. a patient who does not wish to go to the hospital

   _____ c. a patient who is in a ski lodge with delayed transport time

   _____ d. a patient who can seek physician follow-up within an hour of rewarming.

4. Which of the following is NOT a sign or symptom of early or superficial cold injury?

   _____ a. white, waxy skin

   _____ b. a tingling sensation when rewarmed

   _____ c. loss of feeling in the area

   _____ d. a history of exposure to the cold

5. Which of the following is an example of passive rewarming techniques?

   _____ a. immersion in lukewarm water

   _____ b. hot packs in the groin, neck, and armpits

   _____ c. raising the temperature in the ambulance

   _____ d. none of the above are passive methods

Fill in the Blank

For each of the following signs and symptoms of hypothermia, write "early" if it is a sign or symptom that would be seen in early stages or write "late" if it would be seen in a late stage.

1. no shivering   _____
2. rapid breathing   _____
3. pale skin   _____
4. joint stiffness   _____
5. shivering   _____
6. shallow breathing   _____
7. slow pulse   _____
8. red skin

Critical Thinking

1. What are the differences between serious and more minor heat emergency patients?

   _____

   _____

   _____

   _____

2. What is the difference in care between serious and more minor hypothermia?

   _____

   _____

   _____

   _____

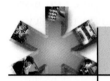

Perspective

Al—The EMT

"There was one important thing we almost forgot. Almost makes me laugh. We got the guy in the ambulance, cut off his clothes, put cold packs in some very personal places—if you know what I mean. I didn't know his name. Sometimes we get into the heat of a serious call like this and forget the most basic thing. We had his medical care right. He trusted us and let us do it. But knowing someone's name from the beginning seems to make the call go better. So we introduced ourselves and kept going and finally asked his name. It is John. When all is done, he won't remember that we may have saved his life—or even the cold packs in the groin. But he will remember that we took good care of him. And a big part of that is knowing and using his name when addressing him."

Other Environmental Emergencies

The outdoors can cause emergencies besides those caused by heat and cold. The remainder of this chapter will discuss emergencies caused by submersion in water and bites and stings from by spiders, snakes, and marine animals.

DROWNING AND NEAR-DROWNING

* **drowning**

death caused by submersion in water.

* **near-drowning**

the condition of having begun to drown but still able to be resuscitated.

Drowning is a term commonly used to describe those submerged in water, but actually it refers to those who have died as a result of submersion. The term **near-drowning** refers to those who have been submerged but who either have vital signs or are resuscitated from a submersion event. There are a variety of factors involved in drowning that ultimately lead to the death of the patient (Figure 23-13).

When a rescue will be attempted around water, safety is the first concern. Emotion may cause rescuers to jump in and become victims themselves. Even strong swimmers, when faced with a panicked patient, very cold water, or fast currents, can succumb to the same hazards faced by the patient.

There are ways to help without entering the water. One way to remember safer methods of rescue without swimming are the terms *reach, throw and tow,* and *row* (Figure 23-14). When close to shore or the edge of a pool, try to reach the patient with a stick or pole. If that fails, throw an item that will float (Figure 23-15) tied to a rope and then tow (pull) the patient to safety. If that fails, row to the patient in a boat. While rowing to the patient is generally safer than trying to swim to him, there are still risks involved, such as capsizing the boat or falling overboard during the rescue.

Assessment considerations for the near-drowning patient include:

4-7.6 Recognize the signs and symptoms of water-related emergencies.

* Considering the possibility of spinal injury

* A thorough initial assessment, including suction and ventilation if necessary

* Identification of cold-water submersions. These patients may be resuscitated even if the time submerged exceeds the limits we would place on normothermic patients in cardiac arrest. Patients have been known to survive

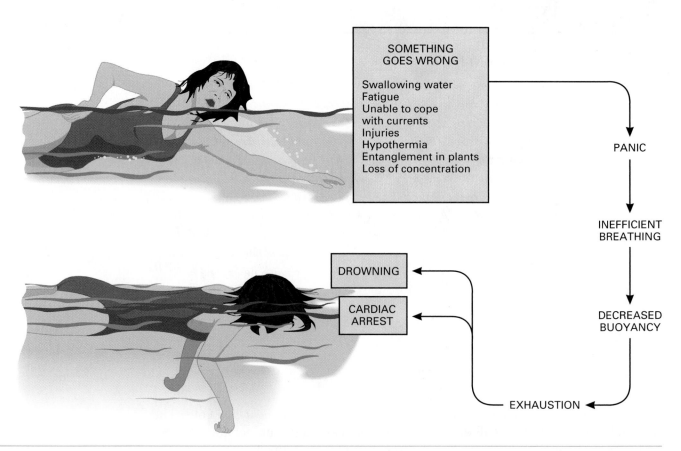

SOMETHING GOES WRONG

Swallowing water
Fatigue
Unable to cope with currents
Injuries
Hypothermia
Entanglement in plants
Loss of concentration

PANIC

INEFFICIENT BREATHING

DECREASED BUOYANCY

EXHAUSTION

DROWNING

CARDIAC ARREST

FIGURE 23-13 Causes of drowning.

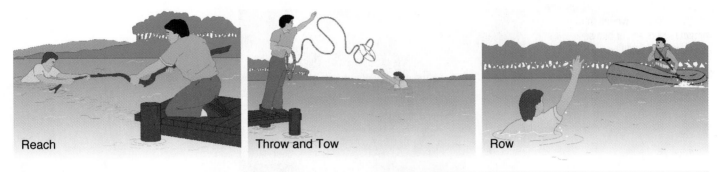

Reach | Throw and Tow | Row

FIGURE 23-14 First try to reach and pull the patient from the water. If that fails, throw him anything that will float, and tow him from the water. If that fails, row to the patient.

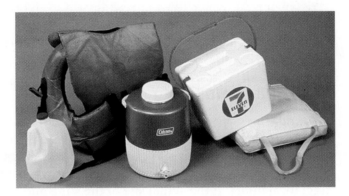

FIGURE 23-15 Throw the patient any object that will float tied to a rope.

after prolonged resuscitation. There are limits, however. In water of any temperature after several hours or if there is extensive freezing, resuscitation is unlikely. Follow your local protocols.

Care for the near-drowning patient includes:

* Removing the patient from the water on a backboard with stabilization of the head and neck if spinal injuries are suspected. If no backboard is available and the patient is in respiratory or cardiac arrest or if you are unable to maintain a patient's airway, remove the patient from the water immediately by the safest method.

* Providing a prompt initial assessment including evaluation of breathing and the need for suction. Suction, ventilate, and provide oxygen as needed

* If the patient is in respiratory or cardiac arrest, provide resuscitation

* Performing a rapid trauma exam

* Initiating prompt transport to an appropriate facility

4-7.7 Describe the complications of near-drowning.

WATER EXTRICATION

Removing patients from the water must be done safely, efficiently, and with the proper priorities. Spinal injuries are possible in many water emergencies, such as diving accidents and rough current injuries. However, the need for spinal care must be balanced with the need for resuscitation. The ability to do adequate and prolonged ventilations in the water is severely limited. Chest compressions in the water are clearly ineffective. Getting a patient to shore and to the hospital are your priorities.

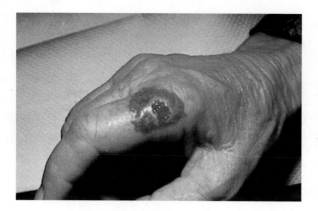

Several methods of immobilization are available for use on patients in the water who have suspected spine injuries. One- and two-rescuer techniques for deep and shallow water are shown in Scans 23-1A and 23-1B on page 600.

BITES AND STINGS

Bites and stings can range from an annoyance to a life-threatening emergency. The life-threatening emergency, anaphylaxis, was covered in chapter 22. This section will cover the assessment and care of bites and stings that are not life threatening.

There are two problems that will present when a patient has received a bite or sting: local injury at the actual site of the sting and the substance (venom) that was injected into the patient's body.

Assessment of the injury site involves an inspection for redness and swelling (Figure 23-16). The patient will usually report feeling pain in the area. If you observe the area of redness expanding, involving hives or increased swelling—especially involving the face, neck, and chest—the patient may be developing anaphylaxis. Be alert for other indications of anaphylaxis such as hoarseness, a feeling of swelling or a lump in the throat, wheezing, and signs of shock.

It will be important to determine if the patient has a history of past reactions to similar stings. In the event the patient has had an allergic reaction to a specific type of bee, remain alert for anaphylaxis even if you are unsure of the type of bee involved in the sting. Since venom may be injected into the patient, other signs and symptoms may develop. These include:

4-7.8 Discuss the emergency medical care of bites and stings.

* ✳ Chills
* ✳ Weakness
* ✳ Dizziness
* ✳ Fever
* ✳ Nausea
* ✳ Vomiting

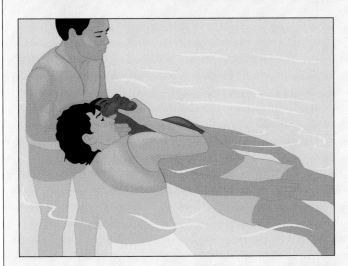

▲ When there are two rescuers present, perform the head-chin support technique to provide in-line stabilization of a patient in shallow water.

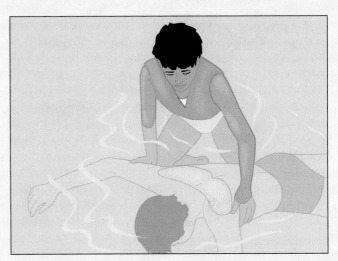

▲ When you find a patient face down in shallow water, position yourself alongside the patient.

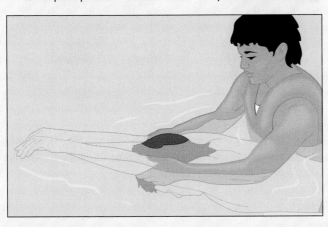

▲ Extend the patient's arms straight up alongside his head to create a splint.

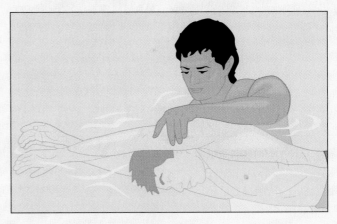

▲ Begin to rotate the torso toward you.

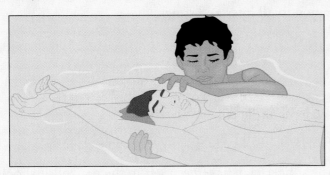

▲ As you rotate the patient, lower yourself into the water.

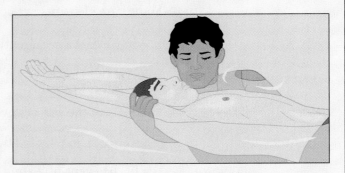

▲ Maintain manual stabilization by holding the patient's head between his arms.

SCAN 23-1B **RESCUE TECHNIQUES FOR DEEP WATER**

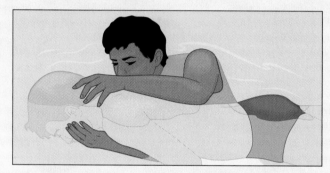

▲ When you find a patient face down in deep water, position yourself beside him. Support his head with one hand and the mandible with the other.

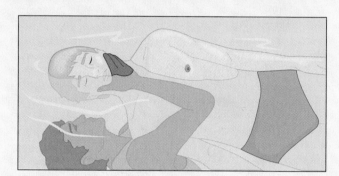

▲ Then rotate the patient by ducking under him.

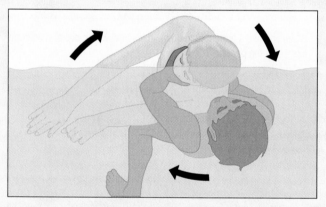

▲ Continue to rotate until the patient is face up.

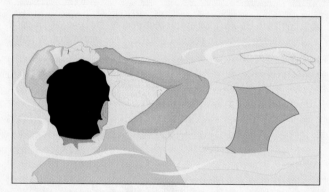

▲ Maintain in-line stabilization until a backboard is used to immobilize the patient's spine.

EMERGENCY CARE FOR BITES AND STINGS

Some care elements are common to all bites and stings:

* ✳ Wash the area gently.
* ✳ Remove jewelry from the area around the bite or sting—before swelling begins, if possible.
* ✳ Place the site below the level of the patient's heart.
* ✳ Monitor the patient carefully for the development of anaphylaxis.

In the event of a sting, the stinger may have been left in the patient. It should be removed. Remove the stinger by scraping it away with the edge of a credit card (Figure 23-17). Do not use tweezers since this might inadvertently squeeze more venom into your patient.

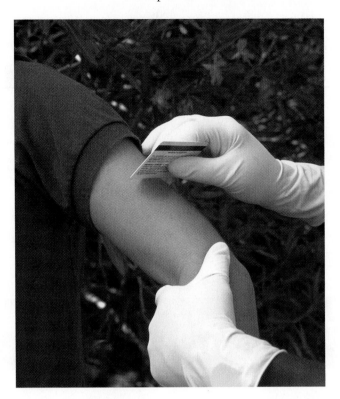

FIGURE 23-17 If the insect stinger is still present, remove it by scraping it away with the edge of a credit card.

In patients who have experienced a snakebite (Figures 23-18A and B), you should be sure that there are no dangerous snakes in the area where you are giving care. Consult medical direction or your local protocols in reference to a **constricting band.** This is a device that encircles an extremity to reduce venous blood return to the body. Avoid applying cold to snakebites.

There are many organisms that may cause bites and stings to humans. Different regions of the country and world see different types of bites and stings. This text provides general concepts of care. Your instructor and local EMS agencies you will work with can provide details on issues common in your area.

* **constricting band**
   a device that encircles an extremity to reduce venous blood return to the body.

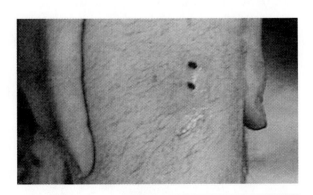

FIGURE 23-18A   Typical rattlesnake bite.

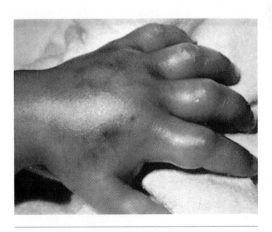

FIGURE 23-18B   Snake bite to the hand.

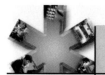

Perspective

John—The Patient

"I don't even know what hit me. It seemed to come on quickly. The next thing I knew there were ambulance guys there. I could barely talk. Later they told me at the hospital that I was close to dying. I'm healthy and young. Didn't think this could happen to me. Maybe I should look for work somewhere air-conditioned."

Stop, Review, Remember!

Multiple Choice

Place a check next to the correct answer.

1. Which of the following is the least safe choice in water rescue?

_____ a. swim

_____ b. row

_____ c. throw and tow

_____ d. reach

2. Which of the following is a correct way to remove a bee stinger from a patient's arm?

_____ a. remove it with your fingers.

_____ b. have the patient remove it with his fingers to prevent contamination.

_____ c. remove it with tweezers.

_____ d. scrape it out with a plastic card.

3. Care for the near-drowning patient includes all of the following EXCEPT:

_____ a. providing resuscitation if necessary.

_____ b. removing the patient from the water with a backboard.

_____ c. pressing firmly on the patient's epigastric region to expel water.

_____ d. suctioning the airway.

4. Cold-water submersions may result in survival of patients who have been submerged 20–30 minutes.

_____ a. true

_____ b. false

5. Near-drowning patients may require spinal precautions when extricating them from the water.

_____ a. true

_____ b. false

Fill in the Blank

For each of the temperature problems below, use the chart in your text to determine the temperature, factoring in wind chill. All temperatures are in Fahrenheit.

1. 5-mph winds at 0 degrees   _____
2. 20-mph winds at 20 degrees   _____
3. 10-mph winds at −10 degrees _____
4. 30-mph winds at 10 degrees   _____

Critical Thinking

1. Why are elevated temperature and humidity factors in patients developing hyperthermia?

   _____

   _____

   _____

   _____

   _____

2. Under what conditions would you press on a near-drowning patient's abdomen to expel water?

   _____

   _____

   _____

   _____

3. What happens when a patient has a severe allergic reaction to a sting?

   _____

   _____

   _____

   _____

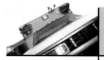

Dispatch Summary

The patient was sufficiently cooled during transport to Atlas Memorial Hospital and was released soon after with orders to rest for 2 days. Based on this and similar events, the oil company began providing air-conditioned trailers at the drilling sites, with orders that the workers be rotated into them for adequate rest periods.

Heat-related emergency calls in Covington County have since dropped by nearly 45 percent.

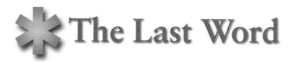

The Last Word

This chapter contained a wide range of emergencies placed together under the heading of "Environmental Emergencies." One significant difference between this chapter and others in the medical module is that, in these emergencies, there is a significant chance that whatever happened to the patient may happen to you. Dangers from water, exposure to heat or cold, or meeting the same insect or animal that stung or bit your patient are risks for you. Safety must always be your first priority.

The other difference in this chapter is that in environmental emergencies patients are often found in a position that isn't safe. They may be out in the cold or heat, in the water, or far away from a road. This poses unique challenges to the EMT.

Finally the extremes in ages (infants and geriatrics) can be more seriously affected by extremes in heat and cold. Remember this information as you assess your patient and then document all appropriate information. The amount of heat or cold that you can tolerate is much more than can be tolerated by patients with limited ability for temperature regulation.

Chapter Review

MULTIPLE CHOICE/TRUE-FALSE

Place a check next to the correct answer.

1. Dehydration can cause the loss of 1 liter of fluid in an hour.

   _____ a. true

   _____ b. false

2. You should break blisters present from cold injury to reduce swelling.

   _____ a. true

   _____ b. false

3. Shivering is not present in late stages of hypothermia.

   _____ a. true

   _____ b. false

4. Patients who have drowned can be resuscitated.

   _____ a. true

   _____ b. false

5. Elderly patients have a reduced ability to regulate body temperature.

_____ a. true

_____ b. false

6. Handling a hypothermic patient roughly could cause abnormal and dangerous heart rhythms.

_____ a. true

_____ b. false

7. You should check the pulse of patients who are severely hypothermic for a maximum of 15 seconds before beginning CPR.

_____ a. true

_____ b. false

CRITICAL THINKING

1. In what situation would you actively warm a deep local cold injury? How would you do it?

_____

_____

_____

_____

2. List three non-weather-related factors that might put a person at an increased risk of hyperthermia.

_____

_____

_____

_____

3. What is the difference between radiation, conduction, and convection?

_____

_____

_____

_____

CASE STUDY

You are out with a group of friends staying in a cabin near the lake. Because it is winter, it is about 20 minutes into the camp by snowmobile and another 2 hours into the town. You and some friends decide to go snowshoeing. While out on what you thought was a field, your friend Thom breaks through the surface of a small pond. His snowshoe gets stuck. By the time he gets his foot out of the water, it is soaked. During the trek back to the cabin Thom tells you that he has lost sensation in his foot. You get back to the cabin and remove his boot. The boot is frozen solid. Thom's foot is white and hard. He tells you he can't feel it. His toes barely move. Thom says they are "stiff."

1. Is this a superficial or deep local cold injury? Why?

   _____

   _____

   _____

   _____

2. What treatment would you provide for Thom?

   _____

   _____

   _____

   _____

3. Would you rewarm the foot? Why or why not?

   _____

   _____

   _____

   _____

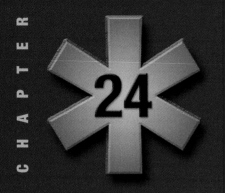

24

Patients with Behavioral Emergencies

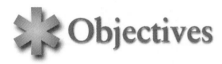

Objectives

Numbered objectives are from the U.S. Department of Transportation 1994 EMT-Basic National Standard Curriculum.

COGNITIVE OBJECTIVES

At the completion of this lesson, the EMT-Basic student will be able to:

4-8.1 Define behavioral emergencies. (pp. 608–610)

4-8.2 Discuss the general factors that may cause an alteration in a patient's behavior. (pp. 610–611)

4-8.3 State the various reasons for psychological crises. (pp. 610–612)

4-8.4 Discuss the characteristics of an individual's behavior which suggest that the patient is at risk for suicide. (pp. 611–614)

4-8.5 Discuss special medical/legal considerations for managing behavioral emergencies. (pp. 619–622)

4-8.6 Discuss the special considerations for assessing a patient with behavioral problems. (pp. 616–617)

4-8.7 Discuss the general principles of an individual's behavior which suggest that he is at risk for violence. (pp. 618–619)

4-8.8 Discuss methods to calm behavioral emergency patients. (pp. 613–614)

AFFECTIVE OBJECTIVES

At the completion of this lesson, the EMT-Basic student will be able to:

4-8.9 Explain the rationale for learning how to modify your behavior toward the patient with a behavioral emergency. (pp. 612–613, 618)

PSYCHOMOTOR OBJECTIVES

At the completion of this lesson, the EMT-Basic student will be able to:

4-8.10 Demonstrate the assessment and emergency medical care of the patient experiencing a behavioral emergency. (pp. 616–618)

4-8.11 Demonstrate various techniques to safely restrain a patient with a behavioral problem. (p. 621)

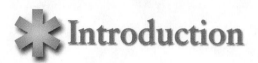

Introduction

Behavioral emergencies are medical emergencies, but unlike many other medical emergencies, the cause and presentation of the condition are different and can be especially challenging. If a patient has diabetes, you can check his blood glucose level. Chest-pain patients can describe their pain and its onset. Not all behavioral emergency patients can do this.

Of course, patients experiencing behavioral emergencies range from those who are depressed or anxious to those who are acting in unusual and potentially dangerous ways. These patients will require your best clinical and people skills.

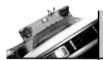

Emergency Dispatch

"You're always talking down to me, Judy!" the man yelled, spittle flying from his lips. "You know how much I hate that!"

"Sir, you need to calm down and my name is Theresa. There's no Judy here." EMT Theresa Hoagland said, feeling fear creeping up from her stomach. The patient had just suddenly—and for no apparent reason—become angry. "We're here to help you . . . just relax on the cot."

Theresa glanced out the back window of the ambulance as it bounced along the dark city streets. Thank God, she thought, only about 3 minutes to the hospital.

"You know what, Judy?" the patient shouted. He was a homeless man and ambulance regular with a history of delusional but nonviolent behavior. "I'm so f**kin' done dealing with you!"

He then began to unbuckle the cot straps and stand up. Theresa's partner, Jerry, saw this in the rearview mirror and quickly pulled the ambulance to the curb and activated the hazard lights.

"Headquarters, 4-54," he said into the radio as he climbed out of the driver's seat. "We're pulled over at Fifth and Walker for an uncooperative patient. I've gotta get Theresa out of the back."

"Ten-four, 54," the dispatcher responded. "P.D. is rolling to your location."

Several minutes later when city police officer Dan Tomlinson arrived, he found Jerry holding an ice pack to Theresa's swollen left eye.

"Where's your patient?" The officer peered into the back of the disheveled ambulance.

"Oh . . . probably about Fifteenth Street by now," Jerry said, pointing down Walker Avenue. "He shouldn't be too hard to find, though. . . he was taking his clothes off as he ran."

4-8.1 Define behavioral emergencies.

∗ **behavioral emergency**
a situation where a patient's behavior becomes intolerable, dangerous, or bizarre enough to cause the concern of family, bystanders, or the patient.

What Are Behavioral Emergencies?

A **behavioral emergency** is defined as a situation where a patient's behavior becomes intolerable, dangerous, or bizarre enough to cause the concern of family, bystanders, or the patient (Figure 24-1).

There are a few points in this definition that must be clarified. The first is that sometimes it is the patient who calls EMS because he feels he is getting out of con-

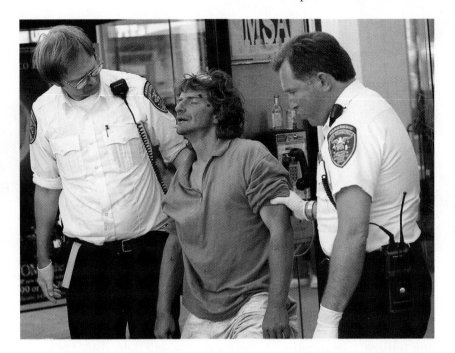

FIGURE 24-1   There are many reasons why a patient may experience a behavioral emergency. (Craig Jackson/In the Dark Photography.)

trol. Patients who have a history of psychiatric problems often recognize when things are getting out of hand.

Did you notice that the definition didn't include the word *normal?* We live in a diverse world where there are many different definitions of "normal." It would be unfair to label or require behavior that only you personally believe is normal.

One thing is sure: As an EMT you will encounter a wide range of patients experiencing psychiatric problems. They will include people from every part of society, every race, every culture, and both genders. Some of these patients will be **withdrawn** and **depressed** while others may exhibit behavior which is considered bizarre or dangerous to themselves or others.

When you receive a call for a psychiatric patient, safety will be a primary concern from the outset of the call. In most areas, it will be the police who make initial contact with the patient and ensure scene safety. Not all psychiatric patients are dangerous—but some can be, so caution is prudent.

You must also think of all patients experiencing behavioral emergencies as having an **altered mental status** caused by trauma or a medical condition until proven otherwise. If you assume that all patients who are acting strangely are "just" behavioral emergencies, you may cause harm to your patient by missing some treatable physical problem.

As you will recall from prior chapters, diabetic patients, patients who are hypoxic, hypo- or hyperthermic, or intoxicated and those experiencing strokes and some types of seizures may present with unusual behavior. You will soon learn that patients in shock or with head injury can display similar behaviors (Figures 24-2A and B on page 610).

* **withdrawn**
   pulling into oneself. Retreating from reality.

* **depressed**
   feeling profound sadness or melancholy.

* **altered mental status**
   change in alertness and awareness.

Clinical Clues: ALTERED MENTAL STATUS

Never assume a patient with an altered mental status is a psychiatric emergency or is simply intoxicated until other medical conditions have been ruled out.

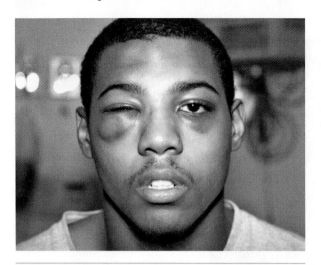

FIGURE 24-2A A closed head injury can cause altered behavior. (© Edward T. Dickinson, M.D.)

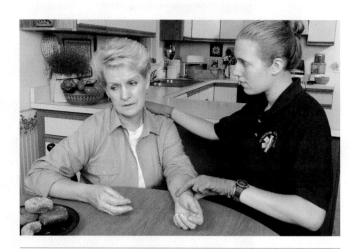

FIGURE 24-2B Medical conditions such as diabetes can cause an altered mental status.

4-8.2 Discuss the general factors that may cause an alteration in a patient's behavior.

4-8.3 State the various reasons for psychological crises.

* **anxiety**

  a state characterized by excess worry or fears.

* **panic attack**

  sudden onset of a fear or discomfort including symptoms such as sweating, trembling, palpitations, feelings of shortness of breath or chest tightness, nausea and/or vomiting, and fears of dying or loss of control.

* **depression**

  profound sadness or feeling of melancholy. May affect major portions of the patient's life including work, relationships, weight changes, sleeping difficulties, feeling of worthlessness and guilt, and occasionally the desire to die.

* **schizophrenia**

  a serious condition that involves unusual or bizarre thoughts, behaviors, and speech. The patient may be very quiet or catatonic in some presentations of the disease.

* **delusions**

  false beliefs.

Of course, psychiatric conditions can also cause these behaviors. Your thorough patient assessment and history taking will help you care for all patients who appear to be having an altered mental status—including those who are experiencing behavioral emergencies.

Types of Behavioral Emergencies

There are many types of psychiatric emergencies. As with many other types of emergency, your role will be to treat the patient and get him safely to the hospital. You won't have to diagnose his condition.

You may, however, hear the patient or a family member relay a history to you that includes a type of psychiatric problem the patient has and the special medications he takes. For this reason, it is helpful to understand some of the more common behavioral, emotional, or psychiatric conditions you may encounter in the field while treating patients. Some of these include:

Anxiety—A very common condition, anxiety is characterized by excess worry or fears. While everyone has occasional fears, patients with this condition have the feelings for a prolonged time, and they interfere with daily activities and functioning.

Panic attack—A sudden onset of a fear or discomfort, it includes signs and symptoms such as sweating, trembling, feelings of shortness of breath or chest tightness, nausea and/or vomiting, and fears of dying or loss of control. It generally occurs for a short time but is quite profound to the patient experiencing it.

Depression—Everyone at some point or another feels depressed. It becomes a problem when it persists for a long time, affects major portions of our lives (e.g., work, relationships), involves weight loss or gain, constant desire to sleep or the inability to sleep, feelings of worthlessness and guilt, and occasionally the desire to die. You will read later that depression is a risk factor for suicide.

Schizophrenia—It is a serious condition that involves unusual or bizarre thoughts, behaviors, and speech, which will be discussed later, including the delusions, paranoia, psychosis and hallucinations. Patients may also be very quiet or catatonic in some presentations of the disease. Some conditions seen in schizophrenia include:

* **delusions**—false beliefs (for example, believing one is a famous person or religious figure).

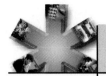

Perspective

Theresa—The EMT

"He hit me! I really don't know what his problem was. I have personally transported that guy at least ten times. Wow! I know he's kind of wacky, but I'd never in a million years guess that he'd get violent! Maybe it goes to show you that you always have to stay alert. I mean, patients can turn on you in an instant. I'm probably lucky that he just used his fist."

* **psychosis**—unusual or bizarre behavior indicating a lack of being in touch with reality.

* **paranoia**—a delusion (false belief) in which the patient believes he is being followed, persecuted, or harmed.

* **hallucinations**—sensory perceptions without an external stimulus. Hallucinations associated with schizophrenia are most commonly auditory. Visual hallucinations are rare.

* **Phobias** are unfounded or intense fears of an object or situation (e.g. snakes, heights)

SUICIDE

Some may say that **suicide** is an epidemic. The facts about suicide are somewhat shocking. According to the Centers for Disease Control and Prevention (CDC), suicide is the third leading cause of death in the 15- to-24-year age group (first is accidental trauma, second is murder) and eighth in the overall population. A dramatic increase in suicide has also been noted in the geriatric population.

It is likely that you will be called to a suicide and to many more patients who have attempted or threatened to take their own life or harm themselves in some way (known as **attempted suicide**). These calls will pose challenges to you in both patient care and the very important "people care."

Several risk factors for suicide have been identified. These include patients who:

* are single, widowed, or divorced

* are depressed

* abuse alcohol or other substances

* have formed a detailed suicide plan (e.g., giving away possessions or purchasing or gathering items to use in the suicide attempt)

* have experienced the prior suicide of a loved one (especially a same-sex parent)

* have made prior suicide attempts

While patients who commit suicide may have one or many of these risk factors, the individual situations will vary from patient to patient. These are

* **psychosis**

   unusual or bizarre behavior indicating a lack of touch with reality.

* **paranoia**

   a delusion (false belief) where the patient believes he is being followed, persecuted, or harmed.

* **hallucinations**

   sensory perceptions without an external stimulus.

* **phobias**

   an unfounded or intense fear of an object or situation.

* **suicide**

   taking of one's own life.

* **attempted suicide**

   attempting or threatening to take one's own life.

4-8.4 Discuss the characteristics of an individual's behavior which suggest that the patient is at risk for suicide.

guidelines to help assess risk. It is usually the role of the EMT to transport a patient to a professional who can formally evaluate the patient for risk and provide appropriate immediate and long-term treatment. If you are in doubt about the intentions of the patient or if a potentially suicidal patient wishes to refuse care, utilize law enforcement, medical direction or community crisis response teams to assist you.

There are many misconceptions about risk factors for suicide. Many experienced EMS personnel may tell you that a patient who is threatening suicide but has threatened many times before may simply be "looking for attention." This is a dangerous attitude, since patients who have attempted suicide before are statistically more likely to commit suicide. Take all threats of suicide seriously—even if they appear "minor" or half-hearted.

Remember that there is an increasing rate of suicide and depression in the geriatric population. The recent loss of a spouse or close friends, decrease in mobility, isolation and related depression, as well as the diagnosis or worsening of a medical condition are additional risk factors for suicide in this age group.

RESPONDING TO THE SUICIDAL PATIENT

When responding to calls where a patient may have attempted harm to himself, you should use an extra level of awareness in your scene size-up. When possible, the police should make initial contact and secure the scene prior to your entry. While most patients expressing suicidal thoughts are not looking to harm you, some may wish to lash out at others. Also, any time a potentially lethal mechanism has been employed (for example, firearms, carbon monoxide) a hazard exists for you as the EMT.

In some cases suicide may be done "by proxy." This means that the person wishing to commit suicide will arrange a situation where someone else will perform a lethal act. One scenario is "suicide by cop," where a person confronts a police officer with a gun (often a toy gun) or other weapon, causing the officer to shoot them. In other cases patients will walk in front of vehicles or trains.

As part of your size-up, look for mechanisms that can cause harm to you or your patient. Note these not only for safety but because they will be important parts of the patient history and documenting the suicide or attempted suicide. You may also see suicide notes or hear statements that will be part of your history and documentation.

Remember that you will bring the patient to the hospital where the mental health professionals will have no knowledge of the scene. It is important that you document and explain pertinent facts, such as the means used in the attempt, whether there was a note, dynamics of family and friends present, and other facts that will help the patient's immediate and long-term care.

Another confounding factor is the complex nature of psychological and suicide emergencies compared to other kinds of emergencies to which you usually respond. For example, if a patient is bleeding, you have been trained to stop it. If the patient has chest pain, you have been taught many possible causes, and you can administer oxygen and assist with medications. Many such emergencies are surprisingly cut and dried compared to psychological emergencies and suicide.

The suicidal patient can cause emotions in you, as an EMT, that may be difficult to deal with. A patient's actions may appear shocking or unbelievable to you. The pain and distress exhibited by the family of a patient who has committed suicide can also be very upsetting.

When dealing with a patient who has attempted suicide, you should treat medical conditions as you would with any patient. Emergencies such as bleeding, carbon monoxide exposure, falls, and others will be treated according to the guidelines for care discussed throughout this text. This chapter will focus on the psychological care of the patient. When dealing with a suicidal patient:

* Be sure to identify yourself and your role.

* Be prepared to spend some time with the patient to develop a rapport. The patient in emotional distress of any type may not open up to you immediately.

* Listen.

* Get down to the patient's level (if safe to do so).

* Use appropriate body language.

* Be calm—regardless of the level of excitement or agitation of the patient.

* Do not speak or act in a judgmental manner.

When you communicate with the suicidal patient, in addition to being polite, it is often a successful strategy to be somewhat direct. It will be part of your assessment to determine the patient's complaint—what they did and why (what was his intent?). You may find it uncomfortable to talk about this with the patient, but it is crucial that you do so. You may wonder how to say "Why did you try to kill (or harm) yourself?" It may seem too direct or insulting. Be direct anyway.

Now consider the alternative. You are the patient in your own house. You are depressed and have just done some sort of harm to yourself. Would you talk to the EMT who couldn't look you in the eye or talk about what you did? Probably not.

Experienced EMTs realize that being direct, yet respectful, is often appreciated by the patient (Figure 24-3). Consider this exchange where an EMT approaches a patient, introduces himself, and tries to identify the chief complaint:

EMT: *My name is Dan, I'm an EMT, and I'd like to help you today, OK?*
Patient: *Sure. Whatever.*
EMT: *I can see you've got some cuts there on your wrist. Are you hurt anywhere else?*
Patient: *No.*
EMT: *Can you tell me what happened?*
Patient: *(pause) I got really pissed off and just wanted to end it all. Just end it.*

The patient here has given you the opportunity to use his terminology. You can now determine his history and use the phrase "end it all" because the patient volunteered it first.

4-8.8 Discuss methods to calm behavioral emergency patients.

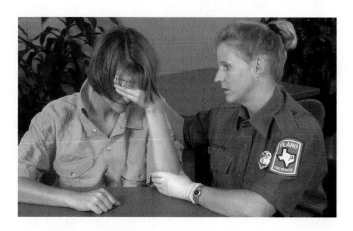

FIGURE 24-3 Talk calmly to a patient who is in crisis.

You can then say, "While I take care of your wrist, can you tell me about your wanting to end it all?" Even though the police may have told you what happened, getting some sort of statement from the patient begins the process of talking. And recall from the assessment chapters that "open-ended" questions like "Can you tell me what happened?" are good to ask rather than yes-or-no statements or questions like "The police say you cut your wrist. Is that true?"

Of course some patients may be angry, others silent, and pose challenges in communication. However, the communications guidelines just discussed, along with some sensitivity and patience, will go far in dealing with your patients.

 Stop, Review, Remember!

Multiple Choice

Place a check next to the correct answer.

1. An unfounded or intense fear is called (a):

_____ a. psychosis.

_____ b. paranoia.

_____ c. phobia.

_____ d. philia.

2. Panic attacks can present with all of the following EXCEPT:

_____ a. low pulse.

_____ b. sweating.

_____ c. chest tightness.

_____ d. vomiting.

3. A patient with unusual behavior should be considered to have a(n) _____ until proven otherwise.

_____ a. psychiatric problem

_____ b. medical problem

_____ c. overdose

_____ d. unusual personality

4. Suicide is the _____ leading cause of death in 15- to-24-year-olds.

_____ a. first

_____ b. second

_____ c. third

_____ d. fourth

5. Patients who are undergoing a behavioral crisis usually act bizarrely and dangerously.

_____ a. true

_____ b. false

6. A patient who has tried suicide several times in the past and tried again today is likely just "looking for attention."

_____ a. true

_____ b. false

7. The most important part of psychiatric assessment is diagnosing the exact psychiatric condition.

_____ a. true

_____ b. false

Short Answer

1. Define behavioral emergency without using the words "normal" or "abnormal."

   _____

2. List five medical conditions that may appear to be a psychiatric emergency.

   _____

3. List five risk factors for suicide.

   _____

Critical Thinking

1. How would your assessment help you to determine the difference between a psychiatric crisis and a medical emergency that causes unusual behavior? List three examples.

   _____

   _____

   _____

   _____

2. You are treating a patient who has attempted suicide. You introduce yourself and ask if you can help. The patient says, "I just took 14 antihistamines because I couldn't take it any more. I don't know, can you help me?" What do you say?

   _____

   _____

   _____

   _____

Behavioral Crisis

Attempted suicide is just one type of behavioral crisis. Consider the following situations—all behavioral emergencies you may encounter:

* You are called to a naked man standing in an intersection yelling at cars.

* You are called to a school for children with emotional problems for a 12-year-old child who has been withdrawn and unwilling to speak to teachers for 2 days.

* You are called to a residence where a man has called because his elderly mother seems depressed and he is very worried about her.

While each of these situations is different, they are all potential behavioral emergencies. Of course each will be considered altered mental status until common causes such as diabetes, injury, overdose, and so on can be ruled out.

The assessment and care of all behavioral emergency patients is essentially the same—even though these patients may present in dramatically different ways.

ASSESSMENT OF BEHAVIORAL EMERGENCY PATIENTS

4-8.6 Discuss the special considerations for assessing a patient with behavioral problems.

You may feel that assessing behavioral emergency patients is different because you can't see the condition, as you could a broken leg. In reality, though, you can't see chest pain either. You must rely on your observation, assessment, and what the patient, family, and bystanders tell you.

Your size-up should ensure that there are no immediate or potential dangers before you approach the scene.

Your assessment of the patient begins with your approach and introduction:

✳ Identify yourself and your role.

✳ Let the patient know what you are doing.

✳ Use a calm, reassuring voice.

✳ Listen.

You will then begin to gather information from a number of sources. Key information you should obtain is sometimes referred to as a "mental status examination." It could actually be considered the focused history and physical exam for the mind. Components of the mental status exam include:

✳ **Orientation**—We perform this exam on all our patients. It includes determining if the patient is oriented to person, place, time, and event.

✳ **Appearance**—The patient's appearance is unusually telling. Observe the patient to determine if he is disheveled or neat. Is his clothing appropriate for the weather conditions? Does his hygiene indicate that he can take care of himself properly?

✳ **Activity**—What is the patient doing? Does it match the environment? Is he active, hyperactive, or catatonic? Does he show aggressive movements or is he withdrawn?

✳ **Speech**—While most patients will be talking to some extent, the volume, urgency, and content of their speech tell quite a bit about the patient's condition and status. Even the fact that the patient will say nothing can indicate anything from depression to anger. Some other speech patterns you may see include:
  • Pressured speech—This patient talks almost constantly. It seems that when his mouth opens, words come out as if they are under pressure. They often don't make sense.
  • Disorganized speech—When someone without a behavioral emergency speaks, the sentences and paragraphs have a logical link and flow. Not so with disorganized speech. Sentence to sentence may not follow a logical flow or order. This is sometimes seen in patients with psychosis or schizophrenia.

✳ **History**—What is the patient's medical history? This will help you identify other potential causes for the patient's behavior (for example, a diabetic emergency) as well as identify any prior psychiatric conditions the patient

TABLE 24-1	COMMON PRESCRIPTION MEDICATIONS TAKEN BY PATIENTS WITH PSYCHIATRIC CONDITIONS

ANTIPSYCHOTIC MEDICATIONS	ANTIDEPRESSANT MEDICATIONS
fluphenazine (Prolixin)	imipramine (Tofranil)
risperidone (Risperdal)	amitriptyline (Elavil)
quetiapine (Seroquel)	desipramine (Norpramin)
chlorpromazine (Thorazine)	nortriptyline (Pamelor)
haloperidol (Haldol)	fluoxetine (Prozac)
lithium (Lithobid)	sertraline (Zoloft)
	paroxetine (Paxil)

may have been diagnosed with. Medications taken by the patient will also provide a clue to his history. Table 24-1 lists common medications taken by patients with psychiatric conditions.

The assessment areas just listed will help you define the "S" in SAMPLE history for the psychiatric patient. The patient's actions, speech, orientation, and appearance will help you identify and document specific signs and symptoms you may find in the psychiatric patient. You will continue to gather appropriate medical history, allergies, and other parts of the sample history as you would in any other patient.

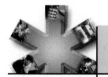

Perspective

Jerry—The EMT

"I've never dealt with that particular guy before, but my first indication that he was a little off was how he looked. I mean, not to be judgmental or anything, but he had this long stringy hair, he stunk, and was wearing a . . . what do you call it . . . like a lady's silk robe type-of-thing over his clothes. When he was first talking to us he was actually kind of funny—the kind of patient who you try your best not to laugh at, but you just can't help yourself. I never would have thought that he'd get violent."

As always, you will also take vital signs as part of your assessment. This is possible on most behavioral emergency patients if you explain what you are going to do. Occasionally, patients may be violent or potentially violent and you will be hesitant to take vital signs. Remember that vitals are a critically important part of the assessment process and they must be taken whenever possible. However, never endanger yourself to obtain vitals if the patient is violent or very uncooperative. You may be able to obtain some vital signs from a safe distance, including respirations, skin color, and level of responsiveness, and document the reasons for not obtaining the other vitals.

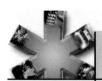

Perspective

The Dispatcher

"I always send the cops for uncooperative patients. Always. Even if the crews say they don't need them. If you tell me that your patient has deteriorated to the point that you have to pull the rig over, then you need back-up. About 11 years ago I was new in dispatch and one of my crews had to pull over for a patient who was going off. The EMT was this ex-football player who competed in Judo and stuff . . . and he tells me not to worry the cops about this 'little guy'. So me, being green, I don't send anybody. Well, that ex-football player is still out on disability. I always send the cops."

DEALING WITH PATIENTS EXHIBITING EXTREMES IN BEHAVIOR

Television has given us some poor examples of psychiatric patients. Such patients are portrayed as extremely violent, anxious, and bizarre. In reality, you will find patients with extremes of behavior—in all directions—as well as some who are simply looking for your help.

A patient's behavior may be placed on a spectrum (Figure 24-4). Your goal is to get the patient to the middle of the spectrum where he is calm, communicative, and cooperative. The following may help you communicate with your patient and gain cooperation:

4-8.7 Discuss the general principles of an individual's behavior which suggest that he is at risk for violence.

✳ Observe your patient's reactions to you and his surroundings. If he becomes more agitated with something you are discussing, talk about something else.

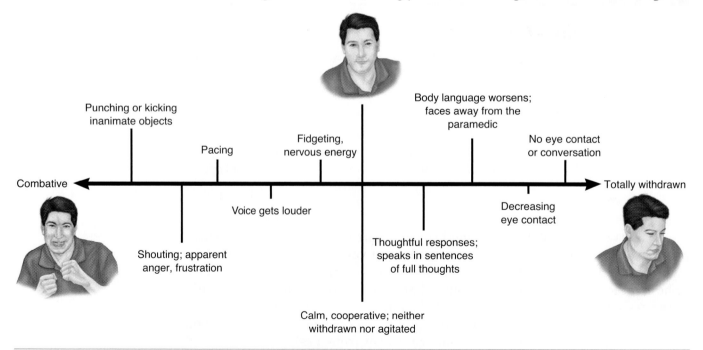

FIGURE 24-4 Continuum of patient responses during behavioral emergency. Whether dealing with a combative or withdrawn patient, you will use your interpersonal skills to bring him to the calm, cooperative state in the middle of the continuum.

If a family member or another person in the patient's presence seems to be agitating the patient, removing this person from the patient's sight may help.

* If you discuss something with your patient and the patient seems to respond (for example, increasing eye contact, improving body language), continue along that course. Similarly, if a patient responds to one person on a call better than another, that person should continue talking with the patient.

* Watch for signs of escalation to behavior that is increasingly agitated or violent. Use the warning signs of louder voice and increasing activity (for example, pacing, violent hand movements) as signs you should retreat and let the police deal with the situation.

Patient Care for Behavioral Emergencies

Your care for behavioral emergency patients will cover two areas:

1. **Providing care for injuries or medical problems.** You may be called for a suicidal patient who has been pulled from a garage filled with carbon monoxide or a patient with wrist lacerations. You may be called for a patient exhibiting bizarre behavior and find him to have low blood sugar. Medical treatment, including life-saving interventions performed during the initial assessment (for example, airway care and oxygen) are vital. Medical conditions must have the same priority for behavioral emergency patients as for patients who are not exhibiting behavioral symptoms.

2. **Care for behavioral issues.** Once care for injuries or medical problems has been provided and medical causes for the behavioral emergency have been ruled out, your care for these patients is largely supportive, using the communication techniques listed earlier in the chapter. Calming the patient, protecting him from harm, and transport to an appropriate facility are the key components of behavioral care.

REFUSAL OF CARE

You will encounter patients who are violent and beyond reason or a danger to themselves or others and wish to refuse care. In these cases you may be asked by the police to transport a patient against his will.

Remember that for a patient to refuse care he must be competent to make an informed decision. Many behavioral emergency patients, as well as those who are intoxicated or drugged, will not be considered competent and therefore cannot legally refuse. In most areas, the police are given the authority to force someone to go to the hospital against his will.

The decision on whether a patient is competent or not is not always clear cut. We would likely be in agreement that a person who has cut his wrists is a danger to himself and should be transported. The same is true for a person who has ingested a quantity of pills. There will be other cases that are less clear. A patient who is disoriented and doesn't know to stay out of traffic can be a harm to himself. A patient who insists on going out on a bitter winter day for a long walk without a coat may also be a harm to himself.

To evaluate these patients, you may wish to call a mobile crisis outreach team if one is available in your area. These teams respond into the community to assist in assessment and care of patients experiencing behavioral emergencies. If a team is not available, you will seek additional help from the police and medical direction.

4-8.5 Discuss special medical/legal considerations for managing behavioral emergencies.

Not all patients who wish to refuse care will be violent. A firm but respectful attitude is often successful. Patients in crisis often respond positively to structure. For example:

"The police have told me that you are going to the hospital. They also told me that you don't want to go. We're going to take you and treat you very well. Now I need you to get on my stretcher . . ."

You will have greater success with firmness than if you send a mixed message about what you are going to do. It may feel uncomfortable or awkward to speak decisively. You may also worry that something you say will cause the patient to act out. If you speak with conviction *and* compassion, you will have the best results.

If the police call you and have the legal authority to force a patient to go to the hospital, avoid asking questions such as "Would you like to go to the hospital?" because there really isn't a choice.

If the patient won't cooperate, restraint will be necessary.

RESTRAINT

Restraint is the process of restricting motion, which allows an unwilling or combative patient to be transported to the hospital. There are many different methods of restraint—and there are some dangers associated with restraint.

Before restraint is begun, be sure to have the legal authority to do so and enough personnel to perform the restraint effectively. The main principle of restraint is to restrain the patient with a minimal amount of force and without injury to the patient or emergency personnel on scene.

The process of restraining a violent patient should be handled by the police. Since there are times you may be called upon to be part of the restraint process, it will be presented here (Scan 24-1). When restraining a patient:

✳ Be sure you have adequate help. Too few people may result in excessive force being used, which may cause injury. Too many rescuers can cause confusion. Generally four or five people is ideal. Each of the first four can take an extremity and the fifth can secure the patient.

✳ When possible, avoid being directly in the path of danger (patient's feet, fists, and mouth) to prevent injury.

✳ Develop a plan. Once the plan is implemented, act quickly. Indecision can cause injury.

✳ Use only the amount of force necessary to effect the restraint. Restraint is never punitive.

✳ Communicate with the patient while you are restraining him.

✳ Use only soft restraints (such as gauze).

✳ Restrain the patient face-up.

✳ Never hog-tie the patient or restrict expansion of the chest cavity in any way.

✳ Reassess the patient frequently during transport.

During restraint, problems may occur. If the patient remains violent and struggling, you will find it best to position the restraints so they prevent the use of major muscle groups (Figures 24-5A and B on page 622). Place a surgical or oxygen mask (with oxygen flowing) over the face of a patient who is spitting at you.

Do not restrain a patient face down. Many will argue it is more efficient, but it prevents you from properly assessing the patient throughout transport.

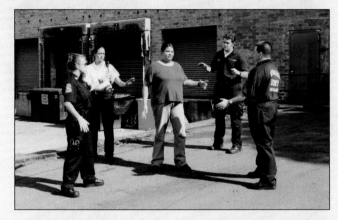

▲ Plan your approach to the patient in advance and remain outside the range of arms and legs until you are ready to act.

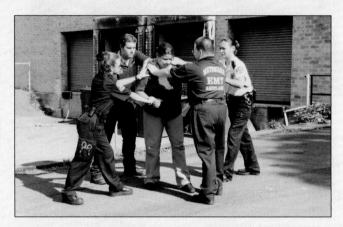

▲ Assign one EMT to each limb, and approach the patient at the same time.

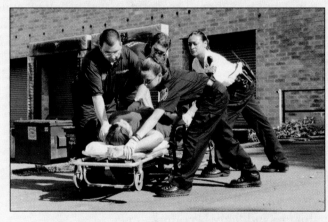

▲ Place the patient on the stretcher as her condition and local protocols indicate. Do not let go until the patient is properly secured.

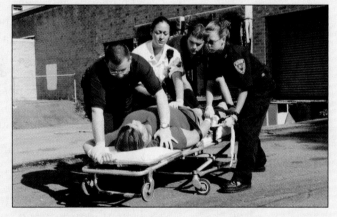

▲ Use multiple straps or other soft restraints to secure the patient to the stretcher.

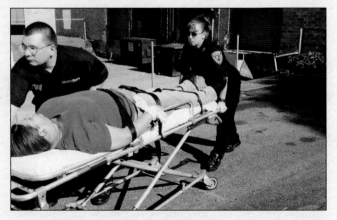

▲ When the patient is secure, assess distal circulation and monitor airway and breathing continually.

All photos: Craig Jackson/In the Dark Photography.

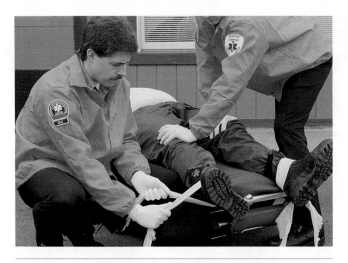

FIGURE 24-5A Place the patient supine on the ambulance stretcher and apply ankle and wrist restraints.

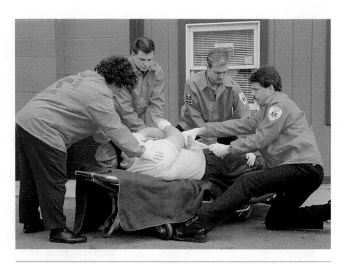

FIGURE 24-5B One method of restraint is to pull arms tightly across the patient's chest and tie on opposite sides of the stretcher frame.

✳ **positional asphyxia**

death of a patient who has been restrained. Often associated with extreme exertion (long foot chases or struggling against restraints), drug or alcohol use, and/or hog-tie or hobble restraints, some patients die while restrained.

✳ **hobble restraints**

a method of restraint in which the legs are secured to the torso to restrict movement.

There is a condition that has been called **positional asphyxia.** It involves the death of patients who have been restrained. Often associated with extreme exertion (long foot chases or struggling against restraints), drug or alcohol use, and/or hog-tie or **hobble restraints,** some patients die while restrained.

The cause isn't exactly known but a common scenario is that a patient who has fought with police and required restraint is transported to the hospital. During the trip to the hospital (or upon arrival) a once loud and combative patient is believed to have calmed down when in fact he has died.

When such a tragic death occurs, there is also significant liability for EMS providers. To prevent positional asphyxia:

✳ Never restrain a patient face down or in a hog-tie or hobble restraint.

✳ Recognize situations where positional asphyxia is likely.

✳ Monitor your restrained patient continuously—especially the ABCs.

✳ Be alert for sudden changes in mental status—especially changes from argumentative and struggling to suddenly becoming quiet.

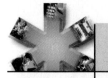

Perspective

Theresa—The EMT

"At first the cop was mad that we let the guy run away. But, come on! There was no way that me and Jerry were gonna get that guy under control. Just the two of us trying to restrain him while he was swinging his fists and yelling at people who weren't there . . . now that's just plain stupid. It isn't safe—and quite frankly it is the police's job."

Stop, Review, Remember!

Multiple Choice

Place a check next to the correct answer.

1. A mental status examination includes all of the following EXCEPT:

    _____ a. appearance.

    _____ b. speech.

    _____ c. history.

    _____ d. occupation.

2. A delusion is a(n):

    _____ a. hallucination.

    _____ b. irrational fear.

    _____ c. false belief.

    _____ d. break from reality.

3. A patient who dies during or as a result of restraint may have experienced:

    _____ a. terminal psychosis.

    _____ b. psychotic asphyxia.

    _____ c. positional asphyxia.

    _____ d. myocardial infarction.

4. Speech that is rapid and seems explosive or forced is called:

    _____ a. disorganized speech.

    _____ b. aphasic speech.

    _____ c. psychotic speech.

    _____ d. pressured speech.

5. Which statement regarding care for behavioral emergencies is correct?

    _____ a. Psychiatric care is performed before care for medical or traumatic conditions.

    _____ b. Restraint is used in most behavioral emergency cases.

    _____ c. EMTs should consider medical problems as a cause of apparent behavioral emergencies.

    _____ d. Knowing the exact diagnosis for the patient's condition will likely change your treatment of the emergency.

6. You are caring for a patient exhibiting bizarre behavior. Which action is least likely to help calm the patient?

    _____ a. introducing yourself and explaining you are there to help

    _____ b. ordering the patient to calm down

    _____ c. using positive body language

    _____ d. listening

Short Answer

Define the following terms:

1. Competent adult: _____

2. Psychosis: _____

3. Soft restraints: _____

Critical Thinking

1. You are transporting a violent patient to the psychiatric center at the request of the police. The patient begins spitting at you. He has been fighting, so he has a bloody lip. List two things you could do to minimize exposure to his blood.

   _____

   _____

   _____

   _____

   _____

2. Why is it important to communicate with the patient while you are restraining him?

   _____

   _____

   _____

   _____

3. Explain positional asphyxia and how to prevent it.

   _____

   _____

   _____

   _____

   _____

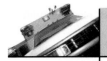

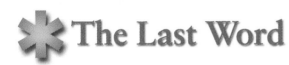

Dispatch Summary

The patient was apprehended, completely naked, on Seventeenth Street, trying to break the window of a parked car with his shoe. He was restrained by law enforcement and transported to St. Luther Hospital, home of the county's mental health unit.

Theresa recovered fully from the assault but now does not hesitate to call for police assistance if her patient is acting unusual in any way.

The Last Word

Patients who are experiencing psychological or behavioral emergencies pose unique challenges for the EMT. Instead of having a list of steps to follow, like the ones you will learn for controlling bleeding, you will have to rely on communication, observation, and some interpersonal skills while treating your patient. Using courtesy and respect will go a long way with these or any patients you encounter.

Just because you can't see the psychological condition doesn't mean that it isn't real. A significant percentage of the population has some sort of psychological condition ranging from depression and anxiety (as much as 10 percent of the population) to schizophrenia (less common). Suicide is the third leading cause of death in the 15- to-24-year age group and increasing rapidly in our geriatric population. So, yes, before long you will certainly deal with patients who have some sort of behavioral emergency.

Chapter Review

MULTIPLE CHOICE

Place a check next to the correct answer.

1. The condition that can lead to a patient dying while restrained is called:

_____ a. positional asphyxia.

_____ b. psychotic asphyxia.

_____ c. terminal asphyxia.

_____ d. myocardial asphyxia.

2. Unusual or bizarre behavior indicating a lack of touch with reality is referred to as:

_____ a. delusions.

_____ b. psychosis.

_____ c. paranoia.

_____ d. hallucinations.

3. Which of the following is a general reason for behavioral emergencies in patients?

_____ a. childbirth

_____ b. depression

_____ c. soft-tissue injury

_____ d. excitement

4. Which of the following statements about patient restraint is NOT correct?

_____ a. Two EMTs restrain most efficiently with less confusion.

_____ b. Communicate with the patient during restraint.

_____ c. The patient must be assessed frequently after restraint.

_____ d. Only soft restraints may be used.

5. To prevent positional asphyxia, which of the following does NOT apply?

_____ a. Never restrain a patient face up.

_____ b. Recognize situations where terminal asphyxia is likely.

_____ c. Monitor your restrained patient continuously—especially the ABCs.

_____ d. Be alert for sudden changes in skin color.

MATCHING

Match the condition or behavior on the left with the correct description on the right.

1. _____ Phobia

2. _____ Psychosis

3. _____ Delusion

4. _____ Depression

5. _____ Panic

6. _____ Paranoia

A. Unusual or bizarre behavior
B. Sudden onset of fear or discomfort
C. False belief one is being followed or persecuted
D. Alteration of mood with feelings of worthlessness, fatigue, guilt, and lack of interest in daily activities
E. False belief
F. Unfounded or intense fear

CRITICAL THINKING

1. Some say that behavioral emergency patients just need restraint and there is nothing you can do to prevent the need. Defend or agree with this statement.

_____

_____

_____

_____

2. You are called to a patient with an altered mental status who has both a diabetic history and a psychiatric history. How might you determine the patient's problem and the care you should give?

_____

_____

_____

_____

3. You are called to a residence for a behavioral emergency. You are met at the curb by a parent who states that her son, who has a history of schizophrenia, has thrown some furniture around. He is calm now. The police are not on scene. Should you enter the residence? Why or why not?

_____

_____

_____

_____

CASE STUDY

Your ambulance is called to the corner of Main and Emmons Streets for a "subject acting strangely." You arrive to find a man talking with a police officer. As you approach, you hear the man tell the officer that he was at the Last Supper and is spreading the word as the Lord told him to. The officer asks for identification to which the man replies, "I am from Heaven. Disciples of God do not need identification."

1. List three ways you would determine if a medical problem is causing this patient's behavior.

_____

_____

_____

_____

2. Why would the belief that this man was at the Last Supper and is from heaven be considered a delusion?

_____

_____

_____

_____

3. The patient is calm until the police tell him he must go to the hospital. What signs might you see that indicate increased agitation?

_____

_____

_____

_____

4. What verbal or interpersonal techniques might you perform to counteract this agitation?

_____

_____

_____

_____

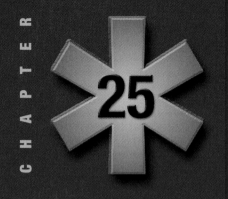

Childbirth and Gynecologic Emergencies

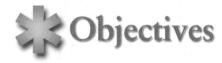

Objectives

Numbered objectives are from the U.S. Department of Transportation 1994 EMT-Basic National Standard Curriculum.

COGNITIVE OBJECTIVES

At the completion of this lesson, the EMT-Basic student will be able to:

4-9.1 Identify the following structures: Uterus, vagina, fetus, placenta, umbilical cord, amniotic sac, and perineum. (p. 630)

4-9.2 Identify and explain the use of the contents of an obstetrics kit. (pp. 633–634)

4-9.3 Identify predelivery emergencies. (p. 647)

4-9.4 State indications of an imminent delivery. (pp. 631–632)

4-9.5 Differentiate the emergency medical care provided to a patient with predelivery emergencies from a normal delivery. (pp. 647–651)

4-9.6 State the steps in the predelivery preparation of the mother. (pp. 632–634)

4-9.7 Establish the relationship between body substance isolation and childbirth. (pp. 632–635)

4-9.8 State the steps to assist in the delivery. (pp. 634–637)

4-9.9 Describe care of the baby as the head appears. (pp. 635–637)

4-9.10 Describe how and when to cut the umbilical cord. (p. 637)

4-9.11 Discuss the steps in the delivery of the placenta. (p. 637)

4-9.12 List the steps in the emergency medical care of the mother post-delivery. (pp. 637–642)

4-9.13 Summarize neonatal resuscitation procedures. (pp. 639–642)

4-9.14 Describe the procedures for the following abnormal deliveries: Breech birth, prolapsed cord, limb presentation. (pp. 643–645)

4-9.15 Differentiate the special considerations for multiple births. (p. 646)

4-9.16 Describe special considerations of meconium. (p. 647)

4-9.17 Describe special considerations of a premature baby. (pp. 646–647)

4-9.18 Discuss the emergency medical care of a patient with a gynecological emergency. (pp. 652–654)

AFFECTIVE OBJECTIVES

At the completion of this lesson, the EMT-Basic student will be able to:

4-9.19 Explain the rationale for understanding the implications of treating two patients (mother and baby). (p. 639)

PSYCHOMOTOR OBJECTIVES

At the completion of this lesson, the EMT-Basic student will be able to:

4-9.20 Demonstrate the steps to assist in the normal cephalic delivery. (p. 636)

4-9.21 Demonstrate necessary care procedures of the fetus as the head appears. (pp. 635–637)

4-9.22 Demonstrate infant neonatal procedures. (pp. 635–637, 639–642)

4-9.23 Demonstrate post delivery care of infant. (pp. 639–642)

4-9.24 Demonstrate how and when to cut the umbilical cord. (pp. 635–637)

4-9.25 Attend to the steps in the delivery of the placenta. (pp. 635–637)

4-9.26 Demonstrate the post-delivery care of the mother. (pp. 642–643)

4-9.27 Demonstrate the procedures for the following abnormal deliveries: vaginal bleeding, breech birth, prolapsed cord, limb presentation. (pp. 643–645, 647–648, 653)

4-9.28 Demonstrate the steps in the emergency medical care of the mother with excessive bleeding. (pp. 647–648)

4-9.29 Demonstrate completing a prehospital care report for patients with obstetrical/gynecological emergencies. (p. 654)

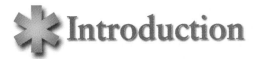

Introduction

Most medical professionals agree that childbirth is not an emergency. It is a natural process that has occurred for centuries outside the hospital. Why, then, does the thought of delivering a baby cause such anxiety?

We realize that it is best to deliver a baby in a hospital when possible. When it is not possible, it is likely you will be called to assist in this natural process. This chapter will help prepare you to deliver a baby and recognize and manage some of the complications you may encounter. You will also learn about pre- and post-delivery emergencies as well as nonpregnancy-related gynecological emergencies.

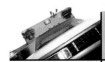

Emergency Dispatch

"Why did the dispatcher say it was an 'O.B. as in baby' call?" Mark asked. He was a new EMT in his second week of field training. "Isn't it kind of obvious that an O.B. emergency will have something to do with babies?"

"Because sometimes over the radio it can sound like O.D., as in overdose," Mark's trainer, Ling, said as she deftly maneuvered the ambulance around cars on the rain-slick roadway. "You obviously don't want to confuse those two calls."

"True."

The patient was a 17-year-old girl who was in the passenger seat of her boyfriend's pick-up truck. A high-

way patrolman had pulled them over for speeding on the interstate and quickly realized what the rush was, so he radioed for an ambulance.

The patrolman approached Ling and Mark as they stepped from their truck and explained why he had called. "Oh, and another thing," he said. "She's deaf and the boyfriend doesn't know sign language."

"Okay, thanks. Mark, pull out your notepad and get a pen," Ling said as she walked up to the truck and peered into the cab. "Oh, hey, never mind! Open the O.B. kit now!"

4-9.1 Identify the following structures: Uterus, vagina, fetus, placenta, umbilical cord, amniotic sac, and perineum.

✳ **uterus**

the muscular organ that contains the developing fetus.

✳ **fetus**

the clinical term for an unborn baby.

✳ **ovum**

an unfertilized egg.

✳ **ovary**

female organ that produces eggs.

✳ **fallopian tube**

structure that extends from the ovary to the uterus.

✳ **fertilization**

union of egg and sperm.

✳ **zygote**

cell produced by union of egg and sperm.

✳ **implants**

becomes imbedded, as a fertilized egg into the wall of the uterus.

✳ **embryo**

stage of fetal development between the zygote and the fetus.

✳ **placenta**

structure that provides nutrition to the fetus and eliminates fetal waste.

✳ **umbilical cord**

structure that connects the fetus to the placenta.

✳ **amniotic sac**

fluid-filled sac surrounding the developing fetus. Also called the "bag of waters."

✳ **bag of waters**

see amniotic sac.

✳ **birth canal**

passageway that extends from the cervix to the vaginal opening through which the baby is born. Also called the vagina.

✳ **cervix**

the opening of the uterus.

Anatomy of Pregnancy

The anatomy of pregnancy and the female anatomy, initially covered in chapter 4, are important to review, because many of the emergencies discussed in this chapter will refer to this anatomy in the explanation. There are also many terms—some medical and some that will be used by the patient and her family—that will be introduced in this chapter.

The **uterus** is the muscular organ that contains the developing **fetus,** the clinical term for an unborn baby.

To become pregnant, the woman's body releases an **ovum** (egg) from an **ovary.** This ovum moves into a **fallopian tube** that transports the ovum from the ovary to the uterus. **Fertilization** with a male's sperm occurs in the fallopian tube. Fertilization creates a **zygote** that travels through the fallopian tube to the uterus where it **implants** in the uterine wall and grows. The zygote becomes an **embryo.** At about 8 weeks, the developing baby is referred to as a fetus.

During pregnancy, the developing fetus receives nutrition and eliminates waste through the **placenta** that also sits within the uterus attached to its wall. This exchange is carried on through the **umbilical cord** that connects the fetus to the placenta. The developing fetus is surrounded by a fluid-filled sac called the **amniotic sac** or **bag of waters.**

A baby is born through the **birth canal.** The muscular uterus begins contracting to expel the baby from the uterus in a process called labor. As the uterus contracts, the baby moves through the **cervix** at the distal end of the uterus. This leads to the birth canal that extends from the cervix to the **vagina,** through which the baby is born. The **perineum** is the skin between the vagina and the **anus.** The perineum can sometimes tear during delivery.

When the baby's head becomes visible at the vaginal opening, it is referred to as **crowning.** The **presenting part** is the part of the baby that first becomes visible. In a vast majority of cases the presenting part is the head, which is normal. It may also be the buttocks (breech presentation) or an extremity (limb presentation). Breech and limb presentations are complications of pregnancy that will be discussed later in the chapter.

There are times when the embryo or fetus does not survive and delivers very prematurely. This is called a **spontaneous abortion.** It is commonly referred to as a **miscarriage.**

A normal pregnancy lasts 40 weeks, measuring from the first day of the last **menstrual cycle** before the pregnancy. Babies will generally deliver at 38 to 42 weeks. Pregnancy is divided into three **trimesters** of approximately 13 weeks each.

Remember that the length of pregnancy can very from person to person and can't be calculated to the exact day. Perhaps this is why we are occasionally called to deliver babies outside the hospital that arrive normally but not within the timeline anticipated by the physician or the mother.

There are some changes in the mother during pregnancy that will affect your assessment and care. By the end of the third trimester, the mother's blood volume can have increased by 40 to 50 percent. Cardiac output also increases. In the second trimester, it is possible to see a normal reduction in blood pressure of about 10 mmHg. The pulse rate may increase by as much as 15 beats per minute during pregnancy, with more dramatic increases during times of exertion. Other changes take place because the baby is growing inside a space that is limited in capacity to expand. Due to added weight in the abdominal area, the mother can become unstable when walking, bending, or moving. The baby can limit expansion area for the mother's lungs and diaphragm, and respirations become shallow and difficult as a result.

Childbirth

This section will concentrate on normal, uncomplicated childbirth. We will explain the **stages of labor** and delivery of a baby. Subsequent sections will explain complications you may see before, during, and after childbirth.

As we discuss the steps of care for the patient about to experience childbirth, it is important to consider the emotional needs of the patient and family. Especially when a baby may be delivered in a location far from the planned hospital, considering the patient's emotional needs is critical. If the mother or father is concerned about complications, or if the baby is a first delivery, or if previous pregnancies have ended tragically, the anxiety level will likely be exceptionally high. You must learn to remain calm, reassuring, and confident as you manage the birth of this child and care of the mother.

You will also be examining the mother for crowning, palpating the abdomen, and completing other tasks that are very personal. Always consider the privacy of the mother during all phases of care. Because this is an emotional time for both mother and father, they need to be treated compassionately. Maintain a high level of professionalism as you complete the tasks associated with this situation. Carefully explain to both mother and father everything you do before you do it.

As we said earlier, childbirth is a natural process. In an uncomplicated delivery you will be there to assist the mother and other family members in delivering a new family member.

Most patients make it to the hospital to deliver their baby. There are times when this doesn't happen. Some are related to logistics—anything from not having a ride to being stranded in a storm; others are by surprise when labor begins and progresses rapidly.

When possible, it is best to deliver a baby in a hospital. There are a series of questions that you may ask to help determine if delivery is imminent. These include:

* How long have you been pregnant?

* Have you had prenatal care?

* Are you having **contractions** or pain?

* Are you aware of any complications with this pregnancy?

* How far apart are the contractions?

* How many times previously have you given birth?

* How long does each contraction last?

* Have you observed any bleeding or discharge? Do you think your water broke? Have you felt a gush of fluid?

* Do you feel pressure in the vaginal area or the need to move your bowels?

* Do you feel the need to push?

* Are you pregnant with twins or triplets (or more)?

The decision on whether to transport the patient, move the patient to the ambulance, or deliver on the scene should be made based on the answers to these questions and following an examination. The actual time until delivery will vary from patient to patient depending on many factors, including how many children the woman has already delivered. Having previous deliveries usually results in

---

* **vagina**

  see birth canal.

* **perineum**

  the skin between the vagina and the anus.

* **anus**

  outlet of the rectum.

* **crowning**

  when the baby's head becomes visible at the vaginal opening.

* **presenting part**

  the part of the baby that first becomes visible.

* **spontaneous abortion**

  when the embryo or fetus delivers naturally before it is able to survive on it's own. Also called a miscarriage.

* **miscarriage**

  see spontaneous abortion.

* **menstrual cycle**

  monthly recurrent changes in the female reproductive system.

* **trimester**

  division of the pregnancy period, usually 13 weeks, or about one-third of the pregnancy.

* **stages of labor**

  divisions of the labor process.

* **contractions**

  tightening of the uterus to expel the baby.

4-9.4   State indications of an imminent delivery.

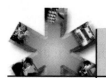

Perspective

The Boyfriend

"I didn't know what to do. I mean, she never told me she was pregnant when we started going out. Then all of a sudden, tonight, she . . . she starts acting like she's sick or hurt. She kept saying that she was fine. And then I thought she like wet herself or something. Then she wrote that I needed to take her to a doctor right away. Man, I freaked out! All I could think of was getting her over to Rogers County Hospital. Now that I think about it, it probably wasn't the closest. But that's where I had my appendix out and I knew how to get there."

shorter labor times in subsequent deliveries. Delivery may be imminent if any of the following is true:

* The patient has contractions less than two minutes apart.

* The patient feels a strong urge to move her bowels.

* The patient has had one or more children previously.

* The baby is crowning. This is the most reliable indication that delivery is imminent.

Furthermore, the distance to the ambulance, terrain, time to the hospital, and other factors will affect your decision to transport. Medical direction may be consulted anytime you have questions or if protocols require you to do so.

If you decide to wait and deliver the baby at the scene and the baby does not deliver in 10 to 15 minutes, initiate transport immediately. Medical direction can also provide guidance in this decision.

STAGES OF LABOR

* **first stage of labor**
stage of labor from the beginning of uterine contractions until full dilation of the cervix.

* **second stage of labor**
stage of labor from full dilation of the cervix until delivery of the baby.

* **third stage of labor**
stage of labor from the birth of the baby until delivery of the placenta.

There are three stages of labor. The **first stage of labor** begins some time before birth as the body prepares for delivery (Figure 25-1). Mild uterine contractions progress to more aggressive contractions. This helps to dilate the cervix. The cervix is usually very narrow. It must prepare to have the large head of a newborn pass through it. The first stage of labor continues until the cervix is fully dilated and ready for birth.

The **second stage of labor** begins with full dilation of the cervix and continues through delivery of the baby (Figure 25-2). Once the cervix is dilated, the contractions will intensify to move the baby through the birth canal. As this begins, the mother may report a feeling of having to move her bowels, a sensation that often indicates birth is imminent.

The **third stage of labor** begins after the birth of the baby when contractions begin again (Figure 25-3). These contractions are to deliver the placenta. This process takes much less time than childbirth, often only 10 to 15 minutes. The third and final stage of labor is over when the placenta delivers.

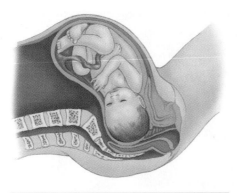

FIGURE 25-1 First stage of labor: beginning of contractions to full cervical dilation.

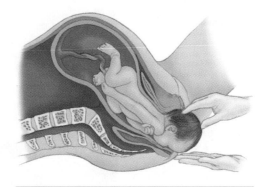

FIGURE 25-2 Second stage of labor: baby enters birth canal and is born.

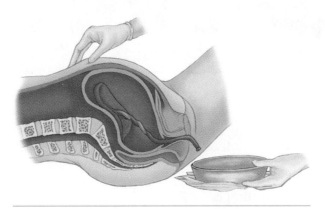

FIGURE 25-3 Third stage of labor: delivery of the placenta.

PREPARATION FOR DELIVERY

There are several things you will do to prepare for a delivery in the field. The first will be to take appropriate BSI precautions. This will include gloves, face protection, and protection for your clothes (gown).

Another portion of your history and assessment will be to determine if the mother is expecting a **multiple birth** (such as twins or triplets) or if any complications were expected or identified during **prenatal** care and evaluations. If you expect any of these issues or if it is a **premature** birth, call for additional ambulances to transport multiple patients—or to have additional staff on hand in the event complications require resuscitation of mother or baby. If the mother hasn't received prenatal care and screenings, consider requesting additional assistance, since problems may be present but not identified.

You will place the mother on her back with her knees drawn up and spread apart. Using materials from your obstetrics (OB) kit (Figure 25-4 on page 634), you will place drapes over the mother's legs and under her buttocks. Table 25-1 on page 634 outlines the contents of the OB kit. This setting will create a sterile (or clean) field in which you will deliver the baby.

Remember the stress the mother will feel in an unexpected home or other nonhospital delivery. She and her family likely had planned for a birth with their obstetrician in a planned setting. The delivery at home is stressful, but may also be frightening and frustrating. Adding to that, it is going to be performed by strangers instead of the obstetrician they know. Be sure to continuously reassure and communicate calmly with the mother and any other family present throughout the preparation, delivery, and transport after delivery. While you do not want to

4-9.6 State the steps in the predelivery preparation of the mother.

4-9.7 Establish the relationship between body substance isolation and childbirth.

✳ **multiple birth**
delivery of more than one baby.

✳ **prenatal**
before birth.

✳ **premature**
born before full development prior to 38 weeks' gestation.

4-9.2 Identify and explain the use of the contents of an obstetrics kit.

FIGURE 25-4 Contents of an OB (obstetric) kit.

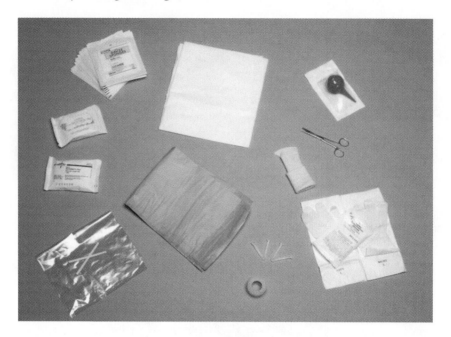

TABLE 25-1 **CONTENTS OF THE OBSTETRICS KIT**
Sterile gloves
Towels or drapes
Scissors (to cut the cord)
Clamps for the umbilical cord
Large gauze pads or sponges
Bulb syringe (for suction)
A blanket for the baby
Sanitary napkins
Plastic bag (for transportation of the placenta)

frighten the family or render medical decisions, if the birth is not progressing well, refrain from promising that the baby will be all right. Say nothing you cannot guarantee to be true, and do not unnecessarily predict problems. If you do not know something, do not promise it.

DELIVERY

It has been mentioned previously and deserves mention again: Childbirth is a natural process that was done for thousands of years before hospitals and EMS existed. Of course, the modern medical system has done much to prevent infection and deal with complications that may occur. In most cases, however, childbirth is an amazing and joyful experience for the parents and their family—and the EMTs.

Complete the preparation we have described when possible. You may, however, be called (or have a car drive into your station) and find a woman who is actually delivering at that moment. In this situation, you will be required to deliver the baby without the drapes and positioning discussed earlier. The follow-

4-9.8 State the steps to assist in the delivery.

ing steps will guide you through the principles of any delivery situation (Scan 25-1 on page 636):

1. Place the patient in a position lying on her back with her knees drawn up and spread apart.

2. Observe the vaginal area. Do not touch this area or do any sort of physical exam of the external or internal **genitalia.**

3. When the head becomes visible (crowning), delivery is imminent. Place gentle pressure on the infant's head to prevent an explosive birth. Avoid placing pressure on the infant's **anterior fontanels** (Figure 25-5) or face.

4. In many cases, the mother will have reported that her "water broke" or that she had a **"bloody show."** These terms refer to the amniotic sac rupturing earlier in labor and/or an initial discharge of blood and mucus at the beginning of labor. Other times, you will find the head of the baby delivering with the amniotic sac still intact. Using your gloved fingers or a clamp, rupture the sac and pull it way from the infant's face. Expect a rush of fluid.

5. After the infant's head is delivered, observe the neck to be sure the umbilical cord isn't wrapped around it. If it is there are two options: If there is enough cord, gently slip it over the baby's head. If the cord is not long enough to allow this to happen, carefully clamp the cord by placing 2 clamps 3 to 4 inches apart. Then cut the cord between the clamps.

6. Once the head has delivered, suction the mouth, then the nose with the bulb syringe from your OB kit. Expel the air from the bulb before placing it in the infant's mouth or nose. Do not touch the back of the mouth with the tip of the syringe.

7. Remember that the infant will be very slippery. Hold the baby carefully and securely.

8. The shoulders, torso and remainder of the infant will come out a bit more rapidly than the head. Be prepared to support the infant.

9. Once the infant is born, again suction the mouth, then the nose. You may also use gauze to wipe away any fluids from around the mouth. Hold the baby's head slightly lower than the torso to allow drainage with gravity.

10. While completing steps 9 and 11, make a note of the time of birth. Hospitals consider this important information for birth records. Do not stop caring for the child while you make note of the time.

* **genitalia**

  organs of reproduction.

* **anterior fontanels**

  soft spot lying between the cranial bones.

* **bloody show**

  referring to the amniotic sac rupturing earlier in labor and/or an initial discharge of blood and mucus at the beginning of labor.

4-9.9 Describe care of the baby as the head appears.

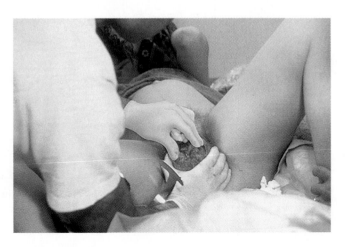

FIGURE 25-5 Place gentle pressure on the scalp as the head presents. Avoid placing pressure on the infant's anterior fontanels or face.

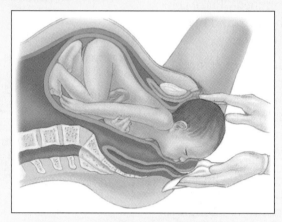

▲ First take BSI precautions. Support the infant's head.

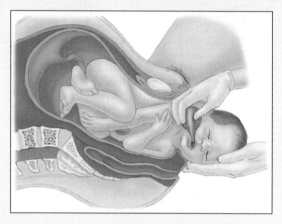

▲ Suction the infant's mouth and then the nose.

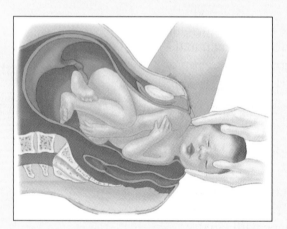

▲ Aid in the birth of the upper shoulder.

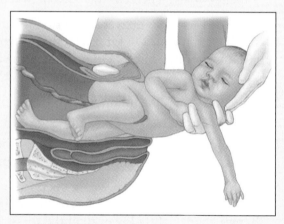

▲ Support the trunk.

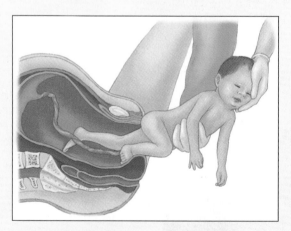

▲ Support the pelvis and lower extremities.

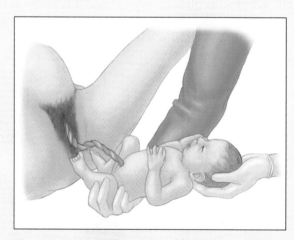

▲ Keep the infant level with the vagina until the umbilical cord stops pulsating.

11. Keep the infant warm. Dry the infant to prevent heat loss and wrap the infant in blankets. Be sure the baby's head is covered. One member of your crew will now be responsible for your second patient, the mothers.

12. The infant should be placed at the level of the vagina until the umbilical cord is cut.

13. The cord must be clamped in two places before it is cut. Place the clamps 3 or 4 inches apart. The clamp closest to the infant should be at least 4 inches away from the infant. Use clamps contained in your kit. Once clamped, cut the cord between the clamps with the scissors contained in your OB kit. If the infant is moving and breathing appropriately, he can be placed in the mother's arms or on the abdomen. Some new mothers may wish to begin nursing.

4-9.10 Describe how and when to cut the umbilical cord.

14. Monitor both patients after the birth for changes in condition.

15. Transport.

4-9.12 List the steps in the emergency medical care of the mother post-delivery.

16. At some point after delivery of the infant, often in a half hour or less, the placenta will deliver. Watch for this while preparing for transport and during transport.

4-9.11 Discuss the steps in the delivery of the placenta.

17. When the placenta delivers, wrap it in a towel and place it in the plastic bag from your OB kit.

18. Place a sterile pad over the mother's vagina, lower her legs, and instruct her to hold them together.

 Stop, Review, Remember!

Multiple Choice

Place a check next to the correct answer.

1. The organ within which the fetus develops is called the:

    _____ a. cervix.

    _____ b. uterus.

    _____ c. placenta.

    _____ d. ovary.

2. The average pregnancy lasts about _____ weeks.

    _____ a. 25–27

    _____ b. 30–32

    _____ c. 34–36

    _____ d. 38–42

3. The second stage of labor is best defined as:

    _____ a. conception to the time actual contractions begin.

    _____ b. from the time contractions begin until full dilation of the cervix.

    _____ c. from full dilation of the cervix to delivery of the baby.

    _____ d. delivery of the baby until expulsion of the placenta.

4. "Crowning" is defined as:

   _____ a. the unusual shape of the head seen in newborns immediately after delivery.

   _____ b. the soft spot on the baby's head.

   _____ c. when the head becomes visible at the vagina.

   _____ d. suctioning the mouth and nose before the baby's shoulder delivers.

5. Which of the following is NOT a sign of impending delivery?

   _____ a. the patient experiencing contractions that last 15–30 seconds

   _____ b. the patient experiencing contractions every 3–5 minutes

   _____ c. the patient having given birth to several children previously

   _____ d. the patient feeling like she has to move her bowels

6. Gentle pressure on the baby's head is required to prevent an explosive birth that could cause injury to the mother or the baby.

   _____ a. true

   _____ b. false

Fill in the Blank

Place a 1, 2, or 3 by each of the following events to represent the correct stage of labor.

1. _____ uterine contractions begin

2. _____ the placenta is delivered

3. _____ mother has a feeling of having to move her bowels

4. _____ delivery of the baby

5. _____ contractions intensify to move the baby through the birth canal

6. _____ cervix is partially dilated

Critical Thinking

1. List five questions to ask a woman who is in labor that may influence your care or decision making regarding, for example, transport or predicting complications.

   _____

   _____

   _____

2. List three things to do in preparation for delivery.

   _____

   _____

   _____

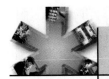

Perspective

Mark—The EMT

"Holy Toledo! I can't believe we delivered a baby! That was amazing. Wow! At first I was really scared, though. You know, one thing they never told me in school is that newborns look kind of dead. I mean, that baby came out and it was grey and purple and just covered with blood and stuff. And it didn't move. It just looked like a rubber doll in Ling's hands. But once she started stimulating it—him—he just came alive, crying and turning pink. That was amazing. Just amazing."

Postdelivery Care

After the delivery you now have two patients. This section will discuss care and evaluation of both of your patients.

Most births are exciting and don't pose critical problems for the mother or newborn. If there are complications with mother or newborn you will find yourself and your crew busy with two patients. This is why many call for a back-up crew early—even if it turns out that mother and baby are doing well. If there are no problems or complications, the mother and baby are transported together. In the event of complications or when resuscitation is necessary a second crew, ALS if available, will transport one patient separately.

POSTDELIVERY CARE OF THE NEWBORN

A newborn infant, also called a **neonate,** requires immediate care after birth. This care is centered around suctioning, drying, and warming the newborn. Since heat can be lost very quickly in the exposed, wet newborn—and the baby's ability to preserve heat and regulate temperature hasn't developed yet—it would take only a few minutes for hypothermia to develop.

Suctioning is important to remove any fluid from the baby's mouth and nose. This suctioning is done with the bulb syringe from the OB kit (Figure 25-6 on page 640). Suction the mouth first, then the nose. Expel air from the bulb syringe before you put it in the baby's mouth and nose.

Remember that evaporation is a cooling process, so you want to prevent evaporation by drying the baby and putting warm, absorbent blankets around it (Figure 25-7 on page 640). Heat loss can occur at an accelerated pace when the head is uncovered, so it is important to keep the top of the baby's head lightly covered.

The suction and drying/warming will take only a short time. After performing these vital tasks, you will turn to an evaluation of the newborn. In short, a pink, crying, moving baby is good. When any of these factors is absent, you may have to take further action. Fortunately this is rare.

If a newborn is not breathing, your first step is to stimulate him. You can do this by flicking the soles of his feet or by rubbing his back. Many times this will be enough to stimulate breathing. If this doesn't work, your steps at resuscitation will be guided by the **inverted pyramid** (Figure 25-8 on page 640). The most common

* **neonate**
    newborn infant up to one month of age.

4-9.13 Summarize neonatal resuscitation procedures.

* **inverted pyramid**
    graphic illustrating the types and frequency of care given to the neonate at birth.

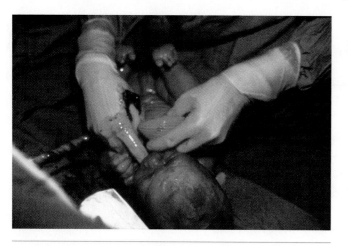

FIGURE 25-6 Suction the mouth and then the nose of the newborn.

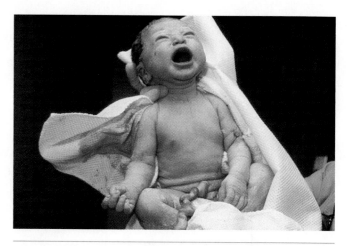

FIGURE 25-7 Before clamping the cord, dry and wrap the infant to keep him warm. (Custom Medical Stock, Inc.)

FIGURE 25-8 Inverted pyramid of neonatal resuscitation. Most infants require only the care listed at the wide, top part of the pyramid. Very few require the care listed at the bottom pointed section.

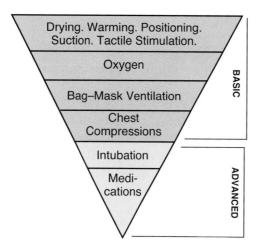

and least invasive techniques are listed at the wide top of the diagram. As you move down the steps in the pyramid, more invasive steps to resuscitate the newborn are presented. Some of these steps are advanced life support procedures. If needed, be sure to request ALS early to the scene or as an intercept.

The steps of the inverted pyramid would be followed in this manner:

1. If a newborn is not breathing immediately after birth and initial suctioning, perform stimulation by rubbing the newborn's back vigorously but not forcefully or flicking the soles of the feet (Figure 25-9). Do not hold the newborn upside down and slap his buttocks. That is only done on television.

2. If breathing hasn't begun or if the breathing appears slow or shallow, you will begin ventilating the newborn. Use a neonatal BVM with small puffs at a rate of 40–60/minute. Overinflation or ventilations that are too fast will cause air to enter the newborn's stomach and actually interfere with breathing.

3. Evaluate the pulse. Listen to the heart with a stethoscope placed near the left nipple. The newborn should have a pulse greater than 100. If the pulse is between 60 and 100, continue artificial ventilation. If the pulse is below 60 or absent, begin chest compressions at the rate of 120/minute. The

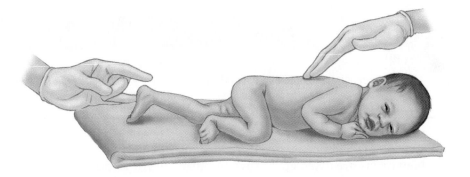

FIGURE 25-9   It may be necessary to stimulate the newborn to breathe.

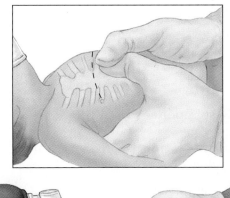

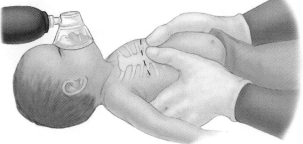

FIGURE 25-10   Deliver chest compressions at 120 per minute, midsternum with two thumbs, at a depth of ½ to ¾ inch. For a very small infant (inset), the thumbs may be overlapped.

two-thumb-encircling-hands method is recommended in CPR for newborns (Figure 25-10).

4. Reevaluate the newborn. If the newborn begins to have more rapid, adequate breathing and a pulse above 100, you should stop compressions. Maintain oxygen delivery by mask or blow-by, especially if the newborn's color remains cyanotic or if the baby is listless or unresponsive.

5. If there is no response to your steps 1 to 4, ALS providers may **intubate** the patient and administer medications.

When a baby is born, it may take up to 30 seconds for breathing to begin as he adjusts to his non-fluid-filled world. It is also common for a baby to have a pink torso but pale or blue extremities initially. This should last for only a few minutes. Remember that the extremities will become pink only when oxygenated blood reaches them, and that takes a few moments to occur. The baby should gradually become pink from its core body outward to the extremities. If the cyanosis does not clear up or if it spreads, ventilations and possibly compressions will be required.

* **two-thumb-encircling-hands method**

  chest compression method which is recommended in CPR for newborns.

* **intubate**

  insert a tube, usually into the trachea.

Clinical Clues: APGAR SCORE

It is quite important to note that the APGAR score is only a tool. *Completing this or any evaluation is secondary to the most important task you have: taking care of the baby!*

✳ **APGAR score**

system for evaluating a newborn's physical condition.

Newborns are assessed by several means, most importantly by their breathing effort, pulse, and appearance. There is a scale used in the medical community called the **APGAR score.** Each letter in APGAR represents one thing to check for:

A – Appearance

P – Pulse

G – Grimace

A – Activity

R – Respiration

Each of the five factors is rated on a scale of 0 to 2, making the total possible score 0 to 10 (Table 25-2).

TABLE 25-2 THE APGAR SCORE			
	APGAR SCORE		
	0	**1**	**2**
Appearance	Blue (or pale) all over	Extremities blue, trunk pink	Pink all over
Pulse	0	<100	>100
Grimace (Reaction to suctioning or flicking of the feet).	No reaction	Facial grimace	Sneeze, cough, or cry
Activity	No movement	Only slight activity (flexing extremities)	Moving around normally
Respiratory effort	None	Slow or irregular breathing, weak cry	Good breathing, strong cry

POSTDELIVERY CARE OF THE MOTHER

In most cases, you will not need to resuscitate or address complications with the mother. Problems are possible, however, and this section will instruct you how to deal with them.

Control Bleeding

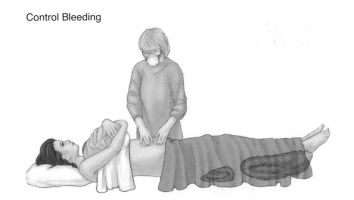

FIGURE 25-11   After delivery of the placenta, massage the uterus to help control vaginal bleeding.

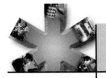

Perspective

The Highway Patrolman

"It's surprising how many people will fake an illness or a pregnancy or something to try and get out of a speeding ticket. The stories that I got after 15 years on the job are unbelievable! But sometimes they're for real. Like that girl today. I was at the births of three of my five kids . . . and while you'll never catch me claiming to be some sort of medical expert, I just knew that that poor kid in the pick-up was in serious trouble."

Postdelivery Bleeding   One of the most common problems with the postdelivery mother is excessive bleeding. Some bleeding is normal and may seem excessive the first time you observe a birth. As much as 500 cc is considered normal. This may look like quite a bit—especially in conjunction with amniotic fluid that will also be present.

If blood loss is excessive, massage the uterus (Figure 25-11). Open your hand and fingers. Place your hand around the uterus, a pronounced grapefruit-sized area on the mother's abdomen above the pubic bone. Use a kneading motion over the area. This will help reduce bleeding. If bleeding continues, treat the patient for shock (raise the legs and apply oxygen). Transport promptly.

Complications during Delivery

In most cases the baby presents head first. When the baby presents with another part of the body, or if the umbilical cord presents first, this is not normal and can be a serious finding.

In all cases of complications in pregnancy, prompt transport will be a major part of your treatment. If you have more than one facility to which you transport, choose the one that is most able to handle pregnancy, neonates, and associated complications.

Complicated childbirth, unlike normal childbirth, cannot be handled most effectively in the field, and often surgical intervention, such as **cesarean section (C-section)** is necessary to best protect both the mother and the child. Decisions that protect both mother and child need to be the priority in emergency medical situations.

4-9.14 Describe the procedures for the following abnormal deliveries: Breech birth, prolapsed cord, limb presentation.

✳ **cesarean section (C-section)**

procedure that surgically removes the baby from the uterus.

FIGURE 25-12 Prolapsed umbilical cord.

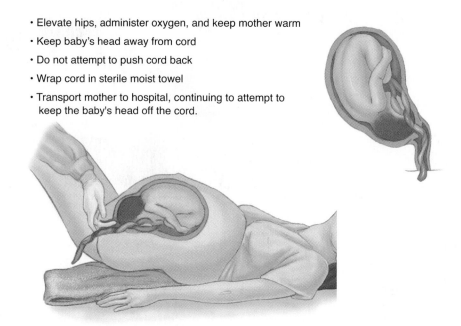

- Elevate hips, administer oxygen, and keep mother warm
- Keep baby's head away from cord
- Do not attempt to push cord back
- Wrap cord in sterile moist towel
- Transport mother to hospital, continuing to attempt to keep the baby's head off the cord.

PROLAPSED CORD

∗ **prolapsed cord**

presentation that occurs when the umbilical cord enters the birth canal before the baby's head.

Prolapsed cord (Figure 25-12) is a presentation in which the umbilical cord enters the birth canal before the baby's head. This creates an extremely serious condition where the baby's head (or other presenting part) occludes blood flow through the cord, which cuts off the baby's supply of oxygen and nutrients.

In addition to your normal size-up, assessments, and vital signs, you will observe the vagina. With a prolapsed cord, you will note that the umbilical cord is visible.

Your care for prolapsed cord will include placing the mother in a supine position with her head lower than her hips. This may relieve some of the pressure on the cord. You will also insert your gloved hand into the vagina to lift the baby's head from the cord. This is the only exception to the rule that you never insert your hand or any item into the vagina. After inserting fingers on each side of the neonate's mouth and nose, split your fingers into a "V" shape to create an opening.

When you insert your gloved hand into the vagina and lift the head, you should feel pulsations in the cord. You must maintain this position throughout your care and transport until you arrive at the hospital. Monitor the cord frequently to ensure that pulsations are present.

BREECH PRESENTATION

∗ **breech presentation**

when the buttocks or both lower extremities are the presenting part.

∗ **ultrasound**

examination technique that uses sound to produce a visual image.

Breech presentation or breech birth (Figure 25-13) is when the buttocks or both lower extremities are the presenting part. If the mother has received prenatal care and **ultrasound** during her pregnancy, she may be aware that this is expected.

If you observe a breech presentation, prepare for transportation immediately. Place the mother in a position where the hips are higher than the head. Administer high-concentration oxygen. Do not wait for delivery.

The mother is at a higher risk of prolapsed cord in a breech presentation. If a prolapsed cord is observed, insert you gloved hand into the vagina and lift the baby off the cord until pulsations resume.

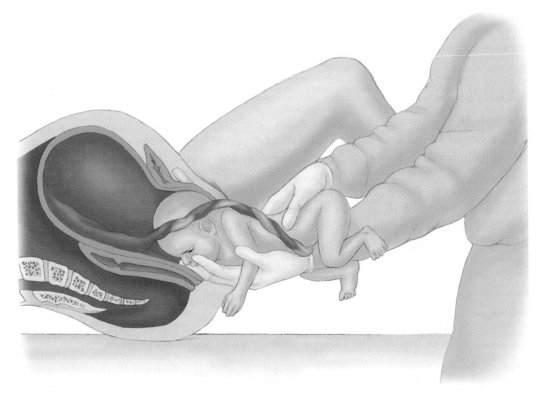

FIGURE 25-13 Breech delivery.

If delivery does occur—and it may—use the steps listed earlier for a normal delivery, and guide the baby as it delivers. Remember that in this case the head will be last. Support the torso while awaiting delivery of the head. You will gently try to prevent explosive delivery as the head emerges. Care for and suction the baby as you would in a normal delivery. Never pull on the legs to stimulate delivery.

LIMB PRESENTATIONS

Limb presentations (Figure 25-14) occur when you observe a single limb presenting from the birth canal. This condition is more serious than when two legs or feet are visible. It is not likely that the baby will deliver, and prompt transportation to the hospital is necessary, preferably one that can handle complications of pregnancy and delivery.

* **limb presentations**
  presentation that occurs when you observe a single limb presenting from the birth canal.

FIGURE 25-14 Limb presentation.

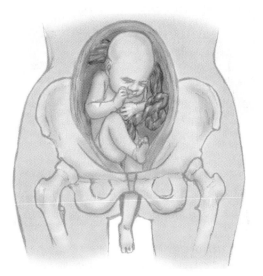
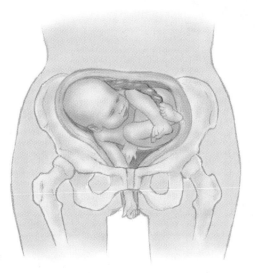

As with other complications of delivery, place the mother in a head-down position (pelvis elevated) and administer high-concentration oxygen. Never pull on an exposed limb to facilitate delivery or for any other reason.

MULTIPLE BIRTHS

4-9.15 Differentiate the special considerations for multiple births.

∗ **multiple births**
> birth of more than one baby.

Multiple births are not necessarily a physical complication. In many cases, twins are delivered in a series of two normal births. Multiple births do have some potential problems, including premature delivery and taxing the resources of rescuers on the scene. Remember that you have two patients with a normal delivery in the field; with twins you will have three, with triplets you will have four, and so on.

Ask the mother if she has received prenatal care. In most cases, when the mother has received prenatal care she will be aware of the fact that she is carrying more than one baby. Without prenatal care, be alert for an unusually large abdomen that does not reduce significantly in size after a first birth.

Twins may share a single placenta or have separate placentas (Figure 25-15). Proceed with cord clamping and cutting as you would with a normal, single gestation delivery.

Be sure to call for help early if you expect multiple births. Something as simple as twins will quickly take you from one patient to three. If one or more patients need continued care or resuscitation, this is even more demanding of resources. When triplets or more babies are expected, risks are substantially higher for premature birth and complications.

4-9.17 Describe special considerations of a premature baby.

PREMATURE BIRTHS

∗ **premature birth**
> birth before the baby has fully developed prior to 38 weeks' gestation.

Premature birth (Figure 25-16) may progress like any other birth as far as stages of labor and delivery. The potential for problems begins when the baby is born.

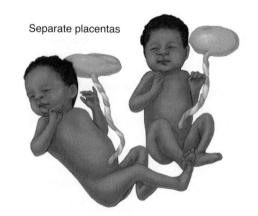

Separate placentas

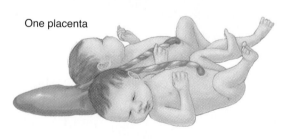

One placenta

FIGURE 25-15   Multiple births.

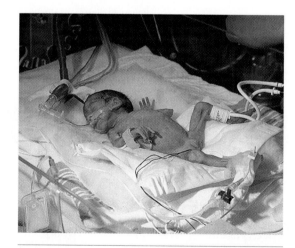

FIGURE 25-16   Premature newborn after 24 weeks of gestation. (Susan Leavines/Photo Researchers, Inc.)

Depending on the number of weeks' **gestation** achieved, the baby may require resuscitation. As noted earlier, pregnancy normally lasts approximately 38-42 weeks or about 9 months. Babies born after about 36 or 37 weeks have much of the development required to thrive after birth. Babies born before this time are more prone to problems. Modern medicine and new technology have been able to stabilize and support babies born after only 23 to 25 weeks, but even then survival is not guaranteed. These babies may weigh only about one pound.

The general rule is to deliver the baby, suction it, and keep it warm and dry. Provide resuscitation according to the inverted triangle as necessary.

You may find that a baby has delivered too long before it is viable to survive outside the uterus. Or you may find that a baby has developed for a significant time in the uterus but has failed to develop properly to survive. If the baby is *clearly* born dead, resuscitation is not required. If there is any doubt, however, begin resuscitative measures immediately and provide prompt transport. Follow local protocols.

MECONIUM

Meconium is fecal matter excreted by the baby while he is still in the uterus. It is often a sign of fetal distress before birth. It appears as a dark, possibly green or yellow-brown substance in the amniotic fluid, which normally should be clear.

If you observe meconium, suctioning becomes an immediate priority—especially suctioning before the baby begins to breathe. Suction thoroughly before stimulating the baby to breathe to be sure the baby does not aspirate meconium. Monitor the airway carefully during transport, and notify the receiving hospital that meconium was observed.

PREDELIVERY EMERGENCIES

Pregnant patients may experience emergencies that do not involve delivery or labor. One of the more common emergencies of this type is vaginal bleeding. Several conditions can cause such bleeding, including ectopic pregnancy, miscarriage, placenta previa, and abruptio placentae.

Emergency care for all of the conditions listed is similar: administer oxygen, treat for shock, and transport promptly. As another critical part of care, be compassionate and considerate. The patient experiencing bleeding while pregnant will have tremendous fear and anxiety about the condition of the baby she is carrying.

ECTOPIC PREGNANCY

An **ectopic pregnancy** is a serious condition. It is a pregnancy that implants and tries to develop in an area other than the uterus. This is usually observed in the first trimester of pregnancy (Figure 25-17 on page 648). Every 28 days, an ovum (egg) is released from an ovary. The egg is guided into the fallopian tube by finger-like projections called fimbrea. As discussed earlier in the chapter, fertilization of the egg occurs in the fallopian tube most of the time. Several days later, the fertilized egg implants into the uterine wall.

If the egg implants anywhere other than the wall of the uterus, for example, the fallopian tube, cervix, within the abdomen, it is called an ectopic pregnancy. It is potentially a life-threatening condition for the mother.

Remember that the usual chief complaint of a patient with an ectopic pregnancy will be vaginal bleeding and/or abdominal pain. In some cases, the patient may not realize that she is pregnant. Any female of childbearing age who complains of abdominal pain and vaginal bleeding is considered to have an ectopic pregnancy until proven otherwise. Because of the amount of blood loss in some

right margin notes:

* **gestation**
length of time from conception to birth.

4-9.16 Describe special considerations of meconium.

* **meconium**
fecal matter excreted by the baby while still in the uterus.

4-9.3 Identify predelivery emergencies.

4-9.5 Differentiate the emergency medical care provided to a patient with predelivery emergencies from a normal delivery.

* **ectopic pregnancy**
pregnancy in which the fetus develops in an area other than the uterus.

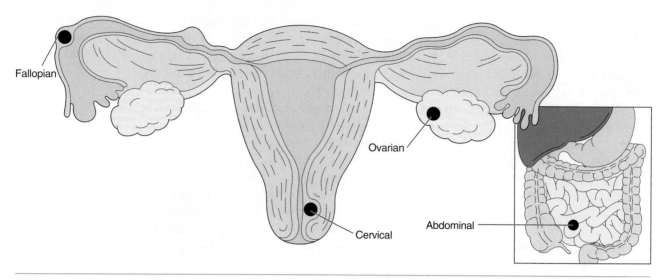

FIGURE 25-17 Various implantation sites in ectopic pregnancy. The most common site is within the fallopian tube, hence the name "tubal pregnancy."

ectopic pregnancies, this must be considered a life-threatening situation, and priorities include rapid transport and care for shock.

It is worth repeating: The care for the patient with abdominal pain and vaginal bleeding from this or any cause is to administer oxygen and treat for shock. This includes the supine position and raising the legs. The patients should be transported promptly to an appropriate hospital.

MISCARRIAGE

As discussed earlier in the chapter—and also called spontaneous abortion or "losing a baby"—a miscarriage is when the fetus delivers before it is able to survive outside the uterus, even with medical intervention. Women who are having a miscarriage often experience cramps, abdominal pain, vaginal bleeding, and possibly the expulsion of fetal tissue from the vagina.

Sometimes these miscarriages are preceded by problems with the pregnancy, such as slight bleeding, and other times the mother may have a history of miscarriages. A significant number of pregnancies end in first-trimester miscarriages, so it is not a tremendously unusual situation. However, it is as painful emotionally to the parents as any other complication of childbirth that results in a nonliving baby. Compassion and caring on the part of the EMT can make this situation much less debilitating for the family. Remember that for couples who experience miscarriage, the words, "You can always have another baby" are not well received at this time.

Treatment is to administer oxygen and position the patient for shock: patient supine with her head elevated. Transport promptly. Bring any expelled fetal tissue to the hospital with you.

ABRUPTIO PLACENTAE AND PLACENTA PREVIA

These two conditions, as their names indicate, involve the placenta. Both occur late in pregnancy, can cause significant bleeding, and are true emergencies for both the mother and the fetus.

In **abruptio placentae** (Figure 25-18) the placenta prematurely separates from the uterine wall and causes pain and bleeding. The placenta may partially or fully (abruptly) or detach from the uterine wall.

✳ **abruptio placentae**

a condition when the placenta prematurely separates from the uterine wall and causes pain and bleeding.

ABRUPTIO PLACENTA

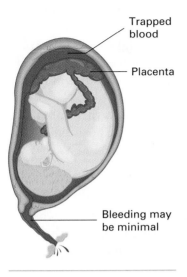

FIGURE 25-18   Abruptio placentae.

PLACENTA PREVIA

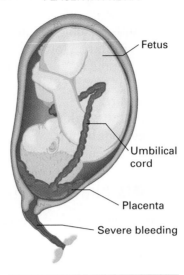

FIGURE 25-19   Placenta previa.

Placenta previa (Figure 25-19) is a condition where the placenta is attached to the uterine wall but in the wrong position. The placenta is near the cervix and is in the way of delivery. As the fetus begins to move down into position for birth and the cervix begins to dilate, the placenta tears and begins to bleed.

Care for both conditions includes oxygen, treating for shock, and prompt transport to an appropriate hospital.

SEIZURES IN PREGNANCY

Pregnant patients undergo many changes in their bodies. There can be changes in fluid balance as well as electrolytes and hormones. Occasionally these changes can cause serious negative effects, including **preeclampsia** and **eclampsia.**

Preeclampsia usually involves high blood pressure, swelling in the face and extremities, and abnormal weight gain.

Eclampsia is a more severe condition that involves the development of seizures in addition to the signs and symptoms of preeclampsia. This condition is an emergency situation that threatens the life of both the mother and fetus.

Treatment involves protecting the patient from harm during the seizure. Administer oxygen and transport the patient promptly. Transport the patient on her left side while carefully monitoring the airway. Transport should be quiet and gentle as rough motion, lights, and sirens can cause or worsen seizures in these patients.

SUPINE HYPOTENSIVE SYNDROME

When a pregnant patient gets into the third trimester of the pregnancy, the growing fetus takes up considerable space in the pelvic and abdominal cavities. One potential negative effect on the mother's body is **supine hypotensive syndrome.** This occurs when the pregnant patient lies flat and the fetus compresses the inferior vena cava. This compression reduces blood flow back to the heart and causes significant hypotension (low blood pressure). This is observed by low blood pressure measurements, dizziness, diaphoresis, and other signs of shock when the patient is supine.

* **placenta previa**

a condition where the placenta is attached to the uterine wall over the opening of the cervix, but in the wrong position.

* **preeclampsia**

pregnancy complication characterized by hypertension (high blood pressure) and edema.

* **eclampsia**

pregnancy complication characterized by severe hypertension (high blood pressure), convulsions, and coma.

* **supine hypotensive syndrome**

a condition that occurs when the pregnant patient lies flat and the fetus compresses the inferior vena cava. This compression reduces blood flow back to the heart and causes significant hypotension (low blood pressure).

The condition can be corrected by having the patient roll onto or lean toward her left side. If the patient is immobilized on a backboard or is unable to follow commands, placing a pillow under her right side will correct the problem. This is because the large, low-pressure inferior vena cava runs to the right side of the spine in the abdomen. When the baby becomes large enough and high enough in the abdomen the compression occurs. Leaning the supine patient to the left will relieve the pressure.

Any time a third-trimester pregnant patient is transported in the ambulance and develops hypotension while supine, suspect this condition and position the patient to prevent it.

TRAUMA DURING PREGNANCY

Trauma may occur to a pregnant patient. If you are called to a situation where a pregnant patient has been injured, you will assess and treat the patient the same as you would any other trauma patient. However, there are some considerations that are unique to a pregnant patient.

Do not transport a third-trimester pregnant patient flat on her back. As mentioned in the prior section on supine hypotensive syndrome, this could cause a serious drop in blood pressure. Roll the breathing, non-spine-injured patient to her left side. If the patient is secured to a backboard, place a pillow under the right side of the backboard to displace the patient slightly to the left.

In the event of unstable traumatic injuries, or when resuscitation may be futile, you may decide to perform CPR to provide some blood to the fetus on the way to the hospital where a cesarean section (C-section) may be performed to surgically remove the baby from the uterus.

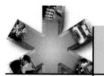

Perspective

Ling—The EMT

"It's kind of weird, delivering a baby. It's really great but such a contrast, I guess. How do I explain it? It's like . . . 95 percent of my job is dealing with sick and dying people. I've honestly lost count of the number of people who I've seen die. I couldn't even guess anymore. And yet today I held a brand new life in my hands. I was the first human being that that little boy encountered in this world. That probably sounds odd, huh? I don't know. Maybe I'm just overly philosophical right now or maybe you just have to be in that situation to understand what I mean."

Stop, Review, Remember!

Multiple Choice

Place a check next to the correct answer.

1. Meconium is:

    _____ a. produced when the mother defecates during the birthing process.

    _____ b. fetal urine in the amniotic fluid.

    _____ c. fetal feces in the amniotic fluid.

    _____ d. foreign particles in the amniotic fluid.

2. Vaginal bleeding in the third trimester is most likely due to any of the following EXCEPT:

    _____ a. placenta previa.

    _____ b. abruptio placentae.

    _____ c. eclampsia.

    _____ d. ectopic pregnancy.

3. The one condition where an EMT must insert a gloved hand into the vagina is:

    _____ a. placenta previa.

    _____ b. breech presentation.

    _____ c. prolapsed cord.

    _____ d. multiple births.

4. Premature separation of the placenta from the uterine wall is called:

    _____ a. placenta previa.

    _____ b. breech presentation.

    _____ c. prolapsed cord.

    _____ d. abruptio placentae.

5. If the heart rate of a baby immediately after birth is less than 100 beats per minute you should ventilate the baby with a BVM or pocket face mask.

    _____ a. true

    _____ b. false

Short Answer

For each of the following history statements by the mother in labor explain any concerns or actions you would take to prepare for delivery:

1. "My doctor told me I am having twins."

    _____

2. "I think I am only 32 weeks pregnant . . . "

    _____

3. "At my last ultrasound the doctor told me the baby was breech. We were hoping he would turn around. They were going to do a C-section next week." _____

4. "I don't believe in prenatal visits. I believe childbirth should be totally natural and I haven't seen a doctor." _____

Critical Thinking

1. What should you assess in the newborn? List an example of each. (Hint: APGAR)

_____

_____

_____

_____

2. Draw the inverted triangle representing the steps of neonatal resuscitation. Label the BLS steps in the triangle.

4-9.18 Discuss the emergency medical care of a patient with a gynecological emergency.

Gynecologic Emergencies

While most of this chapter has been concerned with obstetric emergencies, you will also encounter patients who have vaginal bleeding or trauma to the genitalia that is not related to pregnancy, which will require your care.

VAGINAL BLEEDING

It may be difficult to distinguish vaginal bleeding in a woman who is of child-bearing age as being pregnancy-related or not. Fortunately, it isn't necessary for an EMT to make that determination. The treatment is the same for this patient.

Give oxygen to any patient with vaginal bleeding, treat her for shock, and transport. We suspect shock in all patients with vaginal bleeding because there is the potential for significant blood loss—much of which can be internal and not visible to us. Minor vaginal bleeding may have gone on for several days prior to the onset of an emergency. Patients sometimes determine that an emergency exists because the bleeding became excessive, the pain became significant, the fear of outcomes became unbearable, or all three. Of course, always follow body substance isolation procedures.

Examine the vagina by observation only to look for trauma and determine the rate of blood loss. Never do any type of internal examination or place anything inside the vagina to stop the bleeding. Absorbent materials should be placed outside the vaginal opening to absorb the fluid and blood. These dressings can be changed as needed during transport and to make the patient comfortable.

TRAUMA TO THE GENITALIA

Trauma to the external female genitalia can occur in a number of circumstances. While sexual assault is the one we think of most, it can occur accidentally as well as from **consensual** sexual activities as well as from other mechanisms of injury such as a sports injury or auto collision.

* **consensual**
mutually agreeable.

After taking BSI precautions, your assessment and care will be both clinical and psychological. Remember that your patient will require compassionate care. Having a stranger examine the genitalia (and this applies to either sex) is probably an awkward and embarrassing experience. Introduce yourself, explain all steps in assessment and care, and reassure her frequently.

Be especially sensitive to providing her privacy and shielding from bystanders. Just because there is an emergency right now does not mean the patient will not return to see those people in a few days and be embarrassed by what occurred. Try to keep in mind that she may feel more scared and hurt than embarrassed at the time, but that can change at a later date.

Care for injuries to the external genitalia is similar to care for soft-tissue injury to other parts of the body. You will take BSI precautions, control bleeding, administer oxygen, and be prepared to identify and treat shock early.

SEXUAL ASSAULT

The care for male or female sexual assault victims differs slightly from that of other trauma patients. While the care for soft-tissue injuries is the same, there are **evidentiary** concerns as well as emotional concerns that must be addressed. In sexual assault patients:

* **evidentiary**
all items and materials pertinent to legal consideration.

* Remember that there may also be injuries to other parts of the body from the assault. Be sure to do a complete assessment.

* The patient has just been assaulted and will require gentle, nonjudgmental emotional care. Having a same-sex EMT deal with the patient can be beneficial. If this is not possible, it is even more important that the care be compassionate and nonjudgmental.

* Recognizing that an assault victim has experienced loss of control over what is done to her is vital to the proper care in these cases. Asking her permission to look, to touch, and to provide care gives the victim control of her surroundings once again.

* Try to prevent the victim from bathing, showering, going to the bathroom, douching, or otherwise cleaning up. This may destroy evidence.

* Your state may have legal requirements for reporting crimes such as sexual assault. If you have these requirements, follow them by reporting your observations to the appropriate authority (for example, police or hospital personnel) as required by law. Document all appropriate information.

Stop, Review, Remember!

Multiple Choice

Place a check next to the correct answer.

1. Vaginal bleeding can be life threatening.

    _____ a. true

    _____ b. false

2. When assessing a patient with vaginal bleeding, you should perform an internal examination to determine if there is internal bleeding.

    _____ a. true

    _____ b. false

3. If a sexual assault patient showers, urinates, or defecates, evidence may be lost.

    _____ a. true

    _____ b. false

4. You may use direct pressure to control external bleeding from the female genitalia.

    _____ a. true

    _____ b. false

5. BSI precautions for moderate vaginal bleeding would include:

    _____ a. gloves only.

    _____ b. gloves and eyewear.

    _____ c. gloves, eyewear, gown, and boot covers.

    _____ d. no BSI requirement.

6. Trauma to the external genitalia from sexual assault can happen to both women and men.

    _____ a. true

    _____ b. false

7. Vaginal bleeding and abdominal pain in a 27-year-old woman would cause you to consider ectopic pregnancy as the cause.

    _____ a. true

    _____ b. false

8. Which of the following is least appropriate for a patient with significant vaginal bleeding?

    _____ a. Place an absorbent pad over the vagina.

    _____ b. Administer oxygen.

    _____ c. Place the patient in the Fowler's position.

    _____ d. Observe the external genitalia for trauma.

Short Answer

1. What is the care for vaginal bleeding?

_____

2. Can vaginal bleeding be a sign of internal bleeding?

_____

3. Why is a full patient assessment important in sexual assault patients?

_____

Critical Thinking

1. You are caring for a woman who has been raped. She wishes to use the bathroom. What would you tell her? Do you have the right to stop her if she insists?

_____

_____

_____

_____

2. Does care for trauma to the genitalia differ from soft-tissue injuries in other parts of the body? Why or why not?

_____

_____

_____

_____

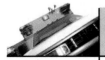

Dispatch Summary

Ling and Mark delivered a healthy 6 lb. 8 oz. baby boy named Nathan Ray in the cab of the pick-up truck and then transported both mother and child to Fleischmann's Hospital on Old County Road.

Two months later, both EMT were surprised to receive invitations to the wedding of Nathan Ray's mother and her boyfriend. Both medics plan to attend.

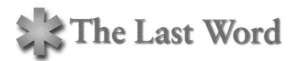

The Last Word

This chapter covered a wide range of situations. Some "natural" emergencies like childbirth are things that you won't see a lot in the field. Many EMTs will go for an entire career and not deliver a baby.

Although not commonly encountered, the topics covered in the chapter will cause you to come in contact with patients who will have a critical need for your assistance. Most parents plan a pregnancy to end at the hospital in a controlled medical setting. When these plans go awry, the calmness, professionalism, and experience you bring to the patient and her family will be remembered long after mother and baby come home from the hospital.

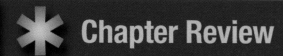

Chapter Review

MULTIPLE CHOICE

1. A fontanel is:

   _____ a. a soft spot on a baby's head.

   _____ b. a twist in the umbilical cord.

   _____ c. an airway obstruction in the newborn caused by fluid or tissue during delivery.

   _____ d. the name for the part of the baby that is visible first at the vaginal opening.

2. When a patient reports "breaking her water" she is referring to:

   _____ a. becoming incontinent of urine due to late stages of pregnancy.

   _____ b. rupture of the amniotic sac.

   _____ c. delivery of the placenta.

   _____ d. vaginal bleeding.

3. You have a patient who has given birth but has consistent vaginal bleeding that does not stop. To control this:

   _____ a. pack the vagina with absorbent dressings.

   _____ b. apply direct pressure to the vaginal opening.

   _____ c. massage the uterus.

   _____ d. clamp the umbilical cord.

4. When suctioning a newborn you should suction the:

   _____ a. mouth first, then the nose.

   _____ b. nose first, then the mouth.

   _____ c. nose only.

   _____ d. mouth only.

5. Which of the following statements is most correct in regard to limb presentation?

   _____ a. The delivery will be relatively normal. Prepare to deliver the baby.

   _____ b. You should gently but firmly manipulate the uterus to get the other limb to present.

   _____ c. Your treatments include transportation of the patient in a head-down position with oxygen.

   _____ d. Transportation of the patient in this condition is too dangerous. Prepare for delivery when the other limb appears.

MATCHING

Match the term on the left with the applicable definition on the right.

1. _____ Meconium
2. _____ Breech presentation
3. _____ Placenta previa
4. _____ Premature birth
5. _____ Multiple birth
6. _____ Prolapsed cord
7. _____ Limb presentation
8. _____ Abruptio placentae

A. The umbilical cord protruding from the vagina
B. More than one fetus
C. A fetus born at 32 weeks' gestation
D. Fetal fecal matter in the amniotic fluid
E. Both legs as the presenting part
F. One arm as the presenting part
G. Vaginal bleeding
H. Separation of the placenta from the uterine wall prematurely
I. Positioning of the placenta near the cervix
J. Ruptured uterus

CRITICAL THINKING

1. Why are most mothers aware that they may have multiple births or potential complications? How will this affect your history taking?

_____
_____
_____
_____

2. Why is it important to dry a newborn and maintain warmth?

_____
_____
_____
_____

3. List five components of an OB kit and what each listed item is used for.

_____
_____
_____
_____

CASE STUDY

You are called to a "woman in labor" in an apartment building in a "bad" part of town. You walk the three flights of stairs because there is no elevator.

Entering the apartment, you find a woman lying on the floor breathing heavily. She is obviously near full term, based on the size of her abdomen. "Hi. We're from the fire department. We're going to help you out." The woman's name is Maria. She is there with her husband, George, in their new apartment.

You determine answers to a few key questions and find that this is Maria's first baby. Labor started only about an hour ago, but the contractions are very intense, long, and close together. She feels the urge to move her bowels. You explain to Maria that you are going to look to see if the baby is coming. You see crowning.

When you ask Maria if she knew of any problems from her doctor visits and ultrasounds, she looks at George who replies, "We have no money. We couldn't afford any doctor visits. None." He looks sad—and to you for help.

1. What does the fact that the patient had no prenatal care mean to your care and decision making at the scene?

   _____

   _____

   _____

   _____

2. How would you handle the fact that you are on a third floor with no elevator?

   _____

   _____

   _____

   _____

3. How would you tell if the patient was having more than one baby?

   _____

   _____

   _____

   _____

4. What resources would you call for? Why?

   _____

   _____

   _____

   _____

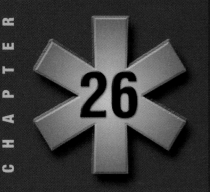
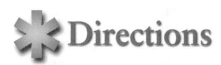 Directions

Assess what you have learned in this module by circling the best answer for each multiple-choice question.
When you are done, check your answers against the key provided in Appendix D.

1. The name of a drug listed in the United States
   Pharmacopoeia is its _____ name.
   a. trade
   b. chemical
   c. proprietary
   d. generic

2. The name given to a drug by the
   pharmaceutical company that markets it is its
   _____ name.
   a. trade
   b. chemical
   c. pharmaceutical
   d. generic

3. Which of the following medications would
   take the longest to have its effect?
   a. an injection of epinephrine
   b. oral glucose gel
   c. a Tylenol tablet
   d. a puff of albuterol

4. The reason a medication is given is its:
   a. action.
   b. indication.
   c. contraindication.
   d. incentive.

5. Undesired consequences of a medication are
   known as:
   a. contraindications.
   b. actions.
   c. side effects.
   d. mis-actions.

6. Once you receive an order to administer
   medication to a patient you should:
   a. repeat the order to the physician.
   b. wait for the physician to verify the order.
   c. write down the order.
   d. all of the above.

7. You are caring for a patient who has been
   stung by a bee and is having a severe allergic
   reaction. You would be most likely to receive
   an order for which of the following
   medications?
   a. epinephrine
   b. nitroglycerin
   c. aspirin
   d. activated charcoal

8. Bronchodilators are given to treat patients
   presenting with which of the following
   problems?
   a. chest pain
   b. poisoning or overdose
   c. difficulty breathing
   d. diabetes

9. Which of the following is an acceptable way to measure a patient's respiratory distress?
   a. how many stairs he can climb without difficulty
   b. how long he can hold his breath
   c. how much oxygen the patient uses at home
   d. the number of words he can speak between breaths

10. Abnormal breathing patterns may be caused by:
    a. stroke.
    b. overdose.
    c. brain injury.
    d. all of the above.

11. _____ is a respiratory illness in which the walls of the alveoli break down and air becomes trapped in the lung.
    a. Asthma
    b. Bronchitis
    c. Emphysema
    d. Tuberculosis

12. Which of the following behavioral changes may be caused by hypoxia?
    a. anxiety
    b. confusion
    c. combativeness
    d. all of the above

13. Which of the following devices delivers tiny droplets of respiratory medication through a mask or mouthpiece over an extended period of time?
    a. small volume nebulizer
    b. metered dose inhaler
    c. spacer
    d. steam vaporizer

14. The ability of the heart to generate its own electrical impulses is called:
    a. conductivity.
    b. contractility.
    c. automaticity.
    d. propensity.

15. Which of the following is NOT one of the links in the chain of survival for cardiac arrest?
    a. early CPR
    b. early aspirin
    c. early defibrillation
    d. early advanced life support

16. The general term applied to patients who present with an emergency related to the heart is:
    a. cardiac compromise.
    b. cardiac arrest.
    c. angina.
    d. myocardial infarction.

17. Another name for a heart attack is:
    a. cardiac arrest.
    b. ventricular fibrillation.
    c. myocardial infarction.
    d. all of the above.

18. Your patient is a 50-year-old male with no previous history of heart problems. He began having pain in his chest and left arm, along with some nausea, after eating some chicken wings while watching a basketball game on television. He took some antacid but didn't get any relief. Over the next hour, his symptoms worsened and he began to feel short of breath. These symptoms are most consistent with:
    a. congestive heart failure.
    b. myocardial infarction.
    c. angina.
    d. asystole.

19. Jugular venous distention is most commonly associated with which of the following conditions?
    a. congestive heart failure
    b. cardiac arrest
    c. myocardial infarction
    d. ventricular fibrillation

20. Which of the following is NOT a contraindication for the administration of nitroglycerin to a patient with chest pain?
    a. The patient took Cialis earlier in the day.
    b. The blood pressure is 88/50.
    c. The patient does not have his own prescription for nitroglycerin.
    d. The patient rates his pain less than a "7" on a scale from 1 to 10.

21. Which of the following patients can be said to have an altered mental status?
    a. a 27-year-old female diabetic who is awake but staring off into space and unable to recall what day it is
    b. an 18-year-old male who is reported to have drunk a large amount of alcohol and responds to painful, but not verbal stimuli
    c. a 38-year-old male reported to have used cocaine who is now awake, alert, and threatening to kill anyone who gets close to him
    d. all of the above

22. When a diabetic patient takes too much insulin and eats too little food, he will experience:
    a. hyperglycemia.
    b. hypoglycemia.
    c. diabetic coma.
    d. insulin effect.

23. A normal blood glucose reading is between _____ and _____ mg/dL.
    a. 40; 80
    b. 80; 120
    c. 100; 120
    d. 120; 150

24. An abnormal surge of electrical signals in the brain is known as a(n):
    a. convulsion.
    b. coma.
    c. seizure.
    d. epileptic fit.

25. The period of time in which a patient has an altered mental status following a seizure is the _____ period or phase.
    a. grand mal
    b. petit mal
    c. postictal
    d. generalized

26. Which of the following is a cause of stroke?
    a. a blood clot in an artery in the brain
    b. high blood glucose level
    c. seizure
    d. all of the above

27. Your patient is a 70-year-old male who experienced a sudden onset of paralysis on his right side and difficulty expressing his thoughts. He is quite frustrated because he cannot make you understand what he wants to say. Which of the following is the best response?
    a. There are new cures for strokes. You'll be good as new in no time.
    b. Don't try to say anything. I know just how you feel.
    c. With physical and speech therapy you may be able to regain a useful life.
    d. Let's get you to the hospital and see what they can do to make you better.

28. The EMT's primary concern in caring for any patient with an altered mental status is:
    a. finding the cause of altered mental status.
    b. getting a good history.
    c. anticipating airway and breathing problems.
    d. stabilizing the cervical spine.

29. Which of the following is/are associated with anaphylaxis, but not with mild or moderate allergic reactions?
    a. airway obstruction
    b. rash
    c. hives
    d. increased heart rate

30. You have just assisted a patient with a severe shellfish allergy in using her Epi-pen. As you are loading her into the ambulance, she becomes anxious and her heart rate increases from 100, initially, to 112. In addition, she tells you she feels like she is going to throw up. Which of the following should you consider?
    a. giving a second dose of epinephrine since the patient is getting worse
    b. reassessing the patient
    c. reassuring the patient that what she is experiencing is a normal reaction to epinephrine
    d. b and c

31. Which of the following is NOT a significant risk factor for heat and cold related emergencies?
    a. old age
    b. female gender
    c. circulatory problems
    d. very young age

32. In which of the following situations is the patient losing body heat primarily by convection?
    a. A 55-year-old male is found lying on the frozen ground without a coat.
    b. A 24-year-old male is wearing wet clothing after falling out of his boat while fishing.
    c. A 32-year-old female is outside in cool, windy weather.
    d. A vapor cloud is created every time your 80-year-old female patient breathes into the cool night air.

33. Which of the following is categorized as a generalized cold emergency?
    a. hyperthermia
    b. frostbite
    c. hypothermia
    d. frostnip

34. Your patient is a 30-year-old male hiker who was lost outside overnight in below-freezing temperatures. He is shivering uncontrollably and has decreased coordination. Which of the following actions is appropriate?
    a. Give him plenty of hot coffee.
    b. Briskly rub his arms and legs to increase circulation.
    c. Have the patient move around as much as possible to generate body heat.
    d. Remove his wet clothing and cover him with blankets.

35. Which of the following is used in active rewarming but not passive rewarming?
    a. giving hot tea, cocoa, or coffee to drink
    b. placing hot packs at the patient's neck, armpits, and groin
    c. covering the patient with a blanket
    d. turning up the heat in the patient compartment of the ambulance

36. Care of a frostbitten extremity includes:
    a. splinting the affected area.
    b. breaking any blisters that form.
    c. applying hot packs to the affected area.
    d. gently rubbing the affected area between your hands.

37. More serious heat-related injuries should be suspected when the patient presents with:
    a. feeling faint.
    b. muscle cramps.
    c. hot, dry skin.
    d. weakness.

38. Your patient is a 25-year-old male who has been working outside in a hot, humid climate. He is alert and oriented, complaining of feeling weak and dizzy. His skin is cool and moist, and he has a heart rate of 104, a blood pressure of 110/70, and respirations of 16. Which of the following is an acceptable treatment?
    a. Place cold packs at the groin, armpits, and neck.
    b. Give the patient some cool water to drink.
    c. Offer the patient some salt tablets.
    d. Wet the skin, turn the air conditioning on high, and vigorously fan the patient.

39. Your patient was hiking in the desert and was bitten on the ankle by a rattlesnake. Which of the following is most appropriate?
    a. keep the foot lower than the level of the patient's heart.
    b. elevate the foot on pillows.
    c. apply a tourniquet above the bite.
    d. apply ice to the area of the bite.

40. Which of the following may be a cause of bizarre behavior?
    a. hypoglycemia
    b. psychiatric illness
    c. head trauma
    d. all of the above

41. Features of schizophrenia may include all of the following EXCEPT:
    a. paranoia.
    b. multiple personalities.
    c. psychosis.
    d. delusions.

42. Which of the following guidelines applies to the patient who is threatening or has attempted suicide?
    a. Directly ask about suicidal thoughts and intentions.
    b. Be prepared to spend some time on the scene with the patient.
    c. Take all threats and attempts seriously, even if they seem designed just to get attention.
    d. All of the above

43. Your patient is a 22-year-old female who is breathing rapidly, clutching her chest, and begging you not to let her die. Her roommate tells you that the patient has a history of panic attacks. Which of the following is an appropriate approach to the patient?
    a. looking the patient directly in the eye and stating, "You need to get a hold of yourself. There's no reason for you to be panicked."
    b. standing back from the patient and asking whether or not she wants to go to the hospital.
    c. getting on the patient's level and stating, "I'm an EMT with the ambulance service. Let's see what we can do to help you."
    d. placing your hand on the patient's shoulder and letting her know that EMTs aren't trained to handle psychiatric problems and that she should contact her psychiatrist.

44. In a pregnant patient, indications of imminent delivery include all of the following EXCEPT:
    a. contractions are two minutes apart or less.
    b. the mother states she needs to urinate.
    c. crowning is present.
    d. the mother has delivered at least one child previously.

45. In a normal delivery, the first part to present is the:
    a. placenta.
    b. buttocks.
    c. head.
    d. feet.

46. You have just assisted with the delivery of a full-term infant. You have suctioned his mouth and nose and have clamped and cut the cord, but the infant is not breathing. Which of the following should you do first?
    a. Insert an oropharyngeal airway and ventilate the patient with a bag-valve mask.
    b. Rub his back.
    c. Perform mouth-to-mask ventilations.
    d. Administer high-flow oxygen.

47. When the placenta separates prematurely from the uterine wall, this is known as:
    a. placenta previa.
    b. ectopic placentae.
    c. preeclampsia.
    d. abruptio placentae.

48. AEDs are designed to help which of the following types of patients?
    a. all patients having a myocardial infarction
    b. all patients in cardiac arrest
    c. patients in ventricular fibrillation
    d. patients with no electrical activity in the heart

49. Which of the following is NOT a contraindication to the use of an AED?
    a. patient experiencing chest pain
    b. 10-year-old patient in cardiac arrest
    c. patient not breathing but has a pulse
    d. unresponsive diabetic

50. For a patient who remains in a shockable rhythm, an AED will deliver ____ shock(s) between prompts to check the patient.
    a. 1
    b. 3
    c. 6
    d. 9

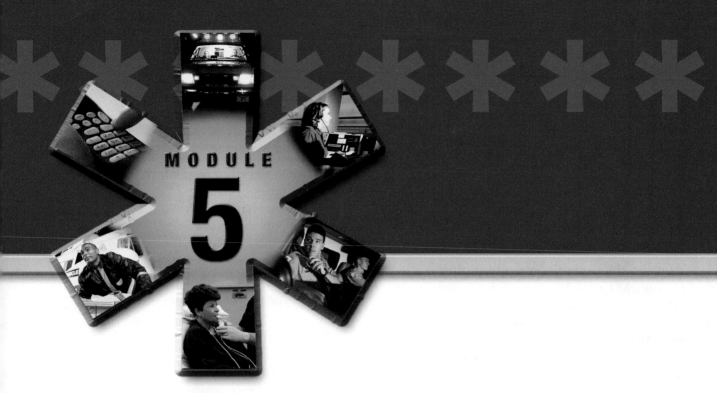

MODULE

5

Trauma

" The smoke, the noise, the flashing lights, the yelling . . . that poor man. I've never in my life seen a person burned so badly . . . His hands and feet peeled off . . . I can't imagine the pain . . . We got him to the burn center as fast as we could. "

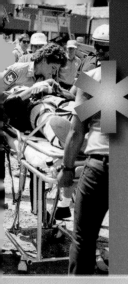

Module Outline

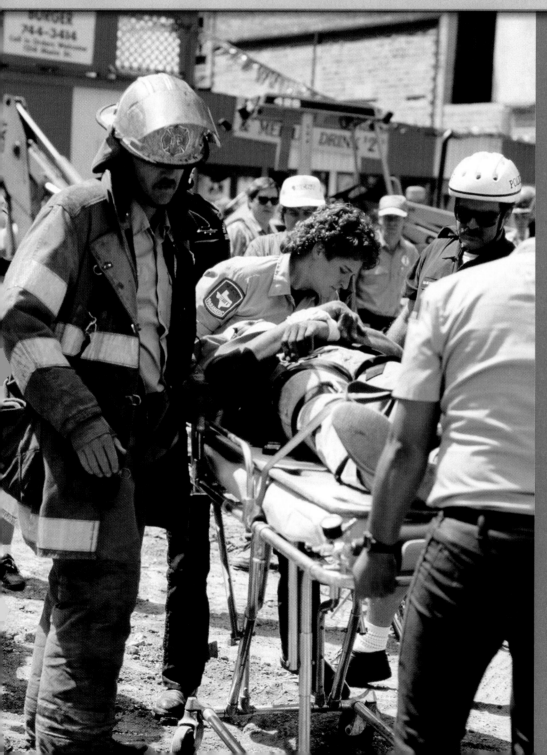

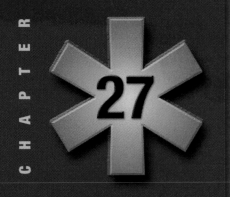

CHAPTER

27

Recognition and Care of the Shock Patient

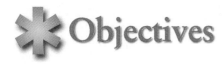

Objectives

Numbered objectives are from the U.S. Department of Transportation 1994 EMT-Basic National Standard Curriculum.

COGNITIVE OBJECTIVES

At the completion of this lesson, the EMT-Basic student will be able to:

5-1.4 Establish the relationship between body substance isolation and bleeding. (pp. 667–668)

5-1.5 Establish the relationship between airway management and the trauma patient. (pp. 679–680)

5-1.6 Establish the relationship between mechanism of injury and internal bleeding. (pp. 670–672)

5-1.7 List the signs of internal bleeding. (p. 672)

5-1.8 List the steps in the emergency medical care of the patient with signs and symptoms of internal bleeding. (p. 680)

5-1.9 List signs and symptoms of shock (hypoperfusion). (pp. 675–678)

5-1.10 State the steps in the emergency medical care of the patient with signs and symptoms of shock (hypoperfusion). (pp. 680–683)

AFFECTIVE OBJECTIVES

At the completion of this lesson, the EMT-Basic student will be able to:

5-1.11 Explain the sense of urgency to transport patients that are bleeding and show signs of shock (hypoperfusion). (pp. 670, 678)

PSYCHOMOTOR OBJECTIVES

At the completion of this lesson, the EMT-Basic student will be able to:

5-1.15 Demonstrate the care of the patient exhibiting signs and symptoms of internal bleeding. (p. 680)

5-1.16 Demonstrate the care of the patient exhibiting signs and symptoms of shock (hypoperfusion). (pp. 682–683)

5-1.17 Demonstrate completing a prehospital care report for patient with bleeding and/or shock (hypoperfusion). (p. 683)

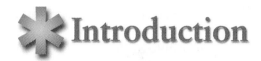

Introduction

We are a very active and mobile society, so it is no surprise that trauma is the leading cause of death among all persons between the ages of 1 and 44. It is safe to say that in most EMS systems nearly half of all the requests for an ambulance are for some type of injury. In this chapter, you will also learn to identify the signs and symptoms of shock (hypoperfusion) and to care for a patient with suspected internal bleeding.

   You will also be reminded of the importance of carefully evaluating the mechanism of injury to help determine the extent of potential trauma.

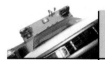

Emergency Dispatch

Johnny, an EMT, and his partner, Greg, had just finished washing their ambulance when the emergency radio crackled to life.

   "Hey guys, I need you to head out to County Line Road. There's been a traumatic injury there at the tire factory."

   "We're on our way, Becky," Johnny replied as he climbed behind the steering wheel and started the engine.

   "Man," Greg said as he shut off the hose and got into the passenger seat. "I hope it's not like the last call we had there. That guy with the amputated leg. Remember?"

   "Yup," Johnny frowned. The road dust that the tires were kicking up was already settling on the glistening truck.

The patient was a 53-year-old machinist who was holding a blood-soaked towel tightly around his right forearm. Johnny immediately noticed that the man's pants were covered with blood and that he was very pale.

   "What happened?" Greg asked as he helped the man onto the stretcher.

   "It was . . . um . . . I was working a hydraulic punch . . . and . . . and . . . " the man's voice trailed off and sweat began to accumulate on his forehead.

   "Quick," Johnny said. "Lay him down. Someone get me a blanket or some jackets."

Appropriate BSI Precautions

Because of the potential for exposure to blood, you must be especially diligent about taking BSI precautions when you care for victims of trauma. A patient with an open wound may be thrashing about in pain, which poses a serious risk of exposure as you attempt to care for him. A patient with facial trauma may splatter blood as he coughs, sneezes, or simply tries to answer your questions. Just because

5-1.4 Establish the relationship between body substance isolation and bleeding.

the patient is not actively bleeding when you get on scene does not mean you won't be exposed to the patient's blood.

Remember that the areas of your body most susceptible to exposure are:

✳ Hands

✳ Eyes

✳ Mucous membranes (nose and mouth)

✳ Open wounds or sores

Use great caution and take appropriate BSI precautions prior to making contact with any trauma patient. There might be times when goggles and/or face shields are necessary and even gowns to protect your clothing. You must anticipate the level of protection that will be necessary, because once you begin treating the patient, it is difficult to stop and add more protective gear. It is also important to properly clean and decontaminate the ambulance and all equipment following the call. And even though you were wearing gloves, don't forget to wash your hands following the removal of gloves and after each and every call.

Perfusion and Shock

✳ **shock**

see hypoperfusion.

✳ **perfusion**

the supply of oxygen to and removal of wastes from the cells and tissues of the body as a result of the flow of blood through the capillaries.

A discussion of **shock** would not be complete without a discussion regarding **perfusion**. Perfusion is the adequate flow of well-oxygenated blood throughout the entire body, especially the vital organs. When the circulatory system is functioning properly, a patient is said to be perfusing well.

Signs of adequate perfusion include:

✳ Normal skin signs

✳ Normal mental status

✳ Normal vital signs

✳ **hypoperfusion**

inadequate perfusion of blood to an organ or organs. Also called shock.

When a person is not perfusing well it is frequently due to a malfunction of one or more of the components of the circulatory system: the heart, the blood, or the blood vessels. A patient who is not perfusing well is said to be suffering from **hypoperfusion** (Figure 27-1). If left untreated, hypoperfusion can quickly lead to shock. Most of the time, the terms *shock* and *hypoperfusion* are used interchangeably, and we will use them that way for our discussion here.

Signs and symptoms of inadequate perfusion include:

✳ Abnormal skin signs (pale, cool, and moist)

✳ Altered mental status (agitation, restlessness, sluggishness, confusion, or decreased responsiveness)

✳ Abnormal vital signs (increased pulse and respiratory rate, decreased blood pressure)

Essential for good perfusion is a properly functioning circulatory system with an adequate blood pressure and a properly functioning respiratory system.

For the most part, the type of shock that we will be discussing in this chapter results from an excessive amount of blood loss and is called hemorrhagic shock.

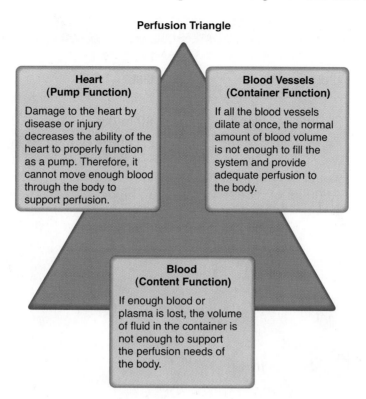

Perfusion Triangle

FIGURE 27-1 The three primary causes of shock: poor heart (pump) function, blood or fluid loss, and dilation of blood vessels.

Heart (Pump Function)

Damage to the heart by disease or injury decreases the ability of the heart to properly function as a pump. Therefore, it cannot move enough blood through the body to support perfusion.

Blood Vessels (Container Function)

If all the blood vessels dilate at once, the normal amount of blood volume is not enough to fill the system and provide adequate perfusion to the body.

Blood (Content Function)

If enough blood or plasma is lost, the volume of fluid in the container is not enough to support the perfusion needs of the body.

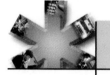

Perspective

Jason—The Patient

"That was weird. I thought that I was doing okay. I've hurt myself worse before and was fine. But this time I got tunnel vision and started feeling really nervous. I knew something was about to happen but I didn't know what, and that's the strangest feeling that I've ever had."

Internal Bleeding

A sudden loss of a significant quantity of blood is dangerous and, if left untreated, life threatening. It is relatively uncommon for a patient to die from external bleeding if there are people at the scene who can assist. Because most external bleeding is obvious, it usually gets the attention of bystanders or rescuers and attempts are quickly made to control the bleeding. See Table 27-1 on page 670 for the approximate total blood volume of an adult, a child, and an infant.

TABLE 27-1	APPROXIMATE BLOOD VOLUME BY SIZE	
ADULT	**CHILD**	**INFANT**
70 ml/kg of blood An average size adult weighing 70 kg (154 lbs) would have approximately 4,900 ml of blood.	80 ml/kg of blood A child weighing 30 kg (66 lbs) would have approximately 2,400 ml of blood.	80 ml/kg of blood An infant weighing 10 kg (22 lbs) would have approximately 800 ml of blood.

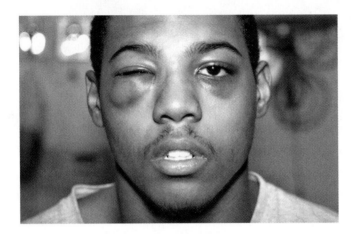

FIGURE 27-2 Blunt trauma can include severe bruising.

In the case of internal bleeding (Figure 27-2), the blood being lost from the circulatory system is contained within the body and cannot be easily detected by rescuers. Even when internal bleeding is suspected, there is little that can be done to stop the bleeding in the field. Patients with internal bleeding generally require surgical intervention to repair the damage and control the bleeding. For this reason, early recognition and rapid transport are essential.

SEVERITY OF BLOOD LOSS

The numerous organs contained within the torso and the many vessels that supply them with blood present a great potential for life-threatening internal bleeding. The areas of greatest concern for internal blood loss are the:

∗ Chest

∗ Abdomen

∗ Pelvis

The volume of blood loss from internal bleeding can exceed several liters. In some larger patients, even injuries to the extremities can conceal enough blood to cause shock (Table 27-2).

PREDICTING INTERNAL BLEEDING

5-1.6 Establish the relationship between mechanism of injury and internal bleeding.

Because internal bleeding cannot be seen, we must use other means to predict the likelihood that it exists. The initial tool used to predict the existence of internal

TABLE 27-2	APPROXIMATE INTERNAL BLOOD LOSS ASSOCIATED WITH UNDERLYING FRACTURES
BONE	**APPROXIMATE BLOOD LOSS**
Rib	125 cc
Radius/ulna	250–500 cc
Humerus	500–750 cc
Tibia/fibula	500–1000 cc
Femur	1000–2000 cc
Pelvis	1000–3000 cc

bleeding is the mechanism of injury. Any significant mechanism, such as penetrating trauma, rapid deceleration, blunt trauma, or crushing injury that affects the chest, abdomen, or pelvis has the potential for causing life-threatening internal bleeding. You must maintain a high index of suspicion for internal bleeding with any of the following mechanisms of injury:

* Falls from a height (Figure 27-3)
* Motorcycle collisions
* Vehicle vs. pedestrian impacts
* Automobile collisions
* Blast injuries
* Penetrating trauma
* Significant blunt trauma

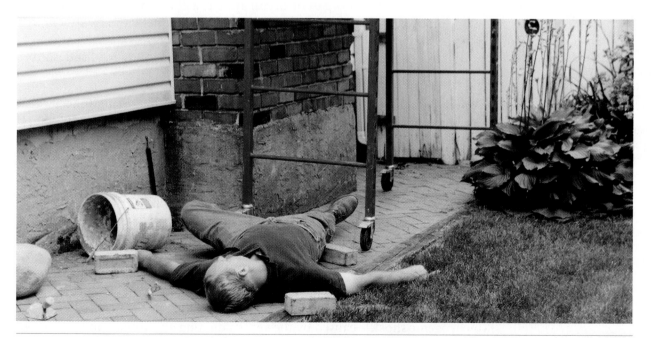

FIGURE 27-3 Maintain a high index of suspicion for internal bleeding with a patient who has experienced a fall from a height. (Craig Jackson/In the Dark Photography.)

In addition to trauma, certain medical conditions can cause sudden internal bleeding. Many of these conditions involve bleeding from the stomach and intestines.

SIGNS AND SYMPTOMS OF INTERNAL BLEEDING

In addition to evaluating the mechanism of injury, you must carefully assess the patient and identify any signs or symptoms that might indicate the presence of internal bleeding. The following is a list of some of the more common signs and symptoms of internal bleeding:

* Rigid, and/or distended abdomen or pelvic region

* Pain, tenderness, swelling, or discoloration on or near the suspected site of injury

* Bleeding from the mouth, rectum, or vagina

* Vomiting bright red blood or dark coffee-ground-colored blood (old blood)

* Bleeding during a bowel movement or stools that are bloody and dark and tarry in color

* Signs and symptoms of shock without external bleeding

Shock

Shock is a progressive condition that occurs when a patient does not receive an adequate supply of well-oxygenated blood to all areas and organs of the body. As already noted, it can occur for several reasons, including damage to the heart, loss of blood, and abnormal dilation of the vessels. Harmful waste products generated by the body that cannot be removed efficiently add to the problem. As a direct result of poor perfusion, the cells of the various organs (liver, kidneys, brain, heart, lungs) begin to starve for oxygen and suffer from the effects of unremoved wastes and can no longer perform their functions. When enough cells within a particular organ have failed, the entire organ or organ system will begin to malfunction and eventually shut down. Without prompt recognition in the field and treatment at a hospital these patients will die.

Not all incidences of shock are caused by bleeding. The following list describes several other types of shock and their root cause:

* **Anaphylactic shock**—caused by an overreaction of the immune system when exposed to an allergen. The severe allergic response causes the blood vessels to dilate, resulting in a decrease in blood pressure and a corresponding decrease in perfusion. Refer to chapter 22.

* **Cardiogenic shock**—caused when the heart can no longer pump blood adequately, resulting in a decrease in cardiac output and thus a decrease in perfusion.

* **Hemorrhagic shock**—caused by loss of blood.

* **Hypovolemic shock**—caused by a sudden decrease in body fluids (blood or other body fluids such as severe diarrhea). The decrease in fluid volume causes a decrease in blood pressure and a corresponding decrease in perfusion.

* **Neurogenic shock**—caused by the vessels dilating abnormally in response to injury to the spinal cord. The dilation of the blood vessels results in a decrease in blood pressure and a corresponding decrease in perfusion.

✳ **anaphylactic shock**
type of shock caused by an overreaction of the immune system when exposed to an allergen.

✳ **cardiogenic shock**
type of shock caused when the heart can no longer pump blood adequately resulting in a decrease in cardiac output and thus a decrease in perfusion.

✳ **hemorrhagic shock**
type of shock caused by loss of blood.

✳ **hypovolemic shock**
type of shock caused by a sudden decrease in body fluids—blood or other body fluids.

✳ **neurogenic shock**
type of shock caused when the vessels dilate abnormally in response to injury to the spinal cord.

* **Septic shock**—caused by severe infections that abnormally dilate the blood vessels. The dilation of the blood vessels results in a decrease in blood pressure and a corresponding decrease in perfusion.

* **Psychogenic shock**—caused by a sudden and temporary dilation of the blood vessels from psychological causes. The dilation of the blood vessels results in a decrease in blood pressure and a corresponding decrease in perfusion.

* **septic shock**

type of shock caused by severe infections that abnormally dilate the blood vessels.

* **psychogenic shock**

type of shock caused by a sudden and temporary dilation of the blood vessels from psychological causes.

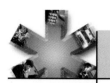

Perspective

Johnny—The EMT

"That guy lost quite a bit of blood. There was a good amount on and around the machine that he was using, who knows how much had soaked into his clothing, and that white towel was all red. I knew right away that shock was going to be an issue in this call, so I started planning for it. You know, going over in my head the steps to follow. Being that Greg and I are EMTs, we can't give IV fluids or anything like that to counter the blood loss, but we can definitely help."

Stop, Review, Remember!

Multiple Choice

Place a check next to the correct answer.

1. Which of the following is NOT a sign of good perfusion?

   _____ a. pink, warm, and dry skin

   _____ b. confused mental status

   _____ c. alert and normal mental status

   _____ d. vital signs within normal limits

2. If left untreated, _____ can lead to shock.

   _____ a. bleeding

   _____ b. high blood pressure

   _____ c. a rapid respiration

   _____ d. an altered mental status

3. In many cases, patients with internal bleeding will require _____ in order to survive.

   _____ a. late detection of shock

   _____ b. surgical intervention

   _____ c. ongoing assessments

   _____ d. a rapid trauma assessment

4. The type of shock that develops when too much blood is lost is known as _____ shock.

_____ a. psychogenic

_____ b. metabolic

_____ c. hemorrhagic

_____ d. anaphylactic

5. _____ shock is caused when the vessels dilate abnormally in response to injury to the spinal cord.

_____ a. Anaphylactic

_____ b. Hemorrhagic

_____ c. Cardiogenic

_____ d. Neurogenic

Fill in the Blank

1. _____ is the leading cause of death among all persons between the ages of 1 and 44.

2. Perfusion is the adequate flow of _____ _____ blood throughout the entire body, especially the vital organs.

3. A patient with adequate perfusion will have normal skin signs, _____ _____, and vital signs.

4. A patient who is not perfusing well is said to be suffering from _____.

5. The areas of greatest concern for internal blood loss are the _____, abdomen, and pelvis.

Critical Thinking

1. Discuss the relationship between mechanism of injury and the likelihood of internal bleeding.

_____

_____

_____

_____

_____

2. Discuss why internal bleeding is frequently more deadly than external bleeding.

_____

_____

_____

_____

_____

3. List as many signs and symptoms of internal bleeding as you can.

_____

_____

_____

_____

_____

Signs and Symptoms of Shock

The signs and symptoms of shock are progressive and develop over time. The speed at which they develop will depend on the extent of bleeding and the care the patient receives. The following is a list of signs and symptoms of shock:

5-1.9 List signs and symptoms of shock (hypoperfusion).

* Increased pulse rate (tachycardia)

* Altered mental status including restlessness and anxiety

* Increased respiratory rate (tachypnea)

* Increased capillary refill time

* Weak peripheral pulses

* Pale, cool, and clammy skin

* Thirst

* Sluggish and dilated pupils

* Nausea and/or vomiting

* Decreasing blood pressure (late sign)

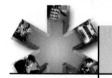

Perspective

Greg—The EMT

"As soon as that guy started to go out I called for the ALS truck, but Becky told us that there had been a rollover accident out on the interstate and Tom wasn't available. So we did what we could do. Do you know what the most effective treatment for shock is on a BLS ambulance with no ALS help available? I call it 'diesel therapy.' It goes something like this: Control any bleeding that you can see, load the patient in the ambulance, and get to the hospital as quickly and safely as possible!"

The signs and symptoms of shock tell us that the body is attempting to compensate for the loss of blood—or heart malfunction, vessel dilation, or other causes—and the inadequate perfusion that results. The presence of the signs and symptoms of shock tell us that the body is working properly to try and save itself. It is making every attempt to compensate for the decrease in perfusion.

Richard: A Case Study for the Progression of Shock

As mentioned before, shock is revealed by specific signs and symptoms that will appear and progress as long as the underlying cause is not corrected. Here is a fictitious patient named Richard to demonstrate how the signs and symptoms of shock progress. Richard is a 44-year-old male who was ejected from a minivan rollover. Richard has suffered significant injury to his abdomen and is bleeding internally. He is responsive and is lying supine on the ground in pain. During your rapid trauma assessment, you discover that Richard was not restrained during the incident and that he is complaining of severe abdominal pain on palpation of both upper quadrants. There is no evidence of external trauma or bleeding, and Richard is alert and oriented × 4.

Richard's vital signs prior to the incident:

TIME	RESPIRATIONS	PULSE	BP	SKIN	PUPILS	MENTAL
1100	16; good tidal volume; unlabored	76; strong; regular	118/76	pink; warm; dry	PERRL	A&O normal

10 minutes into the incident—loss of approximately 500 cc of blood:

TIME	RESPIRATIONS	PULSE	BP	SKIN	PUPILS	MENTAL
1110	18; good tidal volume; unlabored	88; strong; regular	126/86	pink; warm; dry	PERRL	A&O normal

Ten minutes following the incident, Richard is still shaken up and experiencing the effects of the adrenaline that was released as a result of the psychological and physical stress of the crash. The rush of adrenaline has caused his respirations, pulse, and BP to increase slightly for the time being. His circulatory system is damaged, and blood is spilling into his abdomen. The increase in pulse rate from the initial rush of adrenaline has managed to compensate for the blood loss—at least for now.

20 minutes into the incident—loss of approximately 1000cc of blood:

TIME	RESPIRATIONS	PULSE	BP	SKIN	PUPILS	MENTAL
1120	22; good tidal volume; labored	110; strong; regular	118/72	pale; warm; dry	PERRL	A&O anxious

Richard has lost a full liter of blood into his abdomen, and the adrenaline rush from the incident has completely worn off. His body must now work extra hard in an attempt to maintain adequate perfusion. His respiratory and pulse rates are up slightly. Considering what he has been through, the EMT finding Richard with these vital signs might not think the situation is that bad. Anyone who has just survived a rollover collision and is in pain could have these vital signs. Unlike the EMT at the scene, we have the luxury of knowing his vitals both before the incident and 10 minutes following. This begins to illustrate just how easy it is to think your patient is doing okay when in reality he has already begun a spiral into shock. Also notice that Richard's mental status and skin signs have changed slightly. The brain is probably the organ most susceptible to changes in perfusion, and his change in mental status reflects this. His skin is pale now, because the vessels in the skin have constricted in an effort to redirect more blood to the core of the body. This decrease in blood flow to the skin causes changes in both color and temperature.

30 minutes into the incident—loss of approximately 2,000 cc of blood:

TIME	RESPIRATIONS	PULSE	BP	SKIN	PUPILS	MENTAL
1130	26; shallow; and labored	140; weak; regular	108/74	pale; cool; clammy	dilated, sluggish	A&O restless and confused

The most obvious change in Richard's condition at 30 minutes is his altered mental status. He can be aroused only by verbal stimuli and knows his name but cannot provide any other meaningful details. His pulse has increased significantly in an attempt to maintain blood pressure, and his respirations have increased in response to the tissues demanding more oxygen. The vessels in the skin and extremities have all constricted as far as they can, causing his pale and cool skin signs. His clammy skin is due to the enormous stress his body is under trying to save itself. His blood pressure is falling now and is the reason for weak and/or absent peripheral pulses. The loss of adequate perfusion is also causing his pupils to dilate and respond sluggishly to light. Up until this point, Richard's body has been able to compensate for the loss of blood and poor perfusion.

Eventually, even the mechanisms that are trying to sustain his life will fail, due to poor perfusion.

40 minutes into the incident—loss of approximately 2,500 cc of blood

TIME	RESPIRATIONS	PULSE	BP	SKIN	PUPILS	MENTAL
1140	8; shallow labored	130; weak regular	60/palpation	pale; cool; clammy	dilated, nonrespon- sive	unrespon- sive

After 40 minutes and a blood loss of 2,500 cc, Richard's body has now lost the ability to compensate for the blood loss and all body systems are beginning to fail. His blood pressure is falling rapidly. Soon he will be in cardiac arrest, and the likelihood of survival will be almost nonexistent.

Compensated Versus Decompensated Shock

One of the points in using Richard as an example of how shock progresses is to show you that sometimes the early signs of poor perfusion are there, and you may not see them. They are hidden behind the pain and stress that are so much a part of most trauma calls. Therefore, you must anticipate shock and maintain a high index of suspicion when the mechanism of injury suggests it. While an increased pulse rate is an early sign, a decreasing blood pressure is a late sign. Do *not* wait for signs/symptoms of shock to be obvious to initiate care and transport.

✳ **compensated shock**

when the patient is developing shock but the body is still able to maintain perfusion.

✳ **decompensated shock**

when the body can no longer compensate for low blood volume or lack of perfusion. Late signs, such as decreasing blood pressure, become evident.

Early signs of shock, such as increased pulse and breathing rates and pale skin, are indications that the body is working to compensate for the blood loss. This is known as **compensated shock**. If the blood loss is allowed to continue, the body's own compensatory mechanisms will begin to shut down due to poor perfusion and the patient will enter a state referred to as **decompensated shock**. A major indication that the patient has entered the decompensated shock state is a significant drop in blood pressure. In addition to the drop in BP, the patient will also present with a significant decrease in mental status. During this phase, the pulse will become very weak until it finally goes away and the patient experiences cardiac arrest. (Table 27-3)

TABLE 27-3	COMPENSATED VS. DECOMPENSATED SHOCK	
VITAL SIGN	**COMPENSATED SHOCK**	**DECOMPENSATED SHOCK**
Respirations	Increased rate	Decreasing rate
Pulse	Increasing rate	Becomes weaker
BP	Normal to low systolic Normal to elevated diastolic	Decreasing to absent
Skin	Pale, cool, clammy	Pale, cool, clammy
Pupils	Sluggish but responsive	Sluggish to fixed and dilated
Mental Status	Altered	Unresponsive

PEDIATRIC PATIENTS

Pediatric patients have an excellent ability to compensate for blood loss. Some pediatric patients are capable of maintaining what appears to be a normal blood pressure until nearly half of their blood volume is lost. Once the child's body can no longer compensate, its condition quickly deteriorates and death may be sudden. It is especially important to anticipate shock with pediatric patients and initiate care and transport as soon as possible.

Assessment of the Shock Patient

SCENE SIZE-UP

Once you have taken the appropriate BSI precautions, you must confirm that the scene is safe. Assure that there are no hazards, such as downed power lines, that may pose a threat to you and others. As you approach the scene, begin evaluating the mechanism of injury. Do your best to determine the exact mechanism or mechanisms the patient may have suffered. For instance, if it is a motor vehicle collision, how much damage is there to the outside of the vehicle? How about the inside of the vehicle? Does it appear that the patient was restrained? Did an airbag deploy? Did the vehicle roll over?

If the mechanism was a fall, how far did he fall? What type of surface did he land on? What position was he in when he hit the ground?

Your evaluation of the mechanism of injury does not end when you discover the patient. It must continue on throughout the time you are with the patient, and you must attempt to gather as many details as possible without compromising patient care. Maintain appropriate spinal precautions for all victims of trauma.

INITIAL ASSESSMENT

Confirm that the ABCs are all intact and that breathing is adequate. Just because the patient looks okay does not mean he won't get worse. Monitor the ABCs carefully, and initiate high-flow oxygen by nonrebreather mask as soon as possible.

If you have enough help at the scene, baseline vital signs should be obtained simultaneously with the initial assessment. Be sure to obtain and document a complete set of baseline vitals that can be used for trending later. Be sure to write down the vital signs in a place where you can easily see them. This will help you spot trends that would otherwise be difficult to identify. It is difficult to keep mental notes of specific numbers at an emergency scene. Since this information can be critical to saving a life, it is important to pay attention to the previous sets of vitals each time you take new ones.

FOCUSED HISTORY AND PHYSICAL EXAM

All patients who have sustained a significant mechanism of injury must receive a rapid trauma assessment. This is a quick head-to-toe exam looking for all obvious injuries and points of pain. This can be done in about 90 seconds and is almost always completed while on scene.

Gather as much history from the patient and bystanders as possible as you complete your rapid assessment. You should already be planning transport, and one of the simplest ways to transport these patients is on a long backboard.

5-1.5 Establish the relationship between airway management and the trauma patient.

DETAILED PHYSICAL EXAM

This more detailed examination is usually completed while en route to the hospital. You will only perform this exam if the ABCs are intact and there are no other immediate life threats that need your attention.

5-1.8 List the steps in the emergency medical care of the patient with signs and symptoms of internal bleeding.

5-1.10 State the steps in the emergency medical care of the patient with signs and symptoms of shock (hypoperfusion).

ONGOING ASSESSMENT

Continuously monitor the patient's ABCs and repeat the vital signs at least every 5 minutes if the patient is unstable. Consider increasing the oxygen flow if appropriate and confirm that all external bleeding is controlled.

Perform the following steps when caring for a patient who you suspect may have internal bleeding or who is presenting with the signs and symptoms of shock (Scan 27-1):

1. Conduct an appropriate scene size-up and take the necessary body substance isolation precautions.

2. Manually stabilize the spine as appropriate for the mechanism of injury.

3. Perform an initial assessment and initiate high-flow supplemental oxygen.

4. Control any external bleeding.

5. If signs of shock are present and there are no contraindications, apply the pneumatic anti-shock garment (PASG) if approved by medical direction. Follow local protocols.

6. Elevate the lower extremities approximately 8 to 12 inches. If the patient has serious injuries to the pelvis, lower extremities, head, chest, abdomen, neck, or spine, keep the patient supine.

7. Conserve body heat by covering the patient with a blanket when appropriate.

8. Place the patient on a long board as appropriate for the MOI.

9. Initiate transport and request an ALS intercept if available.

10. Perform ongoing assessments as appropriate and be alert for changing vital signs (trending).

Remember that victims of trauma may have suffered a spinal injury. Evaluate the mechanism of injury and take the appropriate spinal precautions with all victims of trauma. If the patient is unresponsive and spinal injury is suspected, use the jaw-thrust maneuver to open the airway. If you are unable to establish an appropriate airway, perform a head-tilt, chin-lift maneuver.

PNEUMATIC ANTI-SHOCK GARMENT

The pneumatic anti-shock garment (PASG) (Figure 27-4 on page 682) is a pair of inflatable trousers designed to care for patients who have suffered specific types of traumatic injury. Originally developed by the military for the treatment of shock, they were once known as Military Anti-shock Trousers or MAST. While somewhat controversial, the PASG is still used today in some parts of the country. Indications for the use of PASG vary from EMS system to EMS system. Check your local protocols.

SCAN 27-1   MANAGING SHOCK

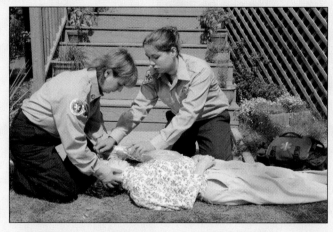

▲ Maintain an open airway, and give high-concentration oxygen by nonrebreather. Control external bleeding. Assist ventilations and perform CPR, if needed.

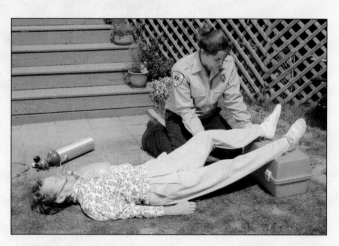

▲ If there is no potential spinal injury, elevate the patient's legs 8 to 12 inches, or . . .

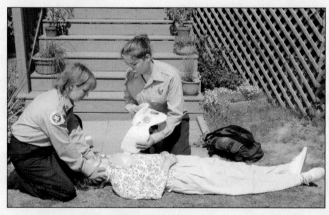

▲ . . . if there is any possibility of spine injury, position the patient with NO elevation of the extremities.

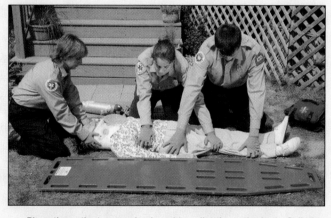

▲ Place the patient on a spine board to splint the entire body. Splinting of individual bone and joint injuries should be done en route.

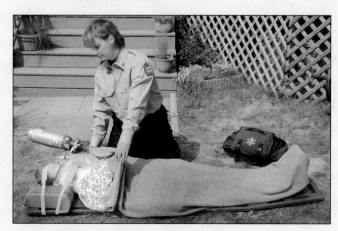

▲ Protect the patient from heat loss.

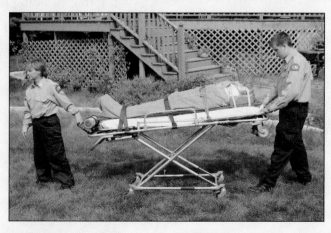

▲ Transport immediately.

FIGURE 27-4 The pneumatic anti-shock garment (PASG).

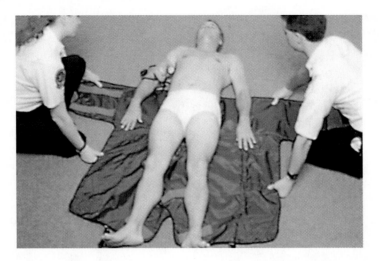

Indications for the PASG may include:

✳ Signs and symptoms of shock due to circulatory collapse from volume loss

✳ Suspected lower extremity fracture(s)

✳ Suspected pelvic fracture(s) with signs of shock

✳ Ruptured abdominal aortic aneurysm (AAA)

In cases of circulatory collapse or volume loss, it has been thought that the garment can be inflated to compress the vessels in the lower extremities and abdomen. This would cause the fluid volume in these areas to be squeezed out and forced into the core of the body where it is needed.

As for the use with suspected extremity and/or pelvic fractures, it is thought that the inflated garment acts as a splint to stabilize these areas. A more stable fracture means less soft tissue damage, less bleeding, and less pain.

The use of PASG and its relative value is controversial, and protocols for its use will vary considerably from system to system. There are a few instances when the use of the PASG is contraindicated. They are as follows:

✳ Cases of known pulmonary edema or increased respiratory difficulty following application

✳ Cardiogenic shock

✳ Internal bleeding of the chest

✳ Impaled objects in the abdomen

✳ Third trimester of pregnancy

✳ Evisceration

✳ May inflate leg sections only if allowed by local protocols

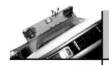

Dispatch Summary

The patient was placed on the stretcher in the Trendelenburg position, covered with a blanket, and placed on 15 lpm of oxygen with a nonrebreather mask. His bleeding was controlled with direct pressure and elevation of the limb. He was then rapidly transported to Farmer's Hospital where he was treated for shock, blood loss, and two 7-centimeter lacerations on his right forearm.

The patient was released several days later and, except for some numbness in two fingers, has recovered fully. He has since returned to work and has joined the factory's emergency response team.

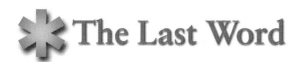

The Last Word

The human body depends on a constant supply of well-oxygenated blood flowing to all tissues. This flow of well-oxygenated blood is known as perfusion. In addition, this flow of blood permits the body to rid itself of the waste products of normal cell metabolism.

When the body senses a decrease in perfusion, it begins to compensate by increasing the pulse rate and decreasing blood flow to less vital areas, such as the skin and extremities. If left untreated, poor perfusion will eventually lead to shock, and the patient will eventually die due to inadequate perfusion to the vital organs.

Early detection based on the mechanism of injury, your patient assessment, and trending of vital signs will lead to early care and rapid transport to an appropriate receiving facility. Many patients with internal bleeding will require surgical intervention to control the bleeding and save their life. Always document all appropriate information in your PCR.

 Chapter Review

MULTIPLE CHOICE

Place a check next to the correct answer.

1. All of the following are signs of shock EXCEPT:

   _____ a. increased pulse rate.

   _____ b. decreasing blood pressure.

   _____ c. pink, warm, moist skin.

   _____ d. altered mental status.

2. The most appropriate method for opening the airway of an unresponsive trauma patient is the _____ method.

   _____ a. jaw-thrust

   _____ b. chin-lift

   _____ c. head-tilt

   _____ d. jaw-tilt

3. Some pediatric patients are capable of maintaining what appears to be a normal blood pressure until _____ of their blood volume is lost.

   _____ a. one-third

   _____ b. nearly half

   _____ c. two-thirds

   _____ d. nearly one-quarter

4. When used for the treatment of suspected pelvic fractures, the PASG helps by:

   _____ a. pushing blood out of the area of the fracture.

   _____ b. redirecting blood back into the area of the fracture.

   _____ c. stabilizing the suspected fracture site.

   _____ d. increasing the patient's heart rate.

5. All of the following are contraindications for the use of the PASG, EXCEPT:

   _____ a. suspected pelvic fracture.

   _____ b. internal bleeding of the chest.

   _____ c. late stage pregnancy.

   _____ d. cardiogenic shock.

6. An adult weighing 70 kg has approximately _____ ml of blood volume.

   _____ a. 2,400

   _____ b. 3,900

   _____ c. 4,200

   _____ d. 4,900

7. Signs of internal bleeding may include all of the following EXCEPT:

   _____ a. rigid abdomen.

   _____ b. the presence of an open wound.

   _____ c. tenderness on palpation.

   _____ d. signs of shock without external bleeding.

8. Shock that results when the heart is damaged and can no longer pump an adequate amount of blood to the body is called _____ shock.

   _____ a. septic

   _____ b. anaphylactic

   _____ c. neurogenic

   _____ d. cardiogenic

9. Which of the following is NOT a sign of hemmorhagic shock?

   _____ a. decreased pulse rate

   _____ b. increased breathing rate

   _____ c. decreased blood pressure

   _____ d. pale, cool, and clammy skin

10. When the body can no longer compensate for the blood loss, the pulse _____ and the blood pressure _____.

    _____ a. increases, increases

    _____ b. decreases, decreases

    _____ c. decreases, increases

    _____ d. increases, decreases

MATCHING

Match the type of shock on the left with the applicable definition on the right.

1. _____ Decompensated shock
2. _____ Cardiogenic shock
3. _____ Anaphylactic shock
4. _____ Hypovolemic shock
5. _____ Neurogenic shock
6. _____ Compensated shock

A. Type of shock caused by an overreaction of the immune system when exposed to an allergen.
B. When the patient is developing shock but the body is still able to maintain perfusion.
C. Type of shock caused when the heart can no longer pump blood adequately, resulting in a decrease in cardiac output and thus a decrease in perfusion.
D. Type of shock caused by a sudden decrease in body fluids (blood or other fluids).
E. Type of shock caused when the vessels dilate abnormally in response to injury to the spinal cord.
F. Occurs when the body can no longer compensate for low blood volume or lack of perfusion. Late signs such as decreasing blood pressure become evident.

CRITICAL THINKING

1. What is the actual cause of death in a patient who is said to have died from shock?

_____

_____

_____

_____

2. Discuss why a low blood pressure is a late sign of shock in a trauma patient.

_____

_____

_____

_____

3. Discuss the difference in the signs and symptoms of internal bleeding and those of shock.

_____

_____

_____

_____

CASE STUDIES

Case Study 1

You have responded to a baseball field for an unknown injury. Upon arrival, you are escorted into one of the dugouts where you find an approximately 35-year-old male. He is dressed in an umpire uniform, and one of the coaches states that he took a direct blow to the chest with a bat as one of the players was warming up. This happened about 45 minutes ago and, after recovering from getting the wind knocked out of him, he decided to go on with the game. At the last break between innings, the man had come into the dugout to rest and get some water when he nearly passed out. He appears a little confused, his skin is pale, cool, and moist, and his pulse is rapid and weak.

1. What are the significant elements of this man's history and current presentation?

   _____

   _____

   _____

   _____

2. How will you care for this patient?

   _____

   _____

   _____

   _____

3. How often will you want to perform ongoing assessments on this patient?

   _____

   _____

   _____

   _____

Case Study 2

You are caring for a 12-year-old boy who was being pulled behind a ski boat on a flotation device and struck something floating in the water. The incident happened just under an hour ago, and the boy is now complaining of increased pain in the left upper and lower quadrants of his abdomen. The only obvious sign of injury is a bright red abrasion down his left side. He is tender to the touch and his vital signs are BP 90/60, pulse 120 weak and regular, respirations 24 with good tidal volume and slightly labored. His skin appears normal and his pupils are PERRL. He has vomited twice in the past 15 minutes prior to your arrival.

1. What are the signs that this boy could be bleeding internally?

   _____

   _____

   _____

   _____

2. Is this patient showing signs of compensated shock or decompensated shock? What made you make this choice?

   _____

   _____

   _____

   _____

3. This boy has pain and abrasions over his left abdomen. What internal structures lie under the skin on the left side of the abdomen that may have been damaged?

   _____

   _____

   _____

   _____

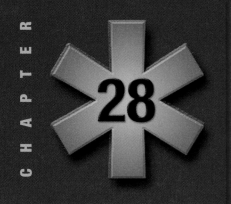

Controlling Bleeding

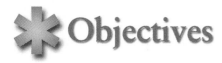 Objectives

Numbered objectives are from the U.S. Department of Transportation 1994 EMT-Basic National Standard Curriculum.

COGNITIVE OBJECTIVES

At the completion of this lesson, the EMT-Basic student will be able to:

5-1.1 List the structure and function of the circulatory system. (pp. 690–691)

5-1.2 Differentiate between arterial, venous, and capillary bleeding. (pp. 698–699)

5-1.3 State methods of emergency medical care of external bleeding. (pp. 699–705)

5-1.4 Establish the relationship between body substance isolation and bleeding. (pp. 703–705)

5-1.5 Establish the relationship between airway management and the trauma patient. (p. 705)

5-1.9 List signs and symptoms of shock (hypoperfusion). (p. 712)

5-1.10 State the steps in the emergency medical care of the patient with signs and symptoms of shock (hypoperfusion). (p. 712)

AFFECTIVE OBJECTIVES

At the completion of this lesson, the EMT-Basic student will be able to:

5-1.11 Explain the sense of urgency to transport patients that are bleeding and show signs of shock (hypoperfusion). (pp. 705, 712)

PSYCHOMOTOR OBJECTIVES

At the completion of this lesson, the EMT-Basic student will be able to:

5-1.12 Demonstrate direct pressure as a method of emergency medical care of external bleeding. (pp. 699–700)

5-1.13 Demonstrate the use of diffuse pressure as a method of emergency medical care of external bleeding. (p. 705)

5-1.14 Demonstrate the use of pressure points and tourniquets as a method of emergency medical care of external bleeding. (pp. 700–705)

5-1.17 Demonstrate completing a prehospital care report for patient with bleeding and/or shock (hypoperfusion). (p. 713)

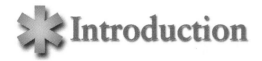 **Introduction**

Bleeding control is one of the most basic of skills that must be mastered by all EMTs. While we all have experience managing minor cuts and scrapes, as an EMT you will encounter major wounds with severe bleeding. You must be able to distinguish between minor and severe bleeding and provide the appropriate care as quickly as possible. Uncontrolled bleeding will lead to shock and even death if not eventually stopped. In this chapter we will review the importance of good perfusion and how to identify and care for all types of external bleeding (Figure 28-1). We will also review the signs and symptoms of shock.

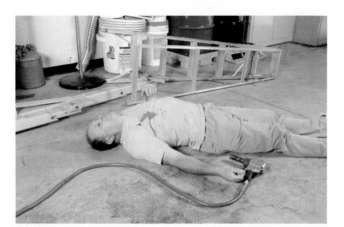

FIGURE 28-1   Bleeding from a traumatic injury.

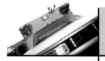 **Emergency Dispatch**

"Ouch! Son of a gun!" EMT Olin Barger pulled his arm from the rear compartment of the ambulance and took a stumbling step backward. Blood poured down the front of his uniform and began pooling on the concrete floor of the ambulance bay.

"What the heck happened, Olie?" His partner, Ken, left the equipment that he had been inventorying and hurried over.

"I don't know." Olin held his forearm tightly with a blood-slick hand. "That backboard was stuck on something . . . and it wouldn't go in . . . so I just shoved it . . ."

"Let me see your arm." Ken grabbed a jump bag from a nearby cot and fished out a handful of gauze packages while donning a pair of exam gloves.

Olin turned his arm toward the other EMT and slowly released his grip. A 15-centimeter laceration, extending from Olin's wrist to mid-forearm, burst open and blood jetted into the air.

"Oh, geez!" Ken quickly covered the wound with wads of gauze and yelled toward the other side of the ambulance bay. "Mark! Mark, get out here, quick! I need you to drive!"

"Oh, wow!" The color began fading from Olin's face. "I don't feel so hot."

5-1.1 List the structure and function of the circulatory system.

Review of the Circulatory System

Before continuing on with this chapter, it will be helpful to review some of the basic anatomy and physiology of the circulatory system (Figure 28-2). Also known as the cardiovascular system, the circulatory system has three components: the heart, the blood, and the vessels that carry the blood throughout the body. Certain illnesses as well as injuries can affect one or all of these vital components, thereby reducing the effectiveness of the circulatory system.

PERFUSION

Review chapter 27 and the information on perfusion and hypoperfusion (shock). Again, perfusion is the flow of well-oxygenated blood throughout the entire body, including the vital organs and other tissues. When the circulatory system is functioning properly, a patient is said to be perfusing well.

FIGURE 28-2 Circulation of blood through the cardiovascular system.

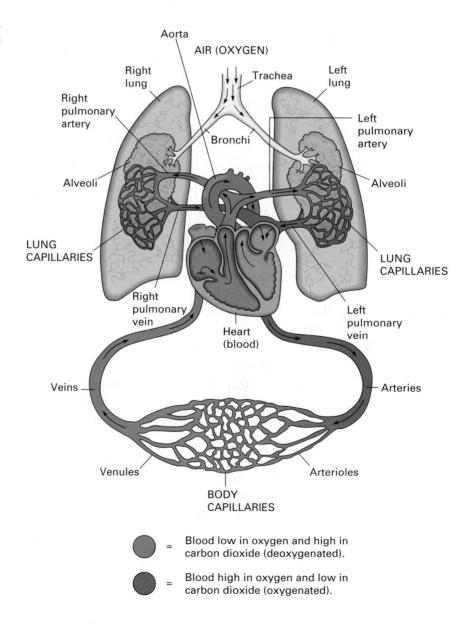

Signs of adequate perfusion include:

＊ Normal skin signs

＊ Normal mental status

＊ Normal vital signs

When a person is not perfusing well, it is frequently but not always due to a malfunction of one or more of the components of the circulatory system. Signs and symptoms of inadequate perfusion include:

＊ Abnormal skin signs (pale color, cool temperature)

＊ Altered mental status (sluggishness, confusion, or decreased responsiveness)

＊ Abnormal vital signs (increased pulse and respiratory rate, decreased blood pressure)

A properly functioning circulatory system, including an adequate blood pressure, is essential for good perfusion.

THE HEART

Be sure to review chapter 4 to refresh your knowledge of circulatory anatomy. The heart is the pump in the system and is responsible for the continuous flow of blood throughout the body. The heart is made up of four interconnected chambers; the top two chambers are the atria and the bottom two are the ventricles. Deoxygenated blood (blood with little or no oxygen) enters the heart at the right atrium and then flows down into the right ventricle. The right ventricle then pumps the blood into the pulmonary arteries for transport to the lungs where it can pick up oxygen. Upon leaving the lungs via the pulmonary veins, the blood reenters the heart at the left atrium, then flows down into the left ventricle. The left ventricle is the largest chamber of the heart because it must then pump blood out to the entire body. Blood leaves the left ventricle, entering the aorta for transport to the body.

THE BLOOD VESSELS

The blood vessels are the "plumbing" or "hoses" of the circulatory system (Figure 28-3 on page 692). They are often described by their function, location, and whether they carry blood to or from the heart. All vessels that carry blood away from the heart are called arteries while vessels that carry blood to the heart are called veins.

Arteries most often begin as larger vessels, branch into smaller ones, and eventually terminate in tiny vessels called arterioles. Conversely, veins begin as tiny venules and eventually merge into large vessels before entering the heart. The tiny vessels that connect arterioles and venules and where oxygen and nutrients are exchanged for waste products from the body's cells are called capillaries.

Following is a list of just some of the major vessels of the body, along with their location and function:

＊ **Aorta**—The largest artery in the body, it is attached directly to the left ventricle. It is responsible for carrying oxygenated blood directly from the heart to the major areas of the body.

＊ **aorta**

the largest artery in the body. It transports blood from the left ventricle to begin systemic circulation.

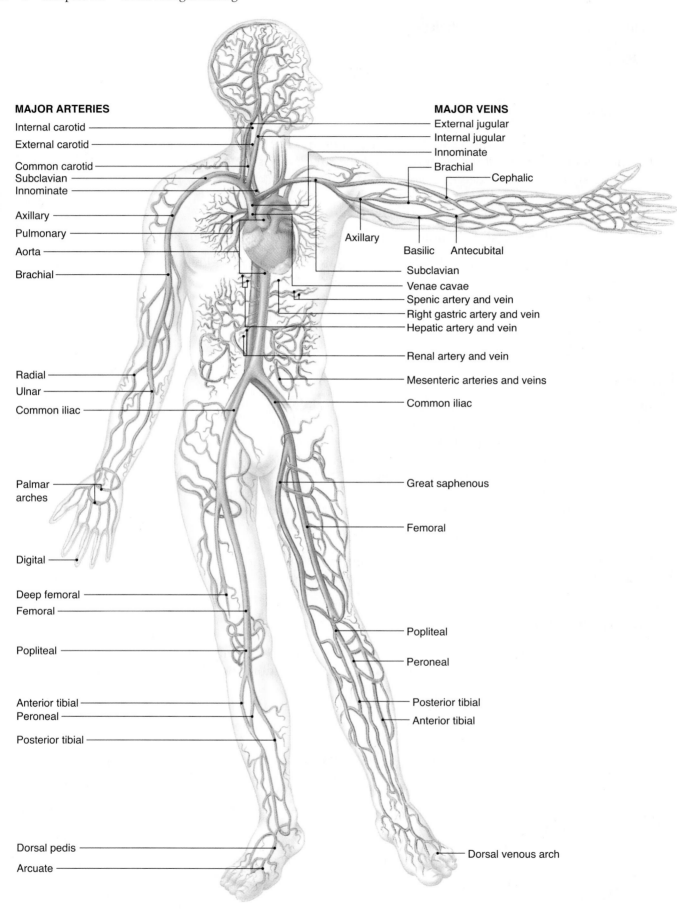

MAJOR ARTERIES

Internal carotid

External carotid

Common carotid
Subclavian
Innominate

Axillary

Pulmonary

Aorta

Brachial

Radial

Ulnar

Common iliac

Palmar
arches

Digital

Deep femoral
Femoral

Popliteal

Anterior tibial
Peroneal

Posterior tibial

Dorsal pedis

Arcuate

MAJOR VEINS

External jugular
Internal jugular
Innominate
Brachial
Cephalic

Axillary

Basilic   Antecubital

Subclavian
Venae cavae
Spenic artery and vein
Right gastric artery and vein
Hepatic artery and vein

Renal artery and vein

Mesenteric arteries and veins

Common iliac

Great saphenous

Femoral

Popliteal

Peroneal

Posterior tibial

Anterior tibial

Dorsal venous arch

FIGURE 28-3 Major arteries and veins.

✱ **Venae cavae**—Either of two major veins that carry oxygen-poor blood from the body to the right atrium. The superior vena cava carries blood from the head; the inferior vena cava carries blood from the lower body. Plural *venae cavae*.

✱ **Coronary arteries**—The small arteries that carry oxygenated blood to the heart muscle itself. A disruption in flow through these arteries can cause chest pain and damage to the heart muscle.

✱ **Pulmonary artery**—Artery that carries oxygen-poor blood from the heart to the lungs.

✱ **Pulmonary vein**—Vein that carries oxygen-rich blood from the lungs to the heart.

✱ **Carotid artery**—The major artery of the neck, a primary supplier of blood to the head. It is palpated to check for a pulse in patients who are unresponsive.

✱ **Brachial artery**—Artery of the upper arm that is palpated to obtain a pulse in infants as well as a pressure point to control bleeding from the arm in all age groups. This is the artery found near the elbow that you listen to when obtaining a blood pressure.

✱ **Radial artery**—Artery that supplies blood to the lower arm. It is palpated on the lateral aspect of the anterior wrist.

✱ **Femoral artery**—A major supplier of blood to the leg. This pulse is palpated near the crease formed by the abdomen, leg, and groin.

THE FUNCTION OF THE BLOOD

Again, please review chapter 4 where this information was initially covered. Blood serves many essential functions as it is carried by the circulatory system and flows throughout the body. Its most fundamental duty is to carry oxygen and nutrients to the cells and to carry away waste products generated by cellular metabolism.

Blood is made up of several components, each with a specialized function or functions. The major components of blood are as follows:

✱ **Plasma**—This is the clear, yellowish fluid portion in which the other components of blood are suspended.

✱ **Red blood cells**—These are disk-shaped cells responsible for transporting oxygen and carbon dioxide to and from the tissues.

✱ **White blood cells**—Any of the colorless or white cells in the blood that help protect the body from infection and disease.

✱ **Platelets**—Irregularly shaped cell fragments that are responsible for promoting blood clotting.

In addition to these very important functions that it provides, blood also must be present in a sufficient quantity to sustain life. There is a direct connection between the volume of blood within the circulatory system, blood pressure, and perfusion. When a patient loses blood from within the circulatory system, blood pressure will eventually fall and perfusion will become inadequate to sustain life.

✱ **venae cavae**

the superior vena cava and the inferior vena cava. These two major veins return blood from the body to the right atrium. (Plural *venae cavae*, singular *vena cava*).

✱ **coronary arteries**

arteries that branch off the aorta and provide blood supply directly to the heart.

✱ **pulmonary artery**

vessel carrying blood from the right ventricle to the lungs.

✱ **pulmonary vein**

vessel carrying blood from the lungs to the left atrium.

✱ **carotid artery**

the large neck artery, one on each side of the neck, that carry blood from the heart to the head.

✱ **brachial artery**

the major artery of the upper arm.

✱ **radial artery**

artery of the lower arm. It is felt when taking the pulse at the wrist.

✱ **femoral artery**

artery located in the anterior groin area, these arteries supply blood to the lower extremities.

✱ **plasma**

the fluid portion of the blood.

✱ **red blood cells**

specialized blood cells containing hemoglobin.

✱ **white blood cells**

specialized blood cells that produce substances that help the body fight infection.

✱ **platelets**

components of the blood; membrane-enclosed fragments of specialized cells.

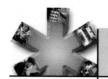

Perspective

Ken—The EMT

"We were getting ready to start our shift and Olie had to put in a new long backboard. Honestly, the crew that had the rig last should've done it. It goes that way sometimes, I guess. But let me tell you, I haven't seen lacerations that bad very often. In that moment before I got it covered with gauze, I could see muscle and tendons, and there was obviously an artery damaged in there somewhere. Man, oh, man. We just couldn't get that bleeding to stop completely. I tried pressure on the cut, a trauma dressing, elevation—even brachial pressure. And then there was shock. I've never run a gnarly trauma call before my shift even started!"

BLOOD LOSS

Whether it's the mechanic who is forever scraping a knuckle, the 5-year-old girl who skins her knee learning to roller skate, or the shipping clerk who cuts his hand opening some boxes, bleeding and blood loss are common. The vast majority of instances are not life threatening.

For example, the average blood loss from a woman's menstrual cycle is 40 to 60 cc (only 8 to 12 teaspoonfuls). Some women can lose up to 400 cc (500 cc is about a pint) and not become symptomatic. People all across the world donate a pint of blood each day and are allowed to drive home shortly after.

Most bleeding occurs to the outside of the body (external) and in most cases is easily controlled with simple first-aid measures. In other instances, bleeding can occur deep within the body (internal) and go unnoticed by the patient or those around them. This type of bleeding has the most potential to be life threatening because it is difficult to detect and difficult to care for in the field. You may hear the term **bleeding out** used in describing a trauma patient. This simply means that the patient is losing a significant amount of blood from within the circulatory system and is not specific to internal or external blood loss.

∗ **bleeding out**

term meaning the patient is losing blood from within the circulatory system and is not specific to internal or external blood loss.

SEVERITY

Blood loss becomes dangerous when it is sudden and rapid and large enough volumes are involved (Figure 28-4). Blood loss becomes even more dangerous when it is complicated by other medical or traumatic problems, such as respiratory compromise or organ damage. Factors that can determine the severity of blood loss are time and quantity.

The sudden loss of the following quantities of blood can be life threatening to their respective age groups:

∗ One liter (1,000 cc) of blood in the adult patient

∗ 1/2 liter (500 cc) of blood in the child (1 to 8 years)

∗ 100–200 cc of blood in an infant (less than 1 year)

THE FOUR STAGES OF HEMORRHAGE

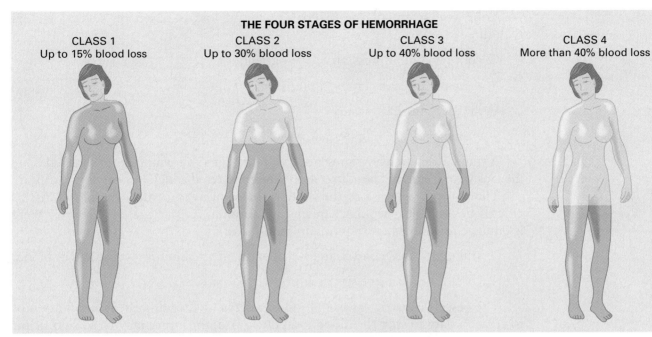

CLASS 1	CLASS 2	CLASS 3	CLASS 4
Up to 15% blood loss	Up to 30% blood loss	Up to 40% blood loss	More than 40% blood loss

HOW THE BODY RESPONDS

The body compensates for blood loss by constricting blood vessels (vasoconstriction) in an effort to maintain blood pressure and delivery of oxygen to all organs of the body.

EFFECT ON PATIENT

• Patient remains alert.
• Blood pressure stays within normal limits.
• Pulse stays within normal limits or increases slightly; pulse quality remains strong.
• Respiratory rate and depth, skin color, and temperature all remain normal.

*The average adult has 5 liters (1 liter = approximately 1 quart) of circulating blood; 15% is 750 ml (or about 3 cups). With internal bleeding 750 ml will occupy enough space in a limb to cause swelling and pain. With bleeding into the body cavities, however, the blood will spread throughout the cavity, causing little, if any initial discomfort.

• Vasoconstriction continues to maintain adequate blood pressure, but with some difficulty now.
• Blood flow is shunted to vital organs, with decreased flow to intestines, kidneys, and skin.

EFFECT ON PATIENT

• Patient may become confused and restless.
• Skin turns pale, cool, and dry because of shunting of blood to vital organs.
• Diastolic pressure may rise or fall. It's more likely to rise (because of vasoconstriction) or stay the same in otherwise healthy patients with no underlying cardio-vascular problems.
• Pulse pressure (difference between systolic and diastolic pressures) narrows.
• Sympathetic responses also cause rapid heart rate (over 100 beats per minute). Pulse quality weakens.
• Respiratory rate increases because of sympathetic stimulation.
• Delayed capillary refill.

• Compensatory mechanisms become overtaxed. Vaso-constriction, for example, can no longer sustain blood pressure, which now begins to fall.
• Cardiac output and tissue perfusion continue to decrease, becoming potentially life-threatening. (Even at this stage, however, the patient can still recover with prompt treatment.)

EFFECT ON PATIENT

• Patient becomes more confused, restless, and anxious.
• Classic signs of shock appear—rapid heart rate, decreased blood pressure, rapid respiration and cool, clammy extremities.

• Compensatory vasoconstriction now becomes a complicating factor in itself, further impairing tissue perfusion and cellular oxygenation.

EFFECT ON PATIENT

• Patient becomes lethargic, drowsy, or stuporous.
• Signs of shock become more pronounced. Blood pressure continues to fall.
• Lack of blood flow to the brain and other vital organs ultimately leads to organ failure and death.

FIGURE 28-4   The patient's signs and symptoms may indicate the severity of blood loss.

Your assessment of the severity of blood loss is based on several factors including:

✳ your general impression of the patient

✳ the patient's signs and symptoms

✳ the mechanism of injury

✳ visible evidence of external blood

A trauma patient who is presenting with the signs and symptoms of shock, despite the lack of any external bleeding, should be considered a high priority for transport.

The natural response of the body to bleeding is to control the blood loss as quickly as possible. Two mechanisms are automatically triggered whenever there is damage to soft tissues resulting in blood loss:

1. Injured vessels constrict (get smaller) in an attempt to slow the loss of blood.

2. A clot forms at the site of injury.

The vessels constrict as the blood binds together and hardens in an attempt to create a dam to stop the blood loss. Of course, the injury may be so significant that these mechanisms are not adequate to control the blood loss. In these instances, the EMT will have to provide specific care to help control the bleeding. These care steps will be discussed later in this chapter. The bottom line is this: Uncontrolled bleeding, no matter how slow, can eventually lead to shock and death.

 Stop, Review, Remember!

Multiple Choice

Place a check next to the correct answer.

1. The largest artery of the body is the:

_____ a. vena cava.

_____ b. aorta.

_____ c. pulmonary artery.

_____ d. femoral artery.

2. _____ are/is responsible for transporting oxygen within the blood.

_____ a. Red blood cells

_____ b. White blood cells

_____ c. Plasma

_____ d. Platelets

3. Which chamber of the heart is responsible for pumping blood to the body?

_____ a. left atrium

_____ b. right atrium

_____ c. left ventricle

_____ d. right ventricle

4. All of the following are factors that will help your assessment of the severity of blood loss EXCEPT:

_____ a. your general impression of the patient.

_____ b. the patient's signs and symptoms.

_____ c. the mechanism of injury.

_____ d. the age of the patient.

5. The sudden loss of _____ cc of blood in a
   child between 1 and 8 years of age is
   considered significant.

   _____ a. 250   _____ c. 500

   _____ b. 300   _____ d. 1,000

Fill in the Blank

1. _____ is the flow of well-oxygenated blood throughout the entire body, including the vital
   organs and other tissues.

2. Signs of good perfusion include normal skin signs, mental status, and _____.

3. A patient who is in shock will have skin that is pale, cool, and _____.

4. The _____ is the largest chamber of the heart and pumps blood out to the entire body.

5. Bleeding that is _____ has the most potential to be life threatening because it is difficult to
   detect and difficult to care for in the field.

Critical Thinking

1. Discuss the relationship between perfusion and blood pressure.

   _____

   _____

   _____

2. Describe how a patient might present who is not perfusing well.

   _____

   _____

   _____

3. Discuss why it might be important to be able to estimate blood loss with a patient who is bleeding
   externally.

   _____

   _____

   _____

5-1.2 Differentiate between
       arterial, venous, and
       capillary bleeding.

External Bleeding

Bleeding that occurs through an opening in the body such as a puncture or laceration is referred to as external bleeding. The amount of blood loss can vary significantly, depending on the mechanism of injury, and range anywhere from very minor (a scrape) to severe and difficult to control. Bleeding is further classified by the types of vessels that are involved. The larger the vessel the greater the chance that there will be significant blood loss and the greater the likelihood that the bleeding will be difficult to control. Review chapter 4 and page 692 for detailed information on arteries, veins, and capillaries. Certain areas of the body tend to bleed more because of their rich blood supply. For example, even a small laceration to the face or scalp can produce heavy external bleeding.

All three types of vessels—arteries, veins, and capillaries—can be damaged and cause bleeding from an open wound. While each may have its own characteristics when damaged, it is often difficult and unnecessary to distinguish between them. In the case of a large wound, you are likely to encounter damage to all three types of vessels.

BLEEDING FROM ARTERIES

Arteries are the vessels that carry blood from the heart and to the tissues and organs of the body. They are under higher pressure than other vessels and for that reason can allow for the loss of a large quantity of blood in a relatively short amount of time. Blood from arteries is generally bright red, due to higher oxygen content, and often can be seen spurting from an open wound with each beat of the heart. Because of the pressure inside arteries, arterial bleeding can be difficult to control. You will not always see arterial blood spurting from a wound, because as a patient loses blood, his blood pressure decreases and so will the amount and intensity of spurting from an injured artery.

BLEEDING FROM VEINS

Veins are the vessels that carry blood back to the heart. Venous flow is under much less pressure than arterial flow and, for this reason, does not spurt from the wound

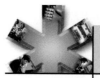

Perspective

Olin—The Patient

"I'm still not sure exactly how or on what I cut myself. I was trying to get that backboard in the slot, and it kept getting hung up on something. I just got mad, I guess, and jammed it in. I remember that it felt like I got punched in the forearm, like a dull pain, you know? It wasn't until I pulled my arm out of the compartment that I saw how bad it really was. You know what's kind of goofy though? The first thought that went through my mind when I saw this huge gash on my forearm was that people would think that I tried to commit suicide. Isn't it odd what goes through our heads during those times? Of course, then I passed out."

Clinical Clues: BODY SUBSTANCE ISOLATION

Always use appropriate barrier devices such as disposable gloves and eye protection while controlling bleeding. If you were to have a small cut or puncture on your hand, the patient's blood could enter your body through this opening in the skin.

but instead flows steadily. The steady, flowing blood from veins may appear darker in color than arterial blood. While it is possible to die from external venous blood loss, it is less likely because the lower pressures make it easier to control than arterial bleeding.

BLEEDING FROM CAPILLARIES

Capillaries are the tiny vessels that connect arterioles and venules. The most common causes of capillary bleeding are scrapes, abrasions, or the classic skinned-knee injury. Capillary bleeding will almost always stop spontaneously and is never life threatening.

Controlling Bleeding

If there is any one skill that has withstood the test of time, it is the skill of bleeding control. The same three progressive steps have been used for decades to control bleeding and save lives. Those steps are:

1. Direct pressure

2. Elevation

3. Pressure points

It is important to understand that these three steps represent a progressive approach to bleeding control. In other words, you do not stop one to begin another. You must begin with direct pressure, continue to hold pressure while elevating the injured limb and then apply a pressure point while maintaining the first two.

DIRECT PRESSURE

Depending on the size of the wound, **direct pressure** can be applied by the EMT using the fingers, palm, or entire surface of one hand (Figures 28-5A and B on page 700). Larger wounds require a larger surface area of pressure and usually more pressure as well. If dressing material is not immediately available, use your gloved hand to initiate direct pressure. As soon as practical, place a sterile or clean dressing between your hand and the wound. For larger wounds, you may have to use several dressings to help absorb the blood while you attempt to control the bleeding.

ELEVATION

Elevation is generally reserved for injuries to the arms and legs (Figures 28-6A and B on page 700). It is thought that elevating the injury site above the level of the

5-1.3 State methods of emergency medical care of external bleeding.

✳ **direct pressure**

pressure applied using the fingers, palm, or entire surface of one hand to help control bleeding.

✳ **elevation**

elevating the injury site above the level of the patient's heart to reduce the amount of pressure at the site and make it easier for bleeding to be controlled.

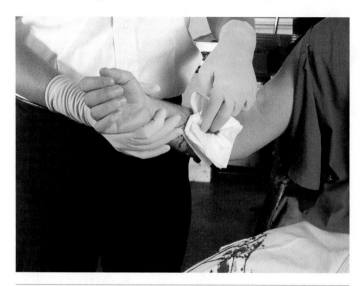

FIGURE 28-5A Apply gloved fingertip pressure over a dressing directly on the point of bleeding.

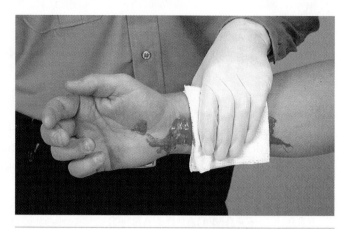

FIGURE 28-5B Apply direct pressure to a bleeding wound with a gauze pad.

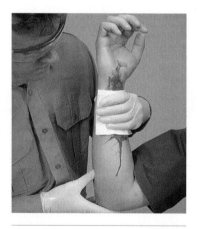

FIGURE 28-6A Elevate a bleeding arm above the level of the heart.

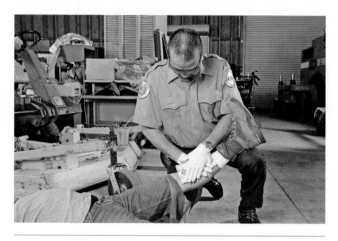

FIGURE 28-6B Elevate a bleeding leg above the level of the heart.

✳ **pressure points**

locations on or near each limb where the major artery supplying the limb lies over a bone. Pressure applied to these points can slow blood flow at the injury site and help facilitate the formation of a clot which will stop the bleeding.

patient's heart will reduce the amount of pressure at the site and therefore make it easier for the bleeding to be controlled. The combination of direct pressure and elevation can control most of the bleeding you might see in the field. Of course elevation should be used only if it can be performed without causing more harm to the patient. For instance, elevation would not be indicated for a wound to the forearm that is associated with a suspected fracture. Elevating an arm that may be fractured will cause severe pain and likely increase the bleeding from the surrounding soft tissues. In most cases, placing the patient in a supine position will make it easier to elevate an injured extremity.

PRESSURE POINTS

There are four main **pressure points** used for the control of severe bleeding from an extremity (Figure 28-7). Pressure points are locations on or near each limb where the major artery supplying the limb lies over a bone. By applying firm pres-

FIGURE 28-7   Location of brachial and femoral pressure points.

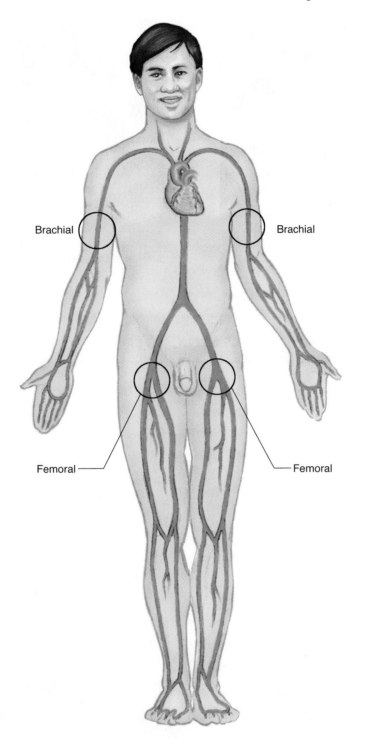

Brachial   Brachial

Femoral   Femoral

sure to these points the EMT can slow the blood flow at the injury site and help facilitate the formation of a clot which will stop the bleeding (Figures 28-8A and B on page 702).

Pressure points are used in conjunction with direct pressure and elevation and must be held long enough for the bleeding to be controlled. It may be necessary to use the assistance of another rescuer, since performing all three steps can be difficult for a single rescuer. It is important to maintain a steady pressure for as long as necessary to control the bleeding. You may have to switch hands or use both hands to maintain a steady pressure.

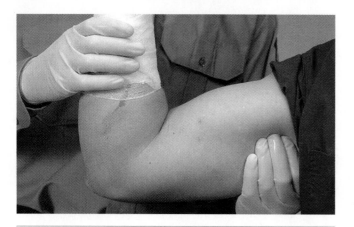

FIGURE 28-8A   If a wound to the arm continues to bleed despite direct pressure and elevation, apply pressure to the brachial artery.

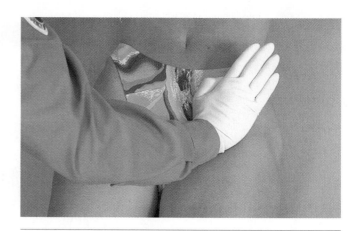

FIGURE 28-8B   If a wound to the leg continues to bleed despite direct pressure and elevation, apply pressure to the femoral artery.

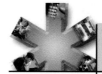

Perspective

Dr. Sanjay—The Emergency Department Surgeon

"Mr. Barger is a very, very fortunate man to have survived. He managed to dissect the artery in a lengthwise manner, preventing it from sealing itself. A severed artery normally has the ability to do that. But, of course, being next to a staffed ambulance when you injure yourself is probably not a bad idea."

✳ **pressure bandage**

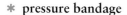

bandage that applies pressure to control bleeding from a wound to an extremity that is still actively bleeding. Also called a pressure dressing.

PRESSURE BANDAGE

A **pressure bandage** is used to help control bleeding from a wound on an extremity. It is comprised of either cravats or roller gauze that is wrapped tightly around a wound, securing a dressing in place (Figures 28-9A and B). The placement of a pressure bandage allows the EMT to use his hands for other important tasks, such

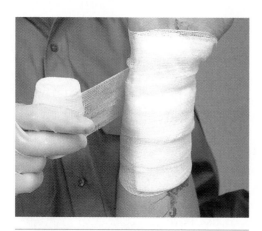

FIGURE 28-9A   Applying a pressure bandage using roller gauge.

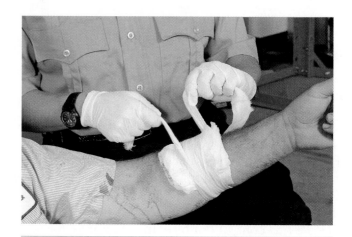

FIGURE 28-9B   Applying a pressure bandage using a cravat.

as elevating the limb or applying a pressure point. Care must be taken not to secure the bandage too tightly and cut off all circulation to the extremity. The objective of the pressure bandage is to slow the flow of blood enough to allow for the formation of a clot at the site of the injury. It is NOT designed to cut off all circulation, as with a tourniquet.

The following steps should be taken as needed to control external bleeding (Scan 28-1):

5-1.4 Establish the relationship between body substance isolation and bleeding.

1. Apply direct pressure with gauze.

2. Maintain direct pressure with elevation.

3. Apply additional dressings.

4. Apply a pressure bandage.

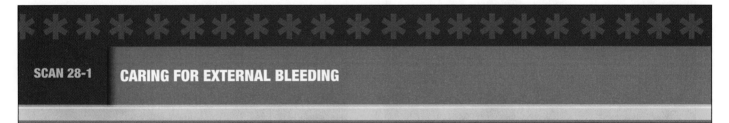

SCAN 28-1   **CARING FOR EXTERNAL BLEEDING**

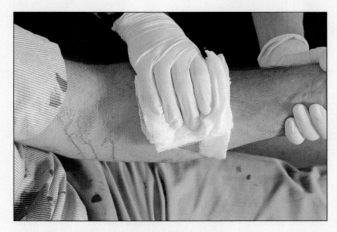

▲ Apply direct pressure with gauze.

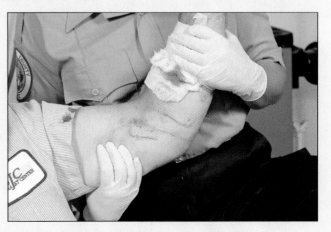

▲ Elevate the extremity and apply direct pressure with gauze.

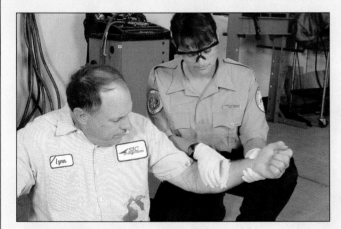

▲ Apply additional dressings.

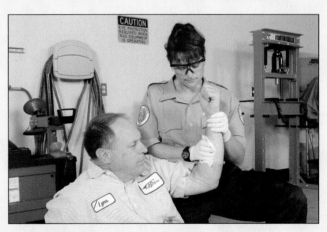

▲ Attempt to control bleeding using pressure points.

(continued on the next page)

CARING FOR EXTERNAL BLEEDING —*(continued)*

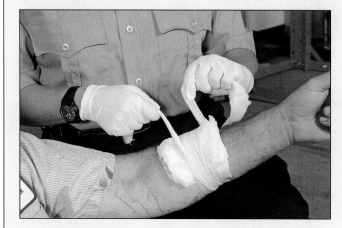

▲ Apply a pressure bandage.

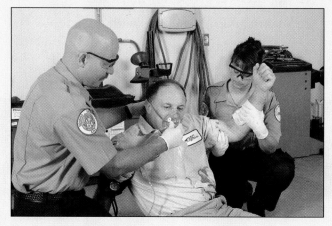

▲ Apply oxygen.

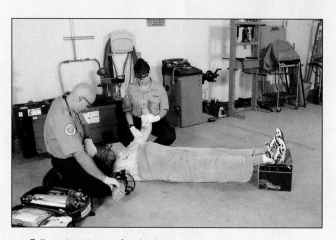

▲ Follow steps to care for shock.

5. Apply firm pressure to a pressure point.

6. Apply oxygen.

7. Care for shock, having the patient lie down with legs elevated and a blanket if appropriate.

Perform the following overall steps when caring for a patient with external bleeding:

1. Take the appropriate BSI precautions and perform a scene size-up.

2. Perform an initial assessment.

3. Attempt to control bleeding using direct pressure, elevation, and pressure points as needed.

4. Initiate oxygen therapy.

5. Perform a rapid or focused trauma assessment as appropriate.

6. Immobilize the injured extremity as appropriate.

7. Initiate transport.

8. Perform ongoing assessments.

9. Watch for signs and symptoms of shock and expedite transport if necessary.

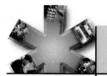

Perspective

Mark—The EMT

"So there I am having a cup of coffee and watching the weather on TV, and all of a sudden Ken's yelling at me from the garage. You gotta understand how suspicious that made me. Last time somebody did that, it was a fellow EMT named Jerry, and when I ran out of the break room, he hit me with a rubber glove completely filled with normal saline. Oh yeah, funny. That was a hoot. But once I saw all the blood and the look on Olie's face, I knew this was a serious situation."

WOUNDS TO THE HEAD AND TORSO

For injuries to the head, neck, and torso you will have to resort to direct pressure or **diffuse pressure** as the primary means of controlling bleeding. The key is to be patient and carefully monitor the flow of blood from the wound. In cases of severe bleeding that cannot be controlled with direct pressure, you may have to expose the wound and use fingertip pressure directly on the bleeding vessel. This should only be attempted if all other attempts to control bleeding have failed. We will discuss more about caring for specific types of wounds in Chapter 29.

Remember that a victim of trauma may have suffered a spinal injury. Evaluate the mechanism of injury and take the appropriate spinal precautions with all victims of trauma. If the patient is unresponsive and spinal injury is suspected, use the jaw-thrust maneuver to open the airway.

> ✳ **diffuse pressure**
> pressure applied over a large area to prevent damage or furthering injuries such as fractures.
>
> **5-1.5** Establish the relationship between airway management and the trauma patient.

Clinical Clues: HEMOSTATIC DRESSINGS

A new classification of dressing now available is called a hemostatic dressing. These are dressings containing agents that promote more rapid and aggressive clotting of the blood and thus better control of the bleeding. Research and field trials will determine the ultimate usefulness of these dressings in prehospital care.

Stop, Review, Remember!

Multiple Choice

Place a check next to the correct answer.

1. The vessel most likely to cause severe bleeding if compromised is an:

   _____ a. artery.

   _____ b. vein.

   _____ c. capillary.

   _____ d. arteriole.

2. Bleeding from arteries is often seen as:

   _____ a. bright red and flowing.

   _____ b. dark red and flowing.

   _____ c. bright red and spurting.

   _____ d. dark red and spurting.

3. Isolated bleeding from capillaries is most often caused by:

   _____ a. lacerations.

   _____ b. abrasions.

   _____ c. contusions.

   _____ d. avulsions.

4. The correct order of the three steps used to control bleeding is:

   _____ a. direct pressure, pressure point, elevation.

   _____ b. pressure point, direct pressure, elevation.

   _____ c. elevation, direct pressure, pressure point.

   _____ d. direct pressure, elevation, pressure point.

5. Wounds to the head and torso are best controlled using which method?

   _____ a. tourniquet

   _____ b. elevation

   _____ c. direct pressure

   _____ d. pressure point

Fill in the Blank

1. _____ are under higher pressure than other vessels and, for that reason, can allow for the loss of a large quantity of blood in a relatively short amount of time.

2. Arterioles and venules are connected by tiny vessels called _____.

3. Bleeding from veins is often steady and flowing and appears _____ in color.

4. It is thought that _____ the injury site above the level of the patient's heart will reduce the amount of pressure at the site and therefore make it easier for the bleeding to be controlled.

5. Pressure points are locations on or near each limb where the major artery supplying the limb lies over a _____.

Critical Thinking

1. Explain why bleeding from arteries is often more difficult to control than bleeding from veins and/or capillaries.

_____

_____

_____

_____

2. Describe how the use of a pressure point helps in controlling bleeding.

_____

_____

_____

_____

3. Explain the dangers of securing a pressure bandage too tightly around an extremity in an attempt to control severe bleeding.

_____

_____

_____

_____

Immobilization

Splints can be helpful in the management of certain wounds, especially if there is a possibility of an underlying fracture (Figure 28-10A on page 708). It may be necessary to straighten an angulated extremity injury in order to immobilize it properly. While it may cause more pain initially, straightening an angulated long bone fracture will make it easier to immobilize and therefore reduce pain and soft tissue damage during transport. If the injury involves a joint and the patient is unable to move the limb, do not attempt to straighten it. Doing so may cause further damage to the joint. In this case, you must get creative and do your best to immobilize the injury in the position you found it.

Air splints (Figure 28-10B on page 708) may help control bleeding because they can maintain a constant pressure when applied properly. Monitor the wound carefully, as it may be difficult to determine if bleeding has stopped with the air splint in place.

The majority of fatalities from pelvic fractures are associated with internal bleeding. Early recognition of a suspected pelvic fracture and appropriate stabilization will help to minimize blood loss from these injuries. While the PASG can be used to help stabilize suspected pelvic fractures, specialized devices such as the

* **air splints**

inflatable splint that can be used to hold a dressing in place on an extremity and control bleeding.

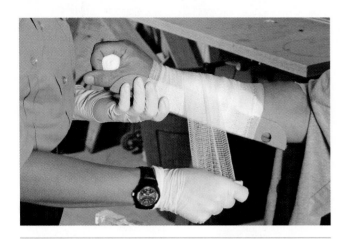

FIGURE 28-10A   Hand and arm that has been bandaged and splinted with cardboard.

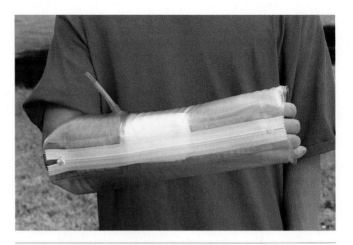

FIGURE 28-10B   An arm injury that has been bandaged and splinted with an air splint.

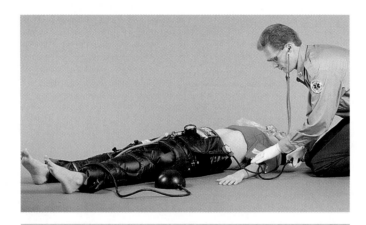

FIGURE 28-11   A pneumatic antishock garment (PASG) can be used to control severe bleeding in the lower extremities, with approval from medical direction.

Traumatic Pelvic Orthopedic Device (TPOD) have been developed specifically for this purpose (Figure 28-11). Once in place, the TPOD maintains circumferential stabilization of the pelvis, reducing pain and minimizing internal blood loss. Check your local protocols regarding recommended devices.

TOURNIQUETS

* **tourniquets**

   method designed to stop all blood flow past the point at which it is applied.

The use of **tourniquets** has long been suggested as a last-resort measure to control severe bleeding from an extremity. While they have a reputation as being dangerous and difficult to apply, this could not be further from the truth. A properly applied tourniquet can be very helpful in controlling severe bleeding from an open extremity wound and will not cause an automatic loss of the limb past the point of application.

   A properly applied tourniquet is designed to stop all blood flow past the point at which it is applied. Follow these steps when applying a tourniquet (Figure 28-12A).

1. Have your partner maintain direct pressure and elevation while you prepare for the application of the tourniquet.

2. Fold a triangular bandage several times until you have a long bandage approximately 2–4 inches wide.

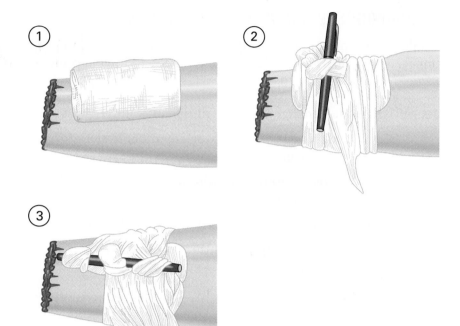

① ② ③

FIGURE 28-12A   Application of tourniquet: (1) Apply pad. (2) Wrap a wide bandage around the extremity twice and tie it off. Then tie a stick-type object to the top. (3) Twist the stick-type object until bleeding stops. Secure it and document the time it was applied.

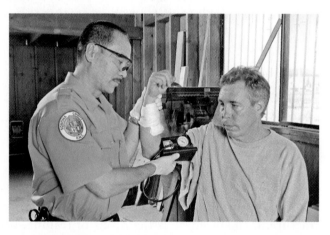

FIGURE 28-12B   Using a blood pressure cuff as a tourniquet.

3. Place the center of the bandage just above the injury site and wrap it firmly around the limb twice. Tie a half knot.

4. Place a stick or similar device over the half knot and tie a full knot over the stick.

5. If possible, locate the distal pulse in the extremity and rotate the stick until the distal pulse goes away.

6. Secure the stick in place using another triangular bandage or similar tie.

7. Document the time the tourniquet was applied and transport immediately. (Some protocols require that the letters *TK* along with the time be written on the patient's forehead.)

It is true that if the tourniquet remains in place for several hours, chances are increased that the limb may suffer permanent damage to nerves, vessels, and soft tissue. The bottom line, however, is that tourniquets are a valuable life-saving tool when all other methods of controlling bleeding have failed.

An alternative method for applying a tourniquet is to place a blood pressure cuff just above the injury site (Figure 28-12B). Palpate the distal pulse and inflate the cuff until the pulse goes away. Confirm through observation that the bleeding appears controlled.

PRECAUTIONS WHEN USING A TOURNIQUET

While a tourniquet can certainly be life saving, if applied improperly it can cause unnecessary pain and tissue damage. Keep the following principles in mind when using tourniquets:

∗ Use a wide bandage (2 to 4 inches) and secure tightly.

∗ Do not use wire, rope, string, or any other material that may cut into the skin and underlying tissue.

∗ Do not remove or loosen the tourniquet once it is applied unless directed to do so by medical direction.

∗ Leave the tourniquet in open view so hospital personnel will know it is there.

∗ If possible, do not apply a tourniquet directly on a joint.

Bleeding from the Nose, Ears, and Mouth

Bleeding from the nose, ears, and mouth may be an indication of more severe underlying trauma. Bleeding from these areas may have any of several causes, such as:

∗ Head trauma

∗ Facial trauma

∗ Digital trauma (nose picking)

∗ Sinusitis and other upper respiratory tract infections

∗ Hypertension (high blood pressure)

∗ Coagulation disorders

Bleeding from the ears or nose may be an indication of an underlying skull fracture. If the bleeding is the result of trauma, do not attempt to stop the blood flow. Instead, cover the areas with a loose dressing.

∗ **epistaxis**

simple nose bleeds.

Simple nose bleeds, or **epistaxis,** are a common occurrence and rarely life threatening. Follow these basic steps when caring for a nontraumatic nose bleed (Figure 28-13):

1. Place the patient in a sitting position and have him lean forward.

2. Use a gloved hand to apply direct continuous pressure by pinching the fleshy portion of the nostrils together.

3. Reassure the patient and keep him calm and quiet.

Many people think that leaning back is the appropriate position for controlling a nose bleed. In fact, this position directs much of the blood to the back of the airway, where it may cause the patient to gag or obstruct the airway. This position also directs the flow of blood to the stomach. Blood is very irritating to the stomach and may cause nausea and vomiting, which will likely make the bleeding worse. These risks may be minimized by having the patient lean forward.

Similar to nose bleeds, bleeding from the mouth is generally easy to control and rarely life threatening. The biggest concern with bleeding from the mouth is the possibility that the patient's airway could become blocked. Responsive patients

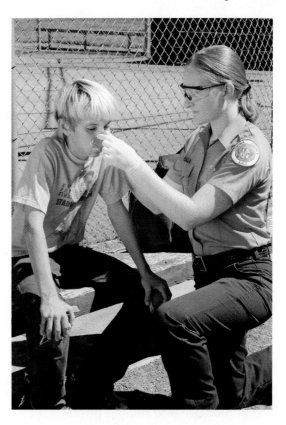

can be allowed to assume a position of comfort and hold clean dressings inside the mouth until the bleeding is controlled. Unresponsive patients can be managed by placing them in the recovery (lateral recumbent) position, if injury permits. It may be necessary to suction the mouth frequently to minimize the chances of an airway obstruction.

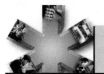

Perspective

Olin—The EMT

"Shock. I can't remember ever going into shock before. It was like my stomach started knotting up, and I got really panicky, like I had to do something but I couldn't think of what it was. Then my vision started closing in and I got cold all over. I could actually feel each drop of sweat popping out on my forehead. Man, that was weird. And right before I blacked out, I remember thinking that I was actually dying. Let me tell you—there was nothing peaceful about it for me! Talk about anxiety! When I came to, I was totally confused and riding in the back of the ambulance with a nonrebreather mask on my face. Now that I look back on that whole thing, though, I'm really glad that it happened. It helped my patient care skills so much. I mean, now I truly know what my patients are going through!"

5-1.9 List signs and symptoms of shock (hypoperfusion).

5-1.10 State the steps in the emergency medical care of the patient with signs and symptoms of shock (hypoperfusion).

Signs and Symptoms of Shock

A patient who has suffered an injury and is presenting with the signs and symptoms of hypoperfusion/shock should be considered a high priority for transport. This patient may have lost a significant amount of blood and his body is attempting to compensate. Remember that not all blood loss is obvious, and victims of trauma may have internal as well as external bleeding. Review chapter 27.

A patient who has signs and symptoms of shock may be in need of surgical intervention. Perform the necessary steps for controlling all obvious bleeding and transport immediately.

Signs and symptoms of shock include:

✳ Increased pulse rate (tachycardia)

✳ Altered mental status including restlessness and anxiety

✳ Increased respiratory rate (tachypnea)

✳ Increased capillary refill time

✳ Weak peripheral pulses

✳ Pale, cool, and clammy skin

✳ Thirst

✳ Sluggish and dilated pupils

✳ Nausea and/or vomiting

✳ Decreasing blood pressure (late sign)

Clinical Clues: SHOCK

Not all patients who are bleeding internally will show signs of shock right away. Do not wait for these signs to appear before transporting. Carefully evaluate the mechanism of injury, assess the patient, and initiate care for shock BEFORE the signs and symptoms appear.

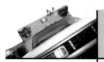

Dispatch Summary

Olie made a complete recovery from his injury. Both he and his partner, Ken, realized more than ever that transport time for a bleeding patient can be critical to his survival.

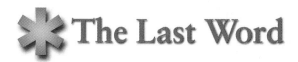

The Last Word

Blood loss due to injury is lost through arteries, veins, and capillaries. The more blood that is lost, the lower the blood pressure eventually falls, resulting in a condition known as shock or hypoperfusion.

Most external bleeding that you will encounter in the field is likely to be minor and therefore easily controlled with direct pressure, elevation and, in rare cases, the use of pressure points. Do not be concerned about completing a thorough patient assessment until all severe bleeding is controlled. Remember that the three primary ways to control external bleeding are direct pressure, elevation, and use of pressure points, in that order.

If the above methods to control severe bleeding fail, consider the use of a tourniquet.

Apply high-flow oxygen to the patient as soon as practical and watch for signs and symptoms of shock. If a patient presents with these signs and symptoms, expedite transport to an appropriate receiving hospital or request an ALS intercept as appropriate. Document all appropriate information in your PCR.

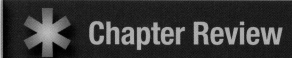

Chapter Review

MULTIPLE CHOICE

Place a check next to the correct answer.

1. Bleeding from _____ is under high pressure and sometimes is found to be spurting from the wound.

   _____ a. the venae cavae

   _____ b. capillaries

   _____ c. veins

   _____ d. arteries

2. This technique involves putting pressure on an artery above the injury site in an attempt to slow the bleeding at the wound.

   _____ a. direct pressure

   _____ b. pressure point

   _____ c. pressure bandage

   _____ d. elevation

3. The purpose of a tourniquet is to:

   _____ a. put pressure directly on the wound.

   _____ b. slow blood flow to the injury site.

   _____ c. stop all blood flow to the injury site.

   _____ d. stop all venous blood flow only.

4. Which of the following represents the most appropriate method for controlling a simple nose bleed?

   _____ a. Pinch the nose and have the patient lean back.

   _____ b. Allow the nose to bleed freely while the patient leans forward.

   _____ c. Allow the nose to bleed freely while the patient leans back.

   _____ d. Pinch the nose and have the patient lean forward.

5. All of the following are signs and symptoms of hemmorhagic shock, EXCEPT:

_____ a. increased pulse rate.

_____ b. increased respirations.

_____ c. decreased blood pressure.

_____ d. decreased pulse rate.

6. The two factors that determine the severity of blood loss are:

_____ a. time and quantity.

_____ b. time and injury.

_____ c. body size and weight.

_____ d. body size and injury.

7. The sudden loss of _____ ccs of blood in the adult patient can be life threatening.

_____ a. 100

_____ b. 500

_____ c. 1,000

_____ d. 2,000

8. Bleeding from _____ is often steady and flowing and appears darker in color.

_____ a. veins

_____ b. arteries

_____ c. capillaries

_____ d. venules

9. Bleeding that occurs from an abrasion will most likely be which type of bleeding?

_____ a. arterial

_____ b. capillary

_____ c. venous

_____ d. severe

10. The most appropriate pressure point for a bleeding wound to the forearm is the _____ artery.

_____ a. carotid

_____ b. radial

_____ c. brachial

_____ d. femoral

MATCHING

Match the term on the left with the applicable definition on the right.

1. _____ Plasma

2. _____ Red blood cells

3. _____ White blood cells

4. _____ Platelets

5. _____ "Bleeding out"

6. _____ Direct pressure

7. _____ Elevation

A. Irregularly shaped cell fragments that are responsible for promoting blood clotting

B. Pressure applied using the fingers, palm, or entire surface of one hand to help control bleeding

C. Disk-shaped cells responsible for transporting oxygen and carbon dioxide to and from the tissues

D. Elevating the injury site above the level of the patient's heart to reduce the amount of pressure at the site and make it easier for the bleeding to be controlled

E. Any of the colorless or white cells in the blood that help protect the body from infection and disease

F. The clear, yellowish fluid portion in which the other components of blood are suspended

G. Term meaning the patient is losing blood from within the circulatory system, not specific to internal or external blood loss

CRITICAL THINKING

1. Describe the type of bleeding you might see from a large wound and the methods you will use in an attempt to control the bleeding.

_____

_____

_____

_____

2. Describe why bleeding from arteries is generally more difficult to control than bleeding from other vessels.

_____

_____

_____

_____

3. List at least three signs and symptoms of shock and their causes.

_____

_____

_____

_____

CASE STUDIES

Case Study 1

You have responded to a business park for a possible amputation. Upon arrival, you are escorted into one of the warehouses where you find an approximately 20-year-old female who is bleeding from the right hand. You can see a large towel wrapped around her right hand that has been completely soaked with blood. One of the workers tells you that they were performing routine maintenance on one of the conveyor belts when it suddenly started, and Monique got her hand stuck in the belt. Monique is lying on her back and in severe pain. She is crying and saying something in Spanish that you cannot understand. One of the workers tells you that Monique is saying that she cannot feel her hand. You can see blood flowing down her arm and onto the cement floor beneath her.

1. What is your priority of care for this patient?

_____

_____

_____

_____

2. You have removed the bloody towel and see that Monique's hand appears to have been crushed. There are several breaks in the skin on both sides of her hand and between the fingers. There is blood spurting from an open wound on her palm. What type of bleeding is present, and how will you manage it?

_____

_____

_____

_____

3. What can you do to treat Monique for shock?

_____

_____

_____

_____

Case Study 2

You have been dispatched to the local hardware store for a possible head injury. Upon arrival, you are met by one of the employees who escorts you to the supply room in the back of the store. There you find an approximately 70-year-old male who is bleeding from the scalp. One of the employees is holding a dressing on the wound, but blood continues to flow down the side of his head. You are told that the man was removing a box from a shelf when a piece of metal fell, hitting him on the head.

1. Other than the bleeding wound, what must you be concerned about with this patient?

_____

_____

_____

_____

2. How will you control the bleeding with this wound?

_____

_____

_____

_____

3. Once bleeding has been controlled, what other care will you provide for this patient?

_____

_____

_____

_____

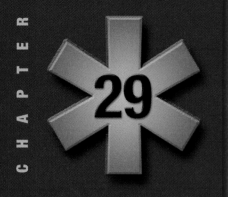

CHAPTER 29

Patients with Soft-Tissue Injuries

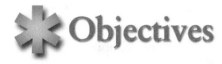

Objectives

Numbered objectives are from the U.S. Department of Transportation 1994 EMT-Basic National Standard Curriculum.

COGNITIVE OBJECTIVES

At the completion of this lesson, the EMT-Basic student will be able to:

5-2.1   State the major functions of the skin. (p. 719)
5-2.2   List the layers of the skin. (p. 719)
5-2.3   Establish the relationship between body substance isolation (BSI) and soft-tissue injuries. (p. 720)
5-2.4   List the types of closed soft-tissue injuries. (p. 720)
5-2.5   Describe the emergency medical care of the patient with a closed soft-tissue injury. (pp. 723–724)
5-2.6   State the types of open soft-tissue injuries. (pp. 724–726)
5-2.7   Describe the emergency medical care of the patient with an open soft-tissue injury. (pp. 729–730)
5-2.21 List the functions of dressing and bandaging. (pp. 739–741)

5-2.22 Describe the purpose of a bandage. (pp. 740–742)
5-2.23 Describe the steps in applying a pressure dressing. (pp. 745–746)
5-2.24 Establish the relationship between airway management and the patient with chest injury, burns, blunt and penetrating injuries. (p. 720)
5-2.25 Describe the effects of improperly applied dressings, splints, and tourniquets. (p. 746)
5-2.26 Describe the emergency medical care of a patient with an impaled object. (pp. 732–734)
5-2.27 Describe the emergency medical care of a patient with an amputation. (pp. 734–736)

AFFECTIVE OBJECTIVES

No affective objectives identified.

PSYCHOMOTOR OBJECTIVES

At the completion of this lesson, the EMT-Basic student will be able to:

5-2.30 Demonstrate the steps in the emergency medical care of closed and open soft-tissue injuries. (pp. 723–724, 729–730)
5-2.31 Demonstrate the steps in emergency medical care of a patient with an open chest wound. (pp. 730, 733)

5-2.32 Demonstrate the steps in emergency medical care of a patient with open abdominal wounds. (pp. 730, 733)
5-2.33 Demonstrate the steps in the emergency medical care of a patient with an impaled object. (pp. 732–734)

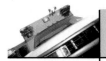 # Introduction

Soft-tissue injuries can be some of the most visually disturbing images an EMT will face in the field. They can also be life threatening to the patient, depending on the extent of the damage and amount of blood loss. While these wounds will certainly require specific care, it will be important not to let the visual impact of an open wound distract you from your priorities of care. Ensuring an open airway, adequate breathing, and pulse are your first priorities. Once these are cared for, you will then control all external bleeding and apply the appropriate dressings and bandages. In this chapter, we will discuss the various types of wounds you are likely to encounter, along with the appropriate care for each.

Emergency Dispatch

"Am I going to die?" The 9-year-old girl named Cassie looked up at EMT, Moe Brenner, tears streaming down her cheeks.

"Honey," he said gently. "We are here to help you."

Moe and his partner, Keenan, had been dispatched to the Running Water Fun Park for "some sort of leg injury" and had arrived to find a young girl with a blood-soaked towel wrapped around her lower left leg. According to witnesses, the girl had struck her leg on an uncovered bolt while on one of the water slides.

"Well," the girl fought to control her sobs. "Is my leg going to look weird when it heals?"

Moe slowly removed the towel, and gasps erupted from the surrounding crowd as a large section of flesh slowly slid away from the girl's leg. The flap was still connected by a 2-inch area of skin and ended up hanging limply above the ground, blood falling to the concrete in bright, red drops.

"I imagine you'll probably end up with a scar," Moe said softly as he replaced the avulsed piece with a gloved hand. "Please try not to worry about that too much right now. Just keep being brave while we wrap this up and get you to the doctor, okay?"

The girl sniffed a little and nodded as Keenan handed Moe a trauma dressing and several rolls of gauze.

A Review of Skin Function

The skin is the largest organ of the body. As you may remember from your study of anatomy in chapter 4, the skin serves many important functions including:

* **Protection**—The skin protects the inner body from a hostile outside environment, which includes extreme temperatures, life threatening pathogens (bacteria and viruses), and impacts from outside forces (blunt trauma).

* **Temperature regulation**—The skin helps the body maintain a consistent internal or core temperature.

* **Sensory**—The skin houses the important sensory nerves that allow us to feel heat, cold, and pain.

* **Fluid Balance**—The skin serves as a barrier against fluid loss and helps maintain a proper fluid balance by controlling evaporation.

The skin is comprised of three layers (Figure 29-1):

* **Epidermis**—the outermost layer of skin

* **Dermis**—the layer just below the epidermis, which contains many of the blood vessels and nerve endings

* **Subcutaneous**—the layer below the dermis, which contains most of the fat and soft tissue of the skin and helps with temperature regulation as well as shock absorption

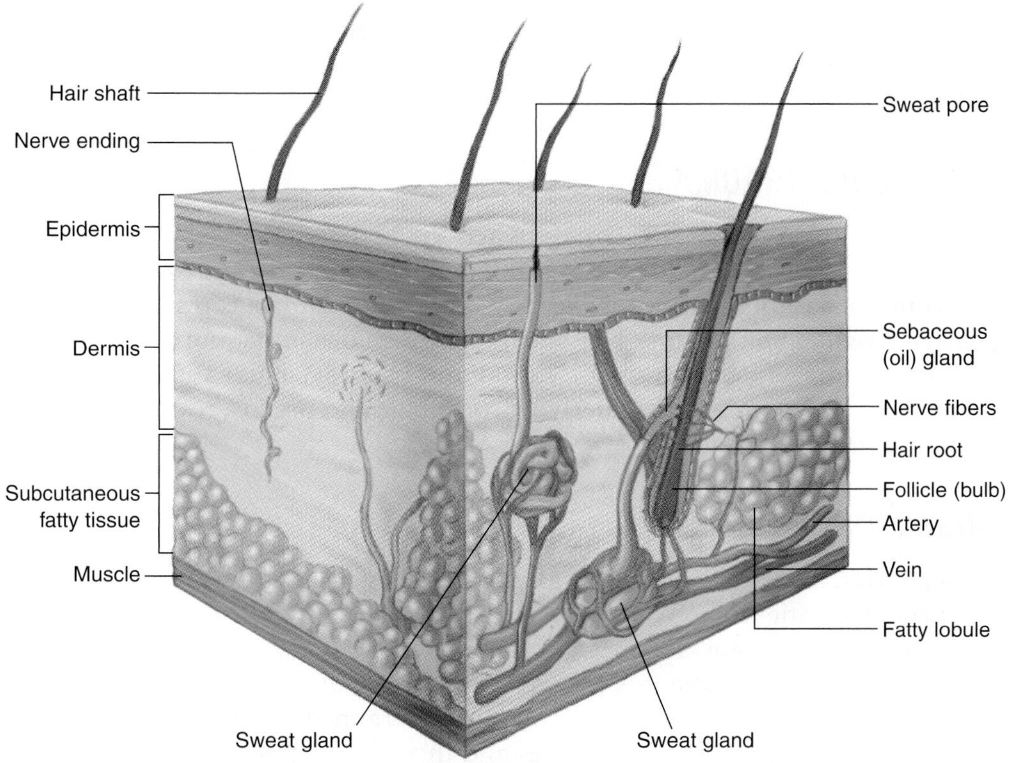

5-2.1 State the major functions of the skin.

5-2.2 List the layers of the skin.

* **epidermis**

  the outer layer of the skin.

* **dermis**

  the inner (second) layer of the skin found beneath the epidermis. It is rich in blood vessels and nerves.

* **subcutaneous**

  the deepest layer of the skin. It is made mostly of fatty tissue and provides shock absorption and insulation for the body.

FIGURE 29-1   A cross section of the skin showing its detailed anatomy.

Hair shaft
Nerve ending
Epidermis
Dermis
Subcutaneous fatty tissue
Muscle
Sweat gland
Sweat pore
Sebaceous (oil) gland
Nerve fibers
Hair root
Follicle (bulb)
Artery
Vein
Fatty lobule
Sweat gland

5-2.3 Establish the relationship between body substance isolation (BSI) and soft-tissue injuries.

Body Substance Isolation Precautions

One of the greatest risks to the EMT when caring for victims of trauma with open injuries is the exposure to blood. As you have already learned, blood is capable of carrying life-threatening pathogens, such as viral hepatitis and HIV. It is especially important to take appropriate BSI precautions and put on the necessary personal protective equipment—such as gloves, facemask, eye protection, and a gown, if necessary—for all trauma patients.

5-2.24 Establish the relationship between airway management and the patient with chest injury, burns, blunt and penetrating injuries.

Injuries to Soft Tissues

Injuries to soft tissues can include damage to the skin, muscles and, in some cases, the underlying organs. Soft-tissue injuries are classified as either open or closed. A closed injury occurs when damage to the underlying tissues occurs without a break in the surface of the skin. Open injuries result when the skin is broken, exposing the lower layers or, in cases of severe injury, the soft tissues and organs that lie below.

Remember your priorities of care when dealing with victims of traumatic injury such as major chest trauma, burns or penetrating injuries. The sight of these injuries can easily distract you from identifying life threatening problems with the airway, breathing or circulation. As with all patients, begin with ensuring an open and clear airway and adequate breathing before attempting to address less life threatening problems.

5-2.4 List the types of closed soft-tissue injuries.

Closed Injuries

Closed injuries to soft tissues can be anywhere from very minor to severe and life threatening. The difference often depends on the amount of tissue damage, how much bleeding there is, and what organs may be affected. There are two mechanisms primarily associated with closed soft-tissue injuries: blunt force and crush force.

BLUNT FORCE TRAUMA

Blunt force trauma is typically caused when the body is struck with a blunt surface, such as the ground following a fall (Figure 29-2) or an object such as a baseball bat or the dashboard of a vehicle. The force of the impact is transferred to the underlying tissues and organs. The outside skin remains intact but may show evidence of the impact, such as discoloration and bruising. Blunt force trauma can easily cause severe damage to underlying soft tissue and organs, resulting in blood loss, shock and even death.

CRUSH FORCE TRAUMA

✳ **crush injuries**

injuries typically caused when a patient or a part of the patient's body becomes trapped between two surfaces and the pressure from both sides causes damage to the soft tissues and/or internal organs.

Crush injuries, also called crush force trauma, are typically caused when a patient or a part of the patient's body becomes trapped between two surfaces and the pressure from both sides causes damage to the soft tissues (Figure 29-3). For example, this can occur when a patient is pinned between a wall and a vehicle, when he is run over by a vehicle or when an extremity gets trapped in a piece of machinery. There are many causes of crush injuries and these are just a few examples. While breakage of the skin is common with crush injuries, they can also occur without damage to the outer layers of the skin. Crush injuries can cause significant organ damage and blood loss, resulting in shock.

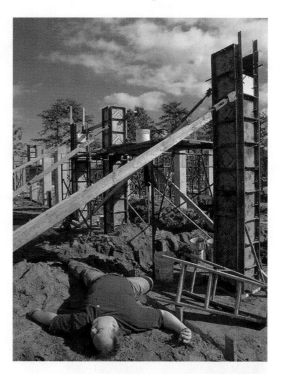

FIGURE 29-2   Blunt force injuries are common in falls from a height.

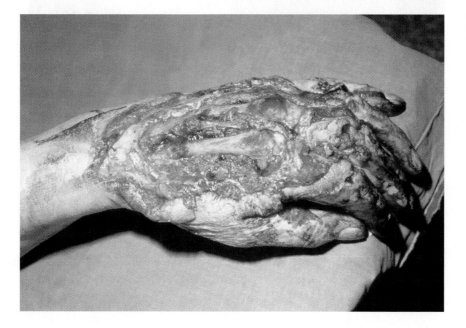

FIGURE 29-3   A crush injury to the hand. (Shout Pictures.)

SIGNS OF CLOSED SOFT-TISSUE INJURY

Aside from pain, there are at least two significant signs of possible closed soft-tissue injury: **contusions** (Figure 29-4 on page 722) and **hematomas** (Figure 29-5 on page 722). Both of these signs are indicative of bleeding beneath the surface of the skin. They can occur alone or together, depending on the amount of force involved.

A simple contusion is rarely life threatening by itself, but it may be the only sign of more significant underlying injury. The outer layer of skin remains intact, but the accumulation of blood below the skin may cause discoloration and swelling that can be detected during the patient assessment. Contusions are typically painful; however the discoloration that so frequently accompanies them may

* **contusions**

  injuries resulting when the tissues below the epidermis are damaged and cause bleeding into the surrounding tissues following a blunt trauma or crushing force. Also called bruises.

* **hematomas**

  areas of localized swelling caused by the accumulation of blood and other fluids beneath the skin.

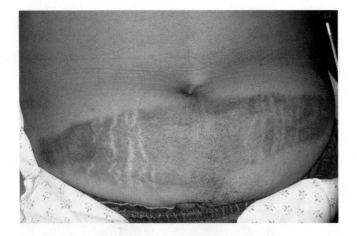

FIGURE 29-5 A hematoma often results when blood accumulates beneath the skin following blunt force trauma. (Dr. P. Marazzi/Photo Researchers, Inc.)

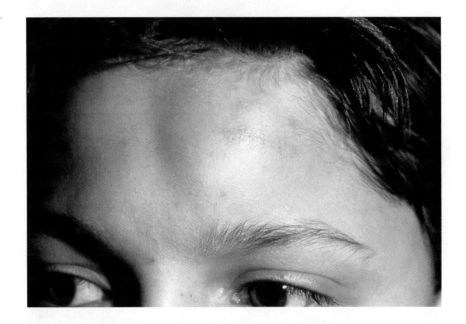

not appear for several hours. Some reddening of the skin at the injury site may be all you will see at the emergency scene.

The presence of a hematoma may indicate a more significant injury involving larger vessels. Depending on the location, a patient can lose up to a liter or more of blood with a hematoma. (See Table 29-1.)

ASSESSMENT OF CLOSED INJURIES

Your assessment of the patient must begin with an evaluation of the mechanism of injury (MOI). This will be especially helpful in patients who are unresponsive and unable to provide any history or offer a response to pain. Maintain a high index of suspicion for internal injuries when the MOI suggests it, even in the absence of obvious signs and symptoms such as contusions, hematomas, or pain.

Your physical exam must be thorough. Use both hands when palpating the chest, abdomen, and pelvis and cover each area well (Figures 29-6A and B). As you palpate, watch the patient's face for grimacing, which usually indicates tenderness and an underlying injury. Expose all areas of tenderness, as appropriate, and observe for evidence of injury. Not all internal injuries will present with external signs.

TABLE 29-1	CONTUSIONS AND HEMATOMAS AND WHAT THEY MAY INDICATE
SIGN	**INDICATION**
Discoloration/bruising of the skin	Tissue damage below the skin. If over the chest, abdomen, or pelvis, suspect injury to underlying organs.
Swelling or deformity at the site of injury	The presence of a hematoma or possible fracture. Consider proper immobilization of injury.
Bruising behind the ears or around the eyes	Trauma to the head and possible skull fracture. Assess for fluid or blood coming from the nose, mouth, or ears. Take proper spinal precautions.

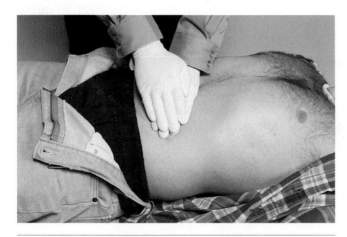

FIGURE 29-6A   Palpate all four abdominal quadrants. Observe the patient's face for grimace indicating pain and potential internal injury.

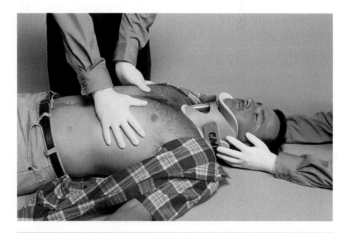

FIGURE 29-6B   Palpate the chest for signs of injury including pain, crepitus and deformity.

Clinical Clues: PALPATION AND PAIN

If you know that pain is present in a certain area, palpate that area last so that the patient does not experience residual discomfort when you examine uninjured areas.

EMERGENCY CARE FOR CLOSED INJURIES

Follow these steps when caring for a patient who presents with the signs and symptoms of a closed soft-tissue injury:

1. Take the appropriate BSI precautions and perform a scene size-up.

2. Perform an initial assessment.

3. Attempt to control any external bleeding, using direct pressure, elevation, and pressure points as needed.

5-2.5 Describe the emergency medical care of the patient with a closed soft-tissue injury.

4. Initiate oxygen therapy as appropriate.

5. Perform a rapid or focused trauma assessment as appropriate.

6. Immobilize the injured extremities as appropriate.

7. Initiate transport.

8. Perform ongoing assessments.

9. Watch for signs and symptoms of shock and expedite transport if necessary.

Open Injuries

Open soft-tissue injuries occur when the mechanism of injury causes a break in the integrity of the skin and the underlying tissue becomes exposed. Bleeding from open wounds is usually obvious and must be controlled as soon as possible. Infection is a serious concern with open wounds; therefore, you must take care to minimize contamination of the wound during your care. This will be discussed in more detail later.

There are several types of open wounds commonly seen in the field. Some of these represent minor injuries with minimal bleeding while others involve major arteries and significant bleeding that may be difficult to control. The following are descriptions of the most common types of open soft-tissue injuries.

✳ **Abrasions**—These are injuries to the skin that involve the wearing down or removal of the superficial layers of the skin (Figure 29-7). Scraped elbows and skinned knees are common examples of abrasion injuries. We have all had them, so we know how painful they can be; however they rarely, if ever, pose a serious threat to life. Bleeding from abrasions is typically minimal and easy to control, as the blood slowly oozes from the wound. Infection is a big concern with abrasions, especially large abrasions, so these wounds must be covered with a clean dressing as soon as possible.

✳ **Lacerations**—These are open wounds that typically have jagged edges, although they can have straight even edges as well (Figures 29-8A and B). Lacerations can be caused by many things, however they are most often caused by sharp objects or forceful impact. Their depth can be shallow or deep, depending on the mechanism. Lacerations have the potential to cause severe bleeding, depending on the vessels that are affected.

5-2.6 State the types of open soft-tissue injuries.

✳ **abrasions**

injuries to the skin that involve the wearing down or removal of the superficial layers of the skin.

✳ **lacerations**

open wounds that can have jagged or straight edges.

FIGURE 29-7 Abrasions are usually the least serious type of open wound. (Charles Stewart, M.D. and Associates.)

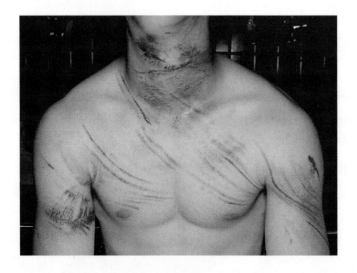

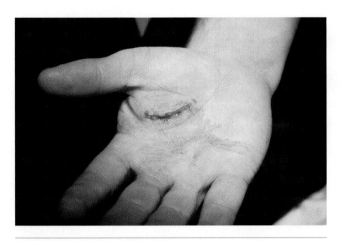

FIGURE 29-8A   An open laceration on the palm of the hand.

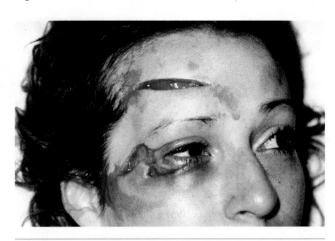

FIGURE 29-8B   Facial lacerations.

* **Avulsions**—These injuries occur when the skin and/or underlying tissue is forcibly torn away by the mechanism of injury (Figure 29-9). In some cases it causes a loose flap of skin, but it can also result in skin being torn completely off. Injuries such as a piece of nose, an ear, and even an eye that is torn from its socket are all described as avulsion injuries. Depending on the involvement of vessels, bleeding from avulsions can be minor to severe.

* **Penetration injuries**—These injuries are typically caused when an object penetrates the skin and underlying soft-tissue or organs (Figure 29-10). While typically caused by sharp objects, such as a knife, some penetrating injuries are caused by bullets and larger blunt objects. Depending on the mechanism of injury, penetrating injuries may have little or no external bleeding. Most of the damage from these injuries is deep within the body and can result in severe internal bleeding. Penetrating injuries will always have at least an entry site and may also have an exit site. An object that has penetrated the skin and remains in the wound is called an impaled object.

* **Amputations**—These injuries occur when the mechanism of injury causes a loss of a limb or part of a limb (Figure 29-11 on page 726). Depending on the mechanism of injury, the bleeding associated with an amputation can be minor or severe. With traumatic amputations, where there is a significant tearing mechanism, the tissues and vessels are pulled to the point of failure.

* **avulsions**
  injuries where the skin and/or underlying tissue is forcibly torn away.

* **penetration injuries**
  injuries caused by an object that passes through the skin or other body tissues.

* **amputations**
  injuries resulting in the loss of a limb or part of a limb.

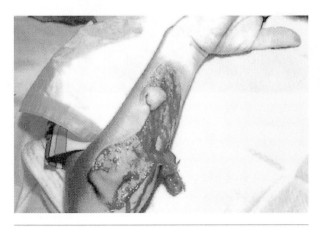

FIGURE 29-9   Avulsion.

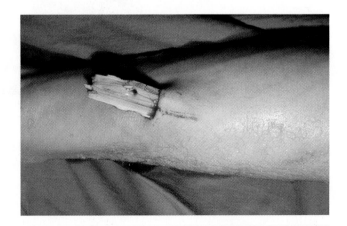

FIGURE 29-10   A penetrating injury to the forearm. (Charles Stewart, M.D., and Associates.)

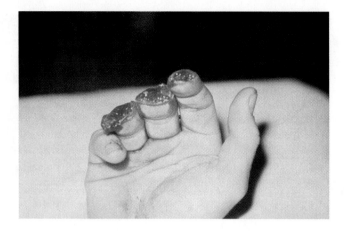

FIGURE 29-11 A hand with three amputated fingers.

For this reason, the blood vessels have a tendency to retract into the wound and bleeding may be minimal.

* **Crush injuries**—As mentioned earlier, these injuries are typically caused when a patient or a part of his body becomes trapped between two surfaces and the pressure from both sides causes damage to the soft tissues and/or internal organs (Figure 29-12). When they involve the extremities, crush injuries frequently cause fractures. Depending on the mechanism and area affected, crush injuries may have minimal external bleeding and major internal bleeding.

FIGURE 29-12 A crush injury to the hand. (Shout Pictures.)

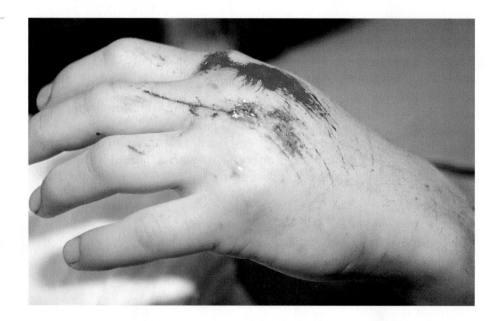

Stop, Review, Remember!

Multiple Choice

Place a check next to the correct answer.

1. The _____ is the outermost layer of skin.

   _____ a. epidermis

   _____ b. dermis

   _____ c. subdermis

   _____ d. subcutaneous

2. Which of the following would NOT be considered a normal function of the skin?

   _____ a. protection from infection

   _____ b. temperature regulation

   _____ c. fluid balance

   _____ d. fluid filtration

3. A patient who has fallen 12 feet onto a hard surface has suffered what is referred to as _____ force trauma.

   _____ a. crush

   _____ b. mild

   _____ c. blunt

   _____ d. severe

4. An injury caused when a patient's leg is run over by a vehicle is an example of _____ force trauma.

   _____ a. crush

   _____ b. mild

   _____ c. blunt

   _____ d. severe

5. The presence of bruising behind the ears may be an indication of:

   _____ a. injury to the eye.

   _____ b. bleeding deep within the brain.

   _____ c. possible skull fracture.

   _____ d. ruptured ear drum.

Matching

Match the definition on the left with the applicable term on the right.

1. _____ The outermost layer of skin

2. _____ The layer just below the epidermis, which contains many of the blood vessels and nerve endings

3. _____ Contains most of the fat and soft tissue of the skin and helps with temperature regulation

4. _____ Result when the skin is broken, exposing the lower layers

5. _____ Caused when the body is struck with a blunt surface

6. _____ Caused when a patient or a part of his body becomes trapped between two surfaces

7. _____ Results when the tissues below the epidermis are damaged and cause bleeding

8. _____ Areas of localized swelling caused by the accumulation of blood

A. Subcutaneous
B. Epidermis
C. Dermis
D. Crush injury
E. Blunt trauma
F. Contusion
G. Open injuries
H. Hematoma

Critical Thinking

1. Describe each of the functions of the skin.

_____

_____

_____

_____

2. Discuss why closed soft-tissue injuries can be more deadly than open soft-tissue injuries.

_____

_____

_____

_____

3. Describe the difference between a contusion and a hematoma and how each may present during a patient assessment.

_____

_____

_____

_____

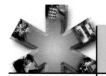

Perspective

Moe—The EMT

"It was kind of weird, actually. I mean, that was probably the worst avulsion that I've ever seen in real life . . . but there was really not much bleeding. I guess that's good, though. Man . . . when I unwrapped that towel and the skin just, sort of, came off . . . it caught me off guard! But that little girl was so scared . . . I really hope that I hid my reaction well enough! I wanted her to feel like . . . like that kind of thing happens every day and that she was gonna be perfectly fine. No big deal, you know? But inside I was like, 'Holy Cow! That's really bad!'"

Emergency Care for Open Soft-Tissue Injuries

SCENE SIZE-UP

Many injuries involving open wounds are caused by a mechanism of injury that may still pose a threat as you approach the scene. Motor vehicle collisions, assaults, and unsafe machinery are just a few examples. Obtain as much information from dispatch as possible prior to arrival, and use extra caution when approaching the scene. If necessary, request additional resources, such as law enforcement, fire department, or utility company to manage any hazards that may exist.

5-2.7 Describe the emergency medical care of the patient with an open soft-tissue injury.

INITIAL ASSESSMENT

Once you have determined that the scene is safe, approach the patient and begin your initial assessment. Do not let the unpleasant site of an open wound distract you from properly addressing the ABCs. Once airway and breathing have been addressed, you must control all external bleeding. If the patient does not have an adequate airway and/or breathing and uncontrolled bleeding is present, you must work with your partner to manage both problems at the same time. One of you must address the airway and breathing while the other controls the bleeding. The specific methods for dressing and bandaging a wound will be discussed later in this chapter. Provide supplemental oxygen as appropriate.

FOCUSED HISTORY AND PHYSICAL EXAM

After the ABCs have been properly addressed, you must continue on with an appropriate history and physical exam. Once again, the specific assessment path will depend on the MOI. A rapid trauma assessment will be required for the patient who has sustained a significant MOI and the focused trauma assessment for the patient with a nonsignificant MOI.

It may be necessary to remove or cut away clothing to expose the wound. This will make it easier to assess and properly care for the wound. Control bleeding using direct pressure, elevation, and pressure points as necessary. Whenever possible, use sterile dressings to minimize further contamination of the wound. Once

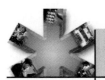

Perspective

Cassie—The Patient

"I was going down the water slide and at this one part I saw a bolt sticking up. I think it's supposed to have some plastic thingy on it, but it didn't. And I just slid over it because I couldn't stop or anything. It hurt, but I didn't know how bad until I got to the bottom. At first it didn't feel nearly as bad as it looked! I wanted my Dad! I got really worried that I could die or that my leg would end up looking all deformed and that everyone would laugh at me when I wore shorts and stuff. The ambulance guys were nice, but I just couldn't stop crying. It hurt so much, and I was really scared!"

bleeding has been controlled, apply an appropriate dressing and bandage. Calm and reassure the patient as necessary. Monitor the patient closely for signs and symptoms of shock and expedite transport.

Follow these steps when caring for a patient with an open soft-tissue injury:

1. Take the appropriate BSI precautions and perform a scene size-up.

2. Perform an initial assessment.

3. Attempt to control any external bleeding, using a sterile dressing with direct pressure, elevation, and pressure points as needed.

4. Administer high-flow supplemental oxygen as appropriate.

5. Perform a rapid or focused trauma assessment as appropriate.

6. Immobilize the injured extremities as appropriate.

7. Initiate transport.

8. Perform ongoing assessments.

9. Watch for signs and symptoms of shock and expedite transport if necessary.

Stop, Review, Remember!

Multiple Choice

Place a check next to the correct answer.

1. In addition to blood loss, _____ is a major concern when caring for open wounds.

   _____ a. CHF

   _____ b. disfigurement

   _____ c. infection

   _____ d. function

2. _____ injuries occur when the skin and/or underlying tissue is forcibly torn away by the mechanism of injury.

   _____ a. Crush

   _____ b. Avulsion

   _____ c. Laceration

   _____ d. Penetration

3. All of the following are reasons that an impaled object may need to be removed in the field EXCEPT to:

   _____ a. make it easier to control the bleeding.

   _____ b. allow for proper chest compressions.

   _____ c. allow for proper airway control.

   _____ d. allow for appropriate transport.

4. The first step in the control of external bleeding is:

   _____ a. elevation.

   _____ b. pressure point.

   _____ c. direct pressure.

   _____ d. application of a tourniquet.

5. A patient who has sustained a significant MOI should receive which type of assessment?

   _____ a. focused medical

   _____ b. rapid medical

   _____ c. focused trauma

   _____ d. rapid trauma

Matching

Match the following steps for the care of a patient with an open soft-tissue injury in the proper order.

1._____

2._____

3._____

4._____

5._____

6._____

7._____

8._____

9._____

A. Perform an initial assessment.
B. Initiate transport.
C. Immobilize the injured extremities as appropriate.
D. Administer high flow supplemental oxygen.
E. Take the appropriate BSI precautions and perform a scene size-up.
F. Perform ongoing assessments.
G. Perform a rapid or focused trauma assessment as appropriate.
H. Watch for signs and symptoms of shock and expedite transport if necessary.
I. Attempt to control any external bleeding, using a sterile dressing with direct pressure, elevation, and pressure points as needed.

Emergency Care for Specific Wounds

Certain injuries may require additional care beyond what has been described. The following segment describes additional care needed for specific types of wounds. Information on the assessment and care for abdominal and chest wounds will be discussed in chapter 31.

5-2.26 Describe the emergency medical care of a patient with an impaled object.

* **impaled object**

  penetrating trauma in which the object remains in the body.

IMPALED OBJECTS

An object that has penetrated the skin and remains embedded in the wound is referred to as an **impaled object** (Figure 29-13). These objects are typically sharp, piercing objects such as knives, steel rods, sharp sticks, and even pieces of glass. In most cases, a portion of the object remains visible outside the wound.

In almost all situations involving an impaled object you will leave the impaled object in the wound and stabilize the object prior to transport (Scan 29-1 and

FIGURE 29-13 An impaled object. (Charles Stewart, M.D., and Associates.)

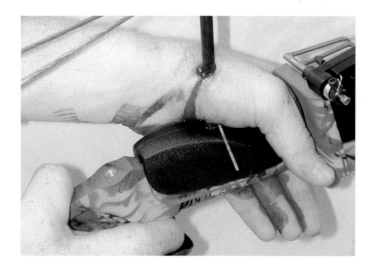

SCAN 29-1   **STABILIZING AN IMPALED OBJECT**

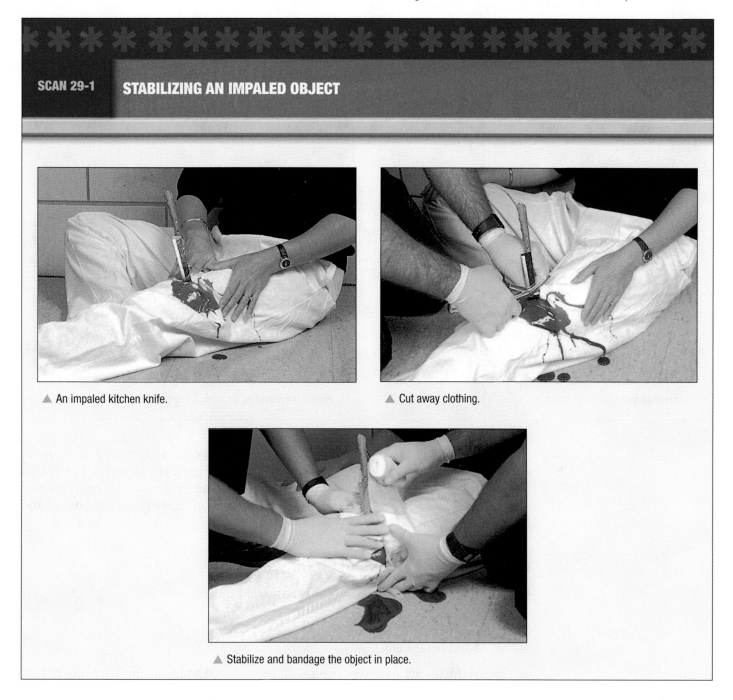

▲ An impaled kitchen knife.

▲ Cut away clothing.

▲ Stabilize and bandage the object in place.

Scan 29-2 on page 734). Removing an impaled object will likely result in an increase in both internal and external bleeding. This is especially true if the object has penetrated an organ or major blood vessel. Do your best to manually stabilize the object with your gloved hands while your partner cuts away clothing to expose the area around the wound. Use sterile dressings and direct pressure to control any external bleeding. You must then attempt to stabilize the object with material such as large bulky dressings, roller gauze, or triangular bandages.

In rare cases, the object may be too long to allow for proper transport, or its position may prevent you from performing appropriate airway care or chest compressions. In these cases, you may attempt to shorten the object or, if that does not work, you may have to remove it prior to transport. Contact medical direction and follow local protocols if you should need to remove an impaled object.

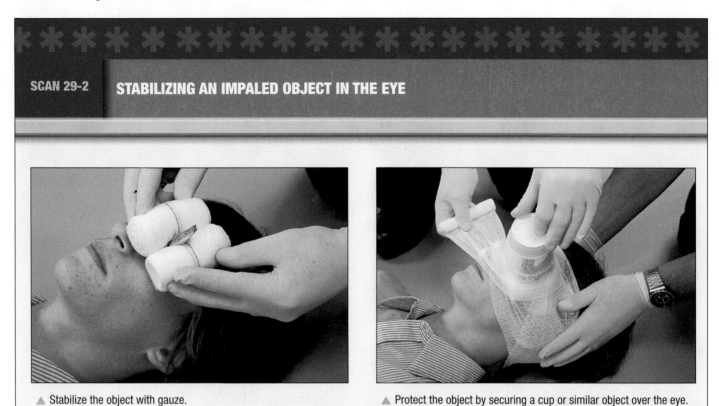

∗ Stabilize the object with gauze.

∗ Protect the object by securing a cup or similar object over the eye.

An object that has impaled the cheek only may be safely removed in the field, especially if leaving it in place could compromise the patient's airway. Objects that have impaled the trachea or are otherwise causing an airway obstruction may be removed as well. Follow local protocols. Have suction ready prior to removal and be prepared to suction the airway to keep it clear.

EMERGENCY CARE: IMPALED OBJECT

Follow these steps when caring for an impaled object:

1. Manage the ABCs as appropriate.

2. Administer high-flow oxygen.

3. Manually stabilize the object with your gloved hands to minimize movement.

4. Have your partner cut away clothing to expose the wound and help control any external bleeding.

5. Attempt to stabilize the object for transport by securing with bulky dressings.

6. Care for shock and transport immediately.

7. Initiate an ALS intercept if available.

5-2.7 Describe the emergency medical care of a patient with an amputation.

∗ **amputation**

injury resulting in the loss of a limb or part of a limb.

Amputations

An **amputation** is the traumatic loss of a limb, organ, or part of the body (Figures 29-14A and B). Amputations commonly seen by EMS include fingers, hands, arms, feet, and legs. Amputations can present special challenges to the EMT be-

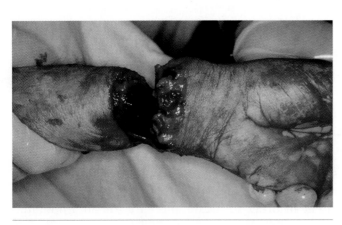

FIGURE 29-14A Amputation of the hand at the wrist. (Charles Stewart, M.D., and Associates.)

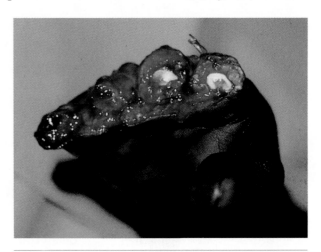

FIGURE 29-14B Finger amputation.

cause, while your primary concern is for the well being of the patient, you must remember to provide appropriate care for the amputated part. The way you manage the amputated part can significantly influence the possibility of reattachment.

Once you have addressed all immediate life threats to the patient, you will direct your attention to the amputated part (Scan 29-3). If necessary, enlist the help of other rescuers to locate the part and provide the indicated care.

Follow these steps when caring for an amputated part:

1. Wrap the amputated part in sterile dressings. If the part is large, such as a leg, cover the damaged open tissue with sterile dressings. Moisten the

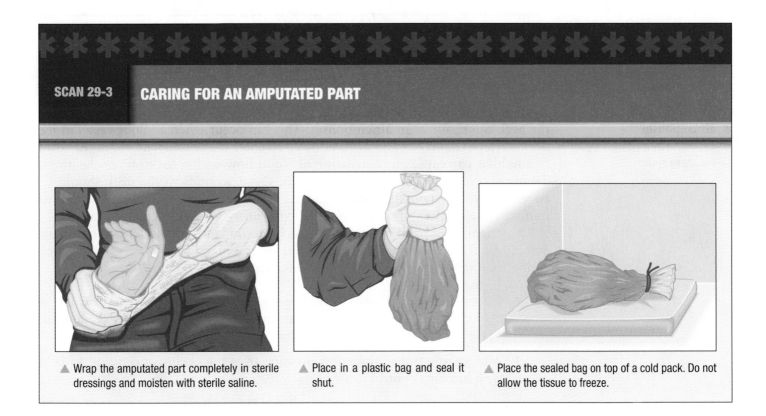

SCAN 29-3   **CARING FOR AN AMPUTATED PART**

▲ Wrap the amputated part completely in sterile dressings and moisten with sterile saline.

▲ Place in a plastic bag and seal it shut.

▲ Place the sealed bag on top of a cold pack. Do not allow the tissue to freeze.

dressings with sterile saline. Follow your local protocols. DO NOT immerse the part in water.

2. Place the wrapped part in a plastic bag or cover the area with plastic to conserve moisture. The common red biohazard bags work well. Properly label the bag with the patient's name so that it does not get thrown away by mistake.

3. Keep the part cool by using cool packs and placing them side by side with the bagged part. Use caution not to overcool or freeze the part. Do NOT place the amputated body part in ice or directly on ice.

4. If possible, always transport the amputated part with the patient to minimize the chances of its becoming lost or getting sent to the wrong hospital. Do not delay transport of a patient in order to locate and care for an amputated part.

Partial or incomplete amputations can present more of a challenge for the EMT. DO NOT attempt to complete the amputation by cutting or tearing away the last pieces of tissue. They may be providing valuable blood supply to the damaged part. Instead, carefully immobilize the entire limb and transport immediately.

Clinical Clues: AMPUTATION AND MEDICAL DIRECTION

It may be appropriate to contact medical direction in cases of amputation. The closest hospital may not be the most appropriate resource for this patient if reattachment is going to be attempted. Medical direction may direct you to the most appropriate receiving facility for this patient. Consider calling a helicopter if transport times will be extended.

Open Wounds to the Neck

∗ **air embolism**

a bubble of air that enters the circulatory system.

Aside from the risk of severe bleeding and airway compromise, open injuries to the neck can result in an **air embolism.** This can occur when a major vessel in the neck becomes damaged and air is allowed to enter the vessel. The air, in the form of a bubble, can cause an obstruction of blood flow within the heart or the lungs. This is a potentially life-threatening event. Open wounds to the neck should be covered as soon as possible with a gloved hand or occlusive dressing in order to minimize the chances of air entering the circulatory system (Figure 29-15).

Any significant open wound to the neck should be considered a risk for an air embolism. To minimize the chances of an air embolism follow these steps when caring for a patient with an open neck wound:

1. Cover the wound with an occlusive dressing as soon as possible. Use a gloved hand, if necessary, until an appropriate dressing can be applied. Make certain that the dressing covers the wound on all sides.

2. Add an additional absorbent dressing over the occlusive dressing to help with bleeding control.

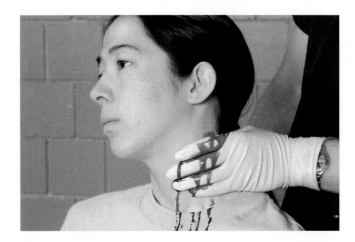

FIGURE 29-15   Place your gloved hand over an open-neck wound until an occlusive dressing can be applied.

3. Use fingertip pressure to control bleeding and minimize pressure on the airway. Compress the carotid artery only if it is necessary to control bleeding. Never compress both carotid arteries at the same time.

4. Monitor the patient's airway and breathing status closely, provide high-flow supplemental oxygen, and transport.

Remember that injuries to the neck are often associated with spinal injury. Carefully evaluate the mechanism of injury as you begin your care and take the necessary spinal precautions as appropriate.

 Stop, Review, Remember!

Multiple Choice

Place a check next to the correct answer.

1. Impaled objects in the _____ may be removed by the EMT in the field.

   _____ a. neck

   _____ b. chest

   _____ c. abdomen

   _____ d. cheek

2. The first step in caring for an amputated part is to:

   _____ a. wrap it with a sterile dressing.

   _____ b. cool the part.

   _____ c. control bleeding from the part.

   _____ d. elevate the part.

3. Whenever possible, it is recommended NOT to remove an impaled object in the field. This is because removing an impaled object may cause:

   _____ a. more contamination.

   _____ b. more damage to soft tissues.

   _____ c. increased internal and external bleeding.

   _____ d. a decrease in pulse.

4. A potentially dangerous complication that can result from an open wound to the neck is a(n):

_____ a. thrombosis.

_____ b. air embolism.

_____ c. pneumothorax.

_____ d. hemothorax.

5. All of the following are reasons to remove an impaled object in the field EXCEPT that the object:

_____ a. interferes with transport.

_____ b. interferes with chest compressions.

_____ c. interferes with proper care of the airway.

_____ d. interferes with rolling the patient.

Matching

Match the term on the left with the applicable definition on the right.

1. _____ Amputation

2. _____ Impaled object

3. _____ Crush injuries

A. Injury typically caused when a patient or a part of his body becomes trapped between two surfaces and the pressure from both sides causes damage to the soft tissues and/or internal organs

B. Injury resulting in the loss of a limb or part of a limb

C. Penetrating trauma in which the object remains in the body

Critical Thinking

1. Describe the unique challenges that the EMT faces with an impaled object and when it may be necessary to remove an object in the field.

_____

_____

_____

_____

2. Describe the complications that can result from an open wound to the neck.

_____

_____

_____

_____

3. Describe how you would care for a partial amputation of the hand.

_____

_____

_____

_____

Proper Dressing and Bandaging of Open Wounds

5-2.21 List the functions of dressing and bandaging.

An important skill that every EMT must learn is the proper way to dress and bandage each of the many types of wounds that you are likely to encounter in the field. There are two main purposes for the application of a dressing and bandage to an open wound. First and foremost is bleeding control. The second purpose is to minimize further contamination of the wound. This section will cover the various types of dressings and bandages and techniques that can be used to apply them.

DRESSINGS

Dressings are typically made of absorbent gauze and are available in both sterile and nonsterile applications. In general, sterile dressings are preferred in wound care. When placed directly over an open wound, dressings help control bleeding by aiding in the formation of a clot. They also help protect against the introduction of contaminants that might cause infection.

Dressings come in a wide variety of shapes and sizes, depending on their intended purpose. The following are examples of some of the more common dressings used in EMS and their intended use:

* **Adhesive dressing**—The brand of dressing most familiar to everyone is Band-Aid®. Self-adhering dressings are also available in a variety of sizes and shapes and are ideal for small cuts and scrapes (Figure 29-16).

* **Gauze pads**—These layered pads come in a variety of sizes such as 2″ × 2″, 4″ × 4″, 5″ × 9″ and 8″ × 10″. Most are available as individually wrapped sterile dressings. However some such as the 4″ × 4″ and 2″ × 2″ come in bulk, nonsterile packages as well. Gauze pads work well for small- to-medium-sized wounds (Figure 29-17 on page 740).

* **Universal/Trauma**—These are similar to the smaller gauze pads just listed but they are bigger (10″ × 30″ and larger), and thicker and are designed for large open wounds. Sometimes called abdominal or ABD pads, these

* **dressings**

  sterile or nonsterile material placed directly over an open wound.

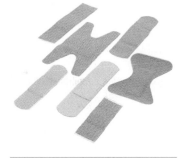

FIGURE 29-16   Examples of adhesive type dressings. (Getty Images—Photodisc.)

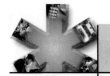

Perspective

Moe—The EMT

"Although it wasn't bleeding that much, I knew that I had to get her leg bandaged right away. Since she had been swimming and sliding at a public water park all day and the injury was caused by what sounded like an old, rusty bolt, I just didn't want to risk any further contamination. I'd hate to have this poor girl lose her leg, or worse, because of infection. I just can't imagine that, you know? Taking a school field trip to a water park to have a fun time with your friends, and then ending up injured! AND to have it deteriorate to the point where one of your limbs, or even your life, is in danger. I hope that she recovers okay. I really do."

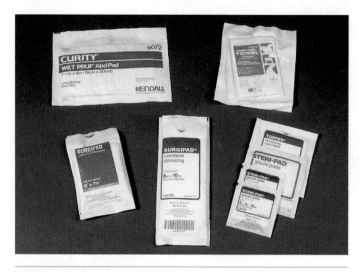

FIGURE 29-17 Several examples of gauze dressings.

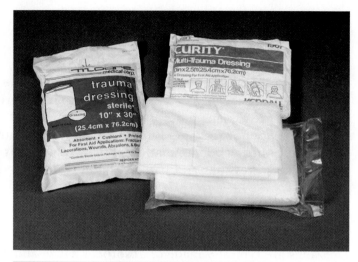

FIGURE 29-18 Universal/trauma dressings.

dressings are well suited for large, open wounds to the chest and abdomen (Figure 29-18).

* **Occlusive**—Just as the name implies, these dressings are typically thin pads of sterile gauze that have been saturated with petroleum jelly or a similar material to occlude, or prevent, air from passing through. These are also available in a variety of sizes (Figure 29-19).

BANDAGES

5-2.22 Describe the purpose of a bandage.

Bandages are typically made of strips of gauze or thin cloth material and are available in both sterile and nonsterile applications. The primary function of a bandage is to hold a dressing or dressings in place over a wound.

Much like dressings, bandages come in a wide variety of shapes and sizes, depending on their intended purpose. The following are examples of some of the more common bandages used in EMS and their intended use:

* **Gauze rolls**—Available in both sterile and nonsterile applications, these are rolls of thin gauze that come in a variety of widths (1″, 2″, 3″, 4″, and 6″). (Figure 29-20).

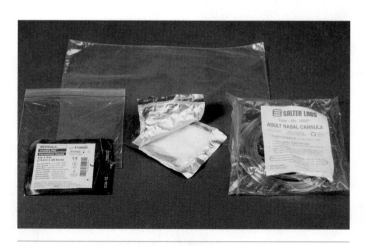

FIGURE 29-19 Occlusive type dressings.

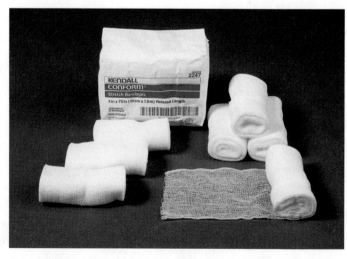

FIGURE 29-20 Gauze roll type bandages.

* **Triangular**—Most commonly thought of as slings, triangular bandages are among the bandages most universally available. They are a fast and easy way to secure dressings to extremities and the head. When folded like a cravat, triangular bandages are ideal for use as pressure bandages (Figure 29-21A–C).

* **Self-adhering**—Commonly called Kling, Kerlix, or, Coban®, these bandages come in a variety of widths and adhere to itself when overlapped, eliminating the need for tape.

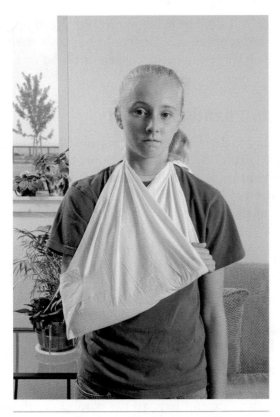

FIGURE 29-21A   A triangular bandage being used as a sling.

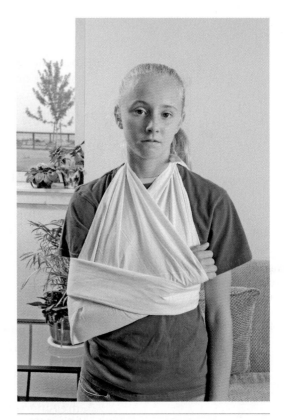

FIGURE 29-21B   A triangular bandage being used as a sling and swathe.

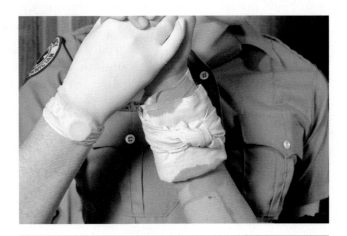

FIGURE 29-21C   A triangular bandage used as a pressure bandage, securing the dressing to the arm.

Clinical Clues: ADHESIVE TAPE ALLERGY

Some patients are allergic to the adhesive on many types of tape. If you are going to use tape directly on the skin, ask the patient if he has an allergy to tape or tape adhesive. Consider using hypoallergenic tape if it is available.

∗ **Air splint**—Only for use on an extremity, the air splint can be used to hold a dressing in place when other methods are not available or not successful.

∗ **Tape**—This universal material is valuable in helping hold dressings to a wound. There are many sizes and types of tape. It should be stated that tape becomes almost ineffective when there is moisture, such as blood or sweat, present on the skin.

APPLICATION OF DRESSINGS AND BANDAGES

Simply put, there is more than one way to dress and bandage wounds. While there are a few simple guidelines that you can follow to ensure the proper application of a dressing and bandage, among your most valuable assets will be your ability to improvise and adapt to the situation at hand.

First and foremost, you need to assess the wound to determine the immediate needs. Is the wound still actively bleeding?—in which case you may need to apply a specific type of dressing called a **pressure dressing**. This will be discussed later. If the bleeding is already controlled, the primary purpose will be to protect the wound from contamination.

Use the following guidelines when applying dressings and bandages:

∗ Remove any jewelry that might get in the way, especially rings that may be difficult to remove once the finger has become swollen.

∗ Choose an appropriate-size sterile dressing and apply it to the wound. If sterile dressings are not available, select the cleanest material available. The dressing should be large enough to extend beyond the wound on all sides. If necessary, apply additional dressings to adequately cover the wound.

∗ If dressings become blood soaked, replace them with fresh dressings. DO NOT however remove the first dressing that is covering the wound. This dressing is helping with the formation of a clot.

∗ Select the most appropriate means to secure the dressing in place. Tape may be appropriate for small wounds or wounds to the torso. For wounds on the head or extremities, roller gauze or triangular bandages work best.

∗ When using a roller bandage, start at the narrowest part of the limb and work your way up from there. To begin the bandage, make two or three wraps directly over one another to ensure a firm foundation for the bandage. Then overlap each spiral approximately one-third to one-half to ensure adequate coverage of the dressing.

∗ The bandage should extend beyond the dressing an all sides. Secure the bandage with tape or by tying it off.

∗ Once the bandage is secured, check distal circulation, sensation, and motor function to ensure that the bandage is not too tight.

∗ **pressure dressing**

dressing that applies pressure to control bleeding from a wound to an extremity that is still actively bleeding. Also called a pressure bandage.

SCAN 29-4 **APPLICATION OF A ROLLER BANDAGE**

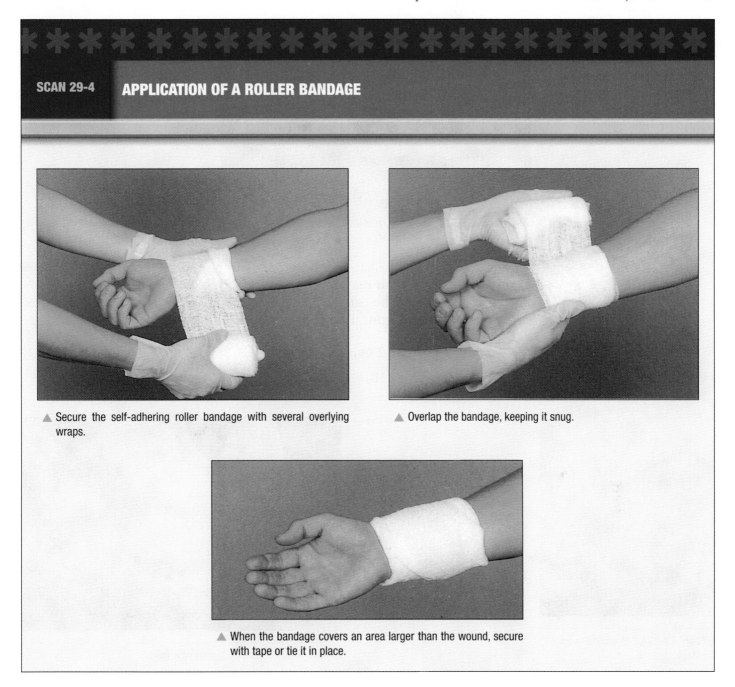

▲ Secure the self-adhering roller bandage with several overlying wraps.

▲ Overlap the bandage, keeping it snug.

▲ When the bandage covers an area larger than the wound, secure with tape or tie it in place.

* If appropriate, immobilize the injured limb and elevate. Watch to see that the bleeding remains controlled during transport.

Scan 29-4 illustrates the simple application of a dressing with a roller gauze.

POSITION OF FUNCTION

When applying dressings and bandages to a hand, it is important to keep the hand in the **position of function** (Figure 29-22 on page 744). This is the position the hand normally takes when it is at rest. You can see this when you let your hands fall relaxed at your sides. Notice how your hand takes a slightly curved shape. You can help to maintain this position during bandaging by placing a roll of gauze in the patient's hand prior to applying the bandage.

* **position of function**

the slightly curved position the hand normally takes when it is at rest.

FIGURE 29-22 Maintain position of function during bandaging by placing a roll of gauze in the patient's hand prior to applying the bandage.

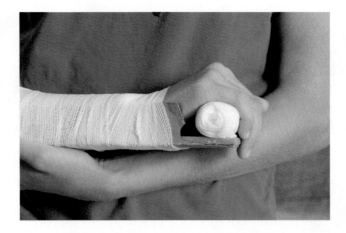

When bandaging the hands and feet, do your best to leave the fingers and toes exposed so that you can reassess circulation, sensation, and motor function following application of the bandage.

Study the following locations of wounds and illustrations:

✳ Scalp (Figure 29-23A)

✳ Eye (Figure 29-23B)

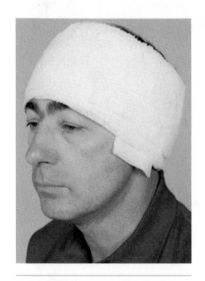

FIGURE 29-23A Head and/or ear bandage.

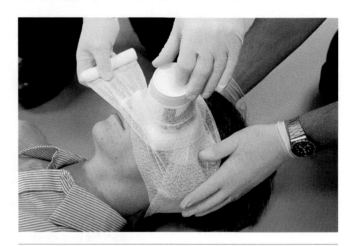

FIGURE 29-23B A bandaged eye wound.

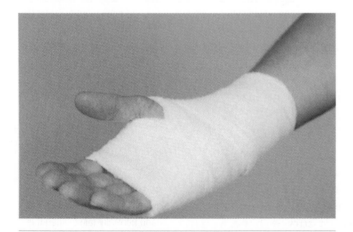

FIGURE 29-23C A bandaged hand wound.

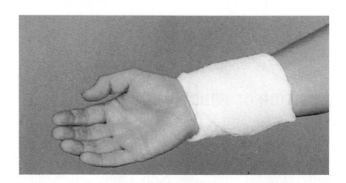

FIGURE 29-23D When the bandage covers an area larger than the wound, secure it with tape or tie it in place.

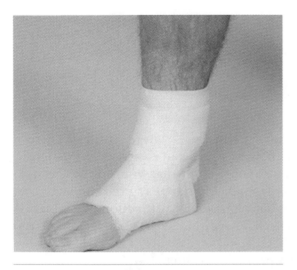

FIGURE 29-23E   Foot and/or ankle bandage.

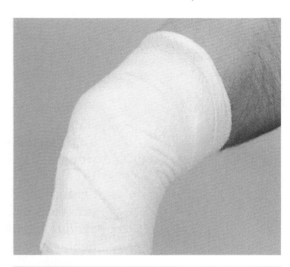

FIGURE 29-23F   Knee bandage.

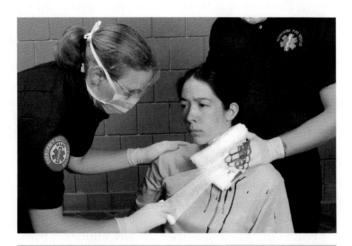

FIGURE 29-23G   To bandage a neck wound, bring the bandage over the dressing and wrap in a figure-eight configuration, winding the bandage under the arm opposite the wound. Never wind the bandage around the neck.

* Hand (Figure 29-23C)
* Arm or leg (Figure 29-23D)
* Foot (Figure 29-23E)
* Knee (Figure 29-23F)
* Neck (Figure 29-23G)

PRESSURE DRESSING

A pressure dressing, sometimes called a pressure bandage, is used to control bleeding from a wound to an extremity that is still actively bleeding. There is less concern for contamination and more focus on establishing a constant force of direct pressure to control the bleeding. By quickly applying a pressure dressing, the EMT is freed to deal with other priorities, such as managing the airway or controlling bleeding from other injuries.

5-2.23 Describe the steps in applying a pressure dressing.

A pressure dressing differs from other types of dressings in these ways:

⁕ It is used on wounds that are actively bleeding.

⁕ More pressure is required.

⁕ It is applied quickly.

You can use either roller gauze or cravats to secure a pressure dressing to a wound. Cravats are preferred because they are faster and easier to secure tightly. Use caution when tying any bandage around a limb that you not secure it so tightly that it cuts off all blood flow to the limb. After applying the bandage to an extremity, recheck distal circulation, sensation, and motor function. If circulation and/or sensation are compromised, check to see that your bandage is not too tight.

Follow these steps when applying a pressure dressing:

1. Place several layers of an appropriate dressing directly on the wound and hold direct pressure while elevating the limb. Use caution when elevating the limb as it may have an underlying fracture.

2. Using a cravat or roller gauze, have your partner begin wrapping the dressing to the wound as tightly as possible without cutting off distal circulation to the limb. Secure the dressing with tape or tie it off.

3. If possible, keep the wound above the level of the heart and maintain direct pressure if you are not needed elsewhere.

4. Monitor the wound closely and add additional dressings and bandages if needed to control the bleeding. Consider the use of a tourniquet only as a last resort.

5-2.25 Describe the effects of improperly applied dressings, splints, and tourniquets.

Following the application of any bandage, tourniquet, or splint to an extremity, it is important to recheck distal circulation, sensation, and motor function. This is to ensure that you have not inadvertently tied something too tight and are cutting off distal circulation to the limb. Bandages and splints that are applied improperly can cause unnecessary pain as well as tissue, nerve, and vessel damage. Monitor the dressing, bandage, and distal extremity throughout transport, and make adjustments as necessary.

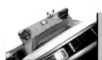

Dispatch Summary

The patient was transported to the Emergency Department at Physician's Hospital where the avulsion was repaired. After several complications caused by post-operative infections, the patient was discharged and sent home with her parents.

The wound has since healed to a very thin V-shaped scar which, according to the patient's doctor, will become even less noticeable as she grows older.

City health inspectors blamed the incident on poor maintenance at the water park. All seven of its water slides have since been replaced and the park now employs a team of off-duty EMTs—including Keenan—to appropriately respond to any future incidents.

The Last Word

The skin serves many important functions, including the protection of underlying tissues, water regulation, temperature regulation, and protection from infection. When the skin becomes damaged, blood loss and infection are the biggest concerns.

Soft-tissue injuries can be both internal and external depending upon the mechanism of injury. Most of the bleeding from open wounds can be managed easily by applying direct pressure, elevation, and pressure points. A pressure bandage can be used for bleeding that is difficult to control.

Dressings are placed directly over a wound and should be sterile whenever possible. Bandages are primarily used to secure dressings to a wound.

Specific types of open wounds such as chest and abdominal wounds require special care beyond the standard dressings and bandages. Remember to carefully evaluate the MOI and maintain a high index of suspicion for internal bleeding if the mechanism is significant. All patients with open or closed wounds must be monitored closely for evidence of shock. Document all appropriate information in your PCR.

✳ Chapter Review

MULTIPLE CHOICE

Place a check next to the correct answer.

1. When placed directly over an open wound, _____ help control bleeding by aiding in the formation of a clot.

    _____ a. bandages

    _____ b. dressings

    _____ c. cravats

    _____ d. tourniquets

2. Which of the following is NOT a common type of dressing used by an EMT?

    _____ a. occlusive

    _____ b. surgical

    _____ c. trauma

    _____ d. adhesive

3. The primary function of a pressure dressing is to:

    _____ a. minimize contamination.

    _____ b. stop all blood flow to the wound.

    _____ c. control active bleeding.

    _____ d. act as a tourniquet.

4. All of the following are commonly used as bandages, EXCEPT:

    _____ a. traction splints.

    _____ b. roller gauze.

    _____ c. tape.

    _____ d. triangular bandages.

5. All of the following are signs or symptoms of an improperly applied dressing and bandage EXCEPT:

    _____ a. excessive pain following application.

    _____ b. loss of distal circulation.

    _____ c. numbness and tingling of the extremity.

    _____ d. good distal circulation.

6. The functions of the skin are protection, temperature regulation, fluid balance, and:

    _____ a. sensation.

    _____ b. excretion.

    _____ c. motor function.

    _____ d. vessel dilation.

7. The layer of skin that consists mainly of fat and connective tissue is the:

_____ a. epidermis.

_____ b. dermis.

_____ c. subcutaneous.

_____ d. cutaneous.

8. Swelling caused by an accumulation of blood beneath the skin is known as a:

_____ a. contusion.

_____ b. bruise.

_____ c. dermis.

_____ d. hematoma.

9. A wound that has a linear cut in the skin is described as a(n):

_____ a. abrasion.

_____ b. laceration.

_____ c. avulsion.

_____ d. contusion.

10. Aside from capillary bleeding, abrasions have a strong likelihood for developing a(n):

_____ a. infection.

_____ b. hematoma.

_____ c. contusion.

_____ d. arterial bleeding.

FILL IN THE BLANK

1. The two main reasons to dress and bandage a wound are to control _____ and minimize _____.

2. When placed directly over an open wound, a _____ helps control bleeding by aiding in the formation of a clot.

3. _____ dressings are ideal for small cuts and scrapes.

4. _____ dressings consist of thin pads of sterile gauze that have been saturated with petroleum jelly to prevent air from passing through.

5. The primary function of a _____ is to hold a dressing or dressings in place over a wound.

6. The _____ is the position the hand normally takes when it is at rest.

CRITICAL THINKING

1. Describe the purpose of a bandage and a dressing.

_____

_____

_____

2. Discuss the reasons for learning to properly apply dressings and bandages.

_____

_____

_____

3. Describe how a pressure dressing differs from other types of dressings or bandages.

_____

_____

_____

CASE STUDIES

Case Study 1

You have been dispatched to a construction sight for a "man down." Upon arrival, you are directed to an adult male lying face up on a concrete slab. Bystanders advise that the man slipped and fell from the roof approximately 12 feet above and landed on a bucket. The patient denies any loss of consciousness and is complaining of severe pain to his right abdomen. Upon examination, you see redness to the right side of his abdomen and severe pain on palpation.

1. Describe your treatment priorities and how you will care for this patient.

   _____

   _____

   _____

2. What type of MOI has this man likely sustained?

   _____

   _____

   _____

Case Study 2

You are caring for an adult male patient who was driving a water-tank truck when it rolled and he was ejected. As the truck rolled, he was caught underneath and sustained significant injury to both legs. His right leg appears to be completely severed above the knee, and the left leg appears to be partially amputated below the knee. He suffered no other injuries or trauma to his torso, neck, or head.

1. What will be your treatment priorities for this man's injuries?

   _____

   _____

   _____

2. Bleeding from the left leg proves difficult to control with direct pressure and pressure point. What will you do next to control the bleeding?

   _____

   _____

   _____

3. How will you care for the injury to the right leg?

   _____

   _____

   _____

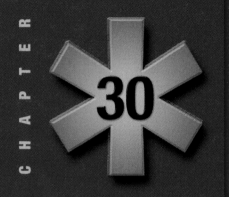

Patients with Burn Injuries

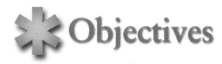 Objectives

Numbered objectives are from the U.S. Department of Transportation 1994 EMT-Basic National Standard Curriculum.

COGNITIVE OBJECTIVES

At the completion of this lesson, the EMT-Basic student will be able to:

5-2.11 List the classifications of burns. (p. 753)
5-2.12 Define superficial burn. (p. 754)
5-2.13 List the characteristics of a superficial burn. (p. 754)
5-2.14 Define partial thickness burn. (pp. 754–755)
5-2.15 List the characteristics of a partial thickness burn. (pp. 754–755)
5-2.16 Define full thickness burn. (pp. 755–756)
5-2.17 List the characteristics of a full thickness burn. (pp. 755–756)
5-2.18 Describe the emergency medical care of the patient with a superficial burn. (pp. 765–767)

5-2.19 Describe the emergency medical care of the patient with a partial thickness burn. (pp. 765–767)
5-2.20 Describe the emergency medical care of the patient with a full thickness burn. (pp. 765–767)
5-2.24 Establish the relationship between airway management and the patient with chest injury, burns, blunt and penetrating injuries. (p. 764)
5-2.28 Describe the emergency care for a chemical burn. (pp. 767–768)
5-2.29 Describe the emergency care for an electrical burn. (p. 768)

AFFECTIVE OBJECTIVES

No affective objectives identified.

PSYCHOMOTOR OBJECTIVES

At the completion of this lesson, the EMT-Basic student will be able to:

5-2.36 Demonstrate the steps in the emergency medical care of a patient with superficial burns. (pp. 765–766)
5-2.37 Demonstrate the steps in the emergency medical care of a patient with partial thickness burns. (pp. 765–766)

5-2.38 Demonstrate the steps in the emergency medical care of a patient with full thickness burns. (pp. 765–766)
5-2.39 Demonstrate the steps in the emergency medical care of a patient with a chemical burn. (pp. 767–768)

Introduction

Severe burns can be among the most traumatic of all injuries. Burns not only affect the skin, they affect many of the body's organ systems as well as the patient's emotional well-being. Aside from the obvious disfigurement, burns can result in severe infection and loss of function to the extremities. Caring for a patient with severe burns can also be a traumatic event for the members of the EMS team.

This chapter will help to prepare you to care for patients with all burns, be they minor or severe. You will learn about the different *sources* of burns and how burns are classified both by *depth of injury* and by *body surface area* (BSA) affected. Through the assessment of these three elements, you will determine the most appropriate care for the burn patient. Definitions of these critical elements are:

1. **Source**—what caused the injury.
2. **Depth**—how deeply the burn has penetrated.
3. **Body surface area (BSA)**—the amount of body surface area affected.

* **source**
  what caused a burn.

* **depth**
  how deeply a burn has penetrated.

* **body surface area (BSA)**
  the amount of body surface area affected.

Emergency Dispatch

"**A**re we just doing a standby then?" Brianna, an EMT with the city ambulance service, asked her partner as they rolled to a stop about two blocks from a fully-engulfed house fire.

"I don't know." Shane rolled the truck to a stop and peered through the windshield at the dark smoke that rose high into the night sky. "But this is as far as we go with the ambulance."

The road ahead of them was blocked by a mass of unoccupied fire and police vehicles, all parked helter-skelter across both lanes, their emergency lights pale in comparison to the fire. Brianna and Shane climbed out, got the cot from the back, and loaded it with their equipment.

"This is for a fire stand-by right?" Shane asked into the portable radio.

"Affirmative," the dispatcher responded through static. "At least. . . I think so. Report to the incident commander."

Brianna and Shane rolled the cot cautiously up the street, straining against the smoke and the intermittent darkness to find the command post.

"Medics!" The shout came from off to their left, toward the rear of the house. "Over here quick!"

There was a small group of firefighters—just silhouettes against the raging house fire—waving their arms and shouting. The EMTs hurried over, struggling to get the cot over the web of hoses that criss-crossed the pavement. As they approached, they saw that the firefighters were standing over a naked man who was lying on the sidewalk.

"I just pulled him out of the house," a fireman shouted breathlessly. "He's alive, but I think I broke his arm!"

The wild-eyed man was severely burned from his scalp down to the bottoms of his feet. Brianna could see the top layers of his skin beginning to slough off in large sheets, exposing the raw, bleeding tissue underneath. The EMTs looked at each other with wide, questioning eyes.

"Get him on the cot and get him out of here!" an older fireman shouted as the group hastily picked the now-screaming man up and set him on the gurney. "Now go! Go!"

Common Sources of Burns

Burns can be caused by several sources and the specific care you provide the patient will be determined by the exact source of the burn. The following are the most common sources of burns:

* **thermal (heat) burn**

  type of burn most commonly caused by exposure to fire, steam, hot objects, and hot liquids.

* **chemical burn**

  type of burn caused when the skin is exposed to substances such as acids, bases, and caustics.

* **electrical burn**

  type of burn caused when the body becomes exposed to an electrical current as it passes through the body.

* **radiation**

  type of burn from sources of radiation such as nuclear fallout or radioactive materials used in medicine.

* **light burn**

  type of burn caused by high-intensity light sources.

* **Thermal (heat) burn**—Thermal burns are most commonly caused by exposure to fire, steam, hot objects, and hot liquids (Figure 30-1).

* **Chemical burn**—These burns are caused when the skin is exposed to substances such as acids, bases, and caustics (Figure 30-2).

* **Electrical burn**—When the body becomes exposed to an electrical current and that current passes through the body, it can cause burns along its path (Figure 30-3)—Electrical burns will vary, depending on the amount of electricity involved, which can cause both entrance and exit wounds as it passes through the body. Electrical sources can be household current, downed power lines, and even lightening. The majority of electrical burns occur deep inside the body and cannot be seen by the EMT.

* **Radiation**—While somewhat rare, burns from sources of radiation such as nuclear fallout or radioactive materials used in medicine may be seen in the field (Figure 30-4).

* **Light burn**—High-intensity light sources are a common source of burns and most often affect the eyes (Figure 30-5). High-intensity lasers and welding are common sources of intense light that can damage the eyes and the skin if exposed.

IMPORTANT: Most sources of burns can present a serious safety risk for the rescuer. Make certain that the scene is safe before attempting to care for the patient. In cases of chemical and radiation burns, caring for the patient may expose the rescuer to the same source that injured the patient. Know your limitations and the limitations of your PPE before providing care. Request additional resources such as the fire department and/or HazMat team as appropriate.

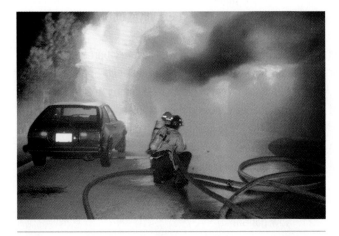

FIGURE 30-1 Fire is a common source of thermal (heat) burn. (David R. Fazier Photolibrary, Inc.)

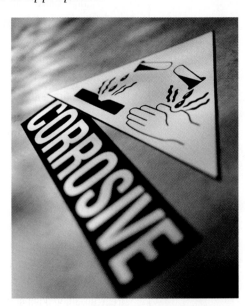

FIGURE 30-2 Corrosives such as acids and alkalis can cause severe burns to the skin. (Getty Images, Inc.-Photodisc.)

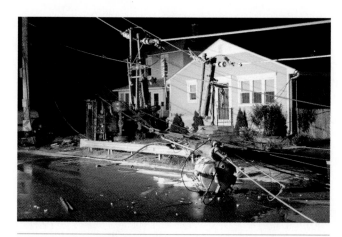

FIGURE 30-3   Downed electric power lines are hazardous and can be a cause of electrical burns. (Mark C. Ide.)

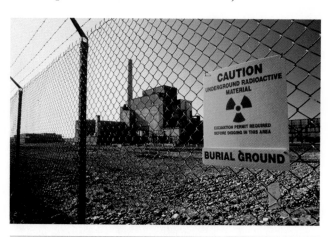

FIGURE 30-4   Although less common, burns from radiation can be deadly. (Getty Images, Inc.-Stone Allstock.)

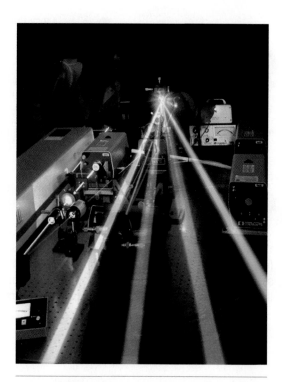

FIGURE 30-5   There is great potential for laser burns in the high-tech environment. (Lawrence Livermore National Laboratory.)

Classification of Burns by Depth

5-2.11 List the classifications of burns.

Regardless of the source or cause of the burn, burns are classified based on the depth of injury (Figure 30-6 on page 754)—in other words, how deep into the tissues the burn has reached. A burn that only affects the outer layer of skin (epidermis) is referred to as a superficial burn. A burn that reaches down to the layers of the dermis is referred to as a partial thickness burn. Any burn that reaches down to or past the subcutaneous layers, even potentially including the muscle, bone, and organs, is referred to as a full thickness burn.

FIGURE 30-6 Classification of burns by depth.

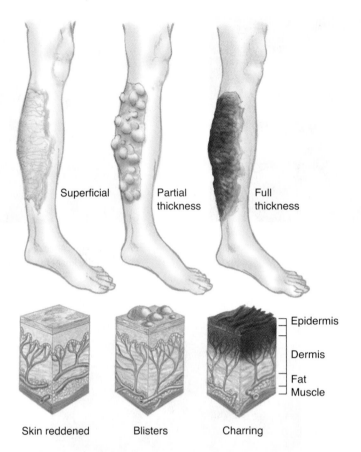

Superficial   Partial thickness   Full thickness

Epidermis
Dermis
Fat
Muscle

Skin reddened   Blisters   Charring

Clinical Clues: BURN CLASSIFICATION

You may remember that at one time burns were classified by degree. They were referred to as first, second, or third degree, depending on the depth of injury. The reference to degree is still seen in the medical literature today. However, the terms superficial, partial thickness, and full thickness are more descriptive of the type of injury and should be used as much as possible.

5-2.12 Define superficial burn.

5-2.13 List the characteristics of a superficial burn.

✳ **superficial burns**
burns that affect the outermost layer of skin, the epidermis.

5-2.14 Define partial thickness burn.

5-2.15 List the characteristics of a partial thickness burn.

✳ **partial-thickness burns**
burns that extend down beyond the epidermis and into the dermis.

SUPERFICIAL BURNS

Superficial burns are burns that affect the outermost layer of skin, the epidermis, and most often present with redness and mild to moderate stinging pain (Figure 30-7). In extreme cases there may be mild swelling. The most common cause of superficial burn is the sun. Superficial burns require no immediate emergency care and will heal completely on their own. Cooling the burn with tap water or a moistened towel will help considerably to ease the pain.

PARTIAL-THICKNESS BURNS

Partial-thickness burns are burns that extend down beyond the epidermis and into the dermis. Partial-thickness burns are characterized by pain, mottled skin color, and the presence of blisters (Figures 30-8A and B). Blisters are formed by the accumulation of fluids that are released from damaged cells and may take several hours to appear. It is important to note that there are likely to be areas of superficial-burns around the perimeter of the partial-thickness burns, adding to the patient's pain and

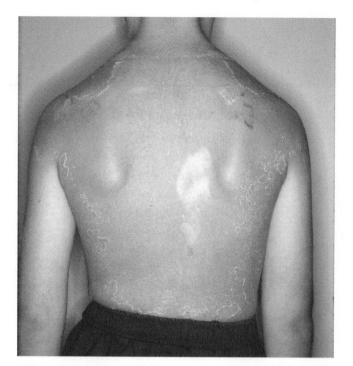

FIGURE 30-7 A patient with a superficial burn. (Charles Stewart, M.D. and Associates.)

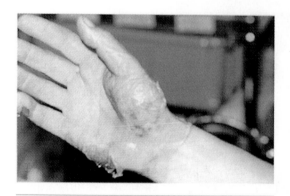

FIGURE 30-8A A patient with a partial-thickness burn to the hand and wrist. (Maria A. H. Lyle/Sarasota Memorial Hospital.)

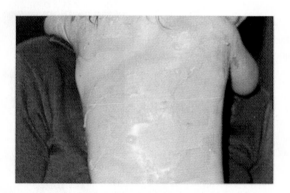

FIGURE 30-8B A patient with a partial-thickness burn of the back. (Maria A. H. Lyle/Sarasota Memorial Hospital.)

discomfort. Providing that the blisters remain intact during the healing process, there is little that needs to be done in the way of emergency care. If blisters break, the risk of infection is great. Provide care for open blisters just as you would for any other open soft-tissue injury.

FULL-THICKNESS BURNS

Full-thickness burns extend beyond all layers of the skin and can even cause damage to underlying muscle, bone, and vital organs (Figure 30-9 on page 756). While there may be little to no pain associated directly with the full-thickness burn, there will be areas of partial-thickness and superficial burns around the perimeter causing severe pain. Full-thickness burns are characterized by a white, dark brown, or charred color and may appear dry and leathery. The color of the burn is often affected by the source. For instance a full-thickness burn caused by steam will be white in color while a burn caused by fire will be dark brown or black. There is a very high risk for infection with full-thickness burns.

5-2.16 Define full thickness burn.

5-2.17 List the characteristics of a full thickness burn.

✳ **full-thickness burns**

burns that extend beyond all layers of the skin and can even cause damage to underlying muscle, bone, and vital organs.

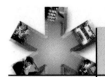

Perspective

Shane—The EMT

"That was unreal. To go from sitting at the post, just watching some stupid TV show, to something like a war zone. The smoke, the noise, the flashing lights, the yelling . . . and that poor man. I've never in my life seen a person burned so badly. It was weird. His hands and feet peeled off and were hanging, literally, by the nails. I can't imagine the pain. And he was conscious and looking at us like he didn't really know what was going on—and the look of pain on his face. We couldn't really even do anything for him but, yeah, we did the basics: administered oxygen, tried to keep him covered with the burn sheet and all, but mostly we just got him to the burn center as fast as we could."

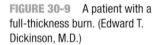

FIGURE 30-9 A patient with a full-thickness burn. (Edward T. Dickinson, M.D.)

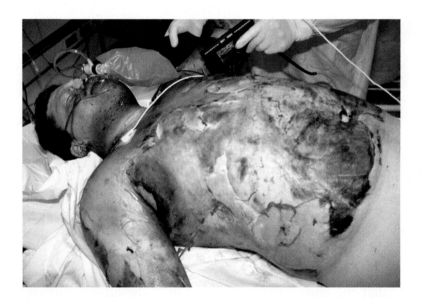

Clinical Clues: BODY TEMPERATURE OF A BURN PATIENT

You must manage the body temperature of a burn patient carefully. This patient is much more susceptible to becoming hypothermic due to the skin's decreased ability to regulate heat. If necessary, cover the patient with a blanket to conserve body heat.

Stop, Review, Remember!

Multiple Choice

Place a check next to the correct answer.

1. A burn affecting the outermost layer of skin that produces a reddish color is described as a _____ burn.

   _____ a. full-thickness

   _____ b. partial-thickness

   _____ c. superficial

   _____ d. subcutaneous

2. The majority of soft-tissue damage from this type of burn is internal and cannot be seen by the EMT.

   _____ a. electrical

   _____ b. radiation

   _____ c. thermal

   _____ d. chemical

3. A burn that appears mottled in color and has developed blisters is described as a _____ burn.

   _____ a. full-thickness

   _____ b. partial-thickness

   _____ c. superficial

   _____ d. subcutaneous

4. These burns are most often caused by fire, steam, hot objects, and hot liquids.

   _____ a. chemical

   _____ b. radiation

   _____ c. electrical

   _____ d. thermal

5. A burn that is black and charred and produces a leathery appearance to the skin is described as a:

   _____ a. full-thickness burn.

   _____ b. partial-thickness burn.

   _____ c. superficial burn.

   _____ d. subcutaneous burn.

Fill in the Blank

1. The appropriate care of all burn patients must include a thorough assessment of the _____, _____, and _____ of the burn.

2. The _____ pertains to the extent of the burn relative to location on the body and the amount of body surface area affected.

3. A _____ burn is most commonly caused by exposure to fire, steam, hot objects, and hot liquids.

4. _____ burns are caused when the skin is exposed to substances such as acids, bases, and caustics.

5. A burn that only affects the outer layer of skin (epidermis) is referred to as a _____ burn.

6. A burn that reaches down to the layers of the _____ is referred to as a partial-thickness burn.

7. A burn that reaches down to or past the subcutaneous layers is commonly referred to as a _____ burn.

Critical Thinking

1. Using your current work environment, list as many potential sources of burns as you can.

_____

_____

_____

_____

_____

2. In reference to your workplace, what safeguards are in place to prevent employees from becoming burned while on the job?

_____

_____

_____

_____

3. Discuss why patients with full-thickness burns are frequently in severe pain, even though the nerve endings have been damaged.

_____

_____

_____

_____

_____

Assessment of the Burn Patient

As an EMT you must learn to quickly assess a burn patient to determine the overall severity of the burns as well as the patient's general condition. An appropriate assessment will assist in the determination of the most appropriate care. In some situations, it may be determined that the patient should be transported directly to an appropriate burn center for definitive care rather than to the closest facility.

An appropriate assessment of a burn patient includes an evaluation of the following factors:

* Airway patency and adequacy of breathing
* Depth of injury
* Percentage of body surface area (BSA) affected
* Location of the injury
* Patient's age
* Preexisting medical conditions

DEPTH OF INJURY

You have already learned the way that burns are classified based on depth of injury. This determination can be difficult at best and requires a careful visual assessment. In many instances, it can be difficult to distinguish between partial-thickness and-full thickness burns. When in doubt, assume the worst and classify uncertain areas as full thickness.

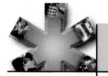

Perspective

Ed Rhome—The Rescue Firefighter

"A neighbor told me he saw all three occupants run out of the house, but when I got into that back bedroom, the smoke cleared for a just a second and I thought I saw a person under a burning bed sheet. Well, the sheet wasn't on fire, like full-on flames or anything, but it was black and the edges were glowing and, you know, moving toward the center. Like when you watch newspaper burn. I felt around until I touched a hand, and then I just yanked the guy over my shoulder and took off. I hope I found him quick enough; I really do."

PERCENTAGE OF BODY SURFACE AREA AFFECTED

When assessing the burn patient, one of the most important factors that must be established is an estimate of body surface area (BSA) affected. The method most commonly used in EMS to estimate BSA is the **rule of nines** (Figure 30-10 on page 760).

The rule of nines is based on dividing the adult body into areas of approximately 9 percent (or multiples of 9 percent) each. These figures allow the EMT to

✳ **rule of nines**

method of determining the body surface area (BSA) burned based on dividing the adult body into areas of approximately 9 percent each.

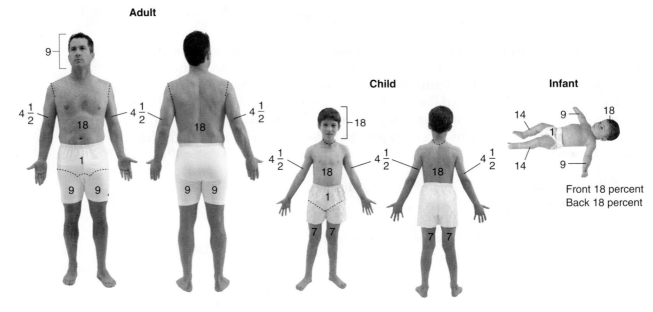

Note: Each arm totals 9 percent (front of arm $4\frac{1}{2}$ percent, back of arm $4\frac{1}{2}$ percent)

FIGURE 30-10 Rule of nines.

quickly arrive at an estimate of BSA affected. A modified version of this method can also be applied to children and infants.

Adults

✳ Head and neck = 9 percent

✳ Each upper extremity = 9 percent

✳ Anterior trunk = 18 percent

✳ Posterior trunk = 18 percent

✳ Each lower extremity = 9 percent × 2 = 18 percent

✳ Genitals = 1 percent

Children and Infants The only adjustment for the pediatric patient is that the lower extremities each represent 14 percent instead of 18 percent and the head represents 18 percent instead of 9 percent.

✳ Head and neck = 18 percent

✳ Each upper extremity = 9 percent

✳ Anterior trunk = 18 percent

✳ Posterior trunk = 18 percent

✳ Each lower extremity = 7 percent × 2 = 14 percent

✳ Genitals = 1 percent

The rule of nines is simply a guideline and not expected to determine the exact percentage of BSA affected. You must learn to use the rule of nines as a tool and understand that it may be necessary to adjust the percentage depending on the area affected. For instance, if only a portion of an arm or a portion of the chest were affected, you would adjust the estimate accordingly.

Another tool that can be used by the EMT to assess BSA is sometimes called the **rule of palm.** It is based on the principle that a patient's palm is equal to approximately 1 percent of his BSA. This can be helpful when trying to assess multiple areas of injury spread over the entire body.

* **rule of palm**

    method of estimating the body surface area (BSA) burned based on the principle that a patient's palm is equal to approximately 1 percent of his BSA.

LOCATION OF BURNS

Specific areas of the body are considered more significant than others when affected by burns. Even partial-thickness burns to certain areas could be considered serious. Burns to the following areas should be considered serious, requiring further care at an appropriate facility:

* **Face**—Burns to the face can affect the eyes and air passages Figure 30-11A and B). If the airways become exposed to heated smoke, steam, or flames, they can begin to swell, causing increased respiratory difficulty. Observe the areas around the mouth and nose for evidence of smoke, soot, or singed hairs that may indicate exposure to heat.

* **Hands and feet**—Burns to the hands and feet are considered serious due to the potential for loss of function if not cared for properly (Figure 30-12A and B on page 762).

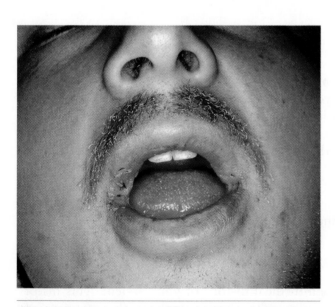

FIGURE 30-11A   A singed mustache and burns to the tip of the tongue signal danger of airway burns. (Charles Stewart, M.D., and Associates.)

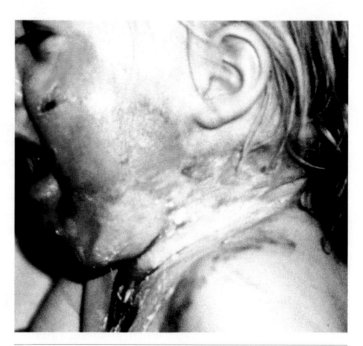

FIGURE 30-11B   Burns to the face and neck may cause airway and breathing problems.

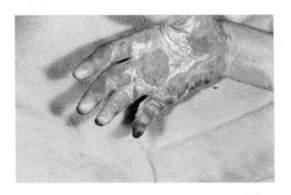

FIGURE 30-12A Burns to the hand may result in loss of function.

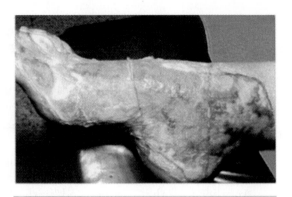

FIGURE 30-12B Burns to the feet could result in loss of mobility.

∗ **Genitalia**—Burns to the genitals are considered serious, as they may affect both form and function if not cared for properly. Burns to the inner thighs and buttocks are more prone to infection.

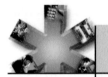

Perspective

Warren Souther, M.D.—The Emergency Physician

"That poor guy isn't going to survive. I did an RSI . . . uh . . . rapid sequence intubation" and when I got the blade in there, his airway was just black. There was soot and burns as far as I could see. I got the endotracheal tube placed and everything, but I'll be surprised if he makes it past 2 days. Four at the outside, even though everybody did their jobs perfectly, from the firefighters to the ambulance crew, to my staff. I truly feel for the guy."

AGE

The age of the patient can play a significant role in the way he responds to an injury caused by burns. The very young (less than 5 years old) and patients over the age of 55 will have more difficulty combating the affects of severe burns.

In children, the body surface area is greater in relation to their total body size. This results in greater fluid loss than in adults. Infants have a higher risk of shock, airway problems, and hypothermia.

In late adulthood, the ability of tissues to heal from any injury is lessened and the time of healing is increased. The body's ability to cope with any injury is reduced by aging tissues and failing body systems.

PREEXISTING MEDICAL CONDITIONS

When possible, obtain a thorough medical history of your patient. This history may reveal preexisting medical conditions that may complicate the treatment and recovery process. Preexisting respiratory conditions may result in an exaggerated response, causing severe respiratory distress. The stress of being burned may cause a patient with a cardiac history to suffer angina or a heart attack. Patients with kidney or immune problems will also have greater difficulty during the recovery process due to the extreme stress on the body. Diabetic patients may have increased problems related to proper healing of burn wounds.

Establishing Patient Priority

Your rapid assessment of the above factors will help to quickly determine both treatment and transport priorities for your patient. Not all burns are life threatening, requiring the care of a specialized burn center. In fact, many burns are considered minor and can be managed appropriately by most hospital emergency departments. Table 30-1 will help you identify the priority of patients with burn injuries.

SCENE SIZE-UP

As always, your safety and the safety of other rescuers and bystanders on the scene is your top priority. Scenes that involve a burn mechanism may present both obvious and unseen hazards to the rescuers (Figure 30-13 on page 764). Keep your eyes and ears open as you approach the scene, and take in as much of the scene as you can. If necessary, stop and remain a safe distance from the scene until the appropriate resources can mitigate the hazards.

If the mechanism causing the burn is still active (fire, steam, chemicals, electricity), you must do what you can to safely stop the burning process. DO NOT

TABLE 30-1   DETERMINING PRIORITY

HIGH PRIORITY (SEVERE)

* Full-thickness burns involving the hands, feet, face, or genitalia
* Burns associated with respiratory injury
* Full-thickness burns affecting more than 10 percent of BSA
* Partial-thickness burns affecting more than 30 percent of BSA
* Burns complicated by an extremity injury such as a fracture
* Moderate burns in young children or elderly patients
* Circumferential burns to the arm, leg, or chest

MEDIUM PRIORITY (MODERATE)

* Full-thickness burns affecting 2 to 10 percent of BSA excluding hands, feet, face, genitalia, and upper airway
* Partial-thickness burns affecting 15 to 30 percent of BSA
* Superficial burns affecting more than 50 percent of BSA

LOW PRIORITY (MILD)

* Full-thickness burns affecting less than 2 percent of BSA
* Partial-thickness burns affecting less than 15 percent of BSA
* Superficial burns affecting less than 50 percent of BSA

FIGURE 30-13 Active fire is a serious risk to rescuers. (Getty Images, Inc. Photodisc.)

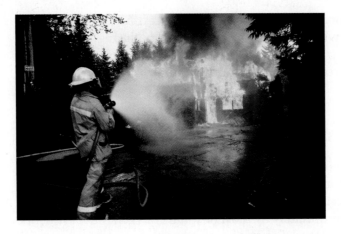

5-2.24 Establish the relationship between airway management and the patient with chest injury, burns, blunt and penetrating injuries.

put yourself at unreasonable risk to accomplish this. Be aware that metal objects such as jewelry, belt buckles, and buttons may remain hot and continue to burn soft tissue long after the heat source has been eliminated. These objects may also pose a hazard to the rescuer. In most instances involving thermal or chemical burns, water can be used to stop the burning process.

INITIAL ASSESSMENT

Once you have determined that the scene is safe and the burning process has been stopped, approach the patient and begin the initial assessment. It may be appropriate to continue cooling the patient as you complete your assessment. If possible, use additional rescuers for this purpose. Your assessment should focus on the patient's airway and ability to breathe adequately. Carefully assess the nose and mouth for evidence of soot or singed hair. This may be an indication that the patient has inhaled super-heated air that may cause swelling of the airway. A hoarse-sounding voice and coughing may also be an indication of a burned airway. A patient who dies early as a result of a burn mechanism does so because of airway swelling and compromise. Do not let the presence of severe burns distract you from managing the patient's ABCs.

Complete the initial assessment by confirming the presence of an adequate pulse and initiating high-flow oxygen by nonrebreather mask. Using the criteria introduced in the previous section, you must make a decision regarding priority for transport.

FOCUSED HISTORY AND PHYSICAL EXAM

Once you have completed your initial assessment and managed any immediate issues relating to the ABCs, complete an appropriate history and physical exam. As with any victim of trauma the specific assessment path you take will depend on the significance of the burns (mechanism of injury). Any patient suffering moderate to severe burns should receive a rapid trauma assessment. Patients with mild burns will receive a focused trauma assessment. When deciding which assessment path is most appropriate, you must consider all aspects of the patient's condition and not only the burns.

Take time during transport to expose as much of the patient as possible and reassess the extent and depth of the burns. When appropriate, based on the patient's condition, obtain a thorough medical history. As you learned above, preexisting medical conditions can be made worse by the trauma of a burn injury.

Remember that infection will be a serious concern during the healing process. Use appropriate BSI precautions and sterile dressings whenever possible.

Care of the Burn Patient

Emergency care for the burn patient is not unlike most care for victims of trauma (Scan 30-1 on page 766). In the case of the burn patient, it is important to confirm that all burning has stopped before beginning emergency care. Once the burning has stopped, complete the following steps:

1. Assure the scene is safe to enter.

2. Take appropriate BSI precautions.

3. Perform an appropriate initial assessment and initiate oxygen therapy.

4. Carefully extinguish and remove smoldering clothing and hot metallic items.

5. Assess burned areas for estimate of BSA affected and depth of injury.

6. Cover burned areas with dry sterile dressings to minimize contamination and minimize heat loss. Some EMS systems recommend moistening the dressings with saline if less than 10 percent BSA.

7. Perform an appropriate history and physical exam.

8. Continually monitor the airway for evidence of compromise.

9. Transport to an appropriate receiving facility.

5-2.18 Describe the emergency medical care of the patient with a superficial burn.

5-2.19 Describe the emergency medical care of the patient with a partial thickness burn.

5-2.20 Describe the emergency medical care of the patient with a full thickness burn.

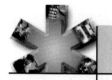

Perspective

Shane—The EMT

"One positive thing that this guy had going for him was where he lived. His house is literally 6 miles from Baptist Hospital, which is the top burn center in the entire state. We notified them that we were en route, and by the time we wheeled him through the doors, there was this team of people that just descended on him. It was actually pretty amazing to watch. I just hope it'll make a difference."

There are several things that should be mentioned as "what not to do" when caring for burns. Despite the fact that some of these have been home remedies handed down from generation to generation, they have no place in prehospital care.

* DO NOT use any type of burn cream, ointment, lotion, or antiseptic on a new burn. These items serve as insulators and cause heat to be retained in the wound, potentially making the burn worse.

* DO NOT intentionally break blisters that may have formed over a burn. Doing so only creates an open wound and greatly increases the risk of infection.

* If possible, avoid the use of a dry chemical or CO_2 fire extinguisher directly on the patient. Both can further worsen soft-tissue injury.

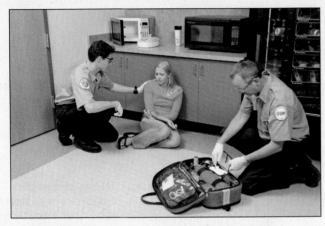

▲ Assure the scene is safe to enter and take BSI precautions.

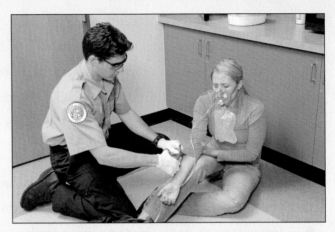

▲ Place the patient on oxygen while your partner cuts away the clothing around the burn.

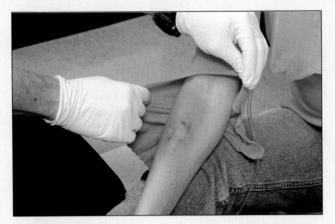

▲ Expose the burned area.

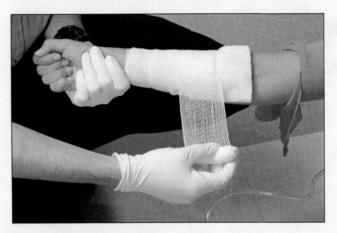

▲ Cover the burns with sterile dressings.

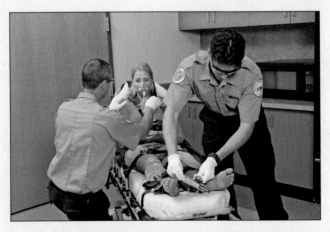

▲ Load the patient onto the stretcher and prepare for transport.

The care of burns, especially severe burns, is a highly specialized skill. One of the best things you can do for your patient is to know the capabilities of the resources within your EMS system to care for burns. Become familiar with the local protocols for the treatment of burn patients and where the nearest specialty burn center is located.

Special Considerations

Certain types of burns require special consideration as they may present unique hazards to both the rescuer and the patient if not cared for properly. Two examples are burns caused by chemicals and burns caused by electricity.

CHEMICAL BURNS

Caring for a patient who has suffered burns from some type of chemical almost certainly presents a hazard to the rescuers who will be providing care (Figures 30-14A and B). Even if the source of exposure has been controlled, there will likely be some residual chemical on the patient that may pose a risk to the EMT. Be sure to conduct a careful and thorough scene size-up before entering the scene and call for additional resources, such as a hazmat team, if necessary.

NOTE: *The typical BSI used by most EMTs may not be adequate when caring for the victim of a chemical burn. If you are not certain, call for additional resources.*

You will certainly want to wear appropriate gloves and eye protection, at a minimum, and you may want to consider donning a protective gown as well. A face mask or even self-contained breathing apparatus may also be appropriate if the source chemical is in a powder form.

Follow these simple guidelines when caring for patients who have been exposed to dangerous chemicals:

* Unless the skin was moist at the time of exposure, dry powders should be carefully brushed off the skin prior to flushing with water.

* When you are able, immediately begin flushing the affected areas with clean water and continue flushing during transport.

* When flushing, be careful not to let the runoff contaminate other areas of the body.

5-2.28 Describe the emergency care for a chemical burn.

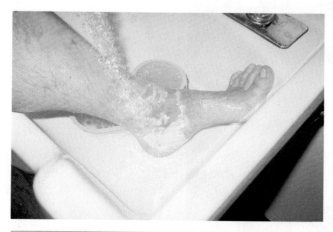

FIGURE 30-14A   An acid burn of the ankle. (Roy Alson, M.D., FACEP)

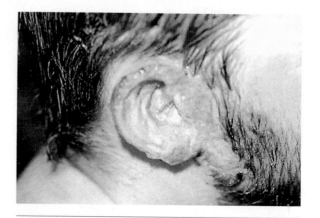

FIGURE 30-14B   A chemical burn to the ear.

✳ If possible, have the patient remove contaminated clothing to minimize the risk of continued contact with the chemical as well as the risk of rescuer exposure.

ELECTRICAL BURNS

5-2.29 Describe the emergency care for an electrical burn.

One of the most dangerous characteristics of electricity is its invisibility. You cannot see the very thing that has injured the patient, and therefore it is a significant risk to rescuers on the scene. When approaching the scene, you and your partner must look up, down, and all around for any evidence of an electrical source. Downed high-power electrical lines can jump around on the ground. Stay well clear of them at all times. Electricity can also jump a considerable distance as it seeks to find a ground. Keeping a safe distance from any electrical source is your best defense. DO NOT attempt to approach or touch a patient until you are absolutely certain that the electrical source has been shut off. In most instances involving high power lines, you must wait for the utility company to shut off the power before you can approach the patient.

Follow these additional guidelines when caring for patients with electrical injuries:

✳ Monitor the patient's respiratory and circulatory status closely. Depending on the path the electricity takes through the body, it can cause either respiratory or cardiac arrest and in some cases both.

✳ In the majority of cases most of the damage is internal, along the path the electricity took as it passed through the body. There may be little or no evidence of injury on the outside.

✳ Some electrical injuries will have an entrance and an exit wound. A thorough assessment should be conducted on all victims of electrical injuries, looking for these wounds.

✳ There may be little or no bleeding at the site of entrance and exit wounds; however they should be cared for, just as for any open soft-tissue injury (Figure 30-15).

✳ **circumferential burns**

burns that completely surround a body part such as a finger, arm, leg, and even the chest.

CIRCUMFERENTIAL BURNS

Circumferential burns are burns that completely surround a body part such as a finger, arm, leg, and even the chest (Figure 30-16). Burns that completely encircle

FIGURE 30-15   An electrical burn to the hand. (Edward T. Dickinson, M.D.)

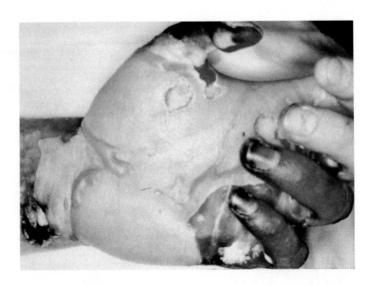

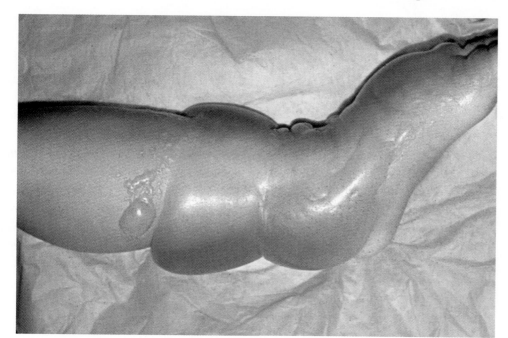

FIGURE 30-16 A circumferential burn. (Trauma Slide Series, Brent Q. Hafen and Keith J. Karren.)

a part of the body can cause swelling, especially with partial- and full-thickness burns. This swelling can cause pressure similar to that of a tourniquet and restrict blood flow to an extremity. Circumferential burns that affect the chest can severely restrict a patient's ability to breathe adequately. The presence of circumferential burns will not necessarily change the way that you care for the patient, but they will make the patient a high priority for transport.

BURNS TO THE HANDS AND FEET

Special care should be provided when caring for burns to the hand and feet. Be sure to remove any jewelry, such as rings and bracelets, that may restrict blood flow should the area become swollen. When bandaging burns to the hands and feet, place sterile dressings between each of the digits before covering the entire area with dressings and bandage (Figures 30-17A–C).

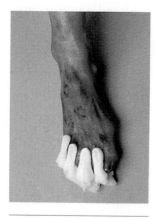

FIGURE 30-17A Separate burned toes with dry sterile gauze.

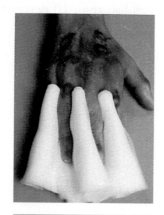

FIGURE 30-17B Separate burned fingers with dry sterile gauze.

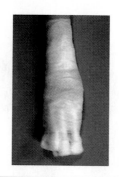

FIGURE 30-17C Cover the burned fingers or toes completely with dry sterile dressings and bandage.

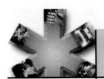

Perspective

Brianna—The EMT

"So as soon as the doctor intubated that guy he shouts that he needs a scalpel and then just sliced right down his chest from his arm pits to the bottom of his ribs. Oh man, that was nasty! I turned to this nurse I know and asked why he did that. She tells me that the guy had a circumferential burn of the chest and the doctor had to reduce the pressure around the chest so he could effectively ventilate the patient. I'm sorry for this man, and I hope never to be burned; I truly think that's got to be the worst."

Pediatric Considerations

Infants and children are particularly susceptible to the affects of burns, even mild burns (Figure 30-18). Due to their greater skin surface area relative to their overall size, they are much more prone to the affects of heat loss and fluid loss. This makes them more susceptible to hypothermia and shock. Burns are also a common form of abuse by adults, and you should always be alert for signs of neglect and abuse when caring for children suffering from burns.

Consider the following guidelines when caring for a pediatric patient with burns:

✳ Any full- or partial-thickness burn greater than 20 percent is considered critical.

✳ Any partial-thickness burn involving the hands, feet, face, airway, or genitalia must be seen by a physician.

✳ Any partial-thickness burn of 10 to 20 percent is considered a moderate burn in a child.

✳ Any partial-thickness burn less than 10 percent is considered a minor burn in a child.

FIGURE 30-18 A pediatric patient with superficial burns.

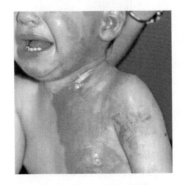

Stop, Review, Remember!

Multiple Choice

Place a check next to the correct answer.

1. A burn affecting the entire right arm and the anterior torso of an adult patient would amount to an approximate BSA of:

   _____ a. 12.5 percent.

   _____ b. 18 percent.

   _____ c. 22.5 percent.

   _____ d. 27 percent.

2. Which of the following is NOT routinely considered a special critical area for burns?

   _____ a. face

   _____ b. hands

   _____ c. chest

   _____ d. genitals

3. Which of the following best describes the appropriate priorities when caring for a burn patient?

   _____ a. ABCs, stop the burning, cover wounds, transport

   _____ b. ABCs, cover wounds, stop the burning, transport

   _____ c. stop the burning, cover wounds, ABCs, transport

   _____ d. stop the burning, ABCs, cover wounds, transport

4. Which of the following would be considered the highest priority for care and transport?

   _____ a. partial-thickness burns affecting more than 30 percent of BSA

   _____ b. full-thickness burns affecting 2 to 10 percent of BSA

   _____ c. partial-thickness burns affecting 15 to 30 percent of BSA

   _____ d. superficial burns of affecting more than 50 percent of BSA

5. Which of the following most accurately represents the amount of BSA affected in a pediatric patient with burns to the front of one leg, the entire back, and half of one arm?

   _____ a. 14 percent

   _____ b. 25 percent

   _____ c. 29.5 percent

   _____ d. 33 percent

Matching

Match the term on the left with the applicable definition on the right.

1._____ Depth of injury

2._____ Rule of Nines

3._____ High priority

4._____ Medium priority

5._____ Low priority

A. Partial-thickness burns affecting less than 15 percent BSA

B. Full-thickness burns involving the hands, feet or genitalia

C. The method used to classify burns.

D. Common method used to estimate body surface area

E. Partial-thickness burns affecting 15 to 30 percent BSA

Critical Thinking

1. List the six factors that must be assessed when determining the overall condition of a burn patient.

_____

_____

_____

_____

2. Describe the role that each of the above factors plays in determining the overall condition of the patient.

_____

_____

_____

_____

3. Identify at least two potential hazards that may exist at the scene of a burn patient and how you might mitigate those hazards before caring for the patient.

_____

_____

_____

_____

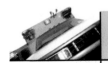

Dispatch Summary

The patient, who remained conscious and able to maintain his own airway, was transported on high-flow oxygen via a nonrebreather mask and admitted to the Baptist Hospital Burn Center. He died 4 days later due to complications from airway burns and injury to his lungs from inhaling superheated smoke and gases.

The incident has been added as a case study to the ambulance company's continuing education program.

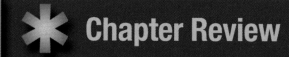 The Last Word

Responding to the scene of a burn patient can present a variety of risks to the EMT. Be extra cautious and perform a thorough scene size-up prior to making patient contact.

In most cases, the burn patient who is critical will need airway and ventilatory care on the scene and en route to the hospital. Do not let the sight of severe burns distract you from the ABCs.

Infection is a major concern with burn patients. Whenever possible use sterile dressings and sterile saline when caring for burns.

Know the capabilities of the receiving hospitals in your area and the location of the nearest specialty burn center. When in doubt, contact medical direction for transport instructions. Always document all appropriate information in your PCR.

* Chapter Review

MULTIPLE CHOICE

Place a check next to the correct answer.

1. Thermal burns are most commonly classified by:

　_____ a. open or closed injury.

　_____ b. cause of injury.

　_____ c. depth of injury.

　_____ d. degree.

2. A superficial burn is best described as a burn that affects the:

　_____ a. epidermis only.

　_____ b. dermis.

　_____ c. subcutaneous layers.

　_____ d. epidural.

3. Superficial burns are characterized by:

　_____ a. dark charred skin.

　_____ b. a leathery appearance.

　_____ c. blisters.

　_____ d. redness and pain.

4. A partial-thickness burn is best described as a burn that affects the:

　_____ a. epidermis only.

　_____ b. dermis.

　_____ c. subcutaneous layers.

　_____ d. epidural.

5. Partial-thickness burns are characterized by:

　_____ a. dark charred skin.

　_____ b. a leathery appearance.

　_____ c. blisters.

　_____ d. redness and pain.

6. A full-thickness burn is best described as a burn that affects the:

　_____ a. epidermis only.

　_____ b. dermis.

　_____ c. subcutaneous layers.

　_____ d. epidural.

7. Full-thickness burns are characterized by:

_____ a. dark or brown charred skin.

_____ b. a mottled appearance.

_____ c. blisters.

_____ d. redness and pain.

8. Care for most chemical burns should include:

_____ a. flushing the area with water.

_____ b. flushing the area with lemon juice.

_____ c. wrapping the area with moist dressings.

_____ d. covering the area with nonsterile dressings.

9. Circumferential burns are burns that:

_____ a. cover the anterior chest.

_____ b. affect the face.

_____ c. involve a foot.

_____ d. encircle a body part.

10. An adult patient who has suffered burns to an entire right arm would have what approximate BSA affected?

_____ a. 4.5 percent

_____ b. 9 percent

_____ c. 13.5 percent

_____ d. 8 percent

MATCHING

Match the term on the left with the applicable definition on the right.

1. _____ Thermal burn

2. _____ Chemical burn

3. _____ Electrical burn

4. _____ Radiation burn

5. _____ Light burn

A. Burns caused when the skin is exposed to substances such as acids, bases, and caustics

B. Burns caused by exposure to fire, steam, hot objects, and hot liquids

C. Burns from sources such as nuclear fallout

D. High-intensity lasers and welders are common sources of these types of burns

E. When the body becomes exposed to an electrical current that passes through the body

CRITICAL THINKING

1. Describe how you would care for a patient with full-thickness burns to both hands and arms.

_____

_____

_____

_____

2. Explain the complications caused by a circumferential burn to the chest or one of the extremities.

_____

_____

_____

_____

CASE STUDIES

Case Study 1

You have responded to a residence for a burn victim. Upon arrival you are met by a family member and directed to the backyard. There you find an approximately 11-year-old boy lying on the ground with his arms and face over the edge of a pool. His mother tells you that he was attempting to light the barbecue when the can of fluid exploded in his hands. You observe what appear to be both partial-thickness and some full-thickness burns to the entire hand and forearm of both arms. You also observe some redness and swelling to his face.

1. What would you estimate the affected BSA to be for this boy?

   _____

   _____

   _____

2. Describe how you will bandage this boy's injuries.

   _____

   _____

   _____

3. What complications could arise as a result of the burns to this boy's face?

   _____

   _____

   _____

Case Study 2

Using the "rule of nines," estimate the BSA affected for each of the following patients.

1. A 55-year-old male with burns over the fronts of both legs and half of his anterior torso.

   _____

   _____

   _____

2. A 4-year-old female with burns over her entire head and entire right arm.

   _____

   _____

   _____

3. A 3-month-old infant with burns over the entire back and the backs of both arms.

   _____

   _____

   _____

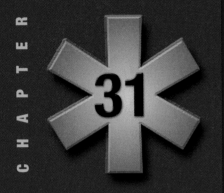

Patients with Injuries to the Chest and Abdomen

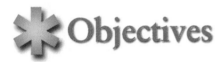 Objectives

Numbered objectives are from the U.S. Department of Transportation 1994 EMT-Basic National Standard Curriculum.

COGNITIVE OBJECTIVES

At the completion of this lesson, the EMT-Basic student will be able to:

5-2.8 Discuss the emergency medical care considerations for a patient with a penetrating chest injury. (pp. 782–785)

5-2.9 State the emergency medical care considerations for a patient with an open wound to the abdomen. (pp. 789–791)

5-2.10 Differentiate the care of an open wound to the chest from an open wound to the abdomen. (pp. 789–791)

5-2.24 Establish the relationship between airway management and the patient with chest injury, burns, blunt and penetrating injuries. (p. 777)

AFFECTIVE OBJECTIVES

No affective objectives identified.

PSYCHOMOTOR OBJECTIVES

At the completion of this lesson, the EMT-Basic student will be able to:

5-2.31 Demonstrate the steps in the emergency medical care of a patient with an open chest wound. (pp. 783–785)

5-2.32 Demonstrate the steps in the emergency medical care of a patient with open abdominal wounds. (pp. 789–791)

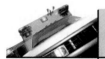 Introduction

Injuries to the chest and abdomen are presented in this separate chapter because they have particular potential to be very serious. This potential arises from the many vital organs and structures that lie within the body and can be damaged from these types of injuries. Your prompt identification and treatment of injuries to the chest and abdomen will be crucial to your patient's survival.

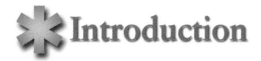

Emergency Dispatch

"You know," EMT Roger Adams sighed and looked over at his new partner, "we're due for either a good trauma call or a full arrest."

Erica stopped picking the lettuce out of her sandwich and looked back at him. "How do you know that?" she asked.

He shrugged and looked up into the overcast sky. "It's just in the air. Maybe after you've done this job long enough you just feel when you're up for a big call."

Erica stared at her partner for a long moment and then laughed. "Yeah. . . okay. . . sure thing."

Roger smiled and returned to the continuing-education article he was reading.

"Unit 9," the radio blared a few minutes later. "Start, code 3, to 1588 Oak Tower Boulevard for a stabbing. This was called in by P.D. and the scene is secure."

"I don't even want to know how you did that," Erica said as she climbed in the cab, fastened her seat belt, and started the truck. Roger just smiled and flipped the emergency lights on.

The patient was a 26-year-old female police officer who had been helping to break up a fight when one of the combatants stabbed her with a folding knife.

"It's in the side. . . of my chest. . . right there next to the edge of the vest." The officer grimaced as she pointed with bloody fingers at the hole in her uniform.

Roger cut the dark fabric of the officer's shirt, careful to avoid cutting through the hole, and pulled it aside.

"Hey, Erica," Roger said calmly as he placed his gloved hand over the bubbling wound. "Grab me an occlusive dressing and some tape real quick. . . and call for an ALS unit. And could you open a nonrebreather before you go?"

Chest Injuries

Due to the proximity to vital organs and major blood vessels, all injuries to the chest should be considered serious and treated accordingly. Injuries to the chest can occur from many types of blunt and penetrating mechanisms, resulting in both open and closed injuries.

Since injury to the chest has the potential to disrupt so many vital organs in both the respiratory and circulatory systems, prompt and efficient airway care, including suction and supplemental oxygenation, are critical.

5-2.24 Establish the relationship between airway management and the patient with chest injury, burns, blunt and penetrating injuries.

ANATOMY AND PHYSIOLOGY

* **thoracic cavity**

the area that lies inferior to the clavicles and superior to the diaphragm.

The chest, or **thoracic cavity**, comprises roughly the upper half of the torso. The thoracic cavity (Figure 31-1) is an area that lies inferior to the clavicles and superior to the diaphragm. The anterior of the upper torso (commonly called the chest) and posterior portion of the upper torso (commonly called the back) are the exterior walls of the thoracic cavity. The contents of the thoracic cavity are protected by the twelve pairs of ribs, the sternum, and the spine.

Since the diaphragm moves with each breath, the boundaries of the chest cavity change accordingly. During a deep exhalation, the diaphragm rises to about nipple-level (the fourth or fifth rib). This means that open wounds to the area of the fourth to tenth ribs may be either chest wounds, abdominal wounds, or both—depending on when the wound occurred in the respiratory cycle.

* **pleura**

two tissue layers that line the chest wall and cover the lungs.

The thoracic cavity is lined with two layers called **pleura.** The parietal pleura lines the chest wall while the visceral pleura lines the lungs. There is a very small space between the pleura that contains fluid. This fluid lubricates the layers to reduce friction during breathing. These pleural layers are critical for maintaining the pressure within the chest.

An example of the relationship between the pleural layers can be seen with a drinking glass on a table. If the table is dry, the glass can be easily picked up. If the table is wet, the glass will stick to the table a bit. It will feel as if there is some suction holding it to the table. This is similar to the relationship of the pleura and the fluid between them.

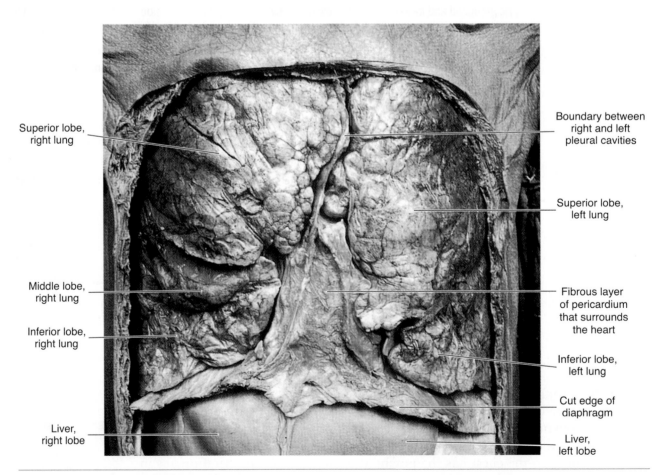

Superior lobe, right lung

Middle lobe, right lung

Inferior lobe, right lung

Liver, right lobe

Boundary between right and left pleural cavities

Superior lobe, left lung

Fibrous layer of pericardium that surrounds the heart

Inferior lobe, left lung

Cut edge of diaphragm

Liver, left lobe

FIGURE 31-1 The anatomy of thoracic cavity.

When the chest wall expands, the pleura move with it, which expands the lungs. If a patient experiences an open chest wound, air is allowed to enter that small pleural space. This prevents expansion of the lung and leads to a collapse of the lung, which will be discussed in more detail later in the chapter.

Within the thoracic cavity are portions of the trachea, the lungs and bronchi, the heart, and the great vessels, which are the aorta and the superior and inferior venae cavae. The heart is covered by a fibrous sac called the pericardium. Damage to any of these key respiratory and circulatory structures can have grave consequences.

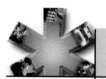

Perspective

Officer Janine Colcord—The Patient

"I can't believe that guy stabbed me! All I was doing was backing up another officer and trying to stop a fight. I mean, where does he get off? And I knew I was bleeding pretty good, but it never even occurred to me that the knife actually went that far into my chest. I'm serious! My first thought, when I found out how bad it was, was 'where's that knife been?' You know? What weird germs or diseases did he just stick in me? That's really messed up!"

Closed Chest Injuries

Closed chest injuries are usually the result of blunt trauma, such as from a fall or a vehicle collision. With enough force, blunt trauma can cause major damage to the organs and vessels of the chest. It is important to thoroughly palpate all areas of the chest for tenderness and deformity.

Chest injuries may be relatively superficial or more serious, involving the organs and structures underneath. Even minor injuries can have serious consequences. For example, bruising can cause pain that prevents a patient from taking a deep breath. This can cause hypoxia in the early stages. A lung that does not expand normally with each breath can eventually develop **pneumonia**, or infection of the lung tissue.

Rib fracture is most commonly caused by blunt trauma. Every rib is connected posteriorly to a thoracic vertebra. The first ten pairs of ribs are connected anteriorly to the sternum, either directly or by cartilage. The last two pairs are called **floating ribs** because they are connected to vertebrae but not to the sternum. Ribs that are connected anteriorly to the sternum are more likely to fracture.

Signs and symptoms of rib fracture include:

* pain made worse by breathing

* deformity

* crepitus

* **pneumonia**
  infection of the lung.

* **rib fracture**
  any break in a rib.

* **floating ribs**
  the two ribs that are connected to vertebrae but not to the sternum.

✳ **flail chest**

  two or more ribs broken in two or more places.

✳ **paradoxical motion**

  movement of a flail segment opposite to the motion of the nonfractured ribs.

✳ **pneumothorax**

  air within the pleural space.

✳ **tension pneumothorax**

  buildup of air under pressure within the thorax. The resulting compression of the lung severely reduces the effectiveness of respirations.

✳ **hemothorax**

  blood within the pleural space.

✳ **spontaneous pneumothorax**

  condition where a pneumothorax develops without a traumatic cause.

✳ **traumatic asphyxia**

  condition where a severe blunt force or weight is placed upon the chest forcing blood from the right atrium up into the circulation of the head and neck.

✳ tenderness to palpation

✳ a mechanism of injury likely to cause the injury

An area of the chest that has sustained two or more ribs broken in two or more places is called a **flail chest** (Figure 31-2). This area of the chest will be very painful and may feel soft or spongy when palpated. Some cases of flail chest may present with **paradoxical motion** of the chest wall and ribs. This means that the flail segment will move in the opposite direction to the motion of the nonfractured ribs. Paradoxical motion is sometimes a late sign. In early stages of the injury, the muscles of the chest wall will contract, creating a splint-like effect, limiting this motion. When the muscles tire, the paradoxical motion will be more noticeable.

Injuries to the chest wall can also cause injuries to the organs underneath. Broken ribs may lacerate or puncture chest or abdominal organs, causing internal bleeding or escape of air from the lungs into the pleural space called **pneumothorax** (*pneumo* referring to air or gas and *thorax* referring to the chest cavity), **tension pneumothorax**, or **hemothorax** (*hemo* referring to blood) (Figure 31-3).

A **spontaneous pneumothorax** is a condition where a pneumothorax develops without a traumatic cause. This can happen when a disease such as COPD has damaged the lung or in some cases without an obvious cause. This happens with some frequency in tall, thin individuals during exertion, such as running. These patients often present with a sudden onset of one-sided sharp chest pain and increasing shortness of breath.

Traumatic asphyxia (Figure 31-4) is a condition where a severe blunt compressive force or weight is placed upon the chest, forcing blood from the right atrium up into the circulation of the head and neck. In this type of injury, you will often see bulging neck veins, dark red or purple discoloration of the head and neck, swelling and discoloration of the lips and tongue, deformity of the chest, and bulging eyes. Respiratory and/or cardiac arrest often develops.

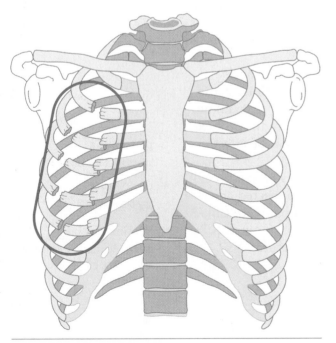

FIGURE 31-2 Flail segment occurs when blunt trauma causes fracture of two or more ribs, each in two or more places.

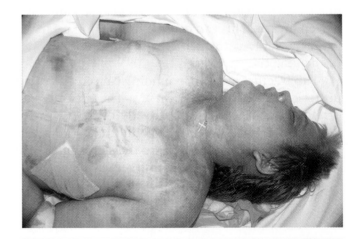

FIGURE 31-3 A patient suffering from traumatic asphyxia.

HEMOTHORAX

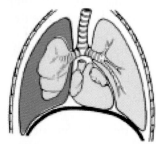

Blood leaks into the chest cavity from lacerated vessels or the lung itself and the lung compresses.

PNEUMOTHORAX

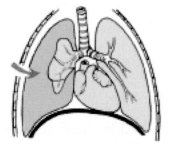

Air enters the chest cavity through a sucking wound or leaks from a lacerated lung. The lung cannot expand.

SPONTANEOUS PNEUMOTHORAX

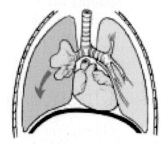

Air leaks into the chest from a weak area in the (nontrauma) lung surface and the lung collapses.

HEMOPNEUMOTHORAX

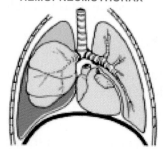

Air and blood leak into the chest cavity from an injured lung putting pressure on the heart and uninjured lung.

TENSION PNEUMOTHORAX

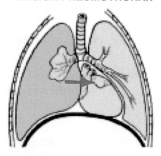

Air continuously leaks out the lung. It collapses, pressure rises, and the collapsed lung is forced against the heart and other lung.

MEDIASTINAL SHIFT

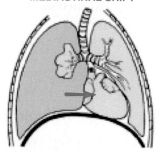

Shifting of the internal chest structures away from the tension pneumothorax.

FIGURE 31-4   Complications of chest injury. (Charles Stewart, M.D., and Associates.)

EMERGENCY CARE

As part of the initial assessment, stabilize the cervical spine and prevent movement of the head, neck, and spine when chest injury is indicated by the mechanism of injury or complaints of pain. Administer oxygen via nonrebreather mask.

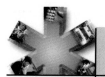

Perspective

Roger—The EMT

"I've only run across a handful of sucking chest wounds like that in my career . . . and it's the only type of trauma that gets to me. I mean, give me amputations, crush injuries, whatever, and I'm fine. But there's something about the sound of the air bubbling out of the chest that I just—oh I just hate it, you know? Maybe it's just me. At least that cop was relatively cool about the whole thing!"

If the patient is responsive, identify the specific injury site by questioning the patient and by palpation. Attempt to splint the injury site by placing a large trauma dressing, folded towels, or a blanket firmly over the site. This will help splint the injury, thereby reducing the pain and allowing the patient to breathe more easily.

5-2.8 Discuss the emergency medical care considerations for a patient with a penetrating chest injury.

* **pleural space**

potential space between the two tissue layers that line the chest wall and cover the lungs.

Open Chest Injuries

Open chest injuries are caused by penetration, as from a knife, a bullet, or any mechanism that pierces the chest wall.

Open chest injuries frequently allow air to enter the **pleural space** around the lung, causing one or more lobes of a lung to collapse. This condition is known as a pneumothorax, as discussed earlier for closed chest injuries. With a penetrating injury, air enters the chest through the open wound during inhalation. This becomes a serious problem when the air entering the chest cavity is not able to escape.

Signs and symptoms of open chest wounds include:

* An open wound to the anterior, posterior, or lateral area of the chest wall. Some of these wounds may bubble or make a sucking noise.

* Difficulty breathing

* Signs of shock, including rapid pulse and respirations, restlessness and anxiety, and decreased blood pressure (late sign)

* A narrowing pulse pressure (the difference between the systolic and diastolic blood pressures)

* Diminished or absent breath sounds over one or more areas of the chest

When enough air has entered the chest cavity and is unable to escape, it causes pressure inside the chest. This buildup of pressure is called a tension pneumothorax and, if left untreated, can cause pressure on the heart and great vessels, compression of the opposite lung, and eventually death.

When trauma to the chest wall or lungs themselves causes bleeding, a certain amount of this blood enters the pleural space. The resulting hemothorax will cause respiratory distress.

In each of these cases, you may auscultate the chest and note absent breath sounds in one or more areas of the lungs. In smaller pneumothoraces, air accu-

---

Clinical Clues: **TENSION PNEUMOTHORAX**

Monitor all patients with open chest injuries very carefully for adequacy of respiratory rate and tidal volume. Just because you have an occlusive dressing in place does not mean pressure cannot build inside the chest. If the patient's respiratory status becomes worse, consider removing the occlusive dressing temporarily to allow pressure to escape. You may have inadvertently induced a tension pneumothorax by sealing the wound. Lift the dressing briefly as the patient breathes out, then place it back down as he begins to inhale. Try this a few times to see if air escapes from the wound.

mulation is seen first in the upper areas of the lungs. The periphery and bases fill next. The center of the lung is the last to be affected. Auscultation will provide some information, but the clinical picture of the patient (respiratory distress, shock, and so on) is the best indicator of serious internal thoracic injury.

The chest cavity can hold several liters of blood. It is possible to bleed to death from internal injuries to the chest without ever losing a drop of blood externally or from any other internal sources.

Often caused by open chest injuries such as knife and gunshot wounds and impaled objects, patients may also experience a condition called **pericardial tamponade** (Figure 31-5). This blood compresses the heart and prevents blood from filling the heart's chambers and, as a result, reduces cardiac output.

* **pericardial tamponade**
collection of blood in the sac surrounding the heart.

EMERGENCY CARE

Open wounds to the chest must be considered life threatening and cared for promptly, along with rapid transport, as detailed in the following section.

Occlusive Dressings Occlusive dressings are dressings that do not allow air to pass through them. Commercially available occlusive dressings are nothing more than pieces of tightly knit sterile gauze that have been saturated with petroleum-based ointment such as petroleum jelly. Other impervious items, such as a rubber glove or plastic bag, can also be used as occlusive dressings.

Trauma to the chest can induce three types of cardiac injury. Determining the nature of the injury is difficult and emergency care in the field is frequently limited to support of vital functions.

FIGURE 31-5 Examples of traumatic cardiac injuries.

	SIGNS AND SYMPTOMS
Cardiac Contusion	Injury to chest Bruising of chest wall Weakness, rapid heart rate — may be irregular Possible sweating Severe nagging pain not relieved with rest but may be relieved with oxygen Usually the result of blunt trauma
Penetrating Wound in Heart	In most cases, patient has a visible chest wound, caused by object like knife or bullet However, heart penetration can occur from bullet entering abdomen or back Chest pain, bleeding Drowsiness, loss of consciouness, possible agitation, combativeness, or confusion (Note: patient may appear intoxicated) Distended neck veins, although these may not be present immediately Pneumothorax or hemothorax (may not develop until several hours after the injury) Shock (hypoperfusion)
Pericardial Tamponade	Cardiac contusion, blunt trauma to anterior chest, penetrating chest wound, or recent cardiac surgery Tamponade may also follow CPR Dyspnea and possible cyanosis Neck vein distention Weak, thready pulse Decreasing blood pressure Shock (hypoperfusion) Narrowing pulse pressure

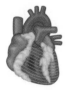
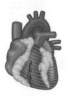

FIGURE 31-6 Seal three edges of an occlusive dressing for an open chest wound.

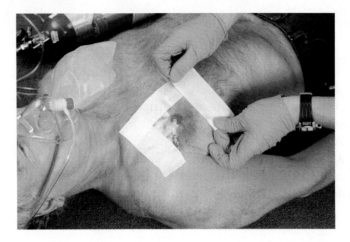

To place an occlusive dressing, follow these steps:

1. Select a commercially available occlusive dressing or other clean, impervious item.

2. If the patient is responsive, ask him to cough. At the end of the cough place the occlusive dressing over the wound.

3. Tape the dressing on three sides (Figure 31-6). The untaped side will seal shut during inhalation but will open and allow air to escape during exhalation.

If blood builds up under the dressing, it may prevent escape of air and increase the chance of tension pneumothorax. If this happens, remove the dressing, clean the blood from the injury site, and reapply the dressing.

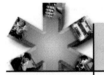

Perspective

Erica—The EMT

"It's kind of funny how you fall back on your training in stressful situations! I'd never seen a stabbing or sucking chest wound before, but I immediately thought, 'Okay, she's got an airway and is breathing because her breaths are still deep—and she's talking to Roger, and she's obviously got circulation because she's, well, she's bleeding.' I kept hearing Mr. Jenkins, my EMT teacher, saying, 'Stop that leak!' over and over in my head. We had to seal that hole in the chest. By the time Roger asked for the occlusive dressing, I already had it halfway out of the package! If you were watching me during that call, you'd have probably thought that I was an old pro! It's a good feeling to look back and know that you did everything just the way that you were taught to, and it actually worked!"

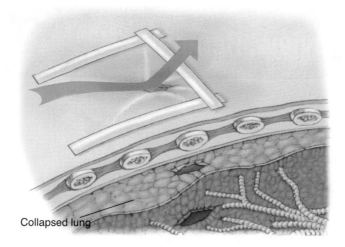

FIGURE 31-7A An occlusive dressing over a chest wound. When one side or one corner is left untaped, inhalation seals the dressing, preventing air entry.

Collapsed lung

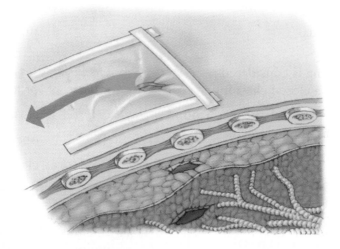

FIGURE 31-7B During exhalation, trapped air escapes through the untaped section of the dressing.

Clinical Clues: SEALING A CHEST WOUND

Seal any chest wound you believe may have penetrated into the thoracic cavity—whether it is actually bubbling or not.

Follow these steps when caring for an open chest injury:

1. Manage the ABCs as appropriate.

2. Cover the wound with an occlusive dressing that is sealed on three sides or, as permitted in some protocols, sealed on four sides with one corner left untaped to serve as a "flutter valve" (Figures 31-7A and B). If necessary, use a gloved hand to seal the wound until an appropriate occlusive dressing can be obtained. Make sure the dressing extends well beyond the wound on all sides and allows air to escape from the chest cavity. Follow local protocols regarding the use of occlusive dressings.

3. Initiate high-flow supplemental oxygen.

4. Treat for shock and transport immediately.

5. Initiate an ALS intercept if available.

Stop, Review, Remember!

Multiple Choice

Place a check next to the correct answer.

1. Which of the following is not located in the thoracic cavity?

   _____ a. larynx

   _____ b. bronchi

   _____ c. alveoli

   _____ d. mitral valve

2. Which of the following is considered appropriate care for a closed chest injury?

   _____ a. Wrap triangular bandages around the chest to splint fractured ribs.

   _____ b. Apply an occlusive dressing.

   _____ c. Splint suspected rib fractures with a bulky dressing such as a folded towel or blanket.

   _____ d. Apply oxygen via nasal cannula.

3. A common complication from an open chest injury is a(n):

   _____ a. evisceration.

   _____ b. perforated ulcer.

   _____ c. pneumothorax.

   _____ d. ruptured aorta.

4. Occlusive dressings taped on three sides are most appropriate for which type of injuries?

   _____ a. closed abdominal wounds

   _____ b. open abdominal wounds

   _____ c. closed chest wounds

   _____ d. open chest wounds

5. It is possible to bleed to death from a single, major injury to the thoracic cavity.

   _____ a. true

   _____ b. false

Matching

Match the condition on the left with the correct definition on the right.

1._____ Pneumothorax

2._____ Hemothorax

3._____ Tension pneumothorax

4._____ Pericardial tamponade

5._____ Flail chest

A. Collection of blood in the thoracic cavity

B. Two or more ribs broken in two or more places

C. Increasing pressure in the thoracic cavity placing pressure on lungs, the heart and great vessels

D. Air in the thoracic cavity

E. A collection of blood in the sac that surrounds the heart

F. Air in the heart and great vessels

Critical Thinking

1. Why does the paradoxical movement seen in flail chest exhibit late in the progression of the injury?

_____

_____

_____

_____

2. What are the differences in care between open and closed chest wounds?

_____

_____

_____

_____

3. Why is an occlusive dressing for an open chest wound sealed on only three sides?

_____

_____

_____

_____

Closed Wounds to the Abdomen

ANATOMY AND PHYSIOLOGY

The abdomen is divided into four quadrants (Figure 31-8 on page 788). The quadrants include the right and left upper quadrants and the right and left lower quadrants. This quadrant system provides a means to identify underlying organs as well as to describe the location of pain and injury.

When assessing the abdomen, note that the lower quadrants extend below the common waistline of most pants. Make sure you don't assess only what is visible, which can be a common error. An accurate and thorough inspection and palpation will involve the four full quadrants—not just what is visible above the clothes.

The organs included in the abdomen are the stomach, small intestine (comprised of the duodenum, ileum, and jejunum), the large intestine or colon, the liver, gallbladder, spleen, appendix, and pancreas. These organs are shown in Figure 31-9 on page 788 and discussed in greater detail in chapter 4.

FIGURE 31-8 The abdominal quadrants.

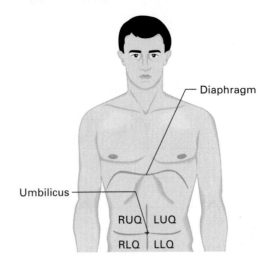

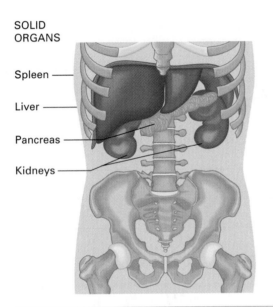

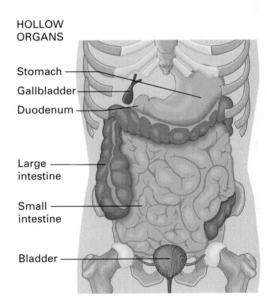

FIGURE 31-9 The structures and organs of the abdomen.

* **retroperitoneal**

  behind the abdominal cavity.

The organs of the abdomen are enclosed within the peritoneum that surrounds the abdominal cavity. Some organs are **retroperitoneal** or behind the abdominal cavity. Although commonly thought of as abdominal organs, the kidneys and portions of the aorta are actually outside the peritoneal space. This is one reason why illness and injury involving the kidneys or aorta often present with pain in the back or flanks.

Injuries to the abdomen can result in significant organ damage and massive internal bleeding. These injuries can be either open or closed, depending on the mechanism of injury.

Closed injuries to the abdomen most frequently result from blunt trauma. This can result from a force such as an assault (punch or strike with an object) or from a seatbelt in a motor vehicle collision.

PATIENT ASSESSMENT

Blunt abdominal trauma can cause considerable pain and may even cause difficulty breathing if the diaphragm is forced superiorly, "knocking the wind out" of the patient. Injuries may be severe if underlying organs are damaged.

If a solid organ, such as the liver, is damaged, internal bleeding can be severe. Hollow organs, such as the intestine, can rupture, spilling contents into the abdomen, causing irritation, pain, and eventual infection. Both solid and hollow organ injuries are serious.

Signs and symptoms of closed abdominal injuries include:

* Pain, spontaneously or on palpation

* Bruising, redness, or discoloration

* Swelling or distention

* Rigidity

* Referred pain to the area of the shoulder

* Signs and symptoms of shock, including rapid pulse and breathing, cool and clammy skin, restlessness or anxiety, and decreasing blood pressure (late sign)

EMERGENCY CARE

Care for closed abdominal injuries is largely supportive. A key element in care is determining if the signs and symptoms and mechanism of injury cause you to suspect serious injury and shock. If you suspect these serious injuries, care for shock and prompt transport to an appropriate facility are critical.

To care for the patient with a closed abdominal injury:

* Ensure the ABCs

* Take spinal precautions if there is a mechanism of injury that suggests spinal injuries are possible.

* If you do not suspect spine injury, place the patient in a position of comfort. This is commonly a recumbent or laterally recumbent position with the knees flexed.

* Administer high-flow oxygen by nonrebreather mask.

* Transport promptly.

Open Wounds to the Abdomen

You should treat a superficial open wound to the abdomen as you would any other open injury, including direct pressure with a sterile dressing to control bleeding. Some rare but serious injuries to the abdomen result in the protrusion of the intestinal organs through the abdominal wall. This is known as an **evisceration** and must be handled carefully to minimize further damage and infection. DO NOT attempt to insert protruding organs back into the abdomen. All eviscerations require prompt surgical intervention once the patient arrives at the hospital.

CARE FOR ABDOMINAL EVISCERATION

Follow these steps when caring for an abdominal evisceration (Scan 31-1 on page 790):

1. Manage the ABCs as appropriate.

2. Administer high-flow oxygen.

5-2.9 State the emergency medical care considerations for a patient with an open wound to the abdomen.

5-2.10 Differentiate the care of an open wound to the chest from an open wound to the abdomen.

* **evisceration**

   injury to the abdomen resulting in the protrusion of the intestinal organs through the abdominal wall.

✳ ✳

SCAN 31-1   **DRESSING AN OPEN ABDOMINAL WOUND**

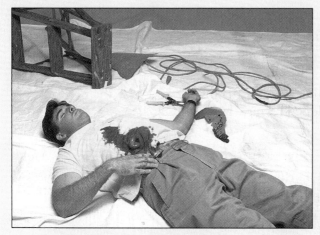

▲ An open abdominal wound with evisceration.

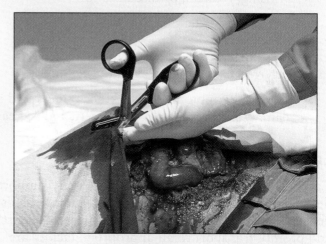

▲ Cut away clothing from wound.

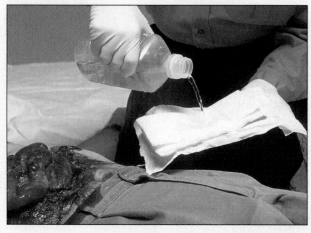

▲ Soak a dressing with sterile saline.

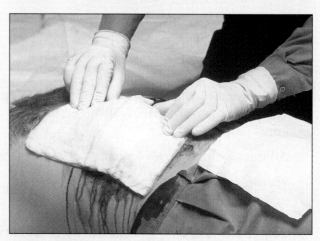

▲ Place the moist dressing over the wound.

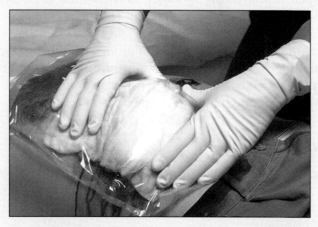

▲ Apply an occlusive dressing over the moist dressing if local protocols recommend that you do so.

3. Do not touch the protruding organs with your hands if it can be avoided. Do not attempt to reinsert the organs into the abdomen.

4. Protect the organs by covering them with a large sterile dressing moistened with sterile saline.

5. Place plastic over the moistened dressings to seal in the moisture.

6. Control external bleeding as appropriate.

7. If appropriate, place the patient in a supine position with the knees bent. This will reduce pressure on the abdominal muscles.

8. Care for shock and transport immediately.

9. Initiate an ALS intercept if available.

 Stop, Review, Remember!

Multiple Choice

Place a check next to the correct answer.

1. An open wound to the abdomen that results in the abdominal contents protruding through the wound is known as a(an):

   _____ a. pneumothorax.

   _____ b. hemothorax.

   _____ c. dissection.

   _____ d. evisceration.

2. Bleeding, open wounds to the abdomen that do not have organs protruding through can be cared for with:

   _____ a. elevation.

   _____ b. a pressure point.

   _____ c. a pressure dressing.

   _____ d. direct pressure.

3. The structure that separates the thoracic cavity from the abdomen is the:

   _____ a. lung.

   _____ b. heart.

   _____ c. diaphragm.

   _____ d. stomach.

4. The organs of the abdomen are enclosed in the:

   _____ a. pleura.

   _____ b. perineum.

   _____ c. peritoneum.

   _____ d. retroperitoneal space.

5. Injury to abdominal organs may present with pain in the shoulder.

   _____ a. true

   _____ b. false

6. The liver is a hollow organ.

   _____ a. true

   _____ b. false

7. You should only palpate areas of the abdomen above the waistline to protect patient privacy.

   _____ a. true

   _____ b. false

Matching

Using information for this chapter and chapter 4 if necessary match the abdominal organ on the left with the function on the right.

1._____ Stomach

2._____ Gall bladder

3._____ Liver

4._____ Pancreas

5._____ Spleen

6._____ Large intestine

7._____ Small intestine

8._____ Appendix

A. Stores bile and aids in fat digestion

B. Removes water from waste and moves waste to the rectum

C. Has no known function

D. Removes nutrients from waste

E. Detoxifies

F. Filters red blood cells

G. Secretes insulin

H. Collects food from the esophagus; acid-secreting organ

Critical Thinking

1. Why is there a difference in care between an open and closed abdominal wound?

   _____

   _____

   _____

   _____

2. For each of the following abdominal quadrants list an organ found within it:

   a. RUQ _____

   b. LUQ _____

   c. RLQ _____

   d. LLQ _____

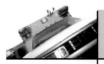

Dispatch Summary

The patient was placed on high-flow oxygen, properly packaged, and transported with lights and siren to the Central County Trauma Center. Erica was able to coordinate with the ALS unit and, at the intersection of 12th and Vancouver, Paramedic Roy Michaels climbed aboard with his jump kit and assumed care of the patient.

Once at the hospital, Officer Janine Colcord underwent emergency surgery and since has recovered fully and returned to patrolling the streets.

The man who assaulted her was later sentenced to a lengthy stint in prison.

The Last Word

This chapter covered injuries to only two parts of the body—but two of the most important parts of the body. When you find a trauma patient in shock without open injuries, it is highly likely that there are injuries to the chest and/or abdomen. These areas contain organs that are vital to our breathing and circulation. They are also very vascular—meaning they have a rich blood supply and will cause profound internal bleeding when damaged. Your recognition of injuries to the chest and abdomen combined with appropriate clinical care and prompt transportation can make the difference between life and death.

Chapter Review

MULTIPLE CHOICE

Place a check next to the correct answer.

1. You have applied an occlusive dressing over an open wound to your patient's chest. About 10 minutes after applying the dressing, the patient's respirations increase, his mental status decreases, and the BP drops. You should:

    _____ a. remove the occlusive dressing.

    _____ b. leave the occlusive dressing in place.

    _____ c. remove the occlusive dressing, wipe away accumulated blood, and reapply.

    _____ d. remove the three-sided occlusive dressing and replace it with a four-sided occlusive dressing.

2. The left lung has _____ lobes.

    _____ a. 1

    _____ b. 2

    _____ c. 3

    _____ d. 4

3. The heart is contained in the thoracic cavity.

    _____ a. true

    _____ b. false

4. Which of the following statements about rib fractures is FALSE?

    _____ a. The pain from rib fractures can cause hypoventilation.

    _____ b. Rib fractures may cause injury to organs that lie beneath.

    _____ c. The floating ribs are more likely to fracture because they are unattached on one end.

    _____ d. Two ribs fractured in two or more places is called flail chest.

5. A patient with a closed abdominal injury may wish to be placed:

    _____ a. in a sitting position.

    _____ b. in a supine position.

    _____ c. recumbent with knees drawn toward the chest.

    _____ d. sitting or supine with legs extended straight.

6. In order to prevent infection, exposed abdominal organs should be gently moved back into the abdomen.

    _____ a. true

    _____ b. false

7. Patients with tension pneumothorax usually have distended jugular veins.

    _____ a. true

    _____ b. false

FILL IN THE BLANK

1. Blood in the sac surrounding the heart is called pericardial _____.

2. Dressings used to cover abdominal eviscerations are moistened with sterile _____.

3. The abdominal aorta and kidneys are located in the _____ space.

CRITICAL THINKING

1. You are caring for a patient who has received a stab wound to the upper right quadrant of the abdomen. In what organs should you suspect injury? What are the implications?

_____

_____

_____

_____

2. You are caring for an adult patient who was jogging and developed a sudden onset of difficulty breathing. If this patient developed a spontaneous pneumothorax, what signs and symptoms would you expect to see?

_____

_____

_____

3. What is the pulse pressure? Would you expect it to widen or narrow in cases of tension pneumothorax?

_____

_____

_____

CASE STUDY

You are called to a patient who has been involved in a motor vehicle collision. He was thrown from the vehicle and found about 20 feet from the car. Your size-up reveals damage to the steering wheel. There was no airbag deployment.

The patient is unresponsive. After opening and suctioning the airway, while spinal stabilization is maintained, you note that the patient is using accessory muscles to breathe and appears to have respiratory distress with very rapid, shallow respirations. You observe a depression on the anterior chest that involves the third through seventh ribs on the left side of the chest that extends from the anterior axillary line to the sternum.

1. What airway and breathing care would this patient receive?

   _____

   _____

   _____

   _____

2. How would you determine if this patient had a flail segment?

   _____

   _____

   _____

   _____

3. What injuries may occur within the chest if a broken rib were to cause damage?

   _____

   _____

   _____

   _____

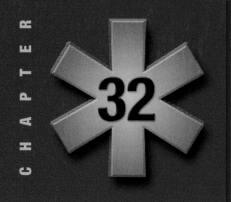

32

Patients with Musculoskeletal Injuries

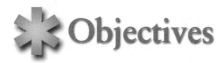 Objectives

Numbered objectives are from the U.S. Department of Transportation 1994 EMT-Basic National Standard Curriculum.

COGNITIVE OBJECTIVES

At the completion of this lesson, the EMT-Basic student will be able to:

5-3.1 Describe the function of the muscular system. (pp. 797–799)

5-3.2 Describe the function of the skeletal system. (pp. 798–799)

5-3.3 List the major bones or bone groupings of the spinal column, the thorax, the upper extremities, and the lower extremities. (pp. 798–799)

5-3.4 Differentiate between an open and a closed painful, swollen, deformed extremity. (pp. 803–807)

5-3.5 State the reasons for splinting. (p. 810)

5-3.6 List the general rules of splinting. (pp. 811–827)

5-3.7 List the complications of splinting. (p. 828)

5-3.8 List the emergency medical care for a patient with a painful, swollen, deformed extremity. (pp. 809–810)

AFFECTIVE OBJECTIVES

At the completion of this lesson, the EMT-Basic student will be able to:

5-3.9 Explain the rationale for splinting at the scene versus load and go. (p. 811)

5-3.10 Explain the rationale for immobilization of the painful, swollen, deformed extremity. (p. 809)

PSYCHOMOTOR OBJECTIVES

At the completion of this lesson, the EMT-Basic student will be able to:

5-3.11 Demonstrate the emergency medical care of a patient with a painful, swollen, deformed extremity. (pp. 809–810, 811–828)

5-3.12 Demonstrate completing a prehospital care report for patients with musculoskeletal injuries. (pp. 828, 830)

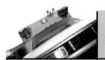 Introduction

Injuries to muscles and bones are some of the most commonly seen injuries encountered by EMTs. While certainly painful, isolated injuries to muscles and bones rarely are immediately life threatening. Since many of these patients will require further orthopedic care, it will be necessary to prepare them properly for transport to an appropriate receiving facility. This includes an appropriate assessment and careful immobilization of the injury to minimize pain and further injury. In this chapter, we will discuss some of the more common types of musculoskeletal injuries and how they occur as well as suggestions for proper immobilization.

Emergency Dispatch

"**D**o you think it's broken?" The young man, still sweating and out of breath, was sitting on the living room floor in obvious pain. "I felt it pop, but it could just be dislocated, right?"

EMTs Jeri Turner and Pat Shipley had been dispatched to a residence for a leg injury. It turned out to be a painfully small apartment crowded with teens, all trying to hide alcohol bottles as the firefighters, EMTs, and police officers squeezed in. One of the teens had wisely called 9-1-1.

"So what exactly happened?" Pat asked as he pulled scissors from his belt and began cutting the patient's pant leg to better expose the injury site.

"David . . . uh . . . was showin' us some new dance moves," a girl said as she tried to hide a smile behind her hand.

"This damn carpet caught my shoe." The patient pointed down angrily. "And it ain't funny!"

Some in the crowd started to laugh and one young man began to lurch around the cramped room, imitating the patient's dance moves. By the time he grabbed his knee and dramatically fell to the floor, everyone, including the patient and many of the emergency personnel, were laughing.

"Okay, okay," the injured teen nodded. "So, it was stupid. But is it bad? Could it just be a sprain or something?"

"Well," Pat palpated the patient's knee. "It is swollen a bit, but it doesn't seem unstable. But that doesn't always mean anything. Let's get you to the hospital so you can get an X-ray. The police officer will give your parents a call to let them know we are on the way to the hospital."

Review of the Musculoskeletal System

You will first want to review the musculoskeletal system (Figure 32-1 on page 798). Please refer to chapter 4 in this text for a more detailed discussion on musculoskeletal anatomy. The muscular system includes the muscles that cover the bones and give us our basic form. It also includes the many **tendons** that connect muscle to the skeleton, allowing for movement (Figure 32-2 on page 799). While

5-3.1   Describe the function of the muscular system.

* **tendons**

tissues that connect muscle to the skeleton.

FIGURE 32-1 The human skeleton.

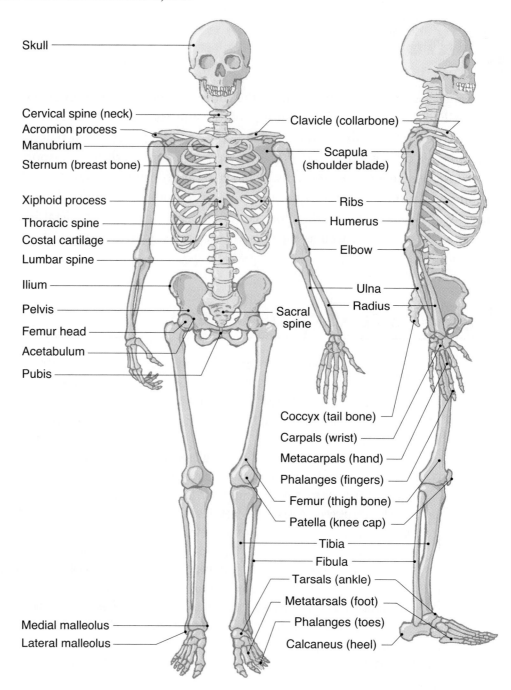

Skull

Cervical spine (neck)
Acromion process
Manubrium
Sternum (breast bone)

Clavicle (collarbone)

Scapula
(shoulder blade)

Xiphoid process
Thoracic spine
Costal cartilage
Lumbar spine

Ribs
Humerus

Elbow

Ilium
Pelvis
Femur head
Acetabulum
Pubis

Ulna
Radius

Sacral
spine

Coccyx (tail bone)
Carpals (wrist)
Metacarpals (hand)
Phalanges (fingers)
Femur (thigh bone)
Patella (knee cap)

Tibia
Fibula

Tarsals (ankle)
Metatarsals (foot)
Phalanges (toes)
Calcaneus (heel)

Medial malleolus
Lateral malleolus

5-3.2 Describe the function of the skeletal system.

✳ **ligaments**

tissues that connect the bones of the skeleton.

✳ **cartilage**

tough elastic connective tissue found in various parts of the body such as the joints, ears, nose, and larynx.

5-3.3 List the major bones or bone groupings of the spinal column, the thorax, the upper extremities, and the lower extremities.

it is not essential that you learn the name of each and every bone in the body, it is important to become familiar with all of the major bones and their functions. This will allow you to better assess, describe, and document injuries you encounter.

The musculoskeletal system is made up of the bones and the muscles of the body. The skeletal system consists of all 206 bones as well as the **ligaments** that help hold the bones of the skeleton together. **Cartilage,** another component of the skeletal system, is a tough elastic connective tissue found in various parts of the body such as the joints, ears, nose, and larynx.

Bones are made up of dense semirigid living tissue and serve many purposes other than just structure and support. They come in many shapes and sizes. Some bones are long and thin (extremities) while others are short and wide (vertebrae). Each has a specific purpose such as movement, protection, or support, based on its specific location and structure.

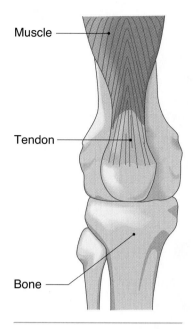

FIGURE 32-2   Tendons connect muscle to bone. The lower muscle and the tendon are not shown.

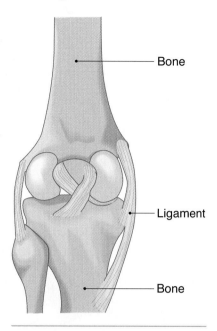

FIGURE 32-3   Ligaments connect bone to bone.

Ligaments are the tough fibrous tissues that connect two or more bones at a joint (Figure 32-3). When joints become injured, ligaments can become stretched or torn, making the joint unstable. An injury to a ligament is commonly referred to as a sprain.

Common Mechanisms of Injury

In most cases, the type and extent of musculoskeletal injury will depend on the mechanism of injury (MOI) and the forces involved. The most common forces responsible for musculoskeletal injuries are direct, indirect, and twisting (Figure 32-4 on page 800).

Direct force is caused by a direct blow to an area of the body. Most blunt trauma is caused by direct force of some kind. An arm struck by a baseball bat and a leg struck by the bumper of a car are examples of direct-force mechanisms. The extent of injury will depend on the amount of force. If the force is significant enough, damage to the bone underlying the point of impact is likely.

An injury caused by **indirect force** occurs when the energy of the force is transferred along a bone, usually proximal to the site of impact. One of the most common causes of indirect-force injury is a person falling on outstretched hands in an attempt to break his fall. This kind of fall can cause a direct-force injury to the wrist. In some cases, it will also cause indirect-force injury to the elbow, clavicle, or shoulder as the energy from the impact is transferred along the arm to the elbow or shoulder. Another common cause of indirect-force injury is the knees of an unrestrained occupant in a vehicle collision striking the dashboard. The knees take the direct force, but the energy is transferred along the femur, frequently causing injury to the hip.

Among the most common **twisting force** injuries is the twisted ankle or twisted neck. The force is applied as the foot, for example, stays firmly planted while the rest of the body twists around the foot, causing damage to the foot, the ankle, and the lower leg.

✳ **direct force**

the force caused by a direct blow to an area of the body.

✳ **indirect force**

the force that occurs when energy is transferred along a bone, usually proximal to the site of impact.

✳ **twisting force**

the force caused by a twisting or turning motion.

FIGURE 32-4 Different types of force can cause different types of injuries.

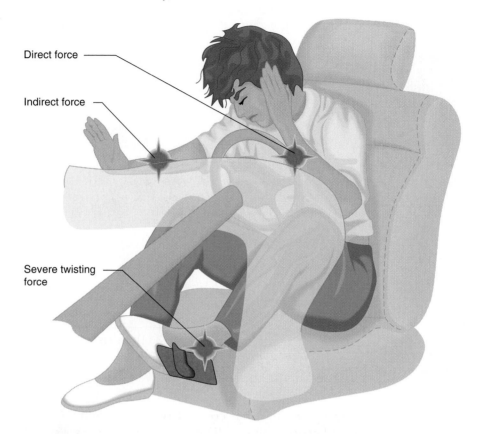

Different types of force can cause different types of injuries.

Direct force

Indirect force

Severe twisting force

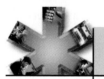

Perspective

David—The Patient

"Oh, man, that hurt! I was just messing around, and I tried to do this spin move, but my sneaker had a better grip on the carpet than I thought. Everything above my knee spun; everything below it didn't. For a split second I actually thought I broke my leg off! And of course it doesn't help when all of your friends are laughing at you too hard to help."

Musculoskeletal Injuries

Injuries to the musculoskeletal system involve damage to soft tissues, bones, joints, or any combination of these.

SOFT TISSUE INJURIES

A **strain** occurs when a muscle is pulled or torn. This is likely to cause severe pain; however, isolated muscle injuries of this kind are not generally the cause for calling an ambulance. A **sprain** is another injury that involves soft tissues. Sprains may occur anywhere there is a joint, resulting in the stretching and/or tearing of the ligaments that support the joint. A sprained ankle is a good example of this type of injury. Most victims of injuries involving the soft tissues of the musculoskeletal system self-treat their injuries, using elevation and ice to help reduce the pain and

✳ **strain**

injury caused when a muscle is pulled or torn, causing severe pain.

✳ **sprain**

injury caused by the stretching and/or tearing of the ligaments and tendons that support the joint.

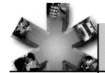

Perspective

Pat—The EMT

"There was definitely swelling around the guy's knee, but I didn't notice crepitus or any glaring instability or anything. Who knows what he did to it. It's hard to respond when patients want a diagnosis. I do not diagnose. Or what's even worse is when you're sure it's a fracture and you say that in your verbal report to the ED, but you turn out to be wrong. Nowadays, unless I can see the end of a bone sticking through the patient's skin, all I ever say is that the injury has 'swelling, pain, and deformity'."

swelling. In some cases, the pain is so great that there is no way to tell if it is a soft tissue injury or a bone injury. In situations such as this, you must assume the worst injury and provide care for a suspected fracture. This will be discussed a little later in this chapter.

Stop, Review, Remember!

Multiple Choice

Place a check next to the correct answer.

1. These structures are made of a tough fibrous tissue that surrounds a joint and connects two or more bones together.

   _____ a. cartilage

   _____ b. tendons

   _____ c. ligaments

   _____ d. metacarpals

2. _____ connect(s) each muscle to the skeleton and allow(s) for movement.

   _____ a. Cartilage

   _____ b. Tendons

   _____ c. Ligaments

   _____ d. Metatarsals

3. An injury to the wrist as a result of a fall onto outstretched hands is caused by which type of force?

   _____ a. direct force

   _____ b. indirect force

   _____ c. twisting force

   _____ d. straight force

4. When a muscle is stretched and torn, the injury is a:

   _____ a. sprain.

   _____ b. fracture.

   _____ c. pull.

   _____ d. strain.

5. _____ may occur anywhere there is a joint and often result in the stretching and/or tearing of the ligaments that support the joint.

_____ a. Sprains

_____ b. Fractures

_____ c. Pulls

_____ d. Strains

Labeling

Using the illustration, correctly label all the major bones of the human skeleton.

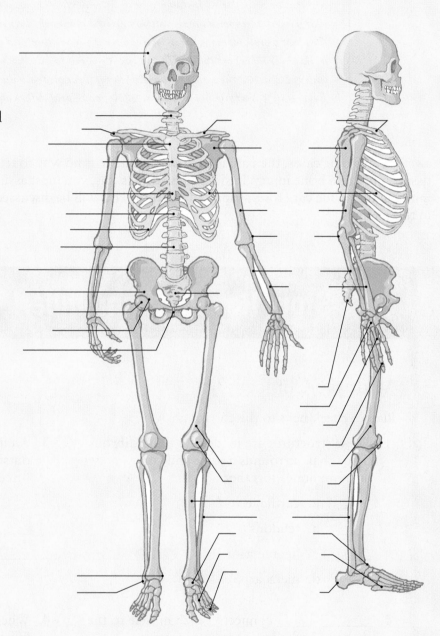

Critical Thinking

1. Describe the difference between a strain and a sprain.

_____

_____

_____

_____

2. What is meant by the term "suspected fracture"?

_____

_____

_____

_____

3. Why is it important for the EMT to care for most complaints of skeletal pain as suspected fractures?

_____

_____

_____

_____

Skeletal Injuries

Skeletal injuries are most commonly **fractures** and/or **dislocations.** Fractures are broken bones and can be as minor as a hairline crack all the way to a badly shattered bone that appears deformed. The most common symptom of a skeletal fracture is pain. For this reason, you should consider all complaints of skeletal pain to be suspected fractures and provide the appropriate care. Dislocations are displacements of the bones that make up a joint, such as the elbow, shoulder, knee, or hip (Figure 32-5 on page 804).

Injuries involving joints can result in sprains, fractures, dislocations, or any combination of these. Injured joints require special attention and care because of the unique function of the joint and the fact that most joints are surrounded by a large supply of vessels and nerves. Damage to joints places these vessels and nerves at great risk of injury as well.

Skeletal injuries are further classified as open or closed (Figure 32-6 on page 804). A **closed skeletal injury** is one that is not associated with any break in the overlying skin (Figure 32-7 on page 804). An **open skeletal injury** occurs when the skin is damaged, causing an open soft tissue wound in connection with the skeletal injury (Figure 32-8 on page 804). For instance, the force of the mechanism can

* **fracture**
  broken bone. Can be as minor as a hairline crack all the way to a badly shattered bone that appears deformed.

* **dislocation**
  displacement of the bones that make up a joint, such as the elbow, shoulder, knee, or hip.

5-3.4 Differentiate between an open and a closed painful, swollen, deformed extremity.

* **closed skeletal injury**
  skeletal injury not associated with any break in the overlying skin.

* **open skeletal injury**
  skeletal injury where the skin is damaged causing an open soft tissue wound in connection with the injury.

Clinical Clues: SUSPECTED FRACTURE

The term "suspected fracture" is used to describe an injury involving the skeletal system. Because, as EMTs, we do not diagnose, we must use terminology that clearly describes our findings without the appearance of a diagnosis. Even when caring for injuries that present as deformed and angulated, we should describe and document them as such and refrain from using the word _fracture,_ which is a diagnostic term. A possible exception may be an obvious open fracture with bone ends protruding through the wound.

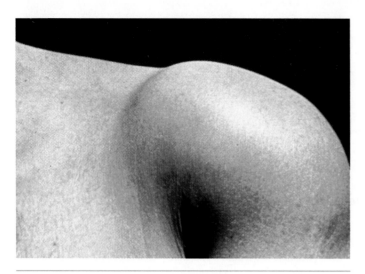

FIGURE 32-5   Deformity caused by dislocation of the shoulder joint.

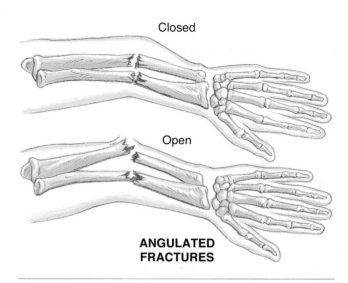

Closed

Open

ANGULATED FRACTURES

FIGURE 32-6   Skeletal injuries may be open or closed.

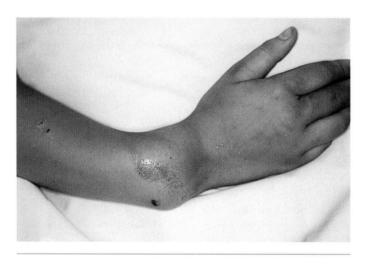

FIGURE 32-7   Deformity caused by a closed injury at the wrist. (Charles Stewart, M.D., and Associates.)

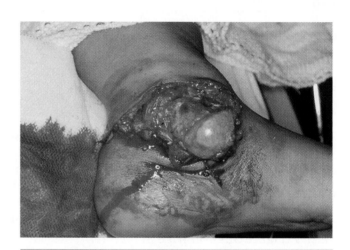

FIGURE 32-8   An open injury of the ankle. (Charles Stewart, M.D., and Associates.)

cause a broken bone end to penetrate the skin, causing an open wound in close proximity to the fracture. Open skeletal injuries can also be caused when a projectile such as a bullet penetrates the skin and the underlying bone. The risk of complication due to infection is very high with open skeletal injuries. It will be important to immediately control any severe bleeding with sterile dressings.

ASSESSMENT OF MUSCULOSKELETAL INJURIES

The assessment of a patient with a suspected musculoskeletal injury begins with an evaluation of the MOI. As you approach the scene, look for evidence that might suggest the mechanism involved. If it is a vehicle collision, assess the extent of damage to both the inside and outside of the vehicle. If the patient is a victim of a fall, do your best to determine how far he fell, how he may have landed, and what type of surface he landed on. All of these factors will help determine the overall mechanism of injury. Remember to consider the need for spinal immobilization if the mechanism of injury suggests it, even if the chief complaint is simply an extremity injury.

Once you have determined that the ABCs are intact and there are no other immediate life threats to the patient, you must focus your assessment on the chief

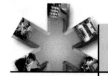

Perspective

Jeri—The EMT

"The patient and his friends told us that he just sat down on the floor after twisting his knee, so there was really no need to worry about spinal immobilization. With most falls, though, I usually use the backboard. I had a patient a few years ago who was hanging a picture in his den, was just standing on his tiptoes, and then lost his balance and fell. He denied any back or neck pain, and we all got a little too focused on this open fracture of his wrist. It wasn't until we were transferring him to the bed in the ED that his extremities started going numb. It turned out that he had actually fractured his neck. He came out of it okay, but I never take chances now."

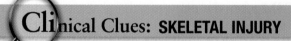

Clinical Clues: SKELETAL INJURY

Do not let the sight of serious skeletal injuries distract you from your priorities of care. Regardless of the injuries you MUST begin with the initial assessment and confirm the adequacy of the ABCs.

complaint. Remember to perform a rapid trauma assessment for any patient who has suffered a significant mechanism of injury. A patient with an isolated injury to an extremity should receive a focused trauma assessment of the affected extremity.

When performing a focused assessment of an injured area, begin by attempting to determine where the pain is centered. To do this, ask the patient to point with one finger to where it hurts the most. Next you must expose the area and observe for any signs of possible skeletal injury.

Signs and symptoms of a musculoskeletal injury include:

* Pain and tenderness

* Deformity (swelling or angulation)

* Discoloration (bruising)

* Open wounds and external bleeding

* Exposed bone

* Crepitation (grating)

* Locked joint (unable to move)

Palpate the area gently to pinpoint the suspected injury site. Palpate beyond the injury site in all directions, assessing for additional injury that may have been caused by indirect force. Be sure to assess any joint that may be distal or proximal to the injury site. A joint that is injured may be stuck in a fixed position and unable to move freely. Ask the patient if he can move the joint on his own. DO NOT force an injured joint that is painful or difficult to move. Severe and permanent damage may result. If the patient is unable to move the joint, you must immobilize it in the position in which it is found. More will be discussed on immobilization later in this chapter.

ASSESSING THE DISTAL EXTREMITY

When assessing extremity injuries you must always check the distal extremity for the presence of adequate circulation, sensation, and motor function (CSM). This can be accomplished by assessing for the presence of a radial pulse in the wrists or the pedal pulse in the feet (Figure 32-9). In some patients it may be difficult to find a distal pulse in the foot. In these cases, it is a good idea to also check capillary refill as a back-up to the pulses. The presence of capillary refill, even in the absence of a pulse, is an indication that the limb has some degree of circulation.

If the injury is angulated and you cannot confirm the presence of circulation either by palpating a pulse or seeing capillary refill, you may have to straighten the extremity. Advise the patient of what you are planning to do before moving the limb. Support the extremity with both hands and carefully straighten the limb while pulling gentle traction. Reassess CSM after the extremity has been straightened. Follow local protocols regarding the straightening of an angulated extremity.

You will then assess sensation by asking the patient if, without looking, he can feel you touching his fingers or toes (Figure 32-10). Have him identify the specific

---

Clinical Clues: DISTAL FOOT PULSE

It is a good idea to mark the location where the distal pulse in the foot is found with a pen. This will be a reminder to keep that area accessible as you splint. It will also make it easier to locate during your reassessment of CSM.

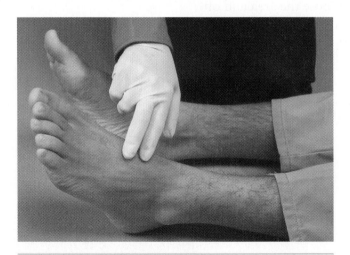

FIGURE 32-9 Assess distal circulation by palpating for a pulse.

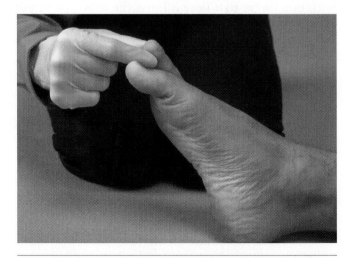

FIGURE 32-10 Assess distal sensation in the lower extremities by asking the patient, "Which toe am I touching?" (Be sure the patient cannot see which toe.)

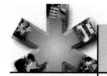

Perspective

Pat—The EMT

"The first thing I did after looking at his knee was to check for a pedal pulse. I tell you, sometimes those are really difficult to find. It can take such a light touch, and just when you think you've got it, it rolls away. I've started drawing a little 'X' on the top of the patient's foot where I found the pulse. It makes it easier to find again during ongoing assessments and it seems that the ED docs appreciate it, too."

toe or finger you are touching. Ask him if he feels numbness or tingling as you palpate the feet and hands.

Check motor function of the feet by having the patient push down against your hands simultaneously with both feet (Figure 32-11). Then have them pull up against your hands. This must be done with both sides at the same time in order to detect slight differences in strength. When assessing the hands, have the patient grip the thumbs or fingers of both your hands simultaneously (Figure 32-12). You should be aware that many times the ability to move the hands and feet on the injured side will be less than the noninjured side. This is commonly due to the pain involved and not always an indication of nerve damage or spinal injury.

Clinical Clues: ASSESSING SENSATION

While most patients can easily tell which finger you are touching without looking, they may have difficulty differentiating which toe is being touched. This is common and normal. When assessing sensation in the feet, choose either the big or little toe when asking the patient which toe you are touching.

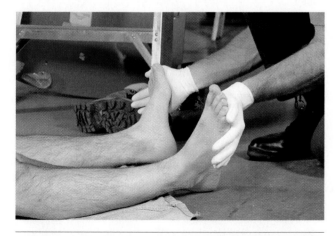

FIGURE 32-11   Check motor function in feet.

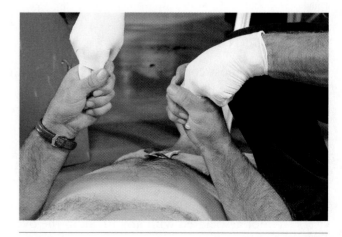

FIGURE 32-12   Check motor function of hands.

Stop, Review, Remember!

Multiple Choice

Place a check next to the correct answer.

1. An injury to the bones of the forearm that was caused by a gunshot would be an example of a(n):

   _____ a. closed skeletal injury.

   _____ b. open skeletal injury.

   _____ c. dislocation.

   _____ d. strain.

2. The risk of complication due to infection is very high with:

   _____ a. long bone splint injuries.

   _____ b. joint ligament injuries.

   _____ c. open skeletal injuries.

   _____ d. closed skeletal injuries.

3. The assessment of a patient with a suspected musculoskeletal injury begins with a(n):

   _____ a. evaluation of the mechanism of injury.

   _____ b. evaluation of the distal extremity.

   _____ c. detailed physical exam.

   _____ d. rapid trauma assessment.

4. Which of the following is specific to an extremity injury and must be assessed *prior to* immobilizing the extremity?

   _____ a. ABCs

   _____ b. distal temperature

   _____ c. mental status

   _____ d. circulation, sensory and motor function

5. _____ may occur anywhere there is a joint and often result in the stretching and/or tearing of the ligaments that support the joint.

   _____ a. Sprains

   _____ b. Fractures

   _____ c. Pulls

   _____ d. Strains

Fill in the Blank

1. The most common symptom of a skeletal fracture is _____.

2. Injuries involving _____ can result in sprains, fractures, dislocations, or any combination of these.

3. A _____ skeletal injury is one that is not associated with any break in the overlying skin.

4. An open skeletal injury occurs when the _____ is damaged, causing an open soft tissue wound in connection with the skeletal injury.

5. The assessment of a patient with a suspected musculoskeletal injury begins with an evaluation of the _____.

Critical Thinking

1. How does the care for a suspected joint injury differ from that of a long bone injury?

   _____

   _____

   _____

2. Discuss your priorities of care for an open skeletal injury.

   _____

   _____

   _____

3. Discuss what it might mean if a patient with a suspected fracture has abnormal distal circulation, sensation, and/or motor function (CSM) findings?

   _____

   _____

   _____

Emergency Care for Musculoskeletal Injuries

As noted earlier, it is not the role of the EMT to determine for certain whether a patient has sustained a fracture or simply a sprain or strain. An evaluation of the mechanism of injury along with an appropriate assessment of the injury site should determine the most appropriate care. In most cases, the injury should be treated as a suspected fracture and immobilized accordingly. Once you have conducted an appropriate scene size-up and initial assessment and cared for any immediate life threats, follow these steps when caring for a suspected fracture:

5-3.8 List the emergency medical care for a patient with a painful, swollen, deformed extremity.

1. Take the appropriate BSI precautions.

2. Expose and assess the injury site and surrounding area.

3. Assess distal circulation, sensation, and motor function.

4. Immobilize the injury site as appropriate.

5. Administer oxygen as appropriate.

6. Elevate the extremity if appropriate.

7. Apply a cold pack to the injury site.

The injured extremity should be elevated only after it has been properly immobilized and only if it does not cause further pain for the patient. Gently place a cold pack over or near the injury site to help minimize swelling.

IMMOBILIZING EXTREMITY INJURIES AND TRANSPORTATION CONSIDERATIONS

5-3.5 State the reasons for splinting.

Most patients with skeletal injuries will need more advanced care than can be provided for them in the field. A thorough evaluation of the injury by a physician and most likely an X-ray will be the minimum care necessary to identify the extent of the injury. For this reason, these patients must be transported to an appropriate receiving facility. Transporting patients by ambulance, of course, means subjecting them to movement. Any movement of a patient with skeletal injuries may result in movement of the injury site. Movement of the injury site may result in more damage and certainly more pain for the patient. That is why immobilizing the injury is an essential element of proper care for these patients.

Within a few seconds following the MOI, a patient will find a position that is most comfortable for his injury. This does NOT mean he is pain free. He is typically self-splinting the injury and has simply found a position that is least painful.

As you approach the patient to begin your assessment, provide care, load him into the ambulance, and transport him to the hospital, you will subject him to movement he cannot control. To minimize complications caused by this movement, you must immobilize the injury prior to transport. The following is a list of complications that can be minimized through proper immobilization of an injury prior to transport:

∗ Movement of the injury

∗ Unnecessary pain

∗ Additional bleeding

∗ Additional swelling

∗ Further damage to soft tissues, nerves, and blood vessels

∗ Creation of an open injury from an existing closed injury

∗ Paralysis caused from a damaged spinal column

Immobilization can be accomplished using one of two methods:

∗ manual stabilization

∗ splinting

Manual stabilization is accomplished by using your gloved hands to stabilize the injury site. This is typically used as an initial step until enough help and supplies are available to properly splint the injury. Splinting involves the application of external devices such as cardboard, wood, or plastic to aid in stabilizing the injury site so that the patient does not have to continue to stabilize it himself.

Splinting does not have to be a complicated process. By following a few simple guidelines, you will be able to quickly and effectively immobilize an injury and minimize discomfort for the patient.

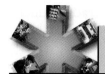

Perspective

David—The Patient

"At first I thought that they were gonna hurt me with that splint! It was just this big, floppy orange thing that they started wrapping around my leg. I didn't know how it would help to hold my leg still. By that time I was in so much pain I really, really needed to keep it still. But then they used this bicycle-pump-looking thing to suck the air out of the splint and, man, it hardened right up and my leg didn't move again until we got to the hospital! My leg was still hurting, but not nearly as much as it had been."

Splinting

The following guidelines should be followed when splinting a suspected skeletal injury:

5-3.6 List the general rules of splinting.

* Properly assess the injury site by exposing it as appropriate.

* Control any bleeding and cover open wounds with sterile dressings.

* Assess distal circulation, sensation, and motor function before and after splinting, and document any changes.

* Immobilize the injury site.

* Immobilize the joint above and below the injury site.

* Pad all splinting material as appropriate for patient comfort.

* If there is a severe deformity or if the distal extremity is cyanotic or lacks pulses, align to the normal anatomical position with gentle traction before splinting.

* Do not intentionally replace any protruding bones.

As a rule, an injured joint with compromised distal circulation, sensation, or motor function should not be moved in an attempt to restore CSM. If the patient is able to move the limb without too much pain, then allow him to do so and recheck CSM status. Otherwise, immobilize the joint in the position found and

Clinical Clues: SPLINT OR NOT?

When caring for a patient who has sustained a significant mechanism of injury, it is important not to waste valuable time attempting to splint all extremity injuries. Patients who have sustained multisystem trauma or who are presenting with the signs and symptoms of shock should be immobilized on a long back board and transported as quickly as possible.

transport immediately. For injuries involving long bones, such as the radius, ulna, tibia, or fibula, with compromised CSM, it is appropriate to attempt to straighten the limb into its normal anatomical position.

POSITION OF FUNCTION

✻ **position of function**

position of the hands and feet when they are at rest without any type of force.

The term **position of function** refers to the position of the hands and feet when they are at rest and not under any type of force. When you are placing a splint, it is important for the patient's comfort to maintain the affected hand and foot in the position of function. This can easily be accomplished by placing a 4-inch roller bandage or similar item in the hand prior to splinting or by allowing the fingers to curl naturally over the end of the splint (Figure 32-13). The foot should simply be allowed to rest in the most natural position, not forced into a flexed or extended position (Figure 32-14).

MATERIALS USED FOR SPLINTING

Just about anything can be used to splint an injury or suspected fracture. The important thing is that you become familiar with the specific tools that will be available to you. By applying the guidelines just outlined, you should be able to utilize any piece of equipment or material at your disposal to properly splint a patient's injuries.

RIGID SPLINTS

As the name indicates, these splints are made of rigid material such as wood, cardboard, metal, or plastic (Figure 32-15). Because they are generally made of a hard material, it is especially important to pad these splints prior to applying them to a patient. Some rigid splints are commercially manufactured and designed for specific injuries. Some of these have integrated padding and Velcro-style closures, making them easier to apply.

PNEUMATIC SPLINTS

Pneumatic splints come in two varieties, the air splint and the vacuum splint. The air splint is a bladder that can be placed completely around an injured extremity

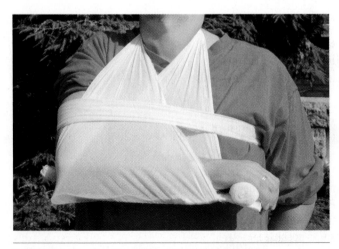

FIGURE 32-13 Hand in position of function on a splint.

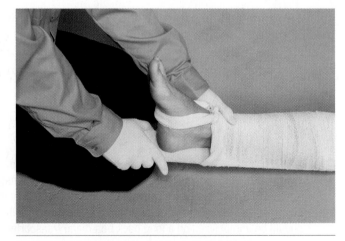

FIGURE 32-14 Secure the foot in position of function.

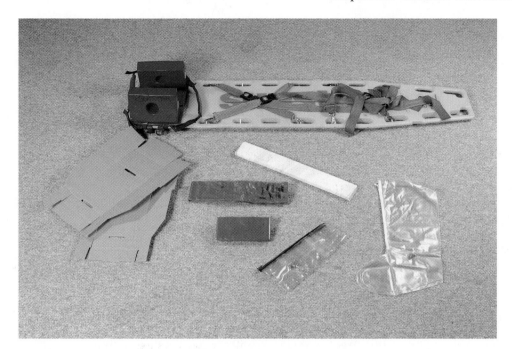

and inflated to provide stability to the area that it covers (Figure 32-16). Air splints are easy to apply; however, they do not allow for further assessment of the injury site since they cover the majority of the limb. Like balloons, air splints are subject to leaks and pressure changes as altitude changes. This is especially important if the patient is transported by air ambulance.

Vacuum splints operate on the opposite principle of air splints. They are comprised of a specially shaped bag filled with tiny beads. When the bag is placed around an injured extremity, a suction pump is used to remove all the air inside the bag. When the air is removed the bag becomes a rigid splint that conforms to the extremity, much like a mold (Figure 32-17). The same disadvantages that apply to the air splint apply here as well. The effectiveness of the splint relies on the bag's ability to remain air tight, and the splint greatly reduces access to the injured extremity for further assessment.

Another pneumatic device that can prove beneficial for patients with suspected pelvic or lower-extremity fractures is the pneumatic anti shock garment or

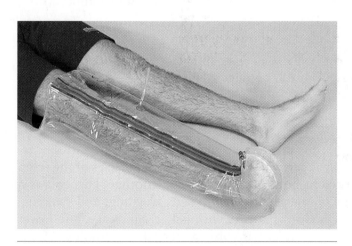

FIGURE 32-16   Immobilization of lower leg injury with air splint.

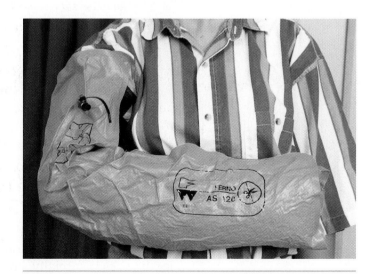

FIGURE 32-17   Immobilization of an elbow injury with a vacuum splint.

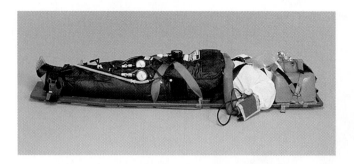

PASG. You must follow local protocols when using the PASG as a splint, and in some instances you may have to contact medical direction prior to applying it (Figure 32-18).

SOFT AND IMPROVISED SPLINTS

Not every splint you apply must be a commercially manufactured splint designed for that purpose. Some of the most effective splints are those that utilize everyday materials such as pillows, blankets, newspapers, and magazines.

One of the most effective devices used to immobilize a shoulder, elbow, or forearm injury is the sling. All by itself, a properly applied sling does an excellent job of immobilizing a bent elbow. When combined with a swathe, it becomes an excellent tool for immobilizing both the elbow and the shoulder.

Follow these steps for the proper application of a sling and swathe (Scan 32-1):

1. Place one end of the base of an open triangular bandage up and over the uninjured shoulder.

2. Ensure that the apex of the triangle is behind the injured elbow and pointing in the same direction of the injured elbow.

3. Now wrap the bottom end of the bandage up and over the shoulder of the injured arm.

4. Be sure the hand of the injured arm is at or above the level of the elbow on the same side.

5. Tie both ends of the bandage at the side of the neck and pad behind the knot as necessary.

6. Secure the apex of the bandage using a pin, tape, or tying in a knot.

7. Secure a swathe as snug and low on the arm as practical.

Pillows and blankets are especially useful for splinting wrist, forearm, elbow, and ankle injuries (Figure 32-19A and B on page 818).

TRACTION SPLINTS

The traction splint is designed specifically to help stabilize a suspected midshaft femur fracture. When a femur is broken and displaced, the large muscles of the thigh begin to spasm, pulling the broken bone ends across one another. This causes a great deal of pain as well as increased soft tissue damage, bleeding, and swelling. Traction splints are contraindicated for patients with pelvic, hip, knee, and lower leg injuries, especially injuries that might involve a partial amputation of the extremity.

SCAN 32-1   **PROPERLY APPLIED SLING AND SWATHE**

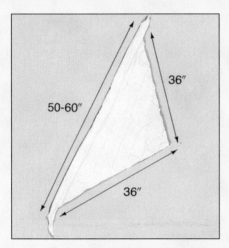

▲ Prepare the sling by folding cloth into a triangle. A triangle bandage makes an ideal arm sling.

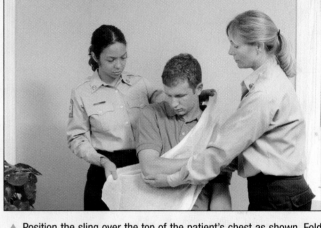

▲ Position the sling over the top of the patient's chest as shown. Fold the injured arm across his chest.

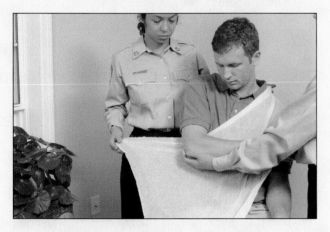

◀ If the patient cannot hold his arm, have someone assist until you tie the sling.

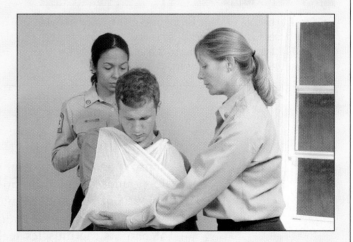

Extend one point of the triangle beyond the elbow on the injured side. Take the bottom point and bring it up over the patient's arm. Then ▶ take it over the top of the injured shoulder.

(continued on the next page)

✳✳✳✳✳✳✳✳✳✳✳✳✳✳✳✳✳✳

PROPERLY APPLIED SLING AND SWATHE—*(continued)*

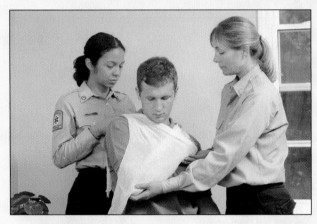

▲ If appropriate, draw up the ends of the sling so that the patient's hand is about 4 inches above the elbow.

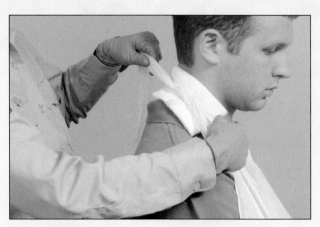

▲ Tie the two ends of the sling together, making sure that the knot does not press against the back of the patient's neck. Pad with bulky dressings. (If spine injury is possible, pin ends to clothing. Do not tie around the neck).

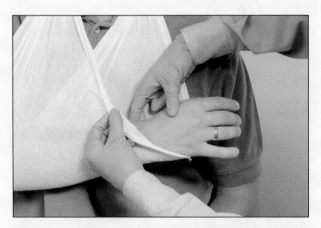

▲ Check to be sure you have left the patient's fingertips exposed. Then assess distal circulation, sensation, and motor function (CSM). If the pulse has been lost, take off the sling and repeat the procedure. Then check again.

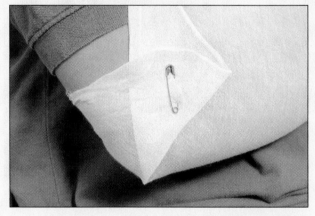

▲ To form a pocket for the patient's elbow, take hold of the point of material at the elbow and fold it forward, pinning it to the front of the sling.

Once applied, gentle traction should be maintained throughout transport (Figure 32-20 on page 818). The rule of thumb is to apply traction force equal to approximately 10 percent of the patient's total body weight up to a maximum of 15 pounds of traction. Some devices (Sager) have a gauge that will indicate the amount of traction being applied. With others, you must estimate the correct amount of traction. Initially, the patient may experience an increase in the amount of pain as the muscles feel the pressure and the bones begin to move. Within a minute or so, the patient will begin to experience some relief as the muscle spasms begin to relax.

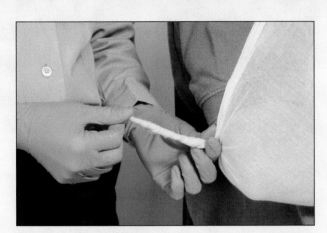

▲ If you do not have a pin, twist the excess material and tie a knot in the point.

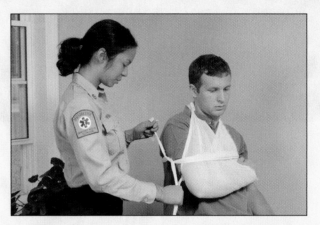

▲ Form a swathe from a second piece of material. Tie it around the chest and the injured arm, over the sling. Do not place it over the patient's arm on the uninjured side.

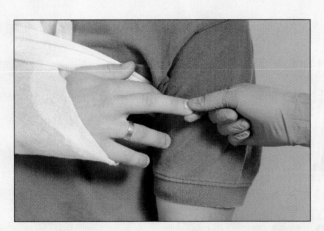

▲ Reassess distal circulation, sensation, and motor function (CSM). Treat for shock, and provide high-concentration oxygen. Take vital signs. Perform detailed and ongoing assessments as appropriate.

SPLINTING SPECIFIC INJURIES

The following section will provide suggested techniques for splinting specific injuries.

Shoulder   Injuries to the shoulder may involve the shoulder joint and or the clavicle and can be splinted the same regardless of which of these structures are involved. The sling and swathe are the main components required for this. Be sure the swathe is placed as low and tight across the arm as possible to minimize movement of the shoulder (Figure 32-21 on page 818).

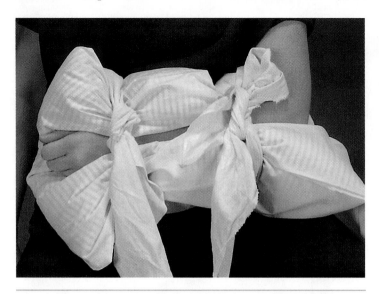

FIGURE 32-19A Soft splinting for wrist and hand injuries.

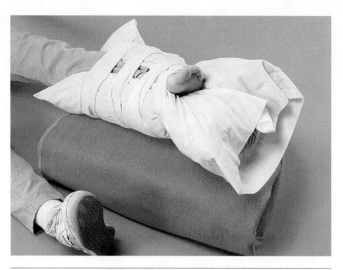

FIGURE 32-19B A blanket used as a pillow to immobilize an ankle injury.

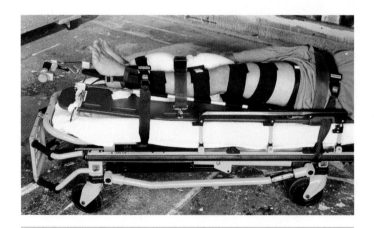

FIGURE 32-20 A patient immobilized with a fraction splint.

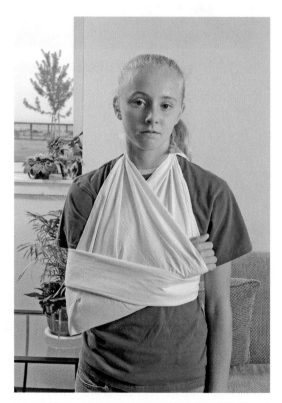

FIGURE 32-21 A properly applied sling and swathe where the swathe is placed low and tight across the arm.

Upper Arm Depending on the extent of injury and position, an injury to the upper arm (humerus) can sometimes be easily managed with a sling and swath. For additional support and protection, a short rigid splint can be applied to the outside (lateral) side of the upper arm and secured with a pair of cravats.

Bent Elbow An elbow found in the bent position is one of the easiest to splint and is ultimately in the most comfortable position for the patient. If the elbow is not found in the bent position, you can ask the patient if he can move it into that position. Do not move the elbow yourself; you must allow the patient to move it for

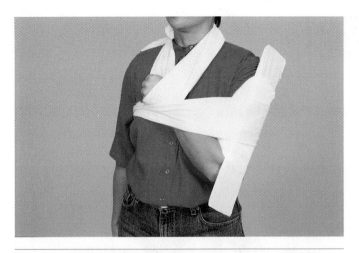

FIGURE 32-22   A suggested method for immobilizing an injury to the upper arm (humerus), immobilize with a rigid splint from the shoulder to below the elbow. Apply a sling and swathe that will elevate and support the limb.

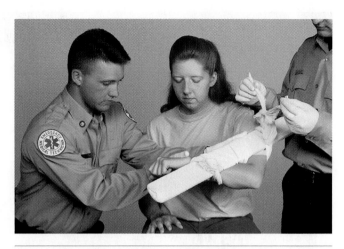

FIGURE 32-23   Application of a pair of rigid splint with sling and swathe to immobilize an injured elbow.

himself. If he is unable to move it, you must immobilize it in the position that it is found. At least two methods can be used to immobilize an elbow injury. The first is a rigid splint in conjunction with the sling and swathe (Figure 32-22) and the second is a method that uses two short rigid splints secured to the arm at 45 degree angles (Figure 32-23). If possible, always incorporate the wrist into one of the splints as it represents the joint below the injury site and must be immobilized.

Straight Elbow   An elbow that is injured and found in the straight position must be managed differently than a bent elbow. First confirm that the patient cannot move the elbow into the bent position. If he cannot, then you must immobilize in the straight position. Immobilize the joint using a rigid splint, then secure the entire upper extremity to the body (Figure 32-24). See Scan 32-2 on page 820 for steps for immobilizing an elbow injury.

Forearm, Wrist, and Hand   Injuries to the forearm, wrist, and hand are some of the most common. A simple rigid or pneumatic splint that extends from the elbow past the wrist will usually suffice. Once the splint is applied the injured extremity should be placed in a sling and swathe. Whenever possible, it is important to maintain the hand on the injured arm at or above the level of the elbow. This will minimize pain caused by throbbing.

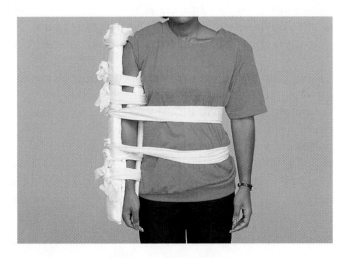

FIGURE 32-24   Fixed splint for elbow in straight position. Suggested method for immobilizing a straight elbow injury.

SCAN 32-2 IMMOBILIZING AN ELBOW INJURY

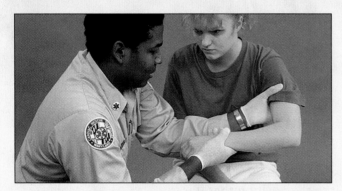

▲ Move the limb only if necessary for splinting or if pulse is absent. STOP if you meet resistance or significantly increase the pain.

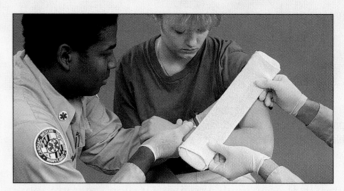

▲ Use a padded board splint that will extend 2 to 6 inches beyond the arm and wrist when placed diagonally.

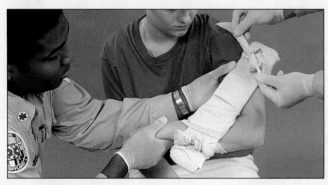

▲ Place the splint so it is just proximal to the elbow and wrist. Use cravats to secure it to the forearm, then the arm.

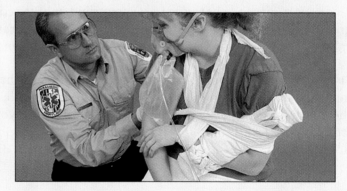

▲ A wrist sling can be applied to support the limb. Keep the elbow exposed. Apply a swathe if possible.

Finger Injured fingers are not typically a reason to be transported by ambulance but can be associated with other injuries and need attention. One of the simplest splints for an injured finger is the tongue blade or bite stick. Pad the splint with gauze and tape or wrap the finger(s) to the splint. Securing the injured finger to an adjacent finger is helpful for additional support (Figure 32-25).

Pelvis The potential for life-threatening blood loss from a pelvic injury is high. Ongoing movement of the unstable pelvic fracture results in increased bleeding from damaged pelvic blood vessels. Traditional treatment of suspected unstable pelvic fractures used to include use of the PASG to minimize movement of the pelvis during transport. Today, there are several devices designed specifically for the stabilization of pelvic fractures in the field. One of those devices is the Trauma Pelvic Orthopedic Device, or TPOD. Devices such as the TPOD are easy to use and have been proven effective in maximizing pelvic stability during transport.

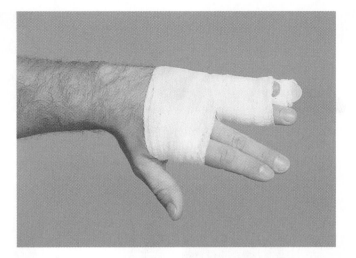

FIGURE 32-25 Finger splinted with a tongue depressor.

Femur Fractured femurs are significant injuries and are best managed using a traction device such as those manufactured by Hare (bipolar device), or by Sager or Kendrick (single pole devices). Regardless of the device, the following steps should be followed when placing a traction splint (Scan 32-3 on page 822).

1. Assess circulation, sensation, and motor function (CSM) distal to the injury and record.

2. Apply ankle hitch.

3. Apply manual stabilization. Apply traction if using a bipolar device.

4. Prepare/adjust splint to proper length using the uninjured leg and position splint on injured leg.

5. Apply proximal securing device (groin strap).

6. Apply distal securing device (ankle hitch).

7. Apply mechanical traction.

8. Position/secure support straps.

9. Reevaluate proximal/distal securing devices.

10. Reassess distal CSM.

Once the splint has been properly applied to the injured extremity, the patient should be secured to a long board for transport. If using a bipolar device, be sure to secure the device to the backboard with tape so that it does not slide around during transport.

Application of a bipolar traction splint should follow these steps:

1. Assess distal CSM.

2. Attach the ankle strap.

3. Stabilize the limb and initiate traction.

4. Prepare and measure splint.

5. Place splint under leg and secure groin strap.

6. Attach ankle strap and initiate traction.

SCAN 32-3   **APPLICATION OF A TRACTION SPLINT (HARE)**

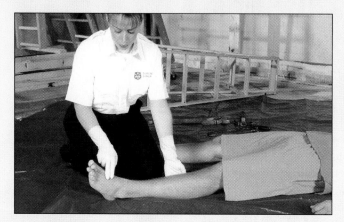

▲ Assess CSM.

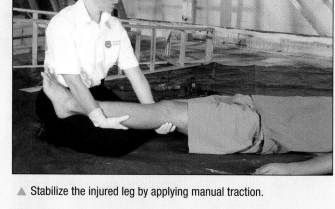

▲ Stabilize the injured leg by applying manual traction.

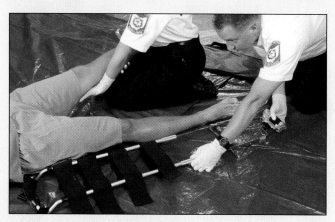

▲ Adjust the splint for proper length, using the uninjured leg as a guide.

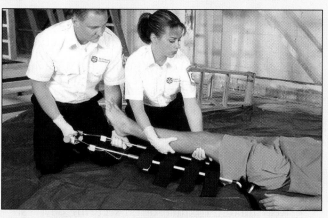

▲ Position the splint under the injured leg until the ischial pad rests against the bony prominence of the buttocks. Once the splint is in position, raise the heel stand.

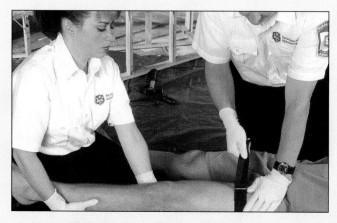

▲ Attach the ischial strap over the groin and thigh.

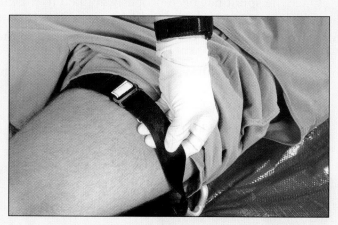

▲ Make sure the ischial strap is snug but not tight enough to reduce distal circulation.

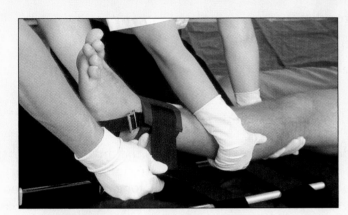

▲ With the patient's foot in an upright position, secure the ankle hitch.

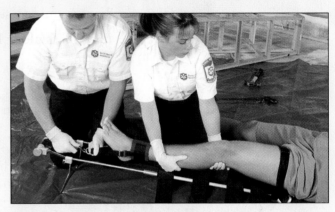

▲ Attach the "S" hook to the "D" ring and apply mechanical traction. Full traction is achieved when the mechanical traction is equal to the manual traction and the pain and muscle spasms are reduced. In an unresponsive patient, adjust the traction until the injured leg is the same length as the uninjured leg.

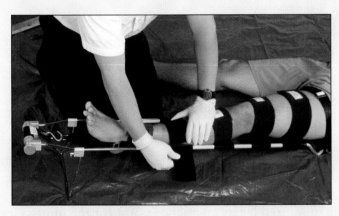

▲ Fasten the leg support straps.

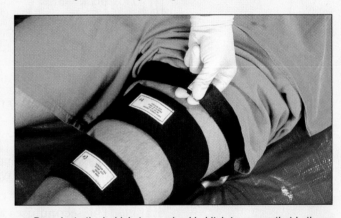

▲ Reevaluate the ischial strap and ankle hitch to ensure that both are securely fastened.

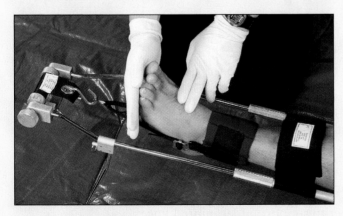

▲ Reassess distal CSM.

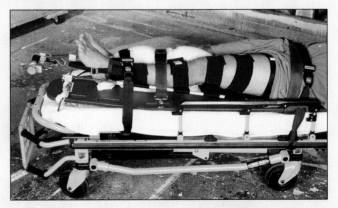

▲ Place the patient on a long board and secure with straps. Pad between the splint and uninjured leg. Secure the splint to the backboard.

7. Reassess CSM.

8. Secure patient and device to long board.

To apply a unipolar traction splint, use the following steps:

1. Assess distal CSM.

2. Attach the ankle strap.

3. Prepare and measure splint.

4. Place splint along leg and secure groin strap.

5. Attach ankle strap and initiate traction.

6. Reassess CSM.

7. Secure patient and device to long board.

Straight Knee and Lower Leg   Injuries to the lower extremities that involve a straight knee or a lower leg can be splinted using the same basic techniques. At the very least, a splint used to immobilize a straight knee should be long enough to extend well beyond the knee in both directions. A splint used for an injury to the lower leg should extend from below the heel to well above the knee (Scan 32-4). You will achieve better support of the extremity if you use a three-sided splint, such as one made of cardboard.

1. Check CSM.

2. Manually stabilize the leg.

3. Slide cravats under leg (2 above knee and 2 below).

4. Measure splint and slide under leg.

5. Secure splint with ties.

6. Reassess CSM.

Bent Knee Injury   A knee that is injured and found in the bent position can be a challenge to properly splint. We will present two options for splinting a bent knee injury. The first uses two rigid splints, one on either side of the leg to create a triangle. The second uses the uninjured leg as an anchor point for the injured leg.
To use the two splint technique, follow these steps (Scan 32-5 on page 827).

1. Check CSM.

2. Pad and secure the splints.

3. Secure the ankle on the injured side to the uninjured leg.

4. Recheck CSM.

To use the anchor point techniques, follow these steps:

1. Check CSM.

2. Secure the injured ankle to the uninjured leg using cravat.

3. Use pillow or blanket to support under injured knee.

4. Recheck CSM.

SCAN 32-4   **RIGID SPLINT OF KNEE AND LOWER LEG**

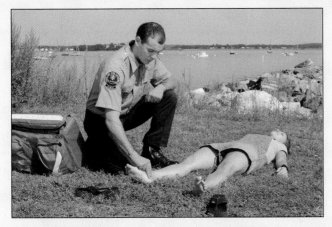

▲ Assess distal CSM function.

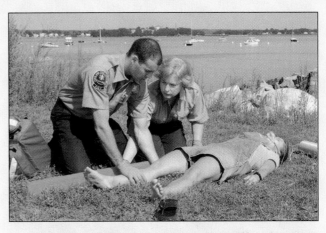

▲ Stabilize. The padded board splint should extend from buttocks to 4 inches beyond heel.

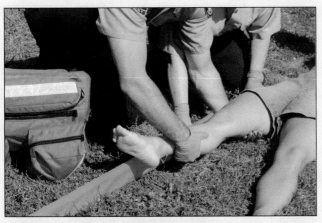

▲ Maintain stabilization and lift limb.

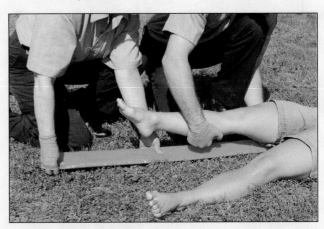

▲ Place splint along posterior of limb.

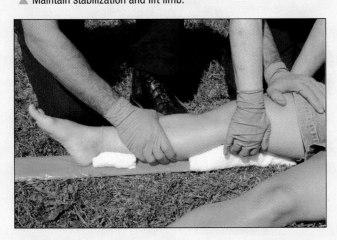

▲ Pad the voids.

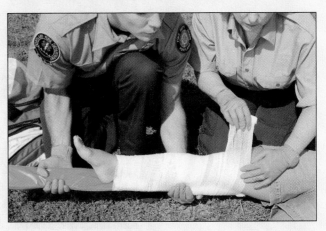

▲ Use a 6-inch roller bandage or cravats to secure injured leg to splint.

(continued on the next page)

RIGID SPLINT OF KNEE AND LOWER LEG—*(continued)*

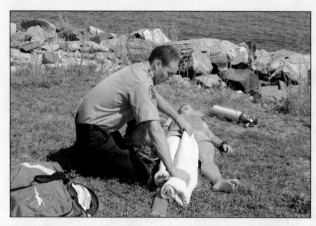

▲ Place folded blanket between legs, groin to feet.

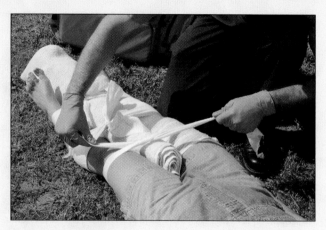

▲ Tie thighs, calves, and ankles together. Do not tie the knot over the injured area.

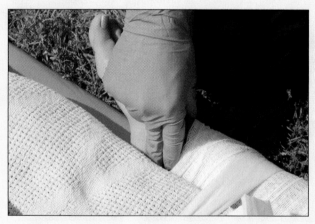

▲ Reassess distal CSM function.

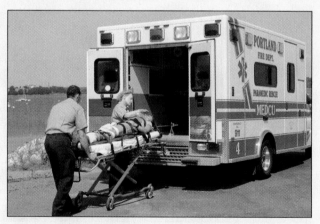

▲ Provide emergency care for shock, and administer high-concentration oxygen.

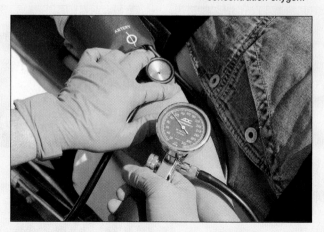

▲ Monitor vital signs during transport.

SCAN 32-5   **USING THE TWO-SPLINT TECHNIQUE**

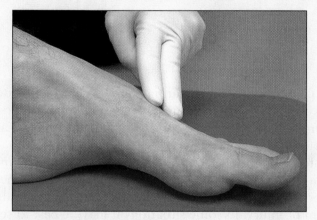

▲ Assess distal CSM function.

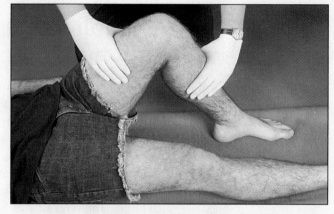

▲ Stabilize the knee above and below the injury site.

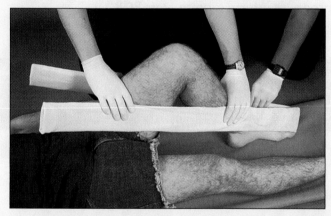

▲ Place the padded side of the splints next to the injured extremity. Note that they should be equal in length and extend 6–12 inches beyond the mid thigh and mid calf.

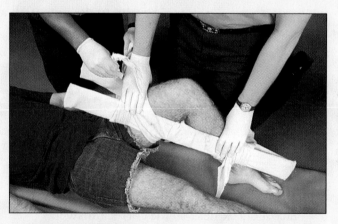

▲ Secure the splints at both ends using cravats or similar material.

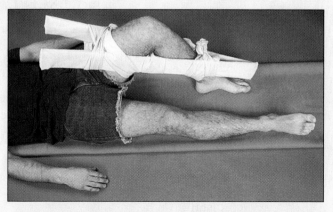

▲ Using a figure-eight configuration, secure one cravat to the ankle and the boards, the second cravat to the thigh and the boards. Reassess distal CSM function.

Ankle and Foot Injuries Ankle and foot injuries can be a challenge to splint, since there are few premanufactured splints for these injuries. One of the best devices for immobilizing the ankle and foot is the folded blanket or pillow. The trick is to fold the blanket in a long narrow fashion and place it under the bottom of the foot and up along both sides of the lower leg for support. Use cravats to secure the blanket or pillow to the extremity. Be sure to keep the toes exposed for easy assessment of CSM.

Complications Caused by Improper Splinting

5-3.7 List the complications of splinting.

An improperly applied splint can do more harm than no splint at all. If it is too tight, splints can cause painful pressure points, compress nerves, and restrict blood flow. If it is too loose, the splint will allow excessive movement of the injury that will cause unnecessary pain, bleeding, and swelling.

Valuable time can be wasted attempting to splint low-priority extremity injuries when the patient may have suffered a more serious injury that needs immediate attention. Before attempting to splint an isolated extremity injury, carefully evaluate the overall mechanism of injury. In some situations it may be best to secure the patient to a long board as a unit and not try and splint isolated injuries. Be sure to document all appropriate information in your PCR.

Stop, Review, Remember!

Multiple Choice

Place a check next to the correct answer.

1. All of the following examples are reasons to immobilize a skeletal injury EXCEPT to:

   _____ a. minimize movement.

   _____ b. minimize pain.

   _____ c. minimize bleeding and swelling.

   _____ d. reduce blood flow to the injury site.

2. Immobilization of a suspected skeletal injury can be accomplished by _____ stabilization and splinting.

   _____ a. manual   _____ c. distal

   _____ b. lateral   _____ d. proximal

3. All of the following are rules the EMT should follow when immobilizing a suspected skeletal injury, EXCEPT:

   _____ a. expose the injury site.

   _____ b. assess CSM before and after splinting.

   _____ c. immediately straighten angulated injuries.

   _____ d. immobilize the injury site.

4. When caring for a patient with a suspected fracture of the femur, what is the best way to immobilize the joint above the injury (hip)?

_____ a. Place patient in the recovery position.

_____ b. Secure patient to a long board.

_____ c. Tie both legs together.

_____ d. Ask the patient to remain still.

5. Which of the following best describes the term "position of function"?

_____ a. the position of comfort

_____ b. the position you find the patient in

_____ c. the way the patient is sitting

_____ d. the position the hand or foot is in when at rest

Fill in the Blank

1. In most cases, a musculoskeletal injury should be treated as a suspected _____ and immobilized accordingly.

2. The injured extremity should be _____ only after it has been properly immobilized and only if it does not cause further pain for the patient.

3. To minimize complications caused by _____, it will be necessary to immobilize the injury prior to transport.

4. Immobilization can be accomplished using one of two methods, _____ _____ and splinting.

5. The _____ refers to the position of the hands and feet when they are at rest and not under any type of force.

Critical Thinking

1. List the most common signs and symptoms of a closed skeletal injury.

_____

_____

_____

_____

_____

2. Describe how you would care for a suspected fracture of the knee if it were locked in a bent position.

_____

_____

_____

_____

_____

3. What is the value of immobilizing the joint above and below a suspected fracture site?

_____

_____

_____

_____

_____

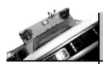

Dispatch Summary

David was transported to University Hospital where he was found to have a dislocated knee. Several attempts to manually reduce it proved unsuccessful, and the joint had to be realigned in surgery. David was released two days later and is currently undergoing physical therapy in an attempt to restore the knee's original integrity.

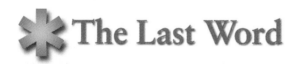

The Last Word

Injuries to muscles and bones, while painful, are rarely life threatening. They can be as simple as a sprained ankle and as severe as an open fracture of the femur.

It is essential to identify and manage all immediate life threats before attempting to splint a skeletal injury.

The basics of splinting are centered around the core steps of assessing distal circulation, sensation, and motor function before and after splinting; immobilizing the injury site; immobilizing the joints above and below the injury site; and making the patient as comfortable as possible. Be sure to document all appropriate information in your PCR.

Chapter Review

MULTIPLE CHOICE

Place a check next to the correct answer.

1. All of the following are examples of rigid splints, EXCEPT:

   _____ a. cardboard.

   _____ b. wood.

   _____ c. air splint.

   _____ d. aluminum.

2. There are two basic types of pneumatic splints, air and:

   _____ a. vacuum.

   _____ b. pressure.

   _____ c. ladder.

   _____ d. balloon.

3. The pneumatic anti shock garment may be used to immobilize a suspected fracture of the:

   _____ a. femur.

   _____ b. pelvis.

   _____ c. spine.

   _____ d. ankle.

4. When caring for a patient with a suspected fracture of the wrist, what is the best way to immobilize the joint above the injury (elbow)?

   _____ a. rigid splint

   _____ b. sling

   _____ c. air splint

   _____ d. vacuum splint

5. Which of the following would be the simplest way to immobilize an injured elbow that is found in the bent position?

   _____ a. air splint

   _____ b. traction splint

   _____ c. swathe

   _____ d. sling

6. Which on of the following would best immobilize an injured shoulder?

   _____ a. air splint

   _____ b. vacuum splint

   _____ c. sling and swathe

   _____ d. rigid splint

7. The bone in the upper arm is called the:

   _____ a. femur.

   _____ b. radius.

   _____ c. ulna.

   _____ d. humerus.

8. Which of the following statements is most accurate regarding the proper care for joint injuries?

   _____ a. Immobilize in the position found.

   _____ b. Straighten prior to splinting.

   _____ c. Treat with manual traction.

   _____ d. Elevate prior to splinting.

9. It is recommended to leave the _____ exposed when splinting a foot injury.

   _____ a. ankle

   _____ b. heel

   _____ c. toes

   _____ d. injury site

10. Which of the following is NOT a complication that can result from improper splinting?

   _____ a. increased circulation

   _____ b. increased bleeding

   _____ c. decreased circulation

   _____ d. increased swelling

MATCHING

You will be given a splinting device on the left and you must list or match as many practical applications for that device on the right. List the bones and or joints that can be immobilized using the device.

1. _____ Long rigid splint
2. _____ Short rigid splint
3. _____ Sling
4. _____ Swathe
5. _____ Blanket
6. _____ Pillow

A. Forearm, upper arm, lower extremity, bent arm (triangle)
B. Foot, ankle
C. Shoulder
D. Elbow, wrist
E. Straight knee, straight arm, bent knee (triangle)
F. Hand, wrist, forearm

CRITICAL THINKING

1. List the most common signs and symptoms of an open skeletal injury.

_____

_____

_____

_____

2. Describe how you would care for a suspected closed fracture of the shoulder.

_____

_____

_____

_____

3. In most cases there is a weakness on the side of injury when you compare both extremities. What is likely the most common cause for this difference?

_____

_____

_____

CASE STUDIES

Case Study 1

You respond to a dispatch for a vehicle collision a few miles outside of town. Upon arrival, you are directed down an embankment by a police officer at the scene. He states that the only patient is the driver of a motorcycle that appears to have hit the guard rail before exiting the roadway. As you approach the patient, you find a bystander holding a bloody towel on the patient's head. The bystander states that he is a first responder and that the patient is unresponsive but appears to have a good airway and is breathing. Your initial assessment finds this to be accurate, and your rapid trauma assessment reveals deformity to the lower right leg, upper left leg, and right forearm.

1. Now that you know his ABCs are okay, what will be your priority for caring for this patient?

_____

_____

_____

2. How will you care for this man's extremity injuries?

_____

_____

_____

3. Is this man a candidate for a traction splint? If so, which leg?

_____

_____

_____

Case Study 2

You are caring for a 14-year-old girl who fell while roller blading and has pain and deformity in her right forearm. She was wearing a helmet and denies hitting her head or any loss of consciousness. She states that she hit her arm on the curb as she fell. Your assessment of the distal extremity reveals numbness, tingling, and the absence of a pulse and delayed capillary refill. The girl's mother is on the scene and has provided consent for treatment.

1. What is your primary concern as you care for this patient?

_____

_____

_____

2. How will you manage the fact that there appears to be no circulation in the distal extremity?

_____

_____

_____

3. Describe exactly how you will immobilize this injury.

_____

_____

_____

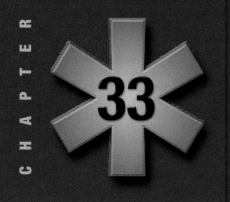

33 Patients with Head Injuries

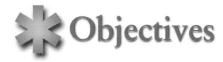

Objectives

Numbered objectives are from the U.S. Department of Transportation 1994 EMT-Basic National Standard Curriculum.

COGNITIVE OBJECTIVES

At the completion of this lesson, the EMT-Basic student will be able to:

5-4.1   State the components of the nervous system. (p. 836)

5-4.2   List the functions of the central nervous system. (pp. 836–838)

5-4.3   Define the structure of the skeletal system as it relates to the nervous system. (pp. 835–838)

5-4.4   Relate mechanism of injury to potential injuries of the head and spine. (p. 847)

5-4.11 Establish the relationship between airway management and the patient with head and spine injuries. (pp. 848–849)

PSYCHOMOTOR OBJECTIVES

At the completion of this lesson, the EMT-Basic student will be able to:

5-4.44 Demonstrate completing a prehospital care report for patients with head and spinal injuries. (p. 856)

AFFECTIVE OBJECTIVES

No affective objectives identified.

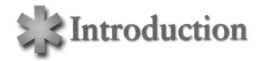

Introduction

Head injuries can range from minor to fatal and occur in a wide range of circumstances. The skull is a closed container without cushioning or room for expansion. Because of this, any trauma to the outside of the head can cause serious trauma to the brain within. And since we can't see inside, the assessment, decision-making, and care we perform will be critical to the patient's survival.

Head injuries associated with spinal injuries are covered in the next chapter, chapter 34. This chapter will detail head injuries only.

Emergency Dispatch

"**H**old on! We're gonna get hit!" EMT Ron Hyde shouted back into the patient compartment as he spun the steering wheel away from the headlights that were rapidly descending toward the ambulance's windshield. The large truck's tires squealed, lost traction, and bounced violently across the pavement toward the freeway median.

The evasive maneuver was enough to prevent the airborne Volkswagen from hitting them head-on. Instead, it impacted the passenger-side of the cab—collapsing it almost right up to where Ron was sitting. The force of the hit tilted the ambulance up onto the left-side tires for a moment before it righted itself with a thundering crash.

For a long moment after the ambulance scraped to a halt on the edge of the median, there was silence, broken only by the hissing of something in the truck's damaged engine.

"What *happened?*" Ron's partner, Barry Luden, called from the patient compartment.

"I'm . . . uh . . . not exactly sure," Ron said, taking off his seatbelt. "How's the patient?"

"I'm okay," Mrs. Lawson, their geriatric patient with shortness of breath said. Her voice was muffled by the nonrebreather mask.

"Dispatch, Medical 9." Ron waited for the dispatcher's response before continuing. "We're on . . . uh . . . 53 . . . just east of . . . the . . . the Merrimac exit. I think I need help."

Ron then pushed his door open and fell, unconscious, onto the pavement.

Anatomy and Physiology of the Head

The bony structure we call the head is actually a series of bones that, joined together, are called the cranium or skull. The skull itself can be divided into the **cranial skull** or **cranial vault** and the facial bones.

The cranial vault is comprised of a series of fused bones including the temporal, frontal, parietal, and occipital bones (Figure 33-1 on page 836). The **basilar skull** forms the floor of the skull. There are many small protrusions or ridges that rise from the basilar skull that can injure the brain when it is moved or compressed.

The basilar skull and **temporal bones** are the weakest areas of the skull and more prone to fracture and subsequent damage to areas adjacent to the brain.

5-4.3 Define the structure of the skeletal system as it relates to the nervous system.

∗ **cranial skull** or **cranial vault**

portion of the skull containing the brain and comprised of the temporal, frontal, parietal, and occipital bones.

∗ **basilar skull**

portion of the skull that forms the floor of the skull.

✳ **temporal bones**

bones that form part of the side of the skull. There is a right and a left temporal bone.

5-4.1   State the components of the nervous system.

5-4.2   List the functions of the central nervous system.

✳ **maxilla**

the upper jaw bone. There are two bones fused together.

✳ **mandible**

the lower jaw bone.

✳ **nasal bones**

the bones that form the upper third, or bridge, of the nose.

✳ **temporomandibular joint**

the movable joint formed between the mandible and the temporal bone, also called the TM joint.

✳ **ethmoid bone**

bone that helps form the nasal cavity.

✳ **lacrimal bone**

bone that helps form the nasal cavity.

✳ **malar bone**

the cheek bone. Also called the zygomatic bone.

✳ **orbits**

the bony structures around the eyes; the eye sockets.

✳ **central nervous system**

part of the nervous system composed of the brain and spinal cord.

✳ **dura mater**

fibrous layer of tissue lining the inside of the cranial vault.

✳ **pia mater**

layer of tissue directly covering the brain.

✳ **arachnoid membrane**

weblike layer of tissue located between the dura mater and the pia mater.

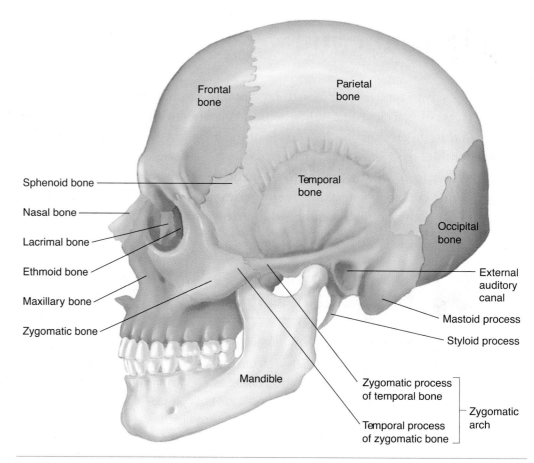

FIGURE 33-1   The bones of the human skull.

The facial bones include the **maxilla, mandible,** and **nasal bones** and form the **temporomandibular joint** (Figure 33-1). There are several smaller bones that make up the nose and sinuses, including the **ethmoid bone, lacrimal bone** and **malar bone.** The **orbits** are the bony structures around the eyes.

The brain is one part of the **central nervous system.** The central nervous system consists of the brain and the spinal cord. This system is responsible for involuntary functions of the body such as heartbeat, breathing, and temperature regulation as well as functions such as sensation and movement throughout the body, thought, and reasoning.

The brain is covered with three membranes or layers (Figure 33-2). The **dura mater** is a fibrous layer that lines the inside of the cranial vault. The **pia mater** lies directly over the brain tissue. Between these two layers is a very thin, weblike layer called the **arachnoid membrane.** These three layers are called the **meninges,** and also cover the spine. **Cerebrospinal fluid** is produced within the brain and resides in the subarachnoid space.

Cerebrospinal fluid is found around both the brain and spinal cord. It acts as a cushion to the brain in the event of trauma. You will see later in this chapter that a clear fluid coming from the nose or ears may indicate a serious head injury. This clear fluid is cerebrospinal fluid that leaks from the normally closed system when a skull fracture occurs.

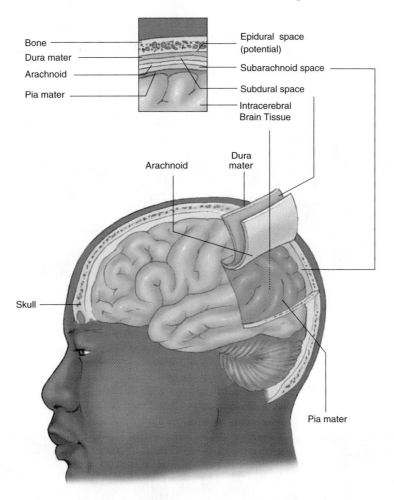

Bone
Dura mater
Arachnoid
Pia mater

Epidural space (potential)
Subarachnoid space
Subdural space
Intracerebral Brain Tissue

Arachnoid
Dura mater
Skull
Pia mater

FIGURE 33-2   Meninges of the brain.

The brain, which takes up the vast majority of the cranial vault, is composed of several regions, each with a specific function (Figure 33-3 on page 838). These include:

* **Cerebrum**—The cerebrum, the largest portion of the brain, is divided into four sections. The cerebrum is responsible for conscious activities, personality, and sensory input.
  * **Frontal**—emotions, speech, motor function
  * **Parietal**—sensory functions
  * **Temporal**—memory, some components of speech
  * **Occipital**—vision

* **Cerebellum**—The cerebellum sits behind and under the cerebrum. It is responsible for coordination, posture, and equilibrium.

* **Brain stem**—The brainstem is at the base of the brain and controls vital activities such as respiration, cardiac function, and blood pressure. There are several parts of the brainstem, including the midbrain, pons, and medulla.

The brain connects with the spinal cord at the base of the skull. The medulla, also known as the **medulla oblongata**, physically connects the brain to the spinal cord through an opening in the base of the skull called the foramen magnum.

* **meninges**

  three membranes that surround and protect the brain and spinal cord. They are the dura mater, the pia mater, and the arachnoid membrane.

* **cerebrospinal fluid**

  fluid found around the brain and spinal cord that helps cushion them.

* **cerebrum**

  largest portion of the brain, responsible for conscious activities, personality, and sensory input.

* **cerebellum**

  portion of the brain that lies behind and under the cerebrum. It is responsible for coordination, posture, and equilibrium.

* **brainstem**

  portion of the brain located at the base, responsible for vital activities such as respiration, cardiac function, and blood pressure.

* **medulla oblongata**

  portion of the brain that directly connects to the spinal cord. Also called the medulla.

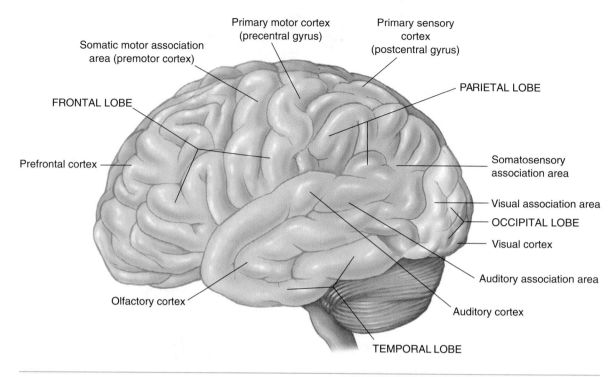

FIGURE 33-3 Regions of the brain.

Stop, Review, Remember!

Multiple Choice

Place a check next to the correct answer.

1. The weakest areas of the skull are the:

     _____ a. temporal and occipital.

     _____ b. parietal and occipital.

     _____ c. frontal and temporal.

     _____ d. basilar and temporal.

2. The layers of the meninges in order from skull to brain are:

     _____ a. dura, arachnoid, pia.

     _____ b. arachnoid, pia, dura.

     _____ c. pia, arachnoid, dura.

     _____ d. dura, pia, arachnoid.

3. Which of the following is NOT a facial bone?

     _____ a. maxilla   _____ c. zygomatic

     _____ b. mandible   _____ d. axis

4. Which of the following statements in reference to cerebrospinal fluid is false?

     _____ a. Cerebrospinal fluid covers the brain and spinal cord.

     _____ b. Cerebrospinal fluid coming from the ears or nose indicates serious head injury.

     _____ c. Cerebrospinal fluid coming from the mouth indicates minor head injury.

     _____ d. Cerebrospinal fluid is clear in color.

5. The portion of the brain responsible for vital functions such as respiration and cardiac activity is the:

_____ a. cerebrum.

_____ b. cerebellum.

_____ c. brainstem.

_____ d. spinal cord.

Matching

Match the function on the left with the portion of the brain responsible for that function on the right.

1. _____ Coordination

2. _____ Vision

3. _____ Speech

4. _____ Emotions

5. _____ Respiration

6. _____ Memory

7. _____ Sensory

8. _____ Equilibrium

A. Cerebrum (frontal)
B. Cerebrum (parietal)
C. Cerebrum (temporal)
D. Cerebrum (occipital)
E. Cerebellum
F. Brainstem

Critical Thinking

1. Why is the cranial skull also called the cranial vault?

_____

_____

_____

_____

_____

2. Explain the dura mater's connection to the other layers of the brain.

_____

_____

_____

_____

_____

Head Injury Classification

✳ **open head injury**

head injury where there is a break in the skull.

✳ **closed head injury**

head injury where there is no break.

✳ **laceration**

a cut; in head injuries, may be a cut to the scalp or to the brain itself.

✳ **crush injury**

mechanism of injury in which tissue is locally compressed by high pressure forces.

There are two types of head injury—**open head injury** and **closed head injury**. Within these two broad classifications there are many types of injuries, some minor and some very serious.

Any injury to the head should be considered serious. In open injuries, in addition to the possibility of direct injury to the brain, injury to the many blood vessels supplying the head can cause profuse bleeding. Closed injuries can cause indirect damage to the brain and swelling within the skull. Brain swelling within the skull is especially dangerous because the rigid skull limits the amount of swelling, which can cause compression of the brain.

An open head injury is one in which there has been a break in the skull (Figures 33-4A and B). The injury can range from relatively minor such as a **laceration** to soft tissue to serious or even fatal (like a **crush injury** that exposes brain tissue through a fractured skull).

Closed head injuries involve damage to the skull and/or brain by a traumatic force that does not cause an open injury of the skull (Figure 33-5). Do not be fooled into thinking that an injury isn't serious simply because there is no bleeding. You will soon learn that dangerously high pressures can develop in a closed head injury—pressures that can cause death if untreated.

These injuries can also be classified by the structure that is injured. Injuries to the scalp involve laceration or bruising from trauma such as the head striking the windshield in a motor vehicle collision.

Injuries to the skull involve damage to the bony structure housing the brain and the bones of the face. Even though the skull is made of bone and is quite durable, it may be fractured by trauma.

Skull fractures may range from undetectable cracks to areas that can be palpated and identified as depressed to major trauma in which brain tissue is exposed.

The brain itself may be injured in both open and closed injuries. In severe skull fractures, brain tissue may be damaged and exposed. This is a grave condition.

Closed head trauma may cause bleeding and/or swelling within the skull that creates pressure on the brain that will compress the brain and alter its function. Excessive bleeding or swelling (discussed in greater detail later in this chapter) within the skull will cause serious injury and often death.

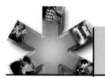

Perspective

Barry—The EMT

"I heard him open the driver's door and thought that he was either checking on the other driver or was going to open the back doors. But then I heard him hit the ground and he didn't respond to my yelling; I got worried. My immediate fear was that it might be some kind of head injury, you know? He seemed a little confused on the radio. But, holy Toledo that was a big, big crash. That other car was actually imbedded in the cab of our truck. I'm actually surprised that none of us were killed. He better be okay. I'd better call his wife."

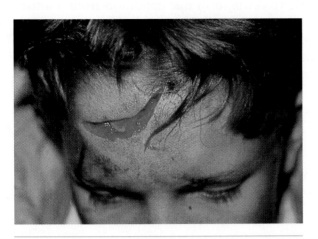

FIGURE 33-4A   A simple scalp laceration.

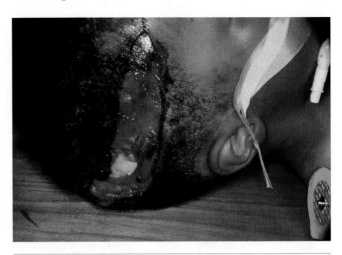

FIGURE 33-4B   A lethal open skull fracture. (Charles Stewart, M.D., and Associates.)

CONCUSSION
• Relatively minor injury, usually with no detectable brain damage
• May have brief loss of consciousness
• Headache, grogginess, and short-term memory loss common

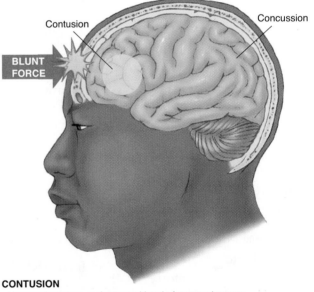

CONTUSION
• Unconsciousness or decreased level of responsiveness
• Bruising of brain tissue

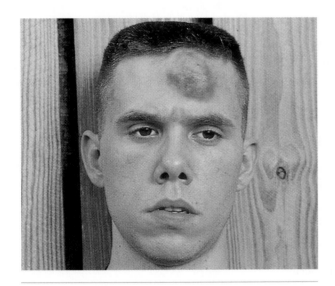

FIGURE 33-5   A closed head injury.

FIGURE 33-6   Concussion and contusion are two types of closed head injury.

You may also hear the terms **concussion** and **contusion** (Figure 33-6). A concussion is an injury that causes jarring to the brain resulting in temporary signs and symptoms. There is usually no permanent damage from a concussion, although it may appear serious at first and symptoms may persist for some time. A concussion may cause loss of consciousness immediately after the injury as well as other forms of altered mental status including loss of memory about the incident, confusion, and headache. If a patient is conscious after the accident without signs and symptoms and develops problems later, the cause is likely a more serious head injury—not a concussion.

A contusion is a bruising of brain tissue. The bleeding in this injury is limited but significant enough to cause altered mental status and other signs and symptoms lasting longer than those of a concussion.

* **concussion**

type of injury causing a jarring to the brain and temporary signs and symptoms including loss of memory about the incident and confusion.

* **contusion**

bruising of the brain tissue.

In the field it will not be possible to distinguish one condition from another. Most importantly, remember that all patients with signs of head trauma of any type should receive hospital examination and care.

Finally, keep in mind that damage to the brain may be due to either primary or secondary factors. The most common primary factor is trauma. Secondary factors may be conditions such as hypoxia, hypoglycemia, and others that can damage the brain as a result of a problem elsewhere in the body.

INTRACRANIAL PRESSURE

Perhaps the most serious problem associated with closed head injury is increasing **intracranial pressure**. When a blow to the head causes injury to the brain or surrounding tissues, bleeding and swelling develop. As little as 20–30 mL of blood can begin to cause intracranial pressure.

Since the skull forms a rigid container, pressure begins to build on the brain. As the pressure continues to rise, the brain is compressed. Eventually the brain begins to shift downward, compressing the brainstem—the part of the brain that controls our most vital bodily functions.

Signs and symptoms of increased intracranial pressure include the following:

* Decreasing mental status

* Vomiting

* Headache

The patient also will exhibit some or all of the following, depending on the amount of pressure inside the cranium.

* Seizures

* Weakness or paralysis on one side of the body

* Abnormal posturing (**decorticate** or **decerebrate**) (Figure 33-7)

* Abnormal breathing patterns

* Decreased pulse rate

* Increased blood pressure

* Nonreactive pupils, dilated pupils, or unequal pupils

* Decreasing Glasgow Coma Score

✳ **intracranial pressure**

increasing pressure within the brain vault due to bleeding and/or swelling.

✳ **decorticate**

patient posture characterized by stiff flexed arms, clenched fists, and extended legs.

✳ **decerebrate**

patient posture characterized by stiff extended arms and pronated forearms.

Clinical Clues: INTRACRANIAL PRESSURE

Not all head injuries cause intracranial pressure. As a matter of fact, most don't. There are a wide range of bumps, scrapes, and lacerations that will cause no permanent damage. The problem is that we can't see inside the skull to look for hidden damage.

When evaluating a patient for potential intracranial bleeding, it is crucial to remember that patients on prescription blood thinners such as Coumadin (warfarin) are at a more significant risk for life-threatening intracranial bleeding, even with an apparently minor mechanism of head injury.

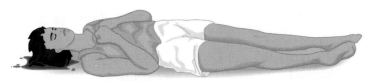

Flexion (decorticate) posturing.

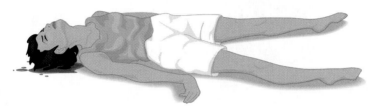

Extension (decerebrate) posturing.

FIGURE 33-7   Nonpurposeful movements: flexion (decorticate) and extension (decerebrate) posturing.

Cushing's triad is commonly taught as an indicator of markedly increased intracranial pressure. The three signs that make up the triad are increased blood pressure, decreased pulse rate, and abnormal respirations. In reality, Cushing's triad is not often seen with all three signs together.

SUBDURAL HEMATOMA

In an injury called **subdural hematoma,** a blow to the head, sometimes as simple as a fall striking the head, causes tearing of small bridging veins between the dura and arachnoid layers inside the skull (Figure 33-8 on page 844). This may most commonly be seen in elderly patients, those in chronically poor health, or alcoholics who have experienced a slight shrinking of brain tissue that causes stretching of these bridging veins. The head injury causes these already vulnerable vessels to rupture. Bleeding begins in the subdural space.

Because the bleeding is venous, it may be slow. Subdural hematomas can begin without symptoms and develop over hours to days. Very slow bleeding may result in a subdural hematoma that produces few or no symptoms for several days or even weeks. Subdural hematomas are the most common type of severe head injury. The slow onset helps us to understand why we insist all patients with head injury go to the hospital—even if the patient seems "OK" at the scene.

EPIDURAL HEMATOMA

With a quicker onset and usually involving arterial bleeding in the brain, an **epidural hematoma** is caused by bleeding between the skull and the dura (Figure 33-9 on page 844). A common scenario for epidural hematoma is trauma to the temporal area of the skull that causes a fracture and damage to an artery in that area. Some patients are unconscious briefly due to the blow to the head (similar to a concussion), regain consciousness, and then lose consciousness again because of the increased pressure in the brain.

Epidural hematomas are rarer than subdural hematomas, but because epidural hematomas often involve arterial bleeding, the onset is quicker and the condition is more severe, requiring rapid neurosurgical care.

Both subdural and epidural hematomas can cause a series of signs and symptoms called **herniation syndrome** (Figure 33-10 on page 844). A **herniation** is when tissue protrudes outside of the area in which it is normally contained. In the case of the brain, since the skull is a closed container, when pressure develops brain

* **Cushing's triad**

  three signs indicative of increased intracranial pressure: increased blood pressure, decreased pulse and abnormal respirations.

* **subdural hematoma**

  collection of blood between the dura mater and the arachnoid membrane.

* **epidural hematoma**

  collection of blood between the dura mater and the skull.

* **herniation syndrome**

  signs and symptoms indicative of a brain herniation, including decreasing mental status, vomiting, and headache.

* **herniation**

  tissue protrusion outside of the area in which it is normally contained.

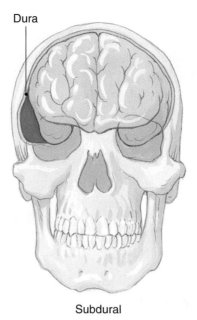

Dura

Subdural

FIGURE 33-8 Subdural hematoma.

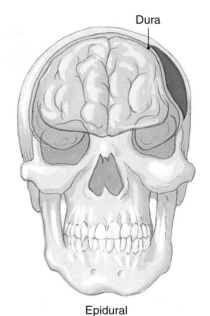

Dura

Epidural

FIGURE 33-9 Epidural hematoma.

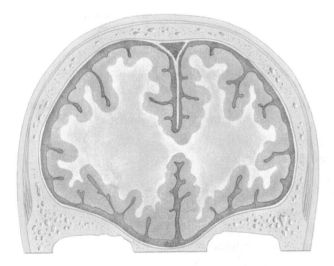

Intracranial pressure begins when trauma causes damage to blood vessels within the layers covering the brain.

Since the brain takes up almost all of the space within the skull, the blood quickly begins to cause pressure which compresses the brain.

As pressure increases, one of the earliest changes you will see is altered mental status.

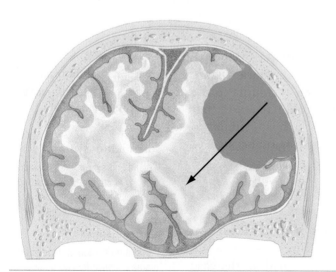

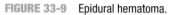

As the hematoma continues to expand it displaces brain tissue. Because of this expansion and displacement the only place for the brain to move is through the foramen magnum at the base of the skull. This movement puts pressure on the brainstem—the area responsible for vital body functions such as respiration. The hematoma forces the brain in the direction indicated by the arrow.

As the pressure continues to build, the mental status decreases further. As pressure becomes severe you will see some combination of slow pulse, increased blood pressure, abnormal pupils and irregular or gasping respirations. You may also see abnormal posturing spontaneously or in response to painful stimulus.

FIGURE 33-10 Progression of herniation syndrome.

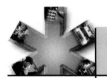

Clinical Clues: HEAD INJURY

It will never be your job as an EMT to determine what type of head injury a patient has sustained (epidural vs subdural). What is important is that you recognize significant MOI and signs and symptoms of head injury. Any patient with a head injury should be encouraged to accept your transport to an emergency department for a complete evaluation.

tissue is compressed. When that can no longer occur the brain is pushed downward causing herniation of brain tissue. Ultimately, the cerebrum and cerebellum may be compressed down onto the brainstem. When the brainstem is compressed, it is forced out of the skull through the foramen magnum, and vital functions such as respiration are compromised.

Perspective

Dr. Mendelez—Emergency Department Physician

"We obviously care for all our patients, but when they bring in somebody in uniform it somehow just changes the mood in the ED. And then I saw it was Ron. I had just talked to him on the phone about 20 minutes before about the patient they were bringing in. That's really tough! And as soon as they came through the doors, I could see he was posturing and . . . oh . . . my heart just sank. Ron's a good guy and he doesn't deserve this kind of thing . . . he just doesn't. It feels different when I know the person."

Stop, Review, Remember!

Multiple Choice

Place a check next to the correct answer.

1. Which of the following is NOT a component of Cushing's triad?

_____ a. increased blood pressure

_____ b. decreased pulse rate

_____ c. fixed pupils

_____ d. abnormal respirations

2. Tissue forced out of an area in which it is normally contained is called:

_____ a. infarction.

_____ b. impalement.

_____ c. compression.

_____ d. herniation.

3. Subdural hematomas form between the:

_____ a. dura and arachnoid layers.

_____ b. arachnoid and pia mater.

_____ c. arachnoid layer and the brain.

_____ d. skull and the dura.

4. The most posterior portion of the brain is called the _____ lobe.

_____ a. temporal   _____ c. occipital

_____ b. frontal   _____ d. parietal

5. The portion of the brain that controls functions such as emotion, speech, and vision is the _____.

_____ a. pons.

_____ b. medulla.

_____ c. cerebellum.

_____ d. cerebrum.

6. EMS providers can always distinguish between a concussion and more serious conditions in the field.

_____ a. true

_____ b. false

7. Damage to the brain cannot be caused by conditions such as hypoxia and hypoglycemia.

_____ a. true

_____ b. false

Labeling

Label the regions and bones of the human skull on the diagram.

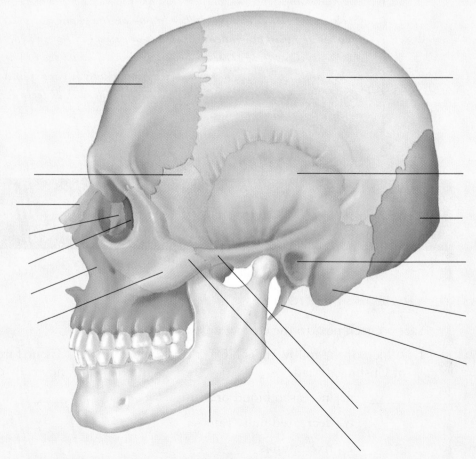

Critical Thinking

1. What is the difference in patient presentation between a patient with a closed injury and a patient with a closed injury and herniation?

_____

_____

_____

_____

2. You are treating a patient who appears to have struck his head on the windshield in a motor vehicle accident. You observe a large hematoma on the forehead. The patient is unresponsive. His pulse is 112, respirations 28, BP 88/52. Are these vital signs caused by his head injury? Why or why not?

_____

_____

_____

_____

Patient Assessment and Care

We have learned thus far that head injuries can be very serious. Head injuries can also pose a significant problem for EMTs in that it is difficult to distinguish the less serious head injuries from the life-threatening head injuries in the field. Since symptoms may vary from person to person and may not show in the patient anywhere from hours to weeks, your thorough and accurate assessment and care of the patient will be critical.

SCENE SIZE-UP

During the scene size-up, safety is always a primary concern. Be sure you are not injured by the same trauma mechanism that injured your patient. Be alert for the mechanism of injury as you approach the scene and the patient. Remember that some patients seem "fine" but may have hidden injuries. Mechanism of injury will be an important indicator to detect possible hidden injuries.

5-4.4 Relate mechanism of injury to potential injuries of the head and spine.

Injuries to the mouth and nose can cause blood to be sprayed when the patient speaks or shouts. Unresponsive patients with these injuries will require suction. Both of these situations will require face protection as part of your BSI determination.

INITIAL ASSESSMENT

Here you will form a general impression as you approach the patient. Combined with the mechanism of injury, this should give you a good starting point for determining the seriousness of the patient. Observe the patient's level of consciousness

5-4.11 Establish the relationship between airway management and the patient with head and spine injuries.

as you approach. An altered mental status or seizures indicate that the patient has a serious injury.

Remember that injuries to the face and head have the potential for significant bleeding. Be prepared to suction the airway—continuously if necessary. This will require someone stationed at the airway for the entire call. This person can administer oxygen and/or ventilate.

Be sure to control severe bleeding. You will also check the pulse and the skin color, temperature, and condition. While you won't check a full pulse rate, a very slow pulse in a patient with an altered mental status and a closed head injury might be the result of increased intracranial pressure.

RAPID TRAUMA ASSESSMENT

Patients with a significant mechanism of injury will receive a rapid trauma assessment. When examining the head, feel the cranium for any signs of injury, including deformity, depression, swelling, or open injury (Figure 33-11).

While palpation of the facial bones for injury and examining the nose and ears for clear (cerebrospinal) fluid is part of the detailed assessment, you may observe these signs as you palpate the head during the rapid trauma examination (Figure 33-12). You will recall from earlier in the chapter that clear fluid from the ears and/or nose may indicate a basilar skull fracture.

You may also observe bruising around the eyes (**raccoon eyes**) (Figure 33-13) or **Battle's sign** (Figure 33–14) indicating a basilar skull fracture. These are late signs of injury and will most likely not be seen in an injury that has just occurred.

VITAL SIGNS AND HISTORY

As with any patient, trends in vital signs over time paint the best picture. Remember that mental status is an important indicator in head-injured patients. Patients

✳ **raccoon eyes**
  bruising around the eyes indicative of a basilar skull fracture.

✳ **Battle's sign**
  bruising behind the ears (over the mastoid process) indicative of a basilar skull fracture.

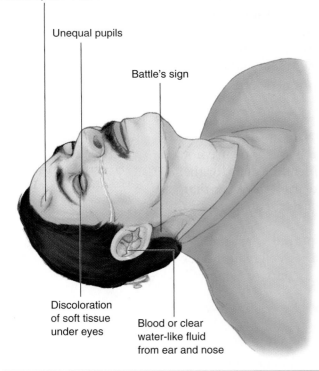

Deformity of the skull

Unequal pupils

Battle's sign

Discoloration of soft tissue under eyes

Blood or clear water-like fluid from ear and nose

FIGURE 33-11   Signs of cranial fracture or brain injury.

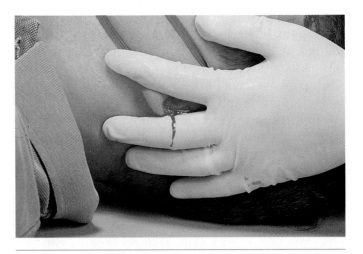

FIGURE 33-12   Blood or fluid draining from a patient's ear suggests basilar skull fracture.

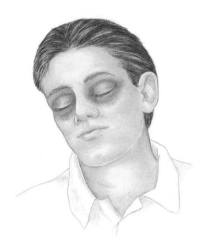

FIGURE 33-13   Bilateral periorbital ecchymosis (raccoon eyes).

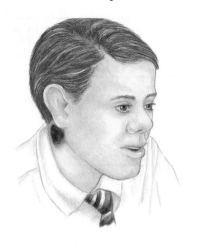

FIGURE 33-14   Retroauricular ecchymosis (Battle's sign).

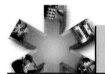

Perspective

Dayna Ridge—The EMT

"I can't believe I was responding to Ron. I mean . . . he's Ron! He's been here longer than anyone I know. He was my first partner after I got out of EMT school and he actually came to my goofy little graduation ceremony when I got my paramedic cert. And there I was tonight—assessing him on the side of the freeway. That's the first time I've ever actually seen Cushing's in real life. That whole call was just wrong. It keeps kind of glossing over in my mind, like it's not real. And then it just jumps back into my face, you know? I don't know what to do right now."

with a concussion may start with unconsciousness or confusion. In many cases these patients gradually regain memory and become less confused. Patients with rising intracranial pressure will have a persistent altered mental status or will have a gradually decreased mental status.

Just as you trend vital signs including blood pressure and pulse, you will need to trend the level of consciousness of patients who have a head injury. The most widely accepted system of trending mental status in patients with a head injury is the Glasgow Coma Score.

GLASGOW COMA SCORE

The **Glasgow Coma Score (GCS)** (Figure 33-15 on page 850) is a numerical scale that rates patients on eye opening, speech, and motor function. This was covered briefly in chapter 21, but we will discuss it in more detail here.

This scale and its scores, which range from 3 to 15, is valuable in monitoring and documenting trends in the patient's neurological status and in determining

✳ **Glasgow Coma Score (GCS)**

numerical score that rates patients on eye opening, speech, and motor function.

FIGURE 33-15 Glascow Coma Score.

GLASGOW COMA SCORE

Eye Opening	Spontaneous	4	
	To Voice	3	
	To Pain	2	
	None	1	
Verbal Response	Oriented	5	
	Confused	4	
	Inappropriate Words	3	
	Incomprehensible Sounds	2	
	None	1	
Motor Response	Obeys Command	6	
	Localizes Pain	5	
	Withdraws (pain)	4	
	Flexion (pain)	3	
	Extension (pain)	2	
	None	1	
Glasgow Coma Score Total			

what care is appropriate for patients with specific types of head injury. The scale is also used in many EMS systems as a triage device to help determine which patients should be transported to trauma centers.

There are three components to the total score that may be obtained on the Glasgow Coma Score:

∗ **Eye opening**—Patients are assigned a score based on whether their eyes open spontaneously (4 points), open to voice (3 points), open to painful stimulus (2 points) or not at all (1 point).

∗ **Verbal response**—Patients are assigned a score based on whether their verbal response is normal and oriented (5 points), confused (4 points), inappropriate words (3 points), incomprehensible (2 points), or none (1 point)

∗ **Motor response**—Patients are assigned a score based on their motor function: patients who follow commands (6 points), localize pain (5 points), withdraw from pain (4 points), display **flexion**/decorticate posturing (3 points), display **extension**/decerebrate posturing (2 points), or no response (1 point).

You will note in the patient care section that follows that your care may depend on the patient's Glasgow Coma Score. If your patient requires constant suction and airway care or has other life-threatening conditions that require your attention, do not spend time obtaining a GCS. This patient already has a high priority for transport.

Remember that the classic pattern of decreasing pulse, increasing blood pressure, and abnormal respirations (Cushing's Triad) only occurs when a patient is experiencing increased intracranial pressure. A patient may have a serious or de-

∗ **flexion**

movement toward a bent position. Opposite of extension.

∗ **extension**

movement toward a straightened position. Opposite of flexion.

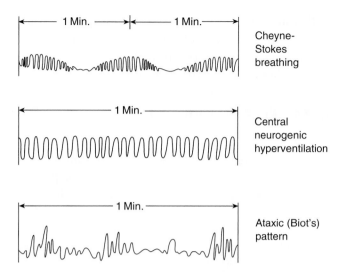

FIGURE 33-16 Abnormal respiratory patterns seen in head injuries.

veloping head injury without these signs, and patients with a severe head injury may not display all signs.

The signs and symptoms of head injury commonly occur immediately after a traumatic event you are called to. In other cases you may be called to a patient with an altered mental status who experienced trauma some time ago and doesn't recall it. A patient may also experience intracranial bleeding from a broken blood vessel without having experienced trauma, although this is less common.

Certain abnormal breathing patterns may be observed in head-injured patients with rising intracranial pressure (Figure 33-16). These patterns indicate serious conditions affecting the brain, including lack of perfusion and oxygen and increasing pressure on brain tissue. It is not critical to memorize or recognize each pattern. What is most important is that irregular patterns such as these generally indicate significant injury.

Abnormal breathing patterns include:

* **Cheyne-Stokes respirations**—a breathing pattern characterized by gradually increasing, then decreasing tidal volume with a period of apnea.

* **Central neurogenic hyperventilation**—deep, rapid respirations (as indicated by the term hyperventilation) caused by damage or injury to the brainstem such as may be seen in herniation syndrome.

* **Ataxic (Biot's) respirations**—a breathing pattern characterized by deep, gasping breaths separated by periods of apnea.

When possible, obtain a medical history from the patient or a family member. Be alert for other conditions that can cause an altered mental status. A patient in a

* **Cheyne-Stokes respirations**

   pattern of respirations characterized by gradually increasing, then decreasing tidal volumes with a period of apnea.

* **central neurogenic hyperventilation**

   pattern of respirations characterized by deep, rapid respirations (as indicated by the term hyperventilation) but the cause is from damage or injury to the brainstem such as may be seen in herniation syndrome.

* **ataxic (Biot's) respirations**

   pattern of respirations characterized by deep, gasping breaths separated by periods of apnea.

Clinical Clues: AVOIDING HYPOXIA OR LOW BLOOD PRESSURE

Brain injury experts have determined that the two things that most negatively affect the recovery of head-injured patients are allowing hypoxia or low blood pressure to develop after the initial injury. Prevention, early recognition and aggressive treatment of airway problems, breathing difficulties and hypoperfusion are the most important prehospital interventions that can be made for the head-injured patient.

collision may exhibit an altered mental status and appear to have a head injury but may be diabetic or have suffered a seizure. Remember that medical and trauma complaints may also occur at the same time in the same patient (such as a seizure that causes a fall resulting in head injury).

DETAILED EXAMINATION

The detailed examination is done en route to the hospital. The detailed exam repeats the areas examined in the rapid trauma examination and adds some examinations very important in the head-injured patient. Here the ears and nose will be examined for blood or clear fluid and the facial bones will be palpated.

Patient Care

From the material presented in this chapter you have learned that there are two types of head injury: open and closed. Head-injured patients may also develop rising intracranial pressure. Your care for the head-injured patient will depend on your assessment.

CARING FOR HEAD INJURIES

Care for a head injury begins during the scene size-up when you take BSI precautions and observe the mechanism of injury. If you suspect spine injury, take spinal stabilization maneuvers as you begin your initial assessment.

Be alert for airway problems. Open head injuries can bleed profusely. If blood is near or flows into the airway, constant monitoring and frequent suction will be required.

Also during the initial assessment you will observe the patient's mental status. An altered mental status is one of the most significant signs of head injury. Note the patient's mental status initially and throughout the call. Decreasing mental status is a serious sign. Time and priorities permitting, you will track changes in the patient during your care using the Glasgow Coma Score.

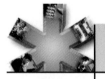

Perspective

Barry—The EMT

"In my head I just keep hearing those really irregular snoring respirations that Ron had. And the sound of tires crunching on broken glass as other cars were driving slowly past the accident scene on their way to wherever they were going, you know? I kept seeing their eyes darting around as they rolled past. The passersby are always curious but not always concerned. It seemed to go on forever. I put a nonrebreather mask on Ron and now I was trying to care for two patients, you know? I didn't know what else to do."

OXYGENATION AND VENTILATION

Head-injured patients require oxygen. It has been mentioned several times in this text that patients who are breathing adequately will receive oxygen by nonrebreather mask; those breathing inadequately will receive assisted ventilation with a pocket face mask or bag-valve mask.

For head-injured patients, there is one additional and very important consideration: the rate of assisted ventilations or artificial ventilation. In the past, EMTs were instructed to hyperventilate all head-injured patients to help reduce intracranial swelling and pressure. Research has demonstrated that ventilating too fast was actually harmful. In this case, more isn't better. Normal ventilations at the rate of 10–12/minute are appropriate in most cases.

If the patient is experiencing the most severe form of head injury, cerebral herniation, however, ventilating at a slightly faster rate has been recommended. Signs of herniation that would cause you to ventilate at a faster rate include:

1. Evidence of a head injury or history indicating head involvement, such as headache before losing consciousness

2. Unresponsiveness

3. Pupillary changes including unilateral (one-sided) dilation, nonreactive, or asymmetrical pupils

4. Decerebrate (extension) posturing

5. Decreasing Glasgow Coma Score (<9)

Ventilation rates for patients experiencing herniation are:

* 20 per minute for adults

* 30 per minute for children

* 30–40 per minute for infants

Ventilate the patient with slow, full breaths as you would for artificial ventilation. The patient may have some respiratory effort or be exhibiting an abnormal breathing pattern (for example, Cheyne-Stokes or ataxic respirations). If so, ventilate during an inspiration, and do not exceed the recommended number of ventilations.

Other care for head injuries includes:

* Ensuring that the airway is open and clear. Be prepared for vomiting.

* Providing cervical spine stabilization

* Administering oxygen to the patient

* Controlling bleeding. Avoid pressure over depressed areas or unstable areas where skull fracture is suspected.

* NOT stopping the flow of cerebrospinal fluid from the nose or ears

* Stabilizing any objects impaled in the head

* Preventing the patient from movement or exertion

* Transporting the patient in a supine position (head neither elevated nor lower than the body)

* Treating for shock

Stop, Review, Remember!

Multiple Choice

Place a check next to the correct answer.

1. A patient has a head injury from a significant MOI with an altered mental status. Which of the following exams would he NOT receive?

   _____ a. initial assessment

   _____ b. focused examination

   _____ c. rapid trauma examination

   _____ d. detailed trauma examination

2. Battle's sign is observed:

   _____ a. around the eyes.

   _____ b. in the cheek.

   _____ c. at the temples.

   _____ d. behind the ears.

3. Patients with a concussion usually:

   _____ a. are unconscious, awaken, then go unconscious again.

   _____ b. are unconscious and never regain consciousness.

   _____ c. have a gradually improving mental status.

   _____ d. have a gradually decreasing mental status.

4. The breathing pattern that involves gradually increasing volume followed by decreasing volume and apnea is called:

   _____ a. Kussmaul's respirations.

   _____ b. Cheyne-Stokes respirations.

   _____ c. Biot's respirations.

   _____ d. central neurogenic hyperventilation.

5. The lowest score on the Glasgow Coma Score is:

   _____ a. 0.

   _____ b. 1.

   _____ c. 3.

   _____ d. 5.

6. Adult patients with suspected herniation should be ventilated at 30 breaths per minute.

   _____ a. true

   _____ b. false

7. A patient may present with symptoms of a head injury one week after the incident that caused it.

   _____ a. true

   _____ b. false

Fill in the Blank

For each of the following patients, determine the appropriate Glasgow Coma Score.

1. Patient opens his eyes when you talk to him, appears confused, and follows commands. _____

2. Patient does not open his eyes, moans briefly, and occasionally and has decorticate/flexion posturing to pain. _____

3. Patient is awake and alert. He appears oriented and follows commands. _____

4. Patient does not respond to any stimulus at all. There is no motor response. _____

5. Patient opens eyes to painful stimulus, mutters sounds you don't understand, and pulls away when you apply the painful stimulus. _____

Critical Thinking

1. You have two hospitals in your area. One is a community hospital that is 20 minutes away. The other is a trauma center that is 35 minutes away. What factors would your protocols likely take into consideration in making a transport decision for a patient with a serious head injury?

_____

_____

_____

_____

2. Your 27-year-old male patient has been involved in a motor vehicle accident. His head struck the "B" post between the driver's and rear passenger door when his car was "t-boned" by a truck into his door. He is awake but somewhat agitated and has the following vital signs: Pulse: 120; Respirations: 28 rapid and a bit shallow; BP: 94/62; skin cool and moist; GCS 15. Is this patient's presentation caused by a head injury?

_____

_____

_____

_____

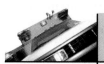

Dispatch Summary

The accident investigation determined that the Volkswagen had been traveling southbound on Highway 53 when it was struck from behind by a tractor-trailer whose driver had fallen asleep. The small car was launched over a three-foot-high concrete barrier and into the northbound lanes—and the ambulance driven by Ron Hyde. The car's driver was killed during the initial collision.

EMT Ron Hyde suffered an epidural hematoma following the impact and required surgery to repair a damaged artery and to release some of the pressure.

He still requires a wheelchair and struggles with aphasia but continues to make positive steps toward recovery.

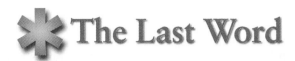

✳ The Last Word

Care for head injuries is about three things: suspicion, setting priorities, and decision making. You should suspect that all patients who have an indication of head trauma have a potentially serious head injury. You will set priorities such as scene time, airway care, and whether you have adequate time and resources to do sequential Glasgow Coma Score determinations. Finally, your decision making will involve determining the rate your patient should be ventilated at and which hospital is best for your patient. Remember to document all appropriate information in your PCR.

✳ Chapter Review

MULTIPLE CHOICE

Place a check next to the correct answer.

1. Meninges are layers:

   _____ a. that cover the brain.

   _____ b. that cover the skull (or cranium).

   _____ c. of the cerebrum.

   _____ d. (components) of the brainstem.

2. The medulla oblongata is part of the:

   _____ a. cerebrum.

   _____ b. cerebellum.

   _____ c. parietal lobe.

   _____ d. brainstem.

3. Increased blood pressure, decreased pulse, and abnormal respirations are collectively called:

   _____ a. Battle's sign.

   _____ b. Cushing's triad.

   _____ c. Starling's law.

   _____ d. Beck's triad.

4. As little as _____ of blood can begin to cause intracranial pressure.

   _____ a. 20–30 mL

   _____ b. 100–150 mL

   _____ c. 200–300 mL

   _____ d. 2–3 liters

5. The three components of the Glasgow Coma Score are:

   _____ a. pulse, respirations, blood pressure.

   _____ b. appearance, pulse, grimace.

   _____ c. speech, facial asymmetry, and motor.

   _____ d. eye opening, verbal, motor.

6. Battle's sign is an early indicator of skull fracture.

   _____ a. true

   _____ b. false

7. Patients with a Glasgow Coma Score of less than 8 are likely to have a good outcome.

   _____ a. true

   _____ b. false

LABELING

Label the following layers of the brain.

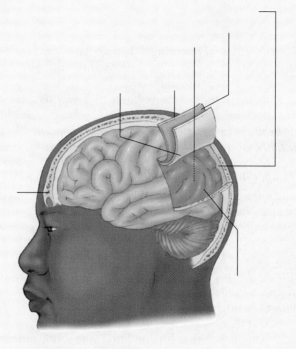

CRITICAL THINKING

1. Explain how to determine the difference between a concussion and a more serious head injury in the field.

   _____

   _____

   _____

   _____

2. What is the most significant indication of head injury you will observe in the field? Why?

   _____

   _____

   _____

   _____

CASE STUDY

You are called to a patient who is "weak and vomiting." You arrive to find the 56-year-old male patient sitting on the closed lid of the toilet, slumped over the sink, and vomiting frequently into a waste basket. The vomitus is light brown and contains obvious food.

The patient is sweaty. His daughter who just came home tells you that her father was supposed to walk a 3-mile benefit walk that morning and, by the looks of the kitchen, had lunch a short time ago. The patient is unable to lift his head, but you believe you hear him mumble "headache" before he vomits again. You ask, "Have you fallen or did you hit your head?" He nods his head "yes."

The daughter explains that your patient has a history of high blood pressure and takes medication for that and also some sort of blood thinner. You obtain a pulse and respirations and find that his pulse is 62 and respirations are 14 and labored. The vomiting seems to cease, and you are able to place the patient on a nonrebreather mask at 15 lpm.

You identify this patient as a high priority and place him on a Reeves stretcher for transport to the ambulance.

En route to the hospital, the patient loses consciousness. His vital signs in the ambulance are pulse 56 strong and regular; respirations 24 and shallow; blood pressure 182/98. After 5 minutes vitals are pulse 48 and regular; respirations about 18 per minute, irregular and gasping; blood pressure 210/105. Pupils do not respond. The patient has begun decerebrate posturing.

1. What indications did the patient give that his condition was serious in the first minute of the call?

   _____

   _____

   _____

   _____

2. En route to the hospital, the patient's condition worsened. Based on the vital signs and other observations, what do you believe the patient's problem is?

   _____

   _____

   _____

   _____

3. What would your care for this patient be?

   _____

   _____

   _____

   _____

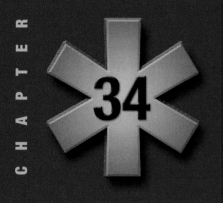

34 Patients with Spinal Injuries

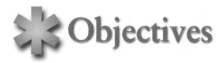

Objectives

Numbered objectives are from the U.S. Department of Transportation 1994 EMT-Basic National Standard Curriculum.

COGNITIVE OBJECTIVES

At the completion of this lesson, the EMT-Basic student will be able to:

5-4.1 State the components of the nervous system. (p. 861)

5-4.2 List the functions of the central nervous system. (pp. 861–862)

5-4.3 Define the structure of the skeletal system as it relates to the nervous system. (pp. 861–862)

5-4.4 Relate mechanism of injury to potential injuries of the head and spine. (pp. 863–867)

5-4.5 Describe the implications of not properly caring for potential spine injuries. (p. 860)

5-4.6 State the signs and symptoms of a potential spine injury. (pp. 867–868)

5-4.7 Describe the method of determining if a responsive patient may have a spine injury. (pp. 870–871)

5-4.8 Relate the airway emergency medical care techniques to the patient with a suspected spine injury. (pp. 871–873)

5-4.9 Describe how to stabilize the cervical spine. (pp. 873–875)

5-4.10 Discuss indications for sizing and using a cervical spine immobilization device. (pp. 873–875)

5-4.11 Establish the relationship between airway management and the patient with spine injuries. (pp. 871–873)

5-4.12 Describe a method for sizing a cervical spine immobilization device. (pp. 875–882)

5-4.13 Describe how to log roll a patient with a suspected spine injury. (p. 888)

5-4.14 Describe how to secure a patient to a long spine board. (pp. 879–882)

5-4.15 List instances when a short spine board should be used. (p. 882)

5-4.16 Describe how to immobilize a patient using a short spine board. (pp. 882–888)

5-4.17 Describe the indications for the use of rapid extrication. (p. 892)

5-4.18 List steps in performing rapid extrication. (pp. 892–894)

5-4.19 State the circumstances when a helmet should be left on the patient. (p. 896)

5-4.20 Discuss the circumstances when a helmet should be removed. (p. 896)

5-4.21 Identify different types of helmets. (pp. 894–896)

5-4.22 Describe the unique characteristics of sports helmets. (pp. 894–896)

5-4.23 Explain the preferred methods to remove a helmet. (pp. 896–898)

5-4.24 Discuss alternative methods for removal of a helmet. (pp. 898–899)

5-4.25 Describe how the patient's head is stabilized to remove the helmet. (p. 896)

5-4.26 Differentiate how the head is stabilized with a helmet compared to without a helmet. (p. 899)

AFFECTIVE OBJECTIVES

At the completion of this lesson, the EMT-Basic student will be able to:

5-4.27 Explain the rationale for immobilization of the entire spine when a cervical spine injury is suspected. (pp. 873–874)

5-4.28 Explain the rationale for utilizing immobilization methods apart from the straps on the cots. (pp. 872–874)

5-4.29 Explain the rationale for utilizing a short spine immobilization device when moving a patient from the sitting to the supine position. (p. 882)

5-4.30 Explain the rationale for utilizing rapid extrication approaches only when they indeed will make the difference between life and death. (pp. 893–894)

5-4.31 Defend the reasons for leaving a helmet in place for transport of a patient. (p. 896)

5-4.32 Defend the reasons for removal of a helmet prior to transport of a patient. (p. 896)

PSYCHOMOTOR OBJECTIVES

At the completion of this lesson, the EMT-Basic student will be able to:

5-4.33 Demonstrate opening the airway in a patient with suspected spinal cord injury. (p. 871)

5-4.34 Demonstrate evaluating a responsive patient with a suspected spinal cord injury. (pp. 872–873)

5-4.35 Demonstrate stabilization of the cervical spine. (pp. 874, 876–877)

5-4.36 Demonstrate the four person log roll for a patient with a suspected spinal cord injury. (pp. 888–889)

5-4.37 Demonstrate how to log roll a patient with a suspected spinal cord injury using two people. (p. 888)

5-4.38 Demonstrate securing a patient to a long spine board. (pp. 879–881)

5-4.39 Demonstrate using the short board immobilization technique. (pp. 882–885)

5-4.40 Demonstrate procedure for rapid extrication. (pp. 893–894)

5-4.41 Demonstrate preferred methods for stabilization of a helmet. (p. 896)

5-4.42 Demonstrate helmet removal techniques. (pp. 896–898)

5-4.43 Demonstrate alternative methods for stabilization of a helmet. (p. 899)

5-4.44 Demonstrate completing a prehospital care report for patients with spinal injuries. (p. 900)

✳ Introduction

5-4.5 Describe the implications of not properly caring for potential spine injuries.

✳ **spinal cord**

central nervous system (CNS) pathway responsible for transmitting sensory input from the body to the brain and for conducting motor impulses from the brain to the body muscles and organs.

✳ **paralyzed**

suffering temporary or permanent loss of muscular power or sensation.

While not all injuries to the spine result in damage to the **spinal cord,** injuries to the spinal cord can be some of the most debilitating injuries a patient can suffer. Many of the most common mechanisms of injury, such as falls, vehicle collisions, blunt trauma, and many sports, have the potential for causing injury to the spine. In the worst case scenario of an injury to the cervical spine, the patient becomes **paralyzed** and may not be able to breathe on his own. These patients must spend the rest of their lives attached to a ventilator. Such was the case with actor Christopher Reeve. In other cases, the patient becomes paralyzed below the point of injury and is unable to move his extremities or care for himself without significant help from others. Whatever the case, spinal injuries have the potential to significantly alter one's life, preventing the person from continuing the level of activity he enjoyed prior to the injury. Proper care and management of patients with suspected spinal injuries is essential for a positive outcome.

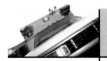

Emergency Dispatch

"How's that look now?" Dan balanced on the top step of the aluminum ladder, trying to hold a satellite dish in place.

"That's perfectly clear, Dan!" His wife called through the open kitchen window. "Leave it right there."

"Okay," he said. "But can I get you to come out for a second? I dropped the wrench."

Tammy walked out into the backyard, drying her hands with a dish towel. "Where is it?"

"Down there." Dan motioned with his head, sweat dripping from the tip of his nose.

She saw the wrench glinting in the dark green of the lawn, picked it up, and held it high above her head. As Dan reached for it, the ladder began to wobble beneath his feet. He let go of the satellite dish, which crashed down to the patio, and tried to grab the edge of the roof to steady himself. The ladder slowed its sway for a second and then suddenly toppled over, sending Dan, arms pinwheeling crazily, to the grass below.

Tammy screamed as Dan hit the lawn face first and then flipped over, landing on his back. He quickly climbed to his feet and stood, dazed.

"Where'd my hat go?" he said, looking around.

"Are you okay, Dan?" Tammy rushed up to him. "You really hit the ground hard."

"I'm fine, Baby," he said, shaking his head. "Just a little. . . surprised, I guess. Oh. . . there it is."

Dan took a couple of shaky steps toward his baseball cap and then slowly began to slump to the ground, coming to rest as a tangle of arms and legs.

"Oh my gosh, Dan! What's wrong?" Tammy ran over and dropped to her knees next to him.

"Please! Call somebody, quick," he said into the grass. "I . . . I can't feel anything."

＊

Anatomy of the Spine and Nervous System

As you learned in chapter 4, one of the primary functions of the spinal column (Figure 34-1 on page 862) is protecting the spinal cord, a major component of the body's nervous system. The nervous system is comprised of the brain and spinal cord and an elaborate network of fibers called nerves that thread throughout the body. The nervous system is the control center for the entire body and coordinates all of the body's actions and reactions by sending impulses between the brain and the nerve endings.

The **central nervous system (CNS)** consists of the brain and spinal cord and the **peripheral nervous system (PNS)** is made up of all the sensory and motor nerves that extend from the brain and spinal cord to all parts of the body (Figure 34-2 on page 863). When this important pathway is interrupted by injury, important bodily functions are affected. The higher the injury to the spinal cord the more body functions affected. The nervous system has far less regenerative abilities than other tissues of the body and therefore damage can be permanent.

The nervous system is housed within a pair of protective bony structures known as the skull and spinal column. The skull protects the brain and the spinal column provides protection for the delicate spinal cord.

The spinal column is made up of 33 irregularly shaped bones stacked or fused together that extend from the base of the skull to what we call the tail bone. The spinal column serves as both a support mechanism for the upper body and a protective structure that surrounds the spinal cord.

5-4.1 State the components of the nervous system.

5-4.2 List the functions of the central nervous system.

＊ **central nervous system (CNS)**

the brain and spinal cord.

＊ **peripheral nervous system (PNS)**

the nerves that enter and leave the spinal cord and those that extend from brain to organs without passing through the spinal cord.

5-4.3 Define the structure of the skeletal system as it relates to the nervous system.

FIGURE 34-1 The spinal column.

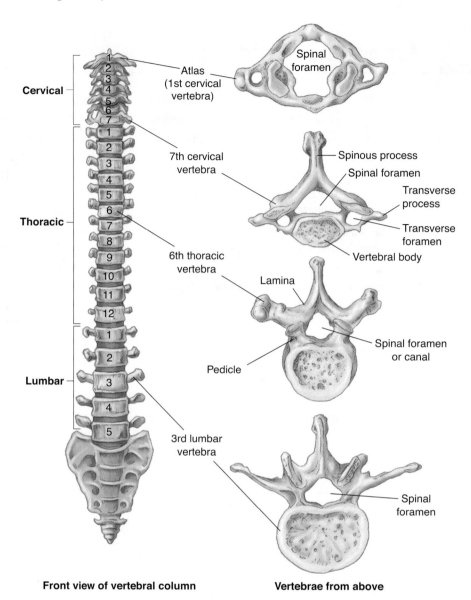

Front view of vertebral column　　　**Vertebrae from above**

＊ **cervical vertebrae**

the seven vertebrae that begin at the head and meet the thoracic vertebrae.

＊ **thoracic vertebrae**

the twelve vertebrae that help form the thoracic cage. A pair of ribs is attached to each thoracic vertebra.

＊ **lumbar vertebrae**

the five vertebrae that form the "lower back" area.

＊ **sacrum or sacral vertebrae**

fused vertebrae that help to form the pelvis.

＊ **coccygeal vertebrae**

fused vertebrae making up the coccyx or tailbone.

　　The spinal column is divided into five sections, beginning at the top. The first seven vertebrae, which are located in the neck, are known as the **cervical vertebrae.** The next section is comprised of twelve vertebrae called the **thoracic vertebrae.** Each of the twelve thoracic vertebrae is attached directly to one of the twelve pairs of ribs located on the sides of the rib cage.

　　Next are the five **lumbar vertebrae.** Below the lumbar region is the triangular shaped bone known as the **sacrum** or **sacral vertebrae.** The sacrum consists of four or five bones during childhood that eventually become completely fused around age 26. The sacrum helps form the posterior wall of the pelvis.

　　Finally we come to the **coccygeal vertebrae** more commonly known as the coccyx or tailbone. The coccyx begins life as four or five bones that eventually fuse together in adulthood. The coccyx is an important attachment point for many muscles in the lower back and pelvis.

　　As noted earlier, injury at any point along the spinal column that causes damage to the spinal cord can result in the loss of sensation and/or function below the site of injury. It will be essential to carefully assess patients with suspected spinal injury and minimize any movement of the spine during care and transport.

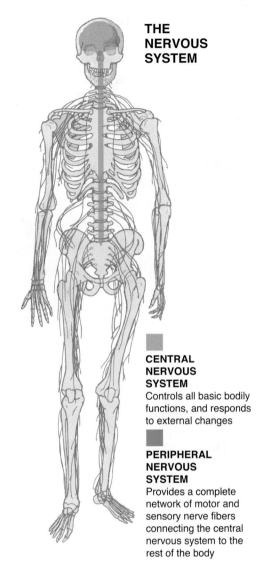

THE NERVOUS SYSTEM

CENTRAL NERVOUS SYSTEM
Controls all basic bodily functions, and responds to external changes

PERIPHERAL NERVOUS SYSTEM
Provides a complete network of motor and sensory nerve fibers connecting the central nervous system to the rest of the body

Common Mechanisms of Injury

One of the most important factors that help us determine the presence of a suspected spinal injury is the mechanism of injury (MOI). Even in the absence of obvious signs and symptoms, it is important to maintain a high index of suspicion for spinal injury if the mechanism suggests it.

The following is a partial list of MOIs suggestive of a spinal injury:

* Motor vehicle crashes

* Pedestrian versus vehicle collisions

* Falls

* Blunt trauma to head, neck, or torso

* Penetrating trauma to head, neck, or torso

* Motorcycle crashes

* Hangings

* Diving into shallow water

5-4.4   Relate mechanism of injury to potential injuries of the head and spine.

FIGURE 34-3 Compression injury.

COMPRESSION INJURY

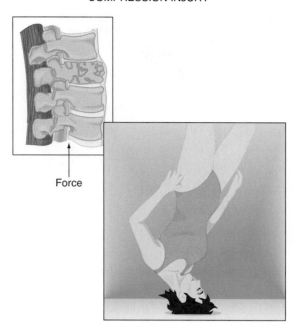

Force

✳ Unresponsive trauma victims

✳ Unresponsive patients with unknown mechanism

The spinal column can be subjected to a wide variety of injuries, depending on the MOI. The following section will discuss the most common MOIs associated with spinal injury.

COMPRESSION

Any force that impacts the spine from the top or bottom has the potential to cause what is referred to as a compression or axial load injury (Figure 34-3). In this kind of injury, the stack of vertebrae compress against one another causing damage (fracture) to one or more of the vertebrae. Common causes of compression injuries are diving into shallow water, falling from a height, and motor vehicle collisions.

FLEXION, EXTENSION, ROTATION, AND LATERAL BENDING

Any mechanism that causes an exaggerated movement of the head in any position can cause a flexion, extension, or rotation injury to the spine (Figure 34-4A–C). The cervical spine is by far the most vulnerable to these forces, as it supports the weight of the head and itself is supported only by muscles and soft tissue. Some of the most common causes of these types of injuries are motor vehicle collisions, diving into shallow water, and falls.

DISTRACTION

Injuries to the spine that cause the individual vertebrae to pull apart from one another are called distraction injuries (Figure 34-5 on page 866). Some of the most common mechanisms that cause distraction injuries are hangings and motor vehicle collisions where the occupant is restrained only with a lap belt.

FLEXION INJURY

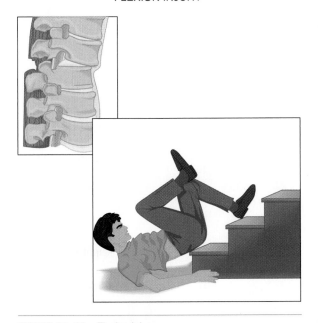

FIGURE 34-4A   Flexion injury.

EXTENSION INJURY

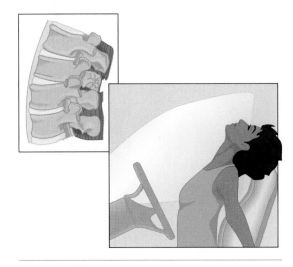

FIGURE 34-4B   Extension injury.

FLEXION-ROTATION INJURY

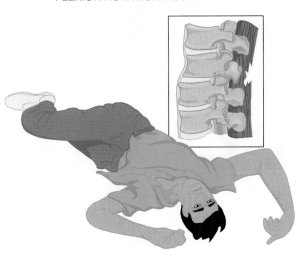

FIGURE 34-4C   Rotation injury.

PENETRATION

Penetration injuries result when something such as a sharp object (knife) or projectile (bullet) penetrates the spine (Figure 34-6 on page 866). Depending on the path of the object, it can result in either an open fracture of the spine and/or injury to the spinal cord.

BLUNT TRAUMA

Anytime the spine is subjected to blunt trauma, injury to the vertebrae and/or spinal cord is possible. Some of the more common causes of blunt trauma injuries are falls, being struck with an object, and vehicle collisions.

DISTRACTION INJURY

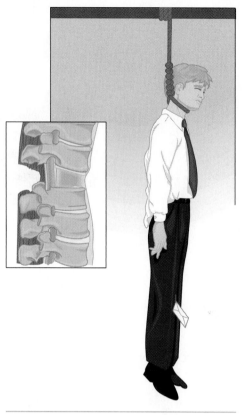

FIGURE 34-5 Distraction injury.

PENETRATION INJURY

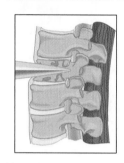

FIGURE 34-6 Penetration injury.

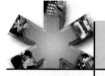

Perspective

Racer Ramirez—The EMT

"Man, as soon as I got into the backyard and saw the ladder on its side and this guy in a heap on the grass, my stomach tightened up. Spinal calls make me really nervous. I mean, if you move a broken arm, it causes pain and maybe some additional soft tissue damage, you know . . . but a neck? If you don't keep a broken neck steady, then the person that you're above, whose scared eyes you're looking down into, may be driving around in a wheelchair for the rest of his life. And that's heavy."

DISPLACED VERSUS NONDISPLACED INJURIES

It is possible and quite common for a patient to suffer a fracture to one or more vertebrae without direct injury to the spinal cord itself. This can occur when the fracture remains in place (nondisplaced), such as a bone that is cracked but not deformed (Figure 34-7). A displaced fracture is one that has some deformity associated with it, and the pieces of bone are separated from one another. The likelihood

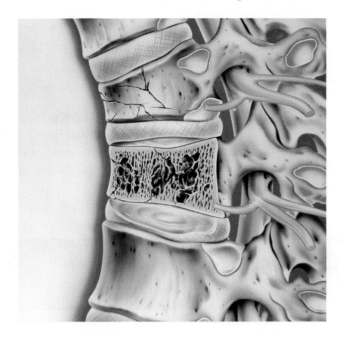

FIGURE 34-7   A nondisplaced fracture of the vertebrae. (Photo Researchers, Inc.)

of spinal cord injury is greater with displaced injuries than with nondisplaced. Whenever possible, it is important to carefully palpate the spine for signs of deformity. It is not your job to try to diagnose a displaced injury in the field. It is, however, extremely important to minimize all movement of the spine during assessment, care, and transport. Your careful handling of the patient will minimize the chances of a nondisplaced injury becoming displaced or a displaced injury penetrating the spinal cord.

Signs and Symptoms of Spinal Cord Injury

As we have already stated, the mechanism of injury will be one of the most important factors in determining the likelihood of a spinal injury. It is very important to understand that the ability of the patient to walk, move his extremities, or feel sensation is not a reason to rule out a spinal injury. The absence of pain should also not be a reason to rule out spinal injury.

The following is a list of some of the more common signs and symptoms of spinal cord injury:

* Tenderness in the area of injury to the spine

* Pain not associated with movement

* Pain associated with movement

* Obvious deformity of the spine upon palpation

* Numbness, weakness, or tingling in the extremities

* Loss of sensation or paralysis below the suspected injury site

* Loss of sensation or paralysis in the extremities

* Incontinence (bowel or bladder)

* **Priapism** (erection of the penis)

5-4.6   State the signs and symptoms of a potential spine injury.

* **priapism**

persistent erection of the penis that may result from spinal injury and some medical problems.

 * Pain along spinal column or lower extremities independent of movement or palpation (may be intermittent)

 * Soft tissue injuries to the head, neck, back, shoulders, or abdomen associated with trauma

In addition to the above signs and symptoms, another serious complication of spinal cord injury is inadequate breathing. Injury to the spinal cord at or above the third cervical vertebra can prevent the diaphragm muscle from assisting with spontaneous respiration. As with all patients, closely monitor the respiratory status and assist if necessary.

 Stop, Review, Remember!

Multiple Choice

Place a check next to the correct answer.

1. Into which two systems is the nervous system divided?

   _____ a. central and peripheral

   _____ b. primary and secondary

   _____ c. vertebral and central

   _____ d. brain and peripheral

2. The spinal column is made up of approximately how many bones?

   _____ a. 7

   _____ b. 12

   _____ c. 22

   _____ d. 33

3. Which part of the spine contains seven vertebrae and is the most vulnerable to injury?

   _____ a. cervical

   _____ b. thoracic

   _____ c. lumbar

   _____ d. sacral

4. Each vertebra of the _____ spine is connected to a pair of ribs that wrap around to form the ribcage.

   _____ a. cervical

   _____ b. thoracic

   _____ c. lumbar

   _____ d. sacral

5. An injury to the spinal cord could result in loss of sensation and function _____ the suspected injury site.

   _____ a. above and below

   _____ b. above

   _____ c. at

   _____ d. below

Labeling

Label the following sections of the spinal column.

coccyx

cervical

lumbar

thoracic

sacral

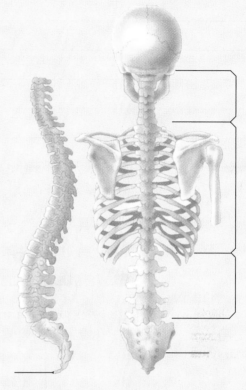

Regions of the spine.

Critical Thinking

1. Discuss the role that mechanism of injury plays in the assessment and care of the patient with a suspected spinal injury.

_____

_____

_____

_____

2. How do the central and peripheral nervous systems differ in function?

_____

_____

_____

_____

3. Discuss why it is so important to minimize the movement of a patient with a suspected spinal cord injury.

_____

_____

_____

_____

_____

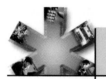

Perspective

Tammy—The Patient's Wife

"I was so scared that he was going to die or something. I just can't believe it. One minute he's putting up our new satellite dish and the next he's getting strapped to a plastic board and . . . and he can't feel me holding his hand. He hit so hard, though. I mean—just bam—like a spear or something into the ground. And then as they were getting him on the stretcher, he . . . wet himself . . . and he didn't even notice. I didn't say anything. Oh my gosh—he would've just died of embarrassment."

Assessment of the Patient with Suspected Spinal Injury

5-4.7 Describe the method of determining if a responsive patient may have a spine injury.

There are some specific techniques you should use when caring for and assessing a patient with a suspected spinal injury. First, you will want to minimize all movement of the spine. In addition to manually stabilizing the patient, advise the patient to remain as still as possible. Instruct the responsive patient to answer your questions with a verbal response only and not to shake or nod his head. You will also want to be gentler when handling the extremities. Do not move the patient in an attempt to elicit a painful response.

In addition to the normal components of your focused history and physical exam, try to pinpoint any pain or tenderness along the spine as best as you can. This can be accomplished by simply asking the patient where the pain is and/or palpating the spine with a gloved hand. If you have help, roll the patient onto his side in order to facilitate a thorough examination of the spine. Be sure to spend a little more time assessing all four distal extremities for adequate circulation, sensation, and motor function (Figure 34-8A and B).

If the patient is unresponsive, rely mostly on the MOI and any obvious signs of trauma. Do your best to obtain additional information from others at the scene

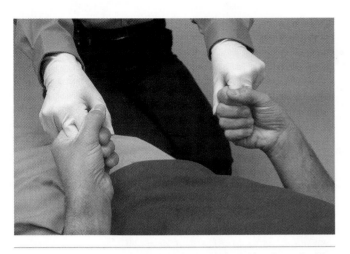

FIGURE 34-8A   Assess strength in the hands by asking the patient to squeeze your fingers.

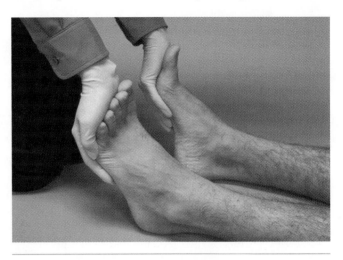

FIGURE 34-8B   Assess strength in the feet and legs by asking the patient to push against your hands.

who may have seen the event or were with the patient prior to your arrival. Try to determine if the patient was responsive at all before you arrived.

SCENE SIZE-UP

Begin to anticipate potential injuries based on the information contained in the initial dispatch. For instance, if you have been dispatched to a vehicle collision, anticipate head and neck injuries and the need for spinal immobilization. You will confirm this when you evaluate the actual mechanism of injury. Ensure that the scene is safe and, if possible, request the appropriate additional resources prior to making patient contact.

Once on scene, look at factors such as the angle of impact, the amount of damage to the vehicle and intrusion into the passenger compartment, and whether or not the patient was wearing a seat belt. Maintain manual stabilization of the spine until the patient can be properly immobilized.

INITIAL ASSESSMENT

While maintaining appropriate stabilization of the spine, ensure that the ABCs are intact and manage any uncontrolled bleeding. Management of the airway must be accomplished using the jaw-thrust maneuver, whenever possible, and the insertion of an appropriate airway adjunct. Maintain the patient's airway and provide manual ventilations with as little movement of the head and neck as possible.

Whenever possible, place the patient's head in alignment with the spine and rest of the body. This usually involves grasping the head with both hands and gently rotating it in line with the spine. Use caution when realigning the head with the rest of the body and stop immediately if resistance is felt.

5-4.8   Relate the airway emergency medical care techniques to the patient with a suspected spine injury.

5-4.11   Establish the relationship between airway management and the patient with spine injuries.

FOCUSED HISTORY AND PHYSICAL EXAM

In most cases of suspected spinal injury the patient will have suffered a significant mechanism of injury, and therefore your next step will be to perform a rapid trauma assessment. As you begin the rapid trauma assessment, have your partner begin obtaining a baseline set of vital signs. Begin gathering the SAMPLE history as you conduct your examination.

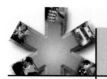

Perspective

Dan—The Patient

"I knew better than standing on that top step. You know, the one that says 'not a step' on it. But nothing bad has ever really happened to me before, so I figured 'what the heck'! I don't remember much! I remember a surge of adrenaline as the ladder started to rock back and forth and then this big, bright flash. And then all I could think of was finding my stupid hat. Everything after that's pretty much a blur. Isn't it odd how a quick decision—like which step do I stand on—can have such far-reaching effects? I am very grateful for the ambulance personnel, though. The doctor told me that if they hadn't done their jobs right, I might have been much worse off than I am."

Once you have completed your assessment of the neck, place an appropriate cervical immobilization device. Be careful not to move the head or neck too much during placement of the collar.

Pay special attention to the circulatory, sensation, and motor function (CSM) status of each extremity. While poor motor function can be a result of pain and not necessarily spinal injury, any amount of numbness or tingling should be investigated further. Move up the arms or legs beginning at the feet to determine how far the numbness or tingling goes. You can simply pinch the skin as you go or use something pointed, such as a pen. Make a mark on the patient's extremity using a pen to signify the point at which normal sensation begins.

The remainder of the patient assessment follows the normal path and covers the standard components. Assess the entire body for DCAP-BTLS and note any abnormalities.

Emergency Care of the Patient with Suspected Spinal Injury

Once the ABCs have been properly managed, focus your care of the suspected spinal injury patient on getting the patient properly secured to an appropriate immobilization device. These devices will be discussed later in this chapter.

Follow these steps when caring for a patient with suspected spinal injury:

1. Take the appropriate BSI precautions and perform a scene size-up.

2. Establish and maintain manual inline stabilization of the spine.

3. Perform an initial assessment and initiate oxygen therapy.

4. Perform a rapid trauma assessment including a thorough assessment of distal CSM in all extremities.

5. Apply an appropriate cervical stabilization device (collar).

6. Place the patient on an appropriate stabilization device, depending on the position found (lying, sitting, standing).

7. Initiate transport.

8. Perform a detailed physical exam as appropriate.

9. Perform ongoing assessments as appropriate.

It should be noted that not all patients with spinal injuries will present with obvious trauma. Any patient who is found unresponsive when you are not able to accurately determine the exact cause of his condition should be treated as though he may have a spinal injury.

Immobilization of the Patient with Suspected Spinal Injury

Patients will be found in one of three possible positions: lying, sitting, or standing. Regardless of the position in which he is found, carefully assess the need for spinal immobilization and secure the patient to an appropriate device.

Several devices are used to properly immobilize a patient with suspected spinal injury. These include cervical collars, head immobilizers, and both long and short spinal immobilization devices.

CERVICAL SPINE IMMOBILIZATION

One of the biggest challenges faced by EMTs is the proper immobilization of a patient's head and neck. When there is a suspected spinal injury, this becomes a very high priority. Properly immobilizing a patient's head and neck can minimize further injury and may even keep him from becoming paralyzed. Unfortunately, not all patients are as cooperative as we would like them to be.

One of the best ways to immobilize a patient's head and neck in the field is through **manual stabilization** (Figure 34-9 on page 874). Firmly grasp the patient's head with both hands and attempt to keep it from moving while another EMT assesses and cares for the patient.

The next step in the immobilization process is to add a device known as a cervical collar (Figures 34-10A–C on page 874). A cervical collar is indicated for

5-4.9 Describe how to stabilize the cervical spine.

* **manual stabilization**
   method of stabilization where the EMT firmly grasps the patient's head with both hands and attempts to keep it from moving.

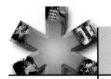

Perspective

Allyson—The EMT

"Back in training, we always practiced holding c-spine on patients who were either sitting perfectly upright or lying flat on their backs. Let me tell you, though, that in 3 years on this ambulance, I have yet to have a spinal call be that simple! Like this guy today. He's in a big heap on the ground . . . and, of course, he's face down. It can be a real challenge to straighten a person's body out and turn them over so you can board them . . . all while maintaining effective immobilization! It takes planning and a lot of direct communication with the people helping you. All in all I think this call went well, though."

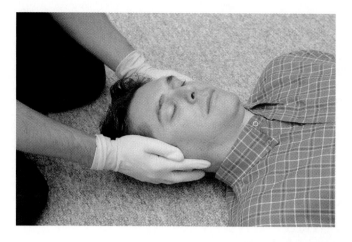

FIGURE 34-9 Bring the head to the neutral in-line position and maintain manual immobilization until the head, neck, and spine are mechanically immobilized.

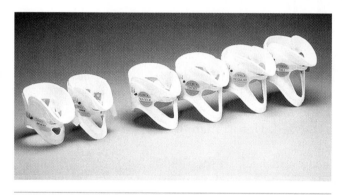

FIGURE 34-10A Stifneck® cervical spine immobilization collars. (Laerdal Medical Corporation.)

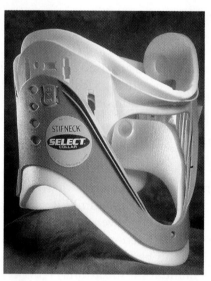

FIGURE 34-10B The Stifneck® Select™ collar can be adjusted to fit many patient sizes. (Laerdal Medical Corporation.)

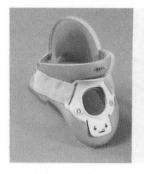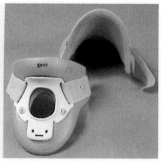

FIGURE 34-10C Philadelphia Cervical Collar assembled and disassembled. (Philadelphia® Cervical Collar Co.)

5-4.10 Discuss indications for sizing and using a cervical spine immobilization device.

any patient who is suspected of having a spinal injury based on the assessment of mechanism of injury and signs and symptoms. Cervical collars are just one piece of the overall immobilization package and DO NOT by themselves ensure proper immobilization of a patient's neck.

To be maximally effective, a cervical collar must fit properly. A collar that is too small can restrict the airway. A collar that is too large will allow excess move-

Clinical Clues: MANUAL STABILIZATION

Manual stabilization of the head and spine MUST be maintained throughout the assessment process, even after the application of a cervical collar. A cervical collar only serves to *"remind"* the patient not to move his neck. Some patients will forget and move anyway. That is why you must maintain manual stabilization until the patient is completely secured to an appropriate spinal immobilization device.

ment of the head and neck, increasing the potential for further injury. Each cervical collar manufacturer has specific guidelines for properly sizing the collar to the patient. Follow the guidelines for the specific device you will be using. Scan 34-1 on page 876 illustrates the steps used to apply an adjustable collar to a seated patient. Scan 34-2 on page 878 demonstrates how to apply a collar to a supine patient.

Even though cervical collars come in a variety of sizes, some patients may still not fit into one. An alternative is to secure the head to the board with adequate stabilization on both sides and tape across the forehead and chin.

5-4.12 Describe a method for sizing a cervical spine immobilization device.

HEAD IMMOBILIZERS

Head immobilizers are simple devices (Figures 34-11A and B) that are used to minimize the side-to-side motion of the head of a patient who is secured to a long spine board (Figure 34-12 on page 879). They can be purchased as premanufactured devices or simply improvised, using rolled up towels or blankets (Figure 34-13 on page 879) or, when other options are unavailable, even the patient's own shoes. Head immobilizers are an important component of the overall spinal package, as they fill the void on either side of the patient's head and minimize side to side movement during transport.

LONG SPINE BOARDS

Also known as long boards and long backboards, these are devices approximately 6 feet by 2 feet and are made of wood, aluminum, or a plastic material

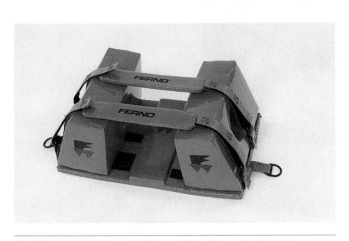

FIGURE 34-11A   Ferno head immobilizer. (Ferno Corporation.)

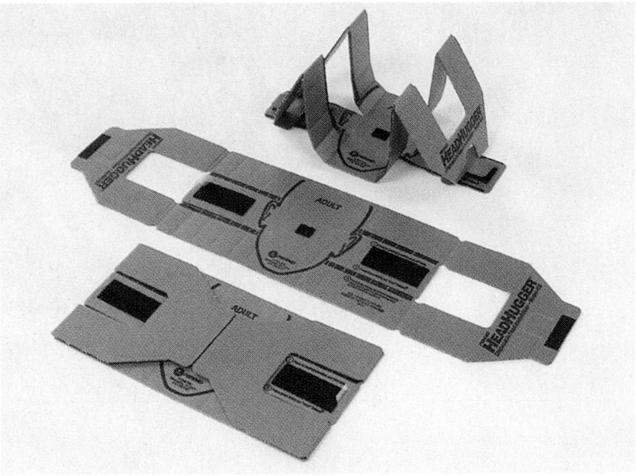

FIGURE 34-11B   Disposable head immobilizer. (Ferno Corporation.)

APPLICATION OF ADJUSTABLE COLLAR TO SEATED PATIENT

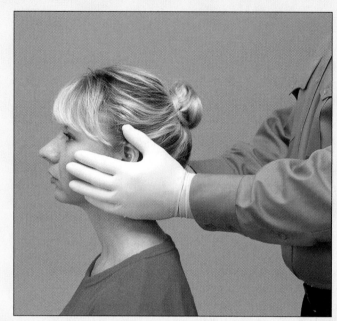

▲ Stabilize the head and neck from the rear.

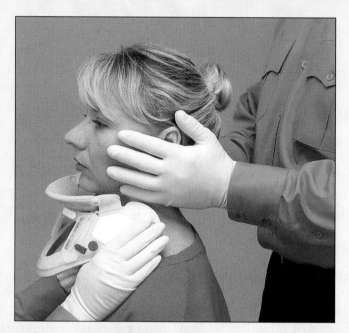

▲ Properly angle the collar for placement.

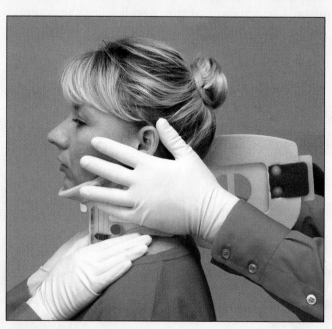

▲ Position the collar bottom.

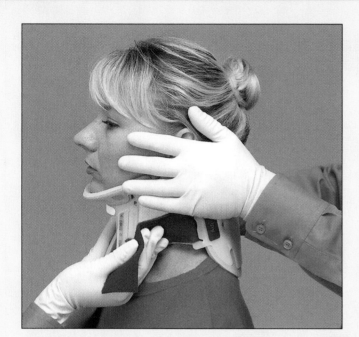
▲ Set the collar in place around the neck.

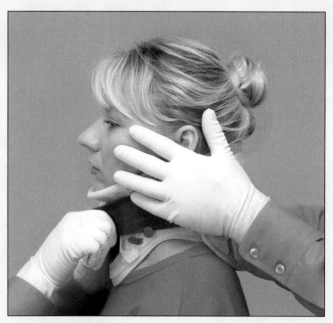
▲ Secure the collar.

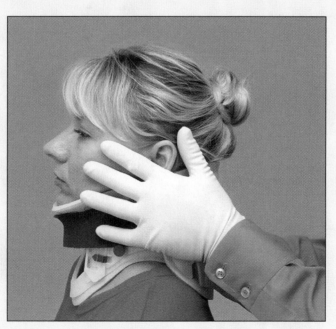
▲ Maintain manual stabilization of the head and neck.

SCAN 34-2 | **APPLICATION OF COLLAR TO SUPINE PATIENT**

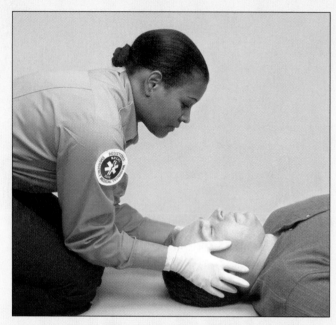

▲ Kneel at the patient's head and stabilize the head and neck.

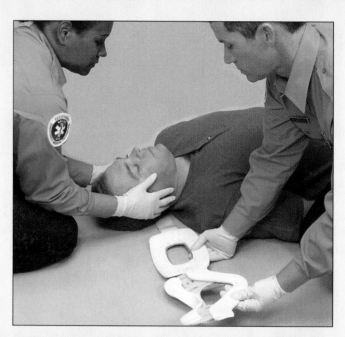

▲ Set the collar in place.

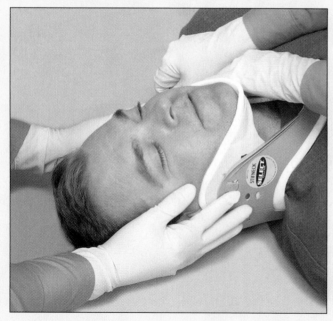

▲ Secure the collar.

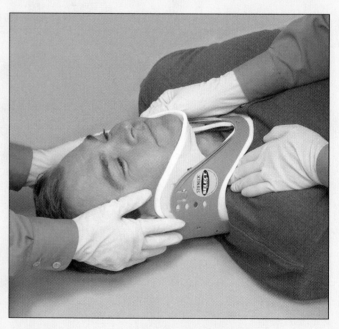

▲ Continue to manually stabilize the head and neck.

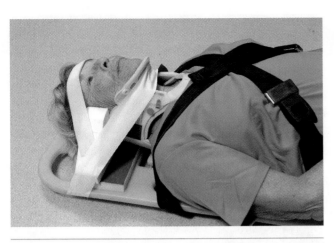

FIGURE 34-12 The patient's head immobilized with a commercial device.

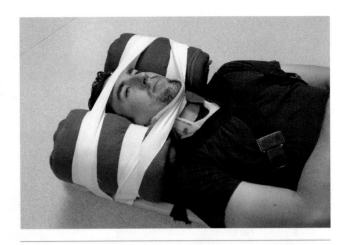

FIGURE 34-13 A patient's head immobilized using towel rolls.

(Figures 34-14A–C). They provide stabilization and immobilization to the head, neck, torso, pelvis, and extremities. Long spine boards are used to immobilize patients suspected of having a spinal injury who are found in a lying or standing position.

If possible, three rescuers should be on hand. Follow these steps to secure a lying patient to a long spine board (Scan 34-3 on page 880):

1. One rescuer maintains manual stabilization of the head the entire time.

2. Check CSM of all extremities and apply an appropriate cervical collar.

3. Position the device at the patient's side ensuring that it is high enough so the patient's head will be on the board once it is placed beneath him.

4. The other rescuers position themselves on the side of the patient, opposite the board.

5-4.14 Describe how to secure a patient to a long spine board.

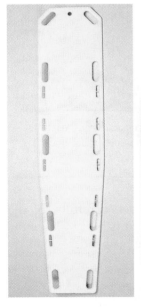

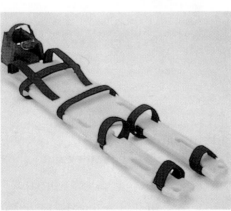

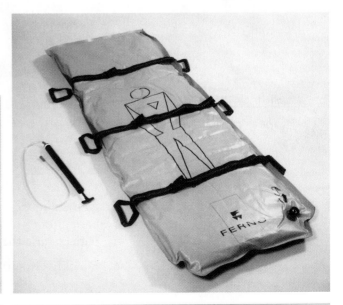

FIGURE 34-14A
Composite backboard.

FIGURE 34-14B A Miller style backboard.

FIGURE 34-14C Full body vacuum splint. (Ferno Corporation.)

※ ※ ※ ※ ※ ※ ※ ※ ※ ※ ※ ※ ※ ※ ※ ※ ※ ※ ※ ※

SCAN 34-3 | **SPINAL IMMOBILIZATION OF SUPINE PATIENT**

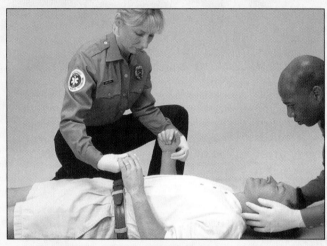

▲ Place head in neutral, in-line position and maintain manual stabilization of the head and neck. Assess distal circulation, sensation, and motor function (CSM).

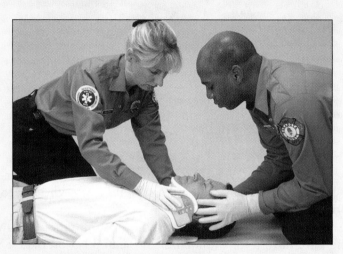

▲ Apply an appropriately sized rigid cervical collar.

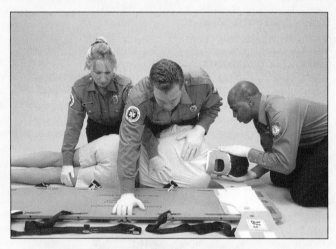

▲ Position an immobilization device.

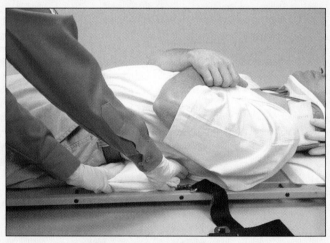

▲ Move the patient onto the device without compromising the integrity of the spine. Once the patient is in position, apply padding to voids between the torso and board.

5. At the direction of the rescuer holding the head, all rescuers carefully roll the patient onto his side (toward the rescuers). If possible, it is best to have the patient raise the arm that he will be rolling onto above his head.

6. Quickly visualize and palpate the patient's posterior side.

7. One rescuer reaches across and positions the board appropriately.

8. At the direction of the rescuer holding the head, all rescuers carefully roll the patient onto the board.

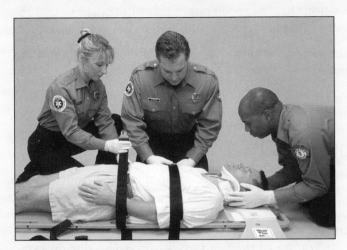

▲ Secure the patient's torso to the board first.

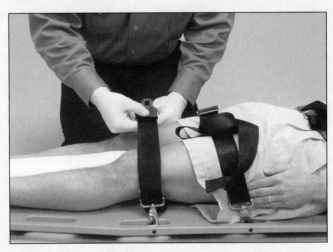

▲ Then, secure the patient's legs (above and below the knee).

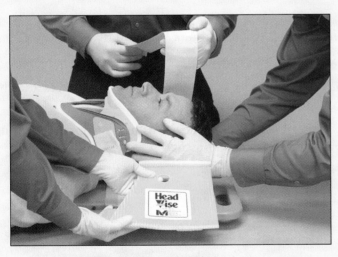

▲ Pad and immobilize the patient's head last.

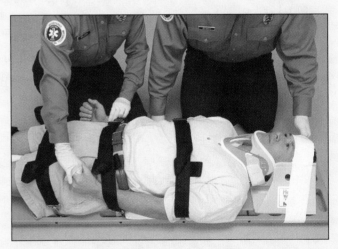

▲ Reassess the patient's distal circulation, sensation, and motor function (CSM).

9. If necessary the patient can be centered on the board using a coordinated up and down movement by all rescuers.

10. Place soft pads under the patient's head and in any voids between the torso and the board.

11. Secure the torso first, then the head and extremities to the board.

12. Reassess CSM after securing to the board.

Follow these steps for securing a standing patient to a long-spine board (Scan 34-4):

1. One rescuer maintains manual stabilization of the head the entire time.

2. Check CSM of all extremities and apply an appropriate cervical collar.

3. Position the device behind the patient, through the arms of the rescuer holding the head.

4. Rescuers 2 and 3 position themselves on either side of the patient and reach with the hand closest to the patient under the arm to grasp the board.

5. At the direction of the rescuer holding the head, all three lay the board down with the patient on it.

The patient can then be secured to the board as normal.

SHORT IMMOBILIZATION DEVICES

5-4.15 List instances when a short spine board should be used.

A short immobilization device is used to immobilize the spine of a noncritical patient found in the seated position such as on a seat of a vehicle. There are essentially two types of short-board immobilization devices, the vest (Figure 34-15) and the rigid short board (Figure 34-16).

Both devices provide stabilization of the head, neck, and torso during extrication and transport.

5-4.16 Describe how to immobilize a patient using a short spine board.

Follow these steps to secure a seated patient to a short immobilization device (Scan 34-5 on page 886):

1. One rescuer maintains manual stabilization of the head the entire time.

2. Check CSM of all extremities and apply an appropriate cervical collar.

3. A second rescuer positions the device behind the patient and secures it to the patient's torso.

4. The second rescuer secures the head to the device using appropriate padding behind the head to maintain proper alignment.

5. Reassess CSM of extremities.

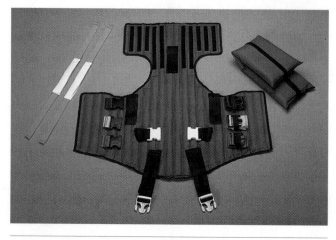

FIGURE 34-15 Ferno KED (Kendrick Extrication Device). (Ferno Corporation.)

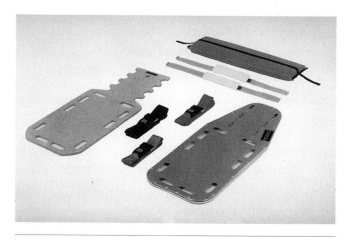

FIGURE 34-16 Short spine board.

SCAN 34-4 **SPINAL IMMOBILIZATION OF A STANDING PATIENT**

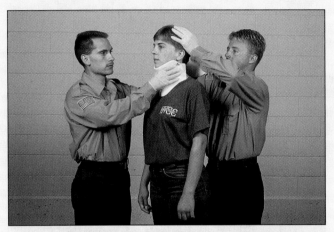

▲ EMT #2 applies a properly sized cervical collar to the patient. EMT #1 continues manual stabilization (collar aids, but does not replace, manual stabilization).

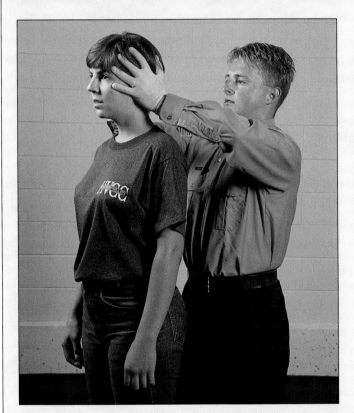

▲ Position your tallest crew member (EMT #1) behind the patient and have him manually stabilize the head and neck. His hands should not leave the patient's head until the entire procedure is complete and the head is secured to the long spine board.

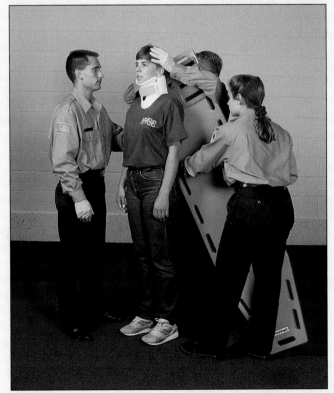

EMT #1 continues manual stabilization, as EMT #2 and another rescuer position a long spine board behind the patient, being careful not to disturb EMT #1's manual stabilization of the patient's head and neck. It will help if EMT #1 spreads his elbows to give the other rescuers more room to maneuver the spine board. ▶

(continued on the next page)

SPINAL IMMOBILIZATION OF A STANDING PATIENT—*(continued)*

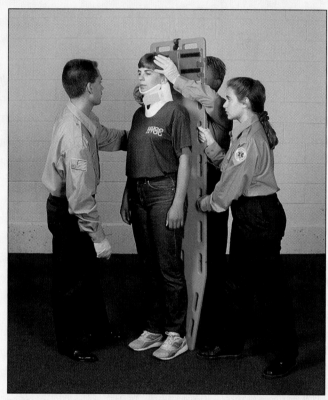

▲ EMT #1 continues manual stabilization. EMT #2 looks at the spine board from the front of the patient and does any necessary repositioning to be sure it is centered behind the patient.

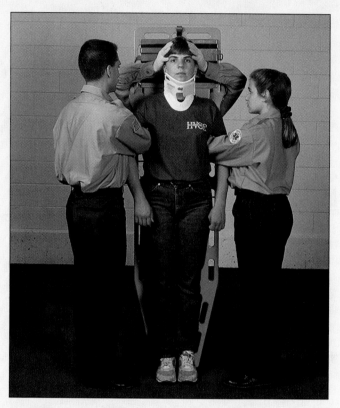

▲ EMT #1 continues manual stabilization. EMT #2 and third rescuer reach arm that is nearest the patient under the patient's armpits and grasp the spine board. (Once the board is tilted down, the patient will actually be temporarily suspended by his armpits.) To keep the patient's arms secure, they will use the other hand to grasp the patient's arm just above the elbow and hold it against the patient's body.

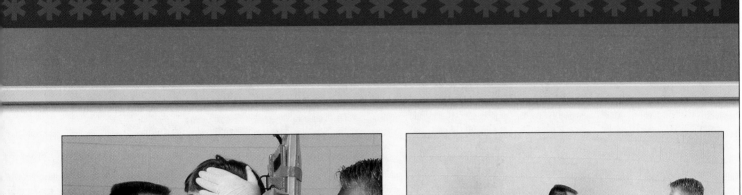

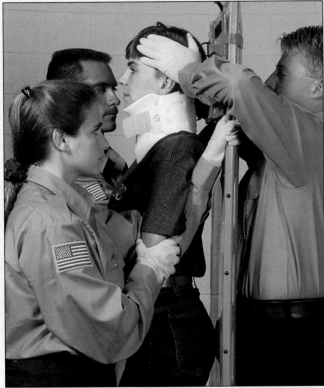

▲ EMT #2 and third rescuer, when reaching under the patient's armpits, must grasp a handhold on the spine board at the patient's armpit level or higher.

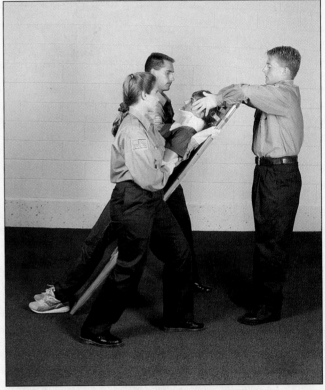

▲ EMT #1 continues manual stabilization. EMT #2 and third rescuer maintain their grasp on the spine board and the patient. EMT #1 explains to the patient what is going to happen, then gives a signal to begin slowly tilting the board and patient to the ground. As the board is lowered, EMT #1 walks backward and crouched, keeping up with the board as it is lowered and allowing the patient's head to slowly move back to the neutral position against the board. EMT #1 must accomplish all this without holding back or slowing the lowering of the board. EMT #1 may need to rotate somewhat so that, once the board is almost flat, he is holding the head down on the board. Once the patient's head comes in contact with the board, it must not be allowed to leave the board, to avoid flexing the neck. The job of the two rescuers doing the lowering is to control it so that it is slow and even on both sides. They should also move into a squatting position as they lower the board to avoid injuring their backs.

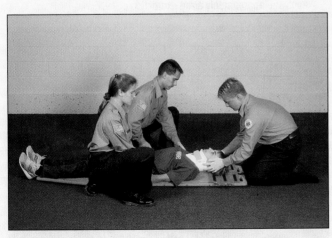

▲ EMT #1 maintains manual in-line stabilization throughout the procedure.

SCAN 34-5 **SPINAL IMMOBILIZATION OF A SEATED PATIENT**

▲ Select an immobilization device.

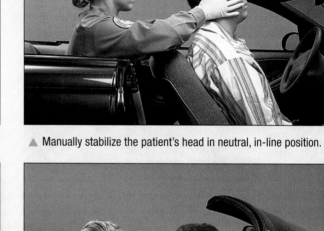

▲ Manually stabilize the patient's head in neutral, in-line position.

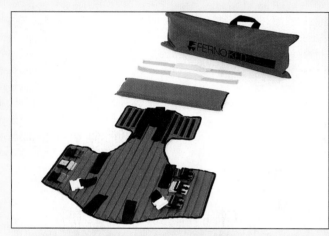

▲ Assess distal circulation, sensation, and motor function (CSM).

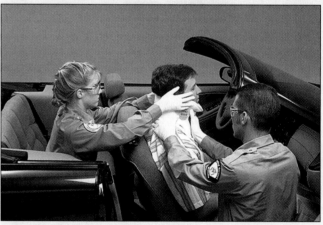

▲ Apply the appropriately sized extrication collar.

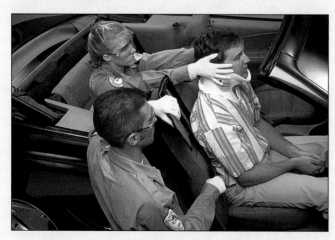

▲ Position immobilization device behind the patient.

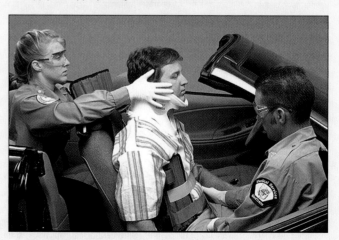

▲ Secure the device to the patient's torso.

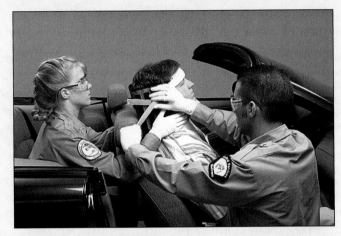

▲ Evaluate and pad behind the patient's head as necessary. Secure the patient's head to the device.

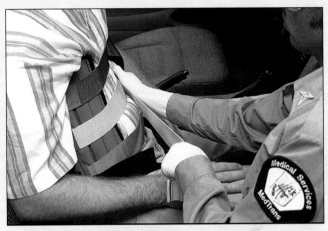

▲ Evaluate and adjust the straps. They must be tight enough so the device does not move up, down, left, or right excessively, but not so tight as to restrict the patient's breathing.

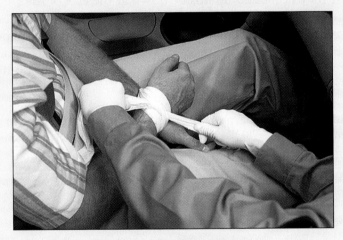

▲ As needed, secure the patient's wrists and legs.

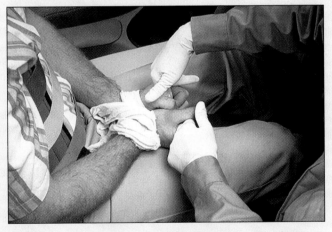

▲ Reassess distal circulation, sensation, and motor function (CSM), and transfer the patient to the long board.

Clinical Clues: EXCEPTION TO SHORT SPINE IMMOBILIZATION

An exception to the application of the short spine immobilization device is for the patient who must be moved due to immediate life threats. In this case, DO NOT waste valuable time placing this device. You must use a rapid extrication technique to move this patient to a long spine board.

In many cases, once a patient has been properly secured to a short immobilization device he will be moved to a long board for transport to the hospital. This can be accomplished by placing a long board under the buttocks of the patient and carefully lowering him onto the board for transport in the supine position.

Repositioning the Patient with Suspected Spinal Injury

5-4.13 Describe how to log roll a patient with a suspected spine injury.

EMS is not an ideal world; our patients are not all found face up and cooperative. Much of the time we must reposition the patient in order to properly immobilize and transport them. Patients with suspected spinal injuries are no exception. If you are fortunate enough to find your patient face up, it will be necessary to roll him onto a backboard. If he is face down, you will have to roll him onto his back and perhaps once again to get him onto the board. Whatever the case, it is essential that you have enough resources and coordinate them well if you are going to minimize movement of the patient's spine.

Ideally, you will have at least three or possibly four rescuers to properly roll a patient from front to back. One rescuer should be at the head, one at the torso, and the last at the hips and legs. To keep the roll coordinated, all movements should be directed by the rescuer holding the head. This will help ensure that the spine stays in alignment with every move. One of the most critical elements of a coordinated roll from the prone position to the supine position is the initial placement of the hands on the patient's head. The rescuer holding the head must place his hands in such a way that they don't end up upside down at the end of the roll. He must place his hands then envision the roll and where his hands will be at the end. It is important for all rescuers to remain balanced and stable throughout the roll to avoid any unexpected movement of the patient.

Follow the steps below to properly roll a patient from the prone to the supine position using three rescuers:

1. Rescuer #1 kneels at the top of the patient and firmly grasps the patient's head with both hands, making certain that the patient's arms will not become twisted during the roll.

2. Rescuer #2 kneels beside the patient's torso and, if possible, has the patient move his arm closest to the rescuer up over his head.

3. Rescuer #3 kneels beside the patient's hips and legs.

4. On the direction of rescuer #1, everyone carefully rolls the patient in the direction of rescuer 2 and 3 and stops once the patient is on his side.

5. All rescuers reposition themselves slightly to accommodate the rest of the roll.

6. On the direction of rescuer #1, the patient is carefully rolled down onto his back.

If a backboard is available, place it in such a way that the patient is rolled directly onto the board, eliminating the need for an additional roll. Be sure to stop briefly to assess the patient's back while he is on his side.

In situations where you are alone or have fewer than three but perhaps two rescuers, you may have to roll the patient as best you can. This is only necessary if there are immediate life threats to the patient and moving him is necessary to address one or more of the life threats.

Special Considerations for Pediatric Patients

Consider using a short spine board for a small child or infant who needs full spinal precautions. Because of the large **occipital** (back) region of the skull, pediatric patients may need additional padding placed from shoulders to feet. This will allow the head to remain in a neutral position when secured to a spinal immobilization device.

There are specialized immobilization devices designed to accommodate the pediatric patient. One such device is a properly sized back board with the head segment lower than the body segment to accommodate the large occipital region in most pediatric patients (Figure 34-17). Other devices address the need for adequate restraint and have built in velcro closures for securing the uncooperative patient to the device (Figure 34-18). Also, consider securing the patient to a board without a cervical collar should you not have the correct size (Figure 34-19). Using a collar that does not fit properly can cause more harm than good.

* **occipital**

posterior (back) region of the skull.

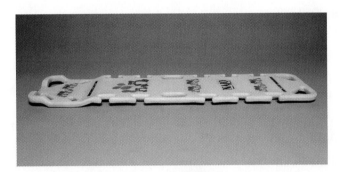

FIGURE 34-17   A pediatric spine board.

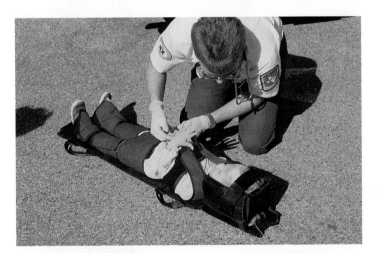

FIGURE 34-18   Pediatric immobilization device. (Craig Jackson/In the Dark Photography.)

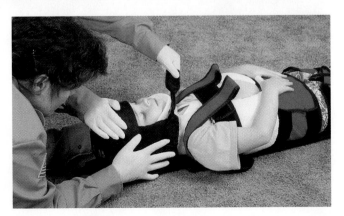

FIGURE 34-19   A child with padding on a spine board with his head secured to the board with a c-collar and with manual stabilization.

Stop, Review, Remember!

Multiple Choice

Place a check next to the correct answer.

1. The most appropriate method for opening the airway of a patient with suspected spinal injury is the:

       _____ a. head tilt-chin lift.

       _____ b. jaw thrust.

       _____ c. sniffing position.

       _____ d. neutral position.

2. In most cases the appropriate assessment path for the patient with suspected spinal injury is the:

       _____ a. rapid medical.

       _____ b. focused medical.

       _____ c. rapid trauma.

       _____ d. focused trauma.

3. Once the ABCs have been properly managed, emergency care of the suspected spinal injury patient will focus on:

       _____ a. vital signs.

       _____ b. proper immobilization.

       _____ c. oxygen therapy.

       _____ d. rapid transport.

4. Which of the following statements best describes the purpose of a cervical collar?

       _____ a. It reminds the cooperative patient not to move.

       _____ b. Once in place, it prevents the neck from moving.

       _____ c. One size collar will fit all patients.

       _____ d. It is not needed unless the patient has pain.

5. The rescuer at the _____ should be the one to direct all movement of the patient.

       _____ a. feet

       _____ b. legs

       _____ c. torso

       _____ d. head

Labeling

Label each photo for the type of MOI.

1. flexion

2. compression

3. extension

4. distraction

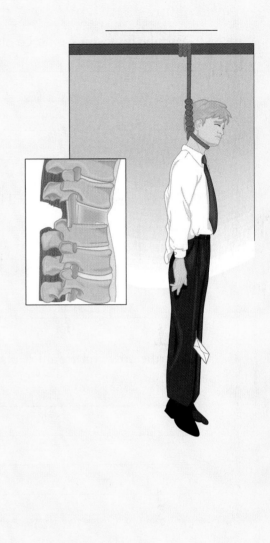

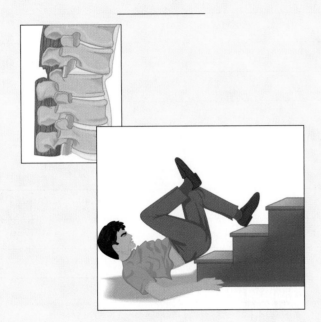

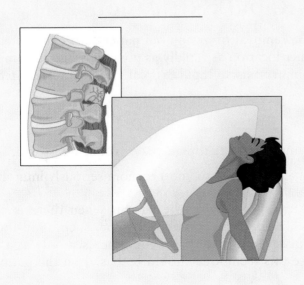

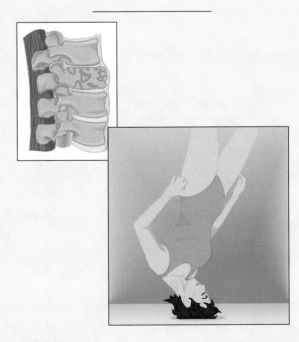

Critical Thinking

1. Describe how you would go about determining if a patient may have suffered a spinal injury.

_____

_____

_____

_____

2. What factors at the scene will help you determine the likelihood of a spinal injury?

_____

_____

_____

_____

3. Describe how you would manage the airway and breathing of a patient with a suspected spinal injury.

_____

_____

_____

_____

Considering Rapid Extrication

5-4.17 Describe the indications for the use of rapid extrication.

* **rapid extrication**

the removal of an injured patient with suspected spinal injuries from a car or other location as rapidly as possible while remaining mindful that a potential spinal injury exists.

Rapid extrication is the removal of an injured patient with suspected spinal injuries from a car or other location as rapidly as possible while remaining mindful that a potential spinal injury exists. Rapid extrication may be indicated in the following situations:

* The scene becomes unsafe.

* The patient has immediate life threats that must be addressed.

* One patient is blocking access to another more seriously injured patient.

Rapid extrication involves moving the patient when there is not enough time to properly stabilize the head, neck, and spine, such as in the case of a compromised airway or severe bleeding. It should be used only as a last resort, and the decision to use this technique should be based on the patient's condition and time.

5-4.18 List steps in performing rapid extrication.

Follow these steps to perform a rapid extrication of a seated patient from a vehicle (Scan 34-6):

1. Rescuer #1 maintains manual stabilization of the head from behind while rescuer #2 places a cervical collar.

2. Rescuer #3 places a long spine board on the seat with one end beneath the patient's buttocks and the other end on the stretcher.

✳✳✳✳✳✳✳✳✳✳✳✳✳✳✳✳✳✳

SCAN 34-6 | **PERFORMING RAPID EXTRICATION OF A SEATED PATIENT FROM VEHICLE**

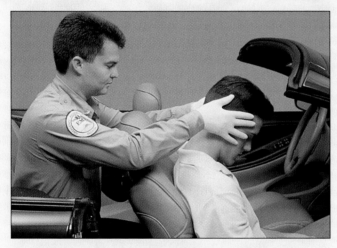

▲ Bring the patient's head into a neutral, in-line position. This is best achieved from behind or to the side of the patient.

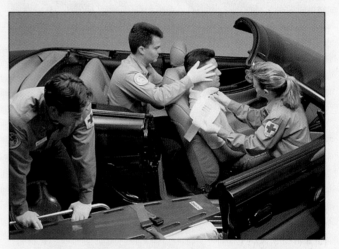

▲ Perform an initial assessment and rapid trauma assessment. Then apply a cervical spine immobilization collar.

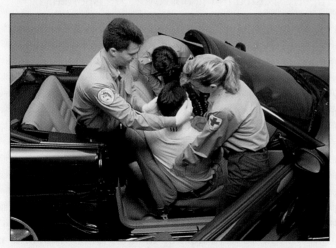

▲ Support the patient's thorax. Rotate the patient until his back is facing the open car door. Bring the patient's legs and feet up onto the car seat.

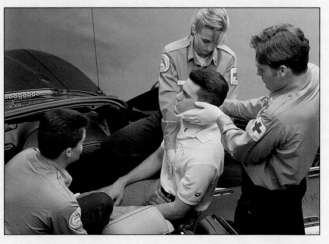

▲ Bring the board in line with the patient and against the buttocks. Stabilize the cot under the board. Begin to lower the patient onto the board.

(continued on the next page)

✳✳✳✳✳✳✳✳✳✳✳✳✳✳✳✳✳✳✳✳✳

PERFORMING RAPID EXTRICATION OF A SEATED PATIENT FROM VEHICLE—*(continued)*

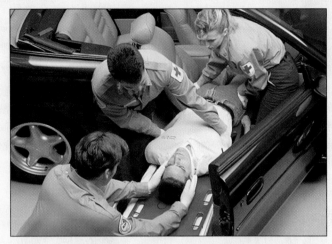

▲ Lower the patient onto the board. Dependent on the structure of the car, it may be necessary to change positions to maintain in-line stabilization while lowering the patient onto the board.

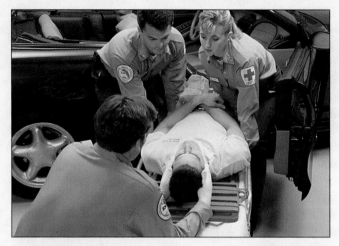

▲ As one EMT maintains in-line stabilization, the other EMTs support the patient as they slide him onto the back board in 6-inch to 12-inch increments.

3. Together rescuer #1 and #2 carefully pivot the patient so his back faces the door opening.

4. As the patient turns, rescuer #2 assumes control of the head while rescuer #1 and #3 assist in laying the patient down on the backboard.

5. The patient is then properly secured to the board and transported.

Dealing with Helmets

The use of protective helmets is becoming more and more common in many sports. This may be because of both state laws and just plain common sense. In any case, you are likely to encounter a patient with a suspected spinal injury who is wearing a helmet, and you will need to know how to deal with the helmet.

TYPES OF HELMETS

5-4.21 Identify different types of helmets.

There are as many types of helmets as there are sports that use them (Figure 34-20A–I). From bicycling to kayaking to field hockey to skiing, helmets come in many shapes and sizes. Most helmets come in two basic varieties: the sports-style helmet that has an open face and opens anteriorly, and the motorcycle style that slips on over the top of the head and encloses the entire face.

5-4.22 Describe the unique characteristics of sports helmets.

As you might expect, the open-face helmets provide easier access to the face and therefore make it easier to both assess and manage the airway without having

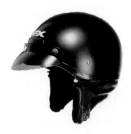

FIGURE 34-20A Half-size motorcycle helmet provides head protection from impact but may not provide face and eye protection, even with a face shield. Easier to remove than a full helmet. (AFX North America, Inc.)

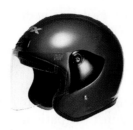

FIGURE 34-20B Three-quarter size motorcycle helmet provides head protection from impact and may provide face and eye protection. Somewhat easier to remove than the full-size helmet. (AFX North America, Inc.)

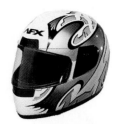

FIGURE 34-20C Full-size motorcycle helmet. In addition to head-impact protection, it provides a measure of facial protection with a face shield. Properly fitting helmets have room beneath the chin bar for a hand to slide under and check for airway and breathing. (AFX North America, Inc.)

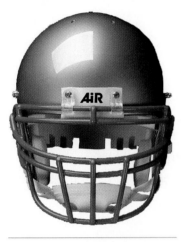

FIGURE 34-20D Football helmet provides a measure of facial protection with a face shield in place as well as head-impact protection. (Schutt Sports.)

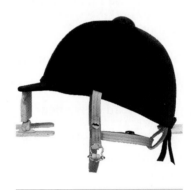

FIGURE 34-20E Horseback riding helmet provides head protection from impact but may not provide face and eye protection. (International Riding Helmets.)

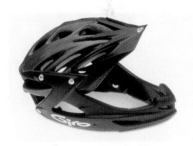

FIGURE 34-20F Mountain bike helmet provides head protection and, with a chin bar, some face protection. (Giro Sport Design.)

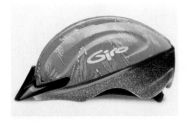

FIGURE 34-20G Youth's bicycle helmet provides head protection if it fits properly and is worn correctly. (Giro Sport Design.)

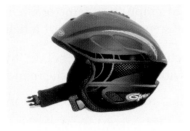

FIGURE 34-20H Snowboarding helmet provided head protection and, with a chin bar, some face protection. (Giro Sport Design.)

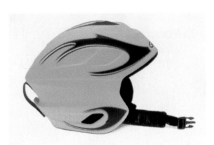

FIGURE 34-20I Downhill skiing helmet provides head protection and, with a chin bar, some face protection. (Giro Sport Design.)

to remove the helmet. Full-face helmets make assessment and management of the patient's airway and breathing much more difficult.

Depending on the situation, you may choose to leave the helmet in place or remove it. The driving factor in deciding to remove the helmet or leave it in place is the adequacy of the patient's airway and breathing. If you are able to assess the airway and breathing and find that it is adequate, look at the fit of the helmet. Does it fit snugly against the patient's head minimizing movement within the helmet? If so, then consider the patient's position. Is the helmet forcing the head into a **hyperflexed** position, putting pressure on the neck? The last factor you must consider is your ability to adequately immobilize the patient with the helmet in place. If the helmet will prevent you from properly securing the patient to an immobilization device, then you may have to remove it.

∗ **hyperflexed**

extreme or abnormal flexion.

5-4.19 State the circumstances when a helmet should be left on the patient.

Leave the helmet in place when:

* There are no immediate or impending airway or breathing problems.

* It does not interfere with ongoing assessment of airway and breathing.

* It provides a snug fit with little movement of head.

* Removal would cause further injury.

Remove the helmet when:

5-4.20 Discuss the circumstances when a helmet should be removed.

* There is inability to assess and/or reassess airway and breathing.

* It prevents adequate management of the airway or breathing.

* Excessive patient head movement is possible within the helmet.

* Proper spinal immobilization cannot be performed due to the helmet.

* Cardiac or respiratory arrest occurs.

GENERAL RULES FOR HELMET REMOVAL

5-4.23 Explain the preferred methods to remove a helmet.

Helmet removal will differ slightly depending on the type of helmet encountered. The primary objective is to minimize any side to side motion and to remove the helmet by pulling in the direction of the spine.

The following is a sequence of steps that can be followed for the proper removal of a helmet. The specific technique that you use will depend somewhat on the actual helmet and may be modified as necessary. Remove the patient's eyeglasses prior to attempting to remove a helmet.

5-4.25 Describe how the patient's head is stabilized to remove the helmet.

Follow these steps for removal of a helmet (Scan 34-7):

1. One rescuer stabilizes the helmet by placing his hands on each side of the helmet with the fingers on the mandible to prevent movement.

2. The second rescuer loosens, cuts, or removes the chin strap, if present.

3. The second rescuer then places one hand on the mandible to stabilize the chin and the other hand posteriorly at the occipital region.

4. The first rescuer then pulls the sides of the helmet apart and gently slips the helmet halfway off the patient's head and then stops.

5. The second rescuer then slides the posterior hand along the back of the patient's head to support the head as the helmet is removed.

6. Following removal of the helmet, the second rescuer assumes normal manual stabilization of the head until full spinal immobilization is complete.

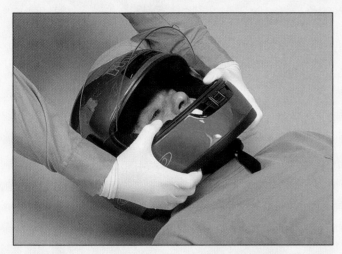

▲ EMT #1 is positioned at the top of the patient's head and maintains manual stabilization. Two hands hold the helmet stable while the fingertips hold the lower jaw.

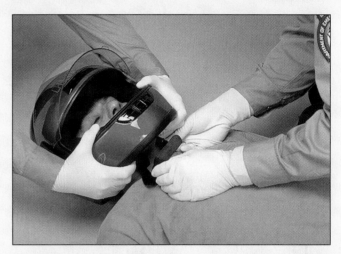

▲ EMT #2 opens, cuts, or removes the chin strap.

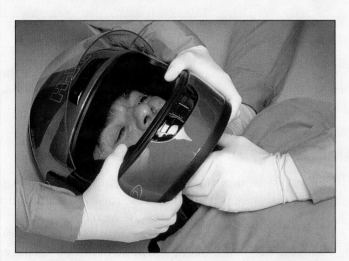

▲ EMT #2 then places one hand on the patient's mandible and, using the other hand, reaches in behind the neck and stabilizes the occipital region. Using the combination of the hand in front of the chin and the hand behind the neck, EMT #2 should be able to hold the head securely. If the patient has glasses on, they should be removed now, prior to removal of the helmet.

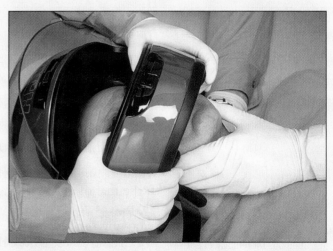

▲ EMT #1 can now release manual stabilization and slowly remove the helmet. The lower sides, or ear cups, of the helmet will have to be gently pulled out to clear the ears.

(continued on the next page)

REMOVAL OF HELMET—(continued)

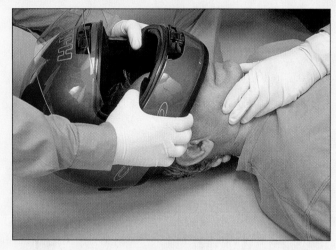

▲ The helmet should come off straight with no backward tilting. A full-face helmet may need to be tilted just enough for the chin guard to clear the nose. EMT #2 must support and prevent the head from moving as the helmet is removed.

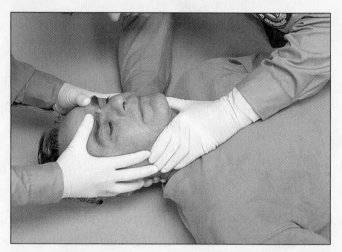

▲ EMT #1, after removing the helmet, reestablishes manual stabilization and maintains an open airway by using the jaw-thrust maneuver.

As the helmet is removed, be certain to support the head so that it does not drop suddenly. After removal of the helmet, gently lower the head onto the board. It is also appropriate to place a thin pad beneath the patient's head for comfort.

FOOTBALL HELMETS AND EQUIPMENT

5-4.24 Discuss alternative methods for removal of a helmet.

When dealing with football helmets, it is important to understand that removing the helmet of a player who is wearing shoulder pads will cause the head to fall into a hyperextended position. This can be prevented by leaving the helmet in place and removing the face guard of the helmet, should access to the airway be necessary. In extreme cases, where the helmet must be removed, it will be helpful to also remove the shoulder pads.

Clinical Clues: REMOVING FOOTBALL EQUIPMENT

Remember that by removing only the helmet and not the shoulder pads, or vice versa, will cause the patient's neck to hyperextend or hyperflex. It is recommended that if you must remove the helmet that you also remove the shoulder pads in order to keep the cervical spine in correct alignment.

OTHER SPORTS HELMETS

An alternative method of removal can be used for sports helmets such as those used for bicycling. Follow these steps for removal of a sports-style helmet (Scan 34-8):

1. The first rescuer establishes manual stabilization of the head in the traditional manner, only the hands will be lower down on the head below the ears.

2. The second rescuer releases the chin strap and removes the helmet.

3. As the helmet is removed the first rescuer gently lowers the patient's head to the board and repositions his hands higher up in the head.

4. The second rescuer then applies a cervical collar.

5-4.26 Differentiate how the head is stabilized with a helmet compared to without a helmet.

When a helmet is left in place, a significant amount of support is required to minimize the side to side movement of the head. This can be accomplished by placing the helmet in a commercial head immobilizer or with towel rolls. It is very likely that you will still need to maintain manual stabilization as the curve and weight of the helmet may be too much for the device to stabilize all by itself.

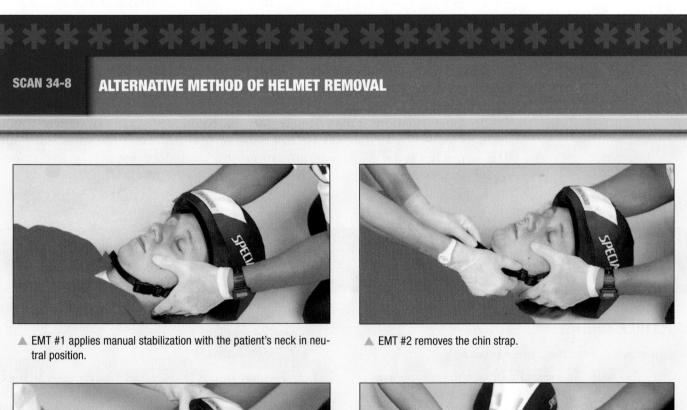

SCAN 34-8   **ALTERNATIVE METHOD OF HELMET REMOVAL**

▲ EMT #1 applies manual stabilization with the patient's neck in neutral position.

▲ EMT #2 removes the chin strap.

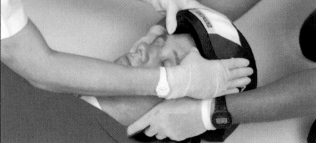

▲ EMT #2 removes the helmet, pulling out on each side to clear the ears.

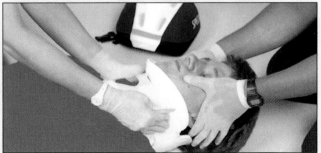

▲ EMT #1 maintains manual stabilization as EMT #2 applies a cervical collar.

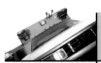

Dispatch Summary

Dan Vandel was secured to a long spine board, administered high-flow oxygen, and transported to the Northeast Medical Center on Green River Parkway. X-rays showed fractures to the C3 and C4 vertebrae, with bone fragments impacting the spinal cord in three places.

Several days after surgery, Dan regained limited use of his arms and some feeling in his lower legs. Dan's doctor anticipates that he will walk again, with the assistance of a cane, but will probably always suffer from numbness and weakness in his extremities.

✳ The Last Word

Injuries to the spinal cord can result in permanent paralysis and loss of function below the injury site. Proper assessment and management of the patient with suspected spinal injury is essential to minimize further damage and long-term paralysis.

Spinal immobilization is not a higher priority than the ABCs, but proper management of the ABCs can be accomplished while being mindful of a suspected spinal injury.

In some situations it may be necessary, based on scene safety or patient condition, to move or extricate the patient without first providing full spinal immobilization. This is called rapid extrication and should be used as a last resort. Remember to complete your PCR with all appropriate information.

✳ Chapter Review

MULTIPLE CHOICE

Place a check next to the correct answer.

1. The brain and spinal cord are the components of the _____ system.

    _____ a. autonomic nervous

    _____ b. skeletal

    _____ c. central nervous

    _____ d. peripheral nervous

2. The network of sensory and motor nerves that extend from the brain and spinal cord make up the _____ system.

    _____ a. autonomic

    _____ b. skeletal

    _____ c. central nervous

    _____ d. peripheral nervous

3. Which of the following mechanisms of injury would be least likely to cause a spinal injury?

_____ a. gunshot wound to the leg

_____ b. motor vehicle collision

_____ c. fall from 20 feet

_____ d. diving into a shallow pool

4. Extreme pulling of the spine is an example of which type of MOI?

_____ a. flexion

_____ b. extension

_____ c. rotation

_____ d. distraction

5. A patient who has fallen from a height and landed in a seated position is likely to experience what type of spinal injury?

_____ a. flexion

_____ b. extension

_____ c. compression

_____ d. rotation

6. Which of the following is least likely to be a sign or symptom of a spinal injury?

_____ a. paralysis on one side of the body

_____ b. numbness and tingling in both legs

_____ c. tenderness along the spine

_____ d. pain along the spine on movement

7. Which of the following is the most serious complication of spinal injury encountered in the field?

_____ a. priapism

_____ b. incontinence

_____ c. inadequate breathing

_____ d. loss of consciousness

8. It is important to assess circulation, sensation, and motor function of all four extremities:

_____ a. before immobilization.

_____ b. before and after immobilization.

_____ c. after immobilization.

_____ d. only during the rapid trauma assessment.

9. When securing a patient with suspected spinal injury to a long spine board, the head must be secured:

_____ a. first.

_____ b. before the torso.

_____ c. before the legs.

_____ d. after the torso.

10. Which of the following best describes the function of a cervical collar?

_____ a. It prevents movement of the neck.

_____ b. It reminds the patient not to move his neck.

_____ c. It provides adequate immobilization of the neck.

_____ d. It must be placed regardless of fit.

11. Which of the following situations is most appropriate for rapid extrication?

_____ a. a patient with inadequate breathing

_____ b. a responsive patient

_____ c. a patient complaining of neck pain

_____ d. none of the above

12. All of the following are indications for leaving a helmet in place on a patient EXCEPT:

_____ a. there are no immediate airway problems.

_____ b. helmet removal would cause further injury.

_____ c. the helmet does not interfere with your assessment.

_____ d. there is excessive head movement within the helmet.

13. When rolling a patient who may have a spinal injury, the rescuer at the _____ should direct all movements.

_____ a. head

_____ b. torso

_____ c. hips

_____ d. legs

14. Which of the following patients would be best suited for a vest-type immobilization device?

_____ a. supine patient on the ground

_____ b. seated patient in a sports car

_____ c. prone patient on the ground

_____ d. standing patient

15. The first step in caring for a suspected spinal injury patient is to:

_____ a. roll the patient.

_____ b. place a cervical collar.

_____ c. place them on an appropriate device.

_____ d. manually stabilize the head and neck.

FILL IN THE BLANK

1. The central nervous system includes the brain and _____.

2. The _____ nervous system is made up of all the sensory and motor nerves that extend from the brain and spinal cord to all parts of the body.

3. The first seven vertebrae located in the neck, are known as the _____.

4. There are _____ vertebrae that make up the thoracic spine.

5. The _____ spine is located in the lower back and is comprised of five vertebrae.

6. Injury at any point along the spinal column that causes damage to the spinal cord can result in the loss of sensation and/or function _____ the site of injury.

7. Any force that impacts the spine from the top or bottom has the potential to cause what is referred to as a _____ injury.

8. Injury to the spinal cord above the _____ cervical vertebrae can prevent the diaphragm muscle from assisting with spontaneous respiration.

CRITICAL THINKING

1. Describe at least two circumstances in which rapid extrication would be necessary.

_____

_____

_____

_____

2. Discuss the priority for proper spinal immobilization in patients needing rapid extrication.

_____

_____

_____

_____

3. Describe how you would manage an unresponsive football player with a suspected spinal injury.

_____

_____

_____

_____

CASE STUDIES

Case Study 1

You have been dispatched to a vehicle collision at a busy intersection in the center of town known for its daily occurrence of collisions. Upon arrival, you find two vehicles, each with substantial damage to the front end. The fire department is on scene and is caring for the patient in the first vehicle. You approach the second vehicle and see no one inside. Just then a police officer calls you over to the curb. He is taking information from a man standing beside him. The man is holding a bloody towel against his forehead and seems to be bleeding from the mouth as well. The officer informs you that this man was the driver of the second vehicle. When asked, the patient denies any neck pain but states only that his head hurts because he hit it on the windshield.

1. Is this patient a candidate for spinal immobilization? If so, why?

_____

_____

_____

_____

2. What additional information will you want to know about this patient?

_____

_____

_____

_____

3. How will you care for this patient?

_____

_____

_____

_____

4. What device is most appropriate for immobilizing this patient?

_____

_____

_____

_____

Case Study 2

You have responded to a motorcycle versus vehicle collision. Upon arrival, you find the rider of the motorcycle lying motionless on his side in the intersection. A passerby is kneeling beside the patient, attempting to get a response. Your assessment reveals that the patient does not appear to be breathing and radial pulses are absent. He has a full-face helmet still in place, and it shows significant damage to the right side. A quick visual also reveals severe deformity to his left lower leg.

1. What is your first priority for this patient?

   _____

   _____

   _____

   _____

2. Will you roll him onto his back? If so, how will you accomplish this with just the bystander as an assistant?

   _____

   _____

   _____

   _____

3. Will you want to remove this man's helmet? If so, how will you accomplish this?

   _____

   _____

   _____

   _____

4. What device would be most appropriate for immobilizing this patient?

   _____

   _____

   _____

   _____

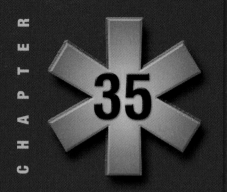

35

Module Review and Practice Examination

✳ Directions

Assess what you have learned in this module by circling the best answer for each multiple-choice question. When you are done, check your answers against the key provided in Appendix D.

1. The largest artery in the body is the:
   a. vena cava.
   b. carotid.
   c. jugular.
   d. aorta.

2. The femoral artery is found in the:
   a. neck.
   b. groin.
   c. arm.
   d. heart.

3. The blood component responsible for carrying oxygen to the cells of the body is:
   a. red blood cells.
   b. white blood cells.
   c. plasma.
   d. platelets.

4. Which of the following factors affects the severity of blood loss and the signs and symptoms associated with it?
   a. rate of bleeding
   b. amount of blood loss
   c. size of the patient
   d. all of the above

5. The body's first response to an injured blood vessel is:
   a. forming a blood clot.
   b. decreasing the blood pressure.
   c. constriction of the blood vessel.
   d. increasing the heart rate.

6. Your patient has cut her hand with a knife and has bright red bleeding that seems to be pumping out under pressure. This is most likely _____ bleeding.
   a. venous
   b. capillary
   c. arterial
   d. mixed venous and capillary

7. The first attempt to control bleeding is always:
   a. applying a tourniquet.
   b. elevation of the affected part.
   c. application of ice to the affected part.
   d. the use of direct pressure.

8. Your patient has a severe laceration to the scalp. Which pressure point should be used to assist in controlling this bleeding?
   a. carotid artery
   b. jugular vein
   c. brachial artery
   d. none of the above

9. Your patient has a gunshot wound to the thigh with severe bleeding. You have tried direct pressure without success. Which of the following is the correct sequence of next steps?
   a. elevation, pressure on the femoral artery, tourniquet
   b. pressure on the femoral artery, elevation, tourniquet
   c. pressure on the femoral artery, tourniquet, elevation
   d. none of the above

10. Which of the following would be the best choice for improvising a tourniquet?
    a. an electrical extension cord
    b. oxygen tubing
    c. a belt
    d. yarn

11. Your patient is a 78-year-old female complaining of a nosebleed that has lasted 1 hour. Which of the following is the most appropriate treatment for this patient?
    a. Have her assume a comfortable position on the stretcher and tilt her head back.
    b. Have the patient sit down and lean forward.
    c. Ask the patient to gently blow her nose.
    d. Apply an ice pack to the back of her neck.

12. Hypoperfusion is often used to mean:
    a. shock.
    b. bleeding.
    c. internal hemorrhage.
    d. adequate circulation.

13. In adults, injury to which area does NOT usually lead to hypovolemia due to blood loss?
    a. pelvis
    b. abdomen
    c. head
    d. chest

14. Which of the following is NOT a typical indication of internal hemorrhage?
    a. vomiting material with a coffee grounds appearance
    b. slow pulse with warm skin and low blood pressure
    c. abdominal pain
    d. bruising or discoloration of the abdominal wall

15. Which of the following statements about shock is true?
    a. Once a patient is in shock, death is inevitable.
    b. Shock is progressive without intervention.
    c. Definitive treatment for the patient in shock is high-flow oxygen.
    d. All blood loss leads to shock.

16. Major functions of the skin include all of the following EXCEPT:
    a. energy production.
    b. protection from the environment.
    c. temperature regulation.
    d. prevention of fluid loss.

17. The blood vessels and nerve endings of the skin are located in the:
    a. subcutaneous layer.
    b. epidermis.
    c. dermis.
    d. percutaneous layer.

18. Your patient is a dockworker who is pinned underneath a forklift that tipped over on his legs. This type of mechanism is most likely to result in which of the following types of soft tissue injury?
    a. blunt force trauma
    b. crush force trauma
    c. penetrating trauma
    d. puncturing trauma

19. Which of the following is a closed soft tissue injury?
    a. laceration
    b. abrasion
    c. puncture
    d. hematoma

20. Which of the following best explains the significance of a contusion to the thigh after a high-speed motor vehicle collision?
    a. Contusions are permanently disfiguring.
    b. Contusions are associated with massive blood loss.
    c. The contusion may be an indication of a femur fracture.
    d. There is a high risk of infection associated with contusions.

21. Your patient is a 12-year-old boy who was not wearing a shirt when he fell off his skateboard while going down a steep incline. As he slid down the incline on his chest, the concrete rubbed off portions of his skin. This type of injury is best described as a/an:
    a. hematoma.
    b. abrasion.
    c. laceration.
    d. avulsion.

22. Your patient is a 35-year-old male who was stabbed in the back with a large knife. When you arrived on the scene, the knife was still embedded in the wound. Which of the following statements regarding this situation is true?
    a. Once airway, breathing, and circulation are assessed and appropriate interventions are performed, the object must be stabilized in place prior to transporting the patient.
    b. It will be necessary to remove the knife in this case because the patient must be placed supine (on his back) in order to care for and transport him.
    c. Impaled objects to the chest must always be removed to prevent a collapsed lung.
    d. The knife should be stabilized with fluffy pillows so that he can be placed supine (on his back) for transport without placing additional pressure on the knife.

23. Your patient is a 44-year-old female whose right lower extremity was amputated just above the knee when the motorcycle she was riding was struck broadside by a car. The patient is pale and her skin feels cool and wet. Her radial pulse is 108 and thready. You have already applied high-flow oxygen to the patient but are having difficulty controlling bleeding from the wound. First responders and the police are looking for the amputated part but have not yet found it. Which of the following is the best course of action?
    a. Apply a tourniquet and wait on the scene, because the patient and the amputated part must always be transported together.
    b. Prepare to transport the patient and advise the police that when they find the body part they should place it in a bag filled with ice and bring it to the hospital.

    c. Ask the patient if she wants to stay and wait for the leg to be found or go ahead to the hospital.
    d. Continue measures to control bleeding and transport the patient without waiting for the part to be found.

24. Absorbent gauze that is placed directly over a wound is best described as a:
    a. bandage.
    b. dressing.
    c. splint.
    d. plaster.

25. Your patient has a 6-inch laceration to the anterior forearm. Which of the following is the correct way to apply roller gauze in the care of this wound?
    a. Place the roll of gauze over the wound and tape it in place.
    b. Starting at the elbow, wrap the roller gauze in overlapping turns around the forearm, moving toward the wrist.
    c. Starting at the wrist, wrap the roller gauze in overlapping turns around the forearm, moving toward the elbow.
    d. Wrap the gauze directly over the wound without extending the wrap beyond the ends of the wound.

26. A burn caused by exposure to hot liquid is classified as a/an _____ burn.
    a. chemical
    b. thermal
    c. electrical
    d. radiation

27. A burn that includes the epidermis and dermis is called a _____ burn.
    a. superficial
    b. partial thickness
    c. full thickness
    d. deep

28. Blisters are associated with _____ burns.
    a. full-thickness
    b. superficial
    c. third-degree
    d. partial-thickness

29. Which of the following is NOT a consideration in determining appropriate care for a burn patient?
    a. depth of the burn
    b. anatomical location of the burn
    c. the patient's gender
    d. the patient's age

30. Your patient is a 16-year-old female with burns to both lower extremities from just above the knees to her feet and her entire right arm. The percentage of body surface area involved is:
    a. 45.
    b. 36.
    c. 27.
    d. 18.

31. Your patient is a 15-month-old male who pulled a deep-fryer full of hot oil off a counter top. He has burns to his entire head, face, and neck. The percentage of body surface area involved is:
    a. 9.
    b. 18.
    c. 24.
    d. 27.

32. Your patient is a 68-year-old female with a burn to her anterior thigh that is about twice the size of her hand. The approximate percentage of body surface area involved is:
    a. 18.
    b. 9.
    c. 5.
    d. 2.

33. Burns are considered more serious if they affect which of the following body parts?
    a. chest
    b. arm
    c. hand
    d. leg

34. Your patient is a 25-year-old male who was soldering two pieces of metal together when the soldering gun slipped and created a full-thickness burn about the size of a pencil eraser on his forearm. This burn would be considered:
    a. severe.
    b. intense.
    c. moderate.
    d. mild.

35. Your patient is a 38-year-old man with a dry chemical powder on his face and hands. Which of the following is most appropriate?
    a. Transport him to the hospital for proper decontamination.
    b. Brush the powder away before flushing with large amounts of water.
    c. Wipe the powder away with a damp cloth.
    d. Find an antidote to the chemical and apply it to the affected areas.

36. Which of the following statements concerning electrical burns is FALSE?
    a. The greatest risk with electrical burns is thermal burns to a large percentage of body surface area.
    b. Electrical burns can be associated with cardiac and respiratory problems.
    c. Exposure to electrical current may cause burns both at the site where the current entered the body and where it exited the body.
    d. Electricity generally travels internally through the body, rather than along its surface.

37. Which of the following is generally NOT a complication of severe burns?
    a. infection
    b. fluid loss
    c. hypothermia
    d. blood loss

38. The pleural layers and the fluid between them are important in providing:
    a. suction between the chest wall and lungs.
    b. friction between the chest wall and lungs.
    c. trapped air in the thorax.
    d. protection from blunt trauma.

39. The EMT should consider a penetrating injury at the level of the eighth rib to be:
    a. a chest injury.
    b. both a chest and abdominal injury.
    c. unlikely to cause serious chest or abdominal injury.
    d. unlikely to cause serious chest injury.

40. Chest trauma may include injury to any of the following EXCEPT the:
    a. aorta.
    b. pancreas.
    c. heart.
    d. bronchi.

41. When two or more consecutive ribs are each fractured in two or more places, this is called:
    a. floating ribs.
    b. a paradoxical segment.
    c. a pneumothorax.
    d. a flail chest.

42. Your patient is a 9-year-old male whose 12-year-old cousin jumped from a fence onto his chest as he was lying on the ground, in an imitation of a television wrestling match. The patient's head and neck are purple in color and his neck veins are distended. His eyes seem to be bulging out of their sockets. This condition can best be described as:
    a. paradoxical motion.
    b. flail chest.
    c. traumatic asphyxia.
    d. hemothorax.

43. Your patient is a 22-year-old male with a gunshot wound to his right side, just below his armpit. In addition to oxygen and transport, which of the following is required in the care of this patient?
    a. a soft, bulky dressing over the site to splint the injury and reduce pain
    b. a circumferential bandage around the chest
    c. a dressing packed tightly into the wound to prevent an air leak
    d. an occlusive dressing taped on three sides

44. The kidneys are located in the:
    a. retroperitoneal cavity.
    b. abdominal cavity.
    c. thorax.
    d. pleural space.

45. The primary concerns with damage to hollow organs of the abdomen are:
    a. irritation of the peritoneum and infection.
    b. bleeding and hemorrhagic shock.
    c. swelling and pain.
    d. vomiting and diarrhea.

46. Which of the following is the appropriate management for an evisceration?
    a. Cover the site with Vaseline-impregnated gauze taped on three sides.
    b. Pack the wound with gauze.

    c. Cover the site with a large sterile dressing moistened with sterile saline.
    d. Rinse exposed organs with sterile saline and place them gently back inside the wound.

47. Bones are connected to one another at joints by:
    a. tendons.
    b. muscles.
    c. ligaments.
    d. marrow.

48. Mrs. Quinn fell forward onto her hands and broke her clavicle. This is an example of an injury caused by _____ force.
    a. pathological
    b. shearing
    c. direct
    d. indirect

49. A strain is an injury to a/an:
    a. bone.
    b. joint.
    c. ligament.
    d. muscle.

50. Your patient is a 17-year-old skater who fell onto the ice and injured her wrist. The most appropriate approach to this patient is a:
    a. detailed history and physical examination.
    b. rapid trauma exam.
    c. focused history and assessment.
    d. detailed history and focused assessment.

51. For which of the following patients would a rapid trauma assessment be appropriate?
    a. 40-year-old female who stepped off a curb, twisted her ankle, and fell to her knees
    b. 9-year-old male who fell 15 feet from a tree house and has a deformed right arm
    c. 75-year-old female who stood up from her chair, felt a "snap" in her hip, and fell back into the chair
    d. 7-year-old female who has a deformed forearm after performing a cartwheel in gymnastics class

52. Your patient is a 45-year-old male cyclist who was forced into a curb to avoid being struck by a vehicle. He was thrown over the handlebars and is complaining of pain to his left forearm. He was wearing a helmet and does not have any other complaints or signs of injury. Your assessment reveals a badly deformed left forearm and no distal pulses in the left lower extremity. You have a 20-minute transport time. Which of the following is most appropriate?
    a. Straighten the extremity with gentle traction and splint at the point where pulses return prior to transport.
    b. Splint the extremity in the position found and transport without delay.
    c. Immediately call for an ALS unit.
    d. Place the extremity in a sling but without using a rigid splint, apply ice, transport.

53. All of the following are reasons for splinting a swollen, painful, deformed extremity EXCEPT to:
    a. prevent unnecessary pain.
    b. prevent the patient from seeing how badly the extremity is injured.
    c. minimize further bleeding.
    d. prevent further damage to nerves, soft tissue, and blood vessels.

54. Your patient has a swollen, deformed, painful ankle. A properly applied splint should start at the patient's _____ and extend to _____.
    a. ankle; the knee
    b. toes; just above the ankle
    c. toes; just below the knee
    d. foot; the mid-thigh

55. A traction splint is designed to be used for which of the following injuries?
    a. open fractures of the tibia
    b. deformed midshaft humerus fractures
    c. injuries to the knee
    d. suspected femur fractures

56. A swathe is a useful adjunct to a sling in splinting which of the following injuries?
    a. dislocated shoulder
    b. fractured pelvis
    c. suspected femur fracture
    d. swollen, deformed, painful finger

57. The first priority in managing the patient with a musculoskeletal injury is:
    a. checking the distal circulation, sensation, and motor function.
    b. immobilizing the injured part.
    c. minimizing the patient's pain.
    d. assessing for and managing life-threatening conditions.

58. The basilar skull best describes which portion of the skull?
    a. the forehead area
    b. the back of the head
    c. the floor of the cranial vault
    d. the facial bones

59. The weakest area of the skull is/are the _____ bone(s).
    a. maxillary
    b. temporal
    c. parietal
    d. occipital

60. The tough, fibrous membrane that lines the inside of the cranial vault is the:
    a. dura mater.
    b. pia mater.
    c. arachnoid membrane.
    d. middle meningeal layer.

61. The largest portion of the brain is the:
    a. medulla oblingata.
    b. cerebellum.
    c. cerebrum.
    d. frontal lobe.

62. The most immediate life-threat in a closed head injury is:
    a. infection.
    b. blood loss.
    c. exposed brain tissue.
    d. increased pressure on the brain.

63. An injury that causes a jarring of the brain with temporary signs and symptoms such as confusion and memory loss is best described as a/an:
    a. cerebral contusion.
    b. concussion.
    c. subdural hematoma.
    d. herniation.

64. Signs of increasing intracranial pressure typically include all of the following EXCEPT:
    a. increased blood pressure.
    b. decreased heart rate.
    c. pinpoint pupils.
    d. seizures.

65. Which of the following is NOT consistent with an isolated closed head injury?
    a. abnormal breathing pattern
    b. shock
    c. vomiting
    d. abnormal posturing in response to pain

66. Of the following, the highest priority in the care of the trauma patient is:
    a. controlling bleeding.
    b. maintaining an open airway.
    c. providing supplemental oxygen.
    d. taking vital signs.

67. In most cases the proper rate of assisted ventilations for a patient with a suspected head injury is _____ per minute.
    a. 8 to 10
    b. 10 to 12
    c. 16 to 20
    d. 24 to 28

68. Which of the following is NOT a reason to increase the rate of ventilations in a patient with a suspected head injury?
    a. unequal pupils
    b. decerebrate posturing
    c. unresponsiveness
    d. confusion

69. The spinal cord is part of the _____ nervous system.
    a. accessory
    b. primary
    c. peripheral
    d. central

70. The seven vertebrae of the neck are known as the _____ vertebrae.
    a. cervical
    b. thoracic
    c. lumbar
    d. sacral

71. A 30-year-old skydiver landed hard on his feet when his parachute malfunctioned. The mechanism by which he may have suffered a spinal injury is:
    a. flexion.   c. distraction.
    b. rotation.   d. compression.

72. The most important consideration in determining the need for spinal immobilization is:
    a. the presence of spinal deformity.
    b. pain on palpation of the spine.
    c. the patient's complaint of numbness or inability to move.
    d. a significant mechanism of injury.

73. The first step in proper spinal immobilization is:
    a. manual stabilization of the head and neck.
    b. placing a properly sized cervical collar.
    c. using a short spinal immobilization device.
    d. logrolling the patient onto a long spine board.

74. Which of the following is a consideration in spinal immobilization of small children?
    a. Cervical collars are not made in pediatric sizes and must be improvised.
    b. Children should never be immobilized unless there are signs and symptoms of spinal cord injury.
    c. It is necessary to pad under the shoulders to prevent flexion of the neck.
    d. It is best to use a cervical collar without a long spine board when immobilizing small children.

75. Which of the following is a reason for rapid extrication of a patient with a possible spinal injury from a vehicle?
    a. The patient is in pain and complaining that it is taking too long to get her out of the car.
    b. The patient is preventing you from accessing another occupant who is more seriously injured.
    c. The patient does not have signs or symptoms of spinal injury and a short immobilization device seems unnecessary.
    d. None of the above

76. Which of the following is an indication for removing the helmet of a patient who requires spinal immobilization?
    a. inability to assess and/or manage the airway
    b. snug fit of the helmet
    c. patient is stable
    d. all of the above

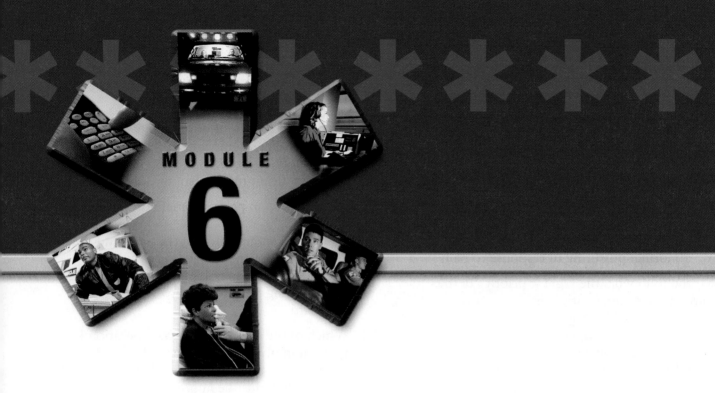

Pediatrics and Geriatrics

"... when I saw that my newborn baby was struggling to breathe, I just panicked and called 9-1-1 ... What a nightmare. "

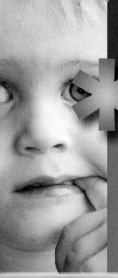

Module Outline

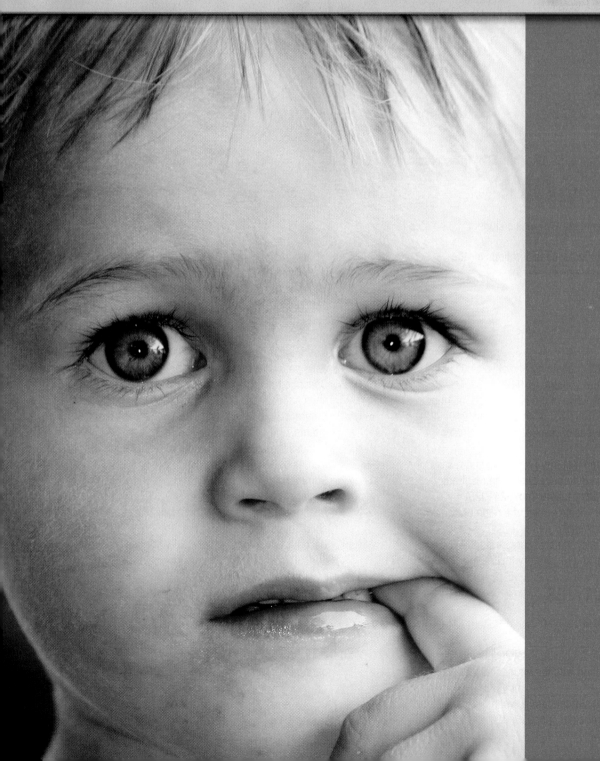

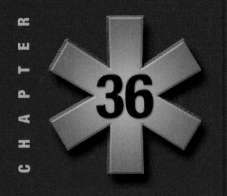

36

Caring for Pediatric Patients

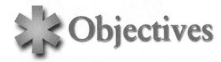 **Objectives**

Numbered objectives are from the U.S. Department of Transportation 1994 EMT-Basic National Standard Curriculum.

COGNITIVE OBJECTIVES

At the completion of this lesson, the EMT-Basic student will be able to:

6-1.1 Identify the developmental considerations for the following age groups: (pp. 916–919)
- infants
- toddlers
- preschool
- school age
- adolescent

6-1.2 Describe differences in anatomy and physiology of the infant, child, and adult patient. (p. 919)

6-1.3 Differentiate the response of the ill or injured infant or child (age specific) from that of an adult. (pp. 919–922)

6-1.4 Indicate various causes of respiratory emergencies. (pp. 924–925)

6-1.5 Differentiate between respiratory distress and respiratory failure. Describe the differences between respiratory distress and respiratory failure. (pp. 924–925)

6-1.6 List the steps in the management of foreign body airway obstruction. (pp. 925–929)

6-1.7 Summarize emergency medical care strategies for respiratory distress and respiratory failure. (pp. 924–925)

6-1.8 Identify the signs and symptoms of shock (hypoperfusion) in the infant and child patient. (p. 931)

6-1.9 Describe the methods of determining end organ perfusion in the infant and child patient. (p. 931)

6-1.10 State the usual cause of cardiac arrest in infants and children versus adults. (pp. 924–925)

6-1.11 List the common causes of seizures in the infant and child patient. (pp. 936–937)

6-1.12 Describe the management of seizures in the infant and child patient. (pp. 936–937)

6-1.13 Differentiate between the injury patterns in adults, infants, and children. (pp. 934–935)

6-1.14 Discuss the field management of the infant and child trauma patient. (p. 934)

6-1.15 Summarize the indicators of possible child abuse and neglect. (pp. 938–939)

6-1.16 Describe the medical legal responsibilities in suspected child abuse. (pp. 938–939)

6-1.17 Recognize need for EMT-Basic debriefing following a difficult infant or child transport. (pp. 940–941)

AFFECTIVE OBJECTIVES

At the completion of this lesson, the EMT-Basic student will be able to:

6-1.18 Explain the rationale for having knowledge and skills appropriate for dealing with the infant and child patient. (pp. 915–916)

6-1.19 Attend to the feelings of the family when dealing with an ill or injured infant or child. (pp. 915, 926, 940)

6-1.20 Understand the provider's own response (emotional) to caring for infants or children. (pp. 915, 940)

PSYCHOMOTOR OBJECTIVES

At the completion of this lesson, the EMT-Basic student will be able to:

6-1.21 Demonstrate the techniques of foreign body airway obstruction removal in the infant. (pp. 925–929)

6-1.22 Demonstrate the techniques of foreign body airway obstruction removal in the child. (pp. 925–926)

6-1.23 Demonstrate the assessment of the infant and child. (pp. 919–923)

6-1.24 Demonstrate bag-valve-mask artificial ventilations for the infant. (pp. 930–931)

6-1.25 Demonstrate bag-valve-mask artificial ventilations for the child. (pp. 930–931)

6-1.26 Demonstrate oxygen delivery for the infant and child. (pp. 929–930)

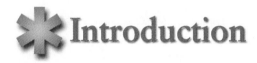 **Introduction**

Calls involving infants and children are often intimidating or frustrating to the EMS provider due to several factors. Their small size, restricted communication skills, and resistance to strangers are just some of the reasons. An additional factor is that quite often these patients are surrounded by highly emotional or distraught parents or caregivers. You must attend to them as well.

Understanding the differences between age groups as well as behaviors common to most young children will help you interact more successfully with these patients and their families. The care pediatric patients require varies enormously, because a newborn baby is as different from a 12-year-old as a 7-year-old is from an adult as a result of their differing stages of psychological, anatomical, and physiological development.

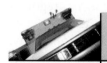 **Emergency Dispatch**

"Four-fifty-three, four-five-three, I need you to respond to an emergency to the Grand Hotel downtown. Room . . . uh . . . two-twenty. This is an infant in respiratory distress."

"Ten-four, show us en route," Jake, an EMT, dropped the microphone into the holder. "Oh man, why a peds call? The shift had been going so well!"

"It'll be fine," Jake's partner, Aaron, said. "Just stay focused."

"They're just so little, and everything's different," Jake blasted the air horn at a car that wasn't pulling off to the right. "I just don't want a little kid to die on me. I don't know how I would handle that."

Aaron sighed and looked out the window as they sped through the glass canyons downtown. He occasionally caught a glimpse of his own somber face,

framed by red and blue flashes, reflected from the darkened windows of shops and office buildings. Sometimes kids don't make it, though, he thought. But after awhile, you do cope with it. That's what he's been told anyway.

The Grand Hotel was a towering structure of mirrored windows and bright lights with a marble driveway leading to a bank of huge glass entry doors. Aaron and Jake rolled the cot into the lobby and were directed to a large service elevator. On the second floor, a security guard led them down a long, carpeted hall and into an open hotel room.

"Oh, thank goodness." An older woman greeted them. "My granddaughter seems to be doing better, but she was having trouble breathing and vomiting. She was born 6 weeks prematurely, so we got really nervous."

A second woman in the room, the infant's mother, held her up so Jake could see her. The baby was tiny, maybe 4 pounds, and was attached to a portable monitor that beeped quietly. A feeding tube protruded from the infant's left nostril and was taped to her cheek.

"Was she just released from the hospital?" he asked.

"They released her and showed us how to feed her and kind of what to watch for on the monitor. We were afraid that something bad would happen. That's why we stayed in town at this hotel instead of heading back home."

"Well," Jake said as he prepared the car seat. "Let's get her over to Children's Hospital and find out what's going on."

Pediatric Development

6-1.1 Identify the developmental considerations for the following age groups:
- infants
- toddlers
- preschool
- school age
- adolescent

The pediatric population ranges from birth through adolescence. Generally, children are divided into five categories according to age.

These are:

＊ Newborn/infant (birth to 1 year old) (Figure 36-1)

＊ Toddler (1–3 years old) (Figure 36-2)

＊ Preschooler (3–6 years old) (Figure 36-3)

＊ School-age (6–12 years old) (Figure 36-4)

＊ Adolescent (12–18 years old) (Figure 36-5)

The ability to estimate age and weight is important, as many of your treatment decisions will depend on these factors. Also, definitions of pediatric age categories vary depending on the context in which they are receiving care, such as in the context of CPR and AED use. Procedures will differ according to the child's anatomy.

A guide to average weights commonly associated with children of different ages can be found in Table 36-1.

The weight used for calculating the size of equipment used with children is always given in kilograms. Learning to estimate age and weight (and translating that weight into kilograms) will help you improve your pediatric assessment skills.

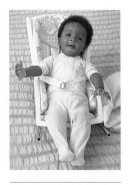

FIGURE 36-1
Newborns and infants, birth to 1 year.

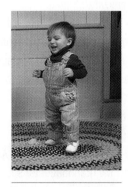

FIGURE 36-2
Toddlers, 1 to 3 years.

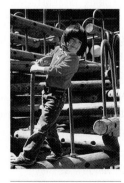

FIGURE 36-3
Preschool children, 3 to 6 years.

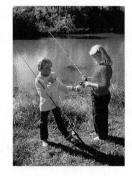

FIGURE 36-4
School age children, 6 to 12 years.

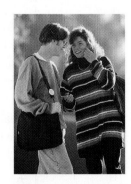

FIGURE 36-5
Adolescents, 12 to 18 years.

TABLE 36-1	AVERAGE PEDIATRIC WEIGHTS	
AGE	**WEIGHT IN KILOGRAMS**	**WEIGHT IN POUNDS**
Newborn	3.5kg	7.7 lb
6 months	7 kg	15.4 lb
1 year	10 kg	22.0 lb
18 months	12 kg	26.4 lb
2 years	13 kg	28.6 lb
4 years	16 kg	35.2 lb
6 years	20 kg	44.0 lb
8 years	25 kg	55.0 lb
10 years	32 kg	70.4 lb
12 years	40 kg	88.0 lb
14 years	48 kg	105.6 lb

Development Characteristics

Children behave differently at different ages, so it is useful to know something about the stages of child development and how you may need to tailor your patient assessment for children of different ages.

NEWBORNS AND INFANTS (BIRTH TO 1 YEAR)

When approaching the newborn or infant, it is important to keep two important ideas in mind: He does not like to be cold, and he does not like to be separated from his parents or primary caregivers. Once infants are crying from discomfort or anxiety, your assessment will become much more difficult to perform.

It is a good idea to look at the baby closely while he is being held by a familiar caregiver. You can evaluate skin color, level of alertness, chest movement, and respiratory rate. To preserve warmth, the infant does not need to be completely undressed. Ask the caregiver to undress the infant enough to give you a good view of the chest. Warm the bell of the stethoscope before applying it to the patient's chest to listen to breath sounds. If the baby is crying, allow the caregiver to attempt to comfort him with a pacifier or similar object. You may also try distracting the baby with a toy or your penlight. If the baby needs oxygen, try having the caregiver hold the mask in front of the baby's face rather than trying to strap it on, as these patients do not like facial stimulation. Lastly, be sure to run your hand over the newborn's head to check the fontanels. These are open areas in the skull where the bones have yet to fuse together. Bulging or depressed fontanels may be an indication of the patient's fluid status—bulging fontanels indicating possible increased intracranial pressure, sunken fontanels indicating possible dehydration.

TODDLERS (1–3 YEARS)

The toddler has developed a sense of independence through walking and talking but still is unable to reason well or communicate complex ideas. The toddler does

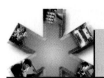

Perspective

Jake—The EMT

"I was so relieved that she was okay when we got there. I had all sorts of horrible scenarios in my head while we were on the elevator. But when I saw that little baby—just alert and looking around at all of us—I was so relieved that she was breathing. It's the first time I've ever seen such a tiny baby outside of an NICU, and yet there she was. I'm just glad that the call turned out okay, and I can see why the mother and grandmother were so nervous! That little kid was so cute—you should've seen her!"

not like to be touched by strangers or separated from his parents. As with the infant, a good part of the assessment can be done visually while you are taking the history from the parent or caregiver. The alert child will be watching you closely. Listen to heart and lung sounds by pulling up the child's shirt and placing the bell of your stethoscope underneath it, rather than trying to undress the child. Examine the chest before the head. Use a quiet, confident, soothing voice, and allow the child to hold a toy or favorite object while being examined. When using a stethoscope, it may be helpful to first place it on a parent or favorite stuffed animal to show the child that it does not hurt. The alert toddler will not tolerate an oxygen mask well, while the toddler who does not resist the mask may be seriously ill. The toddler may understand injury, illness, or separation from family as punishment, so they need lots of reassurance that they are not to blame and that their parents or caregivers are with them or know where they are.

PRESCHOOLERS (3–6 YEARS)

Preschool children have developed concrete thinking skills that allow them to understand and follow instructions. It is important to ask them for their version of how they feel and what happened. Like toddlers, preschoolers may believe they are being punished for wrongdoing by illness or injury. They are very frightened of potential pain, the sight of blood, and permanent injury. They need lots of reassurance and respond well to simple explanations that avoid medical or complicated terminology. Separation causes them anxiety, so allow the parent or caregiver to hold or sit near the child as you begin your examination. In an effort to build trust, begin your examination with the extremities and then the trunk, followed by the head. The preschooler is typically quite modest, so replace items of clothing after taking them off, or allow the child to help you by pulling up his own shirt or exposing the area of injury.

SCHOOL-AGED CHILDREN (6–12 YEARS)

By the time children reach school age, they have a basic understanding of the body and its functions, and they usually try to cooperate with the physical exam. They are able to communicate and understand more complex ideas. However, they are

Clinical Clues: BEHAVIOR

Pay close attention to the way the child behaves and responds to your presence. A child responding inappropriately to his environment may be seriously ill.

very literal, so avoid using confusing language and be aware that they are listening to every word you say, even if you are not talking to them. School-aged children, just like adults, are aware of and afraid of death and dying as well as pain, deformity, blood, and permanent injury. They benefit from reassurance as well as inclusion in discussions involving their care.

ADOLESCENTS (12–18 YEARS)

The adolescent child has a more thorough understanding of anatomy and physiology and is able to process and express complex ideas. Adolescents are frequent risk takers but are often poor judges of consequence. They are afraid of disfigurement and permanent injury yet often believe they are immortal or indestructible. They want to be treated as adults, but they may need the same level of support and reassurance as a younger child. By speaking to the adolescent respectfully and non-judgmentally, you will improve your ability to obtain an accurate history. Protecting their privacy and modesty will help gain their trust. It may be helpful to interview or examine them away from parents or caregivers.

The Pediatric Airway

The most important focus of prehospital care for infants and children is airway, breathing, and oxygenation. A cardiac event in an infant or child is almost always preceded by an obstructed airway or inadequate respirations.

6-1.2 Describe differences in anatomy and physiology of the infant, child, and adult patient.

ANATOMICAL AND PHYSIOLOGICAL CONCERNS

The head of the child is proportionately larger and heavier relative to its body than that of an adult, and the neck muscles are less developed. Because of these factors, the head of a supine child will likely tilt forward possibly occluding the airway. The tongue is also larger in proportion to the lower jaw than in an adult and often falls back, blocking the airway. The trachea is thinner and more elastic, and can close off more easily with hyperextension of the head. Infants primarily breathe through their noses, which are easily blocked with secretions. Also, the infant and child have a higher respiratory rate and breathe mainly by using their abdominal muscles, which tire quickly when stressed. All of these factors contribute to the difficulty of obtaining and maintaining an adequate airway and breathing in the pediatric patient. Refer to Table 36-2 on page 920.

Assessment of the Pediatric Patient

The initial pediatric assessment triangle involves observing the general appearance, breathing, and circulation (skin signs) of the child (Figure 36-6 on page 920).

6-1.3 Differentiate the response of the ill or injured infant or child (age specific) from that of an adult.

TABLE 36-2	SPECIFIC ANATOMICAL CHARACTERISTICS OF CHILDREN
CHARACTERISTICS	**SIGNIFICANCE**
Infants breathe through their noses.	Secretions can cause airway obstruction.
The head is large in proportion to the body.	When the child is supine the head is flexed forward.
The tongue is large in proportion to the mouth.	The tongue can easily obstruct the airway when the child is supine.
Muscles between the ribs are immature.	Children experiencing respiratory distress tire quickly.
Abdominal breathing is common in children.	Excess gas in the stomach can impede chest expansion.
The trachea is thin and flexible.	The airway is more likely to collapse if the neck is flexed or extended.
Neck muscles are immature.	The head is more likely to flop forward.
The nose does not have much supporting cartilage.	Nasal flaring is an early indicator of respiratory distress.

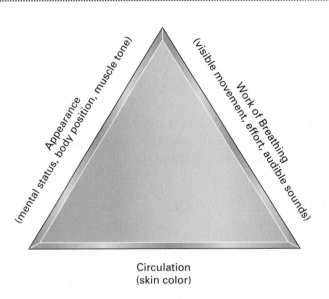

FIGURE 36-6 Pediatric assessment triangle. (American Academy of Pediatrics.)

Observe the child's overall appearance as you approach him. You will get an impression of a well versus a sick child (Table 36-3).

APPEARANCE AND ENVIRONMENT

Observe the general surroundings.

∗ Is the scene safe?

∗ Is there an obvious mechanism of injury?

∗ Is the environment safe for a child?

∗ Is the child active and attentive?

TABLE 36-3 QUICK PEDIATRIC ASSESSMENT CLUES					
APPEARANCE		**WORK OF BREATHING**		**CIRCULATION TO SKIN**	
Assessment	Indication	Assessment	Indication	Assessment	Indication
Does the child make eye contact?	Poor eye contact can indicate respiratory distress, and/or shock.	Is the respiratory rate too fast?	Rapid breathing is a sign of respiratory distress.	Is the skin pink?	Pale or mottled skin can indicate shock.
Is the child afraid of strangers?	Lack of stranger anxiety is unusual in the healthy child.	Are the child's respirations noisy?	Noisy respirations indicate lower or upper respiratory obstruction.	Are the mucous membranes moist and pink?	Pale dry mucous membranes indicate shock.
Can the child hold its head up?	Decreased muscle tone can be the result of respiratory distress and/or shock.	Is the child using accessory muscles to breathe?	Retractions and nasal flaring indicate respiratory distress.	Is the child crying tears?	Absence of tears indicates dehydration, which can lead to shock.

✳ Can the child make eye contact?

✳ Does the child respond to his parent's voice?

WORK OF BREATHING

Look for symmetrical chest movement and note the respiratory rate. Barky or noisy breathing, **stridor,** and grunting sounds during exhalation are signs of increased work of breathing. **Retractions,** caused by immature chest wall muscles, will appear as muscles pulling in between the ribs and above the sternum with inspiration. Infants breathe mainly through their noses, and **nasal flaring** indicates increased respiratory effort. If the child is talking or crying, listen for the quality of those sounds. Observe the color of the skin for paleness or mottling, indicating poor circulation. Is the child consolable or inconsolable? How is he responding to you, the stranger? How is he positioned, and how is his muscle tone?

Begin your hands-on assessment with the chest, listening with the stethoscope for the presence or absence of breath sounds, stridor, and **wheezing.** Determine if the breath sounds are equal on both sides of the chest. Note the quality of a cough, if present, and the amount of secretions in the airway. Remember that respiratory disorders are the primary cause of cardiac arrest in children.

CIRCULATION

Assess **central perfusion** by palpating brachial and femoral pulses. In the smaller child and infant, **peripheral pulses** are more difficult to palpate; if the radial pulse

✳ **stridor**
a harsh high pitched sound that can occur during inhalation or exhalation. Indicative of partial upper airway obstruction.

✳ **retraction**
muscles pulling in between the ribs and above the sternum with inspiration.

✳ **nasal flaring**
the extended opening or flaring of nostrils.

✳ **wheezing**
high-pitched sounds created by air moving through narrowed air passages in the lungs.

✳ **central perfusion**
the supply of oxygen to and removal of wastes from central circulation. May be assessed by palpating brachial and femoral pulses.

> ### Clinical Clues: RETRACTIONS
>
> Expose the child's bare chest to observe for retractions. The presence of retractions is a sign of significant respiratory distress.

✳ **peripheral pulses**

pulses in the distal circulation such as the radial pulse, the pedal pulse found on the top of the foot.

✳ **capillary refill time**

how long it takes for the normal pink color to return after pressing on the fingernail and releasing it. Normally, this takes no more than 2 seconds.

✳ **decompensate**

become unable to compensate for low blood volume or lack of perfusion.

is hard to find, the pedal pulse on the top of the foot is usually easier to feel. Assess **capillary refill time** by squeezing the forearm or kneecap or end of a finger, fingernail, or toe until the nail bed blanches. Expect the capillary fill time to be less than 2 seconds centrally and peripherally in the well child. Any delay indicates poor perfusion. At this time, you can also assess the skin temperature, color, and moisture.

Blood pressures are often difficult to obtain in children under the age of 3, especially if the child is fussy or crying. Your assessment of circulation will need to rely on the mental status, the quality of pulses, and capillary refill. In children over 3, be sure to use the right size blood pressure cuff for the patient. It should cover two-thirds of the upper arm. Be aware of variations of vital signs with age in the pediatric and infant population. It is very important to realize that children can compensate for poor respirations and circulation, and vital signs may remain normal until they suddenly **decompensate** and deteriorate very quickly.

✳ Stop, Review, Remember!

Multiple Choice

Place a check next to the correct answer.

1. When examining a toddler, start with the:

_____ a. head.

_____ b. feet.

_____ c. arms.

_____ d. eyes.

2. When examining the adolescent, it is important to:

_____ a. respect his privacy.

_____ b. include parents in all aspects of the exam.

_____ c. question his ability to tell the truth.

_____ d. expect him to behave like an adult.

3. Initial assessment of the pediatric patient includes:

_____ a. appearance.

_____ b. work of breathing.

_____ c. circulation to skin.

_____ d. all of the above.

4. If you have trouble listening to respiratory sounds because the child is talking or crying, you should:

_____ a. tell the child to be quiet.

_____ b. tell the parent to quiet the child.

_____ c. try distracting the child with a favorite toy or sound.

_____ d. place the child on your gurney, away from caregivers.

5. Children experiencing respiratory distress tire easily because they:

_____ a. eat less.

_____ b. use their abdominal muscles to breathe.

_____ c. do not sleep well.

_____ d. have a more rigid trachea.

Fill in the Blank

1. The most important focus of prehospital care for infants and children is on _____, _____, and oxygenation.

2. Any child showing signs of respiratory distress, respiratory failure, or shock should receive _____.

3. Assess _____ by palpating the brachial and femoral pulses.

4. A child's vital signs may remain within normal limits until he _____ and deteriorates very quickly.

Critical Thinking

1. At what age would you expect a pediatric patient to be able to give a reliable history?

_____

_____

_____

_____

2. How can you assess the level of responsiveness and respiratory status of an infant before you begin a hands-on exam? Of an 8-year-old?

_____

_____

_____

_____

3. How is the pediatric airway different from the adult airway?

_____

_____

_____

_____

✳ **respiratory distress**

an abnormal physiologic process (airway obstruction, asthma, shock) that prevents adequate gas exchange.

✳ **compensates**

makes up for a deficiency; maintains perfusion while developing shock.

✳ **respiratory failure**

the inability of respirations to maintain adequate oxygenation and ventilation.

✳ **respiratory arrest**

the absence of breathing.

✳ **cyanosis**

a blue or gray color resulting from lack of oxygen in the body.

Common Problems in Infants and Children

RESPIRATORY EMERGENCIES

Respiratory illness is common among pediatric patients. The most common cause of respiratory distress among these patients is asthma, but other causes include chronic lung disease, airway obstruction, congenital heart disease, foreign body aspiration, and chest wall trauma. *The most frequent cause of cardiac arrest in children, other than trauma, is respiratory failure.* Early identification of respiratory distress and prompt treatment can avert decompensation, respiratory failure, and arrest.

Respiratory distress occurs in the child experiencing an abnormal physiologic process (airway obstruction, asthma, shock) that prevents adequate gas exchange. The child will show signs of increased work of breathing. The increased work of breathing **compensates** for the inadequate gas exchange. However, as the child becomes fatigued, respiratory distress will decompensate very quickly to respiratory failure. See Table 36-4.

Respiratory failure occurs when the child can no longer maintain adequate oxygenation and ventilation. This may be because of exhausted chest wall muscles or from failure of the central respiratory drive, as seen in head injury and coma. Successful intervention before respiratory distress proceeds to respiratory failure prevents respiratory arrest.

Respiratory arrest is the absence of breathing. If adequate ventilation and oxygenation are not restored, respiratory arrest will rapidly progress to full cardiopulmonary arrest. Survival rates following a full cardiac arrest in children are very low.

It is very important to differentiate between respiratory distress caused by airway disease and distress caused by airway obstruction, because the management priorities are different. The patient with upper airway obstruction, may have stridor on inspiration or, in the case of complete obstruction, no crying, no speaking, no coughing, and **cyanosis.** The patient with lower airway disease may have wheezing and prolonged, labored exhalations with a rapid respiratory rate and no stridor. Actions taken to clear an obstructed airway could be very harmful to a child with respiratory disease.

The child experiencing respiratory distress will be breathing rapidly and have increased work of breathing. The child may have obvious retractions in the chest wall and above the sternum, or, in younger children, may be using the diaphragm to assist chest expansion. The skin is still pink, and the child is alert but not ac-

---

TABLE 36-4   SIGNS OF RESPIRATORY DISTRESS IN CHILDREN

* Altered mental status
* Flared nostrils
* Pale or cyanotic lips or mouth
* Noisy respirations (stridor, grunting, gasping, wheezing)
* Respiratory rate greater than 60
* Retractions
* Use of abdominal muscles for breathing (see-saw breathing)
* Poor peripheral perfusion
* Decreased heart rate

tive. The child may have assumed a position that best supports his respiratory efforts, such as the tripod position (leaning forward, hand on knees) or the sniffing position (chin raised or thrust forward).

As respiratory distress progresses to respiratory failure, the child will have a decreased mental status and seem distant, making poor eye contact with parents or caregivers and not responding to voice. The child will become pale, cyanotic, and floppy, with a delayed capillary fill time and weak pulses. You may hear audible grunting with exhalation. The infant may have a pronounced head bobbing with respiration. The child will appear visibly fatigued. Without immediate intervention, this child will progress to an inadequate respiratory rate of less than ten, he will become unresponsive and limp, and his heart rate will begin to decrease to bradycardia and eventually cardiac arrest.

Clinical Clues: "FROM THE DOOR"

It is said you can assess a pediatric patient "from the door" as you approach. Observe whether the child is active or limp, how he responds to parents and strangers, or has an increased work of breathing. The patient's color can tell you that he is unstable before you get to him. If you see signs the pediatric patient is unstable, prepare to provide aggressive airway care, oxygenation, transport promptly, and call ALS if available.

AIRWAY MANAGEMENT

The first priority of airway management is maintaining an open airway. For infants and children, the head-tilt chin lift method is modified slightly. The airway must be neutrally aligned, avoiding **hyperextension** or **flexion** of the neck. This can be maintained by placing a small folded towel under the patient's shoulders. As the age of the child increases, slight extension of the neck may be helpful. Note the difference in the child's position with and without the towel in Figures 36-7A and B.

If there are secretions or vomit in the airway, the patient needs to be suctioned. A flexible bulb-type suction device is preferred when suctioning the nose and mouth of an infant. To suction, deflate the bulb prior to inserting it into the infant's nose. Once inserted, release the bulb to initiate gentle suction. For larger children, use a thin flexible plastic catheter to suction thin secretions, inserting it just inside the **nares**. A large-bore rigid plastic catheter is better for removing thick

∗ **hyperextension**

extreme or abnormal extension or increase in the angle between bones of a joint; tilting the head backward.

∗ **flexion**

decrease in the angle between the bones forming a joint; tilting the head forward.

∗ **nares**

external openings in the nasal cavity; nostrils.

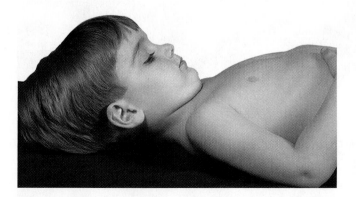

FIGURE 36-7A   When an infant or young child is supine, the head will tip forward, obstructing the airway.

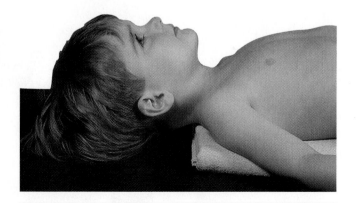

FIGURE 36-7B   To keep the airway aligned, place a folded towel under the shoulders.

FIGURE 36-8 A toddler being held by his caregiver.

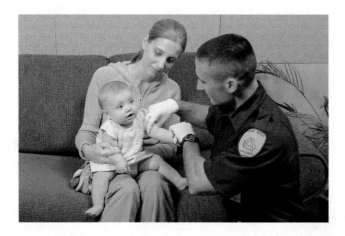

6-1.6 List the steps in the management of foreign body airway obstruction.

* **blow-by technique**

    providing supplemental oxygen by holding the mask or tubing near the child's face if he cannot tolerate wearing a mask.

secretions such as vomit. Administer 100 percent oxygen prior to suctioning, and do not suction for more than 5 seconds at one time to avoid further respiratory compromise. Do not allow the suctioning device to touch the back of the throat, as this can slow the heart rate and cause soft-tissue trauma.

When the airway becomes partially obstructed by foreign material or secretions, some air can move past the obstruction, making respirations noisy. The child may also demonstrate increased work of breathing, including retractions around the ribs and sternum, but still be alert with pink mucous membranes and good peripheral perfusion. This child should be allowed to assume a position of comfort, which will likely be sitting up. Try not to upset the child, as anxiety and crying can worsen the airway obstruction. Allow the child to sit with a parent or care provider (Figure 36-8). Provide oxygen therapy via a nonrebreather mask or via the **blow-by technique.** (Figure 36-9).When possible allow the parent or caregiver to hold the oxygen device (Figure 36-10).

FIGURE 36-9 Oxygen delivered to an infant by the blow-by method. Pushing the oxygen tubing through the bottom of a paper cup is less frightening than using a mask.

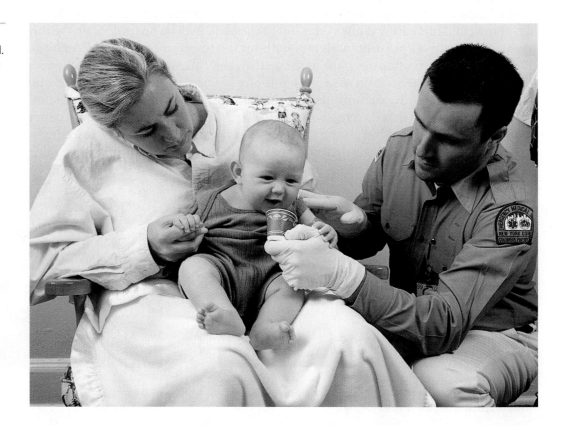

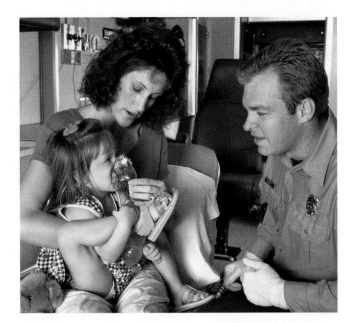

FIGURE 36-10   If possible, let a young child sit in the parent's lap during assessment and care. (During transport, the child should be in a car seat, secured to a stretcher, or immobilized to a back board.)

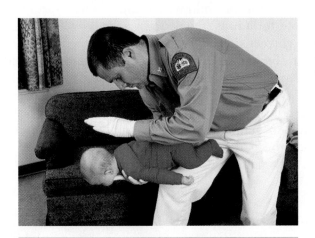

FIGURE 36-11A   For complete airway obstruction in an infant, alternate back slaps shown here with chest thrusts.

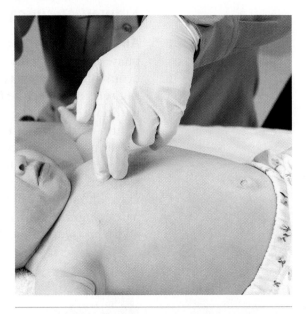

FIGURE 36-11B   The back slaps are alternated with chest thrusts shown here, five times each until the object is cleared.

In the event of partial or complete obstruction of the airway with absence of speaking or crying, ineffective cough, altered mental status and/or respiratory arrest, the obstruction must be removed. If, after opening the airway with the tongue-jaw lift, ventilation is ineffective or impossible, you must perform airway clearance techniques.

In children less than one year this is done by delivering five back slaps followed by five chest thrusts. If a foreign object is visible, a finger sweep may be used to remove it, but do not perform blind finger sweeps as this could force an object further into the airway. The back slaps are alternated with the chest thrusts, five times each, until the object is cleared (Figures 36-11A and B).

For children ages one year to adolescence, open the airway, position properly, and attempt to ventilate. Do not perform blind finger sweeps. Perform abdominal thrusts as you would on an adult.

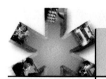

Perspective

Aaron—The EMT

"Man, that was a tiny baby! I've seen preemies before when we transfer them from the helicopter to the ED and they're in those big traveling incubators. I've never seen one out of the medical setting. That mom and grandmother must have been so scared. Heck, I was scared. I don't think that any of our neonate equipment would have even fit that kid. Well, as my EMT teacher used to say, we would have had to 'improvise, adapt, and overcome.' Working on an ambulance makes you good at that, though!"

AIRWAY ADJUNCTS

An oral or nasal airway helps maintain an open airway in the child that has adequate respiratory drive but is unable to maintain his own airway. As in adults, an oropharyngeal airway (OPA) is used for the child who is unresponsive and has no gag reflex. Unlike the method used for adults, the pediatric oral airway is inserted without rotation. To choose the correct size OPA, measure from the corner of the mouth to the tip of the ear lobe (Figure 36-12). A tongue depressor inserted to the back of the tongue with downward pressure may be used to control the tongue while inserting the airway. The nasopharyngeal airway (NPA), or nasal trumpet, may be used in the responsive child who cannot maintain an open airway. Choose an NPA whose lumen diameter is slightly smaller than the child's nares (Figure 36-13). The child who is developmentally appropriate for his age and who tolerates an NPA is a very sick child.

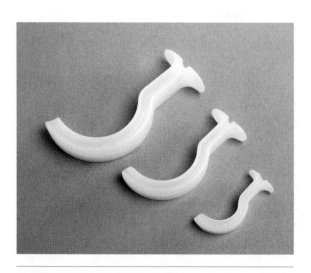

FIGURE 36-12 Oropharyngeal airways come in a variety of sizes.

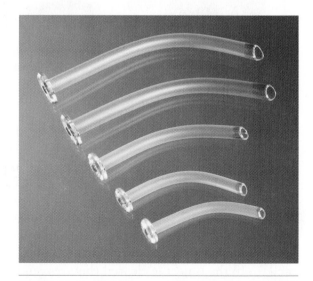

FIGURE 36-13 Nasopharyngeal airways come in a variety of sizes.

Follow these steps for insertion of an OPA:

1. Take appropriate BSI precautions.

2. Measure the airway for the appropriate size (corner of mouth to tip of earlobe).

3. Using a tongue depressor or similar tool, place downward pressure on the tongue while directly inserting the airway.

4. Make certain that the flange of the airway remains visible outside the patient's lips.

Follow these steps for insertion of an NPA:

1. Take appropriate BSI precautions.

2. Measure the airway for the appropriate size (nostril to the **tragus**). Also confirm that the diameter is appropriate.

3. Lubricate the airway before gently inserting it into the child's nose.

4. Make certain that the flange of the airway remains visible outside the patient's nose.

Remember that NPAs should not be used if the patient has sustained severe facial trauma.

* **tragus**
the projection of skin-covered cartilage in front of the meatus of the external ear.

OXYGEN THERAPY

Oxygen starvation, or hypoxia, can quickly lead to a slowed heart rate (bradycardia) and/or altered mental status in the infant or pediatric patient. Any infant or child showing signs of respiratory distress, or who has inadequate respirations, or who is showing signs of shock, should receive high-concentration oxygen. Any infant or child with bradycardia should also receive high-concentration oxygen. This can be delivered via nasal cannula, a nonrebreather mask, or using the blow-by technique.

The nasal cannula should be used when the child will not tolerate a mask. Remember that infants breathe primarily through their noses. Placing a nasal cannula without oxygen flowing will severely restrict the flow of air breathed in by the patient. Oxygen should be administered at 2 to 4 liters per minute through the nasal cannula (Figure 36-14 on page 930).

The nonrebreather mask provides a higher concentration of oxygen than the cannula. It should be used for the infant or child showing signs of respiratory distress, if he will tolerate it. Oxygen should be administered at 10 to 15 liters per minute. Unfortunately, most babies and young children are afraid or intolerant of the mask. As noted earlier, these patients can receive oxygen via the blow-by technique. Use oxygen tubing and hold the end of the tubing close to the patient's face (about two inches) or disguise the end of the tubing with a favorite toy or by running it through the bottom of a paper cup. Have the caregiver or parent hold the object and follow the face as it turns so the child gets as much oxygen as possible.

If the patient is receiving high-concentration oxygen and remains cyanotic with an altered mental status, remains limp or floppy, or has inadequate respiratory rate, you will need to begin assisted ventilations.

FIGURE 36-14 A nasal cannula in place on a pediatric patient.

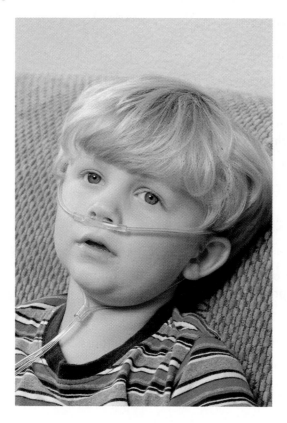

ASSISTED VENTILATIONS

The presence of cyanosis, altered mental status, severe respiratory distress, respiratory failure, or arrest in an infant or child means that assisted (artificial) ventilation is required. Remember, prior to beginning ventilations for infants and children, to make sure the airway remains in a neutral position by not flexing or hyperextending the neck. Choose a mask for the patient that will seal well over the mouth and nose. Use a pediatric-sized resuscitation bag for smaller children (less than 8 years of age) to avoid overinflating the lungs. If the patient is a victim of trauma, maintain cervical spine precautions while opening the airway with the modified jaw-thrust maneuver.

One or two hands may be used to maintain an airtight seal of the mask on the child's face (Figure 36-15). Using two hands will seal the mask more tightly but requires a second person to deliver ventilations. The one-hand technique can be used by a single rescuer. In either case, avoid pressing on the neck with your fingers, which can occlude the airway. Squeeze the bag-valve device slowly and evenly over 1 second so the chest rises adequately, but avoid hyperinflation. The best rate of ventilation for infants and children is 12 to 20 per minute. Whenever possible, use a bag-valve device with a reservoir that can be attached to 100 percent oxygen.

You can also deliver ventilations via a pocket face mask with a one-way valve. Maintain a good seal with the mask and use enough air to make the chest rise adequately.

6-1.8 Identify the signs and symptoms of shock (hypoperfusion) in the infant and child patient.

6-1.9 Describe the methods of determining end organ perfusion in the infant and child patient.

SHOCK

Some of the common causes of shock or hypoperfusion in children are vomiting and diarrhea, infection, trauma, and blood loss. Less often, shock may be caused by allergic reactions or poisoning. In infants and children the presence of shock is very

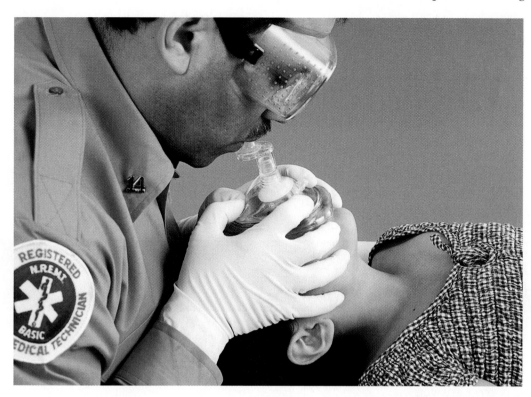

FIGURE 36-15   Proper hand placement for optimal mask seal.

rarely cardiac in origin. Rarely, you may encounter children born with congenital and/or chronic heart disease who present with the signs and symptoms of shock.

The signs and symptoms of shock in infants and children are similar to those of adults (Table 36-5). Some of the most important questions to ask the caregiver of the very young child or infant are whether the child has had vomiting or diarrhea and how frequently they have changed wet diapers. In the early stages of shock, the child becomes inactive and floppy. The child may have no tears with crying and appear pale. As shock progresses, the child's mental status further deteriorates. The skin becomes cool and clammy, and it may be pale, ashen, or mottled. The child has a rapid heart rate, peripheral pulses are difficult to palpate and may be absent, and capillary refill is delayed.

The child who has deteriorated to late shock is a very sick child and needs to be transported immediately. Children compensate in the early stages of shock by

TABLE 36-5   SIGNS AND SYMPTOMS OF SHOCK
* Rapid heart rate
* Rapid respiratory rate
* Cool extremities
* Pale skin, dry mucous membranes
* Delayed capillary fill time
* Weak central pulse
* Weak or absent distal pulse
* Decreased response to environment
* "Floppy" muscle tone

maintaining their heart rate and blood pressure. If shock is allowed to progress without intervention, they deteriorate very quickly.

EMERGENCY MEDICAL CARE

If you suspect shock in an infant or child, expedite transport or consider an ALS backup. Do not delay to complete a detailed physical exam on scene, but complete it in route. Control any obvious bleeding. Deliver high concentration oxygen by nonrebreather mask (not resisting the oxygen mask can be an ominous sign), and be prepared to assist respirations. Keep the patient warm by turning up the heat in the ambulance and using blankets. Elevating the legs may help to perfuse the vital organs of head and chest.

 # Stop, Review, Remember!

Multiple Choice

Place a check next to the correct answer.

1. The first priority of care for the child in respiratory distress is:

_____ a. 100 percent oxygen via nonrebreather mask or blow-by technique.

_____ b. oxygen via nasal cannula.

_____ c. removing the child from the caregiver.

_____ d. keeping the child cool.

2. Signs of shock in an infant or child include:

_____ a. increased respiratory rate.

_____ b. increased heart rate.

_____ c. decreased responsiveness.

_____ d. all of the above.

3. It is important to keep infants and children warm because:

_____ a. they wear less clothing.

_____ b. hypothermia can lead to decreased blood sugar.

_____ c. they lose most of their heat through their heads.

_____ d. they will feel more comfortable.

4. Which child is in shock?

_____ a. the child who clings to her mother and cries tears

_____ b. the child with a high fever who is sucking on his bottle

_____ c. the child who is limp and pale with mottled extremities

_____ d. the screaming child with a laceration to the forehead

5. The nasal cannula should be used when:

_____ a. the blow-by technique is used.

_____ b. a non-rebreather mask is not available.

_____ c. the pediatric patient will not tolerate a mask.

_____ d. the pediatric patient will not breathe through his mouth.

Critical Thinking

1. How can you assess the respiratory rate of a crying child?

   _____

   _____

   _____

   _____

2. What kind of distracting techniques could you use to calm the crying child in order to assess breath sounds?

   _____

   _____

   _____

   _____

3. Determine the best mode of oxygen delivery for each of these patients:

   a. the alert 1-month-old with retractions but good perfusion

   _____

   _____

   _____

   b. the wheezing 8-year-old who can only speak in short sentences

   _____

   _____

   _____

   c. the 6-year-old who fell out of a tree and is not breathing, after the airway is opened while the spine is immobilized

   _____

   _____

   _____

   d. the quiet toddler with decreased lung sounds, fever, and coughing

   _____

   _____

   _____

Trauma

6-1.13 Differentiate between the injury patterns in adults, infants, and children.

6-1.14 Discuss the field management of the infant and child trauma patient.

Traumatic injury is the number one cause of death for infants and children. Most of these fatal injuries are the result of blunt trauma. Motor vehicle crashes are the most common cause of blunt trauma in children. Some aspects of motor vehicle crashes are different for infants and children than they are for adults. The child is always a passenger who may or may not be restrained. The unrestrained child will most likely sustain head and/or neck injuries because of the relative heaviness of the head and weakness of the neck muscles. The restrained child may sustain injury to the abdomen and lower spine, because the abdominal wall is still undeveloped and the musculature is relatively weak compared to adults.

Another common cause of traumatic injury in children is motor vehicle versus bicycle, resulting in head, spine, and abdominal injuries for the same reasons as just mentioned (Figure 36-16). Children may be unaware of traffic and are difficult to see because of their size, resulting in pedestrian versus vehicle incidents. Classically, the bumper of the car will impact the abdomen or upper legs, and then the child will be thrown to land on the head. In toddlers, the bumper will likely impact the head or neck area. Abdominal, head, upper leg, and pelvic injuries occur frequently in this scenario.

Other causes of traumatic injury in infants and children include falls from a significant height or diving into shallow water, burns, sports injuries, and child abuse.

HEAD INJURIES

Care of the child who has sustained a head injury starts with securing an open airway using the modified jaw-thrust maneuver. The most common cause of hypoxia in the head-injured patient is the tongue obstructing the airway, which is why the modified jaw-thrust maneuver is critically important. Injury to the head may result in respiratory failure and arrest that may be delayed and occur during transport. Nausea and vomiting are the most common signs of head injury. If the child has sustained significant blunt force to the head, other injuries are often present, including internal injuries that may result in shock (hypoperfusion). Secondary injuries should always be considered in the child presenting with head injury and

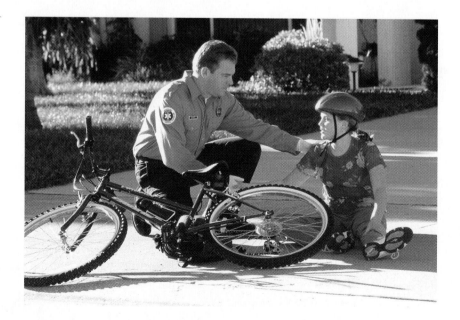

FIGURE 36-16 Bicycles are a common cause of injury in the child.

shock. Remember not to use sandbags to stabilize the head of the infant or child, because the weight can cause further damage, especially if the backboard needs to be rolled if the child vomits.

CHEST INJURIES

The ribs of children are less developed and more pliable, meaning they can bend farther than adults' ribs before breaking. Because of this, there may be significant internal injury without obvious external signs, such as abdominal bruising.

ABDOMINAL INJURIES

Abdominal injuries are more common in infants and children than in adults. The abdominal muscles of infants and children are weaker than in adults, and the internal abdominal organs are less securely anchored. It may be very difficult to detect abdominal injury, especially in the crying child, but abdominal injury must be suspected in the trauma patient who is deteriorating without outward signs of injury.

It is important to remember that air can accumulate in the stomach during assisted ventilations, and a large amount of air may make it more difficult for the child to breathe or may interfere with assisted artificial ventilations.

INJURIES TO THE EXTREMITIES

While isolated limb injuries may occur more frequently in the pediatric population, they are rarely life threatening and are managed in the same manner as for adults.

Some EMS agencies use the pneumatic antishock garment (PASG) to improve perfusion in the event of very low blood pressure and pelvic instability. Use of the pneumatic antishock garment, also known as military antishock trousers (MAST), is *prohibited* in the infant and young child. It may be possible to use the device if it fits the child, but do not inflate the abdominal compartment, which could interfere with breathing. Check with medical direction.

BURN INJURIES

The burn patient of any age is always at risk for hypothermia because of impaired skin integrity and exposure. Be sure to keep these patients warm. Body surface assessment in children and infants with burns is slightly different because of their relatively large head and chest. Burns should be covered with sterile gauze or a sterile sheet, preferably a nonsticking burn sheet. Candidates for burn centers should be identified according to local protocol.

EMERGENCY MEDICAL CARE

As with every patient, the traumatically injured infant or child requires a patent, well-positioned airway. Open the airway using the modified jaw-thrust maneuver while maintaining cervical spine immobilization. Be prepared to assist in protecting the airway by suctioning. Provide oxygen and use the bag-valve mask to assist ventilations in the patient experiencing respiratory distress, respiratory failure, or respiratory arrest. Secure the patient to a backboard for spinal immobilization. Transport immediately to the most appropriate facility.

Other Pediatric Emergencies

HYPOTHERMIA

The pediatric patient has more body-surface exposure relative to mass than an adult. Infants lack the kind of fat the adult body uses for insulation. Infants and children have smaller stores of glucose in their bodies. Because of these differences, these patients are more affected by environmental conditions, especially cold. Hypothermia decreases perfusion and increases glucose consumption, resulting in decreased blood sugar. It is always important to keep these patients warm (Figure 36-17).

Emergency Medical Care For infants, much of their heat is lost through the head, so using a cap or a blanket around the top of the head will help keep the patient warm. Exposing patient assessment areas such as the chest or a limb one at a time and replacing clothing or covering before exposing another area can also conserve heat. In the ambulance, turning the heater on will improve ambient temperatures. The child with a fever should not be exposed to aggressive cooling techniques that will cause further physiologic stress and increased glucose consumption.

SEIZURES

6-1.11 List the common causes of seizures in the infant and child patient.

Seizures may be caused by infections, poisoning, hypoglycemia, hypoxia, or head trauma. By far the most common cause of seizures in infants and children is a sudden rise in core temperature associated with a viral illness. These are commonly referred to as febrile seizures. Many children suffer from chronic seizure disorders controlled by medications that need to be constantly adjusted as they grow. When these children have seizures, it is rarely life threatening. Nonetheless, seizures in children, including febrile seizures, and seizures in the chronic seizure patient should be taken seriously by the EMT. The seizure will usually be over by the time the EMT arrives, and the patient may show typical postseizure signs, such as decreased respiratory rate and unresponsiveness.

As you approach the patient, ask the caregiver how many seizures the child has had, how long they lasted, and what part of the body, if any, was convulsing. Ask the caregiver if the child has a recent history of a fever or chronic seizure disorder and what medication the child takes. Assess the child for the presence of injuries that may have occurred during a seizure.

6-1.12 Describe the management of seizures in the infant and child patient.

Emergency Medical Care Treatment of the seizure patient is similar in adults and children: Maintain a patent airway, protect the cervical spine as necessary, provide oxygen

FIGURE 36-17 Proper warming of an infant to prevent hypothermia.

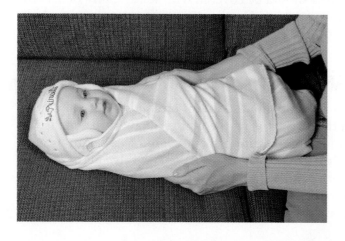

and, if needed, provide assisted ventilations. Be prepared with suction in case the child vomits. All infants and children who have had a seizure with no prior history require medical evaluation and should be transported to an appropriate facility.

ALTERED MENTAL STATUS

Many conditions, including hypoglycemia, poisoning, postseizure, infection, head trauma, hypoxia, shock, and fatigue can result in an altered mental status in the infant or child. It is very important to try to discover the underlying cause; however, this should not delay the prompt delivery of appropriate care.

Emergency Medical Care   Maintain a patent airway, be prepared to suction and provide assisted ventilations, and transport any infant or child presenting with an altered mental status.

POISONING

Accidental ingestion is a common reason for ambulance calls for infants and children (Figure 36-18). Children are notoriously poor historians, but you may be able to discover the suspected substance and its container, which you should try to bring to the receiving facility.

   If the patient is responsive, contact medical direction. You should administer oxygen and transport while continuing to observe the patient closely for changes. If the patient is unresponsive, maintain a patent airway, provide oxygen, be prepared to suction and provide assisted ventilations, and attempt to rule out the possibility of trauma.

Emergency Medical Care   Contact medical direction and transport.

FEVER

Another common reason for ambulance calls in the infant and pediatric population is complaint of fever. This is very seldom life threatening in and of itself, although the underlying disease process causing the fever could be serious, as in the case of meningitis, which presents as fever and a rash. Most often, the underlying cause is infectious. The numerical value of the child's temperature does not reflect the severity of the disease process.

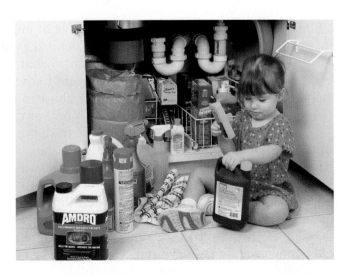

FIGURE 36-18 Poisoning is the number one cause of accidental death among children.

Emergency Medical Care   Transport and be alert for seizures, especially in those patients under 4 years of age.

NEAR DROWNING

Near drowning is defined as a submersion resulting in respiratory or cardiac arrest that has responded to resuscitative efforts. Near-drowning incidents involving children most commonly involve prolonged submersion in the bathtub or swimming pool. Neck and head trauma from falling or diving may be a factor in some near drownings. In older children and adolescents, alcohol ingestion may have contributed to the incident. The child may be in severe distress or pulseless and apneic. The child may have swallowed a lot of water and may vomit during assisted ventilations. Some children may present in moderate respiratory distress after a brief period of submersion or may have a period of breathing followed by **apnea.** These patients may become the victims of **secondary drowning syndrome,** which can occur minutes to hours after the event because of compromised lung tissue.

Emergency Medical Care   All children who have experienced submersion should be transported to a hospital. Providing artificially assisted ventilation in children with absent or inadequate breathing is the first priority. Maintain cervical spine immobilization at all times. Provide supplemental oxygen to patients with adequate breathing. Be prepared to suction to protect the airway. Keep the child warm.

SUDDEN INFANT DEATH SYNDROME

The sudden death of healthy infants in the first year of life is called **sudden infant death syndrome (SIDS).** While there are many theories, the causes of this syndrome are poorly understood. The infant is often discovered in the morning, or after an ordinary nap period, by the caregiver. The infant is apneic when found. The caregiver is often hysterical from extreme emotional distress, guilt, and remorse. (It is never appropriate to suggest neglect or blame to the caregiver.)

Emergency Medical Care   Unless the child is stiff with **rigor mortis** or shows **morbid lividity** (the pooling of blood in the lower parts of the body after death), you must provide CPR. Maintain the airway, assist ventilations, and transport rapidly to the nearest hospital.

Child Abuse and Neglect

Child abuse is defined as the use of excessive or improper action so as to cause injury or harm to a child. Child neglect is defined as failing to give sufficient attention or respect to a child that has claim to that attention. Being aware of the conditions of neglect and abuse is important to the EMT, who should learn to develop an **index of suspicion** of neglect or abuse in the presence of certain signs or symptoms during the assessment of the infant or child.

Signs and symptoms of abuse include fresh burns or bruises in multiple stages of healing. Infants who have been violently shaken (shaken baby syndrome) may have a high-pitched cry or be unresponsive because of undetected brain injury. The story describing the mechanism of injury may not match with the injuries themselves, and different caregivers may tell different stories. There may have been many previous requests for emergency response from the same address. Caregivers may appear unconcerned or otherwise behave inappropriately. The child who is old enough to talk may avoid discussing how the injury occurred.

＊ **apnea**

absence of breathing.

＊ **secondary drowning syndrome**

respiratory distress or apnea that can occur minutes to hours after a near-drowning event because of compromised lung tissue.

＊ **sudden infant death syndrome (SIDS)**

the sudden death of healthy infants in the first year of life.

＊ **rigor mortis**

body stiffness or rigidity that occurs in dead bodies.

＊ **morbid lividity**

pooling of blood in the lower parts of the body after death.

6-1.15 Summarize the indicators of possible child abuse and neglect.

6-1.16 Describe the medical legal responsibilities in suspected child abuse.

＊ **index of suspicion**

awareness that there may be injuries, abuse, or neglect.

Signs and symptoms of neglect often are less obvious. There may be an apparent lack of adult supervision of the infant or child. The living environment may be unsafe. The infant or child may appear malnourished. Children with chronic illnesses such as diabetes or asthma may have no medication.

Do not delay transport to accuse or confront a suspected negligent or abusive caregiver. Be sure to alert the receiving facility of your suspicions and provide them with objective information. State laws require reporting suspected abuse or neglect, and the EMT should be familiar with local regulations. Remember to report objectively, identifying specific things you saw or heard, not what you think might have happened.

Infants and Children with Special Needs

Advances in medical technology have allowed many infants and children with different types of chronic disease not only to survive but to live at home. Often these patients are dependent on specific supportive equipment, including tracheostomies, ventilators, central intravenous lines, feeding tubes and pumps, or cerebral spinal fluid shunts. It is important to be aware of basic complications that may occur with these devices. Always include the caregiver of the chronically ill infant or child in your assessment and care of the patient. The caregiver will be familiar with the patient's unique medical needs, medications, and devices.

Tracheostomy tubes come in a variety of types and are usually secured around the neck with twill tape (Figure 36-19). The caregiver will know the type and size.

* **tracheostomy tube**
   tube placed through a surgical opening in the neck to provide an airway.

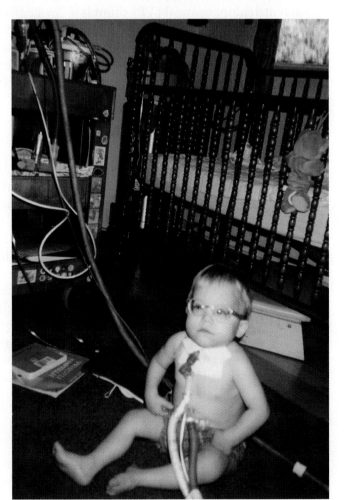

FIGURE 36-19   Children who have complicated medical problems are often dependent on various technologies. (Family Voices.)

The tube may become obstructed, dislodged, or infected. Other complications include bleeding or air leaking around the cuff of a cuffed tracheostomy tube. Emergency medical care includes maintaining an open airway, providing oxygen, and suctioning as needed to improve respiratory effort. Transport the patient in a position of comfort to minimize stress.

* **home ventilator**

  a mechanical device that moves air in and out of the lungs.

Home ventilators also come in a wide variety of types. The caregiver will be familiar with operating the device. Emergency care includes ensuring that the airway is open and that the ventilator is providing adequate ventilations, or providing assisted ventilations via bag-valve tube in the event of ventilator failure. Transport the ventilator with the patient.

* **central venous line**

  intravenous catheter placed close to the heart for long-term fluid or medication administration.

Central venous lines are intravenous catheters placed close to the heart for long-term fluid or medication administration. Complications of these lines include cracking or leaking of the line, clotting of the line, bleeding from the line or from around it, or infection at the insertion site and along the line. Emergency medical care includes applying pressure to stop bleeding, if present, and transporting the patient.

* **gastrostomy tube (G-Tube)**

  tube placed directly into the stomach or upper small intestine through the abdominal wall to provide nutrition to a patient who cannot eat or swallow.

Gastrostomy tubes (G-Tubes) are placed directly into the stomach or upper small intestine through the abdominal wall to provide nutrition to those patients who cannot eat or swallow. These tubes come in many shapes and sizes. They can become dislodged or infected. Patients with feeding tubes are at risk for vomiting and aspiration or the inhaling of gastric contents. Emergency medical care includes maintaining the airway, providing oxygen, suctioning as necessary, and transporting with the head up and lying on the right side, if possible, to minimize further risk of aspiration.

* **ventriculoperitoneal (VP) shunt**

  a device that drains excess cerebral spinal fluid from the brain to the abdomen.

A **ventriculoperitoneal (VP) shunt** is a device that drains excess cerebral spinal fluid from the brain to the abdomen. The shunt line is often visible or palpable on the side of the skull. Shunts may become occluded or infected. Emergency medical care: These patients may present with an altered mental status and it is important to remember that they are prone to respiratory arrest. Maintain and manage the airway, be sure assisted ventilations are adequate for oxygenation, and transport.

Family Response

Care of the infant or child does not occur in isolation from the family, and the family or caregivers may feel anxious, helpless, and afraid for the well-being of the child. They may react to the EMTs with anger or hysteria. If the caregiver is anxious and upset, the infant or child is more likely to respond in the same way. Calm, supportive interaction with the family will often improve interactions with the patient. Allowing parents or caregivers to remain with the child unless the child is unaware or seriously unstable will increase trust and feelings of usefulness. The parent or caregiver should be instructed to calm the child. He can assist in maintaining a position of comfort for the child or by holding the blow-by oxygen. Most parents have no medical training, but they are the experts on what is normal or abnormal for their child, and they know best what will be calming and comforting to their child. Listen to their concerns and explain your interventions.

Provider Response

6-1.17 Recognize need for EMT-Basic debriefing following a difficult infant or child transport.

Many emergency medical care providers are intimidated by their perceived or actual lack of experience in the care of infants and children. They may be intimidated by a fear of failure or distracted and distressed by identifying the patient with a

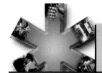

Perspective

The Mother

"It was the apnea alarm on the portable monitor that actually woke us up. And when I saw that Adrianna was struggling to breathe, I just panicked and called 9-1-1! The nurse had given us so many directions when we left the hospital that I just couldn't remember what to do, so I just picked her up and she vomited and started crying. I did remember that crying was good, since it meant that she was breathing again. I'm so angry and scared right now. I really wanted Adrianna to stay in the hospital like her twin sister Alexis did. I just shudder when I think of what might have happened if that monitor alarm didn't wake me or my mom up. What a nightmare. I just want my babies to be healthy and at home with me and Mike."

child of their own. However, emergency medical skills can be learned and applied to children. Much of what the provider learns about adults can be applied to children, but it is important to remember the differences. Exposure to the care of children in all settings, getting as much practice as possible with assessing the infant and child, and becoming familiar with the equipment used in their care, will improve provider confidence.

Stop, Review, Remember!

Multiple Choice

Place a check next to the correct answer.

1. In the case of accidental ingestion and your pediatric patient is responsive, provide all of the following care EXCEPT:

   _____ a. maintain a patient airway.

   _____ b. provide activated charcoal.

   _____ c. contact medical direction.

   _____ d. be prepared to suction.

2. When assisting the child who has experienced a near-drowning incident:

   _____ a. roll him to the rescue position.

   _____ b. always maintain cervical spine immobilization.

   _____ c. raise his feet on towels.

   _____ d. perform the Heimlich maneuver.

3. Which child is mostly likely to be suffering from abuse or neglect?

_____ a. the school child who develops lice

_____ b. the withdrawn, emaciated child

_____ c. the ventilator-dependent, chronically ill child

_____ d. the child from a poor neighborhood

4. The best way to interact with the infant or child's caregiver is to:

_____ a. gently take the child away to be examined.

_____ b. ask him to step outside while you examine the young child.

_____ c. listen carefully to what he thinks is wrong.

_____ d. ask him to write down his questions.

Fill in the Blank

1. A child with a rapid heart rate and respiratory rate with decreased responsiveness could be in _____.

2. The _____ is the most common cause of airway obstruction in the head-injured child.

3. First priority care of the traumatically injured child includes maintaining an open _____ while also maintaining cervical spine.

4. A rapid rise in core temperature could result in a _____ seizure.

Critical Thinking

1. How are hypothermia and hypoglycemia related? How can you help avoid them for your patient?

_____

_____

_____

_____

2. How will you respond when you are assessing a child you believe has been abused?

_____

_____

_____

_____

3. What opportunities do you have to practice your assessment infants and children?

_____

_____

_____

_____

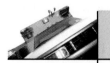

Dispatch Summary

Adrianna was transported with her mother to Children's Hospital, where she was admitted for observation. About 3 weeks later, both Adrianna and her twin sister Alexis were sent home, where they have continued to develop normally with no further incidents.

EMTs Jake and Aaron used this call to convince their ambulance service to provide more continuing education and training scenarios focusing on pediatric patients. As a result, the service's overall success rate with pediatric patients has increased and many of the EMTs and medics have expressed much less anxiety when confronted with sick or injured children.

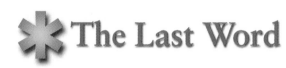

The Last Word

The most important focus of prehospital care for infants and children is airway, breathing, and oxygenation. Cardiac events in infants or children are almost always preceded by an obstructed airway or inadequate respirations. A rapid assessment that focuses on responsiveness, work of breathing, and perfusion begins as soon as you encounter the pediatric patient. Recognizing respiratory distress, respiratory failure, and the signs and symptoms of shock, then intervening quickly, best improves the outcomes in these patients.

Calls involving infants and children are often intimidating to the EMS provider, but using the information provided in this chapter to better understand the differences between age groups as well as to recognize behaviors common to most young children will help you interact more successfully with these patients and their families. Often, pediatric patients are surrounded by highly emotional or distraught parents or caregivers. Calm, supportive interaction with the family will help you improve interactions with the child.

Chapter Review

MULTIPLE CHOICE

Place a check next to the correct answer.

1. When assessing the infant or child it is important to keep him:

   _____ a. quiet.

   _____ b. warm.

   _____ c. undressed.

   _____ d. well fed.

2. The child with nasal flaring, retractions, and decreased responsiveness is experiencing:

   _____ a. respiratory distress.

   _____ b. an asthma attack.

   _____ c. respiratory failure.

   _____ d. a choking episode.

3. If you suspect there is a foreign body in the airway of a child less than 1 year old, you should:

_____ a. perform a blind finger sweep.

_____ b. try to ventilate with a BVM.

_____ c. perform five back blows followed by five chest thrusts.

_____ d. assist the child to a position of comfort.

4. The first interventions for a child with a slow heart rate are:

_____ a. open the airway, give 100 percent oxygen.

_____ b. ask the parents about any allergies.

_____ c. roll the child to the rescue position.

_____ d. apply the AED.

5. The child in shock may:

_____ a. have warm extremities.

_____ b. have a slow heart rate.

_____ c. floppy muscle tone.

_____ d. be drooling and crying tears.

MATCHING

Match the definition on the left with the applicable term on the right.

1. _____ Retractions

2. _____ Stridor

3. _____ Wheezing

4. _____ Cyanosis

5. _____ Apnea

6. _____ Decompensate

A. Absence of respiration
B. Barky or noisy breathing
C. Whistling breath sound
D. Deteriorate rapidly
E. Pale, bluish skin
F. Pulling in of muscles between the ribs with inspiration

CRITICAL THINKING

1. Why is it important to understand the developmental differences of children?

_____

_____

_____

_____

2. Why is it important to differentiate between respiratory distress and respiratory failure in the pediatric patient?

_____

_____

_____

_____

3. What is the most common cause of death for infants and children?

_____

_____

_____

_____

4. What is the most common cause of cardiac arrest for infants and children?

_____

_____

_____

_____

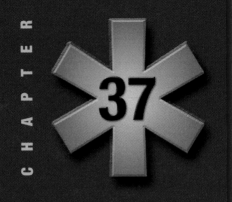

37

Caring for the Geriatric Patient

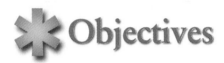

Objectives

There are no objectives in the U.S. Department of Transportation 1994 EMT-Basic National Standard Curriculum that pertain to this chapter.

Introduction

* geriatric

a person aged 65 or older.

In this chapter, you will learn about special considerations in assessing and providing care for geriatric patients. There are nearly 35 million elderly or **geriatric** persons in the United States. The segment of the population aged 65 and older is the fastest growing of all age groups (U. S. Census Bureau, 2000). The elderly are living longer, healthier lives than ever before, but age-related changes in anatomy and physiology continue to make certain types of emergencies more common among the elderly.

These changes also alter the way elderly patients respond to illness and injury, often changing the assessment findings that would be expected in a younger person. You will likely be called upon routinely to care for elderly patients.

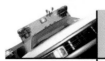

Emergency Dispatch

"Oh, hey! Watch out!" EMT Janis Burns grabbed onto the door of the ambulance and steadied her feet. "It's a solid sheet of ice from here over to the steps."

Janis and her EMT partner, Leroy Purcell, inched their way to the back of the truck, eased the cot out, and continued on to the steps of the single-wide trailer. It was a clear January afternoon, and although the sun stood brightly in the sky, the temperature just wouldn't rise above thirty degrees.

"I'm so glad that you're here!" A man in his mid 50s answered the door after one brief knock. "It's my mom. You need to take her to the hospital."

"Okay." Janis struggled to get the cot through the narrow doorway. "What's your mom's name and what is she having trouble with today?"

"Her name is Pauline and it's her leg." The man fumbled with his thick glasses, and motioned toward the back of the trailer. "She fell about 2 weeks ago and it's. . . it looks infected or something."

The EMTs left the cot in the small living room and carried their bags back to the patient.

"Do you smell that?" Leroy said quietly as they entered the bedroom.

"The nose always knows," Janis replied, stopping at the bedside of an elderly woman who appeared to be asleep. "Ma'am? Are you awake?"

The woman stirred and her eyes fluttered open. "Darn it, Ralphie!" She pulled the covers up to her neck. "I told you not to call the ambulance people!"

"But Mom," he stammered. "There's something wrong with your leg. Even Doris thought so, remember?"

"I haven't been to a doctor in my entire life," the woman hissed at her son. "And I'm not going to go to one now!"

"Ma'am," Leroy smiled broadly. "Tell you what. Let us just look at your leg and tell you what we think. We can't take you anywhere against your will. You're totally in control, and it won't cost you anything for me to look at it. I just want to see how bad it is. Okay?"

The woman stared at Leroy for a moment, shifted her gaze to the ceiling, and then slowly slid her leg out from under the sheets.

The Geriatric Patient

Many of your patients will be older. There are many terms that describe the older population, including senior citizen, elderly, geriatric, simply "old," and more. Each definition may technically be a bit different, but these terms are used interchangeably by our patients and their families and friends.

We have some major misconceptions about our older patients. Some things remain constant, however: that this population is growing, that it poses significant challenges to EMTs when presenting as a medical or traumatic emergency, and that there are some physiological changes that make this population different from younger patients.

MISCONCEPTIONS ABOUT THE ELDERLY

Since EMS providers often see elderly patients who are chronically ill, and since we respond frequently to extended-care facilities, it is easy to develop a distorted view about the elderly population as a whole. The majority of elderly persons in the United States are in good health, live independently, and enjoy active life styles. It is often assumed that elderly patients have difficulty hearing and cannot give reliable information. This is true of some elderly patients and must be taken into consideration, but it is certainly not true for the majority of elderly patients. Do not assume that elderly patients cannot hear or answer questions about their own health. However, the elderly have unique life experiences and psychosocial concerns that may not be well understood by younger persons. Older patients must be treated with respect and regarded as unique, dignified individuals.

Age-Related Physical Changes

The way we age is related to our genetic blueprint, our environment, and our life style. Aging proceeds at variable rates from individual to individual, but some changes are fairly predictable (Figure 37-1 and Table 37-1). It is important for EMS providers to understand how changes in the organ systems of elderly patients can predispose them to certain illnesses and injuries and how these changes can affect physical examination findings.

RESPIRATORY SYSTEM CHANGES

As we age, our lung capacity decreases, lung tissue becomes less elastic, and the chest wall is less compliant. The mechanisms that help the body detect low oxygen levels and high carbon dioxide levels in the blood are not as sensitive. This means that the elderly patient can be quite hypoxic before the body recognizes the

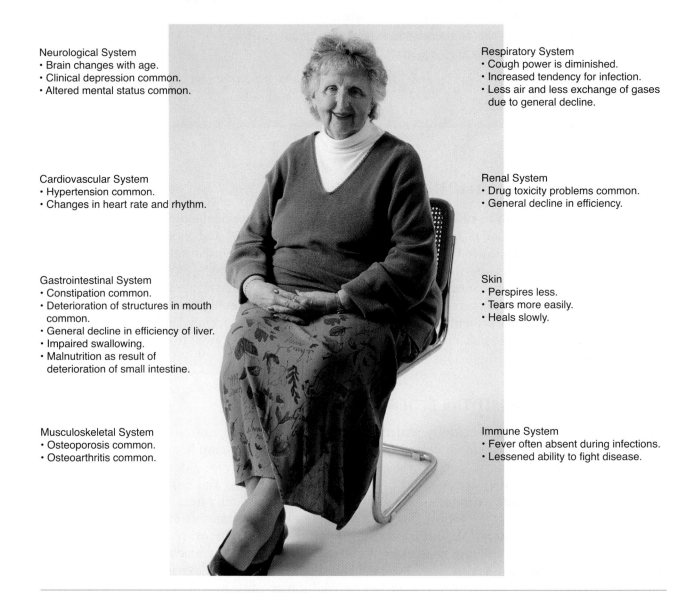

Neurological System
• Brain changes with age.
• Clinical depression common.
• Altered mental status common.

Cardiovascular System
• Hypertension common.
• Changes in heart rate and rhythm.

Gastrointestinal System
• Constipation common.
• Deterioration of structures in mouth common.
• General decline in efficiency of liver.
• Impaired swallowing.
• Malnutrition as result of deterioration of small intestine.

Musculoskeletal System
• Osteoporosis common.
• Osteoarthritis common.

Respiratory System
• Cough power is diminished.
• Increased tendency for infection.
• Less air and less exchange of gases due to general decline.

Renal System
• Drug toxicity problems common.
• General decline in efficiency.

Skin
• Perspires less.
• Tears more easily.
• Heals slowly.

Immune System
• Fever often absent during infections.
• Lessened ability to fight disease.

FIGURE 37-1 Changes in the body systems of the elderly.

TABLE 37-1 PHYSIOLOGICAL EFFECTS OF AGING AND IMPLICATIONS FOR ASSESSMENT

CHANGE	RESULT	IMPLICATION FOR ASSESSMENT
Depositing of cholesterol on arterial walls that have become thicker	Increased risk of heart attack and stroke, hypertension	Heart attack and stroke more likely
Decreased cardiac output	Diminished activity and tolerance of physical stress	More prone to falls; more complaints of fatigue
Decreased elasticity of lungs and decreased activity of cilia	Decreased ability to clear foreign substances from lungs	Higher risk of pneumonia and other respiratory infections
Fewer taste buds, less saliva; less acid production and slower movement in digestive system	Difficulty chewing and swallowing; less enjoyment of eating; difficulty digesting and absorbing food; constipation; early feeling of fullness when eating	Weight loss; abdominal pain common
Diminished liver and kidney function	Increased toxicity from alcohol and medications; diminished ability of blood to clot	Need for reduced doses of medication; bleeding tendencies
Diminished function of thyroid	Decreased energy and tolerance of heat and cold	Increased risk of hypothermia and hyperthermia
Decreased muscle mass, loss of minerals from bones	Decreased strength	Fall more likely; minor falls more likely to cause fractures
Multiple medical conditions	Many different medications, sometimes prescribed by different physicians	Increased risk of medication error; potentially harmful medication interactions common
Deaths of friends and family	Depression; loss of social support	Increased risk of suicide
Loss of skin elasticity, shrinking of sweat glands	Thin, dry, wrinkled skin	Increased risk of injury (The EMT must handle the patient gently to avoid injuring skin and subcutaneous tissues.)

situation and tries to compensate by increasing the respiratory rate and tidal volume. If there is any reason to suspect that the elderly patient may have a problem that could decrease oxygenation, don't rely on the typical signs of hypoxia to guide your care of the patient. Apply high-concentration oxygen early in the patient's care.

Aging also leads to a decrease in the number of **cilia,** the tiny structures that help sweep mucus and foreign particles, including infectious bacteria, upward in the respiratory system. This makes the elderly more prone to respiratory illnesses, such as pneumonia. Cough and gag reflexes are diminished as well, so that the elderly patient is not as able to protect the lower airway from **aspiration.** Some elderly patients may have difficulty swallowing due to a prior stroke or other medical problems. If this is the case, monitor the patient's airway carefully and be prepared to suction secretions.

* **cilia**

  tiny hairlike structures that help sweep mucus and foreign particles, including infectious bacteria, upward in the respiratory system.

* **aspiration**

  inhaling foreign material, such as vomitus, into the lungs.

CARDIOVASCULAR SYSTEM CHANGES

* **cardiac output**

  the amount of blood pumped by the heart in 1 minute.

* **dysrhythmia**

  a disturbance in heart rate or rhythm.

* **atherosclerosis**

  a build-up of fatty deposits on the inner walls of arteries.

* **aneurysm**

  the dilation, or ballooning, of a weakened section of the wall of an artery.

* **syncope**

  fainting.

* **near syncope**

  near fainting.

The effects of aging on the heart include decreased **cardiac output,** impaired ability to increase the heart rate, and increased likelihood of **dysrhythmias,** heart failure, and sudden cardiac death. The blood vessels also change with age, becoming less elastic and more likely to be narrowed by **atherosclerosis.** These changes can lead to high blood pressure and decreased organ perfusion. The elderly patient is more prone to stroke, heart attack, and **aneurysms** because of these changes in the blood vessels. Poor peripheral circulation may cause the hands and feet to be cold.

Medications for heart conditions or high blood pressure can prevent the heart rate from increasing or the blood vessels from contracting as they normally would. This results in a decreased ability to compensate for changes in blood volume. Often, decreased mental status may be the first sign of inadequate perfusion. If there is reason to believe that an elderly patient has significant blood loss, he should be treated for shock, even though the heart rate and respiratory rate may not be increased.

Additionally, age-related changes and medications can make it hard for the cardiovascular system to adjust when the elderly patient rises from a lying or sitting position. Gravity causes blood to pool in the lower extremities upon standing. The body is unable to constrict the blood vessels and increase cardiac output as it normally would to compensate. Under these conditions, the brain is not perfused, causing **syncope** or **near syncope.** Abnormal heart rhythms are another major cause of syncope in the elderly.

URINARY SYSTEM CHANGES

Elderly men may develop blockage of urine flow due to an enlargement of the prostate gland. This causes urine to be retained in the bladder, making urinary tract infection more likely. Elderly women are also at risk for urinary tract infections. At times, the elderly patient with a urinary tract infection may be very ill without specific symptoms of urinary tract infection. The elderly may not have a fever with severe infection. Overwhelming infection may occur, leading to septic shock. Urinary **incontinence** can be a problem for both men and women.

* **incontinence**

  inability to retain urine or feces because of loss of sphincter control.

NERVOUS SYSTEM CHANGES

Decreases in the number of nerve fibers and the speed of impulse conduction and changes in the chemical balance of the brain may lead to decreased sensory perception, decreased motor reaction time, changes in balance and coordination, and alterations in sleep patterns. These changes lead to an increased likelihood of injury in the elderly. There are many ways the homes of the elderly can be made safer to compensate for these changes. EMS providers are in a unique position to note safety issues in the homes of the elderly and to provide education about making their homes safer.

Impairments in thinking and memory are not normal results of aging but are indications that there is an abnormal condition. It is not uncommon for the elderly to present with altered mental status, such as decreased responsiveness, agitation, or confusion. There may be a variety of underlying causes. The effects of medication or acute illness can be a temporary cause of altered mental status. It is important to find out from the patient's family or caregivers what the patient's usual behavior and mental status are. Changes in mental status may be long-standing and progressive due to chronic disease, such as Alzheimer's disease or a prior stroke. A sudden change in mental status indicates a serious underlying problem.

Depression is a common condition among the elderly, with both situational and biochemical causes. It is not uncommon for the elderly to attempt suicide. According to the Centers for Disease Control, suicide rates are on the rise for our elderly population. Signs of depression are numerous, and include poor hygiene, poor eating habits, and a disorderly living environment.

Changes in the Senses   Aging generally leads to a decrease in the acuity, or sharpness, of the senses. Changes in vision include increasing farsightedness, cataracts, poor night vision, impaired depth perception, decreased peripheral vision, and less tolerance for glare. These changes make it difficult to read medication labels or tell the color of one pill from another, which may lead to medication errors. Visual changes also contribute to many unintentional injuries, such as motor vehicle crashes and falls. Hearing may decrease, especially for higher-pitched sounds. The senses of taste and smell diminish, as does the ability to feel pain. Sensory changes contribute to a decreased ability to be aware of one's environment and potential dangers in it. Since the sensation of pain diminishes, any complaint of pain in the elderly should be regarded as a symptom of serious illness or injury. The lack of a complaint of pain in the elderly patient does not, however, rule out the possibility of serious illness or injury.

MUSCULOSKELETAL SYSTEM CHANGES

As we age, we lose muscle mass and are at risk for **osteoporosis**. Due to thinning of the discs between the vertebrae, we may lose 2 to 3 inches in height. Musculoskeletal changes also lead to changes in posture, mobility, and balance. These changes factor significantly in falls in the elderly population. Because of the accompanying loss of bone mass, even minor falls may lead to fractures. Bone fractures are much more serious in the elderly, leading to a number of health complications. Age-related changes of the spine result in a curvature of the spine that may make airway management and spinal immobilization challenging.

✳ **osteoporosis**
  softening of bone tissue due to the loss of essential minerals, principally calcium.

DIGESTIVE SYSTEM CHANGES

With age, the digestive system slows and produces less of the secretions needed to break down food. The sense of taste is diminished, making eating less pleasurable, and the loss of teeth or poorly fitting dentures may make eating difficult.

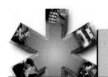

Perspective

Janis—The EMT

"Leroy is always so good with the older patients. Especially the ladies! He's got this big smile and a low voice, you know? And I think he talks to them not only with a lot of respect, I guess, but about the things that worry them. Like the money. It was good that he built rapport, though. She had a serious case of gangrene. It won't surprise me if she loses part of that leg. Yet she was just stubborn enough that she might have refused to go with us if Leroy hadn't immediately made that connection with her."

These factors can lead to poor nutrition, frequent heartburn, excessive gas production, and constipation. Since the stomach empties more slowly, vomiting of stomach contents may occur during illness or injury. Tooth loss, no teeth, or poorly fitting dentures may make it difficult for an elderly patient to communicate. If the patient is not wearing dentures and you are having difficulty understanding him, ask if he has dentures he can put in. Lack of teeth or poorly fitting dentures can also make it difficult to maintain a good seal with a bag-valve mask or pocket mask.

Ulcers and disorders of the intestinal tract may lead to bleeding. Bleeding from the upper gastrointestinal tract (the esophagus and stomach) may result in vomiting blood. Blood that has been exposed to the digestive secretions of the stomach may take on a "coffee grounds" appearance. Bleeding in the lower gastrointestinal tract can lead to blood in the stools. Generally, blood from an upper gastrointestinal source will result in dark (tarry), sticky stools, while blood from lower in the gastrointestinal tract will not undergo these changes and will appear as maroon or bright red in color.

CHANGES IN THE SKIN

Some of the more noticeable age-related changes are those that affect the skin. The skin develops more darkly pigmented areas, sometimes called "age spots" or "liver spots." This change is most noticeable in lighter-skinned individuals. The skin secretes less oil, making it drier and flakier. The skin secretions that normally help protect against infection decrease as well. Perspiration decreases, making heat-related emergencies more likely in the elderly as they lose this important cooling mechanism. The elderly may not exhibit the excessive perspiration called diaphoresis that is associated with shock in younger patients. Loss of fat and weakening of the connective tissues of the skin cause it to become looser, thinner, and more fragile. The skin of elderly individuals tears quite easily. This also makes the elderly more prone to bedsores when they are confined to bed or spend long periods of time sitting.

IMMUNE SYSTEM

The immune system does not function as well when we age. Common illnesses such as influenza and pneumonia have a higher fatality rate in the elderly. Because the body's ability to respond to infection is lessened, fever may not be present, even when the elderly patient has a serious infection. The diminished function of the immune system means that the elderly do not recover as well from trauma, surgery, and illness.

RESPONSE TO MEDICATION

Changes in the digestive system, liver function, kidneys, and body composition mean that the elderly respond to and process medications differently than younger individuals. Elderly patients may have exaggerated responses to medications and more profound side effects. Since the elderly often take several medications, both over-the-counter and prescription, interactions between medications can occur (Figure 37-2). EMS providers should always consider medication reactions as a possible cause of unexplained physical illness and behavioral changes in the elderly.

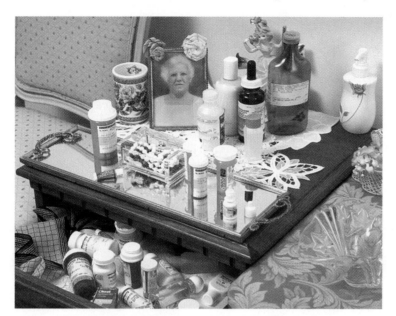

FIGURE 37-2   Older patients often take multiple medications.

 Stop, Review, Remember!

Multiple Choice

Place a check next to the correct answer.

1. Which of the following is an age-related change of the skin?

   _____ a. loss of pigmentation

   _____ b. decreased ability to prevent infection

   _____ c. oiliness

   _____ d. increased thickness

2. Which of the following decrease(s) the elderly patient's ability to compensate for blood loss?

   _____ a. diminished ability to increase the heart rate

   _____ b. decreased cardiac output

   _____ c. decreased elasticity of the blood vessels

   _____ d. all of the above

3. Which of the following is NOT a typical age-related change in vision?

   _____ a. farsightedness

   _____ b. impaired depth perception

   _____ c. unequal pupils

   _____ d. cataracts

Fill in the Blank

For each body system, list at least one age-related change.

Body System	Age-Related Changes
1. cardiovascular system	
2. respiratory system	
3. musculoskeletal system	
4. digestive system	
5. nervous system	

Critical Thinking

1. How do changes in the cardiovascular system affect the signs and symptoms of shock in the elderly patient?

_____

_____

_____

_____

2. Why are burn injuries more serious in the elderly than they would be in a younger patient?

_____

_____

_____

_____

Psychosocial Concerns of the Elderly

* **psychosocial**
related to a patient's personality, style, dynamics of unresolved conflict, or crisis management methods.

Many **psychosocial** and economic concerns impact the lives of the elderly. They include loneliness, alcoholism, substance abuse, physical and psychological abuse, neglect, and poverty. These factors can all have a significant impact on the health of elderly individuals. Being aware of these factors is important in developing empathy and compassion for elderly patients.

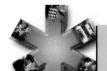

Perspective

Pauline—The Patient

"I just hadn't been feeling right for awhile, I guess. Ever since my Raymond passed away, maybe. Raymond was my middle boy. I've lost my husband, a child, and my best friend since grade school—all in a span of 2 years. It's hell getting old. I don't know if I'd wish this on my worst enemy. So when I fell and hurt my leg, staying in bed just didn't seem like a bad idea at all. I kind of thought that I might. . . maybe just. . . pass on. Or something. But instead I got Ralphie, my youngest, running around like a darn Chicken Little. Calling out those ambulance folks. That boy! But I do know my leg isn't in good shape."

DEPRESSION

Depression is common among the elderly. It may be a result of chemical changes in the brain or of a number of situational factors. Friends and relatives may have died, leaving the elderly person living alone and feeling isolated and lonely. Loss of independence and having to rely on others for help with daily activities may be a factor in depression as well. Some patients may feel shame, self-disgust, or embarrassment at the loss of body functions, such as incontinence, or at changes in appearance. Depression can be treated with medication and/or therapy, yet suicide and attempted suicide remain significant issues for the elderly population.

SUBSTANCE ABUSE AND MEDICATION ERRORS

Healthcare providers may not think to suspect abuse of alcohol and other substances in the elderly. It may seem strange to think of an older adult as having a substance abuse problem, but a person who was in his 20s or 30s in the 1960s, when illicit drug use was popular across socioeconomic groups, is now a person in his 60s or 70s. Alcohol and substance abuse may contribute to deterioration of physical and mental health, may be a cause of altered mental status in the elderly person, and can contribute to injuries due to falls and motor vehicle crashes.

Always ask the patient or caregiver about medications taken recently or that day. Is there a possibility of confusion regarding when and if medications were taken properly—or not frequently or too frequently—due to memory loss or confusion?

ELDER ABUSE AND NEGLECT

Abuse and **neglect** of the elderly often go unrecognized and unreported. Abuse may be physical, psychological, sexual, or financial. Neglect may either be due to the patient's inability to take care of himself (self-neglect), or because the patient's caregiver is failing to provide adequate care. EMS personnel are in a unique position to

* **abuse**

physical or psychological injury by another person.

* **neglect**

a person's inability to care for himself or a person's caregiver providing inadequate care.

FIGURE 37-3 When you encounter evidence of serious head injury, maintain a suspicion of geriatric abuse until proven otherwise.

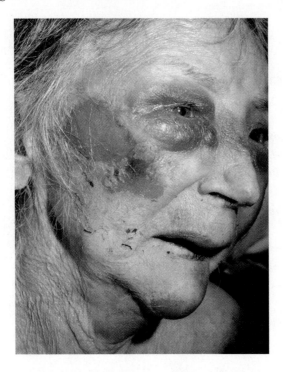

detect abuse and neglect of the elderly. All 50 states have laws pertaining to the reporting of elder abuse. Most states have laws requiring EMS personnel to report geriatric abuse and neglect (mandatory reporting laws) (Figure 37-3).

Regardless of whether the elderly patient lives with a spouse, grown children, or in an extended-care facility, there are a number of factors that increase the risk of abuse. An elderly person who requires assistance with daily activities, has trouble sleeping, has lost bowel or bladder control (incontinence), or who exhibits bizarre behavior is more likely to be abused or neglected.

Abuse should be suspected when an injury seems inconsistent with how it was reported to have happened or when there are multiple injuries in various stages of healing. The patient may be reluctant to discuss the nature of the injury in the presence of the abuser because of fear of punishment. The patient may also feel shame or embarrassment. The neglected patient may be deprived of food, water, needed medications, or hygiene activities such as bathing or changing clothes. If you suspect abuse, do not confront the abuser. Make every attempt to transport the patient to the hospital, and follow state laws and system protocols concerning reporting suspected abuse.

FINANCIAL CONCERNS

Many older adults live on limited incomes. As a result, they may not have adequate medical care, food, safety, or shelter. They may not be able to secure their homes against crime or make necessary repairs and modifications for safety. The elderly may not be able to afford to heat or cool their homes to maintain an acceptable environmental temperature and may suffer heat- or cold-related emergencies in their homes. Using alternative sources of heating such as a space heater or an open oven can lead to fires, burns, or carbon monoxide poisoning. A frequent reason why the elderly patient does not take medications as needed is the inability to afford prescription medications. The patient may take less than needed or may not take the medication at all in order to save money. The elderly may also be exploited financially by individuals who prey on the elderly or even by their own family members.

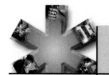

Perspective

Ralph—The Son

"Mom's on a fixed income. Isn't that what it's called? Where she only gets social security and Dad's pension each month? Everything's about money with her, you know? 'How much is this costin' me?' or 'How much is that costin' me?' Get this: She once called me because a pan had caught fire on her stove and she asked me if she'd get charged for calling for a fire truck. I said, 'Momma, is the pan still burnin' right now?' and she says, 'Oh, yeah, and the drapes by the sink too.' Do you believe that? After that, I've watched for her safety, too."

Common Illness and Injuries in the Elderly

Common illnesses in the elderly include pneumonia, chronic obstructive pulmonary diseases such as **chronic bronchitis** and **emphysema,** pulmonary embolism, heart attack, heart failure, cardiac dysrhythmias, aortic aneurysms, hypertension, stroke, **Alzheimer's disease, Parkinson's disease,** diabetes, gastrointestinal bleeding, urinary tract conditions (infection, incontinence), and medication reactions. The elderly are also prone to heat-related emergencies and hypothermia.

Trauma in the Elderly

Trauma remains a leading cause of death as we age. In the elderly, trauma often includes burns, falls, and motor vehicle collisions. It takes a less significant mechanism of injury to result in trauma to the elderly person than it does the younger person. Medications taken by the elderly to prevent abnormal blood clotting may make controlling bleeding from even relatively minor wounds difficult. The effects of aging alone make the elderly trauma patient up to three times more likely to die than he would have from the same injury when he was younger. Injury prevention is important among the elderly population. The risk of burns and falls can be reduced by taking safety measures in the home, such as reducing the temperature of the hot water heater, using nonskid rugs, and installing hand holds in the shower.

Assessment of the Geriatric Patient

SAFETY AND SCENE SIZE-UP

Ensuring your own safety is no less important when responding to an elderly patient than it is with any other patient. An elderly patient with an altered mental status or a condition such as Alzheimer's disease may become violent. There are special considerations, too, for the scene size-up when responding to an elderly patient. Look for the following:

* Conditions that suggest abuse or neglect

* Potential hazards, such as loose or missing handrails on porches or stairs, and loose carpets or rugs

* **chronic bronchitis**

   long-term inflammation of the bronchi; a form of chronic obstructive pulmonary disease.

* **emphysema**

   disease that causes a loss of elasticity of the alveoli; a formal chronic obstructive pulmonary disease.

* **Alzheimer's disease**

   a progressive, degenerative disease that attacks the brain and results in impaired memory, thinking, and behavior. It affects 4 million American adults.

* **Parkinson's disease**

   chronic, degenerative nervous disease characterized by tremors, muscular weakness and rigidity, and a loss of postural reflexes.

✳ Poorly functioning heat or cooling systems

✳ Inadequate food, shelter, or hygiene

As you approach the elderly patient, focus on him rather than on family members or caregivers who may be anxious to speak for him. This demonstrates respect for the patient and gives him more control over the situation. Make eye contact. Get on the patient's level if he is sitting down or in bed, rather than standing over him (Figure 37-4). Introduce yourself. Address the patient by title and last name— "Mrs. Fox" or "Mr. Popejoy"—rather than by terms such as "honey," "sweetheart," "dear," or "partner." Offering a handshake during your introduction helps establish rapport and allows you to determine the patient's skin temperature and ability to move. Determine the patient's chief complaint by asking why EMS was called. Asking "what's wrong" may elicit a lengthy explanation of medical complaints—both current and past—as well as nonmedical complaints. If the patient offers a number of complaints or the onset of the complaint is difficult to determine, "What is different today?" or "What happened today?" can be a helpful question.

COMMUNICATING WITH THE ELDERLY PATIENT

The principles of communication you learned about earlier in the text apply to the elderly, as well. Age-related changes may interfere with the ability of the elderly patient to communicate with others. It is important not to assume that elderly patients have a hearing deficit. Make eye contact with the patient and speak clearly in a normal tone. Make sure the patient can see you. Speak louder only if it becomes clear that the patient is having difficult hearing you. If the patient seems to be having difficulty hearing you, ask if he has a hearing aid. Give the elderly patient a chance to answer your question before assuming he cannot hear you. It sometimes takes an elderly person a moment to give a response. Sometimes the elderly patient has difficulty communicating due to a stroke. This can be very frustrating for the patient. If the patient's speech is difficult to understand, determine if the patient is able to write. This may help you communicate with the patient.

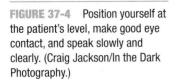

FIGURE 37-4 Position yourself at the patient's level, make good eye contact, and speak slowly and clearly. (Craig Jackson/In the Dark Photography.)

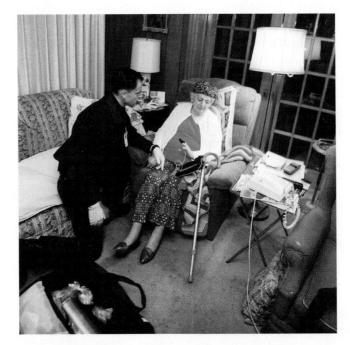

Clinical Clues: PSYCHOSOCIAL ISSUES

This chapter has used the word *psychosocial*, which very appropriately describes issues you may face when caring for an elderly patient. Patients may be stoic and not admit they are sick, may not be able to afford care or medications, may be depressed or neglected by their families. These are some of the many psychosocial issues you will face when caring for the elderly patient. Considering these and others as you care for the patient will make your assessment and care more successful. It may also allow you to identify problems and allow you to notify appropriate people in the hospital or community to overcome these issues for your patient.

Elderly patients may deny symptoms of illness or injury for many reasons. They may fear leaving home, going to a hospital, or losing independence. They may have concerns about the cost of medical care, ambulance transportation, and possible admission to the hospital. They may also be afraid to leave behind a spouse, sibling, or pet for which they provide care. Remember that the elderly person who is refusing to be transported may have a number of fears. Try to find out what the fears are and assist in finding a solution. This may be as simple as making a phone call or contacting a neighbor.

GENERAL CONSIDERATIONS FOR ASSESSMENT

With any patient, your assessment is vital and will guide your care. Your assessment of an elderly patient will include some special considerations and practices to increase the accuracy and efficiency of your assessment.

The following considerations are important when examining the elderly patient:

* The elderly patient can be easily fatigued by the physical exam.

* The elderly patient may have multiple layers of clothing, making examination difficult.

* Respect the modesty and privacy of the elderly patient, just as you would a younger patient.

* Explain what you are going to do before you do it.

* Handle the patient gently.

Recall that age-related changes may reduce the elderly patient's ability to respond to injuries and illness. They may not have the expected signs and symptoms of specific illnesses and injuries. The elderly may present with generalized weakness or a change in mental status in response to illness. It is often difficult to determine the cause of illness until a physician has examined the patient and ordered diagnostic tests.

PHYSICAL ASSESSMENT AND VITAL SIGNS

While the procedures and steps for assessment will not change when assessing an elderly patient, you will have certain cautions and considerations that may not be present in a younger patient. These include the following:

* The pain tolerance of an elderly patient will be highly variable. Some patients have decreased pain sensation that could mask a broken bone. Others may

experience severe pain when a bone isn't broken. This is due in some part to changes in the nervous system.

✳ The patient's skin is often drier and less elastic than that of younger patients. This will require more careful palpation of injuries and gentle application and inflation of the blood pressure cuff.

✳ The patient's pupils may no longer be round and can be less reactive due to diseases such as glaucoma and medications used to treat the disease.

✳ The blood pressure may be higher. Hypertension is common in older adults.

Clinical Clues: ASSESSMENT IN THE ELDERLY

Elderly patients are a series of contradictions when it comes to assessment and determining severity of injury. They can develop infections—but often don't have a fever. They can be injured—but not feel the pain a younger patient would. And they may have trouble communicating their symptoms and concerns to you. Take time to assess your patient. Obtain a history. Listen to what the patient says and what the patient doesn't say, (for example, body language). And remember the differences between the elderly and younger patients.

OBTAINING A HISTORY

Communication and accuracy are both vital parts of the history—and both may be problematic in the elderly patient.

Hearing loss, difficulty speaking, and chronic altered mental status (dementia) may prevent you from communicating effectively. If you complete your initial assessment and vital signs and do not find life-threatening issues, you will be able to take a bit more time. When obtaining a history:

✳ Speak slowly and clearly.

✳ Ask one question at a time.

✳ Listen attentively.

✳ Position yourself where the patient can easily see you.

It is important to accurately determine the patient's chief complaint as well as any past medical history. Patients who have difficulty communicating (hearing, seeing, or speaking) will find it difficult to relate this information.

Many elderly patients have multiple medical conditions. These may include cardiovascular disorders, such as prior heart attacks and hypertension; respiratory problems, such as chronic obstructive pulmonary disease (COPD) and congestive heart failure (CHF); and neurological conditions, such as stroke and Alzheimer's disease. It will be challenging to get an accurate list of these conditions and sift through the information for facts important to the patient's current condition.

The patient's medications will also provide vital information. You will ask if a patient takes medications. With many elderly patients, there will be so many medications that the patient will show you a list or offer to show you his medications. The medications are commonly found in a location convenient to the patient such as the kitchen or a nightstand. There may be dozens of medications.

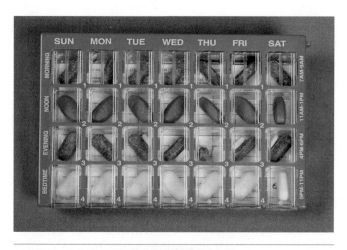

FIGURE 37-5A   Many elderly persons use a pill organizer to help them remember when to take his medications.

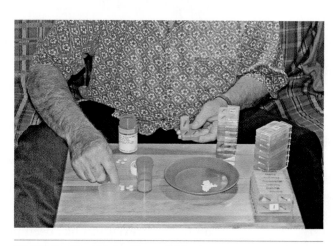

FIGURE 37-5B   There are many kinds of devices that enable the elderly person to keep track of his medications.

These medications provide clues to existing medical conditions. A pocket drug reference will help you identify medications used for certain conditions. This will help you determine or confirm a history of these conditions. You should also be alert for the possibility that medications have been taken inappropriately. Overdosing or not taking enough of a medication may actually have caused the problem you were called for.

There are many reasons elderly patients take medications improperly. Most commonly they fail to understand the instructions and/or can't read the small print on the prescription bottles. Because of limited income, some patients will intentionally reduce a dose to make a prescription last longer. Finally, as mentioned earlier in the chapter, depression in the elderly population is significant and a suicide attempt should be suspected if prescription or other medication bottles that are new or recently filled appear empty.

It may be difficult to determine the amount of medication left in a prescription, since medications are often transferred to different containers. There are many containers designed to assist patients in remembering doses (Figure 37-5A and B).

✳ Stop, Review, Remember!

Multiple Choice

Place a check next to the correct answer.

1. Which of the following regarding depression in the elderly patient is FALSE?

_____ a. Depression may be treated with medication.

_____ b. Elderly patients may feel isolated leading to depression.

_____ c. Increased independence associated with aging prevents depression.

_____ d. Physical changes associated with aging can cause depression.

2. Which of the following statements regarding trauma in the elderly is TRUE?

_____ a. Bones heal more quickly because there is less bone mass.

_____ b. Blood-thinning medications help stop bleeding.

_____ c. The risk of death from a traumatic injury is three times higher than in younger adults.

_____ d. Injury prevention has been proven ineffective for the elderly population.

3. Which of the following would be LEAST valuable when assessing a patient with Alzheimer's disease?

_____ a. speaking loudly

_____ b. getting a list of the patient's medications

_____ c. asking a caregiver to compare the patient's current mental status to the usual mental status

_____ d. obtaining two or more sets of vital signs

4. Elderly patients are less prone to hyperthermia than younger adults.

_____ a. true

_____ b. false

5. Elderly patients may not take medications correctly because they:

_____ a. fail to understand instructions.

_____ b. can't afford them.

_____ c. fail to read the labels' small print.

_____ d. all of the above.

6. Elderly patients may abuse alcohol and drugs.

_____ a. true

_____ b. false

Fill in the Blank

For each of the following write in "more" or "less" to complete the statement correctly.

1. The elderly patient's skin is _____ elastic.

2. The elderly patient is _____ able to compensate for shock.

3. Elderly patients have _____ medical problems than younger adults.

4. Elderly patients are _____ likely to die from trauma than a younger adult.

5. Elderly patients usually take _____ medications than younger adults.

6. Elderly patients are _____ likely to have a fever with an infection.

7. Elderly patients have _____ cilia in their airway.

Critical Thinking

1. You are treating a generally healthy 84-year-old female who, according to her daughter, seems a bit confused today. What could you do to make communication with this patient effective?

   _____

   _____

   _____

2. You are taking the blood pressure of an elderly man. As you pump the cuff up he begins to scream in pain. You look at the gauge and note that it is only at about 120 mmHg. What might be some causes of this discomfort?

   _____

   _____

   _____

Transport Considerations for the Elderly Patient

Typically, the elderly patient should be transported in a position of comfort. It is important to keep in mind that the elderly patient's skin is fragile and to protect the patient by using padding to prevent pressure and abrasion to the skin. Some elderly patients develop a curvature of the spine due to musculoskeletal changes. When immobilizing an elderly patient on a long backboard, use enough padding under the head to maintain the head in the position that is normal for the patient, rather than trying to fit the patient to the backboard. It is also important to pad the long backboard. Pressure on the patient's skin from being compressed between the skeleton and a hard surface like a backboard reduces the blood flow to that area. Although a bedsore will not be immediately apparent, the damage that causes it can occur in as little as 20 minutes.

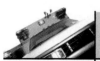

Dispatch Summary

Leroy was able to persuade the patient to see a doctor and, due to the ice outside of the home, Janis requested lift assistance from the local fire station. The patient was then transported, in a position of comfort, to County General, where the ED physician recommended immediate surgery on her leg.

The patient declined all treatment and, against the physician's advice, had her son take her back home.

She succumbed to sepsis less than a week later.

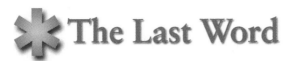 **The Last Word**

The number of elderly persons in the United States is growing quickly. Since most EMTs will routinely respond to care for elderly patients, it is important to have an understanding of the unique physical and psychosocial characteristics of the elderly. Although the majority of the elderly lead healthy, active lives, many illnesses become more common with age. Age-related changes make the elderly prone to injuries from falls and motor vehicle collisions and leave them less able to compensate for illness and injury. Because of this reduced ability to respond and compensate, the patient's illness or injury may be much more serious than it appears. In addition to the physical changes of aging, financial concerns, isolation, substance abuse, and depression can impact the health of the elderly patient.

 Chapter Review

MULTIPLE CHOICE

Place a check next to the correct answer.

1. In reference to physiological changes in the respiratory system, all of the following are true EXCEPT:

   _____ a. lung tissue becomes more elastic.

   _____ b. gag reflexes may be diminished.

   _____ c. elderly patients are more prone to pneumonia.

   _____ d. strokes and nervous system diseases can cause difficulty swallowing.

2. Medications for high blood pressure and heart conditions may:

   _____ a. prevent the heart rate from increasing to compensate for shock.

   _____ b. cause severe coughing fits.

   _____ c. cause unequal pupils.

   _____ d. cause a build-up of fluid in the sac surrounding the heart.

3. Which of the following is true regarding the senses in the elderly?

   _____ a. All elderly patients have hearing deficits.

   _____ b. A slightly delayed response to a question indicates a hearing problem.

   _____ c. A prior stroke may cause problems with speech.

   _____ d. If the patient cannot see, you should try writing your questions on a piece of paper.

4. Patients may take reduced doses of their medication because they cannot afford to take the full dose.

   _____ a. true

   _____ b. false

5. Suspected elder abuse legally must be reported by:

   _____ a. EMT's.

   _____ b. neighbors.

   _____ c. family members.

   _____ d. All of the above.

6. People can lose 2 to 3 inches in height as part of the aging process.

   _____ a. true

   _____ b. false

7. Suicide rates are increasing in the elderly population.

   _____ a. true

   _____ b. false

CRITICAL THINKING

1. You are called to the residence of an elderly patient who has fallen out of bed. She is not injured and refuses transport. You consider this an opportunity to prevent further falls and injury. List three things you can check that might prevent injury in the future.

   _____

   _____

   _____

2. If you were to respond to an elderly patient several times and the complaint always seems minor, what would you look for to determine if the patient is experiencing depression?

   _____

   _____

   _____

CASE STUDY

You are called to an 89-year-old female patient who has an altered mental status. You were called by her daughter who says she checked on her mother the night before and she was fine.

You arrive to find the patient sitting quietly in a chair. She tells you she feels "fine, but tired." Her daughter is concerned because of the sudden change in mental status. You perform a history and physical examination for a medical patient. She denies falls or injury, is not diabetic and has eaten, shows no signs of neurological problems, and has no problems completing all components of the Cincinnati Prehospital Stroke Scale. Her vitals are within normal limits. She has a history of high blood pressure and is on a blood thinner because she had a "mini-stroke" several months ago.

1. Based on the information in this chapter and throughout the book, choose two or three possibilities of what could be wrong with this patient.

   _____

   _____

   _____

   _____

2. For each of the possibilities chosen in question 1, list two ways to examine or explore that problem.

   _____

   _____

   _____

   _____

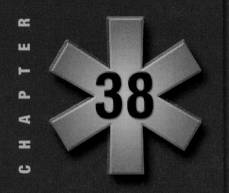

CHAPTER 38

Module Review and Practice Examination

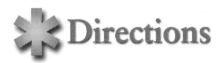

Directions

Assess what you have learned in this module by circling the best answer for each multiple-choice question. When you are done, check your answers against the key provided in Appendix D.

1. The bones of the skull are not yet fused at the suture sites in patients who are in which of the following age groups?
   a. infants, toddlers, and preschoolers
   b. infants and toddlers
   c. infants
   d. none of the above; the bones are fused at birth

2. Believing that injury or illness is a punishment for bad behavior is characteristic of which of the following age groups?
   a. infants and toddlers
   b. toddlers and preschoolers
   c. preschoolers and school-aged children
   d. school-aged children and adolescents

3. When a pediatric patient suffers cardiac arrest, it is most often due to:
   a. a respiratory problem.
   b. birth defect.
   c. poisoning.
   d. electrical shock.

4. The pediatric assessment triangle includes all of the following EXCEPT:
   a. observing the safety of the environment.
   b. general appearance of the patient.
   c. work of breathing.
   d. circulatory status as noted by skin signs.

5. How long should it take for capillary refill after blanching the back of the hand of the patient?
   a. less than 10 seconds
   b. less than 7 seconds
   c. less than 5 seconds
   d. less than 2 seconds

6. The absence of tears in the crying pediatric patient should be considered by the EMT to be a/an:
   a. sign of dehydration.
   b. variation of normal.
   c. indication that the illness or injury is not serious.
   d. sign of psychiatric illness.

7. Which of the following statements concerning respiratory emergencies in pediatric patients is true?
   a. Pediatric patients gradually decompensate, providing warning of impending respiratory failure.
   b. The presence of nasal flaring is unlikely to occur in the pediatric patient in respiratory distress.
   c. Grunting with exhalation is a sign of respiratory distress in pediatric patients.
   d. Respiratory distress is always accompanied by cyanosis in the pediatric patient.

8. To maintain an open airway in an unresponsive pediatric patient, the head must be in a _____ position.
   a. hyperextended
   b. neutral
   c. flexed
   d. saggital

9. To maintain the airway of an unresponsive pediatric patient, it may be necessary to place a folded towel under the:
   a. head.
   b. neck.
   c. shoulders.
   d. back.

10. Which of the following devices is preferred for nasal suctioning of a newborn infant?
    a. bulb syringe
    b. 30-mL medicine syringe
    c. flexible suction catheter
    d. rigid suction tip

11. Which of the following devices is preferred for oral suctioning of a newborn infant?
    a. bulb syringe
    b. 30-mL medicine syringe
    c. flexible suction catheter
    d. rigid suction tip

12. Inserting a suction tip too far into the mouth of a pediatric patient may result in:
    a. slowing the heart rate.
    b. inducing gagging.
    c. trauma to the soft tissue.
    d. all of the above.

13. You have responded to a report of a child choking. Your patient is a 20-month-old male who is coughing and has stridorous breathing. He was playing with a toy car when his mother went to the kitchen to get him some juice. When she returned, he was coughing and having some difficulty breathing. The patient is alert, his skin color is normal, and his skin is warm and dry. Which of the following is appropriate for this patient?
    a. Visualize the mouth and perform a finger sweep.
    b. Transport, allowing the mother to give him some oxygen by "blow-by" technique.

    c. Place him across your lap and perform back blows.
    d. Place him on the floor and perform abdominal thrusts.

14. Your patient is a 16-month-old female whose grandmother gave her some canned peaches for lunch. The patient started choking while eating and is now limp and pale with cyanotic lips. Her respiratory effort is ineffective. Which of the following is appropriate for this patient?
    a. Place her across your lap and perform back blows.
    b. Alternate back slaps and chest thrusts.
    c. Perform abdominal thrusts.
    d. Perform a finger sweep if you cannot see the obstruction.

15. Which of the following is true concerning the use of oropharyngeal airways in pediatric patients?
    a. They are measured from the center of the mouth to the earlobe, rather than from the corner of the mouth as in an adult.
    b. The airway must be rotated as it is inserted.
    c. Oropharyngeal airways are contraindicated for children under 12 years old.
    d. Correct head position must be maintained, even with a properly inserted oropharyngeal airway.

16. Which of the following is NOT a common cause of shock in pediatric patients?
    a. blood loss
    b. vomiting
    c. diarrhea
    d. cardiac problems

17. Which of the following is a late sign of shock in a pediatric patient?
    a. pale skin color
    b. lack of activity
    c. weak peripheral pulses
    d. lack of tears when crying

18. Your patient is a 9-month-old male with a 3-day history of fever and refusing food and fluids. He is pale and limp and does not take note of your presence. His skin is mottled and clammy. Which of the following describes the appropriate sequence of care for this patient?
    a. apply high-concentration oxygen, perform a rapid physical examination, take vital signs, begin transport, perform on-going assessment
    b. perform a detailed physical examination, take vital signs, apply high-concentration oxygen, begin transport, perform on-going assessment
    c. take vital signs, perform a rapid physical examination, apply high-concentration oxygen, begin transport
    d. apply high-concentration oxygen, take vital signs, perform a detailed physical examination, begin transport

19. The leading cause of death in children is:
    a. sudden infant death syndrome.
    b. poisoning.
    c. trauma.
    d. asthma.

20. The most common cause of blunt trauma in children is:
    a. falls.
    b. motor vehicle crashes.
    c. child abuse.
    d. recreational injuries.

21. Which of the following is NOT a factor in the increased risk of hypothermia in the pediatric population?
    a. less body fat
    b. greater body surface area
    c. few glucose reserves
    d. slower metabolism

22. When documenting suspected child abuse, all of the following are appropriate EXCEPT:
    a. describing the appearance of injuries.
    b. quoting statements made by caregivers.
    c. reaching conclusions based on the history and injuries.
    d. describing the behavior of the child.

23. Which of the following devices is used to provide nutrition to the pediatric patient who cannot eat or swallow?
    a. gastrostomy tube
    b. ventral-peritoneal shunt
    c. tracheotomy tube
    d. central venous line

24. The fastest-growing segment of the U. S. population is those aged _____ years.
    a. 1 to 25
    b. 30 to 55
    c. 55 to 80
    d. 55 and older

25. Geriatric patients are those aged _____ years and older.
    a. 40
    b. 65
    c. 70
    d. 85

26. Which of the following changes occurs with aging?
    a. The body is less able to detect changes in oxygen levels.
    b. The body is less able to detect changes in carbon dioxide levels.
    c. Lung capacity decreases.
    d. All of the above.

27. Which of the following statements regarding the majority of elderly persons in the United States is true?
    a. They live in extended care facilities.
    b. Their health is generally poor.
    c. They enjoy active lifestyles.
    d. They suffer severe problems with memory and thinking.

28. The elderly may be less able to compensate for blood loss due to which of the following factors?
    a. decreased elasticity of the blood vessels
    b. taking medications for heart conditions or high blood pressure
    c. taking blood-thinning medications
    d. all of the above

29. The elderly may be less able to compensate for blood loss due to which of the following factors?
    a. taking medications to prevent stroke or heart attack
    b. decreased number of cilia
    c. increased elasticity of the heart
    d. all of the above

30. Which of the following is NOT a normal age-related change in the nervous system?
    a. decreased sensory perception
    b. decreased motor reaction time
    c. inability to learn new things
    d. altered sleep patterns

31. Which of the following increases the risk of injury in the elderly?
    a. decreased sensory perception
    b. thinning of the skin
    c. changes in vision
    d. all of the above

32. Which of the following statements is true regarding depression in the elderly?
    a. The elderly suffer from a high rate of depression, but suicide is rare.
    b. Depression may have both biochemical and situational causes.
    c. There are no warning signs of depression in the elderly.
    d. All of the above.

33. Musculoskeletal changes in the elderly include all of the following EXCEPT:
    a. curvature of the spine.
    b. changes in posture.
    c. decreased height.
    d. increased bone density.

34. Which of the following may contribute to malnutrition in the elderly?
    a. decreased sense of taste and smell
    b. poorly fitting dentures
    c. depression
    d. all of the above

35. Which of the following is NOT a normal age-related change of the skin?
    a. increased fat deposit under the skin
    b. liver spots
    c. decreased oil secretion
    d. decreased perspiration

36. Which of the following is NOT a normal age-related change in the senses?
    a. increasing farsightedness
    b. decreased ability to hear, especially for lower-pitched sounds
    c. loss of peripheral vision
    d. increased sensitivity to pain

37. Which of the following is a psychosocial concern among the elderly population?
    a. substance abuse
    b. poverty
    c. psychological abuse
    d. all of the above

38. Which of the following is NOT related to depression among the elderly?
    a. living independently
    b. needing help with activities of daily living
    c. loss of body functions
    d. changes in appearance

39. Which of the following would be a form of neglect among the elderly?
    a. exploitation of the elderly person's finances
    b. restraint
    c. food deprivation
    d. degrading comments

40. Which of the following may prevent an elderly person from reporting or admitting to being abused or neglected?
    a. altered mental status
    b. fear of retribution
    c. shame or embarrassment
    d. all of the above

41. Which of the following conditions in the elderly may result from living on a limited income?
    a. injuries in the home
    b. environmental emergencies
    c. malnutrition
    d. all of the above

42. Which of the following is NOT a common illness or injury among the elderly population?
    a. measles
    b. trauma
    c. aneurysm
    d. diabetes

43. Which of the following is NOT an injury-prevention measure in the home of an elderly person?
    a. installation of smoke detectors
    b. reducing the hot water temperature
    c. using throw rugs on hard tile or vinyl floors
    d. installing railings on steps and stairways

44. Which of the following should be part of the scene size-up when responding to an elderly patient?
    a. looking for indications of violence or potential violence
    b. looking for household hazards
    c. noticing the temperature of the environment
    d. all of the above

45. You have just introduced yourself to a 71-year-old female. She responds with, "My name is Inez Goldsmith." You should then address her as:
    a. Inez.
    b. Mrs. Goldsmith.
    c. Sweetie.
    d. Any of the above is acceptable.

46. You have just introduced yourself to an 87-year-old male patient. He responds with, "What's that? I can't hear you." All of the following would be appropriate EXCEPT:
    a. making sure the patient can see your face when you speak.
    b. asking if the patient has a hearing aid.
    c. turning off any background noise, such as a radio or television.
    d. shouting.

47. Your 85-year-old female patient is obviously short of breath but is refusing to be transported to the hospital. Which of the following should you do FIRST?
    a. Find out if a family member has power of attorney to consent to the patient's transport.
    b. Contact medical direction for advice.
    c. Find out why the patient does not want to go to the hospital.
    d. Have the patient sign a refusal of treatment and transport form.

48. Which of the following may hamper the history and physical examination of the elderly patient?
    a. They often respond to a question so quickly that you need to ask them to slow down.
    b. They may not exhibit the expected signs and symptoms of an illness.
    c. In general, they are not able to give a reliable history.
    d. Pain is not an important finding or complaint in the elderly patient.

49. Failure to provide adequate padding when immobilizing an elderly patient on a long backboard may result in which of the following?
    a. abnormal positioning of the spine
    b. increased pain
    c. bed sores
    d. all of the above

50. When maintaining the airway and ventilating an unresponsive elderly patient, all of the following may be necessary EXCEPT:
    a. padding under the head.
    b. keeping dentures in place.
    c. taking dentures out.
    d. extreme hyperextension of the neck.

51. Your patient is a 16-month-old female who has experienced a seizure. She takes no medications, has no significant past medical history, and has no signs of trauma. Which of the following questions is most meaningful in this patient's history?
    a. "Was the patient born full-term?"
    b. "Has the patient had a fever or illness recently?"
    c. "Does the patient have any allergies?"
    d. "Is there a family history of seizures?"

52. Your patient is a 12-year-old male with a history of asthma. He experienced the onset of an asthma attack while at football practice. He is awake, noticeably short of breath with audible wheezing, use of accessory muscles, and a respiratory rate of 28. Which of the following is correct in the management of this patient?
    a. Assist the patient with his metered-dose inhaler, if he has one with him.
    b. Contact the parents before taking any other action.
    c. Insert an oropharyngeal airway and begin BVM ventilations.
    d. Transport but do not initiate treatment unless you are able to contact the parents.

53. Your patient is a 4-year-old female who was run over by a vehicle as she was playing in her driveway. The patient has a capillary refill time of 3 seconds. The most likely explanation for and safest assumption about this finding is:
    a. She is hypothermic.
    b. This refill time is normal for a 4-year-old.
    c. She has internal injuries.
    d. She is frightened.

54. Your patient is a 78-year-old male who was the unrestrained driver of a classic car (no airbags) that struck a tree. There is about 12 inches of intrusion into the hood. The patient is awake, seems "dazed" (awake, but not exactly sure what happened), has dry, cool skin, a heart rate of 72, and respirations of 24. You note that your patient has an irregular pulse. Which of the following statements about this patient is/are true?
    1. An irregular heart beat is not unusual in elderly patients and is nothing to worry about.
    2. Given his presentation, there is no reason to suspect internal hemorrhage.
    3. The patient may be hypoperfusing.
    4. The patient may have a cardiac injury due to the collision.
    a. 1, 2
    b. 2, 4
    c. 3
    d. 3, 4

55. Your patient is an 80-year-old female resident of an extended care facility. Facility staff called 911 to report that the patient had fallen out of bed. The patient is agitated and combative. She has a hematoma on her forehead, a deformity of her right forearm, and a large skin tear on the back of her right hand. Which of the following statements concerning this situation is/are true?
    1. The patient may have fallen out of bed because she was agitated.
    2. The patient may be agitated because she received a head injury when she fell.
    3. The facility staff may have abused the patient because of her agitation.
    4. Agitation is a normal finding for this age group and not likely related to the current situation.
    a. 4
    b. 1, 4
    c. 1, 2, 3
    d. 1, 2

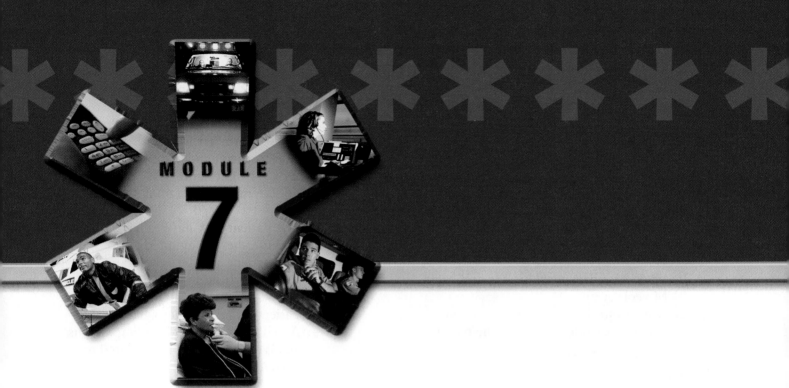

MODULE
7

Operations

“ *I didn't know where to start . . . then all at once I remembered something my instructor told me. She said, 'Start where you stand.' So I did. I began to triage.* ”

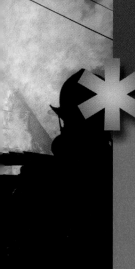

Module Outline

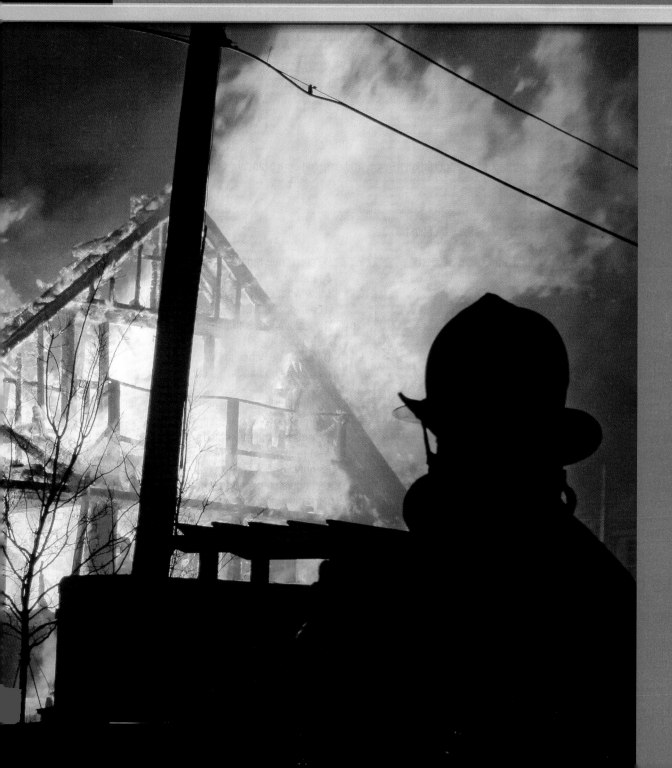

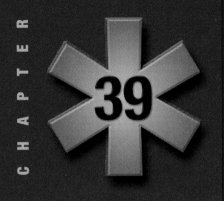

Operating and Maintaining Your Ambulance

39

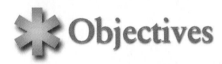

Objectives

Numbered objectives are from the U.S. Department of Transportation 1994 EMT-Basic National Standard Curriculum.

COGNITIVE OBJECTIVES

At the completion of this lesson, the EMT-Basic student will be able to:

7-1.1 Discuss the medical and nonmedical equipment needed to respond to a call. (pp. 976–983)

7-1.2 List the phases of an ambulance call. (p. 976)

7-1.3 Describe the general provisions of state laws relating to the operation of the ambulance and privileges in any or all of the following categories: (pp. 989–993)
- Speed
- Warning lights
- Sirens
- Right-of-way
- Parking
- Turning

7-1.4 List contributing factors to unsafe driving conditions. (p. 990)

7-1.5 Describe the considerations that should be given to: (pp. 990–991)
- Request for escorts
- Following an escort vehicle
- Intersections

7-1.6 Discuss "due regard for the safety of all others" while operating an emergency vehicle. (p. 989)

7-1.7 State what information is essential in order to respond to a call. (pp. 986–987)

7-1.8 Discuss various situations that may affect response to a call. (pp. 990–991)

7-1.9 Differentiate between the various methods of moving a patient to the unit based upon injury or illness. (pp. 993–996)

7-1.10 Apply the components of the essential patient information in a written report. (p. 998)

7-1.11 Summarize the importance of preparing the unit for the next response. (p. 998)

7-1.12 Identify what is essential for completion of a call. (p. 998)

7-1.13 Distinguish among the terms cleaning, disinfection, high-level disinfection, and sterilization. (p. 998)

7-1.14 Describe how to clean or disinfect items following patient care. (pp. 998–1001)

AFFECTIVE OBJECTIVES

At the completion of this lesson, the EMT-Basic student will be able to:

7-1.15 Explain the rationale for appropriate report of patient information. (pp. 955–998)

7-1.16 Explain the rationale for having the unit prepared to respond. (pp. 975, 976)

PSYCHOMOTOR OBJECTIVES

No psychomotor objectives identified.

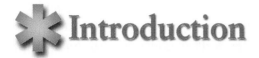

Introduction

Perhaps not as exciting as some of the assessment or clinical chapters, the *material in this chapter will be used on every call.* As a matter of fact, without the preparation discussed in this chapter, the more exciting calls can go poorly. Your ability to be ready at any time for any call with clean, charged, and properly functioning equipment is vital to that mission.

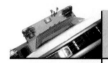

Emergency Dispatch

"Quick, turn up the portable," EMT Rollie Engmeyer said to his partner Marianne. "I think they just called us."

"Oops, sorry," She grinned and adjusted the radio volume before answering the dispatcher.

"Three-three," the dispatcher said. "I need you to respond code three to a rollover MVA on the I-77 service road just south of Vintner."

"10–4 we're on our way," Marianne said as they hurried to the ambulance.

"First call of the day, and it's a good one!" Rollie hit the lights and siren and inched out into the heavy morning traffic.

The cars, full of well-dressed, coffee-sipping people on their way to the financial district, pulled this way and that in front of the ambulance but never quite cleared the way. The drivers' heads were shooting from side to side with confused looks on their faces.

"Come on! Move!" Rollie shouted over the siren, hitting the air horn several times. "How difficult is it to just pull to the right?"

"This is weird," Marianne looked at the clotted traffic. "It's almost like . . . hmm."

"Like what?" Rollie pressed and held the air horn button in an attempt to get the attention of the cars in front of him.

"Like they don't know where we are." Marianne moved her spotlight to look for reflection of the emergency lights in the chrome. Nothing. "We've got no emergency lights."

"What?" Rollie shouted, flipping the console switch off and on. "Look again."

"Still nothing," Marianne said. "Did you check the lights when we got the truck?"

"Yes, I checked the lights!"

Phases of the Ambulance Call

7-1.2 List the phases of an ambulance call.

Each time you report for duty and respond to a call, there is a specific sequence of events that occurs. This can be referred to as the *phases of an ambulance call.* These phases are:

＊ **Preparing for the Call**—You must check and restock the supplies and equipment you may use during your shift as well as check the ambulance for readiness.

＊ **Receiving and Responding to the Call**—The emergency medical dispatcher (EMD) relays important information about the call and provides instructions to the caller. You must operate your vehicle safely and with due regard to others.

＊ **Transferring the Patient to the Ambulance**—After you assess your patient, make important decisions, and provide care, you will transfer the patient to the ambulance. This must be done safely, efficiently, and with regard to the patient's condition.

＊ **Transporting to the Hospital**—The patient in the ambulance is transported to the hospital—sometimes with lights and sirens, sometimes not. In any event, operation of the emergency vehicle must be done with regard to safety. The emergency vehicle operator must also be aware of the ongoing patient care and how operation of the vehicle can affect the care.

＊ **Transferring the Patient to Hospital Staff**—The patient is brought into the hospital and care is transferred to the hospital personnel. This involves transfer of important patient information as well as physically transferring the patient from your stretcher to the hospital gurney.

＊ **Terminating the Call**—After transferring the patient the final stages of the call involve completing your documentation, cleaning and disinfecting equipment, and restocking the ambulance.

The remaining sections of this chapter will discuss each of these phases in detail.

Preparing for the Call

7-1.1 Discuss the medical and nonmedical equipment needed to respond to a call.

Simply stated: Your ambulance has a lot of equipment. Much of this you have spent quite a bit of time on in class (e.g., airway supplies and equipment for taking vital signs). Other things, for example, triage tags and the OB kit, you most likely saw in only one or two classes. The EMT must be familiar with all of this equipment, know its proper place on the ambulance, and how to use it. Table 39-1 is a detailed list of equipment carried on most ambulances.

Some of this equipment includes basic first aid supplies such as bandages and splints. Since not all patients are able to walk, due to their injury or illness, items such as scoop stretchers, stair chairs, long backboards, and other items for moving patients from the incident to the stretcher will be needed.

Specific equipment to provide airway control such as oro- and nasopharyngeal airways must be included as well as portable and mounted suction units to remove fluids that could occlude the patient's airway. Along these same lines, devices like the pocket face mask and bag-valve-mask devices will be important. Oxygen masks and nasal cannulas for both adult and pediatric patients should also be a part of your oxygen delivery system.

TABLE 39-1 PATIENT INFECTION CONTROL, COMFORT, AND PROTECTION SUPPLIES

The following supplies should be carried in the ambulance:
* Two pillows
* Four pillow cases
* Two spare sheets
* Four blankets
* Six disposable emesis (vomit) bags or basins
* Two boxes of facial tissues
* Disposable bedpan, urinal, and toilet paper
* One package of drinking cups
* One package of wet wipes
* Four liters of sterile water or saline
* Four soft restraining devices (upper and lower extremities)
* Packages of large and small red biohazard bags for waste or severed parts
* One package of large yellow bags for used linens or garbage (or otherwise color-coded or labeled according to your service's Exposure Control Plan)
* EPA-registered, intermediate-level disinfectant (which destroys mycobacterium tuberculosis)
* EPA-registered, low-level disinfectant such as Lysol
* An empty plastic spray bottle with lines at the 1:100 level, a plastic bottle of water, and a plastic bottle of bleach for cleaning up blood spills (Measure a fresh mixture of 1 part bleach to 100 parts water each day as needed.)
* Eye shields or other protective eyewear for each crew member
* Sharps container for the vehicle (BLS or ALS unit) and (for ALS unit) drug box
* Disposable latex, vinyl, or other synthetic gloves: a box of each size
* N-95 or HEPA respirator for each crew member

INITIAL AND FOCUSED ASSESSMENT EQUIPMENT

Portable first-in kits come in all shapes and sizes, in hard cases or soft bags. A first-in kit should include supplies for:
* *Airway.* Airways, suction, infection control, personal protective equipment; if permitted for EMT use by local protocols, equipment for adult and pediatric orotracheal intubation
* *Breathing.* Stethoscope, pocket mask with one-way valve and oxygen inlet, bag-valve mask, oxygen, oxygen delivery devices
* *Circulation.* Blood pressure cuff, bandages and dressings, occlusive dressings, automated external defibrillator (AED)
* *Neck and spine stabilization.* Set of rigid cervical collars
* *Exposure.* Scissors and blankets to expose and deal with exposure

(continued)

TABLE 39-1 *CONTINUED*

∗ *Vital signs:*
- Sphygmomanometer kit with separate cuffs for average-size and obese adults as well as child sizes
- Adult and pediatric stethoscope
- Thermometer and a hypothermia thermometer that goes down to at least 82° Fahrenheit
- One penlight
- Many services carry a pocket guide with pediatric vitals and other quick resource information.

EQUIPMENT FOR TRANSFER OF PATIENT

The following carrying devices should be included:

∗ Wheeled ambulance stretcher is designed so that a sick or injured person can be transported in the Fowler's (sitting), supine, or Trendelenburg position. Also called a cot or gurney, the wheeled stretcher should have a number of features. It should be adjustable in height and have detachable supports for intravenous fluid containers. Restraining devices should be provided so that a patient can be prevented from falling off the stretcher or sliding past the foot end or head end.

∗ Reeves stretcher for carrying a patient who must lie supine down stairs when a cot is too heavy or wide

∗ Folding stair chair for moving patients down stairs in a sitting position

∗ Scoop stretcher, also called an orthopedic stretcher, for picking up patients found in tight spaces with a minimum of movement

∗ Stokes or basket stretcher for long-distance carries, high-angle, or off-the-road rescues

∗ Child safety seat for transporting infants and small children in the ambulance (optional)

EQUIPMENT FOR AIRWAY MAINTENANCE, VENTILATION, AND RESUSCITATION

A number of devices should be carried for maintaining an open airway and assisting breathing:

∗ Oropharyngeal airways in sizes suitable for adults, children, and infants

∗ Soft rubber nasopharyngeal airways in sizes 14 through 30

∗ Two pocket face masks with one-way valves and filters for times when ventilation is necessary or when you are the only person ventilating a patient who does not have an endotracheal tube inserted

∗ Three manually operated, self-refilling bag-valve-mask units (infant, child, adult) capable of delivering 100 percent oxygen to a patient by the addition of a reservoir. Masks of various sizes should be designed to ensure a tight face seal and should have an air cushion. The masks should be clear so you can see vomitus and the clouding caused by exhalations.

TABLE 39-1   *CONTINUED*

OXYGEN THERAPY AND SUCTION EQUIPMENT

An ambulance should have two oxygen supply systems (one fixed, one portable) so oxygen can be supplied to two patients at once:

* Fixed oxygen delivery system supplies oxygen to a patient in the ambulance. A typical installation consists of a minimum 3,000-liter reservoir, a two-stage regulator, plus yokes, reducing valve, and non-gravity-type flow meter. Oxygen delivery tubes, transparent masks, and controls should all be located within easy reach when you are sitting at the patient's head. The system should be capable of delivering at least 15 liters of oxygen per minute and adaptable to the bag-valve-mask units carried on the ambulance.

* Two portable oxygen delivery systems that have a capacity of at least 350 liters. Each system should have a regulator capable of delivering at least 15 liters of oxygen per minute. Many ambulances are equipped with multiple-function regulators that can be used for liter-flow oxygen, suctioning, and positive pressure ventilation. In addition, an ambulance should have the following:

* Spare D, E, or jumbo D oxygen cylinders with a current hydrostat test date seal imprinted on the tank

* Six adult and four pediatric nonrebreather masks

* Six adult and four pediatric nasal cannulas

* One flow-restricted, oxygen-powered ventilation device

* One automatic transport ventilator (ATV) (optional)

* One plastic comic cup for administering blow-by oxygen to a child

The fixed suction system should be sufficient to provide an air flow of over 30 liters per minute at the end of the delivery tube. A vacuum of at least 300 mmHg should be reached within 4 seconds after the suction tube is clamped. The suction should be controllable. The installed system should have a large-diameter, nonkinking tube fitted with a rigid tip. There should be a spare nonbreakable, disposable suction bottle and a container of water for rinsing the tubes. There should be an assortment of sterile catheters. The suction system should be usable by a person seated at the head of the patient.

The portable suction unit can be one of the many models powered by battery, hand or foot action, oxygen, or compressed air. The unit should be fitted with a nonkinking tube as well as a large-bore Yankauer tip.

EQUIPMENT FOR CARDIAC RESUSCITATION

The following equipment for assisting with cardiopulmonary resuscitation and defibrillation should be carried on the ambulance:

* Short or long spine board to provide rigid support during CPR efforts

* An automated external defibrillator (AED)

(continued)

TABLE 39-1 *CONTINUED*

SUPPLIES AND EQUIPMENT FOR IMMOBILIZATION OF SUSPECTED BONE INJURIES

The ambulance should carry a variety of devices for immobilization of injured extremities and suspected spine injuries:

* Adult and pediatric traction splints (e.g., Sager or Hare) for the immobilization of a painful, swollen, or deformed thigh
* Padded board splints for the immobilization of upper and lower extremities. Recommended are 2 × 54-inch splints, 2 × 36-inch splints, and 2 × 15-inch splints.
* Variety of splints: air-inflatable splints, vacuum splints, wire ladder splints, cardboard splints, soft rubberized splints with aluminum stays and Velcro fasteners, padded aluminum (SAM) splints, and splints that are inflated with cryogenic (cold) gas
* Tongue depressors to use to immobilize broken fingers
* Triangular bandages for use with splints and for making slings and swathes
* Several rolls of self-adhering roller bandage for securing the various splints
* Six chemical cold packs for use on injured extremities
* Two long spine boards for full-body immobilization, preferably with speed clips or Velcro straps. The long spine board can also be used for patient transfer
* Rigid cervical collars in a variety of adult and child sizes
* One KED, XP1, Kansas Board, or LSP halfback board for seated persons with possible spinal injuries
* Six 9-foot-by-2-inch web straps with air-craft-style buckles or D-rings for securing patients to carrying devices
* Head immobilizer device such as the Headbed, Bashaw CID, Ferno Head Immobilizer, or a rolled blanket

SUPPLIES FOR WOUND CARE AND TREATMENT OF SHOCK

A variety of dressings and bandaging materials should be carried on the ambulance:

* Sterile gauze pads (2 × 2 inches and 4 × 4 inches)
* 5 × 9 inch combine dressings
* Sterile universal dressings (multi-trauma dressings) approximately 10 × 36 inches
* Self-adhering roller bandages in 4- and 6-inch width × 5 yards
* Occlusive dressings (Vaseline gauze) for sealing open (sucking) chest wounds and eviscerations
* Aluminum foil (sterilized in a separate package) for various uses such as occlusive dressings and also to maintain body heat or to form an oxygen tent for a newborn infant
* Sterile burn sheets or prepackaged burn kit

TABLE 39-1 *CONTINUED*

* Adhesive strip bandages for minor wound care 1 × 3/4 inch and 1 × 1/2 inch), individually packaged
* Hypoallergenic adhesive tape (1- and 3-inch rolls)
* Large safety pins for the securing of slings and swathes
* Bandage scissors
* Pneumatic anti-shock garments (PASG) in sizes for adults and children
* Aluminum blankets (survival blankets) for maintaining body heat

SUPPLIES FOR CHILDBIRTH

A sterile childbirth kit, either provided by a local medical facility or a commercially available disposable kit, as mandated by your system, should contain the following:

* Several pairs of sterile surgical gloves
* Four umbilical cord clamps
* One pair of sterile surgical scissors
* One rubber bulb syringe (3 oz.)
* Twelve 4 × 4 inch gauze pads
* Four pairs of sterile disposable gloves
* Five towels
* One baby blanket (receiving blanket)
* Infant swaddler
* Sanitary napkins
* Two large plastic bags
* Two stockinet infant caps

Also carry items that you can wear to minimize contamination of or by the mother and baby during and after childbirth:

* Two surgical gowns
* Two surgical caps
* Two surgical masks
* Two pairs of goggles or eye shields

SUPPLIES, EQUIPMENT, AND MEDICATIONS FOR THE TREATMENT OF ACUTE POISONING, SNAKEBITE, CHEMICAL BURNS, AND DIABETIC EMERGENCIES

A number of poison control kits are available from emergency care equipment suppliers. Whether purchased intact or hand-made, a poison control kit should include these items:

* Drinking water to dilute poisons
* Activated charcoal
* Paper cups and other equipment for oral administration
* Equipment for irrigating a patient's eyes or skin with sterile water

(continued)

TABLE 39-1 *CONTINUED*

* Constriction bands for snakebites
* Instant glucose paste

SPECIAL EQUIPMENT FOR PARAMEDICS AND PHYSICIANS

Depending on state laws and your medical director, some ambulances are provided with locked kits of supplies and equipment that can be used by paramedics or physicians, especially in rural areas. This equipment may include supplies for:

* Endotracheal intubation, orotracheal and endotracheal suctioning, and pediatric nasogastric intubation (In some areas EMTs will be trained to perform these procedures.)
* Chest decompression
* Drug administration
* Advanced airways such as the esophageal obturator airway (EOA), esophageal gastric tube airway (EGTA), or Combitube airway
* Cricothyrotomy
* Cardiac monitoring and defibrillation

SAFETY AND MISCELLANEOUS EQUIPMENT

Ambulances should also be provided with personal protective equipment for you; equipment for warning, signaling, and lighting; hazard control devices; and tools for gaining access and disentanglements including:

* *North American Emergency Response Guidebook*
* Binoculars
* Clipboard, prehospital care reports (PCRs), and other documentation forms
* Ring cutter
* Portable radio
* Multiple-casualty incident management logs
* Triage tags and destination logs
* Command vests
* Tarps in red, green, black, and yellow for multiple-casualty incident field treatment areas
* Disposable Tyvek jumpsuits
* Flares
* Jumper cables
* Set of turnout gear (coat, helmet, protective eyewear, gloves) for each crew member
* Large floodlight/spotlight
* Concentrated sports drink (for example, Gatorade) and a cooler for rehabilitation sector (optional)
* Self-contained breathing apparatus (SCBA) (optional)

TABLE 39-1   *CONTINUED*

* Spring-loaded center punch
* Glas-Master or flathead ax
* Small sledge hammer, pry bar, Biel tool, and other tools for gaining access
* Wheel chocks
* Utility rope
* Stuffed animal for child patients

In addition to these items, an automated external defibrillator (AED) must be included in your ambulance. Early CPR and defibrillation are key to the survival of cardiac arrest, and the AED is an essential tool in this work. Less frequently used but important equipment such as an obstetric (OB) kit are also included.

Next, crews should have maps or street books to provide them with the ability to quickly find an address to which they are dispatched. Most states will require safety equipment such as fire extinguishers, road flares or cones, and tools to assist the crew in the event of a mechanical or other vehicle emergency.

Some agencies have begun to use GPS-based programs that provide on-board directions to calls. Some of these satellite-based systems also communicate with dispatch centers to identify ambulance locations, ensuring that the closest ambulance is dispatched to a call. Continue to carry maps or street books in case a GPS-based program isn't working.

CHECKING THE VEHICLE

The mechanical functioning of the ambulance and all systems should be checked at the beginning of every shift (Scan 39-1 on page 984). The ambulance transports you to each call and allows you to transport the patient to the hospital. Mechanical failures can be tragic.

At a minimum, the following items should be checked:

* Fuel
* Oil
* Engine cooling system
* Battery
* Brakes
* Wheels and tires
* Headlights
* Stoplights
* Turn signals
* Emergency warning lights
* Wipers
* Horn

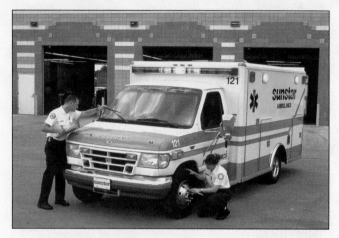

▲ Check the ambulance body, wheels, tires, and windshield wipers.

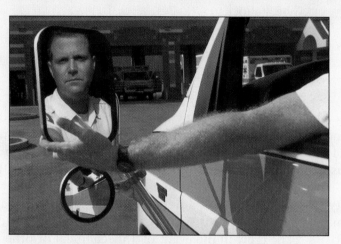

▲ Check windows, doors, and mirrors.

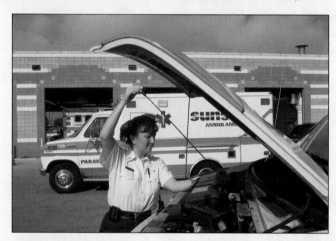

▲ Check all fluid levels.

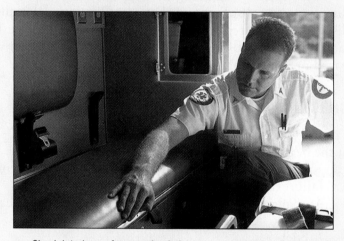

▲ Check interior surfaces and upholstery.

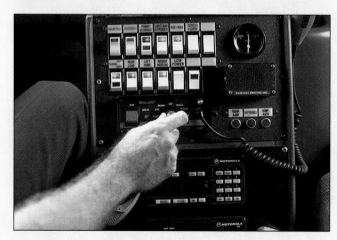

▲ Check dash instruments and communications equipment.

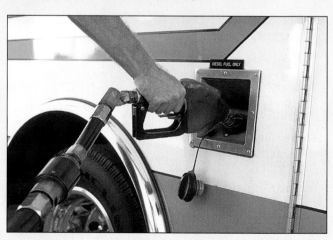

▲ Check the fuel level and fill up.

* Siren

* Doors closing and latching

* Communication system

* Air conditioning/heating system

* Ventilation system

Figure 39-1 is a sample vehicle checklist from Kennebunk Fire Rescue in Maine.

Finally, ambulances should be staffed according to state, regional, or local protocol, but at least one certified EMT should be available to treat the patient in the patient compartment. In many places a minimum of two is required and that is the preferred staffing level for basic life support ambulances. They must be available for emergency calls whether they are stationed at a rescue squad, fire department, or other station.

FIGURE 39-1 Truck check list. (Kennebunk Fire Rescue.)

RESCUE
CIRCLE ONE:

1   2   3

KEENEBUNK FIRE RESCUE
TRUCK CHECK SHEET

	SUN	MON	TUES	WED	THURS	FRI	SAT
DATE							
MILEAGE							
FUEL							
CHECK OIL							
WIPER FLUID							
LIGHTS IN/OUT							
HEAT/AC							
INTERIOR CABINETS							
EXTERIOR CABINETS							
MAIN O2 LEVEL							
PORTABLE O2 LEVEL							
PORTABLE O2 LEVEL							
SPARE TANKS X 3							
MONITOR							
DEFIB PADS, PAPER							
BATTERIES SWAPPED							
USER TEST COMPLETED							
IN-HOUSE SUCTION							
PORTABLE SUCTION							
BLS BAG							
ALS BAG							
PEDIATRIC BAG							
BURN KIT							
IV TRAY							
IV FLUID/EXP							
SIGN DRUG LOG							
CLOSET DRUG LOG							
SIGNATURE							
SIGNATURE							

COMMENTS, CONCERNS, QUESTIONS, PROBLEMS, DEFICIENCIES: _____
_____
_____

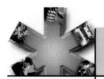

Perspective

Rollie—The EMT

"I can't believe that happened. The crew before us said the lights had cut out on them but had come back on. I tested them and they were OK this morning. Wait'll I see them. They should've done more testing before the next shift. Maybe because they didn't want to drive to the shop—or miss lunch or something—we couldn't get to the patient. But I get a trip to the repair shop and someone else took our call. Next time when it comes to lights, I'll be checking and rechecking. And we've got to work more like a team across shifts."

Receiving and Responding to the Call

7-1.7 State what information is essential in order to respond to a call.

The wheels of the EMS system begin spinning well before you hear the tones that signal your dispatch for a call.

The reporting party is able to dial 9–1–1 and access the closest communications center. Many EMS systems provide education to people in their community on warning signs of serious conditions and when and how to contact EMS. In the event of a cardiac arrest, your system's ongoing involvement in the community could ensure that CPR is being performed, a defibrillator is present, and EMS has been activated at the earliest possible moment.

EMERGENCY DISPATCH

The dispatcher is able to obtain key initial information from the caller including (Figure 39-2):

✳ The nature of the request for emergency assistance

✳ The location of the patient

✳ The call-back number at the location

FIGURE 39-2 Communications play a vital role in the Emergency Medical Services (EMS) system.

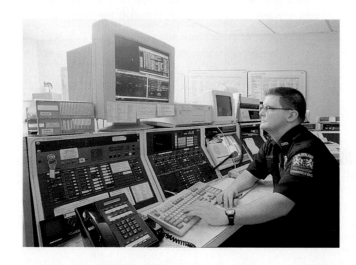

This information is critical in the event the caller loses consciousness or is disconnected from the dispatcher. Even though enhanced 9–1–1 centers display the number the patient is calling from, it is always verified to prevent errors in data entry or technology.

The dispatcher then begins to obtain information on the reason the patient (or family member, coworker, or bystander) called. A few additional focused questions are now asked of the caller. These include:

* Further information in reference to the nature of the call

* The current condition of the patient. For example, is he responsive and breathing?

* Are there hazards on the scene, such as pets, traffic, or a crime in progress?

* Will the EMTs be able to get to the patient in the current location? Are car or house doors unlocked? For an EMS call at an apartment complex or large building such as a factory, dispatchers will obtain detailed location information and instruct the caller to send someone to meet the ambulance.

These questions take a relatively short time. In a single-dispatcher center, the dispatcher will dispatch the ambulance to begin the response. In a multiple-dispatcher center, the call information will be transferred to another dispatcher who will dispatch the call while the original dispatcher stays on the line with the caller.

Some dispatch centers have a policy allowing dispatchers to provide pre-arrival instructions to callers. These instructions may include proper patient positioning, artificial ventilation and CPR, how to stop bleeding, and more. Emergency Medical Dispatchers providing this information receive special training and use a series of cards with prompts determining which questions to ask and the instruction to provide.

The information obtained by dispatchers will also help to determine the priority of EMS response, the need for first response (such as a local engine company for serious calls) and whether additional apparatus (for example, fire, heavy-rescue, or hazmat) will be required.

Dispatchers are a valuable asset to the EMS system. Their actions provide critical information which begins the EMS call in the most efficient way possible.

RESPONDING TO THE CALL

Responding to the call is the next phase of the EMS response. This is perhaps the most visible part of what we do. During the response, the crew should consider who will be responsible for what tasks at the scene. Based on the dispatch information, the crew may also discuss possible causes of the emergency. If your patient is experiencing chest pain, is that chest pain an acute myocardial infarction or angina or is it being caused by asthma or other trouble breathing? Did the patient fall down or get assaulted? Considering different reasons for the call will help prepare you for the questions you may want to ask on scene of the patient.

Additionally during the response, the crew should consider whether or not there are any scene hazards or need for police resources. One rule for crew protection states that if you call for police and stage away from the scene, do so at least two turns away from the incident so that if the dangerous incident starts to come to you, there will be time for you to get away.

Finally, inform your dispatcher that you are responding to the call. Upon your arrival on the scene notify the dispatcher of both your arrival and any specific information other units may need such as an updated address or obvious hazards.

Stop, Review, Remember!

Multiple Choice

Place a check next to the correct answer.

1. Which of the following is not a phase of the ambulance call?

_____ a. transfer to hospital staff

_____ b. preparing for the call

_____ c. training for the call

_____ d. transport to the hospital

2. Which level of training is designed to be the minimum level to staff an ambulance?

_____ a. First responder (Emergency Responder)

_____ b. EMT-Basic

_____ c. EMT-Intermediate

_____ d. EMT-Paramedic

3. Vehicle maintenance checks should be performed at least:

_____ a. daily. _____ c. biweekly.

_____ b. weekly. _____ d. monthly.

4. Specially trained dispatchers can instruct callers over the phone how to perform CPR.

_____ a. true

_____ b. false

5. The following is NOT an important part of the vehicle check.

_____ a. fuel level

_____ b. exterior surfaces

_____ c. wipers

_____ d. fluid levels

Matching

Match the event on the left with the phases of the ambulance call on the right.

1. _____ Moving the patient from your stretcher to the hospital gurney

2. _____ Placing the patient on your stretcher and wheeling it to the ambulance

3. _____ Your morning vehicle checks

4. _____ Completing your documentation

5. _____ Disinfecting the ambulance after an MVC with a patient bleeding

6. _____ Driving to the hospital

7. _____ Stocking the rig after a call

8. _____ The dispatcher radios you with a call

9. _____ Verbally advising the hospital staff about your patient

A. Preparing for the call
B. Receiving and responding to the call
C. Transferring the patient to the ambulance
D. Transport to the hospital
E. Transfer to hospital staff
F. Terminating the call

Critical Thinking

1. You are in a patient's home working a cardiac arrest. You reach for the suction and find that the battery is dead. What do you do? Why did this happen?

   _____

   _____

   _____

   _____

2. The emergency medical dispatcher gets a few pieces of information initially. These include the patient's location, the complaint, and the callback number. They are very important. Why?

   _____

   _____

   _____

   _____

OPERATING AN EMERGENCY VEHICLE

Responding to a call in your ambulance is performed daily. This can be one of the more dangerous tasks performed by EMTs, and extreme care must be used during the response. Many states require that EMTs who operate ambulances on state roads have completed a state-approved driver's course that covers topics such as road hazards, defensive driving, and weather-related traffic issues.

In most states, **warning lights** and **sirens** on an ambulance are allowed to be operated when responding to a call or responding from the scene to the hospital. In some cases, the lights and sirens provide the ambulance driver a **right of way**, or permission to travel through traffic without delay. Some states will allow ambulance drivers going to the scene or leaving for the hospital to use the shoulder, restricted lanes, and other privileges not accorded to nonemergency drivers. However, the lights and sirens of your ambulance never give you a free pass to drive recklessly or at a high rate of speed through traffic. Since each state is different, EMT students should research their local and state rules on these matters before attempting to drive an ambulance.

The term **due regard** (or *due caution*) for the safety of others is the term often used to describe the responsibility of the emergency vehicle operator. Ambulances must not be operated recklessly. Ambulance collisions are a cause of injury and death to EMS providers—and a cause of lawsuits against EMS systems and the operators themselves. Excess speed, failure to use caution at intersections (especially when proceeding against a red light), and operating in poor weather conditions are significant causes of crashes—and the liability that follows.

Ambulances are far too often involved in line-of-duty deaths. The ambulance operator should operate the vehicle in a calm, relaxed manner. Be sure to allow for adequate reaction time (between 4 and 12 seconds) to react in an appropriate and

7-1.3 Describe the general provisions of state laws relating to the operation of the ambulance and privileges in any or all of the following categories:
- Speed
- Warning lights
- Sirens
- Right-of-way
- Parking
- Turning

* **warning lights**

  visual warning devices used on an emergency vehicle.

* **sirens**

  audible warning devices used on an emergency vehicle.

* **right of way**

  permission to travel through traffic without delay.

7-1.6 Discuss "due regard for the safety of all others" while operating an emergency vehicle.

* **due regard**

  functioning in a manner that is precise, cautious, and does not injure anyone else; also called *due caution*.

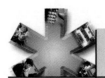

Perspective

Marianne—The EMT

"I was trying to shrink into my seat as all those people were glaring and shouting at us. We stupidly tried to drive through a big glut of cars that didn't even know where we were. This kind of thing just cannot happen. And it's a safety issue for everyone involved! Any time lost getting to the patient is wrong. Just plain wrong."

7-1.4 List contributing factors to unsafe driving conditions.

7-1.8 Discuss various situations that may affect response to a call.

safe manner (e.g., when a car pulls out in front of you or fails to yield to your lights and siren). Remember that few of the calls we respond to are true life-threatening emergencies. Therefore, there is no reason for us to create a life-threatening emergency by responding in an unsafe manner.

Other factors that can contribute to collisions include poor weather conditions, heavy traffic, and smaller roadways such as those found in construction areas, on bridges, and in tunnels. The time of day and day of the week will likely play a role in safety too. For example, cities experience peak traffic during rush hours Monday through Friday. During the day there may be an increase in pedestrian traffic in some areas.

Weather—including rain, snow, sleet, and ice storms—can both limit visibility and make the road surface slippery, causing longer stopping distances.

Heavy traffic and traffic back-ups can change the availability of lanes for turns. Drivers may also stop in the driving lane because they have nowhere to pull over to let you pass.

Construction areas, bridges, and tunnels all have smaller lanes associated with them. They can make driving, turning, and operating your vehicle an increased challenge. The prepared ambulance operator will know of construction plans in his area and will know alternate routes to get to various locations and hospitals without going through these highly congested areas.

Even simple, nonemergent actions such as turning (which requires a much larger radius than for typical vehicles), or simply backing up the ambulance and parking, are all situations where the ambulance has limited visibility for the driver, making accidents more likely. Use a spotter (Figure 39-3) when backing to prevent accidents.

SPECIFIC DRIVING SITUATIONS

7-1.5 Describe the considerations that should be given to:
- Request for escorts
- Following an escort vehicle
- Intersections

In general, ambulances should not receive escorts to the hospital. This is because the danger of the procedure usually outweighs the benefits. Motorists will see one vehicle moving through an intersection and think that it is safe to proceed, never expecting the second vehicle to come through. It is the vehicle being escorted that usually ends up in a collision.

In very few cases are escorts warranted. Some examples of appropriate escorts might include if the driver is lost in an unfamiliar district or if the ambulance is transporting a priority patient and loses power to its warning devices, including the sirens and warning lights.

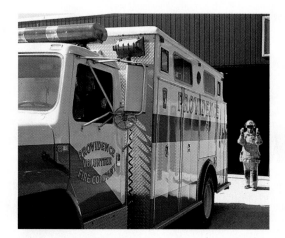

FIGURE 39-3 Use a spotter to help guide the ambulance when backing up.

When following an escort vehicle, give the lead vehicle appropriate distance to navigate through traffic without becoming involved in a collision should they have to stop suddenly. Use the warning systems you have available to you (if any), and drive much more cautiously.

Intersections are another problem area. When responding to a call with a stop sign or red light at an intersection, ambulance operators should stop and check both directions prior to entering the intersection. Many times traffic will hear an ambulance but not see it and will race through intersections hoping to beat the ambulance wherever it is going. It does your patient no good if you do not make it to the call or wind up going to the hospital with them.

Another problem with intersections is that separate emergency units may be responding to a call from different directions. In these cases, an emergency vehicle that does not stop for the red light may inadvertently hit another emergency responder. This creates a two-fold problem as two units responding to the incident are now unavailable, their crews possibly injured, and the original call is still in place but understaffed.

If you know that multiple units have been dispatched to a call and will be traveling through the same intersection, use the radio to notify other units that you are approaching the intersection. Use additional caution as you approach the intersection, as your siren will drown out the sirens of other emergency vehicles.

Every ambulance is marked with a visual display for the organization that operates that ambulance. Reckless behavior and collisions involving ambulances are disastrous for these organizations from a public relations and public trust perspective, even when it is not the ambulance operator who was at fault and even when nobody is hurt. The public takes note of how you operate your vehicle, and it will reflect on both you and your organization.

PARKING AT EMERGENCY SCENES

Parking at an emergency scene, entails many considerations. When responding to calls at residences or businesses, you will park in a place clear of traffic. The position you choose should be convenient to the scene in the event a crew member needs additional equipment and because transfer of the patient between the scene and ambulance should be over the shortest distance safely possible.

When responding to motor vehicle collisions, the ambulance operator will want to park at least 100 feet away from the collision (Figure 39-4 on page 992). This can be one hundred feet in front of or behind the accident.

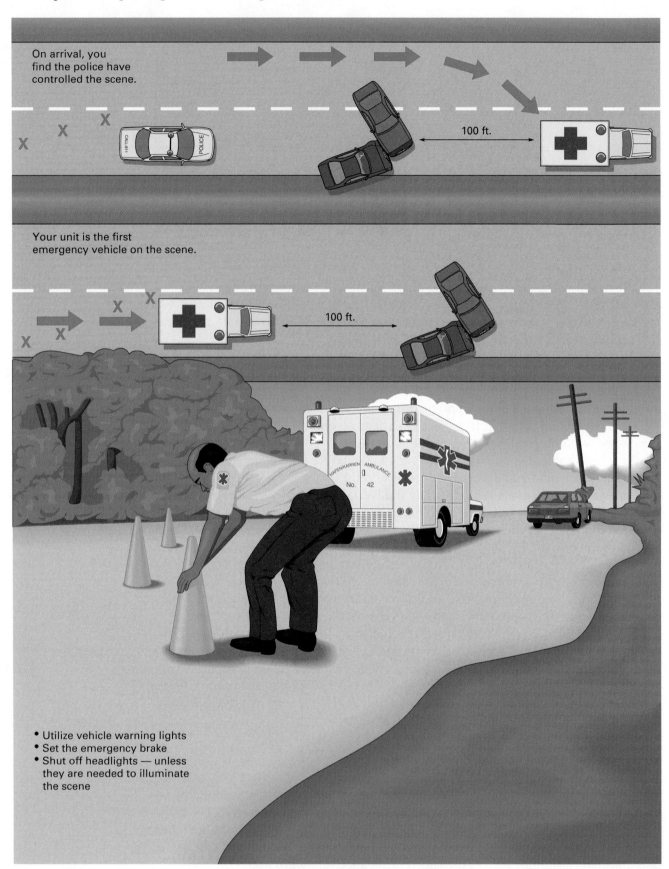

On arrival, you find the police have controlled the scene.

100 ft.

Your unit is the first emergency vehicle on the scene.

100 ft.

- Utilize vehicle warning lights
- Set the emergency brake
- Shut off headlights — unless they are needed to illuminate the scene

FIGURE 39-4 Proper procedure when arriving on the scene.

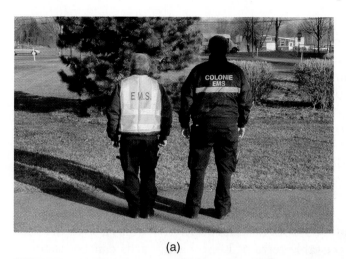
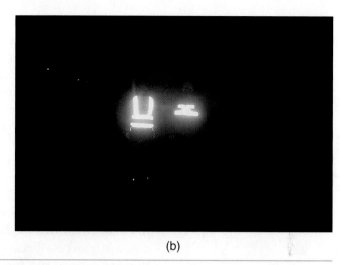

(a)   (b)

FIGURE 39-5   EMTs working in traffic should be dressed for both daytime and nighttime visibility. Photo (a) shows EMTs dressed for daytime visibility. Photo (b) shows how the same clothing would appear in approaching headlights at night. (Both: Jon Politis.)

If you elect to park behind the collision (between oncoming traffic and the collision) because you are the first vehicle on scene, additional care must be given to traffic coming up from behind. Traffic cones or reflective devices should be set up to direct traffic away from the collision scene and give direction to oncoming drivers of the need to change lanes away from where you are working. If the collision scene is over the crest of a hill or beyond a curve, you must place warning devices at the other side of the hill or curve to allow proper stopping time for approaching vehicles.

If you park in front of the collision with other vehicles, maintain the 100-foot safety distance. In the event that someone strikes the police or collision vehicles, they will not be pushed into your ambulance.

Whether you park in front of or behind the collision scene, extreme caution must be used. Motorists are often watching the collision scene and not paying attention to activities in the roadway. Add inattention from cellular phones and other in-car distractions to this mix and it is quite possible that you or your ambulance could be struck at a roadside scene. Be sure all personnel wear reflective vests (Figure 39-5) at roadside scenes.

In situations involving hazardous materials, park approximately one-half a mile away from the incident. Park your ambulance uphill and upwind of a hazardous materials scene to avoid becoming sick from noxious or otherwise dangerous chemicals. Use binoculars to survey the scene from a distance before approaching. Further information on hazardous materials can be found in chapter 42, Responses Involving Hazardous Materials.

At incidents that are not motor vehicle collisions or hazmat spills, the EMS crew should still fully consider the possibility of the scene becoming unstable and park the vehicle to provide for a rapid exit if needed.

Transferring the Patient to the Ambulance

Multiple ways are available to the EMT and ambulance crew to move patients. The method selected will depend on terrain and the condition of the patient.

The stretcher is a mobile bedlike device that can be used to move patients in a supine or semisitting position across flat distances. It should be used with caution, as it may easily tip over due to the high center of gravity when wheeled with the

7-1.9   Differentiate between the various methods of moving a patient to the unit based upon injury or illness.

patient in the elevated position. One safety consideration is to only use stretchers when you can keep the wheels on the floor or ground; otherwise, there is likely a better way to move the patient.

The stair chair, as the name implies, works particularly well over stairs. The stair chair is for patients who will be sitting or semisitting during transport but who need to be moved down steps prior to being placed on the stretcher. See chapter 5 for more information on the stair chair.

Unconscious patients or those being transported supine can be moved using any number of devices including long backboards, scoop stretchers, and Reeves stretchers. Each of these devices has its own benefits and drawbacks that must be considered before their use.

The Reeves stretcher is a flexible, hard plastic, litter-type stretcher that can move unconscious medical patients from upstairs and across areas a stretcher cannot easily access because of unstable terrain. Long backboards can be useful in these situations too but sometimes require additional time to get the patient fully secured to the board.

Once the patient is loaded into the ambulance and secured with seatbelt straps, you will be ready to go to the hospital. Before departing for the receiving hospital, secure any loose equipment, such as oxygen cylinders or pulse oximetry devices. Make sure that any family member who is riding with the patient is secured in the appropriate position in the ambulance per your local guidelines. The ambulance operator should drive to the hospital in such a way as to create a sense of comfort for the patient. Remember, in many cases the patient is not in a typical riding position but is either semisitting or supine and *backwards*. The driver should keep this in mind as he departs for the receiving facility. As you leave the scene, once again notify dispatch of your change in status. They should know your unit identifier, where you are going, how many patients you are transporting, and your mode of transport—with or without lights and sirens.

Transporting the Patient to the Hospital

Transport to the hospital is performed with the same due regard as discussed earlier. The difference is that during response to the hospital the vehicle will be operated while there are a patient and crew in the patient compartment. If you allow a family member to ride in the ambulance (often in the front seat), this may cause a distraction to you. The rider may also have anxieties caused by a lights-and-siren response.

The ride in the back of the ambulance is much different than the ride the driver will experience. The center of gravity for those in the patient compartment is high. This causes considerable swaying of the box, which can throw EMTs around. It is safest for EMTs to remain seated and belted during the trip to the hospital. Many times this is not possible, for example when CPR and airway maneuvers must be performed or when moving close to the patient to obtain vital signs. When not belted, the EMT should have "three points" anchored in the ambulance. For example, if you are standing to adjust the oxygen flow rate, you should have both feet on the floor and one hand holding onto the grab rail above the patient.

TRANSPORTING THE PATIENT

There are many important steps to be taken en route to the hospital (Scan 39-2 on page 996). The patient should be belted to the stretcher. The stretcher should be properly secured to the ambulance by the mounting system on the floor. Be sure to check this system periodically to ensure that all connecting bolts and latches are secure.

The ride for the patient also has its share of discomforts. Since the patient will be supine on the stretcher (sometimes on a rigid backboard), sitting, or somewhere in between, there is a significant portion of the patient in contact with the ambulance floor (via the stretcher). When we EMTs ride in the ambulance, our buttocks touch the seat or bench. A supine patient on a backboard feels bumps in the road over his entire body through a rigid piece of plastic.

The patient also acutely feels any swerves or quick turns in an exaggerated fashion. Be sure to avoid last minute turns, lane changes, and abrupt stops unless necessary to avoid a collision.

Perform ongoing assessments en route to the hospital. These are performed at least every 5 minutes for the unstable patient and at least every 15 minutes for the stable patient. During this assessment be sure to check the oxygen, including transfer of the oxygen from the portable cylinder to the inboard oxygen unit.

Be sure to reassure the patient during transport. This will help calm the patient, who is likely anxious from the transport process in addition to the condition that caused his ride to the hospital.

You will also provide a radio or cell-phone call-in to the receiving hospital. The exact content of this report is covered in chapter 15, Communication in EMS. The report should paint the picture of the patient's condition (generally the patient's signs, symptoms, vital signs, and severity). Should the patient's condition change significantly en route, you should recontact the receiving hospital to advise them of the change.

Communication between the driver and the EMT in the patient compartment is also important en route to the hospital. The driver may need to notify the EMT in back of traffic delays or construction, poor road conditions, or mechanical problems with the ambulance. The EMT in the back may need to communicate changes in the patient's condition, requests to either begin or discontinue use of lights and sirens, or a request to pull to the side of the road in cases such as defibrillation, where the ambulance should be stopped to effectively analyze the heart rhythm.

Not all responses to the hospital require lights and sirens. When determining the need for lights and sirens consider:

* The condition of the patient (stable or unstable)

* The patient's injuries (e.g., bumps cause extreme pain in a fractured leg)

* The effect of lights and sirens on the patient's condition (e.g., anxiety worsening chest pain)

* The distance to be traveled

* The traffic along the route

* The type of roadway (e.g., highway, urban, rural)

TRANSFERRING THE PATIENT TO THE HOSPITAL STAFF

On arrival at the receiving location or hospital, the ambulance operator should inform dispatch so that they know the ambulance has reached its destination.

A core concept in transfer of care is to do so to a person with equal or higher training as your own. Failure to assure that patient care has been assumed by hospital staff would be considered **abandonment**—even though you left the patient at the hospital. An example of this situation would be sliding a patient over to a

* **abandonment**

leaving a patient after care has been initiated and before the patient has been transferred to someone with equal or greater medical training.

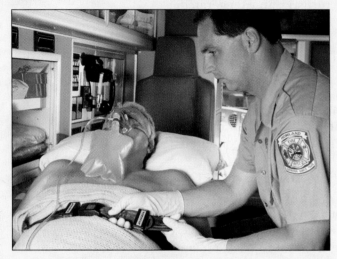

▲ Ensure that the patient is secure.

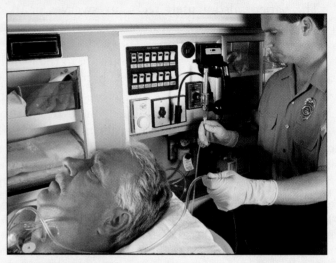

▲ Change to on-board oxygen.

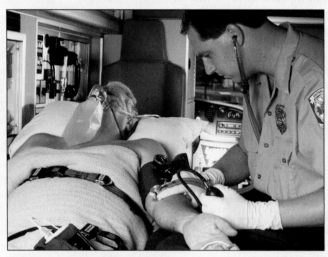

▲ Perform ongoing assessment.

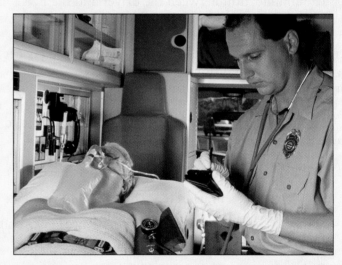

▲ Document your history and other assessment findings.

hospital gurney and leaving him without providing a report or ensuring that staff has taken control of the patient. If you were to leave and complete your report while the patient developed an airway problem, you would likely be considered liable for harm that came to the patient. Generally, a nurse will take your written and verbal report of the situation you found, your assessment, the care you provided, and the patient's responses to your interventions. Make sure you transfer all of the patient's personal belongings that you may have transported, including jewelry, medications, and clothing.

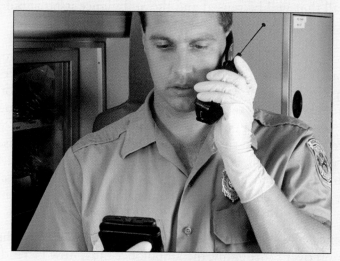

▲ Communicate with medical direction and the receiving medical facility.

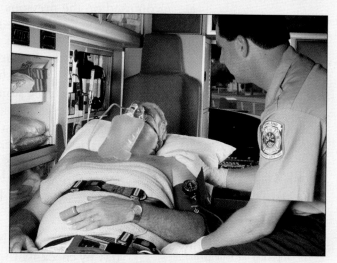

▲ Make the patient comfortable and reassure him.

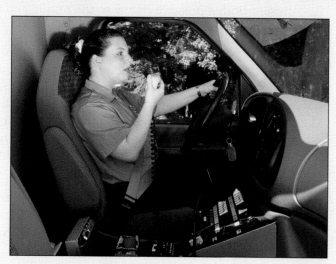

▲ Notify dispatch when you are en route and when you have arrived at
the receiving medical facility.

Terminating the Call

While this section is called "terminating the call," it could quite reasonably be
called "making sure your next call goes well" because the tasks included in this
section not only terminate the current call but assure that your ambulance is ready
for the next call. It is by far *not* the most exciting part of EMS, but the few moments it will take to prepare is a large investment in your next call—and a sign of
integrity and pride in what you do.

* **At the Hospital**—After you have transferred care, you should prepare for your next call. Preparation for the next call starts with washing your hands. Hand washing is the single best way to avoid disease transmission. It is vital for you to not carry any germs from your first patient to future patients or, just as important, to your crew or family.

At the hospital, the ambulance should be restocked with any equipment that is replaced or exchanged from hospital stock. This varies widely by area. Anything you used on the previous call that will be reused and the ambulance itself should be cleaned and disinfected.

* **The Written Report**—The EMT should also complete the patient care report, and a copy should be provided to the receiving facility staff. The report should be complete and accurate, describing the patient's condition upon your arrival and any changes in the patient's condition en route. You should document all vital signs, the patient's medical history, the results of your assessment, care you provided the patient, and the patient's response to that care. Other fields including run data, mileage, and agency-specific information will also be recorded. Further information on documentation requirements may be found in chapter 16, Documenting Your Assessment and Care.

* **Preparing for the Next Call**—Just as you prepared for the first call of the day by checking the unit over thoroughly, the ambulance must now be readied for the next patient. The ambulance should also be cleaned as needed to present both a positive image to the public and a clean environment for you and your crew and the next patient.

* **Equipment**—Many tasks may not be completed at the hospital and are completed while en route to quarters or when you arrive back at quarters (Scan 39-3). When you leave the hospital, you should notify the dispatcher of your status. You may be ready for the next call or remain out of service because necessary equipment is not available or ready for use. Before completing the call, the ambulance should be fully restocked, and refueled as necessary.

* **Disinfection and Sterilization**—You and your partner must wash your hands both after finishing with the patient and after cleaning the ambulance. On the way back from the call, many crews will debrief even minor calls to provide an assessment of the call and consider ways to make the next call go better.

* cleaning

wiping up blood, body fluids, dirt, or grime that may have come from the patient or the scene.

* disinfecting

killing some of the microbes that may be on a piece of medical equipment.

* sterilization

controlled process that, like disinfection, requires its own specific equipment and is usually done under controlled circumstances. In sterilization, all organisms on the piece of equipment are killed.

Regarding cleaning the ambulance, several different terms are sometimes used interchangeably. It is important to note the difference, though, so that proper decontamination can occur. **Cleaning** means to wipe up, as with blood or vomitus that may have come from the patient. **Disinfecting** is killing some of the microbes that may be on a piece of equipment.

Sterilization is a controlled process that, like disinfection, requires its own specific equipment and is usually done under controlled circumstances. In sterilization, organisms on the piece of equipment are killed. This is usually done in the hospital by autoclave in which steam is used to sterilize equipment. Occasionally, dry heat or gas systems will be used instead of steam. A few EMS systems use this type of sterilization equipment, but more often they use a chemical to sterilize equipment.

SCAN 39-3   **TERMINATING ACTIVITIES IN QUARTERS**

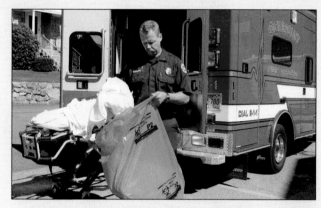

▲ Place contaminated linens in a biohazard container, noncontaminated linens in a regular hamper.

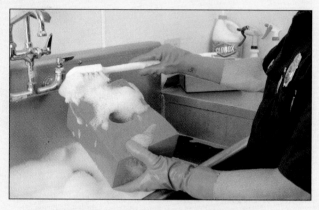

▲ Remove and clean patient-care equipment as required.

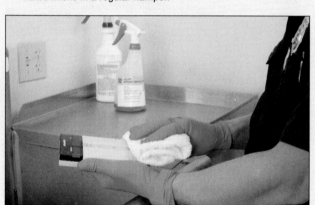

▲ Clean and sanitize respiratory equipment as required.

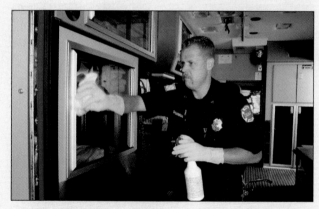

▲ Clean and sanitize the ambulance interior as required. Use germicide on devices or surfaces that were in contact with blood or other body fluids.

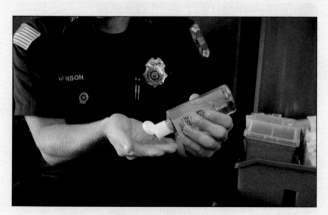

▲ Wash hands thoroughly, and change soiled clothing. Do this first if exposed to a communicable disease.

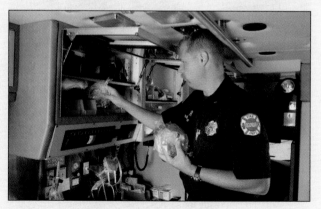

▲ Replace expendable items as required.

(continued on the next page)

TERMINATING ACTIVITIES IN QUARTERS—*(continued)*

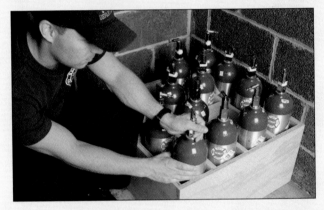

▲ Replace oxygen cylinders as necessary.

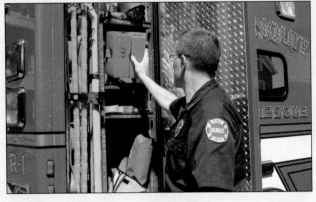

▲ Replace patient-care equipment as needed.

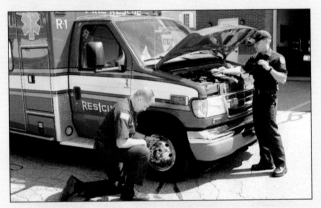

▲ Maintain the ambulance as required. Report problems that will take the vehicle out of service.

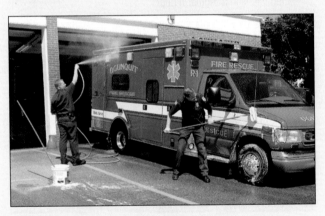

▲ Clean the ambulance exterior as needed.

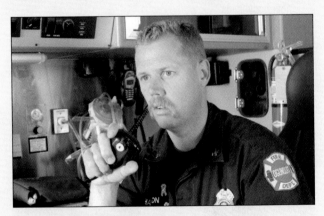

▲ Report the unit ready for service.

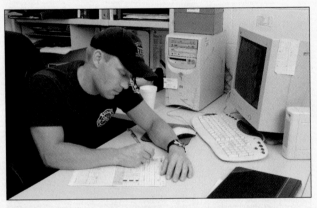

▲ Complete any unfinished report forms as soon as possible.

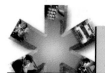

Perspective

Russ—The Commuter

"What the heck was wrong with those guys? I'm just on my way to work and hear this siren somewhere really close by. I'm looking all over the place and all I can see is a bunch of other people just as confused as me! The guy I carpool with thought that maybe it was just a car alarm that went crazy or something. So everyone else and I on 45th St. didn't know if we were pulling over or just moving on! So finally, as I'm turning onto Bryant, this ambulance squeezes past me with the siren blaring but no flashing lights or anything. Talk about creating confusion! I wonder what was up with that ambulance."

First and foremost, the crew must protect themselves by using gloves. If there is any possibility of splashing fluids, eye and face protection must also be used. Additionally, if there is a large amount of body fluid, footwear that is impervious to fluid is important. Footwear should also be equipped with steel toes and non-slip soles.

Basic disinfection can occur with a 1:10 household-bleach-to-water mixture. Clean anything that is visible, and then clean the area again. Towels should be disposable and should be discarded once the cleaning is completed.

High-level disinfection is usually applied to equipment involving the airway, such as laryngoscope blades and handles. Generally, these need to be cleaned by special chemicals or cleaned with boiling water for half an hour or more. This will kill most microbial organisms but not necessarily bacterial spores.

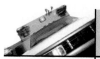

Dispatch Summary

The equipment failure on Rollie and Marianne's truck resulted in their inability to respond safely and quickly. The Post 15 ambulance had to be called in to cover the rollover MVA. Time was lost.

Because of this resource move, and concurrent emergency calls around the city, dispatch wasn't able to back-fill Post 15. A subsequent call in the Post 15 area resulted in a 24-minute response time with a patient who should have received care much sooner but did survive.

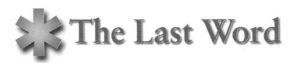

The Last Word

You are nearing the end of this textbook—and your EMT course. The fact that this material is at the back of the textbook and doesn't contain interesting patient-care information doesn't mean, however, that it is any less important. The material in this chapter will be used on *every call*—unlike some of the patient-care material you have learned in other chapters.

Your attention to the details of preparation for and terminating calls may well define you as an EMT. Will you be prepared and thoughtful—or will you rush from call to call without preparation? Which EMT would you want to respond to you if you were ill or injured?

Chapter Review

MULTIPLE CHOICE

Place a check next to the correct answer.

1. You are called to the scene of a multiple-vehicle collision involving a tanker truck. You note a placard on the truck. To quickly and safely determine the substance and its characteristics, you would refer to the:

    _____ a. emergency response guidebook.

    _____ b. textbook for a hazmat course.

    _____ c. company that owns the truck.

    _____ d. shipping papers in the cab of the truck.

2. After transferring the patient to the hospital staff, the most important thing you can do to prevent the spread of disease is to:

    _____ a. wash your hands.

    _____ b. sterilize the ambulance.

    _____ c. continue to wear gloves while at the hospital.

    _____ d. disinfect the ambulance.

3. When operating an emergency vehicle with lights and sirens activated, the operator must exercise _____ for the safety of other motorists and pedestrians.

    _____ a. some caution

    _____ b. due regard

    _____ c. reasonable caution

    _____ d. determinant prudence

4. When cleaning up blood from the floor of your ambulance, which is the correct procedure to use?

    _____ a. Wipe the blood up with a towel.

    _____ b. Use a spray cleaner or bleach solution.

    _____ c. Wipe up the visible material and then use a spray cleaner or bleach solution.

    _____ d. Take the ambulance out of service for sterilization at the ambulance garage.

5. Ambulance collisions are a major source of lawsuits against EMS providers and systems.

    _____ a. true

    _____ b. false

6. All patients must be transported to the hospital using lights and sirens.

    _____ a. true

    _____ b. false

7. Lights and sirens provide an ambulance a legal "right of way."

    _____ a. true

    _____ b. false

8. Which statement is most correct in relation to transporting patients to the hospital?

_____ a. Patients don't care how fast you drive as long as they get to the hospital.

_____ b. The ride on the stretcher is usually the smoothest since the patient is lying down.

_____ c. The patient can utilize the three-point restraint system to be comfortable in the stretcher.

_____ d. The patient may suffer anxiety from quick turns or excess bumps.

CRITICAL THINKING

1. What is the difference between disinfection and sterilization?

_____

_____

_____

2. Which do you do when you clean a blood stain on a long backboard: disinfection or sterilization?

_____

_____

_____

CASE STUDY

You are operating an ambulance with lights and sirens activated en route to a call for a "child choking" at a local day care. The following questions are based on this statement.

1. Does the fact that you are responding to a "child choking" change your driving at all compared to other responses? Would it be different if it were a call for a fall or a "sick person?"

_____

_____

_____

2. What are three considerations you will make in choosing your route to the scene?

_____

_____

_____

3. You are driving to the hospital with lights and sirens while your crew is performing CPR on the child in the back of the ambulance. What driving considerations do you have in regard to the crew working in the back?

_____

_____

_____

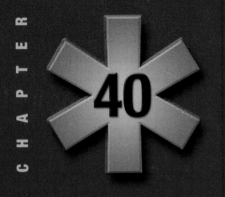

40

Overview of the Incident Management System

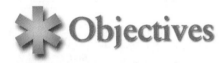

Objectives

Numbered objectives are from the U.S. Department of Transportation 1994 EMT-Basic National Standard Curriculum.

COGNITIVE OBJECTIVES

At the completion of this lesson, the EMT-Basic student will be able to:

7-3.11 Describe basic concepts of incident management. (p. 1006)

7-3.13 Review the local mass casualty incident plan. (pp. 1006–1023)

AFFECTIVE OBJECTIVES

No affective objectives identified.

PSYCHOMOTOR OBJECTIVES

No psychomotor objectives identified.

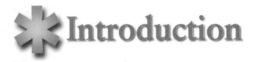

Introduction

* **multiple casualty incident (MCI)**

incidents resulting in illness or injuries that exceed or overwhelm the EMS and hospital capabilities.

At some point in your career as an EMT you will respond to an incident involving more than one patient and that exceeds or overwhelms the resources of the EMS system—a **multiple casualty incident (MCI)**—or you will be called to assist at a major event in which an Incident Management System (IMS) is in operation (Figure 40-1). The multiple-patient incident typically involves a motor vehicle collision (MVC), a fire scene, or any number of other situations. The success of dealing with that incident or event will depend on the EMT and other rescuers following established procedures. This chapter will teach you the principles of an incident management system and the key EMS positions employed by an Incident

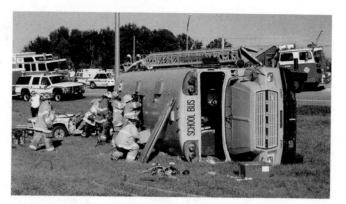

FIGURE 40-1   A multiple-casualty incident.

Commander (IC) to help victims of such events. Your actions and training will have a tremendous impact on the safety of the EMS personnel and affect the outcome of people who require emergency medical services at major events or disasters. More detailed information on multiple-casualty incidents will be covered in chapter 41.

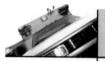

Emergency Dispatch

"Unit six, come in." There was a hint of uncharacteristic panic in the dispatcher's voice. "Unit six, I need you to cancel off that call and proceed, priority one, to Barker and 12th Avenue. Please advise once on scene."

"OK, ten-four," EMT Jeffrey Clark responded as his partner, Kelli Barnaby, spun the wheel and sped toward the new call.

"That's odd," Kelli said, checking her mirrors and changing lanes. "Didn't they already send Mark's truck there for that motorcycle crash?"

"Yeah, I think you're right," Jeffrey said, pulling two exam gloves from the box between the seats.

As Kelli navigated the final corner onto Barker Street, her jaw fell slack and Jeffrey whistled quietly through his teeth.

There were people hurrying around the roadway, swirling through a haze of smoke that just hung in the still air. There was a smashed car over to the left, huge chunks of pavement torn up in front of them, and an ambulance resting on the sidewalk on the right—its front wheels and much of the engine compartment gone. Farther down the road a city bus was sitting di-agonally across both lanes with a small green car buried beneath it and about 50 feet past that, in the next intersection, there was a motorcycle down in the street. A figure lay motionless next to it, blood running like a wide, shining ribbon across the intersection and down into a storm drain.

"Hey," Jeffrey's voice broke the silence in the cab. "There's Mark!"

Paramedic Mark Gainer walked shakily toward their truck, carrying his blood-soaked uniform shirt limply in one hand. Jeffrey got out and hurried over to meet him while Kelli grabbed the cot and equipment from the back.

"What happened, man?" Jeffrey asked. Mark looked at him, moved his mouth several times—as if to speak—and then just threw his arms around him in a tight hug.

Just then, a firefighter ran over from the direction of the bus, sweat soaking his dark t-shirt. "Hey! We got criticals everywhere! One in that car, two in the green one, about four on the bus, a little girl on the sidewalk just past the ambulance and . . . uh . . . I think the motorcycle guy's a black tag. We need more help, quick!"

✳ **National Incident Management System (NIMS)**

system implemented in 2004 by the Department of Homeland Security that provides a consistent nationwide approach for incident management and requires federal, state, tribal, and local governments to work together before, during, and after incidents.

✳ **Incident Management System (IMS)**

system developed to assist with the control, direction, and coordination of emergency response resources. It provides an orderly means of communication and information for decision making and accountability of resources.

✳ **freelancing**

situation when a person on an emergency scene takes action without the knowledge or permission of the incident commander or commanders of the incident.

✳ **Incident Command System (ICS)**

the first management system that was developed by an interagency task force working in a cooperative local, state, and federal interagency effort called FIRESCOPE (Firefighting Resources of California Organized for Potential Emergencies). Initial ICS applications were designed for responding to disastrous wildland fires in southern California.

National Incident Management System (NIMS)

The **National Incident Management System (NIMS)** was established in 2004 by the U.S. Department of Homeland Security. It is a system that provides a consistent nationwide approach for incident management and requires federal, state, tribal, and local governments to work together before, during, and after incidents. It involves preparing for, preventing, responding to, and recovering from domestic incidents of all sizes and complexities.

Within NIMS, the **Incident Management System (IMS)** has been developed to assist with the control, direction, and coordination of emergency response resources. EMTs, firefighters, and police officers are all required to operate under an incident management system at the scene of a multiple-casualty or disaster situation. It provides an orderly means of communication and information for decision making and accountability of resources. Interactions with other agencies are easier because of uniform procedures, common terminology, and coordination using business management principles.

Incident management also seeks to ensure there is no **"freelancing."** Freelancing is when a person on an emergency scene takes action without the knowledge or permission of the incident commander or commanders of the incident. This behavior is dangerous and disruptive to the incident.

Long before NIMS was established, the first incident management system, known as the **Incident Command System (ICS)**, was developed by an interagency task force working in a cooperative local, state, and federal interagency effort called FIRESCOPE (Firefighting Resources of California Organized for Potential Emergencies). Initial ICS applications were designed for responding to disastrous wildland fires in southern California. Early in the development process, four essential requirements became clear:

1. The system must be organizationally flexible to meet the needs of incidents of any kind and size.

2. Agencies must be able to use the system on a day-to-day basis for routine situations as well as for major emergencies.

3. The system must be sufficiently standard to allow personnel from a variety of agencies and diverse geographic locations to rapidly meld into a common management structure.

4. The system must be cost effective.

ICS is now widely used throughout the United States by EMS and fire agencies and is increasingly used for law enforcement, other public safety applications, and for emergency and event management. When NIMS was established in 2004, ICS was incorporated as the backbone of the wider-based federal system.

Homeland Security Presidential Directive 5

To prevent, prepare for, respond to, and recover from terrorist attacks, major disasters, and other emergencies, the United States Government shall establish a single, comprehensive approach to domestic incident management. The objective of the United States Government is to ensure that all levels of government across the Nation have the capability to work efficiently and effectively together, using a national approach to domestic incident management.

Stop, Review, Remember!

Multiple Choice

Place a check next to the correct answer.

1. Which agency was responsible for developing the National Incident Management System?

   _____ a. Department of Homeland Security.

   _____ b. Office of Domestic Preparedness.

   _____ c. local fire department.

   _____ d. local ambulance company.

2. Interaction with other agencies is accomplished using an incident management system because _____ principles are used to manage resources and tasks.

   _____ a. uniform

   _____ b. unified

   _____ c. infamous

   _____ d. numerous

3. The pneumonic NIMS stand for:

   _____ a. Nationally Inventoried Business Management System.

   _____ b. National Incident Management Sequencing.

   _____ c. National Incident Management System.

   _____ d. National Institute of Medicine System.

4. Freelancing can result in:

   _____ a. an EMT injury.

   _____ b. a patient death.

   _____ c. a disorganized incident.

   _____ d. all of the above.

5. The NIMS system incorporates:

   _____ a. an incident guidance system.

   _____ b. an incident control system.

   _____ c. an incident command system.

   _____ d. both a and b.

Fill in the Blank

On the lines at right, write the terms represented by the abbreviations at left.

1. NIMS   _____ _____ _____ _____

2. ICS   _____ _____ _____

3. IMS   _____ _____ _____

4. MCI   _____ _____ _____

5. IC   _____ _____

Critical Thinking

1. When multiple injuries occur at large events, such as a ride collapse at a carnival, use of an incident management system may be necessary. Do you have events such as this in your community? Discuss this list with your instructor.

_____

_____

_____

_____

2. Why would freelancing be the wrong decision on an MCI?

_____

_____

_____

_____

* **Incident Commander (IC)**

  the person in overall charge of an incident under the Incident Command System or Incident Management System.

* **General Staff**

  the key staff positions that oversee the sections in a fully expanded ICS or IMS system.

* **Command Staff**

  the incident commander's staff consisting of the liaison officer, the safety officer, and the information officer.

* **Liaison Officer**

  command staff officer responsible for communicating with other agencies. The liaison officer may be the person making the initial contact with an EMS agency.

* **Safety Officer**

  command staff officer who ensures that the incident safety considerations are recognized and has the power to stop activity or remove people immediately from hazardous situation.

ICS Organization

Every incident or event has certain major management activities or actions that must be performed. Even if the event is small, and only one or two people are involved, these activities will still always apply to some degree. The organization of the Incident Command System (ICS) is built around five major management functions: Command, Operations, Planning, Logistics, and Finance/Administration (Table 40-1).

These five ICS functions apply whether you are handling a routine emergency, organizing for a major event, or managing a major response to a disaster. On small incidents, these major activities may be managed by one person, the **Incident Commander (IC)**. Large incidents usually require that the Incident Commander set up separate sections to organize resources and services. A fully expanded ICS system has several **General Staff** positions. Each member of the General Staff overseas one of the ICS major functional elements and is given the title section chief: the Operations Section Chief, the Planning Section Chief, the Logistics Section Chief, and the Finance/Administration Section Chief.

At each level in the ICS organization, individuals with primary responsibility positions have distinctive titles. Those titles are a key component of the NIMS system that requires emergency responders to be familiar with common titles and common terminology. These positions are staffed only when needed and demonstrate the flexibility of the ICS and IMS system.

The Incident Commander also has a **Command Staff**. The Command Staff is composed of the Liaison Officer, the Safety Officer, and the Information Officer. The **Liaison Officer** is responsible for communicating with other agencies. The liaison officer may be the person making the initial contact with an EMS agency. The **Safety Officer** ensures that incident safety considerations are recognized and

TABLE 40-1   MANAGEMENT ACTIVITIES OF THE INCIDENT COMMAND SYSTEM

COMMAND

* Sets objectives and priorities
* Has overall responsibility at the incident or event

OPERATIONS

* Conducts tactical operations to carry out the plan
* Develops the tactical objectives
* Organization
* Directs all resources

PLANNING

* Develops the action plan to accomplish the objectives
* Collects and evaluates information
* Maintains resource status

LOGISTICS

* Provides support to meet incident needs
* Provides resources and all other services needed to support the incident

FINANCE/ADMINISTRATION

* Monitors costs related to incident
* Provides accounting, procurement, time records, cost analyses

has the power to stop activity or remove people immediately from a hazardous situation. The **Public Information Officer** is the only one authorized to release information to the news media after approval by the Incident Commander (Figure 40-2). Additional positions that may be required for a specific incident can be established by the Incident Commander.

* **Public Information Officer**

  command staff officer who is the only one authorized to release information to the news media after approval by the incident commander.

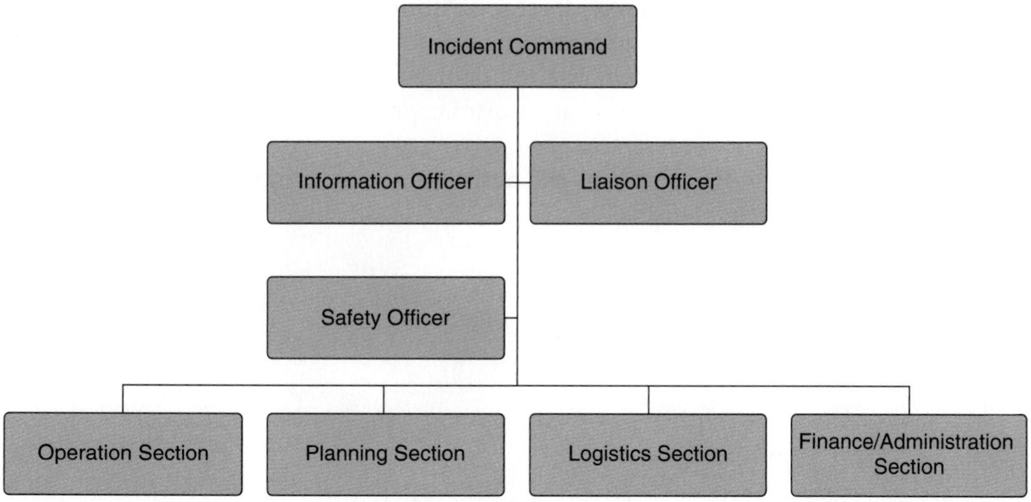

FIGURE 40-2   The command staff organizational chart.

FIGURE 40-2   The command staff organizational chart.

Stop, Review, Remember!

Multiple Choice

Place a check next to the correct answer.

1. The five major activities around which the ICS is organized are:

      _____ a. command, liaison, operations, communications, and logistics

      _____ b. command, planning, operations, communications, and logistics

      _____ c. command, operations, planning, logistics, and finance/administration

      _____ d. command, liaison, safety, operations, and planning

2. In a fully expanded ICS system, the general staff consists of the:

      _____ a. section chiefs.

      _____ b. liaison officers.

      _____ c. operations officers.

      _____ d. planning staff.

3. Name the three major activities of the command staff.

      _____ a. safety, information, and logistics

      _____ b. information, safety, and planning

      _____ c. safety, information, and liaison

      _____ d. planning, logistics, and safety

4. What is the one ICS position staffed at all incidents?

      _____ a. division supervisor

      _____ b. incident commander

      _____ c. task force leader

      _____ d. operations section chief

Matching

Match the term on the left with the applicable definition on the right.

1. _____ Command

2. _____ Operations

3. _____ Planning

4. _____ Logistics

5. _____ Finance/Administration

A. Conducts tactical operations to carry out the plan
B. Has overall responsibility at the incident or event
C. Provides resources and all other services needed to support the incident
D. Provides accounting, procurement, time records, cost analyses
E. Develops the action plan to accomplish the objectives

Critical Thinking

1. You have been assigned the role of Safety Officer during an MCI involving a 15-passenger van. What are some of the things that you should look for?

   _____

   _____

   _____

   _____

2. You are approached by members of the media about your role in an MCI. What would you do?

   _____

   _____

   _____

   _____

   _____

Management of Multiple-Casualty Incidents

An EMT's first exposure to the Incident Command System will likely occur at a multiple-casualty incident. Refer to chapter 41 for more information on multiple-casualty and mass-casualty incidents (MCIs).

An MCI will need to be managed with a heightened response that includes requesting additional resources from other agencies. When personnel or resources are provided by other jurisdictions, this is called **mutual aid.** Multiple-casualty incidents typically do not overwhelm the hospital capabilities of a jurisdiction and/or region, but they may exceed the capabilities of one or more hospitals within a locality. There is usually a short, intense peak demand for health and medical services.

* **mutual aid**
  assistance provided by other jurisdictions.

Components of an Incident Management System

Large-scale events will typically have a written or oral **incident action plan (IAP).** The Incident Commander will make the decision on whether the IAP is written or verbal. On large-scale incidents, the Planning Section creates and puts together the written action plan with the approval of the Incident Commander. Essential elements in any written or oral incident action plan are:

* **incident action plan (IAP)**
  plan for the management of a specific component of incident operations.

* **Statement of objectives**—Appropriate to the overall incident.

* **Organization**—Describes what parts of the ICS organization will be in place for each operational period.

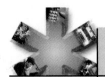

Perspective

Kelli—The EMT

"At first that was just complete pandemonium! Everyone was confused . . . and the firefighter and Mark's partner, Dave, were kind of just jumping around from patient to patient. I knew, at that point, that Mark should have probably been in charge since he is the only paramedic on scene and all, but he was in no condition to do it. So, after calling for, like, seven more ambulances and the helicopter, I got on the PA and told all of the people with minor injuries to get over in one place. Oh man, I was so nervous and just on auto pilot, you know? There were so many injured people and so much to keep track of, I was so glad when the other ambulances started arriving. Then when that fire captain showed up and put on the Incident Commander vest and said, 'Okay, what do you have for me?' I almost just hugged him."

✳ **Assignments to accomplish the objectives**—These are normally prepared for each division or group and include the strategy, tactics, and resources to be used.

✳ **Supporting material**—Examples can include a map of the incident, communications plan, medical plan, traffic plan, and so on.

Span of Control is another principle of an ICS system. Span of control refers to how many organizational elements or people may be directly managed by another person. Maintaining adequate span of control throughout the ICS organization is very important. Effective span of control may vary from three to seven, although a ratio of one to five reporting elements is commonly recommended.

Unity of command is another essential organizational aspect. The principle of unity of command dictates that each individual in an organization has only one supervisor. This helps to ensure accountability and safety of resources. The principle of unity of command should not be confused with a unified command, which will be discussed later.

COMMON RESPONSIBILITIES

If you respond to a large incident or disaster where ICS is in place, there are certain common responsibilities or instructions that everyone assigned to an incident should follow. Following these simple guidelines will make your job easier and result in a more effective operation. Receive your incident assignment from your organization. This should include, at a minimum:

✳ a reporting location and time

✳ likely length of assignment

✳ **span of control**

the number of organizational elements or people that may be directly managed by another person. Effective span of control may vary from three to seven, although a ratio of one to five reporting elements is commonly recommended.

✳ **unity of command**

the principle that each individual in an organization has only one supervisor. The principle of unity of command should not be confused with a unified command.

* brief description of assignment

* route information

* a designated communications link, if necessary (Different agencies may have additional requirements.)

Bring any specialized supplies or equipment required for your job. Be sure you have adequate supplies to last you for the expected stay. Upon arrival, follow the check-in procedure for the incident. Check-in locations may be found at:

* Incident Command Post (at the Resources Unit)

* staging areas

* bases or camps

* helibases

* division or group supervisors (for direct assignments)

COMMUNICATIONS

Radio communications on an incident should use **clear text** also known as plain text or common language, that is, no radio codes. Refer to incident facilities by their incident name, for example, Broadway Command Post, or Second Street Staging Area. EMTs should refer to personnel by ICS title, not numeric code or name of the unit. For example, when calling the treatment area being managed by Medic 4, the title "treatment group" would be used instead of Medic 4. Good communication practice at an ICS scene includes repeating information or assignment. For example, if you arrived on scene as Rescue 18 and Command gives you an assignment to report to the treatment group, you would repeat the assignment, "Rescue 18 copies reporting to treatment group." This practice ensures that the Incident Commander knows you understood your assignment.

Once the incident appears to require more radio traffic, the Incident Commander will move the incident onto a tactical frequency or secondary channel. Using a tactical or secondary channel allows other demands in the EMS system to be met without interrupting the communication at the incident.

* **clear text**
  communications using plain language, that is, no radio codes.

VERBAL COMMUNICATION

Obtain a briefing from your immediate or group supervisor. Be sure you understand your assignment. Acquire necessary work materials, locate, and set up your work station. Organize and brief any other EMS personnel assigned to you. Brief your relief at the end of each operational period. Operational periods are usually 12 hours on large incidents. Complete required forms and reports and give them to your group or division supervisor before you leave. Demobilize according to plan.

Stop, Review, Remember!

Multiple Choice

Place a check next to the correct answer.

1. A written incident action plan, if activated at an incident, will be the decision of the:

   _____ a. Division Leader.

   _____ b. Incident Commander.

   _____ c. Section Chief.

   _____ d. Branch Director.

2. When communicating on the radio in an ICS system, the EMT should use:

   _____ a. clear text.

   _____ b. 10 Codes.

   _____ c. 400 Codes.

   _____ d. secret codes.

3. The concept of unity of command means that:

   _____ a. two agencies share command functions.

   _____ b. one supervisor has no more that seven subordinates.

   _____ c. one person has one supervisor.

   _____ d. the incident is divided into functional blocks.

4. The optimal span of control is:

   _____ a. 5:1.

   _____ b. 3:1.

   _____ c. 7:1.

   _____ d. 4:1.

Matching

1. _____ Span of control

2. _____ Unity of command

3. _____ Mutual aid

4. _____ Incident action plan

A. The principle that each individual in an organization has only one supervisor.

B. Assistance provided by other jurisdictions.

C. Plan for the management of a specific component of a management plan.

D. The number of elements or people that can be effectively managed by one person.

Critical Thinking

1. Think about your community. List the annual events could be organized with an incident action plan and why.

   _____

   _____

   _____

   _____

2. What areas in your community have the capacity to generate a large number of patients or victims?

_____

_____

_____

_____

Scene Size-Up

It is important for the first on-scene EMS unit to conduct a scene size-up on which a brief initial report can be based. When conducting the scene size-up, the EMT should systematically look at:

* Scene safety and appropriate personal protective equipment needed

* Exact location or address of the incident

* Nature of the event and severity

* Number of injuries if known

* Risk factors for EMS responders, such as hazardous material or contamination

* Possibility of a crime scene and requirements for scene safety

* Additional resource(s) required

* Actions you are taking

INITIAL REPORT

After completing a scene size-up, the first arriving EMT will need to transmit a brief initial report to the communications center and for other responders. Often other first responders are on scene first and may have already transmitted a brief initial report with important safety information. The EMT's brief initial report should be transmitted in a short, calm, clear, and concise message. The brief initial report should follow the standardized format:

* On arrival at the location, confirm the address and exact location

* Describe the event and the situation, including safety issues

* Confirm and designate a command

* State the action you are taking

* Request additional resources

* Locate the Command Post

Perspective

Carl Becker—The Dispatcher

"Kelli did such a great job on that call! The only thing that I knew about it was that I had dispatched another unit for a truck versus motorcycle accident and then, about 5 minutes later, I got a cell phone call from them saying that they had been in a collision. I had no idea the extent of it until Kelli got on the radio to call for more units. I've been doing this job for 7 years this coming June, and I must say, not until today have I had a medic get on the radio at an MCI and give me such a perfect initial report!"

ORGANIZING AN INCIDENT

Once the initial report has been transmitted, command will be established. It is important to understand that a more senior command officer will arrive on scene and assume the responsibilities for the management of the incident. This process is known as transfer of command and is completed when the first-arriving unit relays the information and current status to a command officer from the fire department, law enforcement, or EMS agency. This places the responsibility of the incident on a formal Incident Commander and makes the EMS resources available to attend to patients.

The structure of the incident management system for an event involving multiple casualties is determined by the goals, objectives, and tasks needed to resolve the incident. When an incident commander establishes command, **units, groups, divisions,** and **branches** are established as needed.

✳ **unit**

    team assigned a specific task.

✳ **group**

    team assigned to functional activities.

✳ **division**

    team assigned to function in a specific geographical area.

✳ **branch**

    management tool for the Incident Commander that can be either geographical or functional and is used to keep a manageable span of control.

* **Units** can function under groups and divisions and are used for a specific task, often involving only one or two people. A unit assignment is staffed by a unit leader or manager; for example, the triage unit is often conducted by one person

* **Groups** are designated for functional activities, for example the treatment group is responsible for treating patients and requesting resources from the transportation group for the patients to be transported to the hospital.

* **Divisions** are geographical in nature; for example an incident at a concert that has produced casualties on the west side of the location would be called the West Division.

* **Branches** are a management tool for the Incident Commander that can be either geographical or functional and are used to keep a manageable span of control. For example, a fire in an apartment complex that produces several patients may be divided into a multi-casualty branch and a fire-suppression branch.

As an EMT, you will be assigned to a particular role in one of the units, groups, divisions, or branches. Upon arrival, the EMT should report to the Incident Com-

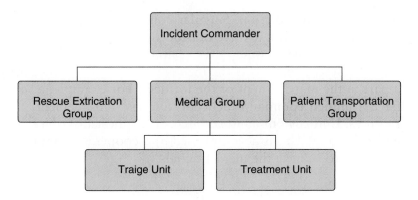

FIGURE 40-3 The medical/multi-casualty branch of the ICS/EMS.

mander, group leader, or division supervisor for specific duties or an assignment. Once assigned a specific task, the EMT should complete the task and report back to the officer in charge of that unit, group, division, or branch.

The medical or multi-casualty branch will have a basic ICS/EMS organization structure. As an EMT you can expect to be assigned to one of the following groups or units (Figure 40-3).

* **Command** directs the overall operation and is responsible for the overall success and safety of the incident.

* **Rescue/Extrication Group** is responsible for all of the operations necessary to remove victim from the hazard zone and to the treatment area. Those assigned should have training in vehicle and special rescue techniques.

* **Triage Group** is responsible for the sorting and tagging of all patients according to the seriousness and extent of injuries.

* **Treatment Group** will establish a treatment area where patient can be treated and collected.

* **Transportation Group** is responsible for obtaining the resources to ensure that all patients are transported to the appropriate hospital.

* **Staging Area** manager directs all incoming resources (e.g., ambulances, rescue equipment, search and rescue teams.)

* **Supply Unit** receives supplies and equipment from staging and issues them to the operational units as requested.

Command

The **Command Post (CP)** is a physical location near the incident that is staffed by the Incident Commander, who is responsible for the overall success and safety of the incident. The Incident Commander implements a strategy for handling all current and potential patients. The safety of ALL responders and citizens is the responsibility of the Incident Commander. It is the incident commander's responsibility to implement an ICS structure for emergency medical services as required by the demands of the incident. Incident Command is commonly set up in the cold zone.

Two types of command are possible at an emergency incident, singular or unified. Most incidents have a single person in command who carries the authority of

* **command**

directs the overall operation and is responsible for the overall success and safety of the incident.

* **Rescue/Extrication Group**

team responsible for all of the operations necessary to remove victim from the hazard zone and to the treatment area.

* **Triage Group**

team responsible for the sorting and tagging of all patients according to the seriousness and extent of injuries.

* **Treatment Group**

team that will establish a treatment area where patients can be treated and collected.

* **Transportation Group**

team responsible for obtaining resources to ensure that all patients are transported to the appropriate hospital.

* **Staging Area**

positions and directs all incoming resources.

* **Supply Unit**

team that receives supplies and equipment from staging and issues them to the operational units as requested.

* **Command Post (CP)**

a physical location near the incident from which the Incident Commander oversees all incident operations. Also called the Incident Command Post (ICP).

∗ **singular command**

method of command used for incidents that are smaller in scope that do not involve outside agencies and often occur within a single jurisdiction.

∗ **unified command**

method of command that is a team effort allowing all agencies with a jurisdictional responsibility for the incident, either geographical or functional, to play a part in the management of the incident.

the agency or jurisdiction. **Singular command** is for incidents that are smaller in scope and that do not involve outside agencies' and often occur within a single jurisdiction. **Unified command** is a team effort that allows all agencies with a jurisdictional responsibility for the incident, either geographical or functional, to play a part in the management of the incident. For example, a school shooting would have a unified command incorporating law enforcement, EMS, and school authorities. Unified command still maintains one set of objectives developed for the entire incident. This is accomplished by a cooperative approach to developing the strategies to achieve the incident goals.

 Stop, Review, Remember!

Multiple Choice

Place a check next to the correct answer.

1. The scene size-up should determine all of the following except:

   _____ a. scene safety and appropriate personal protective equipment needed.

   _____ b. exact location or address of the incident.

   _____ c. place for the media to stage.

   _____ d. nature of the event and severity.

2. The process of transmitting the scene size-up to the communications center and other first responders is known as:

   _____ a. opening report.

   _____ b. initial report.

   _____ c. establishing command.

   _____ d. triage.

Matching

Match the term on the left with the applicable definition on the right.

1. _____ Command

2. _____ Rescue/extrication group

3. _____ Treatment group

4. _____ Transportation group

5. _____ Triage group

A. Is responsible for the all of the operations necessary to remove victims from the hazard zone and to the treatment area and should have training in vehicle and special rescue techniques

B. Directs the overall operation and is responsible for the overall success and safety of the incident

C. Is responsible for the sorting and tagging of all patients according to the seriousness and extent of injuries

D. Is responsible for obtaining resources to ensure that all patients are transported to the appropriate hospital

E. Will establish a treatment area where patient can be treated and collected

Critical Thinking

1. Why is the Incident Commander ultimately responsible for the overall operation of the incident?

_____

_____

_____

_____

2. Why might it be advantageous to locate the Command Post away from the site of the incident?

_____

_____

_____

_____

3. Why is it necessary for the first arriving unit to give an accurate size-up of the incident?

_____

_____

_____

_____

Triage, Identification, and Tracking

Triage is the process of sorting patients based on the severity of their injuries and prioritizing them for treatment and transport. You will take a detailed look at triage in the next chapter.

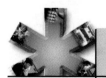

Perspective

Jeffrey—The EMT

"That whole incident almost doesn't seem real now that I look back on it, you know? It was my first real MCI and one that actually needed an Incident Commander. I'm really very impressed with how effectively that whole Incident Command System works! All of the pieces that began as a mass of confusion just fell into place. We didn't lose any patients . . . well, except for the guy on the motorcycle, but he was gone when we arrived on scene."

As an EMT, you realize by now that all of your actions require documentation. Most triage tags have perforated tabs to remove based on patient severity. Some tags have serial or identification numbers on the corner and on the perforated tags that can be detached and left at the location where the patient was found.

Transportation

The Department of Homeland Security under the Federal Emergency Management System's support function for medical incidents has classified emergency medical services resources by two designations: **EMS Task Forces** (Figure 40-4) and **Ambulance Strike Teams** (Figure 40-5).

A task force or strike team should be self-sufficient for 12-hour operational periods, although it may be deployed longer, depending on need. Support elements needed include fuel, security, resupply of medical supplies, and support for personnel. Table 40-2 provides an overview of the U.S. Department of Homeland Security and Federal Emergency Management Agency's classification of ambulance resources.

✳ **EMS Task Force**

any combination of resources within span of control of 3 to 7 units (e.g., ambulances, rescues, engines, and squads) assembled for a medical mission, with common communications and a leader (supervisor).

✳ **Ambulance Strike Team**

a group of five ambulances of the same type with common communications and a leader.

FIGURE 40-4 Vehicular components of an EMS task force.

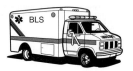
BLS Ambulance

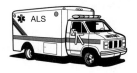
ALS Ambulance

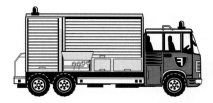
Heavy Rescue Truck

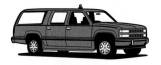
Supervisor

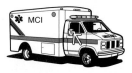
Specialized MCI Truck

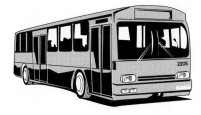
Bus

FIGURE 40-5 Vehicular components of an ambulance strike team.

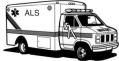
ALS Ambulance

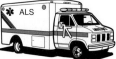
ALS Ambulance

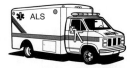
ALS Ambulance

ALS Ambulance

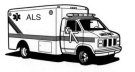
ALS Ambulance

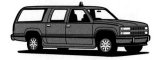
Supervisor

TABLE 40-2	U.S. DEPARTMENT OF HOMELAND SECURITY AND FEDERAL EMERGENCY MANAGEMENT AGENCY CLASSIFICATION OF AMBULANCE RESOURCES

Resource: Ambulances (Ground)
Category: Health & Medical (Emergency Support Function #8)
Kind: Team; Equipment; Personnel; Supplies; Vehicles

MINIMUM CAPABILITIES	TYPE I*	TYPE II	TYPE III*	TYPE IV	OTHER
Emergency medical services team with equipment, supplies, and vehicle for patient transport (Type I-IV) and emergency medical care out of hospital	Advanced Life Support; Minimum 2 staff (paramedic and EMT); Transport 2-litter patients	Advanced Life Support, Minimum 2 staff (paramedic and EMT); Transport 2-litter patients, nonHazMat response	Basic Life Support Minimum 2 staff (EMT and first responder); Transport 2-litter patients	Basic Life Support operations; Minimum 2 personnel (I EMT and first responder); Transport 2-litter patients	Nontransporting emergency medical response; Minimum 1 staff; BLS or ALS equipment supplies

*Type I and Type III: Training and equipment meets or exceeds standards as addressed by EPA, OSHA, and NFPA 471, 472, 473 and 29 CFR 1910, 120 ETA 3–11 to work in HazMat Level B and specific threat conditions; all immunized in accordance with CDC core adult immunizations and specific threat as appropriate

Each team unit can work 12-hour shifts. Backup supply and some equipment required according to number of patients and type of event. Communication equipment may be programmable for interoperability but must be verified. Fuel supply and maintenance support must be available. Plan for augmenting existing communication equipment. Environmental considerations related to temperature control in patient care compartment and pharmaceutical storage may be necessary for locations with excessive ranges in temperature. Security of vehicle support required for periods of standby without crew in attendance. Decontamination supplies and support required for responses to incidents with potential threat to responding services or transport of infectious patients. (U.S. Department of Homeland Security and Federal Emergency Management)

Incident Facilities

ICS facilities will be established depending on the kind and complexity of the incident or event. It is important to know and understand the names and functions of the principle types of ICS facilities. Not all of those listed here will necessarily be used.

The **Incident Command Post (ICP)** is the location from which the Incident Commander oversees all incident operations. There is only one ICP for each incident or event. Every incident or event must have some form of an Incident Command Post. On a map it is marked by a square with a diagonal darkened on the lower half.

* **Incident Command Post (ICP)**

a physical location near an incident from which the Incident Commander oversees all incident operations. Also called the Command Post (CP).

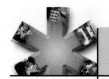

Perspective

Mark

"What an absolute nightmare. I could see the fire truck just up the road at the motorcycle crash, I was putting my gloves on and, you know, going over protocols in my head. Then suddenly there was a car in front of us. I don't know what that driver was thinking! She looked right at us and just turned anyway. When we hit her, all I could see for a few seconds was the blue sky through the cracked windshield, and then we crashed back down and rolled to a stop. I guess there was some sort of chain reaction also. The car we hit crashed into another car, which hit a bus or something. And a little girl got hit on her bike, too. Just a mess. I must've hit my head in there somewhere. I ended up with a pretty good headache and I remember being so confused! At first I did try to treat the lady in the car that we hit. I got my IV start-kit out, but—and this is really weird—I couldn't remember how to start an IV. It's kind of a blur after that."

✳ **staging area**

location or locations at an incident where incoming resources report.

✳ **base**

location at an incident at which primary service and support activities are performed.

✳ **camp**

location where resources may be kept to support incident operations.

✳ **helibase**

location in or near an incident area at which helicopters may be parked, maintained, fueled, and equipped for incident operations

✳ **helispots**

temporary locations where helicopters can land and load and off-load personnel, equipment, and supplies.

Staging area locations are marked by a circle with an "S." Most large incidents will have a staging area, and some incidents may have several staging areas. A **base** is a location at the incident at which primary service and support activities are performed and is marked with a circle with a "B." There will only be one base for each incident. A **camp** is a location where resources may be kept to support incident operations marked with a circle and a "C." A camp differs from a staging area in that essential support operations are done at camps, and resources at camps are not always immediately available for use. Not all incidents will have camps.

If air operations are conducted at the scene of an MCI, activities involved with the take-off and landing of helicopters are organized under the Air Operations Branch. The Air Operations Branch utilizes **helibases** and **helispots.** A helibase is a location in or near an incident area at which helicopters may be parked, maintained, fueled, and equipped for incident operations. They are marked with a circle with an "H." Helispots are temporary locations where helicopters can land and load and off-load personnel, equipment, and supplies. Large incidents may have several helispots, and they are marked by a completely darkened circle.

Treatment and triage areas do not have specific symbols. When an ambulance arrives at the scene of a large incident where maps with symbols are being used, EMTs can expect to be sent to a Base, a Camp, or an assignment. If the EMS crew remains at the Base location, they are often assigned to Logistics or the Medical Unit. The Medical Unit is staffed at large incidents to provide medical care for the responders.

Stop, Review, Remember!

Multiple Choice

Place a check next to the correct answer.

1. Helibases differ from helispots in that:

   _____ a. helibases have maintenance supplies for helicopters.

   _____ b. helispots have fuel for helicopters.

   _____ c. helibases are temporary locations for helicopters to land.

   _____ d. helispots are marked on the map with a circled "H."

2. Triage patients are tagged based on:

   _____ a. severity of their injuries.

   _____ b. time of death.

   _____ c. both a and d.

   _____ d. priority for treatment and transport.

3. An Ambulance Strike Team is a group of _____ ambulances of the same type with common communications and a leader.

   _____ a. two

   _____ b. four

   _____ c. three

   _____ d. five

4. The Incident Command Post is signified on a map with a:

   _____ a. square with a diagonal darkened on the lower half.

   _____ b. circle with a "B."

   _____ c. circle with a "C."

   _____ d. circle with an "S."

5. Some incidents may have more than one staging area.

   _____ a. true

   _____ b. false

6. A large incident can have more than one base.

   _____ a. true

   _____ b. false

7. A large incident may have more than one camp.

   _____ a. true

   _____ b. false

8. Every incident will have a Command Post.

   _____ a. true

   _____ b. false

Critical Thinking

1. Why is it necessary to be able to track patients in an MCI?

   _____

   _____

   _____

   _____

2. Think about your community. What locations could serve as a helibase or helispot in the event that an earthquake, snowstorm, flood, or tornado temporarily disrupts the transportation network?

_____

_____

_____

_____

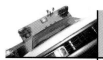

Dispatch Summary

Eight ambulances from several area agencies along with the University Hospital's Life-Flight helicopter, cooperating under the ICS, treated and transported a total of eight critical and six noncritical patients to local hospitals. All of the patients survived, with all but two being discharged within twelve days of the accident. Many are still undergoing physical therapy and/or reconstructive surgeries.

The incident has been hailed as a shining example of the effectiveness of both multi-agency MCI training and the Incident Command System.

EMTs Kelli Barnaby and Jeffrey Clark have been nominated for a special Mayor's Award for their actions during the incident.

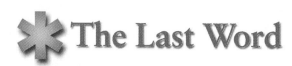

The Last Word

Multiple-casualty and mass-casualty incidents (MCIs) are some of the most challenging calls you will experience in your career. Due to the serious nature and legal implications of MCIs, the federal government has mandated that all first responders be managed by the National Incident Management System (NIMS).

When a structured incident management system is in place EMTs will have a safer more efficient environment in which to function. EMS and first responders will be able to provide the best patient care when a systematic approach to the sorting and movement of victims is accomplished.

EMTs can be expected to function in part of a large-scale incident. The minimum requirement for first responders is some understanding of the command and general staff responsibilities under an incident command system. As an EMT you should look for opportunity to acquire additional ICS or IMS training. The federal government maintains several resources and training programs on the Internet at NIMS.gov.

Chapter Review

MULTIPLE CHOICE

Place a check next to the correct answer.

1. The five major activities around which the ICS is organized are:

   _____ a. command, liaison, operations, communications, and logistics.

   _____ b. command, planning, operations, communications, and logistics.

   _____ c. command, planning, operations, finance/administration, and logistics.

   _____ d. command, liaison, safety, operations, and planning.

2. The General Staff consists of:

   _____ a. Operations, Planning, Logistics, and Information.

   _____ b. Operations, Command, Planning, and Logistics.

   _____ c. Operations, Finance/Administration, Planning, Liaison.

   _____ d. Operations, Planning, Logistics, and Finance/Administration.

3. Name the three major activities of the Command Staff.

   _____ a. safety, public information, and logistics

   _____ b. public information, safety, and planning

   _____ c. safety, public information, and liaison

   _____ d. planning, logistics, and safety

4. What is the one ICS position staffed at all incidents?

   _____ a. Division Supervisor

   _____ b. Incident Commander

   _____ c. Task Force Leader

   _____ d. Operations Section Chief

5. Air Operations, if activated at an incident, will be at what organizational level?

   _____ a. division

   _____ b. unit

   _____ c. section

   _____ d. branch

6. The Incident Commander may have one or more deputies from the same agency or from other agencies or jurisdictions.

   _____ a. true

   _____ b. false

7. When would Branches be used in the Logistics Section?

   _____ a. in place of units

   _____ b. to reduce span of control

   _____ c. to maintain unity of command

   _____ d. to place personnel with their day-to-day supervisors

8. Each individual reporting to only one supervisor defines:

   _____ a. unified command.

   _____ b. unity of command.

   _____ c. span of control.

   _____ d. consolidated command.

9. The _____ is responsible for tracking incident costs.

   _____ a. finance/administration section

   _____ b. command section

   _____ c. public Information section

   _____ d. planning section

10. _____ is responsible for providing facilities, services, and materials for the incident.

____ a. Finance

____ b. Logistics

____ c. Liaison

____ d. Staging

11. An organizational level responsible for operations in a specified geographic area defines:

____ a. group.

____ b. division.

____ c. section.

____ d. branch.

12. The ICS position that oversees the removal of patients from the wreckage is the:

____ a. Treatment Group Supervisor.

____ b. Transportation Group Leader.

____ c. Rescue/Extrication Group Supervisor.

____ d. Medical Unit Deputy.

13. The Information Officer is responsible for:

____ a. bypassing the chain of command when talking with the press.

____ b. coordinating all incident decisions.

____ c. establishing the staging area.

____ d. interfacing with the press and disseminating public information.

14. Effective span of control in ICS may vary from:

____ a. one to three.

____ b. two to seven.

____ c. three to seven.

____ d. five to seven.

15. The decision to have a written Incident Action Plan is made by the:

____ a. Operations Chief.

____ b. Incident Commander.

____ c. Planning Section Chief.

____ d. Safety Officer.

16. Operational periods are how long?

____ a. one hour

____ b. six hours

____ c. twelve hours

____ d. no fixed length

17. Groups have _____ responsibility, while divisions have _____ responsibility.

____ a. functional; geographic

____ b. more; less

____ c. outside; inside

____ d. geographic; functional

CRITICAL THINKING

1. Locate your local area disaster plan and identify the role of the EMS provider in the event of a disaster involving large numbers of patients. Who is in charge and what are the capacities of the hospital resources that are listed in that plan?

_____

_____

_____

2. Read and analyze the following scenario. Outline the incident in an organizational chart format that reflects your system. Be specific about the organizational position titles you would fill and who would fill them. Next make a list of potential problems, additional resources needed, and issues and how you would address them.

After completing this as an individual, you will be assigned to a small group to build a consensus. In this group, each member will discuss his approach to the incident. Make a final organizational chart and present it to the class with all groups taking turns to ask questions and present their organizational charts.

It is 2:00 on a Wednesday afternoon in January, and you and your EMT partner are responding to a reported traffic collision with at least three vehicles involved at a busy downtown intersection. Also dispatched to this incident are the following:

Rescue 10   A fire department transporting paramedic unit staffed with 2 EMT-paramedics.
Engine 2   A fire engine staffed with 3 EMT-firefighters, including the company officer.
Medic 11   An ambulance with 2 EMTs from the local private ambulance company.

You arrive on scene first. Your size-up gives you a total of eight patients. Three are critical trauma victims, two have moderate injuries, and three have minor injuries. The two moderate injuries are trapped inside an overturned vehicle. There is a gas leak from one of the vehicles. All the hospitals are within 10 minutes of the scene.

_____

_____

_____

3. As a group activity locate a piece of plywood and create a small scene using premade plastic buildings that can be purchased in a hobby shop and typically used for model railroading. Configure streets and parking lots. Locate small model cars including a fire truck, ambulance, and any vehicles of interest. As a group, create a model incident and employ the principles described for proper incident management.

_____

_____

_____

CASE STUDY

You are the first arriving ambulance to the scene of an MVC. You must take the role of Incident Commander on the scene of an MCI involving a pickup truck and a 15-passenger van from the local high school carrying band members. Your partner is acting as Triage Officer. He has performed a survey of the scene and found 10 passengers in the van and one driver in the pickup who is obviously DOA. Four of the passengers were crawling out of the overturned van on your arrival. The next ambulance to arrive on scene you assign to treat the wounded. You call the four passengers to a treatment area away from the hot zone. The remaining passengers are pinned or entrapped in the vehicle. The fire department arrives on the scene and begins extrication of the victims. They estimate it will take 10 to 15 minutes to free the remaining patients. You have called for a helicopter to transport two of the most critically injured patients. You have requested two additional transport units to transport the remaining victims. Your supervisor has just arrived on scene and has requested that you turn over command to him. To follow procedure you must give a summation of your efforts thus far.

Write out a verbal report that you would give to your supervisor.

_____

_____

_____

_____

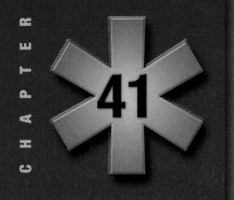
Responses Involving a Multiple-Casualty Incident

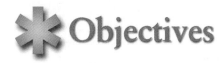

Objectives

Numbered objectives are from the U.S. Department of Transportation 1994 EMT-Basic National Standard Curriculum.

COGNITIVE OBJECTIVES

At the completion of this lesson, the EMT-Basic student will be able to:

7-3.7 Describe the criteria for a multiple-casualty situation. (pp. 1030–1031)

7-3.8 Evaluate the role of the EMT-Basic in the multiple-casualty situation. (pp. 1031–1034)

7-3.9 Summarize the components of basic triage. (pp. 1036–1038)

7-3.10 Define the role of the EMT-Basic in a disaster operation. (pp. 1036–1040)

AFFECTIVE OBJECTIVES

No affective objectives identified.

PSYCHOMOTOR OBJECTIVES

At the completion of this lesson, the EMT-Basic student will be able to:

7-3.16 Given a scenario of a mass-casualty incident, perform triage. (pp. 1036–1040)

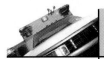 **Introduction**

The facts about **multiple-casualty incidents (MCIs)** may surprise you. Before reading this chapter, you may think of large incidents such as a plane crash or terrorist strike with hundreds or thousands of patients as representative of this type of incident. You are actually more likely to respond to a multiple-casualty incident with three to ten patients. Interestingly, both types of MCIs use the same principles but on different scales. This chapter will provide the critical information you will need to respond to multiple-casualty incidents of any size.

* **multiple-casualty incident (MCI)**

incident resulting from man-made or natural causes resulting in illness or injuries that exceed or overwhelm normal EMS and hospital capabilities. A large multiple-casualty incident may be called a mass-casualty incident.

Emergency Dispatch

"**D**ispatch to fourteen; dispatch to fourteen, do you copy?"

"Go ahead for fourteen," EMT Bill Franks said, trying to keep an ice cream cone from dripping onto his uniform pants.

"Fourteen, I need you to respond to a code three for a small airplane versus a car on Horizon Boulevard. Fire and PD are both en route."

"Ten-four." Bill put the microphone back into its holder, thought for a moment, and then looked over at his partner, Tammy Bursar. "Did he say a small airplane?"

"Yes! Now can we get moving?"

Bill tossed his ice cream into a garbage can outside the truck, activated the emergency lights, and headed toward Horizon Boulevard.

A single fire truck was already on scene and the crew was attempting to extricate the pilot from the small Cessna plane, which was heavily damaged and sitting awkwardly across several traffic lanes.

"How many patients do we have here?" Tammy shouted into the small group of firefighters after climbing from the ambulance and seeing a car and a pickup with extensive body damage pulled off to the side of the road.

One of the firefighters looked over at her, shrugged, shook his head as if to say, "I don't know," and went back to trying to free the lifeless pilot.

"Tammy!" Bill called from the opposite side of the chaotic roadway. "There's a van from Sunflower Preschool on its side down in this ditch. I can see movement!"

Multiple-Casualty Incidents

Multiple-casualty incidents are incidents that result from man-made or natural causes, resulting in illness or injuries that exceed or overwhelm normal EMS and hospital capabilities. A large multiple-casualty incident (or mass-casualty incident) is likely to impose a sustained demand for health and medical services rather than

7-3.7 Describe the criteria for a multiple-casualty situation.

the short, intense peak demand for these services typical of less-extensive multiple-casualty incidents. Examples of multiple-casualty incidents include:

* ✳ Major vehicular crashes with multiple victims

* ✳ Fires with burn or smoke-inhalation victims

* ✳ Environmental disasters

* ✳ Public transportation accidents (e.g., aircraft, train, bus)

* ✳ Mining or construction accidents

* ✳ Industrial accidents

* ✳ Building collapses

* ✳ Hazardous materials incidents

* ✳ Chemical, biological, radiological, nuclear, or explosive (CBRNE) incidents

* ✳ Planned events, such as celebrations, parades, concerts, or **mass gatherings**

✳ **mass gathering**

any collection of more than 1,000 people at one site or location. The term applies to all types of events, including concerts and sporting or other large-scale events.

Multiple-casualty incidents are events that involve multiple patients. While one patient may seem a challenge for the new EMT, a multiple-casualty event (Figure 41-1) can create an entirely new set of challenges for both the new and the experienced EMT. These events will stress the resources of a jurisdiction and, in some cases, a region beyond those normally available for a given call.

Although the terms *multiple-casualty incident* and *mass-casualty incident* are sometimes used synonymously, there is a difference in meaning, and it will be useful here to distinguish between them. A multiple-casualty incident may be defined as one that cannot be handled by the normal responding units but can be handled by a single system's resources. An example of this kind of event would be a three-car crash in which the ambulance and engine company first on the scene call for additional units from within their jurisdiction to assist with scene clean-up and transport of patients. These types of calls usually involve ten or fewer patients.

A mass-casualty incident may be defined as one that cannot be handled by responding units from within the jurisdiction but will require the resources of multiple jurisdictions or even a region. These events are often extensive operations that may require dozens of EMS units and involve more—usually many more—than ten patients.

In general, MCIs do not have to be airplane crashes or terrorism events, but can be a family injured in a house fire, or a three-car collision with two patients

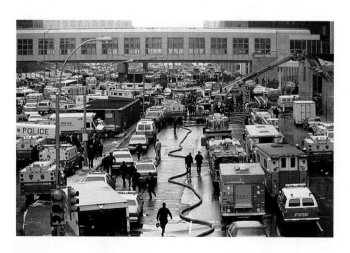

FIGURE 41-1 A multiple-casualty incident. (Black Star.)

in each car. How we approach the airplane crash is very similar to how we approach the three-car collision, as you will see.

MCIs by their very nature are different from our everyday calls. Usually when we handle a call, we go to a single patient. Whether the patient is experiencing chest pain or fell and broke his arm, most of the time it is just one patient you will treat until he is either transported for care or refuses treatment and transport.

MCIs, in which you handle or help handle large numbers of patients, are infrequent. Because of this, day-to-day systems will not work, and your procedures must change to facilitate rapid, yet effective, treatment of numerous patients.

Another issue with MCIs is that, more often than not, there is no anticipation that the event will happen. While some mass-casualty incidents are the result of predictable weather events, such as hurricanes, most are unpredictable, including tornados, earthquakes, fires, vehicle crashes such as trains, planes, and automobiles and, occasionally, acts of terrorism or other criminal acts. This unpredictability factor makes the EMS job that much harder and necessitates preplanning on the part of EMS organizations for a mass-casualty event.

Preplanning can take many forms, but most often it consists of the development of a response plan for future expected or possible events that would require a large response of multiple units, personnel, and leadership. Response plans developed during preplanning are often trialed during MCI drills and then revised based on post-drill debriefing.

As you can see, every call has the possibility of being a multiple-casualty event, and even what seems like a mundane car crash could be an MCI if it involves more patients than you and your crew can handle.

* **preplanning**

developing a plan for future possible events which would require a large response of units, personnel, and leadership.

Goals of MCI Management

When, as a new EMT, you arrive on scene of a mass-casualty event, you should keep three overall goals in the forefront of your mind:

* Do the best for the most.

* Manage very limited resources.

* Avoid relocating the disaster.

These goals may seem easy enough, but each has a significant challenge associated with it.

7-3.8 Evaluate the role of the EMT-Basic in the multiple-casualty situation.

DO THE BEST FOR THE MOST

Doing the best for the most means that the goal is to save the greatest possible number of patients, often allowing mortally injured patients to die rather than to exhaust limited resources.

Every day we respond to medical emergencies with two to eight emergency medical responders for a single patient. In a mass-casualty event, the ratio is reversed, and one provider may be treating up to eight patients. How would a single EMT treat four patients, all with significant airway issues? The answer is—with great difficulty. Understand that a single paramedic, nurse, or physician would also have difficulty in this situation.

This task may seem impossible, but the first-arriving EMT may initially have responsibility for all of the patients who are having difficulty breathing. In these cases, when there aren't enough hands to go around, we must concentrate on doing the most we can for those we can. This means that some patients with conditions we might normally treat will not receive the extensive resources we normally use for them. This may include children who are not breathing and are **tagged** as deceased because they cannot maintain their own airway. It may mean that a person who is in extreme pain from two broken legs is not cared for until some time later because he has been triaged into a low-priority category.

✳ **tagged**

placed in a triage category with a triage tag affixed.

MANAGE VERY LIMITED RESOURCES

The second goal of mass-casualty management is to manage scarce or limited resources. Whether it is ambulances, personnel, trauma dressings, oxygen masks, or even Band-Aids, all will be in short supply on a mass-casualty event. The only thing that will be in abundance will be patients. Ultimately, short supplies will include hospital beds and space, which leads to our third goal.

AVOID RELOCATING THE DISASTER

In a catastrophe, you must not let the incident overtake the team and as a result "relocate the disaster." In an MCI event, there will be a certain number of "walking wounded." These patients will have various injuries but, depending on the event, they may be able to self-refer to a hospital. In general, these patients will not only self-refer to a hospital, but they will go to the closest hospital. This hospital may become inundated with patients from an event, even as rescuers continue to perform the initial scene size-up. Even if patients don't self-refer to the nearest hospital, it is inappropriate for EMS crews to send all of the event's patients to a single location unless they know that the facility can handle the increased patient load. Concise communication between on-scene EMTs and the hospital or hospitals are an essential part of MCI management.

This is a critical point to understand, because if disaster strikes your community, whether it is a bus accident, a train derailment, or any other event, your local hospital must still be available for the patients who would normally go there with shortness of breath, chest pain, and other illnesses and injuries.

Initial Actions: The Five Ss

Many providers have felt overwhelmed by being the first unit to arrive at a mass-casualty event. Some have described feeling drowned by a "sea of patients" and unsure about their first steps. The goals of mass-casualty management may be common sense, but how can an EMT attain the most desirable outcome in events like these?

To help providers limit these normal stress responses and take some charge over the scene, the *Five Ss* were developed, which are a set of systematic actions to start handling a mass-casualty event.

SAFETY

The first S is *Safety*. Whether the call is an auto collision, house fire, or criminally inspired terrorist event, a mass-casualty event by definition, has too many patients. Initial EMS responders must take extra time to make sure they are considering their own safety as they approach an MCI scene. Adding patients to an incident never makes sense. In this case it is absolutely unacceptable.

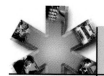

Perspective

Tammy—The EMT

"That was intense! Oh my gosh! We ended up getting seven patients transported from that scene! And that doesn't include the pilot, because he didn't make it. Surprisingly, we were able to handle it all within our agency. It's weird. Sometimes when something big is going to happen there is a kind of lull around the rest of the city, you know? Like when the air gets really still and quiet just before a tornado? I couldn't believe it when I gave my initial report to dispatch and he had about five trucks that he was able to free up and send our way immediately. I think that made a huge difference in the outcome."

SIZE-UP

Size-up is the second S and means to consider the event in its entirety. The initial on-scene report must include a description of the event so that other crews and personnel will have an idea of how big and how bad it may be. Is this a large airliner crash or a small bus crash? How many victims are obvious? What issues will there be with the event that incoming responders need to know?

SEND INFORMATION

The follow-up for sizing up a scene is to *send information,* the third S. Knowing the characteristics of an event without telling other responders does no good. The initial crew on an MCI must not only assess the scene, as they would assess a patient, but must also inform incoming crews so they will be able to begin work as soon as they arrive.

Inform dispatch of your unit designation, the nature of the event, and its correct location. Are there any obvious hazards such as fire, entrapment, or lack of structural integrity? Then request additional units that will assist with the scene or who have specialized rescue capability. Some EMS systems have specific protocols for enlarged EMS responses, such as an EMS Task Force or a One-Alarm Medical assignment that provides specific transport, treatment, and mass-casualty assistance.

SET UP THE MEDICAL SECTOR

The fourth S is *Set up the Medical Sector* using the Incident Command System, as discussed in chapter 40. While setting up a medical command sector may seem a waste of time versus immediately treating patients, the first arriving unit should do this. By starting the event with this mindset, there will be a direction for the event instead of ambulances just showing up, scooping up patients, and going to the closest hospital, which will quickly be overloaded. An organized response leads to a more efficient use of personnel and resources, which will lead to more patients being treated and treated better.

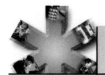

Perspective

Bill—The EMT

"I've never had to triage anybody in real life before. At first I asked myself, 'Where do I start?' There was an injured lady in the pickup, a guy next to the car, the pilot, and a whole group of little kids in that van. I really got overwhelmed. I hate to say it, but I actually started to panic a little. I mean, I was afraid that one of the kids would die if I didn't start with the van, but I'd have to walk right past other patients to get to it. I keep remembering the look in that one lady's eyes. It was the one in the pickup. Her eyes showed just terror and confusion, you know? I couldn't just walk past her! But then, all at once I remembered something my instructor said back in my EMT class. She said, "Start where you stand." So I did. It's amazing. Once you get moving, everything just falls into place."

START TRIAGE

Finally, we must know how many patients we have and how badly injured they are right now. This is accomplished with the fifth S—*START triage*. START stands for Simple Triage And Rapid Transport. Triage enables the Incident Commander to determine how many patients will need to be transported to how many hospitals and how much personnel will be required to accomplish this task.

Stop, Review, Remember!

Multiple Choice

Place a check next to the correct answer.

1. The first and most important of the "five Ss" is:

_____ a. scene size-up.

_____ b. safety.

_____ c. send information.

_____ d. START triage.

2. An incident that will overwhelm the initial responding units but *not* the resources of their system is known as a(n) _____ incident.

_____ a. multi-casualty

_____ b. controlled

_____ c. mass-casualty

_____ d. unmanageable

3. After giving dispatch the initial details of a mass-casualty event, the first responding unit should immediately:

_____   a. size up the scene.

_____   b. initiate START triage.

_____   c. evaluate safety concerns.

_____   d. set up a Medical Sector.

4. Developing a plan for future possible events that would require a large response of units, personnel, and leadership is called:

_____   a. forward incident control.

_____   b. resource management.

_____   c. preplanning.

_____   d. preemptive logistics.

5. The fourth S is *Set up the Medical Sector.*

_____   a. true

_____   b. false

Fill in the Blank

Put the following "Five Ss" in their proper order by placing the order number in the blank space.

1. _____ size-up

2. _____ safety

3. _____ START triage

4. _____ send information

5. _____ set up the Medical Sector

Critical Thinking

1. What are the three primary goals of EMS during an MCI?

_____

_____

_____

_____

2. Explain the difference between a *multi*-casualty incident and a *mass*-casualty incident.

_____

_____

_____

_____

Triage

7-3.9 Summarize the components of basic triage.

7-3.10 Define the role of the EMT-Basic in a disaster operation.

∗ **triage**

the process of sorting patients based on the severity or their injuries and prioritizing them for treatment and transport.

Triage is a French word that means "to sort." As an EMT, you can use any accepted triage system but one of the most dominant at this time is the START system developed in California during the 1980s. The START system (Figure 41-2) uses elementary patient assessment to rank the nature of injuries and the need for care using a color-coded system to identify patient priority categories. As noted earlier, START stands for Simple Triage And Rapid Transport. The colors associated with triage most often are red, yellow, green, and black as summarized in the boxed copy.

Triage should start with the first on-scene unit using a public-address or other system to ask those patients who can move to go to a designated area where another person from the unit can start to treat and identify them. When these patients move they do several things for your incident, one of which is to tell you by their actions that they are "walking wounded" and have minor injuries.

These patients will not be self-referring to the closest hospital because they are receiving medical attention on scene. This supports two MCI goals: not relocating the disaster and doing the most good for the most patients. These patients do not have to be relocated to a serene pasture; they can be moved to any easily locatable position or building where a group can receive basic medical care. These patients are immediately classified as GREEN.

FIGURE 41-2 START triage.

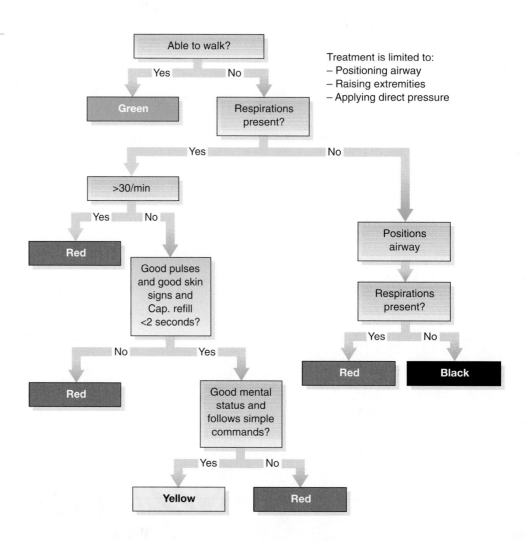

When triaging patients, EMTs should remember to work systematically to make sure that everyone is triaged and tagged (Figure 41-3). Triage time is kept to a minimum because each patient encounter should last only 15 to 30 seconds. Only the most basic care is performed during triage—generally limited to opening airways and controlling gross bleeding.

A final critical note is to be accurate in your patient count. Many EMS systems will utilize colored surveyor's tape tied to patient's wrists to indicate that patient's triage status. One way of keeping track of a large number of patients is to then tear off another section and place it in your pocket. At the conclusion of triaging your area, all these small pieces of triage tape will be in your pocket and will allow you to quickly divide them by color and provide Command with an accurate count of patients in each category.

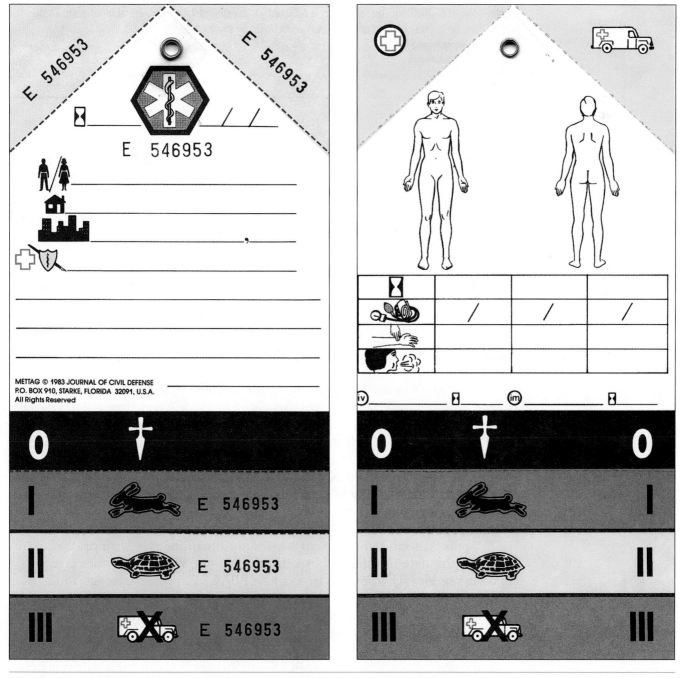

FIGURE 41-3   Triage tag (front and back) used to identify Priority 1, 2, 3, and 0 patients.

✳ **immediate patients**

patients who are at risk for early death, usually due to shock, an airway problem, or a severe head injury.

✳ **delayed patients**

patients who are injured but whose triage findings are more stable than those of the immediate patient.

✳ **minor patients**

patients with minor injuries. Sometimes referred to as walking wounded.

✳ **deceased patients**

patients who are not breathing after opening their airway.

START Triage

Patients are classified in to one of four classes.

Immediate - Red

IMMEDIATE patients, are at risk for early death—usually due to shock, an airway problem, or a severe head injury.

Delayed - Yellow

DELAYED patients are injured and these injuries may be serious. They were placed in the *delayed* category because their triage findings were more stable than those of the immediate patient.

Minor - Green

Patients with **MINOR** injuries, sometimes referred to as walking wounded, are still patients. Some of them may be frightened and affected psychologically by the incident.

Deceased - Black

Patients who are not breathing after opening their airway are tagged as **deceased.**

The START triage system itself is simple to use and relies on a condition-based, not an injury-based, system of classification. For instance, a badly burned patient might be tagged black, red, or yellow depending on how they fit into the criteria. This helps get treatment for the most seriously injured patients and allows resources to be managed more effectively.

JUMPSTART

While doing so may be a source of controversy and emotion, pediatric patients are triaged like anyone else. There are, however, important variations to consider when triaging them. One method for doing this is the JumpSTART system. Developed by Lou Romig, MD, JumpSTART recognizes that pediatric patients experience cardiovascular compromise differently from adults and prioritizes them accordingly.

JumpSTART begins like START triage for adults by trying to move those pediatric patients who can walk on their own to a GREEN sector where they will be triaged a second time. Those patients who do not move are first assessed for breathing.

If a child is not breathing, first reposition his airway. If the child starts to breathe, he is classified as RED. If he is still apneic, check for a pulse. If one is not found, tag the patient BLACK and move to the next patient you can help. Again, this is controversial and, while pediatric cardiac arrest is a very disturbing event for most responders, you must work within the system and move onto the next patient.

If a pulse is found on a patient who is not breathing, give five rescue breaths to try to stimulate the child to breathe on his own. If the child does breathe on his own, tag him RED, otherwise tag him BLACK. In either case, go to the next patient.

If the patient was breathing independently, then check the rate. If the respiratory rate is greater than 40 or less than 15, then tag the patient RED and go to the next patient.

If the respiratory rate is between 15 and 40, again check for a palpable pulse. If one is not found, tag the child RED and go to another patient.

If the breathing patient does have a palpable pulse, then do a disability scale. If the child is alert, responsive to voice, or responsive to pain, tag him YELLOW. If he postures to pain or is unresponsive, tag him RED. Because the use of multiple triage systems can cause confusion at the scene of an MCI, JUMPStart or other variation of START triage should only be used if it has been approved for use in your region.

SECONDARY TRIAGE

After initial attempts to triage all the patients, they should be brought to a central area where they are retriaged. In secondary triage, a more thorough assessment will be made of the patient to include locating specific injuries and providing additional life-threatening-injury treatment. Generally, the secondary triage position will be occupied by an advanced life support provider such as a paramedic or physician.

This part of triage will take longer than the first triage, but it will still last only minutes as patients are moved onto the appropriate treatment sectors.

As noted earlier, patients who are classified as RED are likely in shock or may have difficulty maintaining their own airway. YELLOW patients, while significantly injured, probably will have incapacitating injuries that can be treated later in the course of the event. GREEN patients are those whose injuries are minor and who will be able to wait hours before treatment. Patients tagged BLACK are those with no cardiorespiratory effort.

While initial triage classifies a patient, the patient may need to be reclassified during secondary triage or during his care on scene. An example might be a patient classified as yellow with a leg fracture who may be reclassified as red if subsequent evaluation reveals internal injuries and progressing shock.

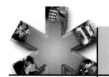

Perspective

Elise—The Preschool Van Driver

"All I can remember is that Randy wasn't breathing . . . and he was this horrible, blue color. Somehow when we rolled over he got stuck underneath one of the seats. I don't understand . . . he was in a booster and was wearing a seatbelt . . . but we just got hit so hard. I think I blacked out, because I didn't know how we ended up in the ditch. Oh, gee, I just keep seeing Randy's little face. And then I see his mom, you know? When she dropped him off this morning, she was wearing this great new leather jacket, and I remember complimenting her on it. And she said, "Please watch out for my little man; he's never been on a field trip without me." And then there he was with his legs and arms all tangled up. I thought he was dead. How would I tell her? How could I? Thank God for that EMT. He reached under the seat and moved Randy's head just a little and he just immediately started gasping for air . . . and crying. You have no idea how wonderful that sound was!"

In some EMS systems, patients tagged as red worsen en route to either secondary triage or the treatment area, resuscitation may take place, depending on the size of the incident and the availability of resources. Patients tagged as deceased on scene during initial triage most likely won't be moved at all. Because of the high probability that there will be investigations of mass-casualty incidents, it is generally better to leave the body in place for investigators, who may include local and state police, the Federal Bureau of Investigation, or the National Transportation Safety Board.

Stop, Review, Remember!

Multiple Choice

Place a check next to the correct answer.

1. The JumpSTART triage system was designed for _____ patients.

   _____ a. unresponsive

   _____ b. critical

   _____ c. "walking wounded"

   _____ d. pediatric

2. The triaging EMT should spend no more than _____ seconds on each patient.

   _____ a. 10

   _____ b. 30

   _____ c. 60

   _____ d. 45

3. Medical interventions during triage should be limited to opening airways and:

   _____ a. controlling severe bleeding.

   _____ b. performing emergency moves.

   _____ c. spinal immobilization.

   _____ d. performing CPR.

4. START stands for:

   _____ a. Selective Transport after Rapid Triage

   _____ b. Safe Transport and Radial Triage

   _____ c. Simple Triage and Rapid Transport

   _____ d. Split Triage and Responsive Transport

5. A triaged patient with no radial pulse is always tagged *black*.

   _____ a. true

   _____ b. false

Fill in the Blank

1. *Triage* is a _____ word that means "_____."

2. Pediatric patients are more likely to have cardiovascular compromise from too _____ breaths than from too _____.

3. During an MCI, more thorough assessments of the patients will be made during the _____ triage.

4. Patients whose injuries are _____ and who can wait an extended period of time before treatment are tagged _____ .

Critical Thinking

1. When triaging, what is the difference between START and JumpSTART?

_____

_____

_____

_____

2. During an MCI, how would you tag a patient who has a strong pulse but is unable to maintain his airway? Why?

_____

_____

_____

_____

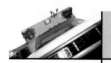

Dispatch Summary

The FAA investigation determined that the pilot had suffered a myocardial infarction just after take-off and had chosen to land on the largest roadway in sight. He suffered an aortic injury during the impact and didn't survive the landing.

Everyone on the ground survived with moderate injuries—with Randy's dislocated femur and mild concussion being the worst.

As a result of the uncoordinated initial response to this incident, a system-wide training program was created that has since greatly improved the ability of law enforcement, fire, and EMS to respond effectively together.

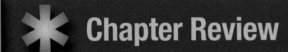

✳ The Last Word

There are differences between a multiple-casualty incident and a mass-casualty incident. One is the number of patients. The other is a mindset. It is the 2-to-10 person MCIs that historically catch EMTs unprepared. When a plane crashes or a passenger train derails, we can all agree we'll need help. But when two cars, each containing three people, collide, or when someone mixes cleaning fluids and eight people get sick, or even when a mother gives birth to premature twins, you have a multiple-casualty incident. Don't be fooled by the small ones.

✳ Chapter Review

MULTIPLE CHOICE

Place a check next to the correct answer.

1. Patients with obvious signs and symptoms of shock will most likely be tagged _____ during an MCI.

   _____ a. black

   _____ b. red

   _____ c. yellow

   _____ d. green

2. A multiple-casualty incident (MCI) is defined as:

   _____ a. an incident with 50 or more patients.

   _____ b. an incident that requires heavy or specialty rescue.

   _____ c. a terrorist or industrial accident.

   _____ d. an incident that exceeds the resources of the EMS system.

3. During the initial triage, rescue breaths should only be provided to _____ patients.

   _____ a. nonbreathing

   _____ b. adult

   _____ c. red-tagged

   _____ d. pediatric

4. You ask all patients who are able to walk to move to a particular area. The patients who do are triaged _____.

   _____ a. green

   _____ b. yellow

   _____ c. red

   _____ d. black

5. The START triage system relies on _____-based classification, not _____-based classification.

   _____ a. injury; condition

   _____ b. patient; incident

   _____ c. condition; injury

   _____ d. system; patient

6. The person responsible for secondary triage will usually be a physician or paramedic.

   _____ a. true

   _____ b. false

7. During large-scale MCIs, the Communications Officer will act as media liaison for the Incident Commander.

   _____ a. true

   _____ b. false

8. Patients marked with black tags should be moved and covered as soon as possible.

_____ a. true

_____ b. false

9. During an MCI, an adequately breathing patient who is responsive to pain should be identified with a yellow tag.

_____ a. true

_____ b. false

10. If possible, "walking wounded" patients should be encouraged to seek help at local hospitals as this will free up on-scene EMS resources.

_____ a. true

_____ b. false

FILL IN THE BLANK

Your ambulance is called to a multiple car collision on a rainy night along the Interstate. You arrive to find five cars all over the road. Traffic is stopped and no hazard from oncoming traffic is present. For each patient, write the correct color code—red, yellow, green, or black—according to the START system.

1. _____ 17-year-old male patient who is sitting in the driver's seat of his car. He has loud, moist gurgling sounds coming from his airway. His pulse is 124 and he responds only to loud verbal stimulus.

2. _____ 42-year-old man who says his neck hurts. He is ambulatory and able to follow instructions.

3. _____ 86-year-old man with a head wound with minor bleeding. He is sitting in his car and appears confused and unable to focus. His pulse is 66. Respirations 24.

4. _____ 79-year-old woman who is the passenger of patient "3." She is unresponsive without respirations or pulse. No obvious injuries. No change when opening her airway.

5. _____ 6-year-old male patient who is unresponsive with a pulse of 140 and respirations of 50.

6. _____ 24-year-old oriented female sitting in her car complaining of neck and abdominal pain. Her pulse is 82 and respirations are 16.

7. _____ 57-year-old female patient who is oriented and ambulatory complaining of shoulder pain.

8. _____ 37-year-old male patient found in the roadway who responds only to painful stimulus. Is breathing irregularly with a slow pulse.

9. _____ 29-year-old male patient sitting at the roadside who does not believe he is injured at all. His pulse is 120 and respirations are 28. He didn't move when ambulatory patients were asked to.

10. _____ 14-year-old alert male patient who believes he has a broken lower leg. Pulse 94, respirations 24.

CRITICAL THINKING

1. You are triaging numerous patients following a structure fire and you find an apneic 4-year-old girl. What should you do?

_____

_____

_____

_____

2. If a large number of green-tagged patients are on scene and they are beginning to get restless or complain about lack of care, what is the Incident Commander's best option?

_____

_____

_____

_____

3. Do you think it would take longer to triage 15 patients on a rolled-over municipal bus or 15 patients injured after a race car hit a wall and peppered the nearby crowd with flying car parts? Why?

_____

_____

_____

_____

CASE STUDY

You are driving home late one evening following a busy day working for the county ambulance service. You are tired and are looking forward to getting home, relaxing in front of the television for a few minutes, and then going to bed. You are suddenly passed by a semi truck that is going much faster than the posted 55 mph speed limit. As you watch in horror, the semi puts on its right blinker and merges directly over the top of a minivan that is about 100 feet ahead of you. The truck's trailer lurches upward and showers the roadway with sparks as it drags the van sideways, finally crushing it under the wide rear wheels. The semi then veers off onto the shoulder and clumsily rolls over, throwing a huge dust cloud up over the road.

1. If you choose to assist in this situation, what is the very first thing that you should do?

_____

_____

_____

2. Would you still follow all five "S's" in this situation?

_____

_____

_____

3. When beginning triage, which vehicle should you approach first?

_____

_____

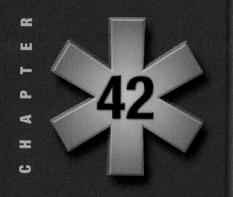

CHAPTER 42

Responses Involving Hazardous Materials

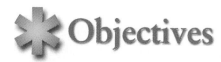

Objectives

Numbered objectives are from the U.S. Department of Transportation 1994 EMT-Basic National Standard Curriculum.

COGNITIVE OBJECTIVES

At the completion of this lesson, the EMT-Basic student will be able to:

7-3.1 Explain the EMT-Basic's role during a call involving hazardous materials. (pp. 1046–1047)

7-3.2 Describe what the EMT-Basic should do if there is reason to believe that there is a hazard at the scene. (pp. 1047–1051)

7-3.3 Describe the actions that an EMT-Basic should take to ensure bystander safety. (pp. 1054–1055)

7-3.4 State the role the EMT-Basic should perform until appropriately trained personnel arrive at the scene of a hazardous materials situation. (pp. 1053–1054)

7-3.5 Break down the steps to approaching a hazardous situation. (pp. 1054–1055)

7-3.6 Discuss the various environmental hazards that affect EMS. (pp. 1056–1059)

AFFECTIVE OBJECTIVES

No affective objectives identified.

PSYCHOMOTOR OBJECTIVES

No psychomotor objectives identified.

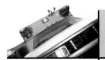 **Introduction**

Every day millions of tons of hazardous materials (HazMats) are processed, transported, and used by business and industry. As an EMT you can expect to be involved in patient care or to function in a support role at the scene of a HazMat incident. An accidental release of these materials presents a potential danger to the public and the environment. Such an incident can be managed more expeditiously when the hazardous materials are specifically identified and characterized. Unfortunately, the contents of storage tanks and trucks may not be properly identified. Records or shipping papers may be inaccessible. Even with such information, an experienced person is needed to define and manage the hazards and the overall safety of the situation.

Emergency Dispatch

"Is this thing even working?" EMT Austin Brace tapped on the ambulance's air conditioning control switch.

"Yeah, it works," his partner, Maya, said as she swept a lock of damp hair from her cheek. "But being that it's 110° outside, it's not gonna do much."

"Eight-oh-two," the radio crackled. "Eight-oh-two, I need you to start emergency care for 4908 County Road Fifty-Three. . . for a. . . standby one."

"Oh, please, let it be a call in a nice air-conditioned office building," Austin pulled his seatbelt on. "Or a swimming pool. Is that too much to ask?"

"Probably," Maya said. "I think the only thing out that far on C.R. Fifty-Three is the. . . ." She was interrupted by the dispatcher.

"Okay, oh-two," the dispatcher added. "It's at the sewage treatment plant at 4908 County Road Fifty-

Three for a man down in the parking lot. . . was called in by a driver who passed by."

"Hmm, the sewage treatment plant," Maya finished, frowning.

As they turned onto the newly paved County Road Fifty-Three, a fire truck rolled to a stop at the sewage plant's entrance gate. Four firefighters spilled out and hurried into the parking lot.

"How do they *do* that?" Austin pulled up next to the fire truck. "They are just so fast."

"Uh-oh, Austin," Maya began jabbing her index finger toward the windshield. "Look!"

All four firefighters were now sprawled motionless on the ground next to the treatment plant worker.

"Oh, shoot—hold on!" Austin slammed the truck into reverse and raced back up the county road as Maya grabbed for the radio.

7-3.1 Explain the EMT-Basic's role during a call involving hazardous materials.

✳ **hazardous material**

any substance or material in a form which poses an unreasonable risk to health, safety, and property.

Hazardous Materials

The U.S. Department of Transportation (DOT) defines a **hazardous material** as "any substance or material in a form which poses an unreasonable risk to health, safety, and property." New hazardous materials are being produced every day, and waste products from chemical manufacturing are reprocessed and disposed of. Even though there are a tremendous number of regulations and safety procedures in place, exposures to hazardous materials do occur. See Table 42-1 for examples of hazardous materials.

TABLE 42-1 EXAMPLES OF HAZARDOUS MATERIALS	
MATERIAL	**POSSIBLE HAZARD**
Benzene (benzol)	Toxic vapors; can be absorbed through the skin; destroys bone marrow
Benzoyl peroxide	Fire and explosion
Carbon tetrachloride	Damages internal organs
Cyclohexane	Explosive; eye and throat irritant
Diethyl ether	Flammable and can be explosive; irritant to eyes and respiratory tract; can cause drowsiness or unconsciousness
Ethyl acetate	Irritates eyes and respiratory tract
Ethylene chloride	Damages eyes
Ethylene dichloride	Strong irritant
Heptane	Respiratory irritant
Hydrochloric acid	Respiratory irritant; exposure to high concentration of vapors can produce pulmonary edema; can damage skin and eyes
Hydrogen cyanide	Highly flammable; toxic through inhalation or absorption
Methyl isobutyl ketone	Irritates eyes and mucous membranes
Nitric acid	Produces a toxic gas (nitrogen dioxide); skin irritant; can cause self-ignition of cellulose products (e.g., sawdust)
Organochloride (Chlordane, DDT, Dieldrin, Lindane, Methoxyclor)	Irritates eyes and skin; fumes and smoke toxic
Perchloroethylene	Toxic if inhaled or swallowed
Silicon tetrachloride	Water-reactive to form toxic hydrogen chloride fumes
Tetrahydrofuran (THF)	Damages eyes and mucous membranes
Toluol (toluene)	Toxic vapors; can cause organ damage
Vinyl chloride	Flammable and explosive; listed as a carcinogen

You will have immediate need for information concerning the material involved when you are called to the scene of a hazardous material incident. For this purpose, two hazardous materials identification systems have been developed, one for building responses and one for transportation responses.

Responses to Hazardous Materials Incidents

Depending on the hazardous material suspected and the location, your response team will need to follow specific protocols to ensure bystander safety and respond appropriately.

7-3.2 Describe what the EMT-Basic should do if there is reason to believe that there is a hazard at the scene.

7-3.3 Describe the actions that an EMT-Basic should take to ensure bystander safety.

RESPONSES TO BUILDINGS

∗ **National Fire Protection Association (NFPA)**

the world's leading advocate of fire prevention and an authoritative source on public safety. NFPA's 300 codes and standards influence every building, process, service, design, and installation in the United States, as well as many of those used in other countries.

∗ **NFPA 704**

a standardized system that uses numbers and colors on a sign to indicate the basic hazards of a specific material being stored in large containers or at a manufacturing site.

∗ **occupancy**

the term used to describe a building that may be used to manufacture or process chemicals.

The **National Fire Protection Association (NFPA)** has devised a voluntary marking system to alert emergency responders to the characteristics of hazardous materials stored in stationary tanks and facilities (Figures 42-1A and B). This system, known as **NFPA 704,** is a standardized system that uses numbers and colors on a sign to indicate the basic hazards of a specific material being stored in large containers or at a manufacturing site.

Occupancy is the term used to describe a building that may be used to manufacture or process chemicals. The occupancy will be marked by a multicolored diamond-shaped sign that indicates characteristics of the stored substance according to the National Fire Protection Association 704 system. Look for the 704 sign to be mounted on the exterior of the building or fencing around the perimeter of a complex.

The diamond-shaped NFPA 704 label is divided into four parts, or quadrants (Figures 42-2 and 42-3).

∗ The left quadrant is *blue,* and contains a numerical rating of the substance's health hazard. Ratings are made on a scale of 4 to 0, with a rating of 4 indicating a severe hazard in which a very short exposure could cause serious injury or death. A zero, or no code at all in this quarter, means that no unusual health hazard would result from exposure.

∗ The top quadrant of the NFPA symbol contains the substance's fire hazard rating. As you might expect, this quadrant is *red.* Again, number

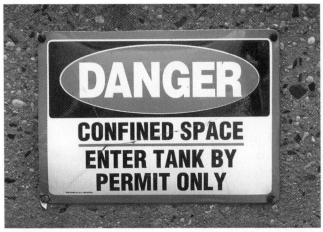

a

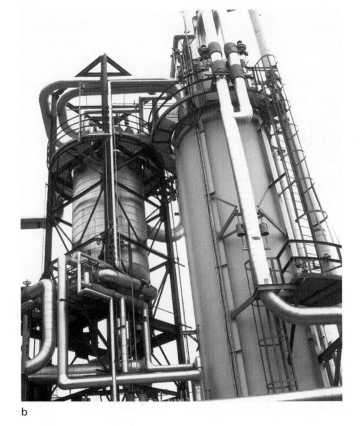

b

FIGURE 42-1A Look for clues, such as signs, to potential hazardous materials.

FIGURE 42-1B Storage tanks often house hazardous materials.

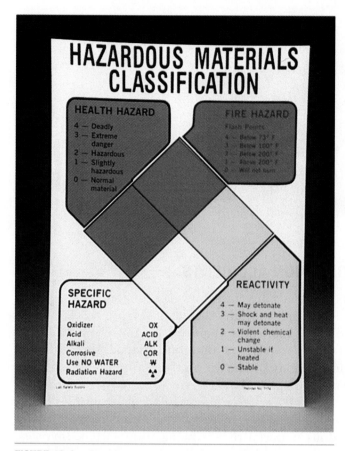

FIGURE 42-2 This is the key to the National Fire Protection
Association (NFPA) 704 system of numeric and color codes to
hazardous materials.

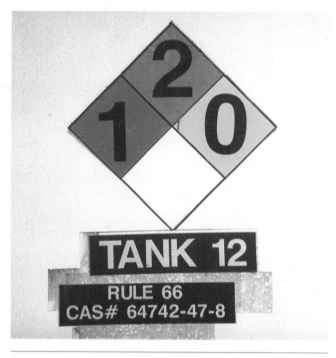

FIGURE 42-3 NFPA 704 labeling on a tank.

codes in this quadrant range from 4 to 0, with 4 representing the highest
level of potential hazard.

∗ The right quadrant, colored *yellow,* indicates the substance's likelihood to
explode or react. As with the health and fire hazard quadrants, ratings from
4 to 0 are used to indicate the degree of hazard. If a 2 appears in this section, the chemical is moderately unstable, and even under *normal* conditions may explode or react violently. A zero in this quadrant indicates that
the material is considered to be stable even in the event of a fire.

∗ The bottom quadrant is *white* and contains information about any special
hazards that may apply. There are three possible codes for the bottom quarter of the NFPA symbol. OXY means this material is an oxidizer. It can easily release oxygen to create or worsen a fire or explosion hazard. The
symbol ₩ indicates a material that reacts with water to release a gas that is
either flammable or hazardous to health. If the material is radioactive, the
usual tri-blade "propeller" symbol for radioactivity will appear.

The EMT needs to pay particular attention to the blue area that denotes the
health hazards of the chemicals inside the occupancy. A 4 rating in the blue area
of the diamond indicates that the building or container contains chemicals that are
deadly.

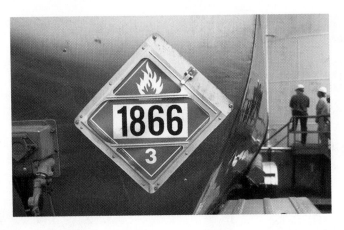

FIGURE 42-4   Vehicles carrying hazardous materials are required to display placards that communicate the nature of their cargo.

✳ **DOT**

   United States Department of Transportation.

✳ **placard**

   diamond-shaped sign placed on cargo tanks, vehicles, or rail cars to display one of nine classes of hazardous materials that is being carried.

✳ **material data safety sheet (MSDS)**

   document from the manufacturer for each hazardous chemical in the workplace. The MSDS contains important safety information about the hazardous chemical.

RESPONSES TO TRANSPORTATION ACCIDENTS

Millions of tons of hazardous materials are transported throughout the country in various containers, packages, and specialty vehicles (Figure 42-4). These containers are required to display markings required by the Department of Transportation (**DOT**). The DOT requires a diamond-shaped sign called a **placard.** The four-digit ID Number may be shown on the diamond-shaped placard or on an adjacent orange panel displayed next to the placard on the ends and sides of a cargo tank, vehicle, or rail car. The placard can display one of nine classes of hazardous materials. Additionally, there may be numbers that show a division of the class of hazardous material that is being transported. Invoices, shipping papers (barges and trains), and bills of lading (trucks) are documents that identify the type, quantity, origin, and destination of the hazardous materials. Often these documents are kept in the wheelhouse of a water-going vessel, the cab of a truck, or with the engineer.

Employers are required to maintain a current **material data safety sheet (MSDS)** from the manufacturer for each hazardous chemical in the workplace (Figure 42-5). The EMT should obtain these materials only if it is safe to do so.

When a patient is transported from a site where an MSDS is maintained, he should be accompanied by the MSDS. Other important information on the number of victims, resources, the manufacturing processes involved, the nature of the exposures, and the specific emergency can be obtained from personnel on leaving the affected area.

THE Clorox Company
7200 Johnson Drive
Pleasanton, California 94566
Tel. (415) 847-6100

Material Safety
Data Sheets

Health	2+
Flammability	0
Reactivity	1
Personal Protection	B

I – CHEMICAL IDENTIFICATION

Name	regular Clorox Bleach	CAS No.	N/A
Description	clear, light yellow liquid with chlorine odor	RTECs No.	N/A

Other Designations	**Manufacturer**	**Emergency Procedure**
EPA Reg. No. 5813-1 Sodium hypochlorite solution Liquid chlorine bleach Clorox Liquid Bleach	The Clorox Company 1221 Broadway Oakland, CA 94612	• Notify your supervisor • Call your local poison control center OR • Rocky Mountain Poison Center (303)573-1014

II – HEALTH HAZARD DATA

• Causes severe but temporary eye injury. May irritate skin. May cause nausea and vomiting if ingested. Exposure to vapor or mist may irritate nose, throat and lungs. The following medical conditions may be aggravated by exposure to high concentrations of vapor or mist: heart conditions or chronic respiratory problems such as asthma, chronic bronchitis or obstructive lung disease. Under normal consumer use conditions the likelihood of any adverse health effects are low. FIRST AID: EYE CONTACT: Immediately flush eyes with plenty of water. If irritation persists, see a doctor. SKIN CONTACT: Remove contaminated clothing. Wash area with water. INGESTION: Drink a glassful of water and call a physician. INHALATION: If breathing problems develop remove to fresh air.

III – HAZARDOUS INGREDIENTS

Ingredients	Concentration	Worker Exposure Limit
Sodium hypochlorite CAS# 7681-52-9	5.25%	not established

None of the ingredients in this product are on the IARC, NTP or OSHA carcinogen list. Occasional clinical reports suggest a low potential for sensitization upon exaggerated exposure to sodium hypochlorite if skin damage (e.g., irritation) occurs during exposure. Routine clinical tests conducted on intact skin with Clorox Liquid Bleach found no sensitization in the test subjects.

IV – SPECIAL PROTECTION INFORMATION

Hygienic Practices: Wear safety glasses. With repeated or prolonged use, wear gloves.

Engineering Controls: Use general ventilation to minimize exposure to vapor or mist.

Work Practices: Avoid eye and skin contact and inhalation of vapor or mist.

V – SPECIAL PRECAUTIONS

Keep out of reach of children. Do not get in eyes or on skin. Wash thoroughly with soap and water after handling. Do not mix with other household chemicals such as toilet bowl cleaners, rust removers, vinegar, acid or ammonia containing products. Store in a cool, dry place. Do not reuse empty container; rinse container and put in trash container.

VI – SPILL OR LEAK PROCEDURES

Small quantities of less than 5 gallons may be flushed down drain. For larger quantities wipe up with an absorbent material or mop and dispose of in accordance with local, state and federal regulations. Dilute with water to minimize oxidizing effect on spilled surface.

VII – REACTIVITY DATA

Stable under normal use and storage conditions. Strong oxidizing agent. Reacts with other household chemicals such as toilet bowl cleaners, rust removers, vinegar, acids or ammonia containing products to produce hazardous gases, such as chlorine and other chlorinated species. Prolonged contact with metal may cause pitting or discoloration.

VIII – FIRE AND EXPLOSION DATA

Not flammable or explosive. In a fire, cool containers to prevent rupture and release of sodium chlorate.

IX – PHYSICAL DATA

Boiling point...................................212°F/100°C (decomposes)
Specific Gravity (H$_2$O = 1).............1.085
Solubility in Water..........................complete
pH...11.4

FIGURE 42-5   A material safety data sheet.

Stop, Review, Remember!

Multiple Choice

Place a check next to the correct answer.

1. The U.S. Department of Transportation (DOT) defines a *hazardous material* as:

    _____ a. a poison or chemical that could harm you.

    _____ b. any substance or material in a form which poses an unreasonable risk to health.

    _____ c. a substance that must be marked with a placard when shipped or stored.

    _____ d. a poison or chemical that is not harmful to you.

2. National Fire Protection Association 704 system is used to mark _____ with a multicolored diamond sign.

    _____ a. occupancy

    _____ b. hazardous materials

    _____ c. flammable material

    _____ d. chemical material

3. You arrive at a building for a medical call. The *red* quadrant of the NFPA symbol contains the number 3. This means there is:

    _____ a. no fire hazard.

    _____ b. a minimal fire hazard.

    _____ c. a serious fire hazard.

    _____ d. a moderate fire hazard.

4. When responding to an motor vehicle collision involving a vehicle that transports hazardous materials, you should look for _____ during your scene size up.

    _____ a. material data safety sheets

    _____ b. invoices, shipping papers, and bills of lading

    _____ c. placards

    _____ d. red diamonds

Matching

Match the following elements of the 704 Placard System.

1. _____ Red
2. _____ Blue
3. _____ Yellow
4. _____ White

A. Reactivity hazard
B. Health hazard
C. Fire hazard
D. Special hazard

Critical Thinking

1. What impact would a hazardous materials incident have on the local high school? What resources does your jurisdiction have to respond to such an incident?

_____

_____

_____

_____

2. What industries within your community have hazardous chemicals in large quantities?

_____

_____

_____

_____

3. What materials are being shipped through your community via all transportation arteries?

_____

_____

_____

_____

General Procedures

One of the most important tasks you may do at the scene of a hazardous materials call is to identify the chemicals involved. Your safety is the primary responsibility when responding to a hazardous materials incident. The ambulance should be equipped with basic equipment for a hazardous materials response, such as the DOT *Emergency Response Guidebook (ERG)* and binoculars (Figure 42-6 on page 1054).

The ERG was developed jointly by Transport Canada (TC), the U.S. Department of Transportation (DOT), and the Secretariat of Transport and Communications of Mexico (SCT), with the collaboration of CIQUIME (Centro de Información Química para Emergencias) of Argentina, for use by firefighters, police, and other emergency services personnel who may be the first to arrive at the scene of a transportation incident involving dangerous goods and hazardous materials. The *Emergency Response Guidebook* provides the names, procedures, physical behavior, medical issues, and evacuation distances for certain chemicals.

7-3.4 State the role the EMT-Basic should perform until appropriately trained personnel arrive at the scene of a hazardous materials situation.

✳ *Emergency Response Guidebook (ERG)*

Department of Transportation quick-information guide to hazardous materials response.

FIGURE 42-6 *Emergency Response Guidebook.*

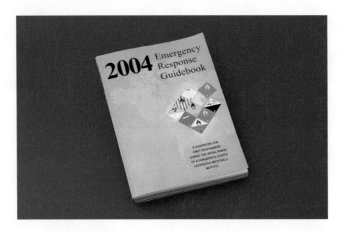

The guidebook is divided into four sections:

✳ The yellow section lists hazardous materials based on a specific identification number.

✳ The blue section lists hazardous materials in alphabetical order based on their name.

✳ The orange section has all the safety recommendations.

✳ The green section, among other things, provides information on safe distances and is further divided into daytime and nighttime incidences.

The ERG is the basic resource for all emergency responders. It is designed to help responders get through the first 20 minutes of an incident.

Approaching the Scene

7-3.3 Describe the actions that an EMT-Basic should take to ensure bystander safety.

When responding to a reported HazMat incident, it is good practice to call for a weather report from the local communications center. It is important to park upwind/uphill from the incident at a safe distance (Figure 42-7). Do not drive through leaking chemicals. Often first responders assess the scene from a distance with binoculars (Figure 42-8).

7-3.5 Break down the steps to approaching a hazardous situation.

As first responders at the scene of a hazardous materials transportation spill, local firefighters and/or police typically have the lead responsibility for:

✳ Identifying the materials involved

✳ Determining the risk or hazard posed by the spill

✳ Calling for additional resources, if necessary, to monitor and contain the spill

✳ Isolating the scene, restricting or rerouting traffic, and conducting evacuation, if necessary

✳ Providing first aid, as needed

✳ Fighting the fire and protecting against explosions

✳ Keeping the public informed of the hazard that exists, the actions being taken, precautionary measures to take, and evacuation routes and destinations (if necessary)

✳ Taking overall scene safety and management responsibilities

Establishing the Danger Zone

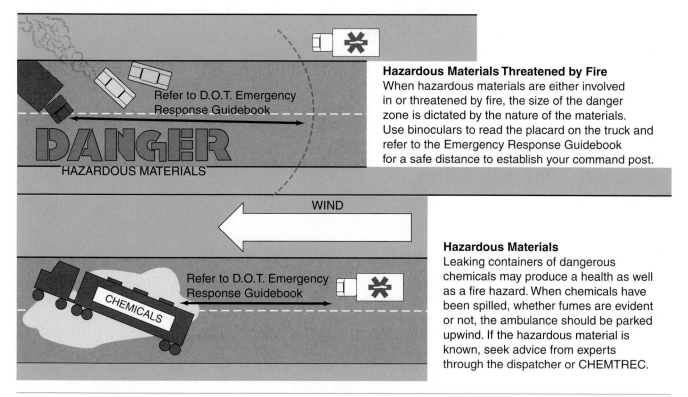

Hazardous Materials Threatened by Fire
When hazardous materials are either involved in or threatened by fire, the size of the danger zone is dictated by the nature of the materials. Use binoculars to read the placard on the truck and refer to the Emergency Response Guidebook for a safe distance to establish your command post.

Hazardous Materials
Leaking containers of dangerous chemicals may produce a health as well as a fire hazard. When chemicals have been spilled, whether fumes are evident or not, the ambulance should be parked upwind. If the hazardous material is known, seek advice from experts through the dispatcher or CHEMTREC.

FIGURE 42-7   Transportation incidents involving hazardous materials.

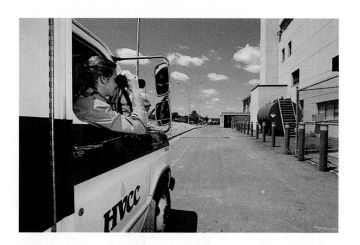

FIGURE 42-8   Binoculars will allow a visual inspection of the hot zone from a safe distance.

The first emergency responders from EMS, fire, or law enforcement that arrive on the scene usually do not have the specialized clothing they would need to rescue personnel in a HazMat emergency without themselves becoming victims. The EMT should keep all unnecessary people away from the area, isolating and denying entry into the area. Remove patients to a safe zone if there is no risk to you as an EMT. In some cases you will need to direct patients to a decontamination area. *Do not enter a HazMat area unless you are trained as a HazMat Tech and have proper training in SCBA and equipment.*

A 24-hour resource available to emergency responders is CHEMTREC. An emergency responder can call 1-800-424-9300 for immediate support on a HazMat emergency. CHEMTREC services are provided to emergency responders by the

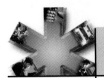

Perspective

John—The Firefighter

"I can't believe we did that. We've been trained and trained and trained about stuff like that, and yet there we were, just running right in. I was thinking the guy was a full arrest or something, you know? I've been with the department for 22 years and there's never been any problems at that plant. I wasn't thinking HazMat. We just didn't consider all the possibilities. I remember climbing out of the truck and for just a split second I thought I smelled rotten eggs. But then it was gone (snaps fingers), just like that. Maybe I imagined it. Well, no, I guess I didn't."

Chemical Manufacturers Association. They will provide notification to the shipper and can obtain emergency information from federal and industry resources.

Sometimes there are *sensory* clues that indicate the presence of hazardous materials. Sensory clues, however, are the least dependable and potentially the most dangerous method of identification. Many materials do not have such warning signals as smell or taste. If you notice that an area has a terrible smell, your eyes water, your skin is irritated, or you begin to cough or feel nauseated, leave immediately and contact your communication center. Police, fire, and local hazardous material response teams should be dispatched. If you encounter a suspicious substance, do *not* handle it yourself. Remove the patient to a safe zone if it is safe to do so, and isolate and deny entry into the area.

DOT Hazard Classification System

7-3.6 Discuss the various environmental hazards that affect EMS.

The hazard class of dangerous substances is indicated either by its hazard class (or division) number or name. For a placard corresponding to the primary hazard class of a material, the hazard class or division number must be displayed in the lower corner of the placard (Figure 42-9). No hazard class or division number, however, may be displayed on a placard representing the subsidiary hazard of a material. For other than Class 7 or the OXYGEN placard, text indicating a hazard (for example, "CORROSIVE") is not required. Text is shown only in the United States. The hazard class or division number must appear on the shipping document after each shipping name.

The DOT hazard classes and divisions are as follows:

Hazard Class 1   **Explosives** (Figure 42-10)

Explosive injuries produce primary, secondary, and tertiary blast injuries.

Hazard Class 2   **Gases** (Figure 42-11)

Gases cause injury by being toxic or displacing oxygen to cause asphyxiation. Toxic gases can kill by causing irritation of the airway and lungs.

Hazard Class 3   **Flammable liquids, combustible liquids [U.S.]** (Figure 42-12 on page 1058)

∗ **Hazard Class 1, Explosives**

cause injuries by the primary, secondary, and tertiary blasts.

∗ **Hazard Class 2, Gases**

cause injuries by being toxic or displacing oxygen to cause asphyxiation.

∗ **Hazard Class 3, Flammable liquids, combustible liquids**

cause injuries by penetrating the skin and attacking internal organs.

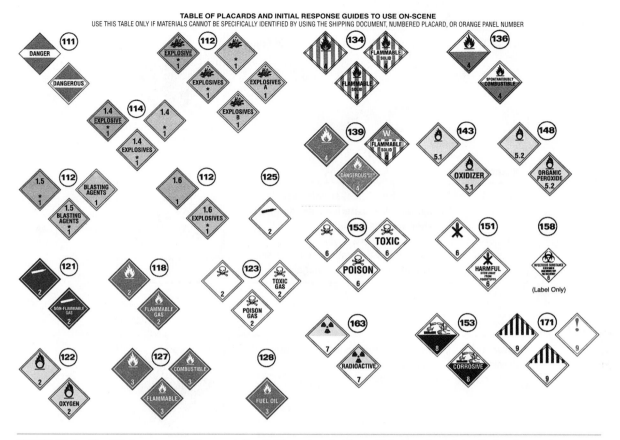

TABLE OF PLACARDS AND INITIAL RESPONSE GUIDES TO USE ON-SCENE
USE THIS TABLE ONLY IF MATERIALS CANNOT BE SPECIFICALLY IDENTIFIED BY USING THE SHIPPING DOCUMENT, NUMBERED PLACARD, OR ORANGE PANEL NUMBER

FIGURE 42-9   The U.S. Department of Transportation (DOT) requires that hazard labels or placards be displayed on packages, storage containers, and vehicles containing hazardous materials.

Hazard Class 1

Class 1	Explosives
Division 1.1	Explosives with a mass explosion hazard
Division 1.2	Explosives with a projection hazard
Division 1.3	Explosives with predominantly a fire hazard
Division 1.4	Explosives with no significant blast hazard
Division 1.5	Very insensitive explosives; blasting agents
Division 1.6	Extremely insensitive detonating articles

FIGURE 42-10   Hazard Class 1.

Hazard Class 2

Class 2	Gases
Division 2.1	Flammable gases
Division 2.2	Non-flammable, non-toxic* compressed gases
Division 2.3	Gases toxic* by inhalation
Division 2.4	Corrosive gases (Canada)

FIGURE 42-11   Hazard Class 2.

Flammable and combustible liquids cause injury by penetrating the skin and attacking internal organs. Vapors or gases can be generated from flammable and combustible liquids that can cause inhalation injury. The ignition of flammable liquids can result in varying degrees of burn injuries.

Hazard Class 4   Flammable solids, spontaneously combustible materials, and dangerous when wet materials (Figure 42-13 on page 1058)

* Hazard Class 4, Flammable solids, spontaneously combustible materials, and dangerous when wet materials

cause injuries by creating severe and deep burns to tissue. Many of the flammable solids are reactive to water.

FIGURE 42-12 Hazard Class 3.

Hazard Class 3

Class 3	Flammable liquids, combustible liquids [U.S.]	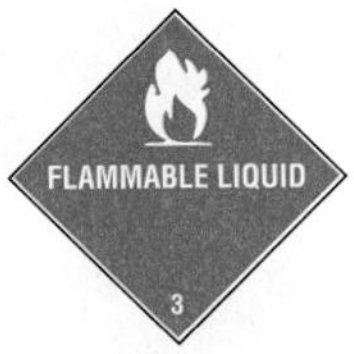
No Divisions		FLAMMABLE LIQUID 3

FIGURE 42-13 Hazard Class 4.

Hazard Class 4

Class 4	Flammable solids, spontaneously combustible materials, and dangerous when wet materials	
Division 4.1	Flammable solids	DANGEROUS WHEN WET 4
Division 4.2	Spontaneously combustible materials	
Division 4.3	Dangerous when wet materials	

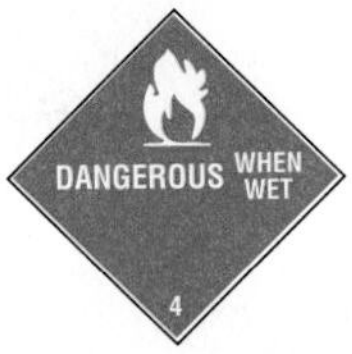

FIGURE 42-14 Hazard Class 5.

Hazard Class 5

Class 5	Oxidizers and organic peroxides	
Division 5.1	Oxidizers	OXIDIZER 5.1
Division 5.2	Organic peroxides	

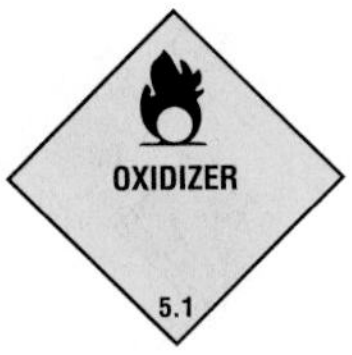

FIGURE 42-15 Hazard Class 6.

Hazard Class 6

Class 6	Toxic* materials and infectious substances	
Division 6.1	Toxic* materials	INHALATION HAZARD 6
Division 6.2	Infectious substances	

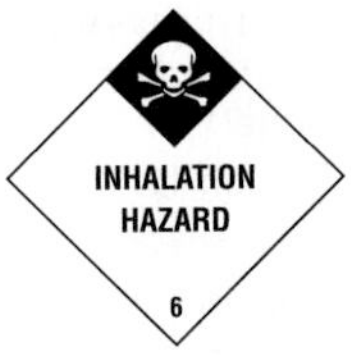

* **Hazard Class 5, Oxidizers and Organic peroxides**

can trigger an explosion and can also act as a corrosive destroying tissue and triggering inflammation in the lungs.

* **Hazard Class 6, Toxic materials and Infectious substances**

involve biological and poisonous substances. Infectious material can include blood products or blood-contaminated materials and plant, virus, bacterial, or other living organisms.

* **Hazard Class 7, Radioactive materials**

injury or kill by disrupting the nervous system or the cellular functions.

Flammable solids cause injuries by creating severe and deep burns to tissue. Many of the flammable solids are reactive to water and create deeper burns when rescuers attempt to flush the material from the skin. Alkaline burns penetrate deep into the tissue and destroy the fat layer under the skin, causing severe tissue destruction. The EMT should contact poison control for treatment procedures and remove powdered or metal materials with a dry brush.

Hazard Class 5 Oxidizers and organic peroxides (Figure 42-14)

Oxidizers can trigger an explosion and can also act as a corrosive, destroying tissue and triggering inflammation in the lungs. Many peroxides can degrade and become explosives that can result in a blast injury.

Hazard Class 6 Toxic materials and Infectious substances (Figure 42-15)

Toxic materials involve biological and poisonous substances. Infectious material can include blood products or blood-contaminated materials and plant, virus, bacterial, or other living organisms. Toxic materials can include cellular poisons or other substances that can injure or kill.

Hazard Class 7 Radioactive materials (Figure 42-16)

Hazard Class 7

Class 7 No Divisions	Radioactive materials	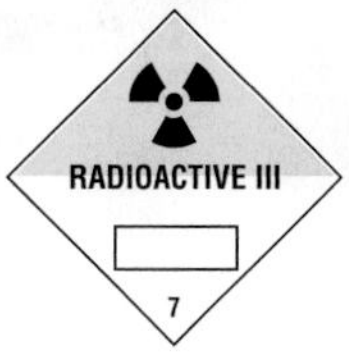

FIGURE 42-16 Hazard Class 7.

Hazard Class 8

Class 8 No Divisions	Corrosive materials	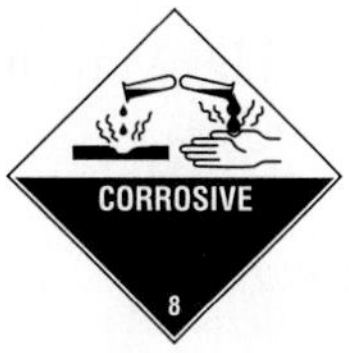

FIGURE 42-17 Hazard Class 8.

Hazard Class 9

Class 9 Division 9.1 Division 9.2 Division 9.3	Miscellaneous dangerous goods Miscellaneous dangerous goods (Canada) Environmentally hazardous substances (Canada) Dangerous wastes (Canada)	

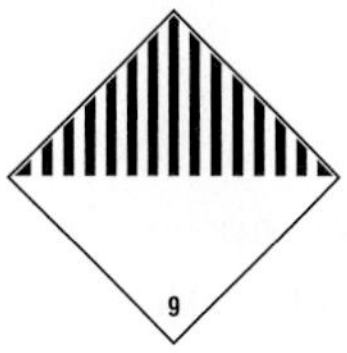

FIGURE 42-18 Hazard Class 9.

Radioactive materials injure or kill by disrupting the nervous system or the cellular functions.

Hazard Class 8   Corrosive materials (Figure 42-17)

Corrosives injure by destroying and dissolving tissue. Corrosives usually involve acids, bases, and some solvents. Alkaline corrosives dissolve fat and connective tissues, creating a waxy appearance. Acids react immediately with the water in the skin and tissue to create acids that may burn or dissolve tissue. Weak acids and bases may only produce signs of irritation or itching.

Hazard Class 9   Miscellaneous dangerous goods (Figure 42-18)

Miscellaneous dangerous goods can be a mixed load of goods that do not require specific labels unless they are in the required amount.

∗ **Hazard Class 8, Corrosive materials**

causes injuries by destroying and dissolving tissue. Corrosives usually involve acids, bases, and some solvents.

∗ **Hazard Class 9, Miscellaneous dangerous goods**

hazardous materials that do not fit into one of the other hazard classes.

Stop, Review, Remember!

Multiple Choice

Place a check next to the correct answer.

1. You should safely evaluate a motor vehicle collision with potential HazMat involvement from a distance, using your _____ to access information on identified placards to set safety and containment zones.

    _____ a. BLS

    _____ b. MSDS

    _____ c. ERG

    _____ d. REG

2. _____ cause injuries by creating severe and deep burns to tissue.

    _____ a. Flammable liquids

    _____ b. Flammable solids

    _____ c. Gases

    _____ d. Flammable gases

3. _____ injure or kill by disrupting the nervous system or the cellular functions.

    _____ a. Radioactive materials

    _____ b. Flammable solids

    _____ c. Corrosive materials

    _____ d. Flammable gases

4. _____ can trigger an explosion and can also act as a corrosive destroying tissue and triggering inflammation in the lungs.

    _____ a. Flammable gases

    _____ b. Toxic materials and infectious substances

    _____ c. Oxidizers and organic peroxides

    _____ d. Flammable solids

5. What class of hazardous materials produce injuries by primary, secondary, and tertiary blast injuries?

    _____ a. gases

    _____ b. explosive

    _____ c. toxic

    _____ d. liquid

6. The first emergency responders to arrive on the scene of a hazardous material incident should enter the scene and begin helping victims.

    _____ a. true

    _____ b. false

7. If you encounter a suspicious substance, do *not* handle it yourself. Remove the patient to a safe zone if safe to do so, and isolate and deny entry into the area.

    _____ a. true

    _____ b. false

8. Many of the flammable solids are reactive to water and create deeper burns when rescuers attempt to flush the material from the skin with water.

    _____ a. true

    _____ b. false

9. Sensory clues are the most dependable method of identification for a hazardous material.

    _____ a. true

    _____ b. false

10. A 24-hour resource available to emergency responders in a hazardous materials incident is CHEMTREC.

_____ a. true

_____ b. false

11. Toxic materials can include cellular poisons or other substances that can injure or kill.

_____ a. true

_____ b. false

12. Gases cause injury by being toxic or displacing oxygen to cause asphyxiation.

_____ a. true

_____ b. false

13. Weak acids or bases are not dangerous; they only cause signs of irritation or itching.

_____ a. true

_____ b. false

Matching

Match the term on the left with the applicable definition on the right.

1. _____ Hazard Class 1

2. _____ Hazard Class 2

3. _____ Hazard Class 3

4. _____ Hazard Class 4

5. _____ Hazard Class 5

6. _____ Hazard Class 6

7. _____ Hazard Class 7

8. _____ Hazard Class 8

9. _____ Hazard Class 9

A. Miscellaneous
B . Corrosive materials
C. Radioactive materials
D. Toxic
E. Oxidizers
F. Flammable solids
G. Flammable liquids
H. Gases
I. Explosive

Critical Thinking

1. Why should you evaluate a potentially hazardous scene from a distance using your ERG and binoculars?

_____

_____

_____

2. You have identified an explosive placard in your ERG guidebook that requires a 1,500-foot safety perimeter. Describe the necessary steps to create this perimeter.

_____

_____

_____

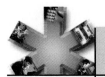

Perspective

Maya—The EMT

"That absolutely scared me to death! You should've seen it! Those fire-fighters were down in a matter of seconds. I really thought they were dead and that Austin and I were next. That HazMat stuff is scary, and it can just sneak up on you, you know? What did I learn? I'll tell you what I learned: To think through all of the possibilities of each call before go-ing in. Heck, if those firefighters had stayed conscious for a little longer before they went down, we would have been lying right next to them! I hate to admit it, but I guess I've been in the habit of just following other people into calls. Police, fire, and even my partner. I swear that my size-ups are going to be much more thorough from now on!"

Operations at a Hazardous Materials Incident

Once a HazMat emergency has been identified, specially equipped responders (HazMat teams) may arrive who are better able to take action. Incident responders who must come into direct contact with hazardous materials (particularly at an incident site) should be wearing appropriate personal protective clothing and equipment.

On hazardous materials incidents requiring protective clothing, a medical unit and medical unit officers will be designated under the Logistics Section in the Incident Command System to support the hazardous materials group. At the direction of the hazardous materials group supervisor, the EMT will provide monitoring services. The Medical Group supervisor is responsible for the medical care of all the personnel operating on the scene. Other EMS personnel in the Medical Group will be responsible for treating civilian patients from the incident.

Hazardous Materials Training

National Fire Protection Association standard 473 details the competencies for EMS providers at hazardous materials incidents. An OSHA standard 29 CFR 1910.120 details the four levels of response for emergency responders. Training is required for all responders who may be called to a hazardous materials incident. The EMT's employer will decide the level of training that the EMT will receive.

The four levels of hazardous materials training for emergency responders are:

✳ The **First Responder Awareness Level,** which is the minimum training an EMT should receive, is designed to protect first responders. The responders are trained to recognize a problem and initiate a response from an agency with operational-level training.

✳ The **Hazardous Materials First Responder Operations Level** training includes procedures to contain and keep hazardous materials from spreading and to

---

✳ **First Responder Awareness Level**

minimum level of training an EMT should receive, designed to protect first responders. The responders are trained to recognize a problem and initiate a response from an agency with operational-level training.

✳ **Hazardous Materials First Responder Operations Level**

level of training that includes procedures to contain and keep hazardous materials from spreading and to prevent exposures to people, property, and the environment. Operations-level training trains first responders to wear and operate in level B protection.

prevent exposures to people, property, and the environment. Operations-level training trains first responders to wear and operate in protection. Operations-level training includes understanding how to decontaminate patients who have been exposed to hazardous materials.

* The **Hazardous Materials Technician Level** training is advanced training that teaches a first responder to control a spill and operate in hazardous environments in chemical protective clothing and suits.

* The highest level of hazardous materials training is the **Hazardous Materials Specialist Level.** Hazardous material specialists have advanced knowledge of monitoring devices, toxicology, and command and control of large-scale hazardous materials incidents.

How Hazardous Materials Harm the Body

Chemicals and hazardous substances may enter the body by several routes, and the nature and onset of signs and symptoms may vary accordingly. The **routes of entry** are:

* Absorption

* Ingestion

* Injection

* Inhalation

ABSORPTION (THROUGH THE SKIN OR EYE)

When a chemical contacts the skin, **absorption** through the skin can occur. This is called **dermal exposure.** If an exterminator is spraying chemicals and the overspray strikes unprotected skin, the chemicals will be absorbed through the skin. This could cause mild skin irritation or more serious problems like burns, sores, or ulcers on the outer layers of the skin. Contact with a substance may also occur by spilling it on the skin or brushing against a contaminated object. When a person is exposed to chemicals or is being decontaminated, it is particularly important never to put hand to eye. Eyes are particularly sensitive to toxic substances; since capillaries are near the surface, the substance can readily enter the bloodstream. Eye contact with toxic substances can cause irritation, pain, or even blindness.

INJECTION

The most familiar example of **injection** is a needle stick, which punctures the skin so that a substance can enter the body. Injection can also occur in other ways. For example, if a contaminated can or a piece of glass that had been in contact with a contaminant cut the skin, the contaminated substance could be injected into the body. This is a very powerful means of exposure because, the contaminant enters the bloodstream *immediately.*

INGESTION

Ingestion occurs when a patient eats a substance that contains a harmful material and the substance enters body by means of the digestive system. An example of this is the child who puts a toxic substance in his or her mouth out of curiosity.

---

* **Hazardous Materials Technician Level**
level of advanced training that teaches a first responder to control a spill and operate in hazardous environments in chemical protective clothing and level A suits.

* **Hazardous Materials Specialist Level**
level of training that includes advanced knowledge of monitoring devices, toxicology, and command and control of large scale hazardous materials incidents.

* **routes of entry**
the way that hazardous materials can enter the body.

* **absorption**
entry through the skin or eye.

* **dermal exposure**
when a chemical contacts and is absorbed through the skin.

* **injection**
entry through a puncture or open skin.

* **ingestion**
entry into the digestive system by eating or drinking.

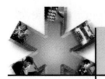

Perspective

Austin—The EMT

"Oh, man! Now that was a helpless feeling. I could see those firefighters and that sewer worker, and I knew that they were either dying or maybe already dead. But all I could do was stay with the ambulance and look at them through the binoculars. I sometimes have to remind myself that I'm not invincible, you know? I kept thinking that if I moved quickly enough or drove right up to them, I could get them out of there and still be okay. Of course, I know that's stupid, and safety is critical, but I'm in this job to help people, right? Not to just stand by and watch them die. It's just a really tough position to be in."

We may also ingest residue from chemicals that have been added to our food to kill germs or parasites.

INHALATION

* **inhalation**

  entry by breathing into the lungs.

It is also possible to be contaminated by **inhalation** when a patient breathes toxic substances into his lungs. Some chemicals have excellent warning properties that let us know when they are in the atmosphere. There is the well-known "rotten egg" smell of hydrogen sulfide, for example. But at high concentrations of this gas, our sense of smell is quickly lost. Many toxic substances, such as carbon monoxide, are both colorless and odorless, providing us with no sensory clues that we are being exposed to anything unusual. Inhalation injuries are the most common of hazardous material exposures and can be the most dangerous.

* **source**

  initial location of the hazardous material.

* **receptor**

  living plant or animal that is exposed to a hazardous substance.

PATHWAY OF EXPOSURE

* **exposure pathway**

  specific route by which a chemical might travel from a source to a receptor.

If we consider these routes of entry, it is possible to think of a number of ways in which contaminants escaping into the environment from their **source** may reach a living plant or animal, or **receptor**. Each specific route a chemical might travel from a source to a receptor is called an **exposure pathway**. The pathway may be either a **direct pathway** or an **indirect pathway**. If an open toxic waste dump were near you, you could inhale the vapors from the toxic material, or your skin could contact toxic contaminants if you walked through the substance. These are direct means of exposure. The substance can also reach you by an indirect pathway. For example, toxic vapors or particles from a site at which hazardous waste has been illegally discarded could be carried some distance in the air or water and deposited on crops or into the water supply.

* **direct pathway**

  exposure resulting from contact with hazardous vapors or substances.

* **indirect pathway**

  exposure resulting from taking in air, water, or food that has been contaminated by hazardous vapors or substances.

Assessing Risk

* **risk**

  the chance of injury, damage, or loss.

How much **risk** is associated with a particular source depends on the characteristics of the source, the availability of pathways for it to reach a receptor, and the characteristics of the receptors. No single piece of information alone is sufficient, and incomplete information can be highly misleading. Among the key questions that must be asked in determining risk are the following:

* What are the **hazardous properties** of the substance? What effects can it have on living things or the environment?

* What is the **concentration,** or how much of the substance exists at the source? A higher quantity or concentration of a toxic substance is more dangerous.

* In what **form** is the substance? Whether the substance is in large blocks or tiny particles, or whether it is a liquid or a vapor, will be important in determining not only how it might travel but also how it could contact and enter the body.

* What are the **chemical and physical characteristics** of the substance? These characteristics determine in what environmental pathways it is likely to move and how rapidly. They include, for example, whether the substance can easily dissolve in water.

* How is the substance **contained**? If a chemical is in old, rusting containers that can leak, the danger is clearly greater than if the container is solid and appropriate to the substance.

* What **pathways of exposure** exist? When scientists study the risk of exposure in any particular situation, they look at all the ways a contaminant could reach the population at risk and make measurements to see how much of it is moving through each identified path. For example, if the source were near a stream, water samples would be taken at several places to see what level of contamination exists at different distances from the source.

* What is the **duration,** or how long did the exposure to the contaminant last? It is another key factor in determining risk.

Toxic Effects

There have been many attempts to categorize or define toxic effects. Generally, the terms *acute* and *chronic* are used to delineate effects on the basis of severity or duration. **Acute exposure** is the exposure to a hazardous substance over a short period of time or at a high dose. A reaction to a chemical can occur at the time of exposure, and might include vomiting, eye irritation, or other symptoms that may be readily linked to a chemical exposure. These are known as **immediate and adverse effects. Chronic exposure** is the exposure to a hazardous substance over a long period of time. If a carpenter used a stripper regularly and breathed in a little of it 8 hours a day for 40 years, this would be a chronic exposure. This type of exposure occurs when a person is repeatedly exposed to the same chemical or hazardous substance at low levels over a long period of time. The term *chronic effect* is often used to cover only the following three effects:

* A **carcinogenic** effect is an increase in an individual's risk of contracting cancer.

* A **mutagenic** effect is a mutation, or permanent change in the genetic material (DNA), which may be passed along to later generations.

* A **teratogenic** effect is an increased risk that a developing embryo will have physical defects.

---

hazardous properties
effects the hazardous materials can have on living things or the environment.

concentration
how much of the substance exists at the source.

form
whether the substance is in large blocks or tiny particles, or whether it is a liquid or a vapor.

chemical and physical characteristics
characteristics that determine in what environmental pathways a hazardous material is likely to move and how rapidly.

contained
stored.

pathways of exposure
all the ways a contaminant could reach the population at risk.

duration
how long the exposure to a contaminant lasted.

acute exposure
exposure to a hazardous substance over a short period of time or at a high dose.

immediate and adverse effects
reactions to a chemical that occur at the time of exposure, such as vomiting or eye irritation.

chronic exposure
exposure to a hazardous substance over a long period of time.

carcinogenic
causing an increased risk of contracting cancer.

mutagenic
causing a mutation, which is a permanent change in the genetic material (DNA) that may be passed along to later generations.

teratogenic
causing an increased risk that a developing embryo will have physical defects.

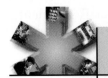

Perspective

Carl—The HazMat Crew Leader

"That's the worst I've seen it. I mean, in my own personal experiences. We got suited up, walked toward the gate, and wham! My H₂S sensor just starts screaming. It showed 500-600 parts per million HYDROGEN SULFIDE?? And it was right there in the parking lot. That's just nuts! No wonder the fire crew crashed so quick. They probably didn't even know anything was wrong until they woke up getting bagged! Well, at least they woke up. Obviously not everyone gets so lucky."

Decontamination

✳ **contaminated**

to have some hazardous material on the person or object.

✳ **cross-contamination**

exposure through contact with a contaminated person or object.

✳ **decontamination**

the process of removing or neutralizing contaminants from a person or object.

A person or item that has been exposed to a hazardous material is **contaminated** and can contaminate other people or items (for example, **cross-contamination**). For example, if you enter your car after being exposed to a toxic substance, you will contaminate your car.

Decontamination is the process of removing or neutralizing contaminants that have accumulated on people and equipment. At hazardous materials incidents, clean areas or "cold" zones must be established and maintained, and materials in contaminated areas must be confined to specific "hot" zones (Figure 42-19). Response personnel who have had to enter the middle area—the "warm" or contamination-reduction zone—must later remove their clothing and equipment, shower in fresh water, be rinsed with neutralizing agents, reshower, and change into clean clothing (Figure 42-20). Station yourself in the cold zone, where equipment and other emergency rescuers should be staged adjacent to the warm zone.

The specific procedure for decontamination will vary according to the chemical the individual was exposed to. Certain items—for example, leather and some plastic and rubber materials—absorb toxic substances so easily that they cannot be completely decontaminated; these items must be discarded. Decontamination methods seek to:

✳ Physically remove contaminants

✳ Deactivate contaminants by chemical detoxification or disinfection/sterilization

✳ Remove contaminants through a combination of physical and chemical methods

If you believe the patient may be contaminated and is in need of immediate medical assistance, remove all of the patient's clothing, shower him thoroughly, and place him in a hospital gown. Advise *all* who come in contact with you that

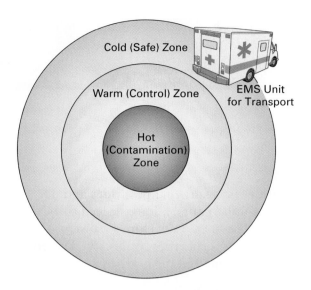

Hot (Contamination) Zone

Contamination is actually present.
Personnel must wear appropriate protective gear.
Number of rescuers limited to those absolutely necessary.
Bystanders never allowed.

Warm (Control) Zone

Area surrounding the contamination zone.
Vital to preventing spread of contamination.
Personnel must wear appropriate protective gear.
Life-saving emergency care is performed.

Cold (Safe) Zone

Normal triage, stabilization, and treatment performed.
Rescuers must shed contaminated gear before entering
the cold zone.

FIGURE 42-19 Establishing safety control zones at the site of a
hazardous materials emergency.

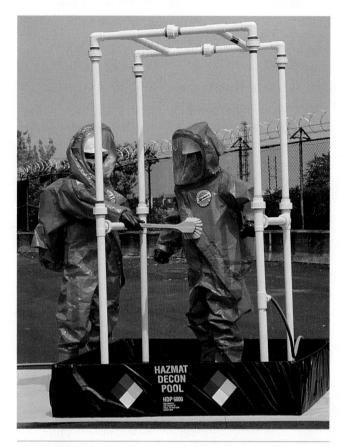

FIGURE 42-20 Rescuer in decontamination process.

you may have been exposed to a toxic substance so they can take proper precautions. To avoid contaminating others, place any exposed clothing in a nonpermeable container without allowing it to contact other materials, and arrange for proper disposal. The steps you must take to decontaminate a patient are:

1. Wash down outer clothing (*unless the chemical is water-reactive*).

2. Remove clothing, working from the top down.

3. Wash down the entire body (*unless the chemical is water-reactive*).

4. Wrap up or dress the patient in clean clothing preferably a hospital gown.

5. Discard contaminated clothing in a well-secured plastic bag.

If you have been or may have been contaminated by contact with the contaminated patient, follow these same steps for yourself.

Stop, Review, Remember!

Multiple Choice

Place a check next to the correct answer.

1. A patient spilled a toxic substance. He coughed, and his eyes immediately began to water. The patient was experiencing what type of exposure?

_____ a. acute

_____ b. chronic

_____ c. septic

_____ d. radioactive

2. You have just learned that a chemical to which a patient was exposed is a mutagen. What effect does this chemical have?

_____ a. increases the risk of cancer

_____ b. increases the risk of physical defects in a developing embryo

_____ c. vauses a permanent change in the genetic material (DNA)

_____ d. irritates the lining of the throat

3. A patient inhaled a substance and became sleepy and slow to respond. The chemical is most likely a substance which is a(n):

_____ a. CNS (central nervous system) depressant.

_____ b. irritant.

_____ c. asphyxiant.

_____ d. corrosive.

4. A farmer was spraying pesticides and not wearing long pants, a long-sleeved shirt, or gloves. The farmer developed nausea, vomiting, and shortness of breath. The poison most likely entered the body by:

_____ a. absorption.

_____ b. injection.

_____ c. ingestion.

_____ d. inhalation.

5. If you inhale the vapors from toxic material, you have been contaminated by which exposure pathway?

_____ a. indirect

_____ b. source

_____ c. multi-direct

_____ d. direct

Matching

Match the term on the left with the applicable definition on the right.

1. _____ Awareness level

2. _____ Operational level

3. _____ Technician level

4. _____ Specialist level

5. _____ Absorption

6. _____ Ingestion

7. _____ Injection

8. _____ Inhalation

A. Includes training in patient decontamination

B. Teaches a responder to operate in hazardous environments

C. The minimum training an EMT should receive

D. When a chemical is absorbed through the skin

E. Has advanced knowledge of hazardous materials

F. The skin is punctured so that a substance can enter the body

G. Route of entry by inhaling into the lungs

H. Enters the body by means of our digestive system

Critical Thinking

1. When transporting a patient from a HazMat scene, it is important to remove all contaminates from the patient prior to transportation. Why?

_____

_____

_____

_____

2. What information is needed to assess risk of a hazardous materials exposure?

_____

_____

_____

_____

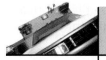

Dispatch Summary

The HazMat crew quickly moved the patients to the green zone where ambulances waited to transport them. They were then able to trace the cause of the leak—an erroneously opened valve—and stop the release of hydrogen sulfide gas.

All four firefighters were in respiratory arrest and transported with ventilatory assistance and oxygen.

The plant worker, who was in cardiac arrest, was transported by an ALS crew, but never regained a pulse.

Fire station twelve recently held a barbecue in honor of the two EMTs, whose quick thinking saved four of their own. And perhaps more.

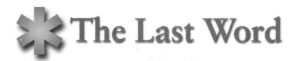

The Last Word

Hazardous materials responses—although rare, do occur in the line of duty. As an EMT you can expect to be involved in patient care or function in a support role in a hazardous materials incident.

Remember that without special training in hazardous materials operations, your primary responsibility is to protect yourself and the public. Secure the scene safely from a distance. Use your binoculars and *Emergency Response Guidebook* to identify placards. Call in the hazardous materials response team. Then prepare to treat and transport decontaminated patients.

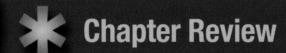

Chapter Review

MULTIPLE CHOICE

Place a check next to the correct answer.

1. Responders can be contaminated at a hazardous materials call by:

   _____ a. being splashed.

   _____ b. contacting vapors or particulate matter in the air.

   _____ c. using contaminated equipment.

   _____ d. all of the above.

2. Decontamination only requires that the exposed victim be hosed-off with water.

   _____ a. true

   _____ b. false

3. Responders should never be allowed into a hazardous sector or decontamination area without:

   _____ a. the proper protective clothing.

   _____ b. monitoring equipment.

   _____ c. an assignment.

   _____ d. all of the above.

4. Decontamination and treatment must always take place in close proximity to the hot zone.

   _____ a. true

   _____ b. false

5. If contaminated victims are transported to the treatment area, medical personnel must:

   _____ a. not treat the patients.

   _____ b. transport the patients without treatment.

   _____ c. be in the proper protective clothing.

   _____ d. none of the above.

6. Department of Transportation placards are used to identify which types of hazard classes?

   _____ a. explosives

   _____ b. flammable solid

   _____ c. poison, poison gas

   _____ d. all of the above

7. The Department of Transportation placard that is approximately half black and half white identifies what hazard class?

   _____ a. poison/poison gas

   _____ b. blasting agents

   _____ c. nonflammable gas

   _____ d. corrosives

8. Hazards like toxic gas will cause:

_____ a. physical discomfort, but usually not permanent injury or death.

_____ b. death, by causing irritation of the airway and lungs.

_____ c. health hazards because they are so poisonous.

_____ d. disease in humans.

9. A number "8" at the bottom of a placard indicates a _____ material.

_____ a. corrosive

_____ b. biohazard

_____ c. explosive

_____ d. radioactive

10. In reference to decontamination of a patient, which statement is false?

_____ a. A contaminated patient can contaminate you and your vehicle.

_____ b. Wash down the patient's contaminated outer clothing.

_____ c. Remove the patient's clothing from the bottom up.

_____ d. Discard contaminated clothing in a well-secured plastic bag.

11. Corrosives may:

_____ a. destroy living tissue upon contact or inhalation.

_____ b. be involved in violent ruptures.

_____ c. splatter in contact with water.

_____ d. all of the above.

CRITICAL THINKING

1. What is the difference between chronic and acute exposure to a hazardous substance?

_____

_____

_____

_____

2. What are the four routes of exposure to a hazardous substance? Briefly describe how exposure through each route occurs.

_____

_____

_____

_____

CASE STUDY

You and your partner have been dispatched to a hazardous materials incident at a local chemical plant to transport victims to the hospital. The scene size-up given over the radio describes a ruptured gas storage tank with about 30 victims.

You arrive at the cold-zone staging area and your unit is then directed to the decontamination treatment area. Your patient is a 33-year-old male, a worker in the chemical plant, who was exposed to hydrogen sulfide gas that was leaking from a storage tank. Hydrogen sulfide is a gas that smells like rotten eggs, that is slightly heavier than air, and that will stratify at or around the head and shoulders. The primary effect of hydrogen sulfide is that it is a cellular asphyxiant, which means that it stops the cell from correctly processing oxygen. The patient has been decontaminated by the HazMat team. He is dressed in the paper dressing gown from the HazMat team's decontamination area. His hair is wet and he is shivering.

Vital signs are respirations 30, pulse 118, blood pressure 138/88. The patient is coughing and complains of difficulty breathing and nausea. His pupils are equal and reactive to light; his mucous membranes are slightly cyanotic. Neck veins are flat, chest has equal rise and fall, breath sounds reveal some crackles, abdomen is soft and nontender. The patient obeys all commands and has good pulses to all extremities.

1. What will be the first steps of care you will provide?

   _____

   _____

   _____

   _____

2. What is your next step in assessment and action?

   _____

   _____

   _____

   _____

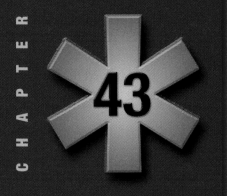

CHAPTER 43

Responses Involving Rescue and Special Operations

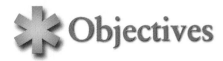 Objectives

Numbered objectives are from the U.S. Department of Transportation 1994 EMT-Basic National Standard Curriculum.

COGNITIVE OBJECTIVES

At the completion of this lesson, the EMT-Basic student will be able to:

7-2.1 Describe the purpose of extrication. (p. 1080)
7-2.2 Discuss the role of the EMT-Basic in extrication. (p. 1080)
7-2.3 Identify what equipment for personal safety is required for the EMT-Basic (pp. 1080–1081)
7-2.4 Define the components of extrication. (pp. 1080–1084)
7-2.5 State the steps that should be taken to protect the patient during extrication. (p. 1080)

7-2.6 Distinguish between simple and complex access. (pp. 1082–1084)
7-3.2 Describe what the EMT-Basic should do if there is reason to believe that there is a hazard at the scene. (pp. 1076–1078)
7-3.3 Describe the actions that an EMT-Basic should take to ensure bystander safety. (pp. 1076–1078)

AFFECTIVE OBJECTIVES

No psychomotor objectives identified.

PSYCHOMOTOR OBJECTIVES

No psychomotor objectives identified.

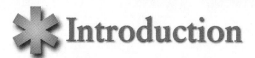 **Introduction**

Rescue and Special Operations are just that: special. You will be involved in some or many during your career, depending on your location. Learning and practicing these operations will be exciting yet challenging.

Classifications

✳ **technical rescue incidents**

rescue situations requiring specialized training and equipment.

There are nine classifications of **technical rescue incidents** according to the National Fire Protection Association (NFPA). Technical rescue incidents can include:

✳ Water rescue

✳ Rope rescue

✳ Rescue from confined spaces

✳ Wilderness search and rescue

✳ Trench rescue

✳ Vehicle and machinery rescue

✳ Dive search and rescue

✳ Collapse rescue

✳ Any other rescue operations requiring specialized training

Interagency cooperation is essential for the successful completion of many technical rescue incidents. When EMS is summoned to a technical rescue incident, the minimum qualifications required of rescuers will be certification at the basic life support (BLS) level and to the rescue awareness level. All personnel at the site need to understand that they must operate under an incident management system.

✳ **consensus standards**

agreed-upon levels of training required for those responding to rescue incidents.

✳ **awareness level**

level of training that represents the minimum capabilities of a responder who, in the course of their duties, could be called upon to respond to or be first on scene of a technical rescue incident.

✳ **operational level**

level of training that is designed for responders who will be responsible for hazard recognition, equipment use, and techniques necessary to conduct a technical rescue.

✳ **technician level**

level of training that is designed for responders who will be capable of hazard recognition, equipment use, techniques necessary to perform, and supervision of a technical rescue incident.

If responding to rescue incidents, **consensus standards** from the National Fire Protection Association identify the need to be trained to the awareness level. The **awareness level** represents the minimum capabilities of a responder who could be called upon to respond to or be first on scene of a technical rescue incident. Awareness-level operations may involve search, rescue, and recovery of victims in technical rescue scenarios. EMTs trained to this level generally do not act as rescuers but rather as support personnel for the operation.

Operational level training is designed for responders who are trained in hazard recognition, equipment use, and techniques necessary to conduct a technical rescue. Rescue operations are usually supervised by a rescuer certified at the **technician level**. Those with technician-level certification are capable of hazard recognition, equipment use, techniques necessary to perform, and supervision of a technical rescue incident.

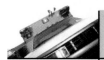

Emergency Dispatch

"**B**e careful!" a firefighter shouted as the second ambulance on scene rolled to a stop. "There's glass everywhere."

EMT Claire Owen stepped from the truck and surveyed the scene while pulling on a pair of exam gloves. She stood in the middle of a notorious intersection known as the "Terrible T" — a location so well-known to local emergency personnel that dispatch would commonly just say, "Accident at the T" when summoning crews.

"It looks like that little car and that glass truck hit head-on." Claire's partner, EMT Ray Parker, pointed as they moved the cot toward the busy rescue crew. "But I've never seen anything like that."

The glass truck, its racks now empty, sat awkwardly off to one side of the road and the small car was overturned, resting partially up the embankment. The car was surrounded in all directions by large shards of broken glass, embedded upright into the soft soil and pointing skyward. Their clear, sharp blades, glinting brightly in the early morning sunlight, prevented access to the car and its injured driver.

"We've got the guy from the truck," EMT Perry Bose said as he and his partner strapped the bloody man onto a long spine board. "You guys are here for the lady in the car. It's gonna be a few minutes. Isn't that the damnedest thing you've ever seen?"

Claire and Ray stopped at the edge of the road and watched patiently as the fire crew dislodged and removed shard after shard of glass, slowly clearing a path to the overturned vehicle.

"Why isn't anyone helping me?" The woman screamed from the car. "I . . . I'm bleeding . . . and my leg is stuck . . . and it really hurts!"

"We're coming, Ma'am," one of the firefighters yelled back, tossing a large piece of glass onto the pile at the edge of the road. "We're going to help you as quickly as we can!"

"Hey Claire," Ray said, peering into the car from different angles. "Can you do me a favor and grab my heavy coat, helmet, and . . . uh . . . leather gloves? Once they get that thing cribbed, I think I'm gonna have to get in through the back window."

Scene Safety

Scene safety at a technical rescue first involves the assessment and analysis of the victim(s) in order to determine if the scenario is a body recovery or a rescue situation. A live victim means a rescue with its associated high level of urgency. A deceased victim, however, is a body recovery that suggests a far less urgent response. You must follow standard safety rescue procedures when making a rescue. As always, it is critical to ensure the safety first and foremost of yourself, your team or partner, and other responders. Several fatalities of emergency responders have occurred when responders rushed to help victims and entered unsafe environments, only to become fatalities themselves.

SPECIAL OPERATIONS SCENE SIZE-UP

Scene size-up in special operations is not much different than what you've already learned. It includes confirming the exact location, the nature, and the seriousness of the incident, the number and condition of victims, and the risks versus benefits that will dictate a rescue or a body recovery. What is different is knowing right away that you will need additional resources.

∗ **scene size-up**

initial evaluation of several scene factors, including confirming the exact location, nature, and the seriousness of the incident; the number and condition of victims; and risks versus benefits that will dictate a rescue or a body recovery.

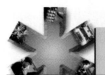

Perspective

Claire—The EMT

"We were the first ones on-scene this morning. Kirk went to check on the guy in the truck and I was gonna check out the overturned car, but all that glass stopped me. I started to kind of kick some of it down but then this one piece cut right through the side of my boot! Oh man, once I saw my sock sticking out, I realized I totally wasn't equipped to do what I was trying to do! So I got on the radio and explained the whole thing to dispatch. They sent out the rescue crew and Claire's ambulance while we started helping the guy in the glass truck. I hope someone got a picture of all that broken glass . . . just standing upright around that car. I've never seen anything like that before!"

✳ **predefined response matrix**

specific set of resources sent to the scene based on the caller's or first responder's information.

You need to know the resources for each type of incident and where they are in your local jurisdictions. Call for available and necessary resources as soon as possible. In some EMS systems a **predefined response matrix** sends a specific set of resources to the scene based on the caller's or first responder's information. This may include fire department resources, specialized rescue teams, and additional EMS resources. Often public works, the utility companies, and law enforcement will be needed at the scene. Lastly, make sure as soon as possible that you verbalize over the radio what actions are being taken, for example conducting triage, and how many victims there are.

VEHICLE AND MACHINERY RESCUE

Rescuing victims from motor vehicles is the most frequent response for emergency medical technicians. The awareness level for vehicle and machinery rescue requires the EMT to conduct a size-up of existing and potential conditions.

When approaching a vehicle collision or machinery incident, note the scope and magnitude of the incident. It is a critical function of the EMT to determine if the incident can be handled by basic life support (BLS) or whether advanced life support (ALS) will be required. The decision must be made whether the condition of the victim(s) warrants a rescue or whether there is a fatal injury or injuries requiring a body recovery.

The number, size of the vehicles, and type of machinery involved are key pieces of information to determine what additional resources are needed. Specialized rescue tools are often required for collisions involving large trucks, school buses, and severely damaged vehicles. The integrity of the vehicle and its stability are important pieces of information. A vehicle on its roof will almost always have a fluid leak, and a vehicle on its side is inherently unstable. The number of victims at the scene will dictate the number of ambulances and additional resources to request.

7-3.2 Describe what the EMT-Basic should do if there is reason to believe that there is a hazard at the scene.

7-3.3 Describe the actions that an EMT-Basic should take to ensure bystander safety.

Report any access problem, for example cars down embankments or vehicles into a building. Report any hazards to other rescuers and responders, such as downed electrical wires or other exposed utilities, fluid leaks, or traffic (Figure 43-1).

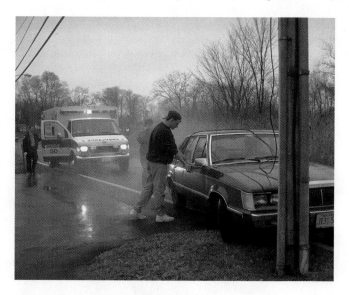

FIGURE 43-1 Downed wires and poles are potential hazards to rescuers and patients. (© Craig Jackson/In the Dark Photography)

Pay special attention to electrical hazards. In older developments there are overhead wire systems. In new developments there are underground systems with pad-mounted electrical transformers set on the ground that, if knocked off their base, can energize a vehicle.

Make sure to note any hazardous traffic conditions. Freeway or highway responses have become one of the most dangerous environments for EMTs and rescue personnel. When placing emergency vehicles at a collision scene, it is important to block approaching traffic with an apparatus parked at a 45-degree angle. In most cases, it is preferred that the blocking vehicle be a fire truck and that the ambulance pull past the blocking vehicle to protect the rescuers who are loading patients. The safety zone should be extended when the emergency scene is on the round of a curve, on the opposite side of the crest of a hill, or in poor weather conditions. Vehicles should be uphill and upwind from any fuel leak or hazardous materials release (Figure 43-2 on page 1078). It is important to request additional resources and alert others to the seriousness of the incident.

All types of vehicle and machinery incidents have the potential for extenuating circumstances. A vehicle collision may involve an unusual vehicle. For example, hybrid electric vehicles present an electric shock hazard, and natural-gas or propane vehicles present explosive hazards.

EMTs must be able to identify the resources necessary to conduct safe and effective operations. As part of the rescue operation, the EMT will implement the emergency response system for vehicle rescue. Scene safety and site control are the responsibility of the EMT at a vehicle or machinery rescue. Ensuring a safe scene requires the EMT to initiate traffic control. It is important for the EMT to be aware of the hazards associated with the vehicle and machinery rescue.

Clinical Clues: ELECTRICAL HAZARDS

Remember that guard rails, other vehicles, and water may conduct electricity if close to the vehicles that are energized. **Do not attempt to move power lines or electrical equipment. Maintain a safe distance and have utility crews cut the power before accessing the vehicle.**

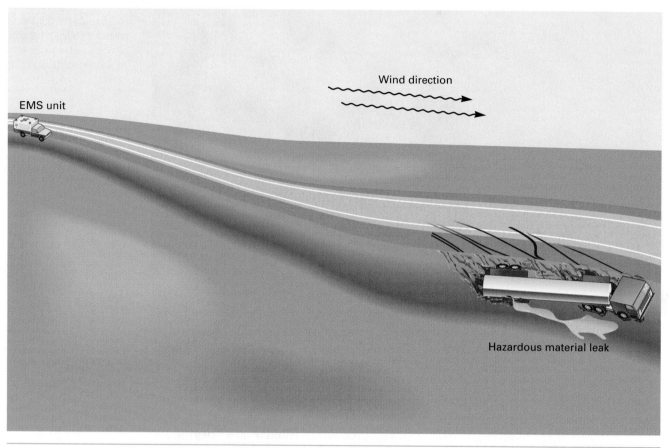

Wind direction

EMS unit

Hazardous material leak

FIGURE 43-2 Park the EMS unit uphill and upwind from any leaking hazardous materials.

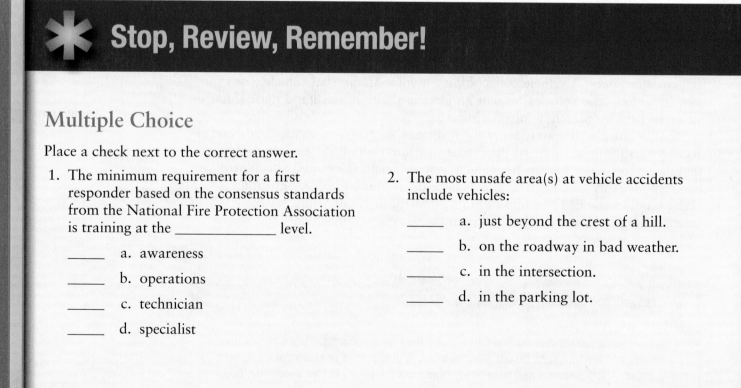

✱ Stop, Review, Remember!

Multiple Choice

Place a check next to the correct answer.

1. The minimum requirement for a first responder based on the consensus standards from the National Fire Protection Association is training at the _____ level.

   _____ a. awareness

   _____ b. operations

   _____ c. technician

   _____ d. specialist

2. The most unsafe area(s) at vehicle accidents include vehicles:

   _____ a. just beyond the crest of a hill.

   _____ b. on the roadway in bad weather.

   _____ c. in the intersection.

   _____ d. in the parking lot.

3. A predefined response matrix is a:

_____ a. priority dispatch.

_____ b. specific set of resources dispatched for a particular incident.

_____ c. set of call numbers for ambulances and fire apparatus.

_____ d. predesignated vehicle accident size.

Fill in the Blank

What are the components of a brief initial report to be transmitted after sizing up a motor vehicle collision?

1. _____

2. _____

3. _____

4. _____

5. _____

6. _____

Critical Thinking

1. Identify the types of vehicles in your community that routinely pose a hazard or may be difficult when conducting a rescue operation?

_____

_____

_____

_____

2. What resources in your community are available to assist in a rescue of a patient from the vehicles identified in the previous question?

_____

_____

_____

_____

7-2.1 Describe the purpose of extrication.

7-2.4 Define the components of extrication.

7-2.5 State the steps that should be taken to protect the patient during extrication.

Fundamentals of Vehicle Rescue

The role of the EMT is to assist rescuers in the process of removing entrapped patients from vehicles, building collapses, and other scenarios that keep a patient from self-extricating. There are 10 phases of a rescue evolution:

1. Preparing for the rescue

2. Sizing up the situation

3. Recognizing and managing hazards

4. Stabilizing the vehicle prior to entering

5. Gaining access to the patient

6. Providing initial patient assessment and a rapid trauma exam

7. Disentangling the patient

8. Immobilizing and extricating the patient from the vehicle

9. Providing a detailed exam, ongoing assessment, treatment and transport

10. Terminating the rescue

7-2.2 Discuss the role of the EMT-Basic in extrication.

7-2.3 Identify what equipment for personal safety is required for the EMT-Basic.

PREPARING FOR THE RESCUE

Your role in a vehicle rescue depends on your agency's responsibility. As an EMT in a non-rescue role, you are responsible for administering patient care prior to the extrication and for assisting the rescue personnel in determining the most appropriate way to remove the patient. Preventing or limiting further injury is a primary responsibility of the EMT. In some cases the EMT is part of the rescue team and, if so, should receive specialized training in vehicle extrication. Vehicle rescue technicians typically receive 40 hours or so of vehicle rescue training. The EMT should cooperate with the activities of the rescuers but not allow these activities to interfere with patient care.

If you are an EMT functioning as part of a rescue team, often you are working under a chain of command and being given direction by fire or rescue squad

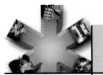

Perspective

Ray—The EMT

"I think that extricating patients from overturned vehicles is probably the toughest thing to do in our line of work. I mean, think about it: You've got this injured person with a busted leg—a possible spinal injury—and just bleeding everywhere. And, oh, guess what? They're hanging upside down. Think about it for a minute. How do we cut them down and get them out of the car—all while trying to keep that closed fracture closed, maintaining spinal immobilization, and not injuring them more than they already are? Or hurting ourselves. Don't forget that one!"

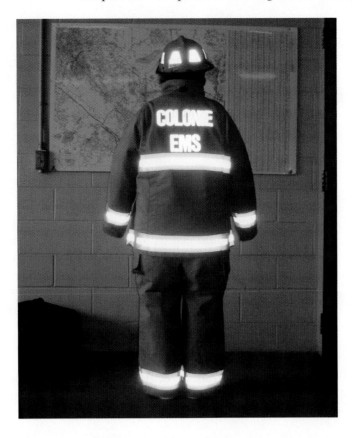

FIGURE 43-3 Full turnout gear with reflective markings should be worn at an extrication. (Jon Politis.)

officers. The chain of command assures that care to the patient before extrication is coordinated with removing the patient in a way to minimize further injury.

Personal safety is the number one priority for you and all EMS personnel. Protective clothing that is appropriate for the situation should be used by rescue and EMS personnel (Figure 43-3). If you are involved with extrication, you should wear firefighter turnout or brush clothing, helmet, and eye protection.

Modern vehicles are made from **composite fibers.** Glass and composite fibers release particles that are hazardous if inhaled. It is recommended that, when cutting these materials, the EMT should wear a particle mask. When using firefighting gloves for extrication and treating a patient, it is important to wear medical gloves under the firefighter gloves to ensure that blood does not soak through and expose the EMT to potential infection. EMTs on the scene who are not involved in the rescue circle should have a high-visibility vest. Since most vehicle collisions are on the roadway, you must be protected and be observant for inattentive or distracted drivers.

* **composite fibers**

combinations of materials used to make vehicle parts.

SAFEGUARDING THE PATIENT

Once measures have been taken to ensure responder safety, you must focus on the patient' safety. Patient care precedes extrication unless delayed movement would endanger the life of the patient. If the patient has an airway compromise or a life-threatening injury, or if there is a hazard that can cause additional injury or death, you should rapidly remove the patient.

The patient should be informed of the aspects of extrication that will involve loud noise and the removal of the vehicle from around them. It is important that the patient be protected from hazards like glass and sharp metal during the extrication processes. Precaution should be taken to ensure that airbags, seatbelt actuators, and power sources are secured in vehicles involved in a collision. Several firefighters and EMTs have been injured when airbags activated during the rescue process. Several techniques or pieces of rescue equipment can be used to protect the patient. Long and short backboards can be positioned as shields. Commercial rescue blankets, and lightweight tarps are all acceptable choices to protect the patient during rescue operations. If the rescue crews are using hydraulic extrication equipment the EMT should monitor the action to ensure that metal and glass do not come in contact with the patient.

STABILIZING THE VEHICLE

Collisions put vehicles in a variety of positions. It is important to realize that even upright vehicles may be unstable because of radial tires or extensive damage to the frame. You should ensure that the vehicle ignition is turned off as part of the size-up. A common practice is to deflate the tires and place the car on **step chocks** or **cribbing** (Figures 43-4 and 43-5). Deflation is best accomplished by pulling the valve stems from the tire to preserve the tire for later investigation. This procedure also prevents any rocking motion created by the rescue efforts. Two 4 × 4 boards or cribbing should be placed on each side of the vehicle. As an added measure of safety cribbing can be placed in the front and rear of the vehicle for additional stabilization.

Keep in mind that a vechicle on its side is inherently unstable and is a real danger to rescuers but can be stabilized with cribbing and/or struts as shown in (Figures 43-6A–C).

ACCESS

Getting to the patient is the next step for the EMT in an extrication scenario. There are two types of access. The first is **simple access,** which does not require equipment. Have the patient unlock doors if possible. Try opening each door. If the doors won't open, roll down the windows.

Complex access requires use of tools or special equipment. In complex access, you and the rescuers will follow a step-by-step process to gain access to the patient. The first step is to survey the vehicle design. New vehicle technologies pose

∗ **step chocks**

wooden blocks or other supportive materials placed in a stair-step pattern to assist in stabilizing a vehicle.

∗ **cribbing**

wooden blocks or other supportive materials placed in a box pattern (crib) to assist in stabilizing a vehicle.

7-2.6 Distinguish between simple and complex access.

∗ **simple access**

means of getting into a vehicle that does not require specialized training, tools, or equipment.

∗ **complex access**

means of getting into a vehicle that requires specialized training, tools, or equipment.

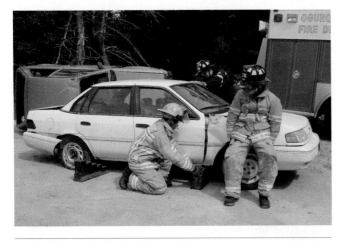

FIGURE 43-4 While placing a step chock, keep hands clear of the vehicle.

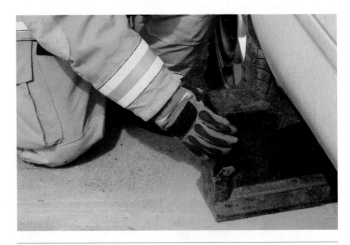

FIGURE 43-5 Stabilize a car on its wheels with cribbing while patient contact is initiated.

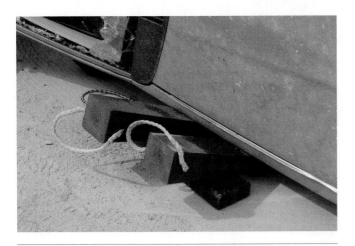

FIGURE 43-6A   A vehicle on its side stabilized with cribbing.

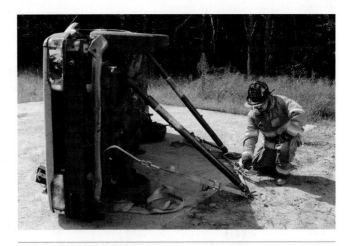

FIGURE 43-6B   A vehicle on its side stabilized with struts.

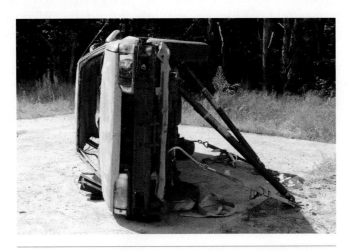

FIGURE 43-6C   A vehicle on its side stabilized with cribbing and struts.

new hazards. The front and rear compartments of modern vehicles have been reinforced. These vehicles have been designed to deflect the wheels, engine, hood, and trunk away from the passenger compartment. **Crumple zones** that absorb energy are now welded into the frame, preventing transmission of crash energy to the passenger compartment. Reinforced dash and side-injury protection bars, designed to encapsulate the passengers, make access difficult.

If simple access methods do not work, removing glass will be the second action taken to gain access to an entrapped victim. Glass is a significant problem to the rescuer. There are two types of glass in vehicles: laminated glass and safety glass. **Laminated glass** is present in the front windshield and occasionally in the rear windshield. Laminated glass has a layer of glue, plastic, or mastic sandwiched between two pieces of glass and must be cut. A flat-head axe, saw, or commercial glass cutter can be used to remove laminated glass. **Safety glass** is present in the side windows and often in the rear windows. When struck, safety glass will break into small rounded pieces—not the sharp shards formed by other kinds of glass. When removing either type of glass, laminated or safety glass, ensure the patient and rescuers are protected.

∗ **crumple zones**

vehicle parts that are designed to collapse, allowing for the crash energy to be absorbed rather than being transmitted to the passenger compartment.

∗ **laminated glass**

type of glass that has a layer of glue, plastic, or mastic sandwiched between two pieces of glass.

∗ **safety glass**

type of glass that, when struck, will break into small pieces. Also called tempered glass.

∗ **Nader pin**

metal pin mounted to the door frame to which the door latching mechanism attaches, designed to prevent doors from flying open and passengers from being ejected in a crash.

If access cannot be achieved by breaking glass, the rescuers will then try to pry open a door. An assortment of tools can be used for this procedure. A pry bar, saw, or hydraulic spreader can be used to force the door open. In most cases, the door is pried or forced open from the **Nader-pin** side by either rolling the door off the pin or forcing the pin out of the latching mechanism. In some vehicles, the side-injury protection bars make it difficult to pry the door open. If it appears there is a delay in the Nader-pin approach, then the rescue team should try to pry open the door from the front hinge side. The metal in the front hinges is weaker than the Nader-pin assembly. In some cases the side-injury protection bar may act as a deadbolt, making it difficult to pry the door from either the hinge or the Nader-pin side.

If forcing the door becomes too time consuming, you and the rescuers may opt to remove the roof and lift the patient out. The A and B posts in modern vehicles are very strong, being designed to support the weight of the vehicle if it turns upside down. So removing the roof requires a hydraulic cutter or reciprocating saw to cut through the "A" and "B" posts with a relief cut to the roof behind the "B" post to fold the roof back. When cutting the "B" post, the rescuers should be cautious not to cut the seatbelt tensioner. The seatbelt tensioner is a pressurized cylinder that can explode if it is cut into. The roof should be secured with rope to prevent the wind from flapping the roof back onto the rescue team. Glass should be removed to prevent injury.

A final procedure that may be necessary for severely trapped patients is a dash roll-up. In some collisions, the dash comes in on the patient and pins the lower extremities and pelvis. The rescue team will make a relief cut to weaken the metal on both sides close to the bottom of the front hinge after the door has been removed. A hydraulic ram is then placed in the door panel and the dash is pushed off the patient. Often this creates an obstruction, and the patient will need to be lifted vertically to a long board.

EMERGENCY CARE

It requires four rescuers to safely remove a patient from a motor vehicle. When removing the patient, it is important to maintain cervical spine stabilization. Before removing the patient, you should complete an initial assessment and provide critical interventions. If the patient is in shock, provide oxygen. You may also need to provide assisted ventilations. Spinal precautions must be taken immediately on gaining access to the patient by applying manual cervical stabilization. Apply a cervical collar as soon as possible. Make sure you maintain the manual stabilization until the patient is moved from the vehicle and secured to a backboard, because even the best cervical collar still allows approximately one-quarter of the movement of the head. Before moving the patient from the vehicle to the backboard, the spine can be immobilized with a short spine board or a Kendrick Extrication Device (KED). If the patient is deteriorating or if there is an immediate threat to the patient's life, rapid extrication is warranted. Remember to "move the patient, not the immobilization device."

Ensure that sufficient personnel are involved with the movement of patients out of a vehicle. A series of coordinated turns and repositioning of rescuers may be necessary to ensure smooth movement of the patient from the vehicle to the long board. Choose the path of least resistance, and avoid dragging the patient over obstacles such as consoles or gear shift mechanisms. Continue to protect the patient from hazards while he is being moved.

Stop, Review, Remember!

Multiple Choice

Place a check next to the correct answer.

1. The metal pin mounted to the door frame to which the door latching mechanism attaches is:

   _____ a. the latch key.

   _____ b. the Nader pin.

   _____ c. the safety hinge.

   _____ d. the B post.

2. A window in a vehicle that has a layer of plastic, glue, or mastic between two sheets of glass is called:

   _____ a. laminated glass.

   _____ b. safety glass.

   _____ c. lexan glass.

   _____ d. impact resistance glass.

3. During a vehicle rescue, the patient should be protected from glass and metal with:

   _____ a. a sheet.

   _____ b. some plastic.

   _____ c. a rescue blanket.

   _____ d. Nothing. You should not cover the patient because they will become frightened.

Labeling

Identify the cut locations on the vehicle to remove a trapped victim.

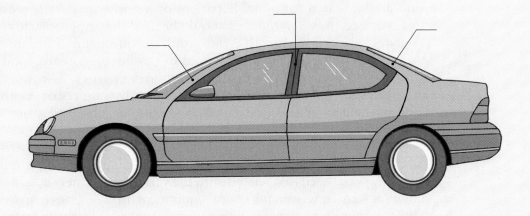

Critical Thinking

1. What are the potential dangers to rescuers that can occur during a vehicle rescue operation?

_____

_____

_____

_____

_____

2. What is the sequence for gaining access to a vehicle?

_____

_____

_____

_____

_____

Wilderness Rescue

Your rescue awareness level allows you to support and assist in a wilderness rescue even if you have never been deployed into the wilderness. Wilderness areas are different around the country and, as an EMT, you must learn the procedures for implementing wilderness search and rescue.

The first on scene EMT at a wilderness rescue should try to determine if there should be a search for a viable patient or a body recovery. An estimate of the time required to search the area should be made and appropriate resources summoned to cover the terrain. It is important to collect and record information necessary to assist operational personnel in a wilderness search and rescue. This includes identifying and isolating the reporting parties. The number of known and potential victims should be confirmed by bystanders or reliable sources. A current weather report and forecast should be obtained from the National Weather Service.

The hazards associated with a wilderness rescue include environmental hazards, terrain hazards, and man-made hazards (Figure 43-7). It is important to realize the special needs associated with the various wilderness conditions. There are limitations to conventional rescue equipment in wilderness environments. You must determine whether specific resources are available for wilderness rescue. Off-road vehicles, aircraft, horseback search teams, search dogs, or other tracking resources should be notified as early as possible. Wilderness environments may generate the need for cave, mine, or avalanche specialty rescue teams. Perimeter control and scene management may also be an EMT role when responding to a wilderness incident.

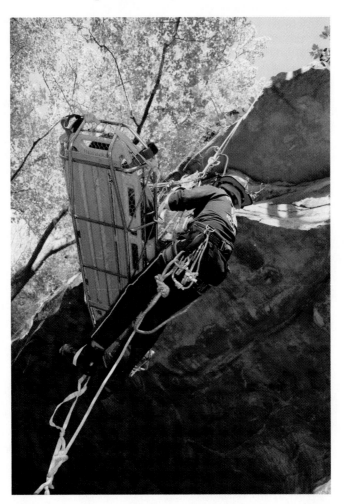

FIGURE 43-7   Dangerous rescue techniques, such as vertical rescue, should be frequently practiced to ensure the utmost safety during actual rescue situations. (© Ken Kerr.)

WATER RESCUE

The need for water rescue can occur suddenly and without warning. In mountainous areas, rain upstream can produce a wall of water in a canyon where the weather may be clear. Normally shallow water and small streams can become dangerous in a matter of minutes. Swift water is water moving at a rate of greater than one knot or 1.15 mph and can occur very quickly. As an EMT, you will need to assess water conditions and conduct a size-up of existing and potential conditions. For public safety, your local EMS must monitor and track severe weather or extreme water conditions.

Water-rescue scenarios may include patients from recreational and commercial diving, ice, and surf-related water environments. Ensure that the scene is safe and that the scene is managed. Make sure to recognize the hazards of a water incident and the procedures necessary to mitigate these hazards in the rescue area. It is important to determine the number of victims and the survivability of people who are in the water or are unaccounted for.

Identify the equipment and resources necessary to conduct a safe and effective water rescue in your local community. The minimum protective equipment includes a personal flotation device, a helmet for water rescue, a cutting device, a whistle, and thermal protection.

Rescuers responding to a water incident must quickly determine what the response will involve. You must not attempt to enter the water unless you are specially trained and properly equipped. This task usually falls to emergency management teams in a local jurisdiction.

✳ **strainer**

a partial obstruction that filters, or strains, the water such as downed trees or wire mesh; causes an unequal force on the two sides.

✳ **hydraulic**

an area of major current changes or reversal due to an obstruction or land formation.

✳ **eddy**

water that flows around an especially large object and, for a time, flows upstream around the downside of an obstruction.

✳ **rip tides**

strong currents that run parallel to the beach between the shore and underwater sandbars until they find a deeper opening and turn to head out to sea where they dump the contents into an undertow.

✳ **undertow**

currents that occur when water is trapped behind sandbars and finds an opening to pull water and anything in the water out to sea.

FIGURE 43-8 Safe ice rescues require proper equipment.

Three potential scenarios may arise:

✳ A person is stranded in the water but at no risk.

✳ A person may be at immediate risk of being washed downstream or caught in a dangerous moving water. Dangerous water scenarios can include a **strainer**, a **hydraulic**, or an **eddy**.

✳ A victim may be not be able to be saved, at which time the strategies turn from rescue to recovery.

SURF RESCUE

Surf-rescue dangers can include tides, **rip tides**, currents, **undertows**, large waves, contamination, debris, and cold water. Due to the changing conditions caused by waves moving onto and off shore, the amount of water in surf-rescue scenario can be deceptive. Recovering victims from surf stirs up the water, sand, and silt and makes a systematic search difficult. You should become familiar with access routes to surf locations in your areas. You may need to summon professional lifeguard, coast guard, or rescue services to rescue or recover victims in dangerous surf.

ICE RESCUE

Ice presents an even more dangerous situation for rescuers and EMS (Figure 43-8). The strength and depth of ice varies greatly, and a victim in the water signals that the ice is unsafe. Cold water will drop body temperature 25 times faster than air and will make victims confused and ultimately unconscious. Some victims have

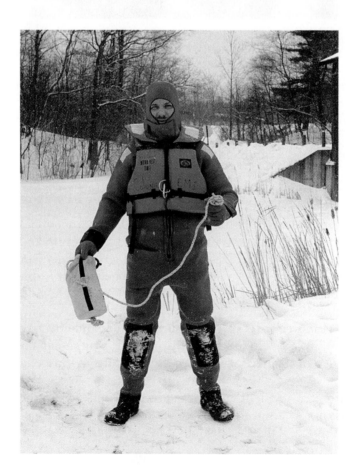

been resuscitated from cold water up to an hour after submersion due to hypothermia and the protective mammalian diving reflex. **Hypothermia** is defined as body temperature below 92°F. The **mammalian diving reflex** is triggered when a person's face is submersed in cold water and can cause the human body to go into a state of extremely low metabolism that preserves the brain, lung, and heart tissue. The patient will have a slow heart rate and low blood pressure and will shunt warm blood to the vital organs.

The clothing most victims wear in a cold environment will cause the victim to be overweight when the clothing becomes saturated with water. Cold water and clothing can also cause frostbite to extremities.

Identify the time the victim went into the water and summon a team that has the appropriate ice rescue equipment. Using a loud speaker or public address system from the vehicle, tell the victim to attempt to stay in the fetal position to conserve body heat. If there are multiple victims, instruct them to huddle together to conserve heat. The treatment for rescued patients should focus on gradual rewarming, minimal movement, and treating for shock. In cases of cardiac arrest, CPR should be continued until the patient is at the hospital and thoroughly rewarmed. Remember the old saying: **A victim is not dead until he is warm and dead.**

DIVE RESCUE

An emergency response to a diving emergency begins with identifying resources in the region that can handle a diving emergency. EMS crews working where there is sport, commercial, or public-safety diving should identify the closest **hyperbaric chamber.** Hypothermia, air embolus, pneumothorax, and decompression sickness are all possible complications from scuba diving.

If a diver ascends to the surface too quickly, an air embolus or pneumothorax can result. The victim may be unable to get out of the water and require a rescue. When a diver stays under water too deep and too long, ascends too rapidly, or dives too many days in a row, nitrogen bubbles form in the blood stream, resulting in a condition call **decompression sickness.** The signs of decompression sickness include chest pain, fatigue, headache, shortness of breath, and joint pain. If a diver is under water when this occurs, he may start to act out of character, exhibiting bizarre behavior. This condition is known as **nitrogen narcosis** and may require rescue. The EMT should treat all diving emergencies with oxygen and care for shock.

∗ **hypothermia**

generalized body cooling to below 92° F.

∗ **mammalian diving reflex**

body response triggered when a person's face is submersed in cold water, causing the body to go into a state of extremely low metabolism that preserves the brain, lung, and heart tissue. Also called the diving response.

∗ **hyperbaric chamber**

pressurized chamber that provides the patient with oxygen under pressure. Hyperbaric oxygen therapy increases tissue oxygenation.

∗ **decompression sickness**

condition resulting from nitrogen bubbles forming in the blood stream. This can happen to a diver who stays under water too deep and too long, ascends too rapidly, or dives too many days in a row.

∗ **nitrogen narcosis**

condition presenting with acting out of character or bizarre behavior resulting when a diver stays under water too deep and too long. Also called raptures of the deep.

Stop, Review, Remember!

Multiple Choice

Place a check next to the correct answer.

1. Hypothermia is defined as a body temperature below:

_____ a. 98 degrees.

_____ b. 94 degrees.

_____ c. 92 degrees.

_____ d. 32 degrees.

2. The mammalian diving reflex in some cases can preserve the body and allow a person submerged greater than _____ minutes to survive.

_____ a. 60 minutes

_____ b. 30 minutes

_____ c. 15 minutes

_____ d. 4–6 minutes

3. You are an EMT in a resort community. As a lifeguard, you are called to a large group of recreational divers returning to port. A 30-year-old female is complaining of shortness of breath after a rapid ascent. She has severe pain in both shoulders and is weak. You suspect a condition called:

_____ a. nitrogen narcosis.

_____ b. pneumothorax.

_____ c. decompression sickness.

_____ d. hyperventilation syndrome.

4. Swift water is defined as water moving at greater than:

_____ a. 5.10 mph.

_____ b. 10 mph.

_____ c. 1.15 mph.

_____ d. 7 mph.

5. When a diver is under water and he starts to act out of character with bizarre behavior, this condition is known as:

_____ a. nitrogen narcosis.

_____ b. pneumothorax.

_____ c. decompression sickness.

_____ d. hyperventilation syndrome.

Fill in the Blank

List the answers to the following questions for your jurisdiction.

1. Where is the closest rescue dive team? _____

2. Where is the closest swift-water rescue team? _____

3. Where is your closest hyperbaric chamber? _____

Critical Thinking

1. With a victim of submersion in cold or ice-covered water, what are the special considerations for treating the responsive patient?

   _____

   _____

   _____

   _____

2. What are the water, surf, or ice hazards in your community? What locations are common response areas for water-related rescues? Where are the access points to safely approach water hazards in your community?

   _____

   _____

   _____

   _____

3. Identify the dive rescue team, swift-water-trained response agencies, and ice-rescue resources in your community.

   _____

   _____

   _____

   _____

TRENCH AND EXCAVATION

The awareness level for trench and excavation emergencies includes sizing up the existing and potential hazards. Upon arrival, report to your incident commander if you are not first on the scene. You will be involved in identifying what is an unsafe trench or excavation site. Any trench that is over 8 feet deep, has an intersection (a place where two trenches intersect), or is compromised by weather-related events is an unsafe environment for you and other EMTs.

Identify local resources necessary to conduct a safe and effective trench or excavation emergency operation.

If you are first on scene, you will need to report the nature of the incident, number of victims, hazards, size of the trench, and access to the scene. Know the local procedures for responding to a trench or excavation emergency and where to call to get additional resources to the scene. Implement site control and scene management by establishing a safety perimeter of 300 feet around the location of the trench or evacuation emergency.

Restrict traffic and other sources of vibration. Zones should be set up similar to a hazardous material incident with a cold, a warm, and a hot zone. Review chapter 42 as needed. The hot zone should be established closest to the hazards and the most dangerous area, where there should be no access except by the rescue team.

Hazards of trench and excavation sites include:

* **Suffocation**—Victims of collapse can succumb to suffocation.

* **Hypoxia**—Victims buried up to shoulder height can have compression of the chest resulting in hypoxia.

* **Hypothermia**—Trenches often are cold and wet, which can lead to hypothermia.

* **Compartment syndrome**—If lower extremities or arms are pinned for greater than 4 hours, the patient can develop compartment syndrome. Compartment syndrome is caused by the build-up of toxins from metabolism in the pinned extremity. When the extremity is freed and circulation is restored, the toxins are circulated into the body and can cause heart rhythm disturbances.

There are several trench collapse patterns; each trench has a unique way that it will collapse. It is also important to understand how a secondary collapse will occur with a trench, excavation, or engulfment. Secondary collapses are likely to occur in unprotected trenches, when there is standing water or seeping water into the trench, when the trench exists in previously disturbed soils, when there is vibration from nearby vehicles, and with exterior cracking of trench walls.

A trench can have other hazards that pose a danger to the rescuer:

* Utilities that can pose a threat to the rescuers include underground electrical services, gas, water or steam lines, sanitary sewer lines, or secondary services like industrial or medical gases. It is important to make sure the rescuer is not entering a hazardous or flammable environment.

* Several mishaps and injuries occur to rescuers, including trips, falls, punctures, strains, and sprains. These can be avoided in situations that allow for a rapid, nonentry extrication of a noninjured or minimally injured victim. It is acceptable for an EMT to place a ladder in the trench to allow a victim to self-rescue (climb out of the trench).

* Certain soils have specific entrapment characteristics. As a general rule, a cubic foot of soil weighs 100 pounds and a cubic yard about 1.5 tons. A person trapped in soils should be treated for traumatic asphyxia due to compression of the chest or crush syndrome if extremities are buried in the soils.

* **compartment syndrome**
a condition that may occur if a large bulk of muscle is crushed or compressed for a long period of time. By-products from the compression of muscle and tissue can trigger life-threatening emergencies and potentially cardiac arrest.

STRUCTURAL COLLAPSE

If you are first on scene at a structural collapse, you will need to evaluate the existing and potential conditions at structural collapse incidents (Figure 43-9). As an

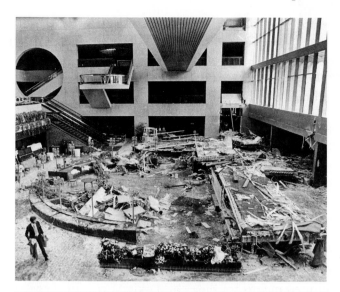

FIGURE 43-9 Incidents involving structural collapse need to be evaluated for existing and potential dangerous conditions. (AP Wide World Photos.)

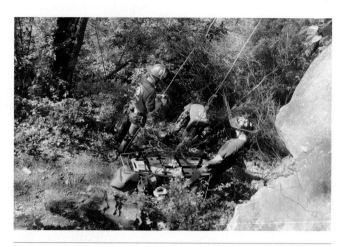

FIGURE 43-10 Rescues in hazardous terrain can be both dangerous and prolonged. (© Ken Kerr.)

EMT you should know the location of resources available to respond to a structural collapse. It is important as a first-on-scene emergency responder to maintain the site control and scene safety. It is important to understand the types of construction and how the components will act.

ROPE RESCUE

The rise in popularity of extreme sports makes the probability of responding to a victim in hazardous terrain a real possibility (Figure 43-10). You will be expected to size up hazardous terrain for a potential rope rescue and identify the resources necessary to conduct safe and effective rope-rescue operations. Rope-rescue scenarios are categorized as either **low angle** or **high angle.**

A rescue that involves accessing terrain at less than a 40-degree angle is considered a low-angle rescue unless the surface is extremely smooth. Low-angle rescues need rescue teams that have harnesses, rope, and safety systems. While an EMT may make access to the scene by scrambling or climbing over the terrain, patient movement and safety of the rescuers will depend on the use of rope systems and litters. Four- to six-person teams can move the patient and the majority of the weight of the rescuers and the patient is on ground.

A **caterpillar pass** is a technique that can be used to negotiate a short section of technical terrain. Rescuers are positioned along the path and the litter is passed through the team. It is important for the rescuers and EMTs to have solid footing and stay in position when passing the litter hand to hand. To be effective, 10 to 12 bearers are desirable and a safety rope is required.

High-angle rescues involve placement of a complex rope and rigging system for situations with a greater than 40-degree angle or a vertical rise. This will require a specialized rescue team proficient at knot tying, ascending and descending rope, packaging a patient in a litter, and using a hauling system and rope to remove the patient from hazardous terrain. High-angle rescue techniques are dangerous and require thorough safety checks as well as qualified personnel. In high-angle or technical rope-rescue scenarios, the majority of the weight of rescuers and the patient is on the rope system. Two-rope systems are required for safety, and the rescuers must be tied into the system.

* **low-angle rescue**
  rescue that involves terrain at less than a 40-degree angle.

* **high-angle rescue**
  rescue that involves terrain at greater than a 40-degree angle.

* **caterpillar pass**
  rescue by which rescuers are positioned along a path and the litter is passed through the team.

Scene control and site safety during a rope rescue may be delegated to the EMT on scene. It is important to restrict the area from bystanders, who could obstruct rope movement or get caught in haul lines. On-scene responsibilities include implementing procedures to carry out the emergency response where a rope rescue is required. When rope is being used to rescue a person, certain hazards exist. Falls are a major concern. The possibility that a rescuer can fall or that something can fall on someone in the rescue party should constantly be evaluated. The rope rescue area should have a 300-foot perimeter. Vehicles should be shut down, access controlled, and hazards removed from the operational area if possible. Certain safety gear is needed for a rope rescue. Rescuers should be equipped with harnesses, gloves, and helmets.

CONFINED SPACE RESCUE

* **confined space**

a space that is large enough and configured so that a person can enter but that has limited means for entry and exit and is not designed for continuous human occupancy.

A **confined space** is defined as a space that is large enough and configured so that a person can enter but that has limited means for entry and exit. A confined space is not designed for continuous human occupancy and may contain a hazardous atmosphere, may have a potential for engulfment or entrapment, and may be configured with downward-sloping walls or walls that narrow into smaller sections that might trap a person. Examples of confined spaces include manholes, mines, tanks, vessels, silos, storage bins, utility vaults, and pits (Figure 43-11). Any commodity that flows, such as grain, plastic beads, or sand can create an engulfment hazard. Certain procedures can be used to retrieve a victim from a confined space without entering the area. Often a victim is tethered to a safety system or harness that the EMT can activate to retrieve the person from the confined space.

EMT functions at a confined space rescue involve assessing the scene and ensuring that the scene is isolated and that nonessential personnel are denied entry into the area. The first-on-scene EMT should attempt to make communication with the patient when possible. A patient who cannot respond may be deceased, and the rescue would now become a recovery operation. The EMT must recognize hazards associated within a confined space. The EMT should assess the perimeter

FIGURE 43-11   Rescuers should never be permitted to enter confined spaces, such as silos, unless they have training, equipment, and experience in this environment. (© Michal Heron)

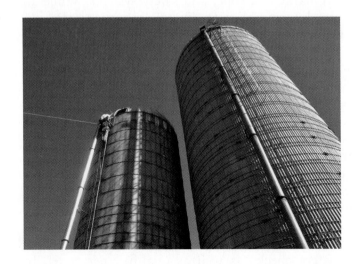

of the confined space to determine the presence of hazards to the rescuers. An attempt should be made to identify the potential hazardous materials or atmospheres through labels on or around the confined space or from information received from on-site manufacturing or rescue teams.

In most cases the patient cannot survive the initial event. If the patient appears to have an injury incompatible with life or is unresponsive and not breathing, without the equipment to perform an immediate rescue the operation will become a body recovery. In the recovery phase, the EMT's role becomes one of support to the rescue team. The procedures for starting an entry include the initiation of the permit process that enables the rescue team to make an entry. Only personnel trained in confined-space rescue to the operations level are permitted to enter a confined space to conduct a rescue operation.

Safety Considerations   There are four deadly chemicals commonly found in a confined space.

* **Carbon dioxide** is slightly heavier than air and will stay at head level. Carbon dioxide displaces oxygen and is classified as an **asphyxiant**. Confinement with carbon dioxide at relatively low levels for as little as 4 to 6 minutes can be fatal. Even if a rescue can be made quickly, they will need to be transported to the hospital, because carbon dioxide decomposes in the body and forms carbon monoxide, which binds to red blood cells and keeps oxygen from getting to the tissues.

* **Carbon monoxide** is slightly lighter than air, will mix with air at all levels, and will displace oxygen. The toxicity occurs as a result of the ability of this product to interfere with oxygen at the cellular level, making this gas a cellular asphyxiant. A cellular asphyxiant disrupts cellular metabolism by interfering with the chemical process of the cell. Any victims who have been in a confined space with carbon monoxide for as little as 4 to 6 minutes will have elevated **Carboxyhemoglobin** levels and, even if rescue can be made quickly, they will need to be transported to a facility with a hyperbaric chamber.

* **Hydrogen sulfide** is slightly heavier than air and will stratify at or around the head and shoulders. Toxicity is the primary danger with hydrogen sulfide because it will displace oxygen, although not as readily as carbon dioxide. Hydrogen sulfide is a cellular asphyxiant that stops the cells from correctly processing oxygen. Hydrogen sulfide is extremely toxic and will produce olfactory fatigue, which means that the ability to smell the odor of rotten eggs generated by hydrogen sulfide goes away over time. Olfactory fatigue can trick a rescuer into thinking the environment is safe to enter to retrieve a victim. If any victims are in the confined space for as little as 4 to 6 minutes with significant levels of hydrogen sulfide, there will be fatalities. Even if rescue can be made quickly, patients rarely recover.

* **Methane** is a saturated hydrocarbon which means that it occurs in nature as the by-product of the breakdown of all organic materials. It exists as a gas, and in this state it is highly volatile. Its physical properties are very simple to address. Out in the open, the primary hazard of methane is flammability, but in a confined space it is toxicity, which can cause asphyxiation.

✳ **carbon dioxide**
slightly heavier-than-air gas that displaces oxygen.

✳ **asphyxiant**
a substance that prevents sufficient intake or use of oxygen.

✳ **carbon monoxide**
slightly lighter-than-air gas that displaces oxygen.

✳ **carboxyhemoglobin**
a compound formed by carbon monoxide and hemoglobin in carbon monoxide poisoning.

✳ **hydrogen sulfide**
slightly heavier-than-air gas that displaces oxygen. It may produce the odor of rotten eggs.

✳ **methane**
a naturally occurring, saturated hydrocarbon that is a by-product of the breakdown of all organic materials.

Stop, Review, Remember!

Multiple Choice

1. Which of the following is NOT considered a confined space?

   _____ a. a grain elevator filled with dried corn

   _____ b. a reactor vessel at a chemical factory used to make solvents

   _____ c. a brewing tank at a microbrewery with mixing blades

   _____ d. a five-foot deep trench

2. Hyperbaric chambers can be used to treat patients with:

   _____ a. diving emergencies and carbon monoxide exposure.

   _____ b. diving emergencies and surf emergencies.

   _____ c. carbon monoxide and hydrogen sulfide exposure.

   _____ d. hydrogen sulfide and carbon dioxide exposure.

3. Which gases are considered cellular asphyxiants?

   _____ a. hydrogen sulfide and carbon monoxide

   _____ b. carbon monoxide and carbon dioxide

   _____ c. carbon dioxide and hydrogen sulfide

   _____ d. methane and carbon dioxide

4. How large should the safety perimeter be around the location of the trench rescue?

   _____ a. 200 feet

   _____ b. 300 feet

   _____ c. 400 feet

   _____ d. 500 feet

Fill in the Blank

1. List the four gases that pose a danger to responders in a confined space.

   a. _____

   b. _____

   c. _____

   d. _____

2. What are the two types of rope rescue?

   a. _____

   b. _____

Critical Thinking

1. What locations or areas in your community have the potential for becoming a confined-space rescue?

_____

_____

_____

_____

2. What resources in your community would be able to conduct a confined-space rescue?

_____

_____

_____

_____

3. At what locations in your community might you have a high- or low-angle rescue?

_____

_____

_____

_____

4. What are the differences between a trench rescue and a confined space rescue?

_____

_____

_____

_____

Medical Issues Related to Technical Rescue Victims

Be ready to provide care related to technical rescue injuries. Victims of a rescue scenario may need cervical and spinal immobilizations. Often patients will have spinal injuries associated with high-energy impacts, falls, and trauma. Cervical and spine precautions may require the patient to be evacuated in a vertical or horizontal position. Be sure to secure the patient on a backboard and into a Stokes basket as appropriate. Often a patient being removed from a confined space or a

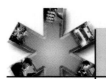

Perspective

The Patient

"That was the worst thing that I've ever gone through. I'm just so thankful that I had already dropped my daughter off at day care. I was just driving to work like I had done a million times before, you know? And I got this weird feeling in my stomach as I came up to that intersection, but I was running late and had spilled my coffee. Just didn't think about it. The next thing I see is headlights and then I was just spinning through the air. It's like it was in slow motion, like a movie or something. The air bag might have been the worst part. I can still smell it. It probably saved my life, though. I don't know. It seemed like it took forever before they got to me in my car. My leg was caught between the steering wheel and the dash and blood just kept dripping from somewhere. I'm still not sure where it all came from! And I heard sirens and men talking and stuff, but no one was helping me. But yet I know they were trying. Did I say that I was so glad that my daughter was already at day care?"

motor vehicle may require the use of a short board or KED to remove him to the stretcher and the ambulance.

Crush injuries are often experienced by patients involved in machinery accidents and building and trench collapses. Crush injuries from entrapment of limbs may initially present as swelling and discoloration. As explained earlier, compartment syndrome can develop. Machinery accidents and vehicle crashes often amputate limbs. This condition is characterized by profound shock. Certain extreme situations may require amputation of a trapped limb in the field to save the patient's life. Be aware of these possibilities and follow local protocols for proper procedures. Call advanced life support before transport, if possible, as the release of pressure on a crushed limb may cause by-products from the injury to enter the blood stream and affect the heart, causing cardiac arrest.

Remember that hypothermia is another common medical condition that an EMT may be required to treat at the scene of a technical rescue. Victims rescued from cold water who appear lifeless must be considered for resuscitation. Remember: **A patient is not dead until he is warm and dead.**

Proper infection control procedures must be followed in a rescue scenario. Often, confined space rescues involve extracting patients from sewers or other areas with bacterial contamination. Other rescue scenarios may involve bloodborne pathogens. The EMT should be familiar with decontamination following possible exposures.

After the incident, it is important for the EMT to be aware of physiological and psychological symptoms that may be triggered by the stress of a technical rescue. Critical incident management should include proper diet and rest, pacing of effort, preconditioning, and personal well-being. During prolonged rescue efforts it is important that EMS and rescue crews are provided proper rehabilitation. The EMT should be on the lookout for the signs and symptoms of critical incident stress.

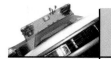

Dispatch Summary

After the glass was cleared, the patient—suffering from an obviously broken right leg and numerous lacerations—was quickly extricated from the vehicle. She was secured to a long-spineboard, placed on high-flow O$_2$, and transported code three to the Dobbs County Memorial Hospital. Once in the ED, she was found to have a pelvic fracture, a ruptured spleen, and a concussion. A precautionary CT scan of her head later showed an acute subdural hematoma.

The patient underwent several surgeries, one to remove her spleen, one to drain the subdural hematoma, and two to reconstruct her leg, and has since been discharged. She is still undergoing daily physical therapy.

The police issued a citation to the driver of the glass truck for failing to stop at the stop sign and for traveling at excessive speed.

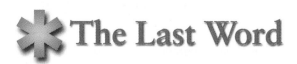

The Last Word

It is important to understand that training over and above the EMT's initial training is required to safely operate in rescue situations. You should strive to achieve awareness-level training in all of the areas of special rescue operations, which will give you the fundamental education you need to operate safely at a rescue. As you know by now, safety is the paramount concern for all responders in any response.

Chapter Review

MULTIPLE CHOICE

Place a check next to the correct answer.

1. You are trained at the awareness level for confined-space rescue. Now you are responding to a confined space incident. What duties might you have to perform at the incident?

_____ a. Enter the confined space search for victims.

_____ b. Assist with the care and transport of recovered victims.

_____ c. Determine if it is safe to enter the confined space.

_____ d. Perform technical rescue of an entrapped victim.

2. You are performing a scene size-up on a motor vehicle collision (MVC). You note that there are two vehicles involved in a T-bone collision; there are two victims, one male, one female, both entrapped; and there are fluids leaking from the front of the van that T-boned the passenger car. Which of the following statements is the best scene size-up to be given over the radio to dispatch?

_____ a. "Unit 14 to dispatch, on the scene with a two-vehicle MVC with two victims."

_____ b. "Unit 14 to dispatch, on the scene of an MVC, T-bone type, with fluids leaking."

_____ c. "Unit 14 to dispatch, on the scene of a two-vehicle, T-bone type MVC, two victims, both entrapped, fluids leaking from one vehicle. Dispatch heavy rescue and fire department to this location."

_____ d. "Unit 14 to dispatch, on the scene of an MVC involving two vehicles, one van and one passenger car. There is one male victim and one female victim, both victims entrapped, fluids leaking from the van. There are no power lines down. Please dispatch heavy rescue to this location."

3. You are inside a vehicle assessing a patient who was involved in an MVC. The fire department is preparing to extricate the patient, and the Fire Captain tells you that they are going to have to pop the windows to access the patient. What precautions should you take to protect your patient?

_____ a. Inform him of what is about to happen, then cover the patient with a rescue blanket.

_____ b. Inform him of what is about to happen, then cover the patient with a sheet.

_____ c. Inform him of what is about to happen, then cover the patient with a plastic bag.

_____ d. Inform him of what is about to happen, then exit the vehicle and let the fire department pop the glass.

4. You have arrived on the scene of a water rescue in late winter to transport the victim, a 14-year-old male who fell through some ice and was rescued by the local fire department. The victim was submerged for 20 to 30 minutes. Assessment reveals the patient is pulseless and not breathing. Which is the most correct course of action to care for this victim?

_____ a. The patient is obviously dead and should be transported to the morgue.

_____ b. The patient should be transported to the hospital for further evaluation.

_____ c. You should call for ALS care, begin CPR, and wait for ALS to transport the patient.

_____ d. You should begin CPR, transport the victim to the hospital, and notify the hospital that the victim is suffering from hypothermic cardiac arrest.

5. Which statement best describes the mammalian diving reflex?

_____ a. When a person's face is submersed in cold water, the body goes into a state of extremely low metabolism that preserves the brain, lung, and heart tissue.

_____ b. When a person's face is submersed in cold water, the heart rate drops to less than 10 beats per minute.

_____ c. When a person's body is submersed in cold water, the body goes into a state of extremely low metabolism that preserves the brain and lung tissue.

_____ d. When a person's body is submersed in warm water, the body goes into a state of extremely low metabolism that preserves the brain, lung, and heart tissue.

6. You have been dispatched to the local airport to meet an inbound flight from the Caribbean. The crew has radioed the tower to report that they have a male passenger who began complaining to the flight attendants of muscle and joint pain in mid-flight. About 20 minutes ago, the patient began to complain of chest pain. The patient is 23 years old and may have been diving while on vacation. What is most likely wrong with this patient?

_____ a. The patient may be suffering from a panic attack.

_____ b. The patient may be suffering from a heart attack.

_____ c. The patient may be suffering from decompression sickness.

_____ d. The patient may be suffering from a pulmonary embolus.

7. You are called to a utility work site at a manhole for a patient suffering from respiratory distress. Your patient states that he entered the tunnel and smelled a strong odor of rotten eggs. He began to have some difficulty breathing and immediately left the work area. You place the patient on high-flow oxygen. What toxic gas was the patient most likely exposed to?

_____ a. carbon dioxide

_____ b. carbon monoxide

_____ c. hydrogen sulfide

_____ d. methane

8. You are at the scene of an industrial incident. Your patient has had his arm pinned in between rollers in a large metalworking machine for about 1 hour. The fire department has just freed the victim from the machine. What condition could your patient begin to suffer as blood flow begins to return to the arm?

_____ a. compartment syndrome

_____ b. crush syndrome

_____ c. fractured arm

_____ d. blood clot due to the lack of blood flow

LABELING

Label the following parts in the diagram:

A post
B post
C post
Nader pin
Crumple zone
Side-injury protection bar

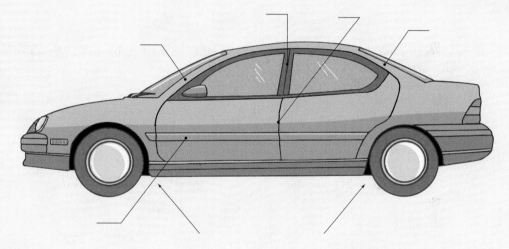

CRITICAL THINKING

1. Your ambulance has arrived on the bridge downstream from a reported incident. Immediately you have identified a man in the water clinging to a tree in the middle of the flood river. What action should you take? What medical considerations apply to this patient?

_____

_____

_____

2. You and your partner are called to assist the sheriff at a local recreation area where two teenagers are reported missing. It is late fall and the temperatures are expected to drop drastically after the sun goes down. You have about 2 hours before dusk. You are the first to arrive on scene. A group of teenagers approaches the ambulance. What steps should you take until the search-and-rescue team arrives?

_____

_____

_____

CASE STUDY

You respond to a neighboring community where a tornado has inflicted severe damage. You are directed by the fire department incident commander to a neighborhood where an apartment complex has been damaged. The search team has assessed the scene and left FEMA markings for collapsed structures. Interpret the markings left on the three damaged apartment buildings.

20 June 06
Truck 10X Biohazard
2 Live
2 Dead

20 June 06
NevadaTF 1X Gas leak
1 Live
1 Dead

21 June 06
E-10X Hazmat
0 Live
2 Dead

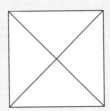

Which of the diagrams indicates an unsafe structure to enter as marked by a FEMA task force using the building marking system?

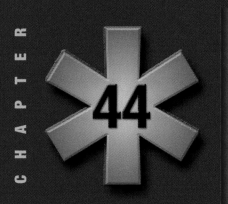

CHAPTER 44

Responses Involving Terrorism

There are no objectives from the U.S. Department of Transportation 1994 EMT-Basic National Standard Curriculum.

Introduction

The new millennium has brought with it a changed nation. Terrorism is now an everyday threat. EMTs are now linked with the Department of Homeland Security and the Office of Domestic Preparedness. Some consider it a matter of *when* our country will have to respond to another terrorist event. The first attack on the World Trade Center in 1993, the Murrah Federal Building in Oklahoma City in April 1995, the devastating attacks of September 11, 2001, and the October 2005 anthrax attacks on U.S. government facilities—these events demonstrate that proper response training for terrorist-related events is critical to your training (Figures 44-1 and 44-2).

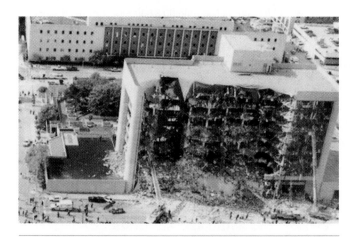

FIGURE 44-1 The scene of the April 19, 1995 bombing of the Alfred P. Murrah Federal Building in Oklahoma City. (Sygma Corbis.)

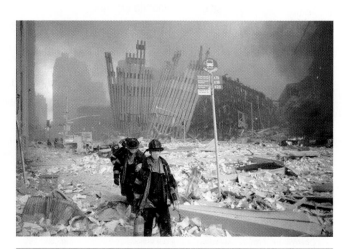

FIGURE 44-2 The Twin Towers of the World Trade Center in New York City were destroyed and thousands were killed on September 11, 2001 when terrorists flew hijacked jetliners into those famous skyscrapers. (Corbis/Sygma.)

Among the most insidious attacks would be an attack using a biological or chemical agent where the first responder will be the sentinel that identifies a terrorist act. EMTs will be among those on the front lines of this new battle and could be faced with life-and-death decisions, in some cases involving hundreds of patients.

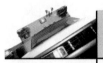

Emergency Dispatch

"**S**tation three, rescue... station three, medical," the dispatcher's voice echoed through the fire station, from the polished concrete floors to the well-stocked kitchen. "Proceed, priority one, to West Avendell, the Cinema 16 building. A semi-truck has apparently hit the building."

The search-and-rescue crew scrambled through the hallways, donning turnouts while piling into the truck, and then disappearing in a cloud of diesel exhaust and screaming sirens.

"Come on, Terry!" EMT Joelle Havens pounded on the bathroom door. "We've got a call!"

"I know! I know!" came the muffled reply. "Get the truck started and I'll be there in 2 seconds!"

Joelle started the ambulance and inched out of the building, nervously tapping on the steering wheel. A minute later Joelle's paramedic partner, Terry Edwards, jumped into the passenger seat, still trying to buckle his belt.

"There's no better way to jinx a nice, quiet afternoon than starting a card game on the computer!" he said. "So, what do we have?"

"A big rig versus the Cinema 16 building," Joelle said, carefully clearing a busy intersection before proceeding.

"Really?" Terry said, suddenly serious. "That's odd. Big trucks aren't even allowed on those downtown streets. How bad is it?"

"I don't know." Joelle sounded the air horn at a taxi that seemed oblivious to them. "But once

Rescue three got there, they called for a lot of fire support."

"Well... just... once we get there... go slow." Terry could just make out the roof of the Cinema 16 building across town and thick, dark smoke was beginning to boil up into the sky above it.

As they turned onto West Avendell, Terry leaned forward and covered his mouth with his hand. "Ooh, brother, there is *no way* that's an accident. "

The box trailer of a semi-truck was jutting from the destroyed lobby entrance of the newly remodeled movie theater, and black smoke poured from the gaping opening. The Rescue Three truck was parked near the rear of the trailer and about seven police cars were situated haphazardly along the road around it. Crowds of screaming movie-goers, blackened from the smoke, streamed from the emergency exits and disappeared in all directions as police officers tried in vain to direct them.

Joelle stopped about a hundred feet from the theater entrance and Terry picked up the radio microphone. Several more fire trucks rounded the corner at the other end of the street. "Something's not right, Jo! I'm serious. Back up, quick!" Terry then keyed the mic. "Headquarters, medical three... we need to set up a perimeter. Don't send anyone else downtown. I repeat...."

The radio transmission ended abruptly as the semi's trailer buckled and then disappeared in a huge explosion that rattled windows nearly 25 miles away.

What Is Terrorism?

It is important to understand the difference between **terrorism** and acts of violence. According to the Department of Justice, terrorism is an illegal act that is dangerous to human life and is against the laws of the United States or any political subdivision. It is performed with intent to intimidate or coerce a government or civilian population in the furtherance of a political or social agenda. The use of violence may need only to be threatened, because it is fear that initiates a change. Terrorists are considered to hold extremist ideas and philosophies and are intolerant of others' viewpoints. They justify their acts by saying and believing that their targets are evil. People develop fear to a degree that the government cannot protect them. There are different types of terrorism, both international and domestic, representing left-wing versus right-winged philosophies. Targets for terrorism can be people, places, or infrastructure.

It is important for you, the EMT, to help conduct an efficient and safe response for the benefit of the victims and to establish trust in government emergency services.

* **terrorism**

    an illegal act that is dangerous to human life, which is against the laws of the United States or any political subdivision, with intent to intimidate or coerce a government or civilian population in the furtherance of a political or social agenda.

Preoperational Considerations

Preparation for responding to a terrorist attack must begin with preplanning and must encompass the entire community. Preplanning is usually addressed in the local disaster response plan. This plan is developed by the local office of Emergency Management with input from local law enforcement, fire service, and EMS. All communities are required to develop a disaster response plan that is required by the federal government to meet the **NIMS** model as discussed in chapter 41 of your text.

* **NIMS**

    National Incident Management System.

SCENE SIZE-UP

Your responsibility in scene size-up in suspected acts of terrorism includes assessing security when approaching the scene and throughout the operation or call. You must develop a high **index of suspicion** or a mental trigger that, when you are called to an event, will help you recognize it as a potential terrorist event.

One key component that should raise awareness is the identification of the building or the location. If the location of the incident has symbolic or historic significance, such as places of public assembly (arenas or stadiums), controversial facilities (some political headquarters), critical infrastructure (for example, the New York Stock Exchange), and government installations are considered common targets for terrorists (Figure 44-3 on page 1106).

Ideally, emergency personnel will have been advised if there has been a threat; however this may not always be the case. Upon arrival or when receiving the dispatch report, look for physical indicators of a potential terrorist incident, such as:

* **index of suspicion**

    mental trigger that, when called to an event, will help an EMT recognize it as a potential terrorist event.

* A report of mass casualties with minimal trauma or without a known traumatic cause.

* Explosions that disrupt the transportation and communication systems, including the emergency services or critical infrastructure.

* A debris field or severe structural damage to a building.

* First-responder casualties, dead animals, or dead vegetation.

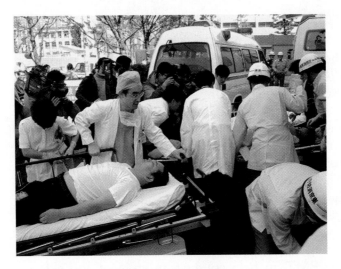

FIGURE 44-3 The scene of a terrorist poison gas attack in the Tokyo subway system. (AP Wide World Photos)

✳ Unusual smells, color of smoke, and vapor clouds indicating the need for immediate respiratory protection and evacuation from the scene.

✳ Incidents that involve large crowds of people, such as concerts or sports events, that begin to have multiple patients injured or showing illness from an unknown cause.

APPROACHING THE SCENE

As you approach the scene, consider the possibility of a terrorist event if there is more than one indicator present. Assess scene safety. If, on approach to the scene, you notice that other first responders, including law enforcement, firefighters, and EMS, have become incapacitated, you should consider that someone has purposely targeted the emergency responders. First responders have sometimes been intentionally targeted, as in the Atlanta Abortion Clinic bombing where **secondary devices** were placed specifically to target the emergency personnel responding to the incident. The best way to minimize the risk of a secondary device is not to do what the terrorists expect of you in a response to a terrorist event (Figure 44-4). Instead of rushing into the scene, stop and consider the best approach.

✳ **secondary devices**

  devices used to intentionally disrupt rescue and to injure emergency responders after an initial attack has taken place.

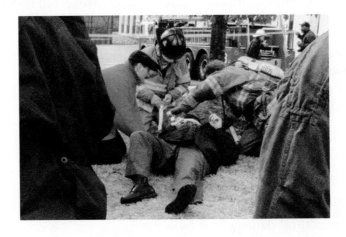

FIGURE 44-4 The scene of a double bombing at an abortion clinic. (Corbis/Sygma.)

Assume command of the scene if no one has done so. Conduct a scene size-up and request resources. Do not park your ambulance in a location closest to the event. Look for suspicious packages, such as back packs, packages, or things that look out of place or appear to be recently left in a location. Secondary devices may be hidden in trash cans, bushes, shrubbery, or planted vehicles. If you identify a secondary device, immediately move to a safe distance; notify dispatch or the incident commander to have the bomb squad neutralize the device.

PRESENCE OF HAZARDOUS MATERIALS

Review chapter 42. It is important for the EMT to identify hazardous substances or the presence of explosions. If multiple indicators exist, you may be on the scene of a terrorist event and should immediately consider the need for respiratory protection and personal protective clothing.

REQUESTING ADDITIONAL RESOURCES

If you suspect a terrorist incident, make immediate contact with law enforcement for coordination. Approach the scene uphill and upwind and ask your dispatch center for a weather report. Make sure you have a quick, unimpeded exit route and are working with a partner. Look for situations in which the response is being funneled into an area that will bottleneck or congest vehicles, making it difficult to withdraw to a safe position if a secondary device or attack on rescue personnel is launched.

Identify a rally point to meet and regroup in the event a secondary device detonates or another attack is conducted on emergency responders. Identify safe staging areas for other EMS, fire, and police units to respond to. Isolate and deny entry to nonemergency personnel, referring to the DOT *Emergency Response Guidebook* (ERG) (Figure 44-5) for a safe minimum distance if an identified hazardous material is present. Consider the need for additional resources and that the site is a potential crime scene. Notify the hospital or hospitals of the situation and the number of patients to expect from the incident.

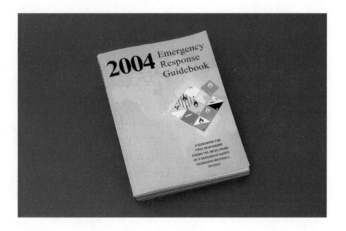

FIGURE 44-5   *Emergency Response Guidebook.*

Stop, Review, Remember!

Multiple Choice

Place a check next to the correct answer.

1. Terrorism can be best defined as:

_____ a. an illegal act that is dangerous to human life and that is against the laws of the United States

_____ b. violence or the threat of violence, because it is fear that initiates a change in behavior in a population

_____ c. the use of a bomb or chemical weapon to kill or injure a population

_____ d. an illegal act of violence to kill or injure a population

2. Which of the following reports would prompt a high index of suspicion of a terrorist attack?

_____ a. a report of a single-vehicle MVC involving a tanker truck

_____ b. a report of multiple victims unresponsive in a train station

_____ c. a report of an explosion in a grain-storage bin in an isolated rural area

_____ d. a report of an explosion of a factory

3. A secondary device is an explosive device designed to:

_____ a. kill bystanders when they come to look at the damage caused by the initial event.

_____ b. injure hospital personnel when victims are transported to their facility.

_____ c. kill first responders when they respond to the initial event.

_____ d. kill those who did not die initially.

Ordering

Indicate the correct sequence—1 to 7—of the following recommended steps in responding to a potential terrorist attack.

1. _____

2. _____

3. _____

4. _____

5. _____

6. _____

7. _____

A. Ask your dispatch center for a weather report.
B. Look for situations in which the response is being funneled into an area that will bottleneck.
C. Make immediate contact with law enforcement for coordination.
D. Identify a rally point to meet and regroup in the event of a secondary device.
E. Identify safe staging areas for other EMS, fire, and police units to respond to.
F. Approach the scene uphill and upwind.
G. Make sure you have a quick, unimpeded exit route.

Critical Thinking

1. Look at your community and identify potential terrorist targets.

    _____

    _____

    _____

    _____

2. When responding to a potential terrorist event, the EMT must be aware of secondary devices. What can you do to minimize the threat to you from secondary devices?

    _____

    _____

    _____

    _____

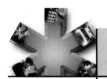

Perspective

Terry—The Paramedic

"I can't believe what happened. I just can't believe it! Right there at the movie theater that I've taken my kids to a hundred times. There were probably kids in there today. Why do this? Why here? Has anyone heard from Rescue Three, yet? I know they couldn't have made it, but I still hope . . . I mean, we were just . . . I can't believe this happened. And why did everyone just rush in? I couldn't have been the only one with that uneasy feeling, could I? It was just all wrong. A semi couldn't accidentally crash into the lobby of that movie theater. There was just no way. Did I know that it would explode? Hell no! I was afraid of some chemical agent in the smoke, actually. I never in a million years thought that it'd blow up."

Nuclear, Biological, and Chemical Weapons

Weapons of mass destruction (WMDs) come in many forms. To this point in the chapter, we have discussed explosive devices. Now we can look at other agents that can be used in a terrorist attack. The other classes of WMDs are **nuclear weapons (NW)**, **biological weapons (BW)**, and **chemical weapons (CW)**. These agents are commonly referred to as **NBCs**. Each NBC has a specific delivery method and accompanying signs and symptoms of the attack.

* **weapons of mass destruction (WMDs)**

variety of explosive, chemical, biological, nuclear, or other devices used by terrorists to strike at government, high-profile, or high-population targets; designed to create a maximum number of casualties.

* **nuclear weapons (NW)**

devices designed to release the energy generated during splitting (fission) or combining (fusion) of heavy nuclei to form new elements that are deliberately distributed to cause harm or death; a weapon that can produce an actual nuclear explosion.

* **biological weapons (BW)**

devices designed to release either living organisms or toxins produced by living organisms that are deliberately distributed to cause disease and death.

* **chemical weapons (CW)**

devices designed to release a range of simple to sophisticated chemicals that are deliberately distributed to cause harm or death.

∗ **NBC**

abbreviation for nuclear, biological, and chemical.

∗ **vapor pressure**

the pressure exerted by a chemical against the atmosphere.

∗ **persistence**

length of time an agent stays in the environment.

∗ **virulence**

the power of infection once started.

∗ **transmissibility**

the ease with which an agent or disease can spread from person to person.

∗ **lethality**

the ability of an agent or disease to cause death; the percentage of those who die from an agent or disease.

∗ **improvised nuclear device (IND)**

a device that can produce a nuclear explosion.

∗ **radiological dispersal device (RDD)**

a conventional bomb laced with radioactive material. Also called a dirty bomb.

∗ **simple radiological device**

device that disperses radioactive particles without explosion.

As an EMT, you must understand the physical principles of the NBC agents. One of the most effective ways to dispense an agent is to disseminate it into the respiratory system. The respiratory system is an easy target because of the vast surface area of the lungs. The smaller the size of the particles the easier it is to aerosolize the agent. Dispersal can occur with explosives, spraying equipment, or natural currents created by the movement of equipment. The heating of agents often creates vapors and that can increase the penetration to the lung tissue. Greater velocity of air movement can move a greater amount of an agent into the lungs, making it more effective.

Vapor pressure, a factor with chemical agents, is the pressure exerted by a chemical against the atmosphere. The higher the vapor pressure the greater the tendency to evaporate (give off a vapor). The higher the vapor pressure the less persistent the agent is in the environment. Biological agents have no vapor pressure and do not vaporize.

How long an agent stays in the environment is known as **persistence**. Persistency depends on exposure to sunlight, temperature, and humidity. **Virulence** is the power of infection once started. The more rapid the onset and the greater the severity of the disease is the more virulent the agent is said to be. **Transmissibility** is the ease with which an agent or disease can spread from person to person. Finally, the EMT must understand the **lethality** of an agent, which is usually expressed as a percentage of those who die from the agent or disease.

Nuclear Agents

Nuclear agents have three basic forms of delivery that the EMT should know about. A nuclear weapon or **improvised nuclear device (IND)** is a device that can produce a nuclear explosion. A nuclear explosion emits gamma, beta, and alpha radiation. A **radiological dispersal device (RDD)** is a conventional (not nuclear) bomb laced with radioactive material. The RDD explosion—although far less powerful than an actual nuclear explosion—spews the radioactive material into the atmosphere, and the contaminated smoke and air will spread downwind from the blast, emitting gamma, beta, alpha, or any combination of these deadly rays. A **simple radiological device** disperses radioactive particles without explosion.

The detonation of a nuclear device would identify itself by the classic mushroom cloud along with radiation that would accompany the event. A radiological dispersal device would appear to be a conventional explosion, but signs of radiation sickness would appear among the victims who were exposed. A simple radiological device would affect a population group that would begin to exhibit signs and symptoms of radiation sickness.

SIGNS AND SYMPTOMS OF RADIATION EXPOSURE AND RADIATION SICKNESS

The blast wave and thermal pulse from an explosion cause burns, injuries, and death immediately. The severity of radiation sickness depends on the total amount of radiation absorbed. Symptoms can vary from loss of appetite, nausea, vomiting, fatigue, and diarrhea with a low-dose exposure to fever, respiratory distress, and increased excitability with a higher dose. This is the stage at which most victims seek medical care.

PROTECTION FROM NUCLEAR THREATS

The best way for the EMT to guard against radiation exposure is to follow the rules of time, distance, shielding, and quantity.

* **Time**—The shorter the time in a radiation field, the less the radiation exposure. Work quickly and efficiently. A rotating-team approach can keep individual radiation exposures to a minimum.

* **Distance**—The farther a person is from a source of radiation, the lower the radiation dose. Do not touch radioactive materials. Use shovels, brooms, and the like to move materials without physical contact.

* **Shielding**—Although not always practical in emergency situations, shielding offered by barriers can reduce radiation exposure.

* **Quantity**—Limit the amount of radioactive material in the working area to decrease exposure.

Biological Weapons

Biological weapons (BW) are accessible to terrorists and are relatively easy to produce. They have often been called the "poor man's nuclear bomb." Their effects usually go undetected for days until large numbers of the population begin to present with a similar pattern of symptoms. There are three types of biological agents: **bacteria** (e.g., anthrax), **viruses** (e.g., smallpox, Figure 44-6), and **toxins** (e.g., botulism or ricin).

Biological agents are dispersed as either wet or dry agents. Dry agents can be dispersed into heating/ventilation/air conditioning (HVAC) systems or appear in packages with no visible evidence. The EMT should be on the lookout for visible foggers, sprayers, or aerosolizing devices. Naturally occurring biological outbreaks start with a few cases and slowly progress to a peak weeks or perhaps a month or more later. A biological terrorism event will have a sudden peak in patients in a very short period of time, because most people will have been exposed at the same time and will become sick within a similar time frame.

Despite the inherent differences among various types of biological agents, bacteria, viruses, and toxins have some common characteristics. Since biological agents are nonvolatile (do not evaporate), they must be dispersed in aerosols as

* **bacteria**

  one-celled organisms without a true nucleus or cell organelles.

* **viruses**

  pathogenic organisms made of nucleic acid inside a protein shell, which must utilize a host cell for growth and reproduction.

* **toxins**

  poisonous substances produced by animals or plants.

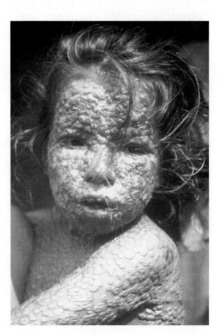

FIGURE 44-6 A young girl in Bangladesh shows the typical raised bumps of the smallpox infection, which she contracted in 1973. In 1977, the World Health Organization announced that smallpox, a potentially fatal disease, had been eradicated from the country. (CDC/Phil, CORBIS-NY.)

1-to-5-micron-size particles (1/30,000 the diameter of a hair follicle), which may remain suspended in the air for hours, depending on weather conditions. The primary route of infection would be inhalation. When inhaled, the particles deposit themselves deep into the alveoli of the lungs, causing disease.

As with agents causing the diseases that you have studied in the medical emergencies section of this textbook (e.g., influenza), a biological agent is a naturally occurring microorganism. The difference is that it has been deliberately altered to be used as a weapon. Biological agents commonly enter the body through one of four routes of entry.

✳ **inhalation**

    entrance of a substance into the respiratory system.

✳ **ingestion**

    entrance of a substance into the digestive system.

✳ **dermal contact**

    entrance of a substance through the skin or mucous membranes.

✳ **vector borne**

    spread by vectors, or carriers, such as animals, insects, or persons who have the disease.

✳ **Inhalation** into the respiratory system—The respiratory system is an easy target because of the vast surface area of the lungs and the warm, wet environment provided by the lungs that allows the organism to grow.

✳ **Ingestion** into the digestive system—Ingestion into the gastrointestinal tract is not as effective as inhalation. Only about 1% of municipal water is consumed and filtration with chlorine or ultraviolet light reduces the threat. More probable is the contamination of food products.

✳ **Dermal contact**—Contact with the skin is another route by which a weapon can be disseminated. While most biological agents are stopped by the skin, the mucus membranes and breaks in the skin can permit absorption and contamination. Remember that intact skin acts as a barrier to biological agents.

✳ **Vector borne** diseases—A vector is an animal, insect, or person that carries a disease. The exposure can occur from a bite, a sneeze, or person-to-person contact. When transmission is human to human, called cross contamination, it becomes a contagious disease.

SIGNS AND SYMPTOMS OF BIOLOGICAL AGENTS EXPOSURE

✳ **incubation period**

    the period of time from exposure until signs and symptoms occur.

Immediately after exposure to a biological agent, there is a period of time before signs and symptoms occur. This is called the **incubation period**. During this period, the agent multiplies and overwhelms the host. At the end of this period, the victim will present with signs and symptoms of the illness. For a bacteria or virus, the incubation period is measured in days. For a toxin, the time frame is much shorter. When compared to chemical weapons, whose effects tend to be immediate, the ill effects from biological weapons are delayed. Therefore, it is more difficult to detect a biological weapon. The EMT who suspects a biological agent should take immediate precautions and obtain the following information from the patient:

    ✳ Travel history: Where has the patient been?

    ✳ Infectious contacts: Has the patient been around any sick people?

    ✳ Employment history: Where does the patient work?

    ✳ Activities over the preceding 3 days: What has the patient been doing?

PROTECTION FROM BIOLOGICAL THREATS

Compliance with the Occupational Safety and Health Administration's (OSHA's) Bloodborne Pathogen Standard (29 CFR 1910.1030) and your organization's exposure control plan will provide adequate protection. Universal precautions include surgical gloves, a high-efficiency particulate air (HEPA) mask of the type used against TB, splash goggles, and an appropriate dermal ensemble. These should be worn when contacting victims of a suspected biological attack.

Chemical Weapons

Terrorists have ample access to chemicals used in the community. For example, chlorine can be found in large quantities in most communities and could be used as a weapon. Chemical agents are classified as nerve agents, blister agents, blood agents, choking agents, and riot control and irritant agents.

Chemical weapons (CW) differ from biologic weapons (BW) in that the chemical agent is a non-living compound. Chemical agents can cause immediate signs and symptoms, unlike biological agents, which require an incubation period. Chemical agents can be aerosolized and cause local or systematic effects. Onset may be rapid from inhalation or ingestion or delayed from agents absorbed through the skin. Victims of a chemical weapons attack can experience a variety of signs and symptoms, depending on the agent used in the attack.

As part of the medical response to a terrorist event, an EMT may be assigned to help with mass decontamination of victims. Decon procedures are broken down into three levels: gross, primary, and secondary decontamination. Gross decontamination is done on scene and is aimed at getting most of the material off the victim. Primary decon is done in a shower area possibly with special chemical agents. Secondary decontamination is conducted at the hospital and includes cleaning wounds and a thorough scrubbing of the skin. Special chemical antidotes may be applied by emergency room staff. The steps for on-scene decontamination include locating the decon area or corridor upwind and uphill from the site.

SIGNS AND SYMPTOMS OF CHEMICAL WEAPONS ATTACK

Several signs and symptoms may indicate a terrorist attack. The EMT should be suspicious of unresponsive victims with minimal or no trauma. Blistered, red, discolored, or irritated skin can indicate exposure to hazardous substances. Are the victims exhibiting **SLUDGEM** signs? SLUDGEM is the acronym for the common signs and symptoms of exposure to nerve agents based on organophosphate pesticides. These chemicals are the basis for nerve agents used in Sarin (GB) gas.

* Salivation

* **Lacrimation**

* Urination

* Defecation

* GI Motility

* Emesis

* Miosis or constricted pupils

PROTECTION FROM CHEMICAL AGENTS

First responders wearing chemical protective gear or firefighting turnout gear with self-contained breathing apparatus (SCBA) may approach the victims to rescue or guide them through the decon corridor. EMTs should avoid direct contact with any liquids, victims' clothing, or other potentially contaminated surfaces. Victims

* **SLUDGEM**

  acronym for the common signs and symptoms of exposure to nerve agents based on organophosphate pesticides: salivation, lacrimation, urination, defecation, gastrointestinal motility, emesis, and miosis.

* **lacrimation**

  abnormal or excessive secretion of tears.

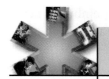

Perspective

Joelle—The EMT

"Terry saved my life. I don't know how we made it. That building collapsed right next to us and, I mean, it totaled the truck. But we walked away from it. I'm numb right now. Just completely numb. I know that many of my friends are still buried out there, and I'll never . . . um . . . never see them again. But it hasn't sunk in yet, you know? It never crossed my mind that that truck was a weapon—even after 9-11, not even a suspicion . . . nothing. I mean, this is still America. And to think that whoever built that thing actually meant for us to get there before it went off. That terrifies me. I don't know what I'm supposed to do with this whole thing. This event. I can't talk anymore right now . . . is that okay?"

should be separated into symptomatic and nonsymptomatic or walking and non-walking. A small number of patients can be decontaminated with a single hoseline from a fire truck, while large number of patients will require a decon corridor to be established. This can be accomplished by placing to two engines side by side.

Stop, Review, Remember!

Multiple Choice

Place a check next to the correct answer.

1. Anthrax is a:

    _____ a. chemical agent.

    _____ b. biological agent.

    _____ c. toxin.

    _____ d. radiological agent.

2. Biological weapons need to:

    _____ a. be dispersed in an aerosol.

    _____ b. enter through dermal or oral routes.

    _____ c. be relatively easy to disseminate.

    _____ d. any of the above.

3. Biological agents that can be used as a terrorist weapon are:

    _____ a. viruses, bacteria, and toxins.

    _____ b. bacteria, chemicals, and toxins.

    _____ c. proteins, bacteria, and toxins.

    _____ d. proteins, viruses, and toxins.

Fill in the Blank

1. S L U D G E M is an acronym for the following:

   S_____

   L_____

   U_____

   D_____

   G_____

   E_____

   M_____

2. List at least 3 things to do when responding to a terrorist attack.

   _____

   _____

   _____

Critical Thinking

1. You have responded to a potential radiological weapons attack. What is the best way to protect yourself?

   _____

   _____

   _____

   _____

2. You are transporting a patient who has possibly been exposed to a chemical weapon during a terrorist attack. He currently has no symptoms. What are the signs and symptoms that you should be alert for that would tend to confirm that the patient has been exposed to a chemical agent?

   _____

   _____

   _____

   _____

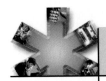

Perspective

Michael—The Local Resident and Survivor

"I was walking my dog to the park over on Bundle Street when I heard all of the sirens. I got kind of curious, and it wasn't really out of my way, you know. So I crossed over to Avendell, about a mile from the theater. I could see the flashing lights and the smoke, but I couldn't really tell what was going on. It definitely was crazy, though. People were running everywhere down there. And then there was this big bright flash. I couldn't see anything else for a second. And then it felt like when you fall on your back and the wind gets knocked out of you—you know? I just couldn't breathe . . . and then I got thrown to the ground really, really hard. Next came the sound. It was so loud that I can't even describe it, but it just seemed to go on forever. I think that was the strangest part for me. I can still hear it, over and over again. That the sound came so long after the blast. Am I making any sense? I think my dog ran away, too. I don't know where he is."

Treatment of WMD Victims

One of the first responsibilities of the EMT when responding to a possible WMD attack is not to become a victim. Once you have assured your personal safety and the safety of the scene, you may proceed to providing patient care. No matter the cause of a WMD attack, there are some basic tenets of patient care that do not change. The primary responsibility of the EMT is to manage the patient's ABCs.

PRIMARY AND SECONDARY BLAST INJURY VICTIMS

In a terrorist attack using explosives, the victims will have many of the injuries that have been discussed in the trauma care module of this text (Figure 44-7). The treatment for these victims is the same as if they had been injured in a motor vehicle crash. In a patient with a traumatic mechanism of injury, cervical spinal precautions must be considered. In a terrorist attack, the EMT must be aware that there will most likely be multiple victims, and the scene will be classified as a multiple-casualty incident (MCI). The EMT must follow the local disaster plan and implement the triage and treatment outlined in it. Remember that during an MCI event, resources are limited and must be used to benefit the maximum number of patients.

CHEMICAL WEAPONS VICTIMS

During a chemical weapons attack, the scene is unsafe and there will be multiple victims suffering from a variety of symptoms. Once the victims have been decontaminated, you may safely begin to treat them. Remember, chemical weapons often target the respiratory system. Therefore most victims of a chemical attack will

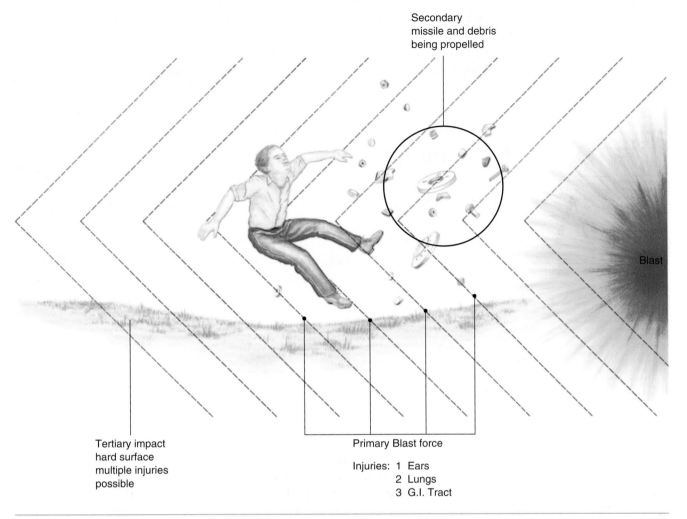

Secondary
missile and debris
being propelled

Blast

Tertiary impact
hard surface
multiple injuries
possible

Primary Blast force

Injuries: 1 Ears
          2 Lungs
          3 G.I. Tract

FIGURE 44-7   Blast injuries can cause injury with the initial blast, when the patient is struck by debris, or by the patient being thrown from the site of the blast.

require aggressive airway management. Chemical weapons can also induce seizures and cause burns to the skin.

Chemical weapons require specific treatments. For example, organophosphate-pesticide-based chemical exposures require a *Mark I* antidote kit, and cyanide-based chemical exposures require a cyanide antidote kit. These antidotes are usually administered by advanced life support (ALS) personnel. Many urban centers that have been listed as potential terrorist targets have these antidote kits stockpiled for distribution in the event of an attack. If you are required to assist in the administration of an antidote kit, you will receive additional training for that responsibility.

BIOLOGICAL WEAPONS VICTIMS

Of all the types of WMDs we have discussed to this point, biological agents will be the most difficult to detect. Many of the common signs and symptoms are similar to those for the flu. As discussed earlier, the biggest clue that you are dealing with a biological agent is the sudden spike in the number and acuity of patients suffering flulike symptoms with a common location of exposure.

Remember that when you are treating potential victims of a biological agent, you should don an approved N-95 respirator and follow universal precautions guidelines. The EMT's care should focus on the ABCs and supportive measures.

As with chemical weapons, the specific treatment depends on the agent used. For example, a bacterium like anthrax requires an antibiotic. Remember that some types of biological agents have no treatment, and the only way to manage the patient is with supportive care at the scene and in the hospital.

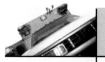

Dispatch Summary

A total of 112 people died that day, including 19 local emergency personnel. Although several foreign and domestic terrorist organizations claimed responsibility for the incident, the F.B.I. has yet to conclude the investigation.

Joelle Havens has become a vocal advocate for terrorism preparedness, speaking at EMS conventions and consulting with educators nationwide.

Terry Edwards remains a paramedic with the city fire department and is happy to see that crews have begun to rebuild the downtown area.

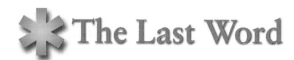 **The Last Word**

In the United States, terrorism is now perceived as an everyday threat. EMTs are on the front line to respond to a terrorist attack. It is important to understand that terrorists use acts of violence to a political or social end, with the intent to intimidate or coerce a government or civilian population in the furtherance of their agenda. Your job as an EMT is to help make the response effective and safe.

Remember that weapons of mass destruction come in many nuclear, biological, and chemical forms. One of your primary responsibilities is to guard against becoming a victim yourself. After you have donned appropriate personal protective equipment, you can safely begin treating patients. Each NBC has a specific delivery method and accompanying signs and symptoms. Your duty is to provide care to the victims of a WMD attack, focusing on the ABCs and providing supportive care.

During your initial EMT training, you may not have the opportunity to train to respond to a WMD attack. However, as an EMT you may have the opportunity to participate in your local community's disaster drill. You should take advantage of the training to prepare yourself for a possible terrorist attack. Additional training is offered free of charge by the Federal Emergency Management Agency (FEMA). This training is available online at *www.fema.gov.*

Chapter Review

MULTIPLE CHOICE

Place a check next to the correct answer.

1. The treatment an EMT would provide for a chemical or biological weapon exposure is:

_____ a. supportive, including the ABCs.

_____ b. not indicated. Pronounce victims dead, because they are very contagious.

_____ c. decontamination.

_____ d. to call the nearest level I trauma center and have the burn center prepared.

2. Biological weapons are:

_____ a. difficult to detect.

_____ b. likely to require a high index of suspicion.

_____ c. likely to initiate patterns of unusual volume of patients with similar complaints or findings.

_____ d. all of the above.

3. Biological agents, could best be described as:

_____ a. very expensive.

_____ b. a rich man's vodka.

_____ c. a poor man's nuclear bomb.

_____ d. a way to control a rushing ambulatory line.

4. Single-celled microorganisms are known as:

_____ a. viruses.

_____ b. chemicals.

_____ c. toxins.

_____ d. bacteria.

5. Bacteria, viruses, and toxins are examples of:

_____ a. drugs found in a doctor's office.

_____ b. weapons of mass destruction that have no treatment options.

_____ c. things a terrorist might be afraid of.

_____ d. biologicals that a terrorist might use as a weapon of mass destruction.

6. Inhalation, absorption, ingestion, and injection, are all:

_____ a. ways a level C suit can be permeated.

_____ b. types of anaphylaxis.

_____ c. routes of exposures.

_____ d. problems you will likely encounter while in a level A suit.

7. A good example of preincident management would be which of the following?

_____ a. Develop a plan of action.

_____ b. Know your community plan.

_____ c. Take part in live exercises and table-top models with realistic scenarios.

_____ d. All of the above.

8. When you identify, isolate, and notify the proper authorities of a hazardous material, you are said to be a(n):

_____ a. informant.

_____ b. task force manager.

_____ c. hazmat technician.

_____ d. hazmat awareness responder.

9. Terrorism is best described as:

_____ a. hijackers on an aircraft with unlawful weapons posing as airline pilots.

_____ b. an intimidation of an entire group of people or government for monetary gain and recognition.

_____ c. the unlawful use of force or violence against persons or property to intimidate or coerce a government or civilian population in furtherance of political or social objectives.

_____ d. a third-world country with disgruntled citizens trying to take control of their government.

10. Miosis, copious secretions, muscle twitching, convulsions, and GI effects are symptoms of:

_____ a. food poisoning.

_____ b. tetanus and diphtheria.

_____ c. nerve agents.

_____ d. hoof and mouth disease.

11. The acronym SLUDGEM means:

_____ a. Slobbering, Lacrimation, Urination, Decreased respirations, Gas, Ecchymosis, Meningitis.

_____ b. Shaking, Loss of bladder control, Urination, Defecation, Gas, Embolism, Miosis.

_____ c. Salivation, Lacrimation, Urination, Defecation, Gastrointestinal motility, Emesis, Miosis.

_____ d. Slurred speech, Lacrimation, Uncontrollable bowels, Decreased respiration, Gangrene, Emesis, Miosis.

MATCHING

Match the definition on the left with the applicable term on the right.

1. _____ Index of suspicion

2. _____ Secondary devices

3. _____ Weapons of mass destruction (WMDs)

4. _____ Nuclear weapons (NWs)

5. _____ Biological weapons (BWs)

6. _____ Chemical weapons (CWs)

7. _____ Fapor pressure

8. _____ Improvised nuclear device (IND)

9. _____ Radiological dispersal device (RDD)

10. _____ Simple radiological device

A. Variety of chemical, biological, nuclear, or other devices used by terrorists to strike at government or high-profile targets; designed to create a maximum number of casualties.

B. Mental trigger that, when called to an event, will help an EMT recognize it as a potential terrorist event.

C. Device used to intentionally disrupt rescue and to injure emergency responders.

D. Devices designed to release either living organisms or toxins produced by living organisms that are deliberately distributed to cause disease and death.

E. Devices designed to release the energy generated during splitting (fission) or combining (fusion) of heavy nuclei to form new elements that are deliberately distributed to cause harm or death.

F. A device that can produce an actual nuclear explosion.

G. Devices designed to release a range of simple to sophisticated chemicals that are deliberately distributed to cause harm or death.

H. The pressure exerted by a chemical against the atmosphere.

I. A device that disperses radioactive particles without explosion.

J. A bomb laced with radioactive material; also called a dirty bomb.

CRITICAL THINKING

1. Create three scenarios of terrorism that might take place in your community or the nearest town of a population of 10,000 or more. Describe the emergency response protocols.

_____

_____

_____

_____

2. Name the three types of biological agents and give an example of how each can be used as an agent of terrorism. What are the signs and symptoms of biological weapons exposure?

_____

_____

_____

_____

CASE STUDY

It is 8:30 A.M. on a Thursday in July in your community. It is partly cloudy, humid, and the temperature is 90 degrees. There have been various militia groups arriving in the city to demonstrate over the weekend and for the July Fourth parade. An EMS unit, a fire engine, and fire investigator have been dispatched to the south end of the city on an "assist the police" call. The information over the mobile data terminal or via a secured transmission indicates this call is for a "suspicious device."

At 8:45 your EMS unit is dispatched to the center of the city at the local government offices for a female short of breath. While responding, you notice heavy traffic and a van disabled in the middle of the driveway entering the government offices complex. Upon arrival, you see approximately 15 people outside the main door to the government building coughing, tearing, and calling for help.

1. What preevent information is important?

_____

_____

_____

_____

2. What recognition during the response is important?

_____

_____

_____

_____

3. What actions should be taken?

_____

_____

_____

_____

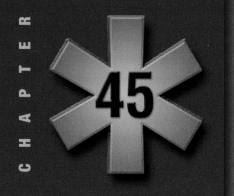

45

Module Review and Practice Examination

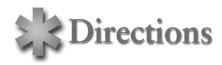 **Directions**

Assess what you have learned in this module by circling the best answer for each multiple-choice question. When you are done, check your answers against the key provided in Appendix D.

1. The phase of an ambulance call in which you complete documentation of your call is called:
   a. preparing for the call.
   b. transfer to hospital staff.
   c. terminating the call.
   d. receiving and responding to the call.

2. Which of the following items is included when checking the mechanical functioning of an ambulance?
   a. AED
   b. maps
   c. bandaging supplies
   d. brakes

3. When responding to a call, which of the following information is LEAST important for an EMT to know?
   a. the patient's ethnic group
   b. the nature of the request for assistance
   c. the current condition of the patient
   d. hazards at the scene

4. Which of the following principles should be followed by EMTs when they are driving the ambulance to respond to a call or transporting a patient?
   a. Have due regard for the safety of all others.
   b. Always pass other vehicles on the right.

   c. Ambulances have the right of way in all circumstances.
   d. EMTs are held harmless from liability due to ambulance collisions.

5. NIMS is best described as:
   a. a consistent nation-wide approach in responding to events requiring coordinated public safety response.
   b. a multiple casualty incident.
   c. EMS personnel "freelancing" at the scene of an emergency.
   d. a designated disaster medical response team.

6. NIMS is overseen by the:
   a. Department of Health and Human Services.
   b. Department of Defense.
   c. Department of Homeland Security.
   d. Justice Department.

7. In an incident command system, the area responsible for developing tactical objectives is:
   a. command.
   b. operations.
   c. planning.
   d. logistics.

8. In an incident command system, the area responsible for providing support and resources is:
   a. operations.
   b. planning.
   c. logistics.
   d. finance/administration.

9. In a smaller incident, the person in charge of all major activities is the:
   a. general staff.
   b. safety officer.
   c. information officer.
   d. incident commander.

10. By definition, an event that exceeds the capabilities of an EMS system is called a/an:
    a. disaster.
    b. MCI.
    c. ICS.
    d. CBRNE.

11. A mass gathering is an assembly of _____ or more people in a single location.
    a. 100
    b. 1000
    c. 10,000
    d. 100,000

12. The number of people or elements that can be effectively managed by a single individual in an ICS is referred to as:
    a. unity of command.
    b. incident action plan.
    c. span of control.
    d. staging.

13. Radio communications in plain language, not using radio codes, is called:
    a. clear text.
    b. regular verbiage.
    c. tactical language.
    d. disaster speak.

14. The incident management element that is geographical in nature is a/an:
    a. division.   c. cluster.
    b. unit.   d. group.

15. Any substance or material that poses an unreasonable risk to health, safety, and property is a/an:
    a. chemical substance.
    b. hazardous material.
    c. inert matter.
    d. vapor compound.

16. Substances stored in stationary tanks and facilities, such as at swimming pools, are marked using a system known as:
    a. DOT placards.
    b. Emergency Response Guides.
    c. NFPA 704.
    d. U.S. Radiologic Survey.

17. You have noted a diamond-shaped sign on a storage tank behind a hospital. The top quadrant of the diamond contains the number 4. This means the substance stored inside the tank poses a/an:
    a. extreme risk of fire.
    b. low risk of fire.
    c. extreme risk of explosion.
    d. low risk of explosion.

18. You have noted a diamond-shaped sign on a storage tank at a farm supply company. The bottom quadrant of the diamond contains a letter "W" with a line through it. This means:
    a. the tank contains an inert substance.
    b. the tank contains a dry substance rather than a liquid or wet substance.
    c. the tank contains an oxidizer.
    d. mixing water with this substance creates a hazard.

19. The diamond-shaped symbol on a transportation container, such as a tanker truck, is called a/an:
    a. bill of lading.
    b. placard.
    c. hazard notice.
    d. material safety data sheet.

20. Employers must keep paperwork on all potentially hazardous substances in the workplace called:
    a. material safety data sheets.
    b. placards.
    c. manifests.
    d. ORM-Ds.

21. The blue quadrant of an NFPA diamond contains information about a substance's:
    a. special considerations.
    b. health risks.
    c. fire hazard.
    d. explosive potential.

22. You have been dispatched to a railroad yard for a "sick person." On your arrival you note that there are three individuals on the ground next to a tank car. Using binoculars to inspect the tank, you should compare the information you find to that found in the:
    a. Emergency Response Guidebook.
    b. HazMat Manual.
    c. bill of lading.
    d. material safety data sheet.

23. Under what circumstances is it permissible for an EMT to approach a hazardous materials scene?
    a. The EMT is a firefighter and is wearing turnout gear.
    b. The EMT is trained as a hazardous materials technician and is wearing SCBA.
    c. The EMT is trained at the hazardous materials awareness level and is wearing a HEPA mask.
    d. The EMT has immediate access to a decontamination shower upon leaving the area.

24. A flammable solid is considered a DOT hazard class:
    a. 1.
    b. 2.
    c. 3.
    d. 4.

25. DOT hazard class 9 indicates:
    a. flammable liquids.
    b. explosives.
    c. miscellaneous dangerous goods.
    d. corrosives.

26. When a chemical substance makes contact with the skin or mucous membranes, it can enter the body through:
    a. injection.
    b. ingestion.
    c. absorption.
    d. amalgamation.

27. Situations calling for wilderness search and rescue, water rescue, rope rescue, and other types of events requiring special training and equipment are called _____ rescue situations.
    a. USAR
    b. operational
    c. tactical
    d. technical

28. The first phase of a rescue operation is:
    a. gaining access to the patient.
    b. preparing for the rescue.
    c. sizing up the situation.
    d. providing initial patient assessment.

29. Devices placed under the deflated tires of a vehicle to stabilize it are called:
    a. cribbing.
    b. props.
    c. jacks.
    d. buttresses.

30. You are able to access a patient entrapped in a motor vehicle following a collision without the use of equipment. This is known as _____ access.
    a. complex
    b. intricate
    c. easy
    d. simple

31. When responding to a victim of a deep-water diving emergency, you should keep in mind the location of the nearest:
    a. hyperresonnance compartment.
    b. hypothermic resuscitation unit.
    c. hyperbaric chamber.
    d. hydrotherapy response team.

32. EMTs without special training should not attempt to rescue a patient from a trench over _____ feet deep.
    a. 5
    b. 8
    c. 12
    d. 15

33. You have been deployed to a large city struck by a hurricane. You note on a building a spray painted "X" with the number 4 at the bottom. This means:
    a. four victims were located in the structure.
    b. FEMA team 4 searched the structure.
    c. 4 FEMA rescuers entered the building.
    d. the building was searched at 0400 hours.

34. You have been deployed to a remote village struck by an earthquake. On the first building you approach you note a large, bright orange, empty square has been spray painted on the exterior. This marking indicates the building:
    a. is structurally unsafe.
    b. has been evacuated of victims.
    c. contains a chemical hazard.
    d. may be entered by rescuers.

35. Terrorism is different from other types of threatened or actual violence in which of the following ways?
    a. Terrorism always involves more victims than other acts of violence.
    b. Terrorism is carried out to further a political or social agenda through intimidation or coercion.
    c. Terrorism relies solely on the use of explosive devices.
    d. Terrorism, by definition, is not committed by U.S. citizens.

36. Which of the following is most suspicious for an act of terrorism being committed?
    a. an explosion at a place of worship
    b. an explosion in a residence
    c. a motor vehicle collision between a car and a tanker truck
    d. a dozen people becoming ill at a wedding reception

37. In regard to a biological agent being released, its persistence is how:
    a. long people becoming infected remain ill.
    b. effective the agent is in producing death.
    c. easily one person can spread the disease to another.
    d. long the agent stays in the environment.

38. A conventional explosive spiked with radioactive material is known as a/an:
    a. improvised nuclear device.
    b. radiologic dispersal device.
    c. simple radiologic device.
    d. smart bomb.

39. Aerosolized anthrax is an example of a _____ weapon.
    a. biological
    b. chemical
    c. nuclear
    d. radioactive

40. An incident involving more than one patient that cannot be managed by the normal responding units but that can be handled by the resources of a single system is a/an _____ casualty incident:
    a. mass
    b. major
    c. multiple
    d. minor

41. Which of the following is a management goal for MCIs?
    a. Relocate the disaster to a controlled environment.
    b. Do the greatest good for the largest number of patients.
    c. Send all patients to the same hospital.
    d. Assign 2 to 3 patients to each provider.

42. Which of the following is the first of the "Five Ss" for initial actions at the scene of an MCI?
    a. scene size-up
    b. send information
    c. start triage
    d. safety

43. The act of sorting patients into categories for treatment and transport based on the severity of their conditions is known as:
    a. triage.
    b. assessment.
    c. classification.
    d. deployment.

44. At the scene of an MCI you encounter a patient who is not breathing. You should first:
    a. open the airway.
    b. tag the patient "BLACK."
    c. tag the patient "RED."
    d. begin rescue breathing.

45. At the scene of an MCI you encounter a patient who is responsive to verbal stimuli, is breathing 28 times per minute, and has a carotid pulse but no radial pulses. This patient should be tagged:
    a. green.
    b. yellow.
    c. red.
    d. black.

46. At the scene of an MCI you encounter a 5-year-old patient who has a pulse but is not breathing. You have opened the airway and the patient is still not breathing. Which of the following should you do next?
    a. Give 5 rescue breaths.
    b. Tag the patient "BLACK."
    c. Tag the patient "RED."
    d. Move on to the next patient.

47. In MCIs, the first patients to be transported are those tagged:
    a. black.
    b. red.
    c. white.
    d. green.

48. In the Incident Command System, the individual responsible for management of the entire scene is the:
    a. public information officer.
    b. safety officer.
    c. triage sector leader.
    d. incident commander.

49. Extrication, triage, treatment, and transportation sectors in an MCI are part of the _____ section.
    a. planning
    b. operations
    c. rescue
    d. finance

50. The individual at an MCI who ensures that ambulances are directed to the appropriate receiving hospital is the _____ officer.
    a. staging
    b. sector
    c. communications
    d. commanding

51. Which of the following is the correct order of the phases of an EMS call?
    1. caring for the patient
    2. dispatch
    3. responding
    4. preparation for the call
    a. 2, 4, 3, 1
    b. 2, 3, 4, 1
    c. 4, 3, 1, 2
    d. 4, 2, 3, 1

52. For which of the following patients is the use of a stair chair appropriate?
    a. 75-year-old male who fell out of bed and is complaining of back and neck pain
    b. 68-year-old male complaining of shortness of breath
    c. 60-year-old female in cardiac arrest
    d. 25-year-old female in hemorrhagic shock

53. You are preparing to return to service following a call for an injured person. The patient you transported had a laceration to his leg, and there is a moderate amount of blood on your stretcher. Which of the following is/are appropriate?
    a. cleaning and disinfection
    b. disinfection only
    c. cleaning and sterilization
    d. cleaning only

54. When rescuers responding to a mass-casualty incident operate outside the incident command system, this is known as:
    a. mutiny
    b. rebellion
    c. freelancing
    d. free contracting

55. Of the following, the greatest benefit of a National Incident Management System is:
    a. It is a commonly understood way of structuring response to large scale incidents.
    b. It allows control of all major incidents by the federal government.
    c. It encourages response by lay rescuers without creating delays caused by unnecessary rules.
    d. It makes it unnecessary for local agencies to create a disaster response plan.

56. In a mass-casualty incident, triage is based on the principle of:
    a. providing the same care as when treating a single patient.
    b. treating the youngest patients first.
    c. transporting to the closest hospital.
    d. providing the best care for the greatest number of patients.

57. You have responded to a small furniture factory. Three employees are experiencing coughing and watering eyes after one of them spilled a can of paint solvent. To find out more about the material spilled, you should locate the:
    a. NFPA 704 placard.
    b. US DOT placard.
    c. Material Data Safety Sheet.
    d. manifest.

58. You have just arrived at the scene of a roll-over motor vehicle collision. There is a sedan on its side in the intersection. You can hear a child crying inside the vehicle. Rescue has a 2 minute ETA. Your obligations as an EMT are best met by which of the following actions?
    1. Stay about 12 feet back from the vehicle and make a better determination of what the situation in the vehicle is.
    2. Check the scene for additional vehicles, patients, and hazards.
    3. Determine the best way to immediately remove the child from the vehicle.
    a. 1, 2
    b. 1
    c. 2
    d. 2, 3

59. You and your partner are responding to a report of an explosion at a doctor's office. Which of the following are appropriate actions?
    1. Park well away from the building.
    2. Consider the possibility of a second explosion in the building.
    3. Enter and search the building for victims.
    4. Consider the possibility of a second explosion outside the building.
    a. 1, 2, 3, 4
    b. 1, 2
    c. 1, 2, 4
    d. 2, 4

60. A simple, home-made explosive device containing radioactive material is best described as a/an:
    a. improvised nuclear weapon.
    b. radiological dispersal device.
    c. simple radiological device.
    d. weapon of mass destruction.

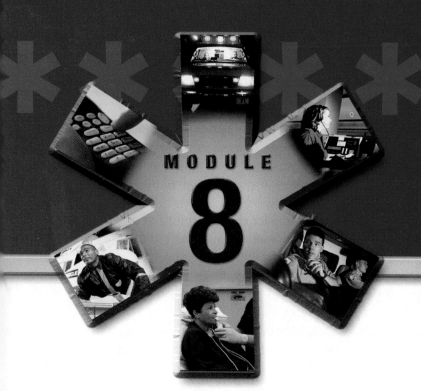

MODULE

8

Advanced Airway

" Two things about that call bothered me. The first was trying to get an airway after a hanging. It can be next to impossible because of the swelling and structural damage and stuff. The other thing, and this is my own deal, is that my brother killed himself back in high school the same way. "

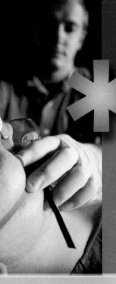

Module Outline

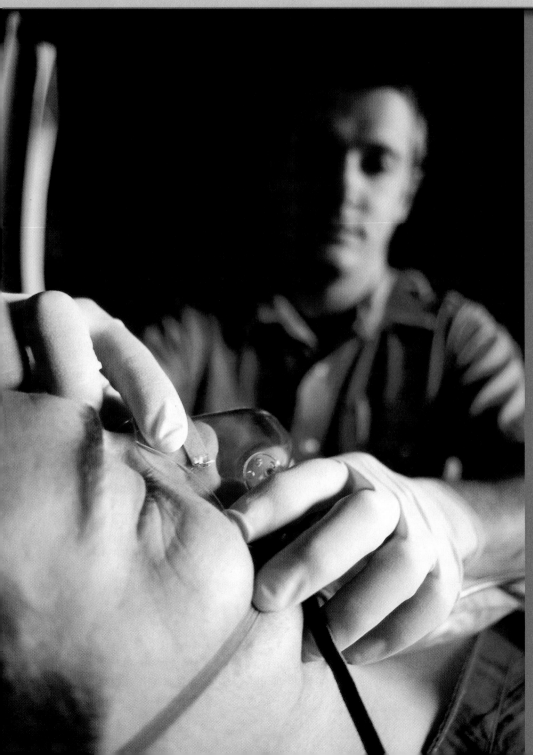

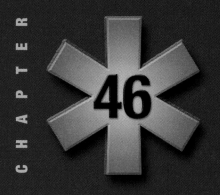
Advanced Airway Techniques

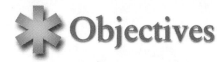 **Objectives**

Numbered objectives are from the U.S. Department of Transportation 1994 EMT-Basic National Standard Curriculum.

COGNITIVE OBJECTIVES

At the end of this lesson the EMT-Basic student will be able to:

8-1.1   Identify and describe the airway anatomy in the infant, child, and the adult. (pp. 1132–1136)

8-1.2   Differentiate between the airway anatomy in the infant, child, and the adult. (pp. 1132–1136)

8-1.3   Explain the pathophysiology of airway compromise. (pp. 1132–1136)

8-1.4   Describe the proper use of airway adjuncts. (p. 1133)

8-1.5   Review the use of oxygen therapy in airway management. (p. 1143)

8-1.6   Describe the indications, contraindications, and technique for insertion of nasal gastric tubes. (p. 1149)

8-1.7   Describe how to perform Sellick's maneuver (cricoid pressure). (p. 1143)

8-1.8   Describe the indications for advanced airway management. (pp. 1131, 1138, 1141)

8-1.9   List the equipment required for orotracheal intubation. (pp. 1138–1140)

8-1.10   Describe the proper use of the curved blade for orotracheal intubation. (p. 1138)

8-1.11   Describe the proper use of the straight blade for orotracheal intubation. (p. 1138)

8-1.12   State the reasons for and proper use of the stylet in orotracheal intubation. (pp. 1140–1141)

8-1.13   Describe the methods of choosing the appropriate size endotracheal tube in an adult patient. (p. 1140)

8-1.14   State the formula for sizing an infant or child endotracheal tube. (p. 1140)

8-1.15   List complications associated with advanced airway management. (p. 1151)

8-1.16   Define the various alternative methods for sizing the infant and child endotracheal tube. (p. 1148)

8-1.17   Describe the skill of orotracheal intubation in the adult patient. (pp. 1141–1142)

8-1.18   Describe the skill of orotracheal intubation in the infant and child patient. (p. 1140)

8-1.19   Describe the skill of confirming endotracheal tube placement in the adult, infant, and child patient. (pp. 1151–1152)

8-1.20   State the consequence of and the need to recognize unintentional esophageal intubation. (pp. 1151–1152)

8-1.21   Describe the skill of securing the endotracheal tube in the adult, infant, and child patient. (p. 1143)

AFFECTIVE OBJECTIVES

At the end of this lesson the EMT-Basic student will be able to:

8-1.22   Recognize and respect the feelings of the patient and family during advanced airway procedures. (pp. 1149, 1156)

8-1.23   Explain the value of performing advanced airway procedures. (p. 1131)

8-1.24 Defend the need for the EMT-Basic to perform advanced airway procedures. (p. 1157)

8-1.25 Explain the rationale for the use of a stylet. (p. 1140)

8-1.26 Explain the rationale for having a suction unit immediately available during intubation attempts. (p. 1150)

8-1.27 Explain the rationale for confirming breath sounds. (p. 1146)

8-1.28 Explain the rationale for securing the endotracheal tube. (p. 1138)

PSYCHOMOTOR OBJECTIVES

At the end of this lesson the EMT-Basic student will be able to:

8-1.29 Demonstrate how to perform Sellick's maneuver (cricoid pressure). (p. 1143)

8-1.30 Demonstrate the skill of orotracheal intubation in the adult patient. (pp. 1141–1142)

8-1.31 Demonstrate the skill of orotracheal intubation in the infant and child patient. (pp. 1141–1142)

8-1.32 Demonstrate the skill of confirming endotracheal tube placement in the adult patient. (p. 1142)

8-1.33 Demonstrate the skill of confirming endotracheal tube placement in the infant and child patient. (pp. 1142–1143)

8-1.34 Demonstrate the skill of securing the endotracheal tube in the adult patient. (pp. 1142, 1146)

8-1.35 Demonstrate the skill of securing the endotracheal tube in the infant and child patient. (p. 1142)

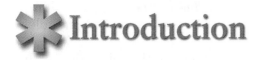 Introduction

You can only be successful with advanced airway management skills after you have mastered the basic skills (positioning, suctioning, oxygen) you've learned in chapters 7 and 19. Since a patent airway is the your highest priority in managing any patient, learning about when and how to use these advanced airway skills will be a benefit to your patients—and a tremendous responsibility for you.

As an EMT, your protocols may allow you to use one or more of the airway devices and procedures covered in this chapter. Use of these skills will require initial training and frequent use in the field or continuous practice to maintain your proficiency in using them.

As you learn and begin to practice advanced airway skills, *never, never, never* forget the importance of basic airway skills.

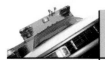

Emergency Dispatch

"Okay, what have we got here?" EMT David Mote asked as he walked through the front door and found a group of firefighters huddled over a man in a small, cluttered living room.

"He hung himself from the shower head." A uniformed woman stood and moved away from the group so David could see the discolored face of the unre-sponsive patient. "We cut him down when we got here about a minute ago. He wasn't breathing and I couldn't find a pulse."

"How long was he up for? Do we know?" Ed Green, David's partner, appeared in the doorway carrying a jump kit and an airway bag.

"Based on what we could get from his wife, about 5 minutes," a sweaty-faced firefighter said as he squeezed the bag on a BVM. The buzzing of the device's pop-off valve made it obvious that the patient didn't have a patent airway.

"Okay Ed." David dropped to his knees at the patient's head. "I need the scope and a . . . uh . . . let's start with an eight-point-oh. We're going to need a backboard and C-collar, too."

"Here you go." Ed quickly handed David an assembled laryngoscope and an endotracheal tube with

the stylet and syringe already in place. "I'll be right back with the other stuff."

David slid the gleaming laryngoscope blade into the patient's mouth, lifted the handle, and peered in. "Oh, man," he exhaled, shaking several beads of sweat from his forehead onto the matted carpet. "There's a lot of swelling, but let's see what we can do."

8-1.1 Identify and describe the airway anatomy in the infant, child, and the adult.

8-1.2 Differentiate between the airway anatomy in the infant, child, and the adult.

8-1.3 Explain the pathophysiology of airway compromise.

✳ **nares**

the opening to the nasal cavity. Also called nostrils.

FIGURE 46-1 Anatomy of the upper airway.

Airway Anatomy Review

In chapters 4 and 7, you learned about general airway anatomy and physiology. To be successful in using advanced airway devices and techniques, you will need to learn and understand even more about upper airway anatomy and physiology (Figure 46-1).

The upper airway extends from the mouth and nose to the epiglottis. The beginning of the nasal upper airway is the **nares,** also known as nostrils. They are

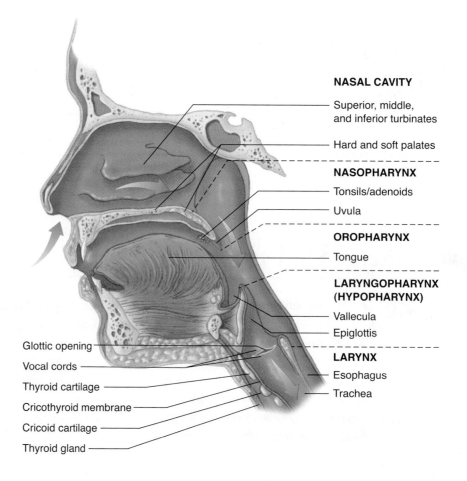

NASAL CAVITY
Superior, middle, and inferior turbinates
Hard and soft palates

NASOPHARYNX
Tonsils/adenoids
Uvula

OROPHARYNX
Tongue

LARYNGOPHARYNX (HYPOPHARYNX)
Vallecula
Epiglottis

LARYNX
Esophagus
Trachea

Glottic opening
Vocal cords
Thyroid cartilage
Cricothyroid membrane
Cricoid cartilage
Thyroid gland

the opening to the nasal cavity. As air enters the nasal cavity, it first passes through the **nasal vestibule.** The nasal vestibule is the anteriormost portion of the nasal cavity and is made up of flexible tissue. Within the nasal cavity there are coarse hairs intended to filter foreign particles and stop them from entering the airway. The nasal cavity also contains **conchae** or what are commonly referred to as turbinates. The conchae are positioned one on top of another and are designed to create a swirling air path across and through each level on inspiration. This swirling of air helps to warm and humidify the air before it enters the lower airways. The conchae are highly vascular and contain multiple nerve endings. Because of this, any procedure involving the nares must be done with an awareness for potential bleeding and pain.

Be cautious of the conchae when using a nasopharyngeal airway or nasogastric tube. Many EMTs insert a nasal airway using an upward and posterior technique. The advised insertion technique is to insert the airway adjunct straight back, because upward insertion will irritate the conchae, causing pain and bleeding.

As air passes from the **nasopharynx,** which is the posteriormost portion of the nasal cavity, it moves toward the **oropharynx.** Prior to reaching the oropharynx, air passes over the **soft palate.** The soft palate is designed to lift up when a person swallows, closing off the oropharynx from the nasopharynx.

From the soft palate, air moves to the oropharynx. The oropharynx is the portion of the pharynx that lies directly behind the oral cavity—specifically, behind the base of the tongue.

Air enters through the mouth as well. As it does, it moves through the mouth and into the oropharynx. As air continues on from the oropharynx, it passes through the **laryngopharynx.** The laryngopharynx is also known as the hypopharynx. From the hypopharynx, air advances to the lower airways.

The lower airway begins with the **epiglottis** and terminates at the **alveoli.** The primary function of the epiglottis, which is a leaf like flap of tissue, is to protect the airway by covering the glottic opening during swallowing. When a person swallows, the muscles of the neck contract, and the **larynx** is elevated. When the larynx moves up, the epiglottis folds back over the **glottis,** and the trachea is covered.

The glottis is the opening from the upper airway that leads into the lower airway. The glottis is at the level of the vocal cords and is at the very top of the trachea.

As air passes through the glottis, it is channeled through the larynx, or voice box. To speak, air passes through the larynx and causes vibration of the **vocal cords.** As the vocal cords vibrate, sound is produced.

On the inferior aspect of the larynx is the **cricoid cartilage.** The cricoid cartilage serves as a protective mechanism for the glottis and trachea and gives support to the larynx. After air moves through the larynx, it advances to the trachea. The cricoid cartilage is sometimes thought of as the first—and only complete—tracheal cartilage.

The **trachea** (Figure 46-2 on page 1134), otherwise known as the windpipe, is a tough but flexible tube with a diameter of about 2½ centimeters or 1 inch and a length of about 11 centimeters or 4¼ inches. The flexibility of the trachea is due to its being made up of about 20 incomplete rings of cartilage, which provide structure and support of the trachea without rigidity. Without these rings, the trachea would constantly expand and contract with inspiration and expiration.

From the trachea, the air will enter the **bronchi.** The mainstem bronchi form two branches, the right and the left. The right mainstem bronchus is much more vertical, having less of an angle, than the left mainstem bronchus. The right mainstem bronchus is approximately 1 inch in length and extends to about the fifth thoracic vertebra. Because there is less of an angle to this bronchus, it is much more likely to receive aspirated foreign matter than the left. Likewise, if an EMS

* **nasal vestibule**

the anteriormost portion of the nasal cavity.

* **conchae**

tissue within the nasal cavity that causes a swirling air path. Also called turbinates.

8-1.4 Describe the proper use of airway adjuncts.

* **nasopharynx**

the section of the pharynx directly posterior to the nose.

* **oropharynx**

the section of the pharynx directly posterior to the mouth.

* **soft palate**

tissue designed to lift up when a person swallows, closing off the oropharynx from the nasopharynx.

* **laryngopharynx**

portion of the pharynx connecting the oropharynx to the larynx. Also called the hypopharynx.

* **epiglottis**

leaf-shaped structure that covers the glottis to prevent food and foreign matter from entering the trachea.

* **alveoli**

the microscopic sacs of the lungs where gas exchange with the bloodstream takes place.

* **larynx**

structure located between the laryngopharynx and the trachea. It houses the glottis and the vocal cords. Also called the voice box.

* **glottis**

opening between the vocal cords that separates the upper airway from the lower airway. Also called the glottic opening.

* **vocal cords**

tissue found within the larynx that opens and closes the glottis to produce sound vibrations.

✳ **cricoid cartilage**

the ring-shaped structure that circles the trachea at the lower edge of the larynx.

✳ **trachea**

the "windpipe"; the structure that connects the pharynx to the lungs.

✳ **bronchi**

the two large sets of branches that come off the trachea and enter the lungs. There are right and left bronchi. Singular bronchus.

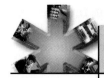

Perspective

David—The EMT

"Two things about that call bothered me. The first was trying to get an airway after a hanging. It can be next to impossible because of the swelling and structural damage and stuff. The other thing, and this is my own deal, I guess, but my brother killed himself back in high school the same way. I found him, and . . . and I can remember just having no clue what to do, you know? I was just a kid, though. The feeling of helplessness that I had back then—just sitting on my brother's bedroom floor holding him—is probably what inspired me to become an EMT more than anything else. I just have this overriding need to know what to do during medical emergencies. While I face that memory over and over again, I think my personal experiences make me a better EMT, though. I really do."

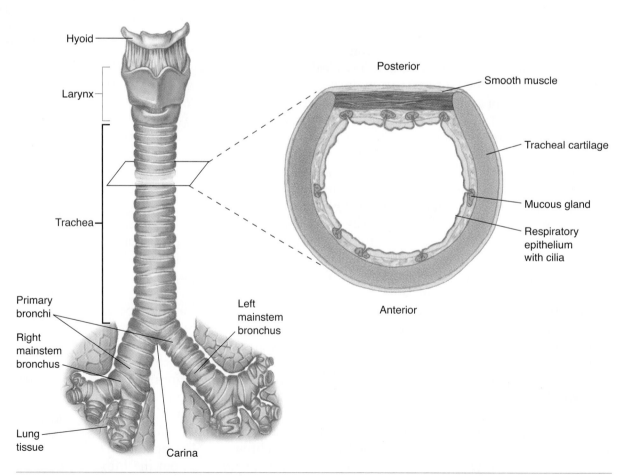

FIGURE 46-2 Anatomy of the lower airway.

provider places an endotracheal tube and advances it too far, it will almost always go down the right mainstem bronchus rather than the left.

The left mainstem bronchus is approximately 2 inches in length, double the length of the right, and extends down to the level of the sixth thoracic vertebrae.

The airways continue to branch from the mainstem bronchi, through the gradually smaller bronchi, then the **bronchioles,** and end at the alveoli, the structures where gas exchange takes place in the lungs.

* **bronchioles**

  the smallest bronchi.

PEDIATRIC AIRWAY VARIATIONS

Pediatric airways are significantly different from adult airways (Figure 46-3). As a result, the equipment you will use for this patient is different as well.

The pediatric differences are:

* The nares are much smaller and constitute the primary route for ventilation in infants. The pediatric tongue is proportionally larger in relation to the size of the mouth.

* The epiglottis is more u-shaped in the child and tends to be more pliable. The adult epiglottis is more leaf-like and rigid, giving it more structure and making it easier to control.

* Another very significant difference between these airways is that the narrowest portion of the adult airway is at the glottic opening and the narrowest portion of the pediatric airway is more inferior at the level of the cricoid cartilage. This is not the case in adults.

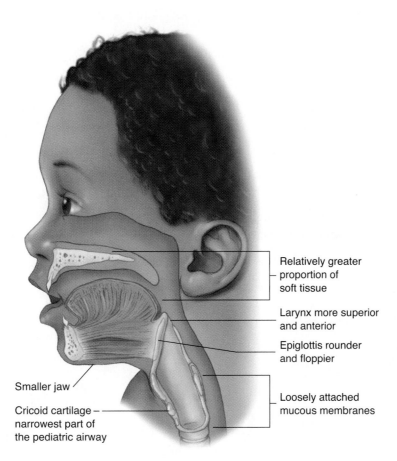

FIGURE 46-3   Anatomy of the pediatric airway.

Relatively greater proportion of soft tissue

Larynx more superior and anterior

Epiglottis rounder and floppier

Loosely attached mucous membranes

Smaller jaw

Cricoid cartilage – narrowest part of the pediatric airway

NASOGASTRIC AND OROGASTRIC ANATOMY

✳ **esophagus**

tube connecting the laryngopharynx to the stomach.

✳ **peristalsis**

motion of the digestive tract that moves food through the system.

✳ **bifurcation**

division into two parts or branches.

Just as in airway anatomy, nasogastric (NG) (*naso-* meaning "nose" and *gastric-* meaning "stomach") anatomy starts at the nares. However, instead of terminating in the lungs, the NG anatomy terminates in the stomach. Orogastric (*oro-* meaning "mouth") anatomy starts at the mouth and terminates in the stomach.

Remember that the nasal cavity contains turbinates, which are very vascular and bleed easily. This is important to remember in NG tube placement, because too much stimulation can cause excessive bleeding.

In digestion, food enters the mouth and moves into the oropharynx. As food is chewed up and swallowing begins, it will pass from the oropharynx to the laryngopharynx. Once at the laryngopharynx, food is moved into the **esophagus** and, eventually, the stomach by **peristalsis**. The **bifurcation** of the airway and digestive structures occurs in the laryngopharynx. The opening of the airway is protected by the epiglottis during the swallowing of foods and liquids.

 # Stop, Review, Remember!

Multiple Choice

Place a check next to the correct answer.

1. An endotracheal tube advanced too far into the trachea will most likely end up in the:

   _____ a. carina.

   _____ b. esophagus.

   _____ c. right mainstem bronchus.

   _____ d. left mainstem bronchus.

2. Which of the following statements about the pediatric airway is false?

   _____ a. The tongue is proportionately larger in relation to the size of the mouth.

   _____ b. The nares are much smaller in the pediatric patient.

   _____ c. The epiglottis is less floppy.

   _____ d. The narrowest part of the pediatric trachea is the area below the glottis.

3. What is the narrowest portion of the adult airway?

   _____ a. the carina

   _____ b. the glottic opening

   _____ c. below the glottis

   _____ d. the fifth tracheal ring

4. What is a major risk associated with the insertion of a nasogastric tube?

   _____ a. bleeding

   _____ b. aspiration

   _____ c. airway obstruction

   _____ d. all of the above

5. The purpose of the epiglottis is to:

   _____ a. cover the glottic opening.

   _____ b. allow the patient to speak.

   _____ c. facilitate aspiration.

   _____ d. cover the esophagus.

Fill in the Blank

1. The nasal cavity contains conchae, which are commonly referred to as _____.

2. The cricoid cartilage surrounds the _____ at the lower edge of the larynx.

3. Once inhaled air has reached the _____, it advances to the lower airways.

4. The bifurcation of the airway and the digestive structures is located in the _____.

5. The left _____ _____ is approximately 2 inches in length, double the length of the right, and extends down to the level of the sixth thoracic vertebrae.

Critical Thinking

1. What is the most important thing to remember about the conchae?

_____

_____

_____

_____

_____

2. How is the first tracheal ring (the cricoid cartilage) different from the rest?

_____

_____

_____

_____

_____

3. Why is the upward-and-posterior technique for inserting nasal airway adjuncts discouraged? What technique is recommended?

_____

_____

_____

_____

_____

Endotracheal Intubation

Endotracheal intubation is the gold standard in airway management. The procedure is performed when an **endotracheal tube (ETT)** is inserted into the trachea in order to provide a direct route for airflow into the lungs for ventilation. **Orotracheal intubation** is the placement of an endotracheal tube orally, that is, by way of the mouth, then through the vocal cords and into the trachea. The greatest benefit to intubation is that the procedure provides definitive airway protection, meaning that it allows direct ventilation of the lungs through the endotracheal tube, bypassing the entire upper airway. Intubation perfomed by an EMT must be accomplished with and by direct visualization of the vocal cords with a **laryngoscope.**

LARYNGOSCOPE

The laryngoscope is an instrument used to lift the tongue off of the posterior pharynx and to move the epiglottis out of the visual field so that the vocal cords are visible. Once the vocal cords are visualized with the laryngoscope it will be possible to pass the distal portion of the endotracheal tube between and past the cords under direct visualization.

The laryngoscope also has a light that illuminates the airway, making it possible to see the airway structures. There are two types of light sources for laryngoscopes: fiberoptic and bulb. Fiberoptic scopes have the light source in the handle, and the light emits from a fiberoptic bundle at the tip of the laryngoscope blade. In bulb-type scopes the light source is a small light bulb at the tip of the device's blade. Because the bulb screws into place, it can become loose and lessen its brightness. Always test the bulb to be sure it is well secured and gives off a bright light— "tight and bright".

Two primary laryngoscope blades are commonly used in the prehospital environment. These blades are the **Macintosh** or curved blade and the **Miller** or straight blade. The curved blade is designed to fit into the **vallecula** (Figure 46-4). When the blade is inserted into the valeculla, it indirectly moves the epiglottis away from the glottic opening, allowing you to see the glottic opening of the vocal cords. The straight blade is designed to slide under the epiglottis and directly

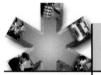

Perspective

Ed—The EMT

"As an EMT, it's pretty fulfilling to be working in a system that allows EMTs to do some advanced airway stuff! Take the call today, for example. Using a BVM to ventilate the guy who hanged himself just didn't work. His airway was way too damaged, and there were no ALS trucks available. But David and I had other options available to us that many EMTs around the country don't have, you know? I really think the advanced airway training made all the difference in the final outcome of that call."

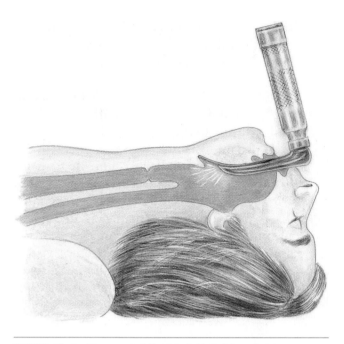

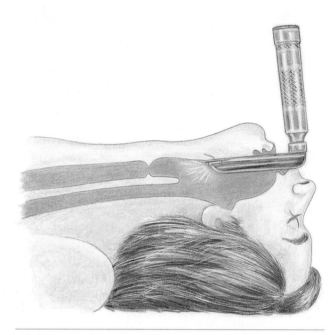

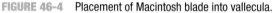

FIGURE 46-4   Placement of Macintosh blade into vallecula.

FIGURE 46-5   Placement of Miller blade under epiglottis.

lift the epiglottis away from the glottic opening (Figure 46-5). Because the straight blade directly manipulates the epiglottis, it is the ideal choice when managing a pediatric airway in which the epiglottis is soft and difficult to move indirectly.

ENDOTRACHEAL TUBE

The endotracheal (ET) tube (Figure 46-6) is a flexible tube that is placed into the trachea to provide ventilation and airway protection. The ET tube is available with internal diameters ranging from 2.5 to 9.0 mm. These diameters represent the tube size.

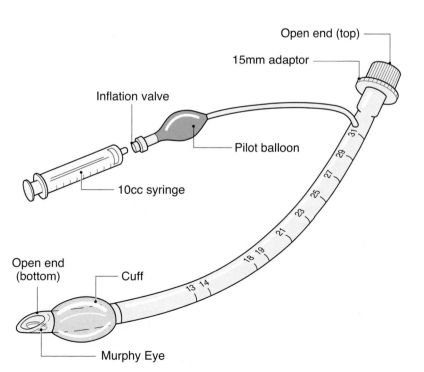

FIGURE 46-6   The endotracheal tube.

8-1.10 Describe the proper use of the curved blade for orotracheal intubation.

Tubes for adults (usually those with an internal diameter of 5.5 mm or greater) have an inflatable cuff on the distal end of the tube. Once the tube is placed in the trachea, this cuff seals the trachea to assure good air delivery to the lungs and to keep foreign material out.

A syringe allows you to inflate the ET tube cuff to prevent air from leaking around the ET tube. Prior to attempting intubation, the ET tube cuff should have been tested by injecting 10 mL of air and ensuring that the cuff holds air and does not collapse as pressure is exerted on it. Once intubation has been completed, the cuff should be inflated until the pilot cuff is rigid and full. If too much air is injected into the cuff, however, pressure will be exerted on the trachea and may cause damage to the lining of the trachea. Once the pilot cuff is inflated, the syringe must be disconnected from the inflation valve to assure the cuff remains inflated.

Air is introduced to inflate the cuff via a port near the proximal end of the tube. Once the tube is placed, the distal end of the tube and cuff are not visible making it difficult to know if the cuff remains inflated. The pilot balloon is a small pouch near the inflation port which represents the status of the cuff. If the pilot balloon is inflated, the cuff likely is, too.

ENDOTRACHEAL TUBE SIZING

8-1.13 Describe the methods of choosing the appropriate size endotracheal tube in an adult patient.

Adult Considerations   As a general rule, most adult males will accommodate between an 8.0 mm and a 9.0 mm ET tube, and most adult females can receive between a 7.0 mm an 8.0 mm ET tube. There are, however, variations to these recommendations. All people are created differently; therefore, it is also wise to have some additional criterion that can be used to select tube size. The EMT can use the diameter of the patient's little finger as a rough gauge for estimating proper ET tube size. The diameter measured is the distance from one side of the internal wall of the tube to the other, called the internal diameter.

Pediatric Considerations   Because the narrowest part of the pediatric airway is inferior to the vocal cords, the endotracheal tubes used on children less than 8 years old do not have inflatable cuffs.

The easiest and most accurate way to initially estimate ET tube size in the pediatric population is to use the following formula:

8-1.14 State the formula for sizing an infant or child endotracheal tube.

$$\frac{16 + \text{Age (in years)}}{4} = \text{ET Tube Size}$$

For example, for a 4-year-old child:

8-1.16 Define the various alternative methods for sizing the infant and child endotracheal tube.

8-1.12 State the reasons for and proper use of the stylet in orotracheal intubation.

$$\frac{16 + 4}{4} = 5 \text{ mm ET tube}$$

* **stylet**

moldable wire that can be inserted into an endotracheal tube to facilitate tube placement.

This formula will allow the EMT to identify the most likely ET tube to be used in a specific age group. Since the pediatric airway does not accommodate a cuffed ET tube, the EMT must also have a larger and smaller tube readily available to be sure of achieving the best fit during intubation.

STYLET

8-1.17 Describe the skill of orotracheal intubation in the adult patient.

8-1.18 Describe the skill of orotracheal intubation in the infant and child patient.

The **stylet** (Figures 46-7A and B) is a moldable wire that can be inserted into the ET tube to stiffen and shape the tube to facilitate tube placement when the airway is narrow or difficult to access. The most common method for stylet manipulation is molding the tube into a hockey-stick shape. Be careful about placing the

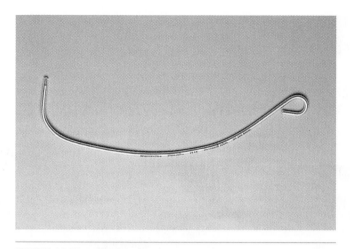

FIGURE 46-7A   A stylet.

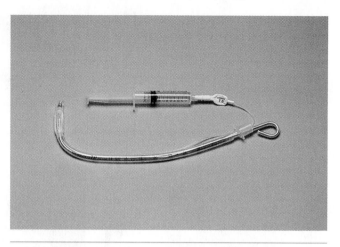

FIGURE 46-7B   An endotracheal tube with a stylet in place.

Clinical Clues: PEDIATRIC INTUBATION SIZING

In some EMS systems, it is still recommended that a standard pediatric measuring device like the **Broselow tape** be used in determining the appropriate ET tube size for a child.

* **Broselow tape**

a measurement tape that provides approximate height/weight ratios in infants and children. Used to estimate ET tube sizes and drug dosages for pediatric patients.

stylet. If the stylet is advanced beyond the distal end of the ET tube, it could cause trauma to the tissue of the airways.

FINAL WORD ON ENDOTRACHEAL INTUBATION

As an EMT you may be permitted by your medical director to perform endotracheal intubation. Endotracheal intubation requires great skill and, if your area allows you to perform endotracheal intubation in your EMS system, you will need hours of additional training beyond your regular EMT course before you will become proficient in the procedure.

Intubation can be a life-saving intervention, but an endotracheal tube that is mistakenly placed in the esophagus will result in your patient's death unless you immediately recognize the misplaced tube. Whenever you are anything less than 100% sure that the endotracheal tube has been properly placed—based on breath sounds, pulse oximetry, end-tidal CO_2 and/or EDD—immediately remove the tube and ventilate the patient with 100% oxygen via a BVM using the solid BLS airway skills you learned earlier in this course.

Orotracheal Intubation Procedure

Follow these steps to perform an orotracheal intubation (Scan 46-1 on page 1142):

1. Gather equipment.
   a. Choose the appropriately sized endotracheal tube. Make certain the cuff (for patients greater than 8 years) holds air and does not leak.
   b. Test the laryngoscope to ensure that the light bulb is "tight and bright."

2. Ensure that BSI precautions have been adhered to.

3. Preoxygenate the patient with bag-valve-mask ventilation with 100% oxygen.

SCAN 46-1 **ENDOTRACHEAL INTUBATION**

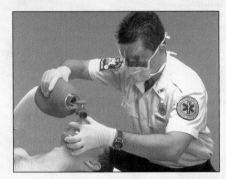

▲ Preoxygenate the patient.

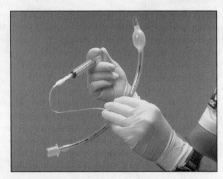

▲ Prepare the equipment.

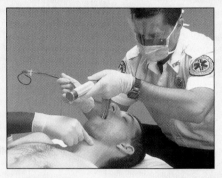

▲ Apply Sellick's maneuver and insert the laryngoscope.

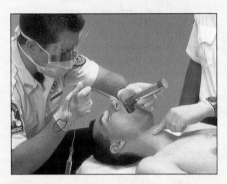

▲ Visualize the larynx and insert the ETT.

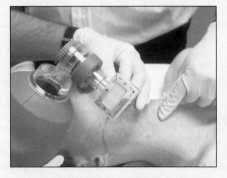

▲ Inflate the cuff and confirm placement with an ETCO$_2$ detector.

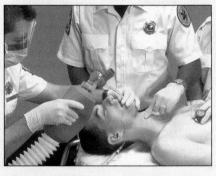

▲ Ventilate and auscultate over the epigastrium and lungs to confirm placement.

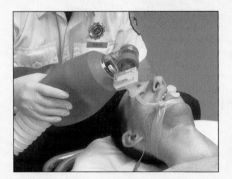

▲ Secure the tube.

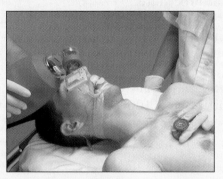

▲ Reconfirm ETT placement.

(All photos © Scott Metcalfe.)

4. Position the patient's head in a sniffing position, assuming there is no trauma. The sniffing position is accomplished by first flexing the neck forward and then extending the head backwards. If there is a suspicion of trauma, the procedure must be performed using an in-line position with manual stabilization of the neck.

5. Perform laryngoscopy.
   a. *Macintosh (curved) blade technique:*
      i. Open the patient's mouth with the right hand, and remove any dentures.
      ii. Grasp the laryngoscope in the left hand.
      iii. Spread the patient's lips and insert the blade between the teeth, being careful not to break a tooth.
      iv. Insert the blade along the tongue, to the right, and rest the tip of the blade at the base of the tongue. This technique should be accomplished with a simultaneous leftward sweeping action. The leftward sweep moves the tongue away from the visual field.
      v. Lift the laryngoscope upward and forward, without changing the angle of the blade, to expose the vocal cords.
   b. *Miller (straight) blade technique:*
      i. Open the patient's mouth with the right hand, and remove any dentures.
      ii. Grasp the laryngoscope in the left hand.
      iii. Spread the patient's lips and insert the blade between the teeth, being careful not to break a tooth.
      iv. Insert the blade directly into the laryngopharynx and lift the laryngoscope upward and forward, without changing the angle of the blade, to expose the vocal cords.

6. After visualizing the glottis and vocal cords, gently advance the tube through the vocal cords and into the trachea. Stop advancing the tube once all of the balloon is just past the cords.

7. Either you or your assistant should carefully hold the ET tube and prevent movement, which could dislodge the tube or force it deeper into the trachea.

8-1.21 Describe the skill of securing the endotracheal tube in the adult, infant, and child patient.

8. Connect an end-tidal CO_2 detector to the tube or use an esophageal detector device (EDD) to verify tube placement.

9. If either device indicates proper tracheal placement of the endotracheal tube, use the syringe to inflate the cuff with 10 ml of air and then detach the syringe from the inflation valve.

8-1.5 Review the use of oxygen therapy in airway management.

10. Attempt ventilation of the patient using 100 percent oxygen and a bag-valve device.

Clinical Clues: OROTRACHEAL INTUBATION

As an EMT, you should only make two attempts at orotracheal intubation. If both attempts fail, insert an oral airway, continue to ventilate the patient with high-concentration oxygen via bag-valve mask, and aggressively suction the airway.

11. Confirm tube placement by auscultating first over the epigastrium and then over the lung fields. If sounds are heard over the epigastrium, immediately stop ventilating the patient and remove the tube.

12. If the initial endotracheal tube placement is unsuccessful, immediately remove the tube, ventilate, and reoxygenate the patient with a BVM. Reattempt intubation and again verify tube placement with an end-tidal CO_2 detector or EDD and then listen for breath sounds and assure there are no sounds over the stomach.

13. Once the tube is properly placed, note the cm mark at the lips. This ensures that the EMT can easily identify a change in tube depth.

14. Secure the tube with tape or a commercial tube-securing device.

SELLICK'S MANEUVER

8-1.7   Describe how to perform Sellick's maneuver (cricoid pressure).

* **Sellick's manuever**

technique of applying downward pressure on the cricoid cartilage, used to help visualize the vocal cords and to reduce the potential for vomiting.

Sellick's maneuver (Figure 46-8)—applying downward pressure on the cricoid cartilage—promotes more effective visualization of the cords during endotracheal intubation. This technique is beneficial in airway management because it also provides compression of the esophagus to reduce the risk of vomiting and, ultimately, aspiration.

BURP MANEUVER

* **BURP maneuver**

acronym for Backward, Upward, Rightward Pressure, a technique of applying such pressure to the thyroid cartilage to help visualize the vocal cords for endotracheal intubation.

The **BURP maneuver** has been steadily rising in popularity and is used to promote more effective visualization of the cords during endotracheal intubation. BURP is an acronym for Backward, Upward, Rightward Pressure. In performing this technique, the intubating EMT should use his right thumb and index finger to apply pressure to the thyroid cartilage (Adam's apple) in a backward (downward) motion, toward the patient's right, and up toward the patient's jaw. The application of this pressure will likely cause the glottis to be compressed posteriorly, allowing the intubating EMT to see the vocal cords or, hopefully, at least the tip of the epiglottis.

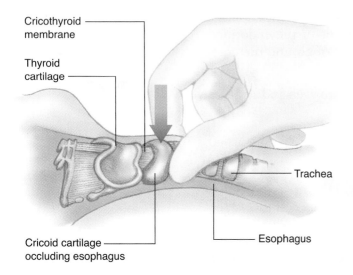

Cricothyroid membrane

Thyroid cartilage

Trachea

Cricoid cartilage occluding esophagus

Esophagus

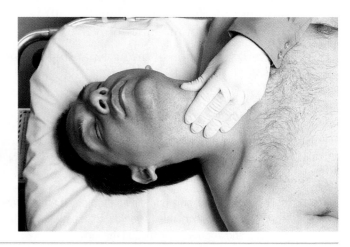

FIGURE 46-8   In Sellick's maneuver, pressure is placed on the cricoid cartilage, pushing it posteriorly against the esophagus. By compressing the esophagus, vomiting is suppressed. The maneuver also helps bring the vocal cords into view.

* Stop, Review, Remember!

Multiple Choice

Place a check next to the correct answer.

1. Sellick's maneuver is beneficial in airway management because it also provides compression of the esophagus to reduce the risk of:

   _____ a. cricoid pressure.

   _____ b. aspiration.

   _____ c. nausea.

   _____ d. epiglottitis.

2. What is the average size ET tube that is used in an adult male?

   _____ a. 6.0–7.0 mm

   _____ b. 7.0–8.0 mm

   _____ c. 8.0–9.0 mm

   _____ d. 9.0–10.0 mm

3. What is the average size ET tube that is used in an adult female?

   _____ a. 6.0–7.0 mm

   _____ b. 7.0–8.0 mm

   _____ c. 8.0–9.0 mm

   _____ d. 9.0–10.0 mm

4. When selecting a laryngoscope, you realize that you need a blade that will fit into the valeculla. Which blade would you choose?

   _____ a. Macintosch

   _____ b. Miller

   _____ c. Wisconsin

   _____ d. none of the above

5. When positioning your patient for intubation, what is the proper position for the patient's head?

   _____ a. neutral

   _____ b. sniffing

   _____ c. flexed

   _____ d. extended

Fill in the Blank

1. The _____ is an instrument used to lift the tongue off of the posterior pharynx and to move the epiglottis out of the visual field so that the vocal cords are visible.

2. Sellick's maneuver involves applying downward pressure on the _____.

3. BURP stands for B_____, U_____, R_____ P_____.

4. The greatest benefit to _____ a patient is that the procedure provides definitive airway protection.

5. The _____ is a moldable wire that can be inserted into the ET tube to facilitate tube placement.

Critical Thinking

1. What is the functional difference between straight and curved laryngoscope blades? Which is preferred for pediatric patients?

_____

_____

_____

_____

_____

2. Why care should be taken when positioning the stylet into the ET tube?

_____

_____

_____

_____

_____

Blind Insertion Airways

This section provides information on several alternatives to the ET tube. These are inserted "blindly" (without a laryngoscope). They may be used in place of ET tubes or as "rescue airways," when attempts at endotracheal intubation fail. Both the Combitube and the laryngeal mask airway (LM) described next require that the patient be unconscious.

ESOPHAGEAL TRACHEAL COMBITUBE

✳ **esophageal tracheal combitube (ETC)**

type of dual-lumen airway used to provide ventilations and help protect the airway

The **esophageal tracheal combitube (ETC)** is a dual-lumen airway (side by side) with a ventilation port for each lumen. One tube is closed-ended but has multiple holes that can be ventilated through. The other tube is open like an ET tube (Scan 46-2).

When inserted, the device will enter the esophagus 90% of the time or the trachea 10% of the time. Regardless of whether the tube enters either the esophagus or trachea, the patient can be ventilated.

There is a large high-volume inflatable cuff near the center of the device. This cuff is designed to be positioned in the oropharynx to prevent air from escaping through the mouth and nose when the device is being used. Near the distal tip of the device is another smaller volume inflatable cuff. When the ETC is placed in the esophagus, this smaller cuff occludes the esophagus preventing both the passage of air into the esophagus and the regurgitation of the stomach contents up into the airway. When the ETT is placed in the trachea, this distal cuff acts like a normal endotracheal tube cuff and fits snugly up against the walls of the trachea.

SCAN 46-2   **VENTILATING WITH THE COMBITUBE**

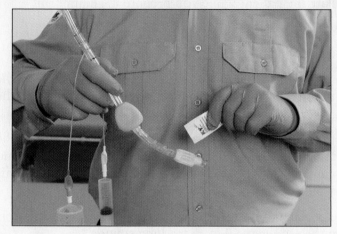

▲ Lubricate the tube generously with water-soluble lubricant.

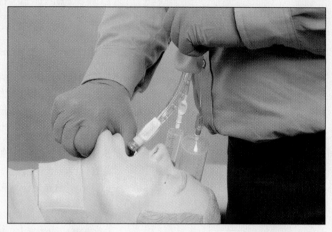

▲ Insert the tube, advancing it down the center and along the natural curve of the mouth and throat. Stop when the teeth are between the two black rings. Do not use excessive force. Inflate the cuffs.

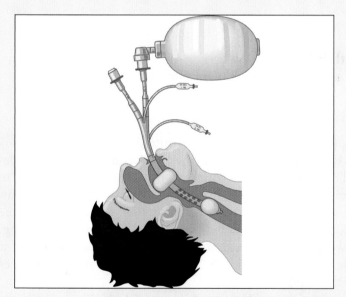

▲ Usually the tube will have been placed in the esophagus. On this assumption, ventilate through tube #1. Listen for the presence of breath sounds in the lungs and the absence of sounds from the epigastrium.

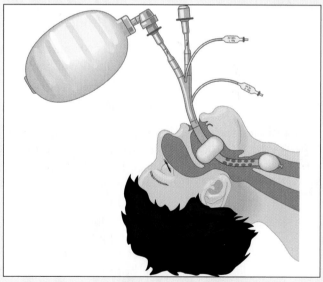

▲ If there is an absence of lung sounds and presence of sounds in the epigastrium, the tube has been placed in the trachea. In this case, ventilate through tube #2. Listen again to be sure of proper placement.

The Combitube is a blind insertion device. It is inserted into the mouth and advanced into the posterior oropharynx and then gently advanced until the teeth rest at the preprinted markings on the device.

Combitubes come in two sizes, 37 French (Combitube SA) for patients from 4 to 6 feet tall, and 41 French for patients from 6 to 7 feet tall.

INSERTING A COMBITUBE

1. Have a partner ventilate the patient while you prepare the equipment.

2. Lubricate the tube with water soluble lubricant.

3. Direct your partner to stop ventilations.

4. Grasp the lower jaw with your left hand and insert the combitube along the natural curve of the mouth and throat. Stop when the teeth are between the two black rings. Do not force the tube into place.

5. Inflate both cuffs. Cuff 1 will be inflated with 100 mL of air (85 mL for the SA combitube). As the cuff inflates, the combitube will be pushed up and into it's proper anatomic position. Cuff 2 will be inflated with 15 mL of air (12 mL for the SA combitube).

6. Ventilate through the port marked #1. Most of the time you will use this port because the tube is in the espohagus. Listen for lung sounds.

7. If you do not hear lung sounds when performing step #6, attach your BVM to the port marked #2 and ventilate. Listen for lung sounds. In this case the tube is in the trachea.

8. Ventilate the patient through the port that provides breath sounds.

9. If ventilation of neither tube results in breath sounds, deflate both balloons, remove the device, and ventilate the patient with a BVM.

LARYNGEAL MASK AIRWAY (LMA)

✳ **laryngeal mask airway (LMA)**

type of airway used to provide ventilations and help protect the airway.

The **laryngeal mask airway (LMA)** (Figure 46-9) was initially designed for use in a controlled environment like the operating room. The LMA is a very different device from the combitube. This device is most commonly used as a rescue device in the prehospital setting as with the combitube. It is imperative that the device is inserted only in a patient who is unconscious with no gag reflex. A large but unique cuff is placed in the laryngopharynx and pointed directly over the glottic opening. The biggest difference between the LMA and an ET tube or combitube is that it does not effectively provide airway protection. LMA masks come in various sizes in both reusable and disposable models.

The LMA comes in various sizes. In general, #3 or #4 LMAs can be used for most adult patients.

To insert the LMA airway (Figures 46-10A and B)

1. Lubricate the posterior side of the cuff with water soluble lubricant.

2. Place the patient's head into the sniffing position.

3. Insert the tube with the open side facing anteriorly, pressing the device against the hard palate as it is being inserted.

4. Advance the tube until the mask is in the hypopharynx and resistance is met. Use your fingers to maintain the shape of the mask as it enters the hypopharynx.

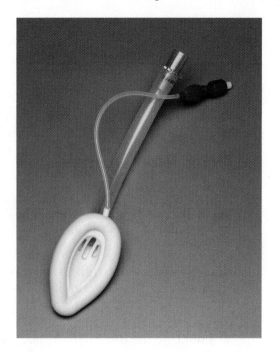

FIGURE 46-9 The laryngeal mask airway (LMA). (LMA North American, Inc.)

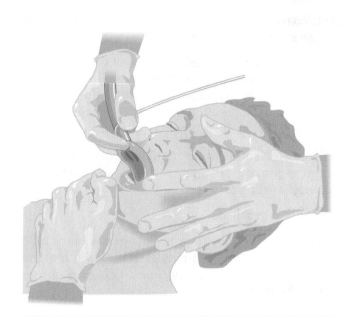

FIGURE 46-10A Inserting the laryngeal mask airway.

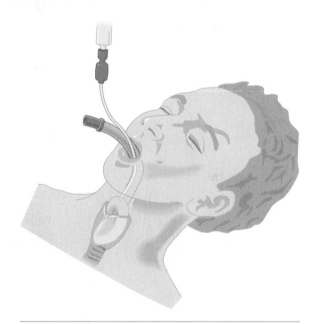

FIGURE 46-10B The laryngeal mask airway in place.

5. Inflate the cuff with the recommended amount of air as directed by the no-tations on the side of the LMA tube. This may cause the appearance that the tube is shifting slightly. This is expected.

6. Ventilate through the tube. Listen for breath sounds in the lungs and the absence of sounds in the epigastrium.

7. Insert an oropharyngeal airway to prevent the patient from biting the tube.

8. Ventilate the patient.

NASOGASTRIC TUBE PLACEMENT

Although not a skill commonly practiced by EMTs, **nasogastric (NG) tube** placement is part of the National EMT curriculum. The most common indications for

8-1.6 Describe the indications, contraindications, and technique for insertion of nasal gastric tubes.

✳ **nasogastric (NG) tube**
a tube designed to be passed through the nose, nasopharynx, and esophagus. It is used to relieve distention of the stomach in an infant or child patient.

placement of an NG tube by an EMT include decompression of gastric air during prolonged bag-mask ventilation or removal of gastric contents. Following NG tube placement, the tube should be attached to low continuous suction.

NG tube placement procedure: (Scan 46-3)

1. Gather equipment.

2. Don nonsterile gloves.

3. If the patient is conscious, explain the procedure and show the equipment to him.

4. If possible, sit the patient upright for optimal neck/stomach alignment.

5. Examine the nostrils for deformity/obstructions to determine the best side for insertion.

6. Measure the tubing from the bridge of the nose to the earlobe, then to the point halfway between the end of the sternum and the navel.

7. Mark the measured length with a marker/tape and note the distance.

8. Lubricate the distal 2 to 4 inches of the tube with water-soluble lubricant. This procedure is very uncomfortable for many patients, so place a squirt of Lidocaine jelly in the nostril and a spray of Cetacaine in the back of the throat to numb the areas if permitted by local protocols.

9. Pass the tube via either nare posteriorly, past the pharynx, into the esophagus, and then into the stomach. Instruct the patient to swallow, and advance the tube as the patient swallows. Swallowing of small sips of water may ease the passage of the tube into the esophagus. If resistance is met, rotate the tube slowly with downward advancement toward the closest ear.

10. Withdraw the tube immediately if changes occur in the patient's respiratory status, if the tube coils in the mouth, or if the patient begins to cough, loses the ability to speak, or becomes cyanotic.

11. Advance the tube until the mark is reached.

12. Check for placement by attaching a 60-mL syringe to the free end of the tube and aspirating a sample of gastric contents. Then inject an air bolus into the tube and listen for the rush of air over the epigastrium to confirm proper placement.

13. Secure the tube with tape.

Following NG tube placement, you must reconfirm proper placement and evaluate functionality. Methods to ensure proper NG tube placement include the auscultation of injected air at the epigastrium or the aspiration of gastric contents. If using the aspiration method of confirmation, it is important to note that normal drainage should be yellow or green. It is not uncommon for minute amounts of blood to be present in the drainage because of the trauma associated with tube placement. After verification of correct placement, the NG tube must be secured to the nose and/or face with tape.

8-1.15 List complications associated with advanced airway management.

Complications can result in NG tube placement. Improper tube placement is the primary cause of these complications, and careful verification must be made to ensure that the tube is properly placed. Misplacement of NG tubes into the lung is a common occurrence.

SCAN 46-3   **NASOGASTRIC INTUBATION—INFANT OR CHILD**

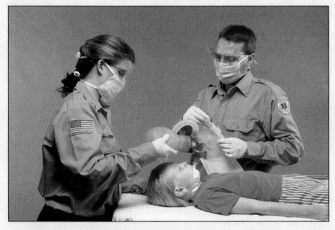

▲ Oxygenate the patient.

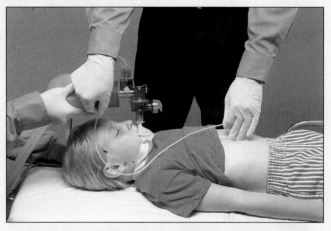

▲ Measure tube from tip of nose, over ear, to below xiphoid process.

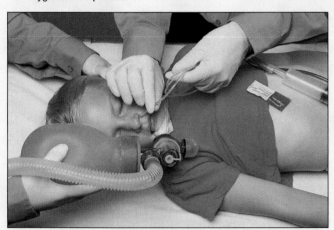

▲ Pass lubricated tube gently downward along nasal floor to stomach.

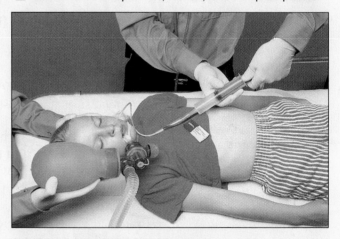

▲ Use suction to aspirate stomach contents.

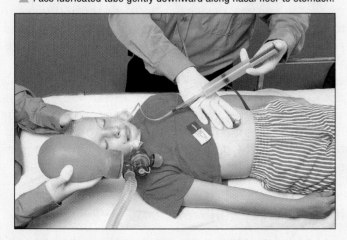

▲ To confirm correct placement, auscultate over epigastrium. Listen for bubbling while injecting 10 to 20 mL air into tube.

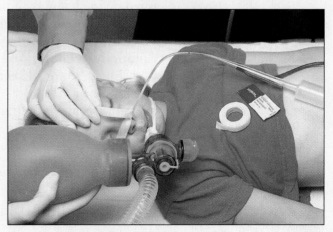

▲ Secure tube in place.

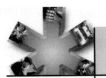

Perspective

Tanya—The Wife

"I don't know what to feel right now. I'm pretty much just numb. We had been arguing about money, like always, you know? Rob has a hard time holding down a job and . . . well . . . it's beginning to cause real trouble for us now that we have a mortgage and kids and all. It just seems like there's been this constant stress that's like a dark cloud over everything. Does that make sense? Not in a million years would I have thought that he'd do that. I really am grateful for the firemen and those guys from the ambulance, though. That one EMT, David, he really seemed to care about Rob and was helpful to me. It's weird, but I also think he could really tell how I was feeling, watching my house fill up with cops and firemen, and just not knowing what to do or how to feel or even what I felt. Oh God, how is this going to affect the kids? How am I supposed to explain this all to them? And how do we just move on from something like this?"

✳

CONFIRMATION OF ADVANCED AIRWAY DEVICE PLACEMENT

> **8-1.19** Describe the skill of confirming endotracheal tube placement in the adult, infant, and child patient.
>
> **8-1.20** State the consequence of and the need to recognize unintentional esophageal intubation.

Confirming placement of an advanced airway device, whether it is an endotracheal tube or a combitube, must be performed consistently and accurately. If an improperly placed device goes unidentified, the patient will certainly die.

There are several methods of confirming proper ET tube placement. The first is watching the tube pass through the vocal cords. After visualizing the tube passing through the cords, the EMT should watch for chest rise and fall. It is also imperative epigastric and lung sounds be auscultated immediately following placement of an advanced airway device. When properly placed, the endotracheal tube will result in equal breath sounds over both sides of the chest and no sounds over the epigastrium. If you listen to the epigastrium first, you may identify an esophageal intubation and be able to stop ventilating the stomach before the patient vomits. Lung sounds that are present on the right side but absent or diminished on the left may indicate that the airway device has been advanced too deeply and has entered the right mainstem bronchus. An end-tidal CO_2 detector or another device approved by your medical director must be used in addition to auscultation to confirm tube placement.

Although rare, absent or decreased lung sounds could indicate a bronchial obstruction or a pneumothorax. Absent lung sounds throughout the chest indicate an esophageal intubation until proven otherwise. Finally, if the patient regains consciousness following placement of a tube into the trachea through the vocal cords, the EMT should understand that the patient will not be able to communicate because the cords cannot move enough to create sound.

> ✳ **end tidal carbon dioxide (ETCO₂) detector**
>
> device used to detect the presence or the amount of carbon dioxide in exhaled air.
>
> ✳ **capnography**
>
> recording or display indicating the presence or quantity of exhaled carbon dioxide concentrations.

END-TIDAL CARBON DIOXIDE DETECTORS

End-tidal carbon dioxide (ETCO₂) detector devices come in the form of simple presence detectors (Figure 46-11) as well as quantifying detectors (Figure 46-12). **Capnography** has been designed to distinguish between esophageal and tracheal

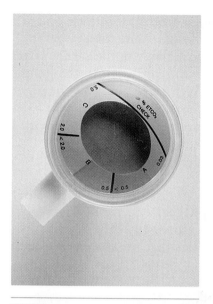

FIGURE 46-11   Colorimetric end-tidal CO_2 detector.

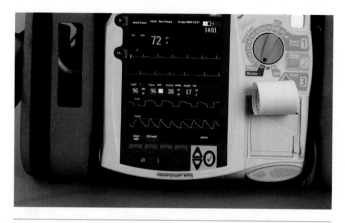

FIGURE 46-12   An electronic end-tidal CO_2 detector built into a cardiac monitor.

intubation. Exhaled carbon dioxide can be present only if the tube has entered the trachea, which leads to the lungs. Exhaled carbon dioxide will not be present if the tube has entered the esophagus, which leads to the stomach.

Disconnection of the tracheal tube from the bag-valve mask, apnea, and equipment failure, can all cause false negatives. In the presence of these false negative readings, there should be no waveform showing on an electronic CO_2 detector's display screen, despite the fact that the tube may be in the trachea. An obstructed ET tube or severe bronchospasm may also give the appearance that the tube is in the wrong place. A normal end-tidal waveform does not necessarily mean that the tube is in the correct place either.

A colorimetric device contains filter paper saturated with a colorless liquid base and a pH-sensitive medium. The color in the device changes when the paper comes into contact with carbon dioxide and returns to normal when the carbon dioxide is gone. Thus a colorimetric device is able to show the presence of CO_2 but not the amount. A **capnometer** is an electronic device that quantifies the amount of carbon dioxide through a probe attached at the end of an endotracheal tube. A **capnographer** will also quantify the amount of carbon dioxide being exhaled, but displays a continuous waveform to indicate levels of carbon dioxide over time.

A capnometer and capnographer work by introducing an infrared light through the exhaled air and measuring the degree of absorption or penetration of the light. The amount of light that penetrates the exhaled gas is proportional to the concentration of CO_2.

✳ **capnometer**
  electronic device that uses infrared light to quantify carbon dioxide in exhaled air.

✳ **capnographer**
  device that uses infrared light to evaluate exhaled carbon dioxide and that displays a continuous waveform to indicate levels of carbon dioxide over time.

Clinical Clues: CAPNOGRAPHY

Capnography can reveal false positive readings and false negative readings. Because of the potential for unreliability, it is essential not to rely solely on capnography to verify or deny proper endotracheal tube placement—just as you would not use auscultation as the sole confirmation of correct tube placement.

The analyzer, or end-tidal CO_2 probe, may be positioned in one of two places: either in-line or out-of-circuit at the end of a sampling tube.

End-tidal CO_2 detectors are not always reliable in the cardiac arrest environment. In the cardiac arrest victim, there is no perfusion to the lungs, so carbon dioxide is not produced. Therefore, the detector will not show the presence of carbon dioxide even if the tube is correctly placed in the trachea.

In most situations, end-tidal CO_2 detectors are of great benefit. It is, however, important to remember that capnography, like pulse oximetry, should be used as just one differential diagnosis tool, in conjunction with the patient's clinical presentation.

Esophageal detector devices or EDDs, (Figures 46-13A–C) are used fairly regularly in the prehospital setting. The esophageal detector device works because of anatomic variations in the trachea and esophagus. The trachea remains rigid and patent because of the cartilaginous rings that run the entire length of it. The

✷ **esophageal detector device (EDD)**

mechanical device that uses negative pressure to differentiate tracheal from esophageal placement of a tube.

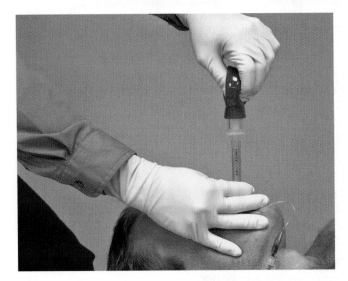

a

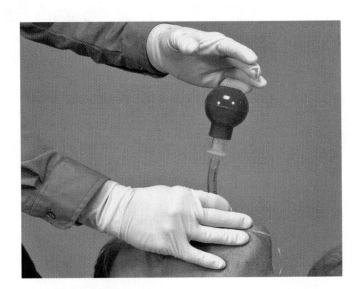

b

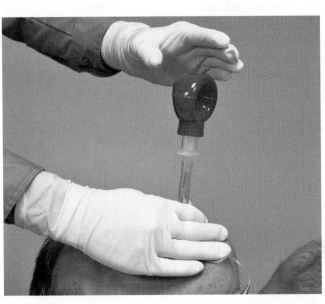

c

FIGURE 46-13 An esophageal intubation detector—bulb style. (a) Squeeze the device and then attach it to the endotracheal tube. (b) If the bulb refills easily on release, it indicates correct placement in the trachea. (c) If the bulb does not refill, the tube is improperly placed in the esophagus.

esophagus, however, has no supporting rings and is therefore collapsible. The principle of the EDDs is that the esophagus will collapse when a negative pressure is applied to its lumen, whereas the trachea will not. There are two common types of EDDs, a syringe type and a bulb type.

The syringe type EDD works by using an adapter to attach a 60-mL syringe to the endotracheal tube. Once the syringe is attached, the EMT should pull back on the plunger to attempt to withdraw air. If resistance is met, then the tube is in the esophagus and the esophagus collapsed as air was removed.

The bulb type EDD is attached to the endotracheal tube while the bulb is fully compressed. If the bulb reinflates when it is released, then the tube is in the trachea. If it does not reinflate, then the tube is in the esophagus and the vacuum created by release of the bulb has collapsed the soft walls of the esophagus.

PULSE OXIMETRY

Pulse oximetry provides a noninvasive and continuous means of determining arterial oxygen saturation. **Pulse oximeters** use infrared light to determine the oxygen saturation of hemoglobin. The oximeter probe is attached to the patient's finger. The infrared light is emitted through the probe, and a sensor placed at the backside of the probe determines how much of the light was able to pass through the capillary beds. Hemoglobin without oxygen bound to it or with low concentrations of oxygen, will allow more light through the capillaries than oxygen-saturated hemoglobin will.

Standard pulse oximeters generally overestimate true arterial hemoglobin oxygen saturation in the setting of carbon monoxide toxicity. By understanding how pulse oximetry works, it is easy to understand how carbon monoxide can produce a false positive reading. Carbon monoxide has a greater affinity to hemoglobin than oxygen does and allows easy passage of infrared light just as oxygen would. Newer co-oximeters can detect both oxygen saturation and hemoglobin bound to carbon monoxide.

Patients with advanced airway devices in place should have their oxygen saturation continuously monitored.

* **pulse oximetry**
  noninvasive and continuous means of determining arterial oxygen saturation.

* **pulse oximeter**
  device that uses infrared light to determine arterial oxygen saturation.

Clinical Clues: PULSE OXIMETRY

It should be understood that pulse oximetry is not the definitive answer to diagnostic tools of respiration. Pulse oximetry should be used as only one differential diagnosis tool, in conjunction with the patient's clinical presentation.

Stop, Review, Remember!

Multiple Choice

Place a check next to the correct answer.

1. You have a 70-year-old female patient in your care who suffered cardiac arrest while working in her yard. The patient was intubated prior to your arrival. As you begin to ventilate the patient, you feel poor bag-valve compliance. Upon direct visualization of the glottis with a laryngoscope, the endotracheal tube appears to pass through the vocal cords. What is the benefit of inserting a nasogastric tube into this patient?

   _____ a. It will provide relief to possible gastric inflation from prolonged ventilation.

   _____ b. It will decrease the amount of stomach secretions and reduce the risk of aspiration.

   _____ c. It will provide an alternative medication route.

   _____ d. It can serve as an additional tube with which to ventilate the patient.

2. What is a disadvantage of an LMA?

   _____ a. It rests over the trachea and esophagus and can lead to aspiration.

   _____ b. It rests over the trachea and does not allow for adequate tidal volume.

   _____ c. It must be used in only patients with no gag reflex.

   _____ d. none of the above.

3. Which device is characterized by a lumen inside of a lumen?

   _____ a. combitube

   _____ b. ET

   _____ c. LMA

   _____ d. none of the above

4. Which device is characterized by two separate lumens side-by-side?

   _____ a. combitube

   _____ b. ET

   _____ c. LMA

   _____ d. all of the above

5. Which device is characterized by an oropharyngeal cuff?

   _____ a. combitube

   _____ b. ET

   _____ c. LMA

   _____ d. all of the above

Fill in the Blank

1. _____ _____ provides a noninvasive and continuous means of determination of the arterial oxygen saturation.

2. Endotracheal intubation tube placement must be confirmed by at least _____ methods.

3. Absent or decreased lung sounds following the correct insertion of an ET tube could indicate a bronchial obstruction or a _____.

4. A _____ works by introducing an infrared light through exhaled air and measuring the degree of absorption or penetration of the light.

5. If an advanced airway device is inserted "_____," it means that no laryngoscope was used.

Critical Thinking

1. You are caring for an unconscious firefighter who was overcome by smoke while fighting a structure fire. Why should you be suspicious of a 98 percent reading on the pulse oximeter?

   _____

   _____

   _____

   _____

2. Why is a laryngoscope unnecessary when inserting an esophageal tracheal combitube?

   _____

   _____

   _____

   _____

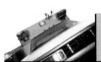

Dispatch Summary

Once the patient had a patent airway, David was able to locate a weak carotid pulse, which grew stronger with each assisted ventilation. The patient was secured to a long spineboard and transported with lights and siren to Our Lady of Peace Hospital on 50th and Eisenhower, where he was further stabilized and admitted to ICU.

Rob has since been released and is undergoing rehabilitation for permanent mental and physical disabilities resulting from his suicide attempt.

During the months following this call, EMT David Mote created a suicide prevention and education program that has been implemented in all of the high schools countywide. He was recently invited to Washington, D.C., to speak about suicide prevention.

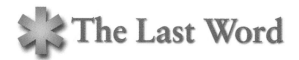
The Last Word

There are very few areas in EMS that are as vital as aggressive, accurate airway management. This chapter highlights some key advanced-level skills that some EMTs may perform. In order to consider having EMTs employ these advanced skills, an EMS service must understand the need to provide regular continuing education. If a decision has been made to implement advanced-level skills for the EMT, there must also be an understanding that the skills must be practiced or performed continuously to maintain proficiency.

✳ Chapter Review

MULTIPLE CHOICE

Place a check next to the correct answer.

1. What is the benefit of using a combitube for airway control?

    _____ a. It can be used for very long periods of time.

    _____ b. It is equivalent to an endotracheal tube.

    _____ c. It works even when placed in the esophagus.

    _____ d. You can confirm placement by direct visualization.

2. You have a 67-year-old male patient in your care that suffered cardiac arrest while jogging. The patient was intubated prior to your arrival. As you begin to ventilate the patient, you feel poor bag-valve compliance. Upon direct visualization of the glottis, the endotracheal tube appears to pass through the vocal cords. On your assessment you note that your patient has no breath sounds on the left side. What is the most a likely cause for the absence of left-sided lung sounds?

    _____ a. pneumothorax

    _____ b. hemothorax

    _____ c. mainstem intubation

    _____ d. obstructed endotracheal tube

3. How many mL of air does the first (large) pharyngeal cuff of a standard endotracheal tube cuff hold?

    _____ a. 10 mL

    _____ b. 20 mL

    _____ c. 60 mL

    _____ d. 100 mL

4. Which is NOT an indicator of correct endotracheal tube placement?

    _____ a. watching the tube pass through the vocal cords

    _____ b. condensation on the ET tube

    _____ c. good lung sounds in all fields

    _____ d. absence of epigastric sounds

5. How many mL of air does the first (large) pharyngeal combitube cuff hold?

    _____ a. 10 mL

    _____ b. 20 mL

    _____ c. 60 mL

    _____ d. 100 mL

MATCHING

Match the advanced airway equipment or technique with the appropriate description.

1. _____ BURP maneuver
2. _____ Macintosh
3. _____ Stylet
4. _____ Miller
5. _____ 10-mL syringe
6. _____ End-tidal CO_2 detector
7. _____ Combitube

A. Used to distinguish between esophageal and tracheal intubation
B. Curved blade used with a laryngoscope
C. Used to inflate the ET tube cuff to prevent air from leaking around the ET tube
D. When inserted, one tube will enter the esophagus and the other will enter the trachea
E. Moldable wire that is inserted into an ET tube to facilitate tube placement
F. Applying pressure to the thyroid cartilage in a backward (downward) motion, toward the patient's right, and up toward the patient's jaw
G. Straight blade used with a laryngoscope
H. Involves simply applying downward pressure on the cricoid cartilage

CRITICAL THINKING

1. What is a "rescue airway" and when should one be used? Name two "rescue airways."

_____

_____

_____

_____

2. Why should you not rely solely on capnography to verify a tube placement?

_____

_____

_____

3. You and your partner arrive on the scene of a cardiac arrest where a firefighter-paramedic has already intubated the patient. Your partner takes over ventilating with the BVM and asks you to confirm proper placement of the tube. How would you do that?

_____

_____

_____

_____

CASE STUDIES

Case Study 1

In this case you will be called upon to make sound clinical decisions, identify patient needs, and deal with bystanders.

You and your partner are dispatched to an address in the ritzy Upper Heights section of the city for an "unresponsive male in his mid forties."

Upon arrival you are quickly ushered by a well-dressed woman into a spacious living room heavily decorated with paintings and marble statues. You immediately recognize the patient as a movie star who (according to the local newspaper's gossip column) had just moved into the area. As you quickly assess the patient, your partner asks the woman what happened. "We were just talking and . . . and he got all pale and fell down. Please tell me that he's going to be okay!" Your assessment reveals that he is pulseless and apneic. Just then, a man appears at one of the room's large bay windows and begins taking photographs while talking excitedly into a cellular phone.

"Ma'am," your partner says. "Can you close the curtains while we see what we can do for him?"

You lie on the floor and insert the laryngoscope blade into the man's mouth but can only see his hard palate. You reposition the blade but get the same result. "I can't see anything in there," You say through clenched teeth as you pull up a little harder. "How long has he been down?" The woman is tearfully pulling the last curtain closed and says, "About five minutes now."

"I just don't think this is going to work," you say, pulling up on the laryngoscope handle again.

1. Would either Sellick's or BURP maneuvers help in this situation? Why or why not?

_____

_____

_____

_____

2. Was it appropriate for your partner to ask the woman to close the curtains? How do you think the photographer knew to show up at the home?

_____

_____

_____

_____

3. After being unable to insert an ET tube, what should you do?

_____

_____

_____

_____

Case Study 2

Answer the following questions based on the case information provided.

You are called to a housing subdivision on the east end of town for a possible carbon monoxide poisoning. You arrive to find two police officers standing over an unresponsive woman who is sprawled on the front lawn of a home. "Her son came over and found her like this in her recliner and the carbon monoxide detector was going off," one of the officers says. "He dragged her out here and she keeps moving a little, but she sure doesn't look good."

1. What is the first step that you should take in caring for this patient?
   a. Intubate her with an appropriately sized tube.
   b. Administer high-flow oxygen via a nonrebreather mask.
   c. Open her airway with the head-tilt, chin-lift maneuver.
   d. Attach a pulse oximeter.

2. This patient would most likely take a _____ ET tube.
   a. 4.5
   b. 8.5
   c. 7.5
   d. 10.5

3. A pulse oximeter reading of _____ would not be unusual for this patient.
   a. 73%
   b. 99%
   c. 85%
   d. all of the above

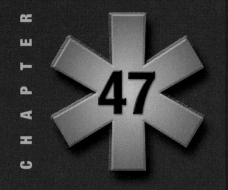

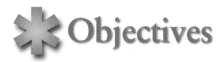

Objectives

There are no objectives in the U.S. Department of Transportation 1994 EMT-Basic National Standard Curriculum that pertain to this chapter.

Introduction

If you are reading this chapter, you are probably about to take your certification exams and are interested in some of the things that EMS has to offer you. Of course you may be anywhere in your training and have a curiosity about what happens after your class. So read on. If you're reading ahead, you are not alone. We are sure that many people in your class have done this as well.

Obtaining certification or licensure as an EMT is the beginning of a journey. You have learned much in your class. There is much more to learn in the field. There are few courses that teach you to do so many vitally important skills in a relatively short time.

The purpose of this chapter is to provide information to help you begin and succeed in EMS and to explore some of the career possibilities that will now be open to you.

EMS is practiced in a number of ways and in a variety of places. Your EMT certification is the beginning of many opportunities.

Success in EMS

Your EMT course taught you many important topics. You listened to lectures, practiced skills, and perhaps did some hospital or ride time as part of your training.

You have likely wondered, "How will I be able to do this on an ambulance?" or "What happens if I get out there and have a horrible accident on my first call?" Or even, "What if I see something gross and puke?" You are not alone. These are questions everyone has. We have prepared a few tips that have helped experienced EMS providers make it through the beginning of their EMS career. We believe they will help you, too.

Before proceeding, it is important to note that there is a strong volunteer component to EMS in the United States. Some EMTs volunteer; some are paid; many do both. The term "career" is used to represent your experience in EMS whether volunteer or paid. Both are done with significant pride and professionalism. Both treat patients using the same skills.

The following tips are designed to help you enjoy EMS for the long haul.

TEN TIPS FOR SUCCESS IN EMS

1. **Find a mentor.**   (Figure 47-1) Beginning any job is stressful. Being an EMT isn't just any job. Many people who succeed in EMS have someone who showed them "the ropes." There are many questions, issues, and feelings you will experience in EMS. A mentor will help you find answers and provide advice to you at important times.

2. **Begin slowly if possible.**   All too often a new EMT is thrown on the street without experience. Nonserious calls may go by uneventfully—but calls can sometimes be serious. Getting in over your head can cause unpleasant experiences, have poor outcomes, and cause you to doubt yourself. When choosing an agency with which to work or volunteer, look for an organization that provides an orientation period and ride time with an experienced EMT.

3. **Strive for confidence.**   Many people feel that they can't ride as the EMT in charge of a call until they know *everything*. You will never know *everything*. Confidence was once defined as knowing how to handle most everything that comes your way and knowing when and where to look for help on the calls that stump you. You won't develop confidence initially. It takes time. Look at people you respect in your EMS service. Those who handle themselves well on calls are most likely confident providers to model.

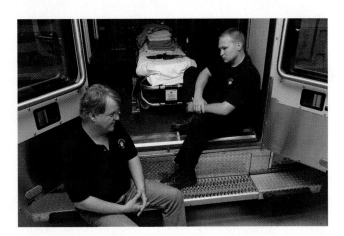

FIGURE 47-1   Finding a mentor can help you in your career. (© Dan Limmer)

4. **Get along.** There is a name for people who act confident without truly being confident or earning the right to be confident. That name is "cocky." When you are a new EMT, demonstrate respect for people who have experience. Pay attention. Ask good questions—the person who is training you will look at thoughtful questions as a sign you are interested. There are many EMTs with great skills and potential who got out of EMS because they couldn't get along with others. It isn't difficult, but it does take some thought.

5. **Be yourself.** It isn't the intent of tip #4 to change you or to say everyone who starts in EMS is a problem. Many come on too strong, try to put up a front of toughness, or pretend to be something they are not. EMTs are people-oriented people. They can spot an act. Be yourself.

6. **Keep learning and practicing.** You have learned a lot in your EMT class. Some of what you learned will be used frequently (e.g., lifting and moving, oxygen administration) while others will be used much less frequently (e.g., traction splinting). Practice these skills to remain sharp. Also keep up with changes in medicine and protocols as research shows us how to do things more effectively.

7. **Remember that EMS isn't all excitement.** As a matter of fact, there will be long stretches of "routine" calls (routine to us but important to our patients). Television portrays EMS as constant heart-pounding, lights-and-siren excitement. It is not! Finding satisfaction in doing all calls well will keep you in EMS longer than if you live for the thrill. No career is always exciting.

8. **Think critically.** You have most likely been introduced to the term "critical thinking." This means that you will assemble all available facts in a given situation, interpret them, and make a correct decision. This is important in patient care. It is also important in career decisions. You will meet many people and have a lot of experiences as you begin EMS. Think critically about the traits you want to have as an EMT. Think about the skills and intentions of the people you work with. Avoid negativity, negative people, and those who seem to have a poor regard for patients.

9. **Remember that EMS is about people.** This profession is about you, the people you work with and, of course, your patients. Regardless of a patient's attitude, odor, socioeconomic class, or medical condition (or apparent lack of same), treating patients well is perhaps one of the most important things we do. We should treat our partners or crews with that same respect.

10. **Be nice.** Our patients may not remember whether we gave them oxygen or checked their distal pulses. But they will remember how they were treated. The act of calming and reassuring a patient is one of the core skills of an EMT. And there are medical benefits to calming your patient. Treating a patient as you would want yourself or a family member treated is a gold standard of EMS (Figure 47-2).

NEXT STEPS

When you read chapter 1 about the four widely accepted levels of EMS certification, you probably weren't thinking about moving up to the next level. (Most

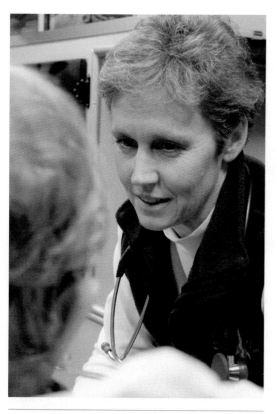

FIGURE 47-2   Treat patients in a calm and respectful manner. (© Dan Limmer.)

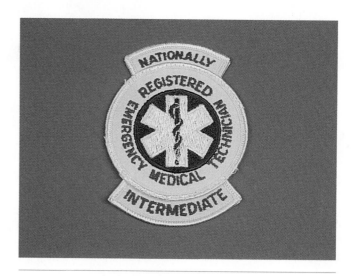

FIGURE 47-3   NREMT EMT-I patch.

are focused on passing the EMT class first.) You may have the opportunity to become an advanced provider such as an EMT-Intermediate (Advanced EMT) or a Paramedic (Table 47-1 and Table 47-2 on page 1166).

The Advanced EMT (AEMT) (Figure 47-3) is, as the name implies, an intermediate step between the EMT and the paramedic. The AEMT level of certification varies widely from state-to-state but generally involves advanced airway techniques, intravenous fluids, and some medications.

The amount of training for the AEMT is significantly less than that for a paramedic. This level is often found in rural areas where recruiting and training personnel is challenging and in cities where transport times to the hospital are very short.

The Paramedic (Figure 47-4 on page 1166) is the highest-trained level of prehospital provider. Training for this level now involves over 1,000 hours and

TABLE 47-1   EMT-INTERMEDIATE SKILLS

EMT-I skills may include:

  * Improved patient assessment and critical thinking skills
  * Advanced airway (ETT, combitube, LMA, etc.)
  * IV insertion and administration
  * Medication administration (may include nitroglycerin, aspirin, epinephrine for anaphylaxis, albuterol by nebulizer, IV dextrose, and others.

NOTE: Skills and medications vary by state and region.

FIGURE 47-4 NREMT
EMT-Paramedic patch.

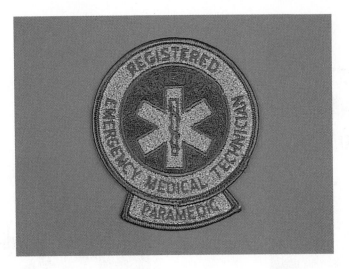

sometimes substantially more. Paramedics can do all the skills of the intermediate but can provide a much larger range of medications and more invasive skills.

It should be noted that the responsibilities of advanced providers are not solely advanced skills. These advanced providers also perform all of the basic skills you will perform as an EMT, including airway maintenance, oxygenation, and the very important reassurance and kindness each patient should receive.

I'M ONLY AN EMT, BUT. . . "

Your authors have been in EMS for many, many years and speak at EMS conferences around the country. One common (and very wrong) thing we hear after presentations is the statement: "I have a question. I am *only* an EMT, but. . . "

EMTs are the foundation of the Emergency Medical Services system. Although there are levels of training above the EMT, it is the EMT who provides the core lifesaving skills such as airway maintenance, ventilation, suction, oxygen administration, early automated defibrillation, spinal immobilization, bleeding control, and more (Figure 47-5). Without these skills being performed, advanced skills wouldn't stand a chance of success. A paramedic uses more EMT skills every day than paramedic skills.

TABLE 47-2 **PARAMEDIC SKILLS**
* Advanced knowledge in anatomy, physiology, pathophysiology, and pharmacology.
* Advanced assessment and decision-making skills
* Advanced airway skills (ETT, combitube, LMA, and in some systems cricothyrotomy and medication-facilitated intubation).
* IV medication administration
* Subcutaneous and intramuscular injections
* Cardiac monitoring
* A wide range of medications including drugs used to relieve pain, treat heart failure, reverse dangerous cardiac rhythms, and treat cardiac arrest.

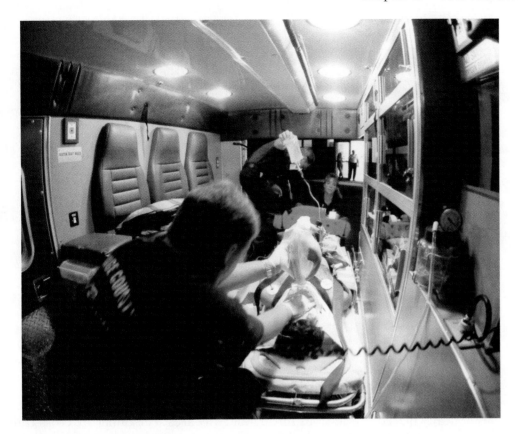

FIGURE 47-5 EMTs work alongside advanced providers in the field.

In response to the statement "I'm only an EMT . . . ," we offer another statement that we have heard in many regions around the country and reflects the pride that EMTs should possess. "Paramedics save patients. EMTs save paramedics." This refers to the fact that advanced skills won't make a difference without a solid foundation of solid basic skills.

WHERE DO EMTs WORK OR VOLUNTEER?

You may think that the answer is simple: on an ambulance. Actually EMTs work and volunteer in a number of settings including:

* fire departments

* industrial response teams

* summer camps and hospitals

* and, of course, ambulances

The EMT training you have taken is one of the few courses that instantly qualifies you for a job upon obtaining your certification. You may choose to begin full-time work, part-time work while a student or at another job, or volunteering. Here are some of the opportunities others who have completed an EMT course have found:

Ambulances—Most people think of EMTs working on ambulances (Figure 47-6 on page 1168). As a matter of fact, when the EMT certification was originally developed it was called "EMT-A" for EMT-Ambulance. In most areas, the EMT is the minimum level of certification required for an ambulance to respond to a call. There are many types of ambulance services including municipal (third service), private, volunteer, and fire-based.

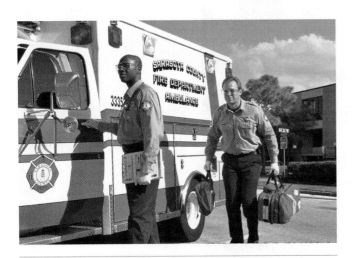

FIGURE 47-6 The EMT is an important member of the prehospital care team.

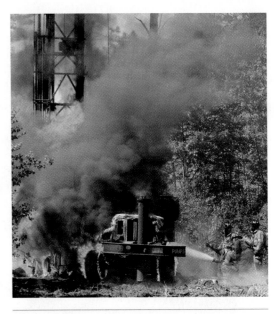

FIGURE 47-7 Many fire departments provide EMS. (© Dan Limmer.)

Fire departments—(Figure 47-7) Many fire departments provide EMS. Many government officials believe that this is an ideal set-up, since there are strategically placed fire stations throughout any area. Personnel are cross-trained as both firefighters and EMTs. In many areas fire service jobs are desirable because of the pay and retirement plans offered. Many, if not most, fire departments require all personnel to be EMTs—some require certification even to take the entrance examination.

Communications—(Figure 47-8) You may find that you are interested in becoming a communications specialist/dispatcher for an EMS or public service agency. Your EMT training will be well regarded in this arena.

FIGURE 47-8 The ideal communications center can communicate with and control the movement of all emergency units within an EMS system.

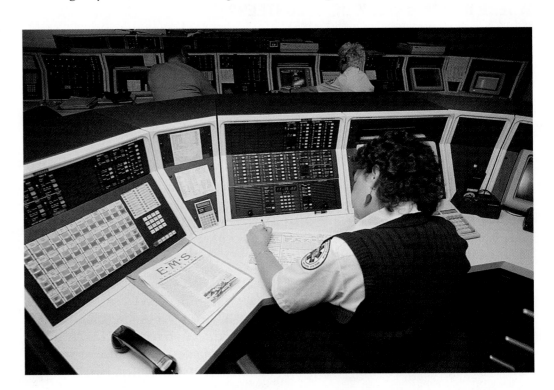

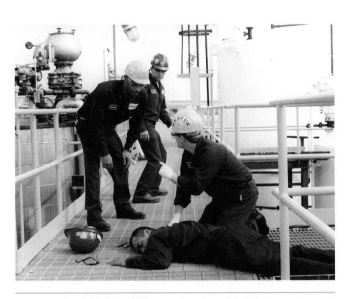

FIGURE 47-9   An EMT working in an urban/industrial setting.

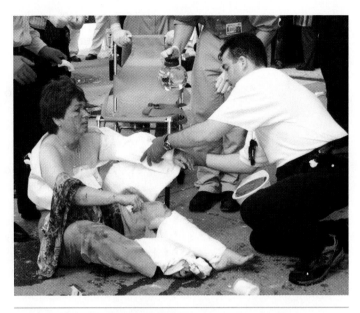

FIGURE 47-10   Providing treatment to a victim of the World Trade Center attack in New York City on September 11, 2001. (Szenes Jason/Corbis Sygma.)

Industrial emergency response—(Figure 47-9) Many employers value EMT certification in their employees. The ability to have someone available to respond in the event of an emergency until the ambulance arrives is beneficial to the employer and the patient. In many professions, there are inherent dangers where a planned emergency response team is created and staffed by EMTs. Examples include industrial plants with heavy equipment, dangerous machinery, or hazardous chemicals.

Disaster response and search and rescue—(Figure 47-10) Over the past several years there have been terrorist incidents, natural disasters, and large-scale accidents where large numbers of emergency personnel have been called from around the country. Many EMTs have taken on additional roles in these situations, including heavy rescue, trench rescue, building collapse, search and rescue (Figure 47-11), and positions on Federal Disaster Medical Assistance Teams (DMATs).

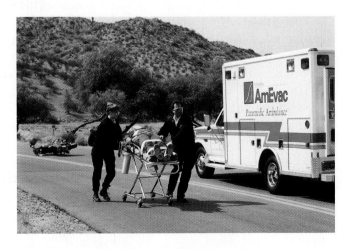

FIGURE 47-11   Career opportunities for the EMT also exist in rural/wilderness settings. (© Michal Heron Photography.)

Hospital jobs—Some of the skills you have learned in EMT class such as taking vital signs, interviewing patients, and providing comfort can translate to the hospital setting. Many hospitals hire EMS personnel as ER Techs. People holding this position were previously called "orderlies" because they moved patients around and generally kept order. Skills have been added to this position, including taking vital signs, processing paperwork, and others. Some hospitals may provide training in additional skills such as drawing blood or obtaining ECGs.

A step toward additional health care training—Many take an EMT course to "test the health care waters" and see if a career in health care is a good fit. Other times it is the EMT course that causes students to realize that they may be interested in another career in health care. There are many programs available that offer advanced standing or additional credit for paramedics toward a nursing degree. Experience in a patient care setting (such as EMS) is generally considered favorably by admissions committees when applying to nursing school or medical school.

Training new EMTs—After you have some experience under your belt, you may choose to help in EMT and First Responder training. Your class had a lead instructor and probably had some guest lecturers and lab assistants. These opportunities may be open to you in the future if you choose.

Not every opportunity listed is for you. Each one has a set of pros and cons that you will have to evaluate. For example, if you only want to provide EMS and not fight fires, the fire service may not be for you.

HITTING THE STREETS

There are a few realities in EMS. It would be unfair if we presented only the positive sides of EMS.

One of these realities is the salary offered to EMTs in some areas. It isn't unusual for students to obtain their certification and find they can't make enough money as a full-time EMT and choose to volunteer or work part time instead. In some cases EMTs work full time and supplement their income with overtime. It is an unfortunate reality that the pay as an EMT isn't always as much as we believe we should be paid—but it is improving.

You can help the salary situation in both local and global perspectives. If you want the status and pay of a professional, you must act like a professional. In the big picture, get involved in national organizations and support legislation and causes that benefit the profession as a whole. **This is EMS.**

You will also find that EMS is a 24-hour-a-day, 7-day-a-week business. Holidays included. And while your training program may have cancelled class because of inclement weather, ambulances are often busier in bad weather. You should plan to work or volunteer on some nights, weekends, and holidays. It's inevitable.

You'll work in very hot or very cold weather . . . in the rain and in the snow. You'll lift patients, be vomited on, and called names. Patients will die. **This is EMS.**

In spite of the issues discussed in this section, never forget the good you can do for your patients and fellow EMTs . . . the fun you can have, the lives you will save. Earlier in the chapter, we told you no job is perfect. EMS is no different.

What EMS offers that many jobs don't is a chance to use what you have learned for the good of others. EMS offers the opportunity to hold the hand of a scared child or an elderly patient . . . to feel the highs of saving a life and the sadness when one is lost . . . to regularly be in the homes of strangers, rich or poor, and see almost every walk of life at their best and worst.

You may be there when something big happens. See yourself on the news at 11 P.M. Deliver a baby on one call and listen to a lonely senior citizen with nothing wrong on the next.

EMS is a profession that can get hold of you and your dreams and hang on—especially if you recognize and embrace the contradictions you will find. Not the best pay but big responsibility. Very sick people and those who abuse the system. Vivid excitement followed by days of monotony. Sincere gratitude from some patients, abuse from others. **This is EMS.**

As the authors of this book, we sincerely welcome you to EMS. We have been involved in EMS for many years, with the good and the bad, and quite frankly we can't imagine not being involved in EMS.

You should be proud of what you have accomplished in your course and look forward to using your skills in the field. We wish you the best. Good luck.

Additional Resources

We would like to conclude this chapter by providing resources for you to obtain further information on the profession of EMS, furthering your education, and using the certification you are about to obtain. The Internet is a source of volumes of information—some of it is reliable.

We also encourage you to subscribe to an EMS journal. You will be able to read current news, clinical updates, and new ideas each month. Some journals provide continuing education (CE) opportunities.

We also encourage you to attend local, regional, state, and national EMS conferences. Your agency or a regional or state EMS agency will have additional information on these.

✳ **For information on the profession of EMS**—The National Registry of Emergency Medical Technicians *www.nremt.org*

✳ The National Association of Emergency Medical Technicians *www.naemt.org*

✳ **EMS Journals**—Journal of Emergency Medical Services (JEMS) *www.jems.com*

✳ EMS Magazine *www.emsmagazine.com*

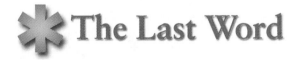 **The Last Word**

This is not the last Last Word you will see: Your training will never end.

EMS is full of opportunities for those who wish to embrace them. Be safe. Treat people well. Think critically. Have fun. **This is EMS.**

✳ Chapter Review

CRITICAL THINKING

This chapter has no formal review. No one will ask to see your homework. These questions are for you. Answering them and writing answers down will help you focus on what you want from EMS and how you may want to practice and further yourself.

1. Are you considering furthering your EMS education? If so, to what certification level?

   _____

   _____

   _____

   _____

2. What programs are available to you to further your EMS education?

   _____

   _____

   _____

   _____

3. How do you plan on maintaining and growing your knowledge and skills once you have been certified?

   _____

   _____

   _____

   _____

4. What EMS conferences are held in your local area, region, or state?

   _____

   _____

   _____

   _____

5. If you decided to move to a neighboring state, how would you obtain EMT certification or licensure there?

   _____

   _____

   _____

   _____

6. What do you think the best part of EMS will be for you?

_____

_____

_____

_____

7. What do you think will be the most challenging part of EMS for you?

_____

_____

_____

_____

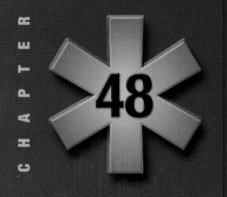

Module Review and Practice Examination

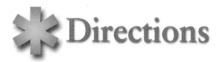 **Directions**

Assess what you have learned in this module by circling the best answer for each multiple-choice question. When you are done, check your answers against the key provided in Appendix D.

1. The boundaries of the upper airway are the:
   a. pharynx and carina.
   b. pharynx and larynx.
   c. nose and epiglottis.
   d. nose and carina.

2. The nasal turbinates serve to:
   a. filter particulate matter from the air entering the lungs.
   b. prevent aspiration of fluids into the nasal conchae.
   c. warm and humidify air entering the lungs.
   d. seal the oropharynx from the nasopharynx.

3. Compared to the insertion of airway adjuncts into the oral cavity, insertion of adjuncts into the nares carries an increased risk of:
   a. bleeding.
   b. infection.
   c. inducing a gag reflex.
   d. failed ventilation.

4. The laryngopharynx is also known as the:
   a. oropharynx.
   b. hypopharynx.
   c. glottis.
   d. soft palate.

5. The term "voice box" refers to the:
   a. glottis.
   b. conchae.
   c. larynx.
   d. carina.

6. Windpipe is the lay term for the:
   a. esophagus.
   b. trachea.
   c. larynx.
   d. bronchus.

7. Because of the difference between the right and left bronchi, the tip of an endotracheal tube that is inserted too far is most likely to end up in the:
   a. right mainstem bronchus.
   b. left mainstem bronchus.
   c. carina.
   d. trachea.

8. Which of the following is an anatomical difference of the pediatric airway, as compared to that of an adult?
   a. This tongue is proportionally smaller.
   b. The epiglottis is "V" shaped.
   c. The narrowest part of the airway is at the level of the cricoid cartilage.
   d. The nares are proportionally larger.

9. The shape of the pediatric airway can be compared to that of a/an:
   a. cylinder.
   b. rectangle.
   c. hexagon.
   d. inverted cone.

10. The division between the airway and digestive structures is at the level of the:
    a. laryngopharynx.
    b. nasopharynx.
    c. oropharynx.
    d. false pharynx.

11. A pediatric patient's airway differs from an adult's in all manner EXCEPT the following:
    a. The chest wall is softer.
    b. The widest area of the airway is the larynx.
    c. All structures are smaller.
    d. The trachea is softer and more flexible.

12. It is recommended to use the _____ _____ in determining the appropriate ET tube size for a child.
    a. ET cuff
    b. stylet wire
    c. ET tube
    d. Broselow tape

13. A manual maneuver in which the EMT presses the cricoid cartilage downward is called the _____ maneuver.
    a. BURP
    b. Sellick's
    c. ELM
    d. MacGyver

14. A manual maneuver in which the EMT presses the thyroid cartilage backward, toward the patient's right, and in the direction of the patient's jaw is called the _____ maneuver.
    a. BURP
    b. Sellick's
    c. ELM
    d. MacGyver

15. An instrument consisting of a blade and handle, used to visualize a patient's airway structures, is called a/an:
    a. ETT.
    b. laryngoscope.
    c. nasogastric tube.
    d. stylet.

16. When visualizing the airway, the tip of a curved blade is placed:
    a. in the vallecula.
    b. in the glottis.
    c. beneath the epiglottis.
    d. between the vocal cords.

17. The size of an endotracheal tube refers to its:
    a. length in centimeters.
    b. circumference in millimeters.
    c. internal diameter in millimeters.
    d. cuff volume in milliliters.

18. On the average, the correct size endotracheal tube for an adult female is between _____ and _____.
    a. 4.0; 5.0
    b. 5.5; 6.5
    c. 7.0; 8.0
    d. 8.0; 9.0

19. When referring to intubation equipment, a Macintosh blade is:
    a. straight.
    b. pointed.
    c. round.
    d. curved.

20. When referring to intubation equipment, a Miller blade is:
    a. straight.
    b. pointed.
    c. round.
    d. curved.

21. If the cuff of an endotracheal tube is overinflated once it is placed in the patient's trachea, it may result in:
    a. tracheal necrosis.
    b. obstruction of airflow through the tube.
    c. air leaking around the outside of the tube.
    d. ischemia of the vocal cords.

22. The BEST way to determine correct endotracheal tube size for a pediatric patient is:
    a. using the formula 16 plus the patient's age in years divided by 4.
    b. choosing a tube the same diameter as the patient's little finger.
    c. using a weight-based resuscitation tape, such as the Broselow tape.
    d. conferring with medical direction.

23. For an adult patient without suspected cervical spinal injury, the recommended head position for intubation is the _____ position.
    a. sniffing
    b. flexed
    c. Macintosh
    d. neutral

24. The laryngoscope is held in the EMT's
_____ hand and inserted from the
_____ side of the patient's mouth.
    a. left; left
    b. left; right
    c. right; right
    d. right; left

25. After the tip of the endotracheal tube passes
through the vocal cords during oral intubation,
the tube should be advanced until the:
    a. BVM adapter on the tube is flush with the
       patient's lips.
    b. 30 cm mark on the tube is at the level of
       the patient's teeth.
    c. resistance is felt.
    d. cuff just passes through the cords.

26. Placement of an endotracheal tube is first
checked by:
    a. auscultating the lungs and epigastrium.
    b. using an aspiration device.
    c. using an end-tidal carbon dioxide detector.
    d. pulse oximetry.

27. Which of the following statements is true
concerning securing a properly placed
endotracheal tube?
    a. The inflated cuff provides adequate
       stabilization of the tube.
    b. Only a commercial endotracheal tube
       securing device is appropriate.
    c. Either tape or a commercially available
       device may be used.
    d. Tape is the only acceptable means of
       securing an endotracheal tube.

28. The esophageal tracheal combitube is known
as a/an _____ airway device.
    a. dual lumen
    b. obturator
    c. visualized airway
    d. laryngeal mask

29. Which of the following statements regarding
an esophageal tracheal combitube is correct?
    a. It requires the use of a laryngoscope if
       tracheal placement is desired.
    b. It will work in either the trachea or the
       esophagus.
    c. It cannot be used in patients over 6'5" tall.
    d. It cannot be used in patients under 5'2" tall.

30. An endotracheal tube is most like a/an:
    a. laryngeal mask airway.
    b. combitube.
    c. nasogastric tube.
    d. lumen tube.

31. The LMA was originally intended for use in
which of the following settings?
    a. advanced prehospital life support
    b. basic prehospital life support
    c. in the operating room
    d. in doctors' offices

32. Which of the following is the most common
indication for placement of a nasogastric tube
in the prehospital setting?
    a. to ventilating the lungs via a nasally placed
       airway
    b. to serving as a rescue or back-up device for
       failed endotracheal intubation
    c. to serving as a route of medication
       administration
    d. to decompression of gastric air during
       prolonged BVM or removal of gastric
       contents

33. Which of the following describes the correct
measurement of a nasogastric tube?
    a. from the nose to the earlobe to a point half-
       way between the xiphoid process and the
       umbilicus
    b. from the nose to the earlobe
    c. from the nose to a point half-way between
       the xiphoid process and the umbilicus
    d. from the corner of the mouth to the earlobe

34. Ideally, the patient will be in a _____
position for insertion of a nasogastric tube.
    a. supine
    b. sitting upright
    c. prone
    d. left lateral recumbent

35. When the tip of a nasogastric tube is placed in
the nostril, it is directed:
    a. superiorly.
    b. posteriorly.
    c. inferiorly.
    d. medially.

36. When a nasogastric tube is being inserted, the
patient should be instructed to:
    a. swallow.
    b. breathe deeply.
    c. hold his breath.
    d. cough.

37. The placement of a nasogastric tube is checked by:
    a. injecting normal saline through the tube.
    b. injecting warm water through the tube.
    c. attaching the tube to high suction.
    d. injecting air through the tube.

38. The most reliable method of confirming endotracheal tube placement is:
    a. pulse oximetry.
    b. end-tidal carbon dioxide monitoring.
    c. seeing the tube pass between the vocal cords.
    d. using a commercial aspiration device.

39. If an endotracheal tube is placed in the esophagus and this is not recognized by the EMT, the patient will:
    a. develop pneumonia.
    b. die.
    c. receive half the normal amount of oxygen.
    d. receive oxygen but not be able to eliminate carbon dioxide.

40. Upon auscultating the lungs of an intubated patient, you hear breath sounds on the right but not on the left. Before intubation, breath sounds were present on both sides. The most likely cause for this is:
    a. laceration of the trachea by the endotracheal tube.
    b. placement of the endotracheal tube in the esophagus.
    c. placement of the endotracheal tube in the right mainstem bronchus.
    d. placement of the endotracheal tube in the left mainstem bronchus.

41. Upon checking placement of an endotracheal tube, you hear bubbling sounds over the epigastrium. This indicates:
    a. correct placement.
    b. placement in the left mainstem bronchus.
    c. placement in the esophagus.
    d. placement in the right mainstem bronchus.

42. Pulse oximetry allows determination of:
    a. saturation of arterial blood with oxygen.
    b. saturation of venous blood with oxygen.
    c. the amount of carbon dioxide present in the blood.
    d. the amount of hemoglobin in the blood.

43. The presence of which of the following in the blood may lead to a falsely high pulse oximetry reading?
    a. carbon dioxide
    b. cyanide gas
    c. carbon monoxide
    d. nitrogen gas

44. Pulse oximetry works by detecting:
    a. the true percentage of oxygen in the blood.
    b. the true pressure of oxygen gas in the blood.
    c. the precise amount of hemoglobin in the blood.
    d. the amount of light that passes through the capillary beds.

45. The measurement of carbon dioxide in a patient's exhaled air is called:
    a. oximetry.
    b. capnography.
    c. pulmonary function testing.
    d. spectrometry.

46. The primary use of an end-tidal carbon dioxide detector in the prehospital setting is to:
    a. determine the quality of bag-valve-mask ventilations.
    b. differentiate between the use of an endotracheal tube and nonvisualized (blindly inserted) airways.
    c. distinguish between endotracheal and esophageal intubation.
    d. determine whether or not a patient can be resuscitated.

47. A colorimetric end-tidal carbon dioxide detector uses:
    a. infrared light.
    b. a temperature sensor.
    c. a humidity sensor.
    d. pH sensitive paper.

48. An end-tidal carbon dioxide detector should NOT be considered reliable in:
    a. patients in cardiac arrest.
    b. patients who are spontaneously breathing.
    c. patients being ventilated by automatic transport ventilators.
    d. any patient.

49. An esophageal detector device works on the principle that:
    a. air does not enter the stomach if the esophagus is intubated.
    b. the esophagus collapses under suction.
    c. the trachea collapses under suction.
    d. air cannot be pulled from the lungs with a syringe.

50. After attaching a compressed bulb-type esophageal detector device to an endotracheal tube that is properly placed, the EMT should expect the bulb to:
    a. remain compressed.
    b. alternately compress and reinflate.
    c. reinflate.
    d. resist negative pressure.

Final Practice Review

MODULE 1

1. Which of the following levels of EMS responder is nationally recognized by the DOT?
   a. First Responder
   b. Cardiac Technician
   c. Advanced Paramedic
   d. Paramedic Specialist

2. EMS personnel staffing the ambulance must be trained to at least the level of:
   a. CPR certification.
   b. paramedic.
   c. cardiac technician.
   d. EMT-Basic.

3. Which of the following components of an EMS system is demonstrated by EMS providers giving training classes and information in their communities?
   a. health education and screening
   b. citizen education resources
   c. public information and education
   d. medical direction

4. The survivor of a disaster experiences an emotional reaction a year after the event. This is an example of a/an _____ stress response.
   a. delayed
   b. atypical
   c. cumulative
   d. tardy

5. In which of the following situations should an EMT wear a HEPA mask?
   a. responding to a hazardous materials incident
   b. caring for a patient with suspected tuberculosis
   c. reporting for duty with a cold, flu, or other respiratory infection
   d. caring for a patient who is spitting at the EMS providers

6. Which of the following is an example of expressed patient consent for treatment?
   a. EMTs treat an unresponsive patient, assuming the patient would consent if she were able.
   b. A patient meets the ambulance at the curb and gets in when the door is opened.
   c. EMTs are unable to contact the parents of a minor prior to transporting the patient.
   d. All of the above.

7. Which of the following patients can be treated under implied consent?
   a. a 22-year-old woman who is confused after hitting her head on the ground during a football game
   b. a 45-year-old man with chest pain who states he smoked some marijuana an hour ago
   c. an 18-year-old high school student who was injured in a motor vehicle collision
   d. a 75-year-old man who knows his name and where he is but is not sure of the day of the week and is complaining of abdominal pain

8. You have just arrived on the scene of a 16-year-old female who reportedly took an overdose of over-the-counter medications. Her eyes are closed and she is not responding to verbal stimuli from bystanders. Your partner believes the patient is just trying to get attention and is not truly unresponsive. He says to you, "Watch this. This will teach her a lesson." He then pinches the patient's arm hard enough to leave a bruise. This constitutes:
   a. battery.
   b. assault.
   c. damages.
   d. abandonment.

9. The primary function of platelets is to:
   a. help blood clot.
   b. carry oxygen.
   c. carry carbon dioxide.
   d. detoxify waste products.

10. The skull is made up of the:
    a. cranium and scalp.
    b. cranium and face.
    c. carpals and metacarpals.
    d. carpals and ilium.

11. Which of the following is a characteristic of a child's airway anatomy when compared to that of an adult?
    a. The tongue is proportionally smaller.
    b. The trachea is rigid and inflexible.
    c. Children primarily use their intercostal muscles to breathe.
    d. The cricoid cartilage is less well-developed.

12. The valve that separates the left atrium from the left ventricle is the _____ valve.
    a. mitral.
    b. tricuspid.
    c. pulmonic.
    d. bilateral.

13. Another word for epinephrine is:
    a. insulin.
    b. glucose.
    c. adrenalin.
    d. bile.

14. You are on the scene of a one-car motor vehicle collision. The vehicle is wedged against a tree at the driver's door. The driver is unresponsive with inadequate respirations. The front seat passenger is alert and oriented with minor complaints, but you cannot get to the driver without first moving the passenger. Which of the following is appropriate in moving the passenger?
    a. emergent move
    b. urgent move
    c. non-urgent move
    d. elective move

15. You have responded to the home of a 60-year-old male who is complaining of nausea and diarrhea and says he gets lightheaded when he stands up. The patient weighs about 350 pounds. The last time you called for assistance in lifting a patient, the responding crew got very upset with you and your partner. Which is the best course of action?
    a. Tell the patient you will help him walk to the ambulance and that if he gets lightheaded, to let you know so he can sit down and rest.
    b. Call for help and deal with the other crew's reaction later if they are upset about it.
    c. Make the patient comfortable on the cot, then, using good communication and body mechanics lift the cot with your partner's assistance.
    d. See if you can find a neighbor or family member to help lift the patient.

MODULE 2

16. The function of the epiglottis is to:
    a. allow food to pass from the pharynx to the stomach.
    b. keep air flowing into the trachea during swallowing.
    c. make the trachea more rigid.
    d. prevent food and liquids from entering the trachea.

17. Respiratory failure is best defined as:
    a. the use of accessory muscles during breathing.
    b. a sensation of shortness of breath.
    c. the inability of the body to compensate for illness or injury, resulting in an inadequate supply of oxygen to the body.
    d. constriction of the bronchioles, resulting in wheezing and coughing.

18. "See-saw" respirations are a sign of respiratory failure that is specific to:
    a. elderly patients.
    b. infants.
    c. very obese patients.
    d. patients with well-developed chest and abdominal muscles.

19. Your patient is a 7-year-old male. You should consider his respiratory rate normal if it is _____ per minute.
    a. 60
    b. 48
    c. 28
    d. 12

20. Which of the following is a disadvantage of mouth-to-mask ventilation?
    a. inadequate volume of ventilation
    b. low delivered oxygen concentration
    c. requires extensive training
    d. difficult to maintain an adequate seal by one rescuer

21. Your patient is an elderly male who is unresponsive and has snoring respirations. The first step in correcting this is:
    a. placing a pillow under his head to flex the neck.
    b. inserting an oropharyngeal airway.
    c. suctioning the mouth and pharynx.
    d. using a head-tilt chin-lift maneuver.

22. Your patient is suspected of taking an overdose of sleeping pills. He is snoring. Which of the following is most likely responsible for this noise?
    a. There is fluid in his lungs.
    b. He has vomited and has fluid in his pharynx.
    c. His tongue is obstructing his airway.
    d. His dentures are obstructing his airway.

23. When suctioning an adult patient's mouth, suction should be applied for no more than _____ seconds.
    a. 5
    b. 10
    c. 15
    d. 20

24. When suctioning the mouth of an infant, suction should be applied for no more than _____ seconds.
    a. 5
    b. 10
    c. 15
    d. 20

25. Which of the following is the correct sequence for suctioning a patient's mouth?
    1. Activate suction on the suction unit.
    2. Place the tip of the catheter in the mouth.
    3. Take BSI precautions.
    4. Cover the side opening of the suction catheter.
    5. Remove the suction tip from the mouth.
    6. Connect the suction catheter to the suction tubing.
    a. 3, 6, 1, 4, 2, 5
    b. 6, 1, 3, 2, 4, 5
    c. 3, 6, 1, 2, 4, 5
    d. 1, 6, 3, 2, 5, 4

26. Which of the following steps are required for nasal suctioning of an adult patient but not for oral suctioning?
    1. Take BSI precautions.
    2. Measure the catheter from the tip of the nose to the earlobe.
    3. Use a water-based lubricant on the suction catheter.
    4. Suction for no more than 15 seconds.
    a. 1, 3
    b. 2, 3
    c. 1, 3, 4
    d. 1, 4

27. A bulb syringe is the device of choice for:
    a. oropharyngeal suctioning of an adult patient.
    b. clearing food, teeth, or other solid objects from the airway.
    c. suctioning the mouth and nose of infants.
    d. inflating the large balloon of a Combitube.

28. Which of the following statements regarding oropharyngeal airways is true?
    a. They must not be used in patients with facial or head trauma.
    b. They eliminate the need for manually opening the airway.
    c. They must never be used in patients with a gag reflex.
    d. They must not be used in patients under 12 years old.

29. The proper way to measure an oropharyngeal airway is from the _____ to the _____.
    a. tip of the nose; earlobe
    b. nostril; earlobe
    c. corner of the mouth; angle of the jaw
    d. center of the mouth; earlobe

30. You are attempting to deliver ventilations to your patient with a bag-valve-mask device, but there is significant resistance to airflow. Which of the following should you immediately do?
    a. Suction the patient's airway.
    b. Remove the oropharyngeal airway you have inserted and replace it with a different size.
    c. Check manual positioning of the airway.
    d. Perform abdominal thrusts.

31. The preferred technique of ventilating a patient is:
    a. one-rescuer bag-valve-mask.
    b. two-rescuer bag-valve-mask.
    c. demand-valve device.
    d. mouth-to-mask.

32. The best device for ventilating through a stoma is a/an:
    a. nonrebreather mask and high-flow oxygen.
    b. Combitube and bag-valve device.
    c. bag-valve-mask device using an infant mask.
    d. oxygen-powered mechanical ventilator using oxygen tubing inserted directly into the stoma.

MODULE 3

33. The best way to protect yourself and your crew from hazards at a scene is:
    a. performing a scene size-up.
    b. always responding with a crew of at least three EMS providers.
    c. wearing body armor.
    d. refusing to respond without law enforcement escort.

34. You should not call for additional resources at a scene until you:
    a. are absolutely certain you need them.
    b. arrive at the scene and begin your scene size-up.
    c. perform a complete assessment of all patients.
    d. consult with medical direction.

35. Which of the following is a patient symptom?
    a. nausea
    b. a deformed extremity
    c. low blood pressure
    d. a laceration

36. Which of the following is a patient sign?
    a. dizziness
    b. nausea
    c. pale skin
    d. itching

37. Trending is best described as:
    a. keeping up on the latest knowledge and skills in EMS.
    b. following a fad in patient treatment without consulting medical control.
    c. a cluster of signs and symptoms related to a specific type of medical problem.
    d. comparing each set of patient vital signs to the sets before it.

38. A patient who breathes 6 times in a 30-second period has a respiratory rate of:
    a. 6.
    b. 12.
    c. 18.
    d. 24.

39. The amount of air that moves in and out of the lungs with each respiration is the _____ volume.
    a. tidal
    b. minute
    c. resting
    d. lung

40. When assessing the pulse of an unresponsive adult, the preferred site is the _____ artery, located in/on the _____.
    a. brachial; neck
    b. radial; wrist
    c. femoral; groin
    d. carotid; neck

41. Blood pressure should be assessed in all patients _____ old or older.
    a. 6 months
    b. 1 year
    c. 3 years
    d. 5 years

42. Which of the following best describes systolic blood pressure?
    a. the reading on the blood pressure gauge when the first sound is heard through the stethoscope as the blood pressure cuff is deflated
    b. the difference between the top number of the blood pressure reading and the bottom number of the blood pressure reading
    c. the reading on the blood pressure gauge when sounds are no longer heard though the stethoscope as the blood pressure cuff is deflated
    d. the lower pressure exerted against arterial walls when the heart is relaxed between contractions

43. Jaundice is best described as:
    a. redness or flushing of the skin.
    b. blueish discoloration of the skin due to poor oxygenation.
    c. yellowish discoloration of the skin.
    d. black, blue, or purple discoloration of the skin due to bruising.

44. When the pupils are described as "dilated," this means they:
    a. are larger than normal.
    b. do not react to light.
    c. are unequal in size.
    d. are smaller than normal.

45. When caring for a patient with significant trauma, the scene time should be kept to a maximum of _____ minutes.
    a. 5
    b. 10
    c. 15
    d. 30

46. Which of the following is NOT performed during the rapid trauma assessment?
    a. taking vital signs
    b. checking the chest for deformities
    c. checking the patient's back for significant injuries
    d. assessing for potentially life-threatening injuries

47. Your patient is a 48-year-old female with pain in the right lower quadrant of her abdomen. Which of the following is the best approach to the assessment and history of this patient?
    a. Perform a rapid physical examination followed by a medical history.
    b. Perform a thorough head-to-toe examination, then obtain a SAMPLE history.
    c. Obtain a medical history and then perform a focused physical examination.
    d. Perform an initial assessment and obtain a history, but defer further assessment to the physician at the emergency department.

48. Which of the following best describes a portable radio?
    a. It is carried by the EMT.
    b. It is mounted in the ambulance.
    c. It is located on a tower to receive and amplify radio signals.
    d. It is used only by ALS personnel to send ECG signals to the physician at the hospital.

49. A patient care report in which events and observations are recorded in the order that they occurred best describes the _____ method of documentation.
    a. SOAP
    b. chronological
    c. CHART
    d. physiological

MODULE 4

50. Which of the following best describes the trade name of a drug?
    a. the name that describes the elemental make up of the drug
    b. the name used in the United States Pharmacopeia to reference the drug
    c. the name used by all companies that market the drug
    d. the name given the drug by the company that first markets it

51. Which of the following medications would have its effect most quickly?
    a. a subcutaneous injection of epinephrine
    b. oral glucose gel
    c. a Tylenol tablet
    d. a puff of albuterol

52. Which of the following best describes contraindications of a drug?
    a. unwanted effects of the drug
    b. reasons why the drug should be given
    c. the desired effects of the drug
    d. reasons why someone should NOT be given a drug

53. The name of a drug that describes its composition is its _____ name.
    a. chemical
    b. official
    c. trade
    d. generic

54. A dangerous side effect of nitroglycerin is that it can cause:
    a. constriction of the coronary arteries.
    b. a drop in blood pressure.
    c. psychotic behavior.
    d. blood clots.

55. For which of the following situations would you most likely receive an order to administer activated charcoal?
    a. a patient who has a known allergy to bees and has just been stung by a bee
    b. a diabetic who has taken his insulin but did not eat lunch
    c. a patient who took an overdose of seizure medications within the last 30 minutes
    d. a patient complaining of chest pain who has a prescription for the drug

56. Asthma is characterized by:
    a. air trapped in the lungs due to breakdown of the walls of the alveoli.
    b. constriction of the small airways leading to the alveoli.
    c. chronic increased mucus production and cough due to smoking.
    d. pockets of pus in the lungs due to bacterial infection.

57. Aspiration is best described as:
    a. drawing air into the lungs during normal breathing.
    b. inhaling foreign material, such as liquids, into the lungs.
    c. air leaving the lungs during breathing.
    d. a fine spray of medication administered into the lungs.

58. Which of the following devices delivers tiny droplets of respiratory medication through a mask or mouthpiece over an extended period of time?
    a. nebulizer
    b. inhaler
    c. aspirator
    d. vaporizer

59. A pulse oximetry reading of below _____ percent indicates severe hypoxia.
    a. 98
    b. 95
    c. 92
    d. 90

60. Cheyne-Stokes respirations are characterized by:
    a. regular, deep, rapid respirations.
    b. alternating cycles of very deep respirations followed by shallow respirations and a period of apnea.
    c. an irregular, chaotic pattern.
    d. shallow, gasping respirations.

61. Fine, crackling sounds in the lungs indicate the presence of which of the following?
    a. thick mucus in the bronchi
    b. swelling in the upper airway
    c. fluid in the alveoli
    d. narrowing of the bronchioles

62. You have just assisted a patient with the use of an albuterol inhaler. Upon reassessing the vital signs, you note the pulse rate has increased from 92 to 112. The patient's hands are shaking, but she is alert and her respiratory rate has decreased from 44 to 30. Which of the following is most likely?
    a. The patient received an adequate dose of the medication.
    b. The patient is becoming hypoxic.
    c. You are making the patient nervous.
    d. She is having an allergic reaction to the medication.

63. A myocardial infarction is a:
    a. cardiac arrest.
    b. heart failure.
    c. heart attack.
    d. stroke.

64. Which of the following is a contraindication for the administration of nitroglycerin to a patient with chest pain?
    a. The patient took Cialis earlier in the day.
    b. The blood pressure is 130/90.
    c. The patient took a nitroglycerin tablet before you arrived.
    d. All of the above.

65. The circulation of well-oxygenated blood to the cells of the body is known as:
    a. perfusion.
    b. metabolism.
    c. distribution.
    d. exchange.

66. Defibrillation is designed to work in which of the following situations?
    a. There is no electrical activity in the heart.
    b. There is chaotic electrical activity in the heart.
    c. The patient is having chest pain.
    d. The patient has an irregular pulse.

67. Most automatic defibrillators are programmed to deliver _____ shock(s) during the first cycle.
    a. 1
    b. 2
    c. 3
    d. 4

68. Prior to being diagnosed, a patient with diabetes will most likely have which of the following conditions?
    a. hyperglycemia
    b. hypoglycemia
    c. diabetic coma
    d. insulin effect

69. A blood clot in, or rupture of, a blood vessel in the brain leading to signs and symptoms such as headache, paralysis, and slurred speech best describes:
    a. seizure.
    b. myocardial infarction.
    c. epilepsy.
    d. stroke.

70. Your patient is a 40-year-old female who is allergic to shellfish. Immediately after eating some stew at a friend's house, she experienced swelling of her face, severe difficulty breathing, lightheadedness, and low blood pressure. This is most likely:
    a. a mild allergic reaction.
    b. hives.
    c. anaphylaxis.
    d. food poisoning.

71. It is a cold morning, but it is clear and there is no wind. Your patient is a 48-year-old male found lying on the frozen ground without a coat. He is losing heat due to:
    a. conduction and radiation.
    b. evaporation and conduction.
    c. convection and evaporation.
    d. convection and radiation.

72. Your patient was hiking in the desert and was bitten on the ankle by a rattlesnake. Which of the following is most appropriate?
    a. Keep the foot lower than the level of the patient's heart.
    b. Elevate the foot on pillows.
    c. Apply a tourniquet above the bite.
    d. Apply ice to the area of the bite.

73. Your patient is a 22-year-old female who is breathing rapidly, clutching her chest, and begging you not to let her die. Her roommate tells you that the patient has a history of panic attacks. Which of the following is an appropriate approach to the patient?
    a. Look the patient directly in the eye and say, "You need to get ahold of yourself. There's no reason for you to be panicked."
    b. Stand back from the patient and ask whether or not she wants to go to the hospital.
    c. Get on the patient's level and say, "I'm an EMT with the ambulance service. Let's see what we can do to help you."
    d. Place your hand on the patient's shoulder and let her know that EMTs aren't trained to handle psychiatric problems and that she should contact her psychiatrist.

74. You have just assisted with the delivery of a full-term infant. You have suctioned his mouth and nose and have clamped and cut the cord, but the infant is not breathing. Which of the following should you do first?
    a. Insert an oropharyngeal airway and ventilate the patient with a bag-valve-mask.
    b. Rub his back.
    c. Perform mouth-to-mask ventilations.
    d. Administer high-flow oxygen.

MODULE 5

75. The aorta is best described as:
    a. a large vein in the neck.
    b. an artery in the chest and abdomen.
    c. the largest vein in the body.
    d. a large artery in the groin.

76. Which of the following factors affects the severity of blood loss and the signs and symptoms associated with it?
    a. rate of bleeding
    b. amount of blood loss
    c. size of the patient
    d. all of the above

77. Your patient has cut her hand with a knife and has bright red bleeding that seems to be pumping out under pressure. This is most likely _____ bleeding.
    a. venous
    b. capillary
    c. arterial
    d. mixed venous and capillary

78. Your patient is a 12-year-old male who cut his anterior elbow when he ran through a glass door with his arms outstretched. The patient is bleeding severely. You have tried direct pressure without success. Which of the following is the correct sequence of next steps?
    a. elevation, pressure on the brachial artery, and tourniquet
    b. elevation, pressure on the popliteal artery, and tourniquet
    c. pressure on the radial artery, tourniquet, and elevation
    d. pressure on the brachial artery, elevation, and tourniquet

79. Shock is best described as:
    a. hypoperfusion.
    b. low blood pressure.
    c. bleeding.
    d. internal hemorrhage.

80. Which of the following statements about shock is true?
    a. Once a patient is in shock, death is inevitable.
    b. Shock is progressive without intervention.
    c. Definitive treatment for the patient in shock is high-flow oxygen.
    d. All blood loss leads to shock.

81. Crush-force trauma would most likely occur in which of the following situations?
    a. A hunter is accidentally shot in the back with an arrow.
    b. A soldier steps on a land mine.
    c. A man falls from a fifth floor balcony onto a parked car below.
    d. A construction worker is pinned by a forklift that rolled over on his legs.

82. Your patient is a 32-year-old male motorcycle rider who struck a parked vehicle and was thrown over the handlebars of the motorcycle. He has contusions on both thighs from contact with the handlebars as he was ejected. Which of the following best explains why you should be concerned with this finding?
    a. The patient is likely experiencing a crush injury.
    b. It indicates the patient is at risk for shock.
    c. Contusions are extremely painful.
    d. The wounds may become contaminated if not properly dressed and bandaged.

83. The purpose of a dressing is to:
    a. cover a wound to control bleeding and prevent contamination.
    b. prevent motion of an injured extremity.
    c. relieve pain and reduce swelling.
    d. hold gauze pads in place over a wound.

84. Partial-thickness burns are characterized by:
    a. redness and swelling.
    b. blisters.
    c. charring.
    d. white, leathery appearance.

85. Your patient is a 15-month-old male who pulled a deep-fryer full of hot oil off a counter top. He has burns to his entire head, face, neck, and anterior torso. The percentage of body surface area involved is:
    a. 9.
    b. 18.
    c. 24.
    d. 27.

86. Burns are considered more serious if they affect which of the following body parts?
    a. chest
    b. arm
    c. hand
    d. leg

87. Your patient is a 25-year-old male who was soldering two pieces of metal together when the soldering gun slipped and created a full-thickness burn about the size of a pencil eraser on his forearm. This burn would be considered:
    a. severe.
    b. intense.
    c. moderate.
    d. mild.

88. Your patient is a factory-worker whose face was splashed with an acid. Which of the following is most appropriate?
    a. Transport him to the hospital for proper decontamination.
    b. Blot the acid away with a sterile towel before flushing with large amounts of water.
    c. Wipe the chemical away with a damp cloth.
    d. Find an antidote to the chemical and apply it to the affected areas.

89. Which of the following statements concerning electrical burns is true?
    a. The greatest risk with electrical burns is thermal burns to a large percentage of body surface area.
    b. Electrical burns can be associated with cardiac and respiratory problems.
    c. Exposure to electrical current does not cause a burn on entry, but causes massive burns where it exits the body.
    d. Electricity generally travels across the skin rather than internally through the body.

90. Your patient is a 15-year-old male who received partial-thickness burns to 50 percent of his body and full-thickness burns to 20 percent of his body. Which of the following should be your greatest concern in the immediate care of this patient?
    a. hypothermia
    b. blood loss
    c. infection
    d. heart failure

91. The pleural layers and the fluid between them are important in providing:
    a. suction between the chest wall and lungs.
    b. friction between the chest wall and lungs.
    c. trapped air in the thorax.
    d. protection from blunt trauma.

92. The EMT should consider an injury to the chest at the level of the eighth rib to be:
    a. a chest injury.
    b. an abdominal injury.
    c. both a chest and an abdominal injury.
    d. unlikely to cause serious chest or abdominal injury.

93. An adult male patient stabbed in the left anterior chest at the nipple-level just next to his sternum with a knife that has a 3-inch blade would be LEAST likely to have injury to his:
    a. kidney.
    b. heart
    c. liver.
    d. bronchus.

94. A flail chest is characterized by:
    a. two or more consecutive ribs each fractured in two or more places.
    b. a collapsed lung.
    c. air entering the pleural cavity through an open wound in the chest wall.
    d. an accumulation of blood in the pleural cavity.

95. The primary concerns with damage to hollow organs of the abdomen are:
    a. irritation of the peritoneum and infection.
    b. bleeding and hemorrhagic shock.
    c. swelling and pain.
    d. vomiting and diarrhea.

96. Which of the following is the best example of injury caused by indirect force?
    a. The driver of a small truck strikes his knees on the dash in a frontal collision and suffers a fractured femur.
    b. An elderly male has bone cancer. He coughs and sustains a fracture of a thoracic vertebra.
    c. A football player has his foot planted when he is struck by another player, causing him to rotate around the planted foot, resulting in a fracture to his tibia and fibula.
    d. A police officer is shot in the thigh with a large caliber projectile that fractures his femur.

97. Overstretching a muscle results in a:
   a. fracture.
   b. strain.
   c. sprain.
   d. dislocation.

98. Your patient is a 30-year-old female who slipped on a wet floor and fell, injuring her wrist. The most appropriate approach to this patient is a:
   a. detailed history and physical examination.
   b. rapid trauma exam.
   c. focused history and assessment.
   d. detailed history and focused assessment.

99. For which of the following patients would a rapid trauma assessment be appropriate?
   a. 40-year-old female who stepped off a curb, twisted her ankle, and fell to her knees.
   b. 9-year-old male who fell 15 feet from a tree house and has a deformed right arm.
   c. 75-year-old female who stood up from her chair, felt a "snap" in her hip, and fell back into the chair.
   d. 7-year-old female who has a deformed forearm after performing a cartwheel in gymnastics class.

100. Which of the following does NOT adequately explain the purpose of splinting a swollen, painful, deformed extremity?
   a. Splinting reduces pain associated with movement.
   b. It makes the patient feel as if you are doing something for him but it serves little medical purpose.
   c. Bleeding can be reduced by splinting.
   d. Stabilizing bone ends reduces the possibility of further tissue damage.

101. Your patient has a swollen, deformed, painful wrist. A properly applied splint should start at the patient's _____ and extend to _____.
   a. hand; just below the elbow
   b. fingers; just above the elbow
   c. hand; the shoulder
   d. wrist; the shoulder

102. A traction splint is designed to be used for which of the following injuries?
   a. open fractures of the tibia
   b. deformed mid-shaft humerus fractures
   c. injuries to the knee
   d. suspected femur fractures

103. A swathe is a useful adjunct to a sling in splinting which of the following injuries?
   a. dislocated shoulder
   b. fractured pelvis
   c. suspected femur fracture
   d. a swollen, deformed, painful finger

104. Your patient is a 12-year-old boy who fell 20 feet from a tree house to the ground. He is sitting up with his back against the tree, crying. He has a badly deformed humerus. Your priority in caring for this patient is:
    a. checking the distal circulation, sensation, and motor function.
    b. immobilizing the injured part.
    c. minimizing the patient's pain.
    d. assessing for and managing life-threatening conditions.

105. The floor of the cranial vault is described as the _____ skull.
    a. frontal
    b. basilar
    c. occipital
    d. parietal

106. The weakest area of the skull is/are the _____ bone(s).
    a. maxillary
    b. temporal
    c. parietal
    d. occipital

107. Of the following, the highest priority in the care of the trauma patient is:
    a. controlling bleeding.
    b. determining the mechanism of injury.
    c. providing manual stabilization of the cervical spine.
    d. ensuring an open airway.

108. The cervical vertebrae are located:
    a. in the back at the level of the ribs.
    b. in the neck.
    c. at the very base of the spine.
    d. at the level of the pelvis.

109. The first step in proper spinal immobilization is:
    a. manual stabilization of the head and neck.
    b. placing a properly sized cervical collar.
    c. using a short spinal immobilization device.
    d. logrolling the patient onto a long spine board.

110. Your patient is a 21-year-old female driver who was involved in a significant lateral-impact collision. She denies neck pain and is stable, but she is crying, she says she is cold, and it is taking you too long to get her into the ambulance. Which of the following is the most appropriate action?
    a. Use rapid extrication to get her out of the vehicle.
    b. Use a short spinal immobilization device, then remove her from the vehicle onto a long backboard.
    c. Contact medical direction for permission to skip spinal immobilization.
    d. Place the long backboard on the stretcher and have the patient place herself on it.

MODULE 6

111. When a pediatric patient suffers cardiac arrest, it is most often due to:
    a. a respiratory problem.
    b. a birth defect.
    c. poisoning.
    d. electrical shock.

112. Which of the following is included in the pediatric assessment triangle?
    a. observing the safety of the environment
    b. general appearance of the patient
    c. parents' reaction to the child's condition
    d. pupillary reaction

113. Which of the following statements concerning respiratory emergencies in pediatric patients is true?
    a. Pediatric patients gradually decompensate, providing warning of impending respiratory failure.
    b. The presence of nasal flaring is unlikely to occur in the pediatric patient in respiratory distress.
    c. Grunting with exhalation is a sign of respiratory distress in pediatric patients.
    d. Respiratory distress is always accompanied by cyanosis in the pediatric patient.

114. Which of the following devices is preferred for nasal suctioning of an infant?
    a. bulb syringe
    b. 30 mL medicine syringe
    c. flexible suction catheter
    d. rigid suction tip

115. Your patient is a 16-month-old female whose grandmother gave her some canned peaches for lunch. The patient started choking while eating and is now limp and pale with cyanotic lips. Her respiratory effort is ineffective. Which of the following is appropriate for this patient?
    a. Place her across your lap and perform back blows.
    b. Alternate back blows and chest thrusts.
    c. Perform abdominal thrusts.
    d. Perform a finger sweep if you cannot see the obstruction.

116. The most common cause of trauma in children is:
    a. falls.
    b. motor vehicle crashes.
    c. child abuse.
    d. recreational injuries.

117. Which of the following is NOT a factor in the increased risk of hypothermia in the pediatric population?
    a. less body fat
    b. greater body surface area
    c. few glucose reserves
    d. slower metabolism

118. A gastrostomy tube is used to:
    a. drain excessive cerebrospinal fluid from the skull into the abdomen.
    b. provide a means of mechanical ventilation through an opening in the neck.
    c. provide nutrition to a patient who cannot eat or swallow.
    d. provide access to the central circulation for the administration of medications.

119. Medically, patients over the age of 65 are referred to as:
    a. old.
    b. geriatric.
    c. seniors.
    d. mature.

120. Which of the following changes occurs with aging?
    a. The body is less able to detect changes in oxygen levels.
    b. The body is more sensitive to changes in carbon dioxide levels.
    c. Lung capacity increases.
    d. All of the above.

121. The elderly may not be as well able to compensate for blood loss due to which of the following factors?
    a. taking medications to prevent stroke or heart attack
    b. decreased number of cilia
    c. increased elasticity of the heart
    d. all of the above

122. Which of the following is a normal age-related change in the nervous system?
    a. increased sensitivity of the skin
    b. decreased motor reaction time
    c. inability to learn new things
    d. altered sleep patterns

123. Your 85-year-old female patient is obviously short of breath but is refusing to be transported to the hospital. Which of the following should you do FIRST?
    a. Find out if a family member has power of attorney to consent to the patient's transport.
    b. Contact medical direction for advice.
    c. Find out why the patient does not want to go the hospital.
    d. Have the patient sign a refusal of treatment and transport form.

MODULE 7

124. NIMS is best described as:
    a. a consistent nation-wide approach in responding to events requiring coordinated public safety response.
    b. a multiple casualty incident.
    c. EMS personnel "freelancing" at the scene of an emergency.
    d. a designated disaster medical response team.

125. Any substance or material that poses an unreasonable risk to health, safety, and property is a/an:
    a. chemical substance.
    b. hazardous material.
    c. inert matter.
    d. vapor compound.

126. Substances stored in stationary tanks and facilities, such as at swimming pools, are marked using a system known as:
    a. DOT placards.
    b. Emergency Response Guides.
    c. NFPA 704.
    d. U.S. Radiologic Survey.

127. You have noted a diamond-shaped sign on a storage tank behind a hospital. The top quadrant of the diamond contains the number 1. This means the substance stored inside the tank poses a/an:
    a. extreme risk of fire.
    b. low risk of fire.
    c. extreme risk of explosion.
    d. low risk of explosion.

128. You have noted a diamond-shaped sign on a storage tank at a farm supply company. The bottom quadrant of the diamond contains a letter "W" with a line through it. This means:
    a. the tank contains an inert substance.
    b. the tank contains a dry substance rather than a liquid or wet substance.
    c. the tank contains an oxidizer.
    d. mixing water with this substance creates a hazard.

129. The diamond-shaped symbol on a transportation container, such as a tanker truck, is called a:
    a. bill of lading.
    b. placard.
    c. hazard notice.
    d. material safety data sheet.

130. Employers must keep paperwork on all potentially hazardous substances in the workplace called:
    a. material safety data sheets.
    b. placards.
    c. manifests.
    d. ORM-Ds.

131. The blue quadrant of an NFPA diamond contains information about a substance's:
    a. special considerations.
    b. health risks.
    c. fire hazard.
    d. explosive potential.

132. You have been dispatched to a railroad yard for a "sick person." On your arrival, you note that there are three individuals on the ground next to a tank car. Using binoculars to inspect the tank, you should compare the information you find to that found in the:
    a. Emergency Response Guidebook.
    b. hazmat manual.
    c. bill of lading.
    d. material safety data sheet.

133. Under what circumstances is it permissible for an EMT to approach a hazardous materials scene?
    a. The EMT is a firefighter and is wearing turnout gear.
    b. The EMT is trained as a hazardous materials technician and is wearing SCBA.
    c. The EMT is trained at the hazardous materials awareness level and is wearing a HEPA mask.
    d. The EMT has immediate access to a decontamination shower upon leaving the area.

134. A flammable solid is considered a DOT hazard class:
    a. 1.
    b. 2.
    c. 3.
    d. 4.

135. DOT hazard class 9 indicates:
    a. flammable liquids.
    b. explosives.
    c. miscellaneous dangerous goods.
    d. corrosives.

136. Situations calling for wilderness search and rescue, water rescue, rope rescue, and other types of events requiring special training and equipment are called _____ rescue situations.
    a. USAR
    b. operational
    c. tactical
    d. technical

137. The first phase of a rescue operation is:
    a. gaining access to the patient.
    b. preparing for the rescue.
    c. sizing up the situation.
    d. providing initial patient assessment.

138. Devices placed under the deflated tires of a vehicle to stabilize it are called:
    a. cribbing.
    b. props.
    c. jacks.
    d. buttresses.

139. You are not able to access a patient entrapped in a motor vehicle following a collision without the use of equipment. This is known as _____ access.
    a. complex
    b. intricate
    c. easy
    d. simple

140. When responding to a victim of a deep-water diving emergency, you should keep in mind the location of the nearest:
    a. hyperresonnance compartment.
    b. hypothermic resuscitation unit.
    c. hyperbaric chamber.
    d. hydrotherapy response team.

141. EMTs without special training should not attempt to rescue a patient from a trench over _____ feet deep.
    a. 5
    b. 8
    c. 12
    d. 15

142. You have been deployed as part of your local disaster assistance team to a large city struck by a hurricane. You note on a building a spray painted "X" with the number 4 at the bottom. This means:
    a. 4 victims were located in the structure.
    b. FEMA team 4 searched the structure.
    c. 4 FEMA rescuers entered the building.
    d. the building was searched at 0400 hours.

MODULE 8

143. Compared to insertion of basic airway adjuncts into the oral cavity, insertion of basic adjuncts into the nares carries a decreased risk of:
    a. bleeding.
    b. infection.
    c. inducing a gag reflex.
    d. failed ventilation.

144. Because of the difference between the right and left bronchi, the tip of an endotracheal tube that is inserted too far is most likely to end up in the:
    a. right mainstem bronchus.
    b. left mainstem bronchus.
    c. carina.
    d. trachea.

145. A manual maneuver in which the EMT presses the thyroid cartilage backward, toward the patient's right, and in the direction of the patient's jaw is called the _____ maneuver.
    a. BURP
    b. Sellick's
    c. ELM
    d. MacGyver

146. On the average, the correct size endotracheal tube for an adult female is between _____ and _____.
    a. 4.0; 5.0
    b. 5.5; 6.5
    c. 7.0; 8.0
    d. 8.0; 9.0

147. The laryngoscope is held in the EMT's _____ hand and inserted from the _____ side of the patient's mouth.
    a. left; left
    b. left; right
    c. right; right
    d. right; left

148. Which of the following best describes the proper use of a nasogastric tube in the prehospital setting?
    a. to ventilate the lungs via a nasally placed airway
    b. to serve as a rescue or back-up device for failed endotracheal intubation
    c. to serve as a route of medication administration
    d. to allow removal of stomach contents

149. The most reliable method of confirming endotracheal tube placement is:
    a. pulse oximetry.
    b. end-tidal carbon dioxide monitoring.
    c. seeing the tube pass between the vocal cords.
    d. using a commercial aspiration device.

150. The primary use of an end-tidal carbon dioxide detector in the prehospital setting is:
    a. to determine the quality of bag-valve-mask ventilations.
    b. to differentiate between the use of an endotracheal tube and non-visualized (blindly inserted) airways.
    c. to distinguish between endotracheal and esophageal intubation.
    d. to determine whether or not a patient can be resuscitated.

Medical Terminology

As an EMT, you will probably never have to use more than a few medical terms in the course of your pre-hospital emergency care activities, and most of them will probably deal with parts of the body. Physicians and nurses prefer EMTs to speak in other than medical terms. But if you are an avid reader, much of what you read is likely to be freely sprinkled with medical terms, and if you cannot translate them, you may not understand what you are reading.

Medical terms are comprised of words, word roots, combining forms, prefixes, and suffixes—all little words, if you will, and each with its own definition.

Sometimes medical terms are made up of two whole words. For example, the word SMALL is joined with the word POX to form the medical term SMALL-POX, the name of a disease. Would that it were all so simple!

Word roots are the foundations of words and are not used by themselves. THERM is a word root that means heat; to use it alone would make no sense. But when a vowel is added to the end of the word root to make it the combining form THERM/O, it can be joined with other words or word roots to form a compound term. THERM/O and METER (an instrument for measuring) combine to form THERMOMETER, an instrument for measuring heat or temperature.

More than one word root or combining form can be joined to form medical terms; ELECTROCAR-DIOGRAM is a good example. ELECTR/O (electric) is joined to CARDI (heart) and the suffix -GRAM (a written record) to form the medical term that means a written record of the heart's electrical activity.

Prefixes are used to modify or qualify the meaning of word roots. They usually tell the reader what kind of, where (or in what direction), or how many.

The term -PNEA relates to breathing, but it says nothing about the quality or kind of breathing. Adding the prefix DYS- qualifies it as difficult breathing.

ABDOMINAL PAIN is a rather broad term; it gives the reader no clue as to exactly where the pain is located either inside or outside the abdomen. Adding the prefix -INTRA to ABDOMINAL pinpoints the location of the pain, for INTRA-ABDOMINAL PAIN means pain within the abdomen. -PLEGIA refers to paralysis of the limbs. The prefix QUADRI informs the reader as to how many limbs are paralyzed. QUADRIPLEGIA means paralysis of all four limbs.

Suffixes are word endings that form nouns, adjectives, or verbs. Medical terms can have more than one suffix, and a suffix can appear in the middle of a compound term affixed to a combining form. A number of suffixes have specialized meanings. -ITIS means inflammation; thus ARTHRITIS means inflammation of a joint. -IAC forms a noun indicating a person afflicted with a certain disease, as for example, HEMO-PHILIAC.

Some suffixes are joined to word roots to form terms that indicate a state, quality, condition, procedure, or process. PNEUMONIA and PSORIASIS are examples of medical conditions, while APPENDEC-TOMY and ARTHROSCOPY are examples of medical procedures.

Some suffixes combine with word roots to form adjectives, words that modify nouns by indicating quality or quantity or by distinguishing one thing from another. GASTRIC, CARDIAC, FIBROUS, ARTHRITIC, and DIAPHORETIC are all examples of adjectives formed by adding suffixes (underlined) to word roots.

Some suffixes are added to word roots to express reduction in size, -OLE and -ULE, for example. An ARTERIOLE is smaller than an ARTERY, and a VENULE is smaller than a vein.

When added to word roots, -E and -IZE form verbs. EXCISE and CATHETERIZE are examples.

Finally, some of what are commonly accepted as suffixes are actually the combination of a word root and a suffix. -MEGALY (enlargement) results from the combination of the word root MEGAL (large) and the suffix -Y (which forms the term into a noun). CARDIOMEGALY means enlargement of the heart.

STANDARD TERMS

The following terms are used to denote direction of movement, position, and anatomical posture.

abduction movement away from the body's midline.

adduction movement toward the body's midline.

afferent conducting toward a structure.

anterior the front surface of the body.

anterior to in front of.

caudad toward the tail.

cephalad toward the head.

circumduction circular movement of a part.

craniad toward the cranium.

deep situated remote from the surface.

distal situated away from the point of origin.

dorsal pertaining to the back surface of the body.

dorsiflexion bending backward.

efferent conducting away from a structure.

elevation raising a body part.

extension stretching, or moving jointed parts into or toward a straight condition.

external situated outside.

flexion bending, or moving jointed parts closer together.

inferior situated below.

internal situated inside.

laterad toward the side of the body.

lateral situated away from the body's midline.

lateral rotation rotating outward away from the body's midline.

left lateral recumbent lying horizontal on the left side.

mediad toward the midline of the body.

medial situated toward the body's midline.

medial rotation rotating inward toward the body's midline.

palmar concerning the inner surface of the hand.

peripheral away from a central structure.

plantar concerning the sole of the foot.

posterior pertaining to the back surface of the body.

posterior to situated behind.

pronation lying face downward or turning the hand so the palm faces downward or backward.

prone lying horizontal, face down and flat.

protraction a pushing forward, as the mandible.

proximal situated nearest the point of origin.

recumbent lying horizontal, generally speaking.

retraction a drawing back, as the tongue.

right lateral recumbent lying horizontal on the right side.

rotation turning around an axis.

superficial situated near the surface.

superior situated above.

supination lying face upward or turning the hand so the palm faces forward or upward.

supine lying horizontal, flat on the back and face up.

ventral the front surface of the body.

PLANES

A plane is an imaginary flat surface that divides the body into sections.

coronal or frontal plane an imaginary plane that passes through the body from side to side and divides it into front and back sections.

midsagittal plane an imaginary plane that passes through the body from front to back and divides it into right and left halves.

sagittal plane an imaginary plane parallel to the median plane. It passes through the body from front to back and divides the body into right and left sections.

transverse plane an imaginary plane that passes through the body and divides it into upper and lower sections.

WORD PARTS

Prefixes are generally identified by a following dash (AMBI-). Combining forms have a slash and a vowel following the word root (ARTHR/O). Suffixes are generally identified by a preceding dash (-EMIA).

a- (not, without, lacking, deficient) afebrile, without fever.

ab- (away from) abduct, to draw away from the midline.

abdomin/o (abdomen) abdominal, pertaining to the abdomen.

-able, -ible (capable of) reducible, capable of being reduced (as a fracture).

ac- (to) acclimate, to become accustomed to.

acou (hear) acoustic, pertaining to sound or hearing.

acr/o (extremity, top, peak) acrodermatitis, inflammation of the skin of the extremities.

acu (needle) acupuncture, the Chinese practice of piercing specific peripheral nerves with needles to relieve the discomfort associated with painful disorders.

ad- (to, toward) adduct, to draw toward the midline.

aden/o (gland) adenitis, inflammation of a gland.

adip/o (fat) adipose, fatty; fat (in size).

aer/o (air) aerobic, requiring the presence of oxygen to live and grow.

af- (to) afferent, conveying toward.

ag- (to) aggregate, to crowd or cluster together.

-algesia (painful) hyperalgesia, overly sensitive to pain.

-algia (painful condition) neuralgia, pain that extends along the course of one or more nerves.

ambi- (both sides) ambidextrous, able to perform manual skills with both hands.

ambl/y (dim, dull, lazy) amblyopia, lazy eye.

amphi-, ampho- (on both sides, around both) amphigonadism, having both testicular and ovarian tissues.

amyl/o (starch) amyloid, starchlike.

an- (without) anemia, a reduced volume of blood cells.

ana- (upward, again, backward, excess) anaphylaxis, an unusual or exaggerated reaction of an organism to a substance to which it becomes sensitized.

andr/o (man, male) android, resembling a man.

angi/o (blood vessel, duct) angioplasty, surgery of blood vessels.

ankyl/o (stiff) ankylosis, stiffness.

ant-, anti- (against, opposed to, preventing, relieving) antidote, a substance for counteracting a poison.

ante- (before, forward) antecubital, situated in front of the elbow.

antero- (front) anterolateral, situated in front and to one side.

ap- (to) approximate, to bring together; to place close to.

apo- (separation, derivation from) apoplexy, sudden neurologic impairment due to a cardiovascular disorder.

-arium, -orium (place for something) solarium, a place for the sun.

arteri/o (artery) arteriosclerosis, thickening of the walls of the smaller arteries.

arthrio (joint, articulation) arthritis, inflammation of a joint or joints.

articul/o (joint) articulated, united by joints.

as- (to) assimilate, to take into.

at- (to) attract, to draw toward.

audi/o (hearing) audiometer, an instrument to test the power of hearing.

aur/o (ear) auricle, the flap of the ear.

aut/o (self) autistic, self-centered

bi- (two, twice, double, both) bilateral, having two sides; pertaining to two sides.

bi/o (life) biology, the study of life.

blephario (eyelid) blepharitis, inflammation of the eyelid.

brachi/o (upper arm) brachialgia, pain in the upper arm.

brady- (slow) bradycardia, an abnormally slow heart rate.

bronch/o (larger air passages of the lungs) bronchitis, inflammation of the larger air passages of the lungs.

bucc/o (cheek) buccal, pertaining to the cheek.

cac/o (bad) cacosmis, a bad odor.

calc/o (bad) calculus, an abnormal hard inorganic mass such as a gallstone.

calcane/o (heel) calcaneus, the heel bone.

calor/o (heat) caloric, pertaining to heat.

cancr/o (cancer) cancroid, resembling cancer.

capit/o (head) capitate, head-shaped.

caps/o (container) capsulation, enclosed in a capsule or container.

carcin/o (cancer) carcinogen, a substance that causes cancer.

cardi/o (heart) cardiogenic, originating in the heart.

carp/o (wrist bone) carpal, pertaining to the wrist bone.

cat-, cata- (down, lower, under, against, along with) catabasis, the stage of decline of a disease.

-cele (tumor, hernia) hydrocele, a confined collection of water.

celi/o (abdomen) celiomyalgia, a pain in the muscles of the abdomen.

-centesis   (perforation or tapping, as with a needle) abdominocentesis, surgical puncture of the abdominal cavity.

cephal/o   (head) electroencephalogram, a recording of the electrical activity of the brain.

cerebr/o   (cerebrum) cerebrospinal, pertaining to the brain and spinal fluid.

cervic/o   (neck, cervix) cervical, pertaining to the neck (or cervix).

cheil/o, chil/o   (lip) cheilitis, inflammation of the lips.

cheirio, chir/o   (hand) cheiralgia, pain in the hand.

chlor/o   (green) chloroma, green cancer, a greenish tumor associated with myelogenous leukemia.

chol/e   (bile, gall) choledochitis, inflammation of the common bile duct.

chondr/o   (cartilage) chondrodynia, pain in a cartilage.

chrom/o, chromat/o   (color) monochromatic, being of one color.

chron/o   (time) chronic, persisting for a long time.

-cid-   (cut, kill, fall) insecticide, an agent that kills insects.

circum-   (around) circumscribed, confined to a limited space.

-cis-   (cut, kill, fall) excise, to cut out.

-clysis   (irrigation) enteroclysis, irrigation of the small intestine.

co-   (with) cohesion, the force that causes various particles to unite.

col-   (with) collateral, secondary or accessory; a small side branch such as a blood vessel or nerve.

col/o   (colon, large intestine) colitis, inflammation of the colon.

colp/o   (vagina) colporrhagia, bleeding from the vagma.

com-   (with) comminuted, broken or crushed into small pieces.

con-   (with) congenital, existing from the time of birth.

contra-   (against, opposite) contraindicated, inadvisable.

cor/e, core/o   (pupil) corectopia, abnormal location of the pupil of the eye.

cost/o   (rib) intercostal, between the ribs.

crani/o   (skull) cranial, pertaining to the skull.

cry/o   (cold) cryogenic, that which produces low temperature.

crypt/o   (hide, cover, conceal) cryptogenic, of doubtful origin.

cyan/o   (blue) cyanosis, bluish discoloration of the skin and mucous membranes.

cyst/o   (urinary bladder, cyst, sac of fluid) cystitis, inflammation of the bladder.

-cyte   (cell) leukocyte, white cell.

cyt/o   (cell) cytoma, tumor of the cell.

dacry/o   (tear) dacryorrhea, excessive flow of tears.

dactyl/o   (finger, toe) dactylomegaly, abnormally large fingers or toes.

de-   (down) descending, coming down from.

dent/o   (tooth) dental, pertaining to the teeth.

derm/o, dermat/o   (skin) dermatitis, inflammation of the skin.

dextr/o   (right) dextrad, toward the right side.

di-   (twice, double) diplegia, paralysis affecting like parts on both sides of the body.

dia-   (through, across, apart) diaphragm, the partition that separates the abdominal and thoracic cavities.

dipl/o   (double, twin, twice) diplopia, double vision.

dips/o   (thirst) dipsomania, alcoholism.

dis-   (to free, to undo) dissect, to cut apart.

dors/o   (back) dorsal, pertaining to the back.

-dynia   (painful condition) cephalodynia, headache.

dys-   (bad, difficult, abnormal, incomplete) dyspnea, labored breathing.

-ectasia   (dilation or enlargement of an organ or part) gastrectasia, dilation (stretching) of the stomach.

ecto-   (outer, outside of) ectopic, located away from the normal position.

-ectomy   (the surgical removal of an organ or part) appendectomy, surgical removal of the appendix.

electr/o   (electric) electrocardiogram, the written record of the heart's electrical activity.

-emia   (condition of the blood) anemia, a deficiency of red blood cells.

en-   (in, into, within) encapsulate, to enclose within a container.

encephal/o   (brain) encephalitis, inflammation of the brain.

end-, endo-   (within) endotracheal, within the trachea.

ent-, ento-   (within, inner) entopic, occurring in the proper place.

enter/o (small intestine) enteritis, inflammation of the intestine.

ep-, epi- (over, on, upon) epidermis, the outermost layer of skin.

erythr/o (red) erythrocyte, a red blood cell.

esthesia (feeling) anesthesia, without feeling.

eu (good, well, normal, healthy) euphoria, an abnormal or exaggerated feeling of well-being.

ex- (out of, away from) excrement, waste material discharged from the body.

exo- (outside, outward) exophytic, to grow outward or on the surface.

extra- (on the outside, beyond, in addition to) extracorporeal, outside the body.

faci/o (face, surface) facial, pertaining to the face.

febr/i (fever) febrile, feverish.

-ferent (bear, carry) efferent, carrying away from a center.

fibr/o (fiber, filament) fibrillation, muscular contractions due to the activity of muscle fibers.

-form (shape) deformed, abnormally shaped.

-fugal (moving away) centrifugal, moving away from a center.

galact/o (milk) galactopyria, milk fever.

gangli/o (knot) ganglion, a knotlike mass.

gastr/o (stomach) gastritis, inflammation of the stomach.

gen/o (come into being, originate) genetic, inherited.

-genesis (production or origin) pathogenesis, the development of a disease.

-genic (giving rise to, originating in) cardiogenic, originating in the heart.

gloss/o (tongue) glossal, pertaining to the tongue.

glyc/o (sweet) glycemia, the presence of sugar in the blood.

gnath/o (jaw) gnathitis, inflammation of the jaw.

-gram (drawing, written record) electrocardiogram, a recording of the heart's electrical activity.

-graph (an instrument for recording the activity of an organ) electrocardiograph, an instrument for measuring the heart's electrical activity.

-graphy (the recording of the activity of an organ) electrocardiography, the method of recording the heart's electrical activity.

gynec/o (woman) gynecologist, a specialist in diseases of the female genital tract.

gnos/o (knowledge) prognosis, a prediction of the outcome of a disease.

hem/a, hem/o, hemat/o (blood) hematoma, a localized collection of blood.

hemi- (one-half) hemiplegia, paralysis of one side of the body.

hepat/o (liver) hepatitis, inflammation of the liver.

heter/o (other) heterogeneous, from a different source.

hidr/o, hidrot/o (sweat) hidrosis, excessive sweating.

hist/o (tissue) histodialysis, the breaking down of tissue.

hom/o, home/o (same, similar, unchanging, constant) homeostasis, stability in an organism's normal physiological states.

hydr/o (water, fluid) hydrocephalus, an accumulation of cerebrospinal fluid in the skull with resulting enlargement of the head.

hypn/o (sleep) hypnotic, that which induces sleep.

hyal/o (glass) hyaline, glassy, transparent.

hyper- (beyond normal, excessive) hypertension, abnormally high blood pressure.

hypo- (below normal, deficient, under, beneath) hypotension, abnormally low blood pressure.

hyster/o (uterus, womb) hysterectomy, surgical removal of the uterus.

-iasis (condition) psoriasis, a chronic skin condition characterized by lesions.

iatr/o (healer, physician) pediatrician, a physician that specializes in children's disorders.

-id (in a state, condition of) gravid, pregnant.

idio (peculiar, separate, distinct) idiopathic, occurring without a known cause.

il- (negative prefix) illegible, cannot be read.

ile/o (ileum) ileitis, inflammation of the ileum.

ili/o (ilium) iliac, pertaining to the ilium.

im- (negative prefix) immature, not mature.

in- (in, into, within) incise, to cut into.

infra- (beneath, below) infracostal, below a rib, or below the ribs.

inter- (between) intercostal, between two ribs.

intra- (within) intraoral, within the mouth.

intro- (within, into) introspection, the contemplation of one's own thoughts and feelings; self-analysis.

ir/o, irid/o (iris) iridotomy, incision of the iris.

ischi/o   (ischium) ischialgia, pain in the ischium.

-ismus   (abnormal condition) strabismus, deviation of the eye that a person cannot overcome.

iso-   (same, equal, alike) isometric, of equal dimensions.

-itis   (inflammation) endocarditis, inflammation within the heart.

kerat/o   (cornea) keratitis, inflammation of the cornea.

kinesi/o   (movement) kinesialgia, pain upon movement.

labi/o   (lip) labiodental, pertaining to the lip and teeth.

lact/o   (milk) lactation, the secretion of milk.

lal/o   (talk) lalopathy, any speech disorder.

lapar/o   (flank, abdomen, abdominal wall) laparotomy, an incision through the abdominal wall.

laryng/o   (larynx) laryngoscope, an instrument for examining the larynx.

lept/o   (thin) leptodactylous, having slender fingers.

leuc/o, leuk/o   (white) leukemia, a malignant disease characterized by the increased development of white blood cells.

lingu/o   (tongue) sublingual, under the tongue.

lip/o   (fat) lipoma, fatty tumor.

lith/o   (stone) lithotriptor, an instrument for crushing stones in the bladder.

-logist   (a person who studies) pathologist, a person who studies diseases.

log/o   (speak), give an account logospasms, spasmodic speech.

-logy   (study of) pathology, the study of disease.

lumb/o   (loin) lumbago, pain in the lumbar region.

lymph/o   (lymph) lymphoduct, a vessel of the lymph system.

-lysis   (destruction) electrolysis, destruction (of hair, for example) by passage of an electric current.

macr/o   (large, long) macrocephalous, having an abnormally large head.

malac/o   (a softening) malacia, the morbid softening of a body part or tissue.

mamm/o   (breast) mammary, pertaining to the breast.

-mania   (mental aberration) kleptomania, the compulsion to steal.

mast/o   (breast) mastectomy, surgical removal of the breast.

medi/o   (middle) mediastinum, middle partition of the thoracic cavity.

mega-   (large) megacolon, an abnormally large colon.

megal/o   (large) megalomaniac, a person impressed with his own greatness.

-megaly   (an enlargement) cardiomegaly, enlargement of the heart.

melan/o   (dark, black) melanoma, a tumor comprised of darkly pigmented cells.

men/o   (month) menopause, cessation of menstruation.

mes/o   (middle) mesiad, toward the center.

meta-   (change, transformation, exchange) metabolism, the sum of the physical and chemical processes by which an organism survives.

metr/o   (uterus) metralgia, pain in the uterus.

micr/o   (small) microscope, an instrument for magnifying small objects.

mon/o   (single, only, sole) monoplegia, paralysis of a single part.

morph/o   (form) morphology, the study of form and shape.

multi-   (many, much) multipara, a woman who has given two or more live births.

myc/o, mycet/o   (fungus) mycosis, any disease caused by a fungus.

my/o   (muscle) myasthenia, muscular weakness.

myel/o   (marrow, also often refers to spinal cord) myelocele, protrusion of the spinal cord through a defect in the spinal column.

myx/o   (mucous, slimelike) myxoid, resembling mucous.

narc/o   (stupor, numbness) narcotic, an agent that induces sleep.

nas/o   (nose) oronasal, pertaining to the nose and mouth.

ne/o   (new) neonate, a newborn infant.

necr/o   (corpse) necrotic, dead (when referring to tissue).

nephr/o   (kidney) nephralgia, pain in the kidneys.

neur/o   (nerve) neuritis, inflammation of nerve pathways.

noct/i   (night) noctambulism, sleep walking.

norm/o   (rule, order, normal) normotension, normal blood pressure.

null/i   (none) nullipara, a woman who has never given birth to a child.

nyct/o (night) nycturia, excessive urination at night.

ob- (against, in front of, toward) obturator, a device that closes an opening.

oc- (against, in front of, toward) occlude, to obstruct.

ocul/o (eye) ocular, pertaining to the eye.

odont/o (tooth) odontalgia, toothache.

-oid (shape, form, resemblance) ovoid, egg-shaped.

olig/o (few, deficient, scanty) oligemia, lacking in blood volume.

-oma (tumor, swelling) adenoma, tumor of a gland.

o/o- (egg) ooblast, a primitive cell from which an ovum develops.

onych/o (nail) onychoma, tumor of a nail or nail bed.

oophor/o (ovary) oophorectomy, a surgical removal of one or both ovaries.

-opsy (a viewing) autopsy, postmortem examination of a body.

opthalm/o (eye) opthalmic, pertaining to the eyes.

opt/o, optic/o (sight, vision) optometrist, a specialist in adapting lenses for the correcting of visual defects.

or/o (mouth) oral, pertaining to the mouth.

orch/o, orchid/o (testicle) orchitis, inflammation of the testicles.

orth/o (straight, upright) orthopedic, pertaining to the correction of skeletal defects.

-osis (process, an abnormal condition) dermatosis, any skin condition.

oste/o (bone) osteomyelitis, inflammation of bone or bone marrow.

ot/o (ear) otalgia, earache.

ovari/o (ovary) ovariocele, hernia of an ovary.

ov/i, ov/o (egg) oviduct, a passage through which an egg passes.

pachy- (thicken) pachyderma, abnormal thickening of the skin.

palat/o (palate) palatitis, inflammation of the palate.

pan- (all, entire, every) panacea, a remedy for all diseases, a "cure-all."

para- (beside, beyond, accessory to, apart from, against) paranormal, beyond the natural or normal.

path/o (disease) pathogen, any disease-producing agent.

-pathy (disease of a part) osteopathy, disease of a bone.

-penia (an abnormal reduction) leukopenia, deficiency in white blood cells.

peps/o, pept/o (digestion) dyspepsia, poor digestion.

per- (throughout, completely, extremely) perfusion, the passage of fluid through the vessels of an organ.

peri- (around, surrounding) pericardium, the sac that surrounds the heart and the roots of the great vessels.

-pexy (fixation) splendopexy, surgical fixation of the spleen.

phag/o (eat) phagomania, an insatiable craving for food.

pharyng/o (throat) pharyngospasms, spasms of the muscles of the pharynx.

phas/o (speech) aphasic, unable to speak.

phil/o (like, have an affinity for) necrophilia, an abnormal interest in death.

phleb/o (vein) phlebotomy, surgical incision of a vein.

-phobia (fear, dread) claustrophobia, a fear of closed spaces.

phon/o (sound) phonetic, pertaining to the voice.

phor/o (bear, carry) diaphoresis, profuse sweating.

phot/o (light) photosensitivity, abnormal reactivity of the skin to sunlight.

phren/o (diaphragm) phrenic nerve, a nerve that carries messages to the diaphragm.

physi/o (nature) physiology, the science that studies the function of living things.

pil/o (hair) pilose, hairy.

-plasia (development, formation) dysplasia, poor or abnormal formation.

-plasty (surgical repair) arthroplasty, surgical repair of a joint.

-plegia (paralysis) paraplegia, paralysis of the lower body, including the legs.

pleur/o (rib, side, pleura) pleurisy, inflammation of the pleura.

-pnea (breath, breathing) orthopnea, difficult breathing except in an upright position.

pneum/o, pneumat/o (air, breath) pneumatic, pertaining to the air.

pneum/o, pneumon/o (lung) pneumonia, inflammation of the lungs with the escape of fluid.

pod/o   (foot) podiatrist, a specialist in the care of feet.

-poiesis   (formation) hematopoiesis, formation of blood.

poly-   (much, many) polychromatic, multicolored.

post-   (after, behind) postmortem, after death.

pre-   (before) premature, occurring before the proper time.

pro-   (before, in front of) prolapse, the falling down, or sinking of a part.

proct/o   (anus) proctitis, inflammation of the rectum.

pseud/o   (false) pseudoplegia, hysterical paralysis.

psych/o   (mind, soul) psychopath, one who displays aggressive antisocial behavior.

-ptosis   (abnormal dropping or sagging of a part) hysteroptosis, sagging of the uterus.

pulmon/o   (lung) pulmonary, pertaining to the lungs.

py/o   (pus) pyorrhea, copious discharge of pus.

pyel/o   (renal pelvis) pyelitis, inflammation of the renal pelvis.

pyr/o   (fire, fever) pyromaniac, compulsive fire setter.

quadri-   (four) quadriplegia, paralysis of all four limbs.

rach/i   (spine) rachialgia, pain in the spine.

radi/o   (ray, radiation) radiology, the use of ionizing radiation in diagnosis and treatment.

re-   (back, against, contrary) recurrence, the return of symptoms after remission.

rect/o   (rectum) rectal, pertaining to the rectum.

ren/o   (the kidneys) renal, pertaining to the kidneys.

retro-   (located behind, backward) retroperineal, behind the perineum.

rhin/o   (nose) rhinitis, inflammation of the mucus membranes of the nose.

-rrhage   (abnormal discharge) hemorrhage, abnormal discharge of blood.

-rrhagia   (hemorrhage from an organ or body part) menorrhea, excessive uterine bleeding.

-rrhea   (flowing or discharge) diarrhea, abnormal frequency and liquidity of fecal discharges.

sanguin/o   (blood) exsanguinate, to lose a large volume of blood either internally or externally.

sarc/o   (flesh) sarcoma, a malignant tumor.

schiz/o   (split) schizophrenia, any of a group of emotional disorders characterized by bizarre behavior (erroneously called split personality).

scler/o   (hardening) scleroderma, hardening of connective tissues of the body, including the skin.

-sclerosis   (hardened condition) arteriosclerosis, hardening of the arteries.

scoli/o   (twisted, crooked) scoliosis, sideward deviation of the spine.

-scope   (an instrument for observing) endoscope, an instrument for the examination of a hollow body, such as the bladder.

-sect   (cut) transsect, to cut across.

semi-   (one-half, partly) semisupine, partly, but not completely, supine.

sept/o, seps/o   (infection) aseptic, free from infection.

somat/o   (body) psychosomatic, both psychological and physiological.

son/o   (sound) sonogram, a recording produced by the passage of sound waves through the body.

spermat/o   (sperm, semen) spermacide, an agent that kills sperm.

sphygm/o   (pulse) sphygmomanometer, a device for measuring blood pressure in the arteries.

splen/o   (spleen) splenectomy, surgical removal of the spleen.

-stasis   (stopping, controlling) hemostasis, the control of bleeding.

sten/o   (narrow) stenosis, a narrowing of a passage or opening.

stere/o   (solid, three-dimensional) stereoscopic, a three-dimensional appearance.

steth/o   (chest) stethoscope, an instrument for listening to chest sounds.

sthen/o   (strength) myasthenia, muscular weakness.

-stomy   (surgically creating a new opening) colostomy, surgical creation of an opening between the colon and the surface of the body.

sub-   (under, near, almost, moderately) subclavian, situated under the clavicle.

super-   (above, excess) superficial, lying on or near the surface.

supra-   (above, over) suprapubic, situated above the pubic arch.

sym-, syn-   (joined together, with) syndrome, a set of symptoms that occur together.

tachy-   (fast) tachycardia, a very fast heart rate.

-therapy   (treatment) hydrotherapy, treatment with water.

therm/o (heat) thermogenesis, the production of heat.

thorac/o (chest cavity) thoracic, pertaining to the chest.

thromb/o (clot, lump) thrombophlebitis, inflammation of a vein.

-tome (a surgical instrument for cutting) microtome, an instrument for cutting thin slices of tissue.

-tomy (a surgical operation on an organ or body part) thoracotomy, surgical incision of the chest wall.

top/o (place) topographic, pertaining to special regions (of the body).

trache/o (trachea) tracheostomy, an opening in the neck that passes to the trachea.

trans- (through, across, beyond) transfusion, the introduction of whole blood or blood components directly into the bloodstream.

tri- (three) trimester, a period of three months.

trich/o (hair) trichosis, any disease of the hair.

-tripsy (surgical crushing) lithotripsy, surgical crushing of stones.

troph/o (nourish) hypertrophic, enlargement of an organ or body part due to the increase in the size of cells.

ultra- (beyond, excess) ultrasonic, beyond the audible range.

uni- (one) unilateral, affecting one side.

ur/o (urine) urinalysis, examination of urine.

ureter/o (ureter) ureteritis, inflammation of a ureter.

urethr/o (urethra) urethritis, inflammation of the urethra.

vas/o (vessel, duct) vasodilator, an agent that causes dilation of blood vessels.

ven/o (vein) venipuncture, surgical puncture of a vein.

ventr/o (belly, cavity) ventral, relating to the belly or abdomen.

vesic/o (blister, bladder) vesicle, a small fluid-filled blister.

viscer/o (internal organ) visceral, pertaining to the viscera (abdominal organs).

xanth/o (yellow) xanthroma, a yellow nodule in the skin.

xen/o (stranger) xenophobia, abnormal fear of strangers.

xer/o (dry) xerosis, abnormal dryness (as of the mouth or eyes).

zo/o (animal life) zoogenous, acquired from an animal.

Glossary

9-1-1 system   a system for telephone access to report emergencies.

A

abandonment   leaving a patient after care has been initiated and before the patient has been transferred to someone with equal or greater medical training.

abrasions   injuries to the skin that involve the wearing down or removal of the superficial layers of the skin.

abruptio placentae   a condition when the placenta prematurely separates from the uterine wall and causes pain and bleeding.

absorption   entry through the skin or eye.

abuse   physical or psychological injury by another person.

accessory muscles   muscles in the neck, chest, back, and abdomen used to assist ventilations in respiratory distress.

actions   desired responses in the body a medication may cause. Also called the desired effect.

activated charcoal   a medication used to treat certain cases of poisoning or overdose.

active rewarming   application of an external heat source to rewarm the body of a hypothermic patient. See also passive rewarming.

acute   sudden-onset. Opposite of chronic.

acute exposure   exposure to a hazardous substance over a short period of time or at a high dose.

adequate breathing   breathing that is sufficient to support life.

adrenaline   see epinephrine.

advance directive   a legal statement of a patient's wishes regarding his own health care.

Advanced EMT, formerly EMT-Intermediate   this level of EMT has completed additional training in order to provide a minimum level of advanced life support, such as the initiation of intravenous (IV) lines, advanced airway techniques, and administration of some medications beyond those the EMT is permitted to administer.

agonal respirations   occasional, gasping attempts at breathing.

air embolism   a bubble of air that enters the circulatory system.

air splints   inflatable splint that can be used to hold a dressing in place on an extremity and control bleeding.

albuterol a medication used to dilate bronchioles in patients with respiratory disorders.

alcohol-based waterless hand cleaner hand cleaner that can be used in the field when soap and water are not available.

allergens substance that causes sensitivity.

allergic reactions the body's exaggerated response when exposed to specific substances to which it has sensitivities.

altered mental status (AMS) appearing abnormally sleepy, confused, violent, or even completely unresponsive; change in alertness and awareness.

alveoli the microscopic sacs of the lungs where gas exchange with the bloodstream takes place.

Alzheimer's disease a progressive, degenerative disease that attacks the brain and results in impaired memory, thinking, and behavior. It affects 4 million American adults.

Ambulance Strike Team a group of five ambulances of the same type with common communications and a leader.

amniotic sac fluid-filled sac surrounding the developing fetus. Also called the "bag of waters."

amputation injury resulting in the loss of a limb or part of a limb.

anaphylactic shock progression of a severe allergic reaction. May result in death.

anaphylaxis sudden, severe allergic reaction.

anatomical position the standard reference position for the body in the study of anatomy. In this position, the body is standing erect, facing the observer, with arms down at the sides and palms of the hands forward.

aneurysm the dilation, or ballooning, of a weakened section of the wall of an artery.

angina literally a pain in the chest. Occurs when one or more of the coronary arteries are unable to provide an adequate supply of oxygenated blood to the heart muscle. Also called angina pectoris.

anterior the front of the body or body part. Opposite of posterior.

anterior fontanels soft spot lying between the cranial bones.

anus outlet of the rectum.

anxiety a state characterized by excess worry or fears.

aorta the largest artery in the body. It transports blood from the left ventricle to begin systemic circulation.

aortic valve a structure between the left ventricle and aorta that opens and closes to permit the flow of a fluid in only one direction.

APGAR score system for evaluating a newborn's physical condition.

apnea absence of breathing.

arachnoid membrane weblike layer of tissue located between the dura mater and the pia mater.

arrhythmias see dysrhythmias.

arteries blood vessels that carry blood away from the heart.

arterioles the smallest arteries.

articulates connects or unites, as bones at a joint.

asphyxiant a substance that prevents sufficient intake or use of oxygen.

aspiration   inhaling foreign material, such as vomitus, into the lungs.

aspirin   medication used both during a heart attack and as a method to prevent heart attacks.

assault   the threat to use force upon another.

asthma   a disease that has attacks involving bronchoconstriction and mucus production with significant difficulty breathing.

ataxic (Biot's) respirations   pattern of respirations characterized by deep, gasping breaths separated by periods of apnea.

atherosclerosis   a build-up of fatty deposits on the inner walls of arteries.

atria   the two upper chambers of the heart. There is a right atrium (which receives unoxygenated blood returning from the body) and a left atrium (which receives oxygenated blood returning from the lungs).

attempted suicide   attempting or threatening to take one's own life.

auscultation   the act of listening for sounds made by internal organs such as the lungs and the heart. Also the technique used to listen for pulse sounds when obtaining a blood pressure

automated external defibrillator (AED)   electrical device that automatically analyzes the heart rhythm and, if appropriate, provides a measured dose of electricity through the heart in an attempt to defibrillate or convert the heart into a normal rhythm.

automaticity   the ability of the heart muscle to generate and conduct electrical impulses on its own.

AVPU   a method for classifying a patient's level of responsiveness, or mental status. The letters stand for Alert, Verbal, Painful, and Unresponsive.

avulsions   injuries where the skin and/or underlying tissue is forcibly torn away.

awareness level   level of training that represents the minimum capabilities of a responder who, in the course of their duties, could be called upon to respond to or be first on scene of a technical rescue incident.

axillae   armpits.

B

bacteria   one-celled organisms without a true nucleus or cell organelles.

bag of waters   see amniotic sac.

bag-valve mask (BVM)   a hand-held device with a face mask and self-refilling bag that can be squeezed to provide artificial ventilations to a patient. It can deliver air from the atmosphere or oxygen from a supplemental oxygen supply.

ball-and-socket joints   type of joint where the ball-shaped head of one bone fits into a rounded receptacle or socket in another bone; type of joint with the greatest range of motion.

base   location at an incident at which primary service and support activities are performed.

base station radio   a two-way radio at a fixed site such as a hospital or dispatch center.

baseline vital signs   the very first set of vital signs obtained on a patient.

basilar skull   portion of the skull that forms the floor of the skull.

battery   the carrying out of a threat to use force upon another.

Battle's sign bruising behind the ears (over the mastoid process) indicative of a basilar skull fracture.

behavioral emergency a situation where a patient's behavior becomes intolerable, dangerous, or bizarre enough to cause the concern of family, bystanders, or the patient.

bifurcation division into two parts or branches.

bilateral on both sides.

bile chemical that assists in the digestion of fat.

biological weapons (BW) devices designed to release either living organisms or toxins produced by living organisms that are deliberately distributed to cause disease and death.

birth canal passageway that extends from the cervix to the vaginal opening through which the baby is born. Also called the vagina.

bladder organ that stores urine until excretion.

bleeding out term meaning the patient is losing blood from within the circulatory system and is not specific to internal or external blood loss.

blood clotting clumping together of blood cells.

blood pressure the pressure exerted by blood against the walls of blood vessels. Usually arterial blood pressure (the pressure in an artery) is measured. Systolic blood pressure is the maximum arterial pressure that occurs during a ventricular contraction. Diastolic blood pressure is the minimum arterial pressure that occurs while the heart is at rest between contractions.

bloody show referring to the amniotic sac rupturing earlier in labor and/or an initial discharge of blood and mucus at the beginning of labor.

blow-by technique providing supplemental oxygen by holding the mask or tubing near the child's face if he cannot tolerate wearing a mask.

blunt trauma injury caused by a blow to the body that does not penetrate the skin.

body mechanics the proper use of one's body to facilitate lifting and moving in such a way as to minimize injury.

body substance isolation (BSI) precautions the practice of using appropriate barriers to infection at the emergency scene, such as gloves, masks, gowns, and protective eyewear.

body surface area (BSA) the amount of body surface area affected.

brachial artery the major artery of the upper arm.

brachial pulse pulse point felt in two locations: on the inside of the upper arm and over the medial aspect of the anterior elbow.

bradycardia a pulse rate below 60 beats per minute.

brainstem portion of the brain located at the base, responsible for vital activities such as respiration, cardiac function, and blood pressure.

branch management tool for the Incident Commander that can be either geographical or functional and is used to keep a manageable span of control.

breech presentation when the buttocks or both lower extremities are the presenting part.

bronchi the two large sets of branches that come off the trachea and enter the lungs. There are right and left bronchi. Singular bronchus.

bronchioles smallest branches of bronchi.

bronchoconstriction   constriction of the bronchioles in the lungs, caused by allergies, respiratory infections, exercise, or emotion.

Broselow tape   a measurement tape that provides approximate height/weight ratios in infants and children. Used to estimate endotracheal tube sizes and drug dosages for pediatric patients.

BURP maneuver   acronym for Backward, Upward, Rightward Pressure, a technique of applying such pressure to the thyroid cartilage to help visualize the vocal cords for endotracheal intubation.

C

camp   location where resources may be kept to support incident operations.

capillaries   thin-walled, microscopic blood vessels where the oxygen/carbon dioxide and nutrient/waste exchange with the body's cells takes place.

capillary fill time   how long it takes for the normal pink color to return after pressing on the fingernail and releasing it. Normally, this takes no more than 2 seconds.

capillary refill test   a test used to assess perfusion status in the extremities.

capnographer   device that uses infrared light to evaluate exhaled carbon dioxide and that displays a continuous waveform to indicate levels of carbon dioxide over time.

capnography   recording or display indicating the presence or quantity of exhaled carbon dioxide concentrations.

capnometer   electronic device that uses infrared light to quantify carbon dioxide in exhaled air.

carbohydrate   source of fuel for the body.

carbon dioxide   waste gas found in the blood. This is exchanged with oxygen in the lungs; slightly heavier-than-air gas that displaces oxygen.

carbon monoxide   slightly lighter-than-air gas that displaces oxygen.

carboxyhemoglobin   a compound formed by carbon monoxide and hemoglobin in carbon monoxide poisoning.

carcinogenic   causing an increased risk of contracting cancer.

cardiac arrest   the stopping of the heart, resulting in a loss of effective circulation.

cardiac muscle   specialized involuntary muscle found only in the heart.

cardiac output   the amount of blood pumped by the heart in 1 minute.

cardiogenic shock   type of shock caused when the heart can no longer pump blood adequately resulting in a decrease in cardiac output and thus a decrease in perfusion.

cardiovascular system   the system made up of the heart (cardio), the blood vessels (vascular) and the blood. Also called the circulatory system.

carotid artery   the large neck artery that carries blood from the heart to the head. There is one carotid artery on each side of the neck.

carotid pulse   the pulse point located on either side of the anterior neck lateral to the trachea.

carpals   the wrist bones.

cartilage   tough elastic connective tissue found in various parts of the body such as the joints, ears, nose, and larynx.

caterpillar pass rescue by which rescuers are positioned along a path and the litter is passed through the team.

cavitation expansion of tissue greater than the size of the bullet that penetrated the tissue. The tissue may stretch, tear, or simply return to its place without injury.

central nervous system part of the nervous system composed of the brain and spinal cord.

central neurogenic hyperventilation pattern of respirations characterized by deep, rapid respirations (as indicated by the term hyperventilation) but the cause is from damage or injury to the brainstem such as may be seen in herniation syndrome.

central perfusion the supply of oxygen to and removal of wastes from central circulation. May be assessed by palpating brachial and femoral pulses.

central venous line intravenous catheter placed close to the heart for long-term fluid or medication administration.

cerebellum portion of the brain that lies behind and under the cerebrum. It is responsible for coordination, posture, and equilibrium.

cerebrospinal fluid fluid found around the brain and spinal cord that helps cushion them.

cerebrum largest portion of the brain, responsible for conscious activities, personality, and sensory input.

cervical vertebrae vertebrae that begin at the head and meet the thoracic vertebrae.

cervix the neck of the uterus at the entrance to the vagina.

cesarean section (C-section) procedure that surgically removes the baby from the uterus.

CHART acronym for Chief complaint, History, Assessment, Rx (or treatment), and Transport. A method of documentation in which each letter stands for a specific portion of the narrative.

chemical and physical characteristics characteristics that determine in what environmental pathways a hazardous material is likely to move and how rapidly.

chemical burn type of burn caused when the skin is exposed to substances such as acids, bases, and caustics.

chemical name the medication name that reflects the chemical structure of the medication.

chemical weapons (CW) devices designed to release a range of simple to sophisticated chemicals that are deliberately distributed to cause harm or death.

Cheyne-Stokes respirations deep respirations alternating with very shallow respirations. There may also be a period of apnea in the cycles. Seen in patients who have brain injury or end-stage brain tumors.

chief complaint the patient's perception of the problem in his own words.

chronic slow-onset or long-term. Opposite of acute.

chronic bronchitis condition where the lining of the bronchiole is inflamed. Excess mucus is formed and remains in the airway. The accumulations become severe as the body is unable to clear the mucus from the airway.

chronic exposure exposure to a hazardous substance over a long period of time.

cilia   tiny hairlike structures that help sweep mucus and foreign particles, including infectious bacteria, upward in the respiratory system.

circulatory system   the system made up of the heart, the blood vessels, and the blood. Also called the cardiovascular system (cardio referring to the heart; vascular referring to the blood vessels).

circumferential burns   burns that completely surround a body part such as a finger, arm, leg, and even the chest.

clavicles   the collarbones.

cleaning   wiping up blood, body fluids, dirt, or grime that may have come from the patient or the scene.

clear text   communications using plain language, that is, no radio codes.

closed head injury   head injury where there is no break.

closed skeletal injury   skeletal injury not associated with any break in the overlying skin.

coccygeal vertebrae   fused vertebrae that make up the coccyx or tailbone.

colon   see large intestine.

command   directs the overall operation and is responsible for the overall success and safety of the incident.

Command Post (CP)   a physical location near the incident from which the Incident Commander oversees all incident operations. Also called the Incident Command Post (ICP).

Command Staff   the incident commander's staff consisting of the liaison officer, the safety officer, and the information officer.

commission   errors of commission are actions done that shouldn't have been done, especially actions that cause harm to a patient.

communication   the exchange of common symbols—written, spoken, or other kinds, such as signing and body language.

compartment syndrome   a condition that may occur if a large bulk of muscle is crushed or compressed for a long period of time. By-products from the compression of muscle and tissue can trigger life-threatening emergencies and potentially cardiac arrest.

compensated shock   when the patient is developing shock but the body is still able to maintain perfusion.

compensates   makes up for a deficiency; maintains perfusion while developing shock.

competent   the ability of an adult to make informed and rational decisions about his own well-being.

complex access   means of getting into a vehicle that requires specialized training, tools, or equipment.

composite fibers   combinations of materials used to make vehicle parts.

concentration   how much of the substance exists at the source.

conchae   tissue within the nasal cavity that causes a swirling air path. Also called turbinates.

concussion   type of injury causing a jarring to the brain and temporary signs and symptoms including loss of memory about the incident and confusion.

conduction pathway   the pathway of electrical impulses through the heart, which causes the heart to beat. The cardiac conduction pathway begins at the sinoatrial node and flows down the center of the heart eventually branching across both ventricles.

conduction system   specialized tissue that provides the electrical stimulus that makes the heart beat.

conductive tissue   a system of specialized muscle tissues that conduct the electrical impulses that stimulate the heart to beat.

confined space   a space that is large enough and configured so that a person can enter but that has limited means for entry and exit and is not designed for continuous human occupancy. Rescues involving confined spaces require specialized training and equipment.

congestive heart failure (CHF)   an overload of fluid in the body's tissues that results when the heart is unable to pump an adequate volume of blood.

consensual   mutually agreeable.

consensus standards   agreed-upon levels of training required for those responding to rescue incidents.

consent   permission from the patient for care or other action by the EMT. See also expressed consent; implied consent.

constricted pupils   pupils that are smaller than normal.

constricting band   a device that encircles an extremity to reduce venous blood return to the body.

contained   stored.

contaminated   to have some hazardous material on the person or object.

contractions   tightening of the uterus to expel the baby.

contraindications   situations where a medication should not be administered because it may do more harm than good.

contusions   injuries resulting when the tissues below the epidermis are damaged and cause bleeding into the surrounding tissues following a blunt trauma or crushing force. Also called bruises.

convulsions   full-body muscle contractions lasting up to several minutes.

coronary arteries   small arteries that carry oxygenated blood to the heart muscle itself. A disruption in flow through these arteries can cause pain and damage to the heart muscle.

crackles   a fine-crackling or bubbling sound heard upon inspiration. The sound is caused as air passes through fluid in the alveoli or by the opening of closed alveoli.

cranial skull or cranial vault   portion of the skull containing the brain and comprised of the temporal, frontal, parietal, and occipital bones.

cranium   the bony structure making up the forehead, top, back, and upper sides of the skull.

crepitation   the grating sound or feeling of broken bones rubbing together. Also called crepitus.

cribbing   wooden blocks or other supportive materials placed in a box pattern (crib) to assist in stabilizing a vehicle.

cricoid cartilage   the ring-shaped structure that circles the trachea at the lower edge of the larynx.

Critical Incident Stress Debriefing (CISD)   a process in which teams of professional and peer counselors provide emotional and psychological support to

EMS personnel who are or have been involved in a critical (highly stressful) incident.

Critical Incident Stress Management (CISM)   a comprehensive, integrated, multicomponent crisis intervention system comprised of seven core components: pre-crisis preparation, support programs, defusing, debriefing, one-on-one intervention, family crisis intervention, and follow-up.

cross-contamination   exposure through contact with a contaminated person or object.

croup   viral illness characterized by inspiratory and expiratory stridor and a sealbarklike cough.

crowning   when the baby's head becomes visible at the vaginal opening.

crumple zones   vehicle parts that are designed to collapse, allowing for the crash energy to be absorbed rather than being transmitted to the passenger compartment.

crush injuries   injuries typically caused when a patient or a part of the patient's body becomes trapped between two surfaces and the pressure from both sides causes damage to the soft tissues and/or internal organs.

Cushing's triad   three signs indicative of increased intracranial pressure: increased blood pressure, decreased pulse, and abnormal respirations.

cyanosis   a blue or gray color resulting from lack of oxygen in the body.

cyanotic   a bluish skin color indicative of poor oxygenation.

D

DCAP-BTLS   a mnemonic used to identify the obvious signs of injury. The letters stand for Deformities, Contusions, Abrasions, Punctures/Penetrations, Burns, Tenderness, Lacerations, and Swelling.

dead space   areas of the lungs outside the alveoli where gas exchange with the blood does not take place.

deceased patients   patients who are not breathing after opening their airway.

decerebrate   patient posture characterized by stiff extended arms and pronated forearms.

decompensate   become unable to compensate for low blood volume or lack of perfusion.

decompensated shock   when the body can no longer compensate for low blood volume or lack of perfusion. Late signs, such as decreasing blood pressure, become evident.

decompression sickness   condition resulting from nitrogen bubbles forming in the blood stream. This can happen to a diver who stays under water too deep and too long, ascends too rapidly, or dives too many days in a row.

decontamination   the process of removing or neutralizing contaminants from a person or object.

decorticate   patient posture characterized by stiff flexed arms, clenched fists, and extended legs.

defusing   small-group discussion held within hours of a critical incident, designed to address acute symptoms of stress.

delayed patients   patients who are injured but whose triage findings are more stable than those of the immediate patient.

delusions false beliefs.

demand valve a device that uses oxygen under pressure to deliver artificial ventilations. It has automatic flow restriction to prevent overdelivery of oxygen to the patient. Also called a flow-restricted, oxygen-powered ventilation device (FROPVD).

dementia condition involving gradual development of memory impairment and cognitive disturbance.

depressed feeling profound sadness or melancholy.

depression profound sadness or feeling of melancholy. May affect major portions of the patient's life including work, relationships, weight changes, sleeping difficulties, feeling of worthlessness and guilt, and occasionally the desire to die.

depth how deeply a burn has penetrated.

dermal contact entrance of a substance through the skin or mucous membranes.

dermal exposure when a chemical contacts and is absorbed through the skin.

dermis the inner (second) layer of the skin found beneath the epidermis. It is rich in blood vessels and nerves.

detoxifies breaks down harmful substances and renders them harmless.

diabetes medical condition that results when a person's pancreas will no longer produce an adequate supply of insulin or when the body loses the ability to utilize insulin properly.

diabetic coma altered mental status resulting from untreated hyperglycemia.

diabetic ketoacidosis a hyperglycemic condition in which an absence of insulin causes the body to metabolize other sources of energy such as fat. The blood becomes acidic and the condition may result in a fruity breath odor and AMS.

diaphoretic perspiring, sweaty, moist. A characterization of skin condition.

diastolic the pressure remaining in the arteries when the left ventricle of the heart is relaxed and refilling.

diffuse pressure pressure applied over a large area to prevent damage or furthering injuries such as fractures.

dilated pupils pupils that are larger than normal.

direct force the force caused by a direct blow to an area of the body.

direct pathway exposure resulting from contact with hazardous vapors or substances.

direct pressure pressure applied using the fingers, palm, or entire surface of one hand to help control bleeding.

disinfecting killing some of the microbes that may be on a piece of medical equipment.

dislocation displacement of the bones that make up a joint, such as the elbow, shoulder, knee, or hip.

distal farther away from the torso. Opposite of proximal.

distention a condition of being stretched, inflated, or larger than normal.

division team assigned to function in a specific geographical area.

do not resuscitate (DNR) order a legal document, usually signed by the patient and his physician, which states that the patient has a terminal illness and does not wish to prolong life through resuscitative efforts.

dorsal referring to the back of the body or the back of the hand or foot. Synonym for posterior.

dorsalis pedis artery artery supplying the foot, lateral to the large tendon of the big toe.

dorsalis pedis (pedal) pulse pulse point located over the anterior foot.

dose how much of the medication is administered.

DOT United States Department of Transportation.

dressings sterile or nonsterile material placed directly over an open wound.

drive to breathe stimulation to breathe. Usually related to the level of carbon dioxide in the blood.

drowning death caused by submersion in water.

due regard functioning in a manner that is precise, cautious, and does not injure anyone else; also called due caution.

dura mater fibrous layer of tissue lining the inside of the cranial vault.

duration how long the exposure to a contaminant lasted.

duty to act a legal obligation to provide care to a patient.

dysrhythmias any variations from the normal rate or rhythm of the heart. Also called arrhythmias.

E

eclampsia pregnancy complication characterized by severe hypertension (high blood pressure), convulsions, and coma.

ectopic pregnancy pregnancy in which the fetus develops in an area other than the uterus.

eddy water that flows around an especially large object and, for a time, flows upstream around the downside of an obstruction.

electrical burn type of burn caused when the body becomes exposed to an electrical current as it passes through the body.

electrolyte a substance that, in water, separates into electrically charged particles.

elevation elevating the injury site above the level of the patient's heart to reduce the amount of pressure at the site and make it easier for bleeding to be controlled.

embryo stage of fetal development between the zygote and the fetus.

Emergency Medical Dispatcher (EMD) specially trained dispatchers who not only obtain the appropriate information from callers but also provide medical instructions for emergency care, including instructions for CPR, artificial ventilation, bleeding control, and more.

Emergency Medical Responder, formerly called First Responder this level of training is designed for the person who is often first at the scene. The emphasis is on activating the EMS system and providing immediate care for life-threatening injuries or illnesses, controlling the scene, and preparing for the arrival of the ambulance.

Emergency Medical Services (EMS) a highly specialized chain of resources designed to minimize the impact of sudden injury and illness on our society.

Emergency Medical Technician-Basic: National Standard Curriculum (NSC) the Curricululm developed by the U.S. Department of Transportation as the foundation for the scope of practice for all EMTs, formerly EMT-Basics.

Emergency Medical Technician, formerly EMT-Basic the curriculum for the EMT deals with the assessment and care of the ill or injured patient and in most areas is considered the minimum level of certification for ambulance personnel. Certification as an EMT requires successful completion of a state approved EMT Training Program or its equivalent and approval by a state EMS program or other authorizing agency.

Emergency Response Guidebook (ERG) Department of Transportation quick-information guide to hazardous materials response.

emergent moves a category of patient moves performed when there is an immediate risk of death or serious injury to the patient or another patient.

emphysema disease that causes a loss of elasticity of the alveoli; a formal chronic obstructive pulmonary disease.

EMS Task Force any combination of resources within span of control of 3 to 7 units (e.g., ambulances, rescues, engines, and squads) assembled for a medical mission, with common communications and a leader (supervisor).

end tidal carbon dioxide (ETCO$_2$) detector device used to detect the presence or the amount of carbon dioxide in exhaled air.

endotracheal intubation technique used to place an endotracheal tube into the trachea in order to provide a direct route for airflow into the lungs.

endotracheal tube (ETT) flexible tube that is placed into the trachea to provide ventilation and airway protection.

epidermis the outer layer of the skin.

epidural hematoma collection of blood between the dura mater and the skull.

epiglottis leaf-shaped structure that covers the glottis to prevent food and foreign matter from entering the trachea.

epilepsy a neurological disorder characterized by sudden recurring attacks of motor, sensory, or psychic malfunction with or without loss of consciousness or convulsive seizures.

epinephrine a hormone produced by the body in response to stress; also called adrenaline. As a medication, it constricts blood vessels and dilates respiratory passages and is used to relieve severe allergic reactions.

epistaxis simple nose bleeds.

esophageal detector device (EDD) mechanical device that uses negative pressure to differentiate tracheal from esophageal placement of a tube.

esophageal tracheal combitube (ETC) type of dual-lumen airway used to provide ventilations and help protect the airway.

esophagus tube connecting the laryngopharynx to the stomach.

ethmoid bone bone that helps form the nasal cavity.

evidentiary all items and materials pertinent to legal consideration.

evisceration injury to the abdomen resulting in the protrusion of the intestinal organs through the abdominal wall.

excretion elimination of waste products from the large intestine.

exhalation a passive process in which the intercostal (rib) muscles and the diaphragm relax, causing the chest cavity to decrease in size and air to flow out of the lungs. Also called expiration.

exposure pathway   specific route by which a chemical might travel from a source to a receptor.

expressed consent   consent given by adults who are of legal age and mentally competent to make a rational decision in regard to their medical well-being. See also consent; implied consent.

extension   movement toward a straightened position. Opposite of flexion.

F

facial bones   bones combined to give us our facial structure as well as to allow breathing and eating.

fallopian tubes   carries the egg and extends from the ovary to the uterus. Female counterpart to the vas deferens.

falsification   documentation of false information in a prehospital care report.

febrile seizures   seizures caused by a sudden increase in fever. Most common in children.

femoral artery   artery located in the anterior groin area, these arteries supply blood to the lower extremities.

femoral pulse   pulse point located deep in the groin between the hip and the inside of the upper thigh.

femur   the large bone of the thigh.

fertilization   the combining of a sperm and an egg. Usually occurs in the fallopian tube.

fetus   the clinical term for an unborn baby.

fibula   the lateral and smaller bone of the lower leg.

fimbria   a fingerlike anatomical part or structure.

First Responder Awareness Level   minimum level of training an EMT should receive, designed to protect first responders. The responders are trained to recognize a problem and initiate a response from an agency with operational-level training.

first stage of labor   stage of labor from the beginning of uterine contractions until full dilation of the cervix.

flail chest   two or more ribs broken in two or more places.

flexible stretcher   a lightweight device used for carrying supine patients down stairs or through tight spaces. Also known as a Reeves stretcher.

flexion   decrease in the angle between the bones forming a joint; tilting the head forward; movement toward a bent position. Opposite of extension.

floating ribs   the two ribs that are connected to vertebrae but not to the sternum.

flushed   a reddish skin color commonly seen when someone is embarrassed or is suffering a heat-related emergency.

form   whether the substance is in large blocks or tiny particles, or whether it is a liquid or a vapor.

Fowler's position   a sitting position.

fracture   broken bone. Can be as minor as a hairline crack all the way to a badly shattered bone that appears deformed.

freelancing   situation when a person on an emergency scene takes action without the knowledge or permission of the incident commander or commanders of the incident.

frostbite local cold injury. Damage to local tissues from exposure to cold temperatures. See also frostnip.

frostnip early or superficial frostbite.

full-thickness burns burns that extend beyond all layers of the skin and can even cause damage to underlying muscle, bone, and vital organs.

fused joints type of joint where bones meet but do not move.

G

gallbladder an organ in the form of a sac on the underside of the liver that stores bile produced by the liver.

gastrostomy tube (G-Tube) tube placed directly into the stomach or upper small intestine through the abdominal wall to provide nutrition to a patient who cannot eat or swallow.

gels jelly-like form of medication.

general impression an element of the patient assessment that includes assessing approximate age, gender, and level of distress.

General Staff the key staff positions that oversee the sections in a fully expanded ICS or IMS system.

generalized tonic-clonic seizure seizure characterized by a loss of consciousness, convulsions. Also called a grand mal seizure.

generic the medication name found in the U.S. Pharmacopoeia.

genitalia organs of reproduction.

geriatric a person aged 65 or older.

gestation length of time from conception to birth.

Glasgow Coma Score (GCS) numerical score that rates patients on eye opening, speech, and motor function.

gliding joints type of joint where one bone end slides upon another.

glottis opening between the vocal cords that separates the upper airway from the lower airway. Also called the glottic opening.

glucose a simple form of sugar that is required by all cells as fuel for metabolic processes; blood sugar.

Good Samaritan laws laws, varying in each state, designed to provide limited legal protection for citizens and some health care personnel when they are administering emergency care.

group team assigned to functional activities.

guarding body defense mechanism, to prevent the movement of an injured part.

gurgling intermittent low-pitched sounds. Indicative of fluids in the upper airway.

H

hallucinations sensory perceptions without an external stimulus.

Hazard Class 1, Explosives cause injuries by the primary, secondary, and tertiary blasts.

Hazard Class 2, Gases cause injuries by being toxic or displacing oxygen to cause asphyxiation.

Hazard Class 3, Flammable liquids, combustible liquids   cause injuries by penetrating the skin and attacking internal organs.

Hazard Class 4, Flammable solids, spontaneously combustible materials, and dangerous when wet materials   cause injuries by creating severe and deep burns to tissue. Many of the flammable solids are reactive to water.

Hazard Class 5, Oxidizers and Organic peroxides   can trigger an explosion and can also act as a corrosive destroying tissue and triggering inflammation in the lungs.

Hazard Class 6, Toxic materials and Infectious substances   involve biological and poisonous substances. Infectious material can include blood products or blood-contaminated materials and plant, virus, bacterial, or other living organisms.

Hazard Class 7, Radioactive materials   injure or kill by disrupting the nervous system or the cellular functions.

Hazard Class 8, Corrosive materials   causes injuries by destroying and dissolving tissue. Corrosives usually involve acids, bases, and some solvents.

Hazard Class 9, Miscellaneous dangerous goods   hazardous materials that do not fit into one of the other hazard classes.

hazardous material   any substance or material in a form which poses an unreasonable risk to health, safety, and property.

Hazardous Materials First Responder Operations Level   level of training that includes procedures to contain and keep hazardous materials from spreading and to prevent exposures to people, property, and the environment. Operations-level training trains first responders to wear and operate in level B protection.

Hazardous Materials Specialist Level   level of training that includes advanced knowledge of monitoring devices, toxicology, and command and control of large scale hazardous materials incidents.

Hazardous Materials Technician Level   level of advanced training that teaches a first responder to control a spill and operate in hazardous environments in chemical protective clothing and level A suits.

hazardous properties   effects the hazardous materials can have on living things or the environment.

head-tilt, chin-lift maneuver   a means of opening the airway by tilting the head back and lifting the chin. Used when no trauma, or injury, is suspected. See also jaw-thrust maneuver.

Health Insurance Portability and Accountability Act (HIPAA)   federal law protecting the privacy of patient-specific health care information and providing the patient with control over how this information is used and distributed.

helibase   location in or near an incident area at which helicopters may be parked, maintained, fueled, and equipped for incident operations.

helispots   temporary locations where helicopters can land and load and off-load personnel, equipment, and supplies.

hematomas   areas of localized swelling caused by the accumulation of blood and other fluids beneath the skin.

hemoglobin   molecule within the red blood cell that carries oxygen to the cells and carbon dioxide away from the cells.

hemorrhagic shock   type of shock caused by loss of blood.

hemothorax   blood within the pleural space.

herniation tissue protrusion outside of the area in which it is normally contained.

herniation syndrome signs and symptoms indicative of a brain herniation, including decreasing mental status, vomiting, and headache.

high-angle situations vertical or above-ground rescue situation requiring specialized training and equipment.

hinge joints type of joint that moves in only one direction.

hives red, itchy, possibly raised blotches on the skin, possibly from insect bites or food allergy.

hobble a method of restraint in which the legs are secured to the torso to restrict movement.

home ventilator a mechanical device that moves air in and out of the lungs.

hormones chemicals involved in regulation of body functions.

humerus the bone of the upper arm, between the shoulder and the elbow.

hydraulic an area of major current changes or reversal due to an obstruction or land formation.

hydrogen sulfide slightly heavier-than-air gas that displaces oxygen. It may produce the odor of rotten eggs.

hyperbaric chamber pressurized chamber that provides the patient with oxygen under pressure. Hyperbaric oxygen therapy increases tissue oxygenation.

hypercarbia excessive carbon dioxide in the blood.

hyperextension extreme or abnormal extension or increase in the angle between bones of a joint; tilting the head backward.

hyperflexed extreme or abnormal flexion.

hyperglycemia abnormally high blood glucose level.

hyperthermia abnormally elevated core body temperature.

hyperventilation breathing that is abnormally rapid and deep.

hypoglycemia abnormally low blood glucose level.

hypoperfusion inadequate distribution of blood to an organ or organs of the body. Also called shock.

hypothermia abnormally low core body temperature.

hypovolemic shock type of shock caused by a sudden decrease in body fluids—blood or other body fluids.

hypoxia an insufficiency of oxygen in the body's tissues.

hypoxic drive when the stimulus to breathe is the amount of oxygen in the blood rather than the normal drive to breathe that is related to the amount of carbon dioxide in the blood.

I

ilium the superior and widest portion of the pelvis.

immediate and adverse effects reactions to a chemical that occur at the time of exposure, such as vomiting or eye irritation.

immediate patients patients who are at risk for early death, usually due to shock, an airway problem, or a severe head injury.

impaled penetrating of the body by an object that remains in the body.

impaled object penetrating trauma in which the object remains in the body.

implantation   the attachment of a fertilized egg to the uterine lining.

implants   becomes imbedded, as a fertilized egg into the wall of the uterus.

implied consent   the consent it is presumed a patient or patient's parent or guardian would give if they could, such as for an unconscious patient or by a parent who cannot be contacted when care is needed. See also consent; expressed consent.

improvised nuclear device (IND)   a device that can produce a nuclear explosion.

inadequate breathing   breathing that is not sufficient to support life.

incident action plan (IAP)   plan for the management of a specific component of incident operations.

Incident Command Post (ICP)   a physical location near an incident from which the Incident Commander oversees all incident operations. Also called the Command Post (CP).

Incident Command System (ICS)   the first management system that was developed by an interagency task force working in a cooperative local, state, and federal interagency effort called FIRESCOPE (Firefighting Resources of California Organized for Potential Emergencies). Initial ICS applications were designed for responding to disastrous wildland fires in southern California.

Incident Commander (IC)   the person in overall charge of an incident under the Incident Command System or Incident Management System.

Incident Management System (IMS)   system developed to assist with the control, direction, and coordination of emergency response resources. It provides an orderly means of communication and information for decision making and accountability of resources.

incontinence   inability to retain urine or feces because of loss of sphincter control.

incubation period   the period of time from exposure until signs and symptoms occur.

index of suspicion   an awareness or suspicion that there may be injuries based on the evaluation of the mechanism of injury.

indication   reason a medication is administered.

indirect force   the force that occurs when energy is transferred along a bone, usually proximal to the site of impact.

indirect pathway   exposure resulting from taking in air, water, or food that has been contaminated by hazardous vapors or substances.

infection   invasion and multiplication of foreign microorganisms within the tissues of the body.

inferior   away from the head; usually compared with another structure that is closer to the head (e.g., the lips are inferior to the nose). Opposite of superior.

ingestion   entrance of a substance into the digestive system.

inhalation   an active process in which the intercostal (rib) muscles and the diaphragm contract, expanding the size of the chest cavity and causing air to flow into the lungs. Also called inspiration.

inhaled bronchodilators   medication used to open up bronchioles that are constricted due to a respiratory disease such as asthma.

inhaler   a spray device with a mouthpiece that contains an aerosol form of a medication that a patient can spray into his airway.

initial assessment a component of the overall patient assessment. The primary objective of the initial assessment is to identify and treat any immediate life threats to the patient.

injection placement of medication in or under the skin with a needle and syringe.

insulin hormone produced by the pancreas and required for the transfer of glucose (sugar) from the blood to the tissues and cells where it can be used for fuel.

insulin shock condition resulting from untreated hypoglycemia.

interventions actions taken to correct or improve a patient's condition.

intracranial pressure increasing pressure within the brain vault due to bleeding and/or swelling.

intubate insert a tube, usually into the trachea.

inverted pyramid graphic illustrating the types and frequency of care given to the neonate at birth.

involuntary muscle muscle that responds automatically to brain signals but cannot be consciously controlled. Also called smooth muscle.

ischium the lower, posterior portions of the pelvis.

islets of Langerhans a group of cells in the pancreas that secrete insulin and other hormones into the blood.

J

jaundice a yellowish color of the skin and whites of the eyes indicative of poor liver function.

jaw-thrust maneuver a means of correcting blockage of the airway by moving the jaw forward without tilting the head or neck. Used when trauma, or injury, is suspected. See also head-tilt, chin-lift maneuver.

jugular vein distention (JVD) bulging of the neck veins.

K

kidneys a pair of organs that filter the blood to remove excess water and waste.

Kussmaul's respirations rapid, deep ventilations usually caused by very acidic blood such as some diabetic conditions and aspirin overdose.

L

lacerations open wounds that can have jagged or straight edges.

lacrimal bone bone that helps form the nasal cavity.

lacrimation abnormal or excessive secretion of tears.

laminated glass type of glass that has a layer of glue, plastic, or mastic sandwiched between two pieces of glass.

large intestine organ that is a muscular tube that removes water from waste products received from the small intestine and removes anything not absorbed by the body toward excretion from the body. Also called the colon.

laryngeal mask airway (LMA) type of airway used to provide ventilations and help protect the airway.

laryngopharnyx portion of the pharynx connecting the oropharynx to the larynx. Also called the hypopharynx.

laryngoscope instrument used to lift the tongue off the posterior pharynx and move the epiglottis out of the visual field so that the vocal cords are visible.

larynx structure located between the laryngopharnx and the trachea. It houses the glottis and the vocal cords. Also called the voice box.

lateral to the side, away from the midline of the body.

laterally recumbent lying on one side.

left referring to the patient's left.

lethality the ability of an agent or disease to cause death; the percentage of those who die from an agent or disease.

Liaison Officer command staff officer responsible for communicating with other agencies. The liaison officer may be the person making the initial contact with an EMS agency.

ligaments tissues that connect bone to bone.

light burn type of burn caused by high-intensity light sources.

limb presentations presentation that occurs when you observe a single limb presenting from the birth canal.

liver produces bile to assist in breakdown of fats and assists in the metabolism of various substances in the body.

lobes sections of the lung. The left lung has two lobes; the right lung has three lobes.

locked-in technique when lifting, locking your back in position, avoiding twisting.

long-axis drag a method used to move a patient while maintaining the body's long axis.

long backboard a rigid device, usually made of a plastic or composite material that is used to stabilize a patient with a suspected spinal injury. Also called a long spine board.

low-angle rescue rescue that involves terrain at less than a 40-degree angle.

low-angle situations "off-road" rescue situation requiring specialized training and equipment.

lumbar vertebrae the five vertebrae that form the "lower back" area.

lung the primary organ of respiration. There is a left lung and a right lung.

M

Macintosh a type of laryngoscope blade. Also called a curved blade.

malar bone the cheek bone. Also called the zygomatic bone.

mammalian diving reflex body response triggered when a person's face is submersed in cold water, causing the body to go into a state of extremely low metabolism that preserves the brain, lung, and heart tissue. Also called the diving response.

mandible the lower jaw bone.

manual stabilization method of stabilization where the EMT firmly grasps the patient's head with both hands and attempts to keep it from moving.

mass gathering   any collection of more than 1,000 people at one site or location. The term applies to all types of events, including concerts and sporting or other large-scale events.

material data safety sheet (MSDS)   document from the manufacturer for each hazardous chemical in the workplace. The MSDS contains important safety information about the hazardous chemical.

maxilla   the two fused bones forming the upper jaw.

mechanism of injury (MOI)   a force or forces that may have caused injury.

meconium   fecal matter excreted by the baby while still in the uterus.

medial   toward the midline of the body.

Medical Direction   oversight of the patient-care aspects of an EMS system by the Medical Director.

Medical Director   a physician who assumes ultimate responsibility for the patient care aspects of the EMS system.

medulla oblongata   portion of the brain that directly connects to the spinal cord. Also called the medulla.

meninges   three membranes that surround and protect the brain and spinal cord. They are the dura mater, the pia mater, and the arachnoid membrane.

menstrual cycle   monthly recurrent changes in the female reproductive system.

metacarpals   the hand bones.

metatarsals   the foot bones.

metered-dose inhaler   device that patients use to breathe in medication.

methane   a naturally occurring, saturated hydrocarbon that is a by-product of the breakdown of all organic materials.

midaxillary   a line drawn vertically from the middle of the armpit to the ankle.

midclavicular   the vertical line through the center of each clavicle.

midline   an imaginary line drawn down the center of the body, dividing it into right and left halves.

Miller   a type of laryngoscope blade. Also called a straight blade.

minor patients   patients with minor injuries. Sometimes referred to as walking wounded.

miscarriage   see spontaneous abortion.

mitral valve   a structure between the left atrium and left ventricle that opens and closes to permit the flow of a fluid in only one direction.

mobile data terminals (MDTs)   computers that are mounted in a vehicle and connected to the base station by radio modem. In addition to full functionality as a computer, the MDT will display dispatch information for calls and may provide the ability to enter information for prehospital care reports.

mobile radio   a two-way radio that is used or affixed in a vehicle.

morbid lividity   pooling of blood in the lower parts of the body after death.

motor   portion of the nervous system that carries information from the brain through the spinal cord and to the body.

mucus   slippery secretion that lubricates and protects airway surfaces.

multi-system trauma   term referring to the multiple organ systems that are generally affected by significant mechanisms of injury.

multiple birth   delivery of more than one baby.

multiple-casualty incident (MCI)   incident resulting from man-made or natural causes resulting in illness or injuries that exceed or overwhelm normal EMS and hospital capabilities. A large multiple-casualty incident may be called a mass-casualty incident.

mutagenic   causing a mutation, which is a permanent change in the genetic material (DNA) that may be passed along to later generations.

mutual aid   assistance provided by other jurisdictions.

myocardial infarction (MI)   occlusion or blockage of one or more of the coronary arteries resulting in damage to the heart muscle. Also called a heart attack.

N

Nader pin   metal pin mounted to the door frame to which the door latching mechanism attaches, designed to prevent doors from flying open and passengers from being ejected in a crash.

nares   the opening to the nasal cavity. Also called nostrils.

nasal bones   the bones that form the upper third, or bridge, of the nose.

nasal cannula   a device that delivers low concentrations of oxygen through two prongs that rest in the patient's nostrils.

nasal flaring   the extended opening or flaring of nostrils.

nasal vestibule   the anteriormost portion of the nasal cavity.

nasogastric (NG) tube   a tube designed to be passed through the nose, nasopharynx, and esophagus. It is used to relieve distention of the stomach in an infant or child patient.

nasopharyngeal airway   a soft flexible breathing tube inserted through the patient's nose into the pharynx to help maintain an open airway.

nasopharynx   the section of the pharynx directly posterior to the nose.

National Fire Protection Association (NFPA)   the world's leading advocate of fire prevention and an authoritative source on public safety. NFPA's 300 codes and standards influence every building, process, service, design, and installation in the United States, as well as many of those used in other countries.

National Highway Traffic Safety Administration (NHTSA)   a division of the U.S. Department of Transportation (DOT). This agency develops the National Standard Curricula for various levels of EMS providers.

National Incident Management System (NIMS)   system implemented in 2004 by the Department of Homeland Security that provides a consistent nationwide approach for incident management and requires federal, state, tribal, and local governments to work together before, during, and after incidents.

nature of illness   what is medically wrong with a patient.

NBC   abbreviation for nuclear, biological, and chemical.

near syncope   near fainting.

near-drowning   the condition of having begun to drown but still able to be resuscitated.

nebulized process of mixing air and medication to produce a mist, which is inhaled.

nebulizers devices that continuously administer a vaporized medication, as opposed to the inhaler that provides a one-time dose.

neglect a person's inability to care for himself or a person's caregiver providing inadequate care.

negligence a finding of failure to act properly in a situation in which there was a duty to act, needed care as would reasonably be expected of the EMT was not provided, and harm was caused to the patient as a result.

neonate newborn infant up to one month of age.

neurogenic shock type of shock caused when the vessels dilate abnormally in response to injury to the spinal cord.

NFPA 704 a standardized system that uses numbers and colors on a sign to indicate the basic hazards of a specific material being stored in large containers or at a manufacturing site.

NIMS National Incident Management System.

nitrogen narcosis condition presenting with acting out of character or bizarre behavior resulting when a diver stays under water too deep and too long. Also called raptures of the deep.

nitroglycerin a medication used to treat chest pain.

non-urgent moves a category of patient moves performed when there is no need to expedite due to the patient's condition or hazards at the scene.

nonrebreather mask a face mask and reservoir bag device that delivers high concentrations of oxygen.

normothermic normal body temperature.

nuclear weapons (NW) devices designed to release the energy generated during splitting (fission) or combining (fusion) of heavy nuclei to form new elements that are deliberately distributed to cause harm or death; a weapon that can produce an actual nuclear explosion.

O

objective information that you have personally observed, can measure, or can attest to.

occipital posterior (back) region of the skull.

occupancy the term used to describe a building that may be used to manufacture or process chemicals.

off-line medical direction consists of standing orders issued by the Medical Director that allow EMTs to give certain medications or perform certain procedures without speaking to the Medical Director or another physician.

omission errors of omission are those where something wasn't done that should have been.

on-line medical direction consists of orders from the on-duty physician or their designee given directly to an EMT in the field by radio or telephone.

ongoing assessment a continuous recheck of the patient's condition to ensure that everything checked previously is still okay.

open head injury head injury where there is a break in the skull.

open skeletal injury   skeletal injury where the skin is damaged causing an open soft tissue wound in connection with the injury.

operational level   level of training that is designed for responders who will be responsible for hazard recognition, equipment use, and techniques necessary to conduct a technical rescue.

OPQRST   a mnemonic for the questions asked to get a description of the present illness. The letters stand for Onset, Provocation, Quality, Region and Radiate, Severity, and Time.

oral glucose   a medication used to treat patients with suspected low blood sugar.

orbits   the bony structures around the eyes; the eye sockets.

oropharyngeal airway   a curved device inserted into the patient's mouth and the pharynx to help maintain an open airway.

oropharynx   the section of the pharynx directly posterior to the mouth.

orotracheal intubation   the placement of an endotracheal tube orally, by way of the mouth, then through the vocal cords and into the trachea.

orthostatic vital signs   a test in which vital signs are measured before and after a patient moves from a supine to a sitting or a sitting to a standing position.

osteoporosis   softening of bone tissue due to the loss of essential minerals, principally calcium.

ovaries   internal gland producing the ovum. Female counterpart to the testicles.

ovulation   the release of an ovum (egg) from the ovary.

ovum/ova   female sex cell. Female counterpart to the sperm; an unfertilized egg.

oxygen   a medication used to increase the amount of circulating oxygen in the blood stream.

P

pacemaker   site within the heart that originates an electrical impulse.

pale   a whitish skin color indicative of poor perfusion.

palmar   referring to the palm of the hand.

palpation   the act of examining by feeling with the hands. Also a technique used for obtaining a blood pressure reading.

pancreas   a gland located behind the stomach that produces insulin and produces juices that assist in digestion of food in the duodenum of the small intestine.

panic attack   sudden onset of a fear or discomfort including symptoms such as sweating, trembling, palpitations, feelings of shortness of breath or chest tightness, nausea and/or vomiting, and fears of dying or loss of control.

paradoxical motion   movement of a flail segment opposite to the motion of the nonfractured ribs.

paradoxical movement   movement of a part of the chest in the opposite direction to the rest of the chest during inhalation and exhalation.

paralyzed   suffering temporary or permanent loss of muscular power or sensation.

Paramedic, formerly EMT-Paramedic   the paramedic receives significant additional training in advanced life support procedures. Paramedics are trained to perform invasive procedures such as the insertion of endotracheal tubes, initiation of IV lines, administration of a variety of medications, interpretation of electrocardiograms, and cardiac defibrillation.

paranoia a delusion (false belief) where the patient believes he is being followed, persecuted, or harmed.

parietal pleura membrane that is attached to the chest wall.

Parkinson's disease chronic, degenerative nervous disease characterized by tremors, muscular weakness and rigidity, and a loss of postural reflexes.

partial-thickness burns burns that extend down beyond the epidermis and into the dermis.

passive rewarming covering a hypothermic patient and taking other steps to prevent further heat loss and help the body rewarm itself. See also active rewarming.

patella the kneecap.

patent in reference to the airway (passage from nose or mouth to lungs), open and clear, without interference to the passage of air into and out of the body.

pathogens organisms that cause infection, such as viruses and bacteria.

pathophysiology the study of how disease affects normal body processes.

pathways of exposure all the ways a contaminant could reach the population at risk.

patient assessment overall evaluation of the patient for life-threatening and non-life-threatening conditions.

patient data all the information about the patient (name, address, date of birth), insurance information, and detailed information on the patient's complaint, assessment, care, and vital signs.

pelvis the basin-shaped bony structure that supports the spine and is the point of proximal attachment for the lower extremities.

penetrating trauma injury caused by an object that passes through the skin.

penetration injuries injuries caused by an object that passes through the skin or other body tissues.

penis external male genitalia that contains the urethra.

perfusion distribution of blood to all parts of the body to deliver oxygen and remove waste products. Hypoperfusion is inadequate perfusion.

pericardial tamponade collection of blood in the sac surrounding the heart.

perineum the skin between the vagina and the anus.

peripheral nervous system (PNS) the nerves that enter and leave the spinal cord and that convey impulses to and from the central nervous system.

peripheral pulses pulses in the distal circulation such as the radial pulse, the pedal pulse found on the top of the foot.

peristalsis motion of the digestive tract that moves food through the system.

peritoneum two thin membranes, one covering the abdominal organs and the other attached to the abdominal wall.

PERRL a mnemonic used to evaluate a patient's pupils. The letters stand for Pupils Equal and Round Reactive to Light.

persistence length of time an agent stays in the environment.

personal protective equipment (PPE) equipment that protects the EMS worker from infection and/or exposure to the dangers of rescue operations.

pertinent negatives questions that are important to know the answers to—even if the answer is no.

pharynx   passageway from nose and mouth to trachea.

phobias   an unfounded or intense fear of an object or situation.

pia mater   layer of tissue directly covering the brain.

placard   diamond-shaped sign placed on cargo tanks, vehicles, or rail cars to display one of nine classes of hazardous materials that is being carried.

placenta   structure that provides nutrition to the fetus and eliminates fetal waste.

placenta previa   a condition where the placenta is attached to the uterine wall over the opening of the cervix, but in the wrong position.

plane   a flat surface formed when slicing through a solid object.

plantar   referring to the sole of the foot.

plasma   the fluid portion of the blood.

platelets   components of the blood; membrane-enclosed fragments of specialized cells.

pleura   two tissue layers that line the chest wall and cover the lungs.

pleural space   potential space between the two tissue layers that line the chest wall and cover the lungs.

pneumonia   infection of the lung.

pneumothorax   air within the pleural space.

popliteal pulse   pulse point located over the posterior aspect of the knee.

portable radio   a handheld two-way radio.

portable stretcher   a lightweight device made of canvas or plastic with two poles extended from each side for easy carrying.

position of function   position of the hands and feet when they are at rest without any type of force.

positional asphyxia   death of a patient who has been restrained. Often associated with extreme exertion (long foot chases or struggling against restraints), drug or alcohol use, and/or hog-tie or hobble restraints, some patients die while restrained.

posterior   the back of the body or body part. Opposite of anterior.

posterior tibial artery   artery supplying the foot, behind the medial ankle.

posterior tibial pulse   pulse point located over the medial ankle just posterior to the ankle bone.

postictal   period following a generalized seizure where patient will remain unresponsive or also may be sleepy or groggy for up to 30 minutes or so.

power grip   gripping with as much hand surface as possible in contact with the object being lifted, all fingers bent at the same angle, hands at least 10 inches apart.

power lift   a lift from a squatting position with weight to be lifted close to the body, feet apart and flat on the ground, body weight on or just behind balls of feet, back locked in. The upper body is raised before the hips. Also called the squat-lift position.

predefined response matrix   specific set of resources sent to the scene based on the caller's or first responder's information.

preeclampsia   pregnancy complication characterized by hypertension (high blood pressure) and edema.

prehospital care report (PCR)   written documentation of the call and patient encounter. Also called a patient care report or a run report.

premature birth birth before the baby has fully developed prior to 38 weeks' gestation.

prenatal before birth.

preplanning developing a plan for future possible events which would require a large response of units, personnel, and leadership.

presenting part the part of the baby that first becomes visible.

pressure bandage bandage that applies pressure to control bleeding from a wound to an extremity that is still actively bleeding. Also called a pressure dressing.

pressure dressing dressing that applies pressure to control bleeding from a wound to an extremity that is still actively bleeding. Also called a pressure bandage.

pressure points locations on or near each limb where the major artery supplying the limb lies over a bone. Pressure applied to these points can slow blood flow at the injury site and help facilitate the formation of a clot which will stop the bleeding.

priapism persistent erection of the penis that may result from spinal injury and some medical problems.

prolapsed cord presentation that occurs when the umbilical cord enters the birth canal before the baby's head.

prone lying face down. Opposite of supine.

proteins source of amino acids, the building blocks of the body.

protocols written guidelines or treatment plans for patient care to help the EMT provide the most appropriate care. Protocols are approved by the Medical Director of an EMS system.

proximal closer to the torso. Opposite of distal.

psychogenic shock type of shock caused by a sudden and temporary dilation of the blood vessels from psychological causes.

psychosis unusual or bizarre behavior indicating a lack of touch with reality.

psychosocial related to a patient's personality, style, dynamics of unresolved conflict, or crisis management methods.

pubis the medial anterior portion of the pelvis.

Public Information Officer command staff officer who is the only one authorized to release information to the news media after approval by the incident commander.

Public Safety Answering Point (PSAP) the agency responsible for answering 9-1-1 calls.

pulmonary arteries vessels that carry blood from the right ventricle to the lungs.

pulmonary edema a condition of fluid in the lungs.

pulmonary vein vessel carrying oxygen-rich blood from the lungs to the left atrium.

pulmonic valve a structure between the right ventricle and pulmonary arteries that opens and closes to permit the flow of a fluid in only one direction.

pulse the pumping of the heart as a pressure wave felt over an artery.

pulse oximeter an electronic device for determining the amount of oxygen carried in the blood, known as the oxygen saturation. The pulse oximeter measures the percentage of hemoglobin molecules that are saturated with oxygen.

pulse oximetry   use of an electronic device, a pulse oximeter, to determine the amount of oxygen carried by the hemoglobin in the blood, known as the oxygen saturation or SpO_2.

Q

Quality Improvement (QI)   a process of continuous self-review with the purpose of identifying and correcting aspects of the system that require improvement.

R

raccoon eyes   bruising around the eyes indicative of a basilar skull fracture.

radial artery   artery of the lower arm. It is felt when taking the pulse at the wrist.

radial pulse   pulse point located over the lateral aspect of the anterior wrist.

radiation   type of burn from sources of radiation such as nuclear fallout or radioactive materials used in medicine.

radiological dispersal device (RDD)   a conventional bomb laced with radioactive material. Also called a dirty bomb.

radius   the lateral bone of the forearm.

rapid extrication   the rapid removal of a patient from a vehicle when the patient's condition or the situation does not permit use of a short backboard or vest-type extrication device.

receptor   living plant or animal that is exposed to a hazardous substance.

red blood cells   blood cells that contain hemoglobin.

referred pain   pain that is felt in a location other than where the pain originates.

repeater   a device that picks up signals from lower-power radio units, such as mobile and portable radios, and retransmits them at a higher power. It allows low-power radio signals to be transmitted over longer distances.

Rescue/Extrication Group   team responsible for all of the operations necessary to remove victim from the hazard zone and to the treatment area.

respiration   inhalation and exhalation. May also be called ventilation.

respiratory arrest   when breathing completely stops.

respiratory distress   the body's attempts to compensate for an inadequate supply of oxygen.

respiratory failure   the reduction of breathing to the point where oxygen intake is not sufficient to support life.

retraction   muscles pulling in between the ribs and above the sternum with inspiration.

retroperitoneal   referring to the area behind the abdominal cavity.

rhonchi   low-pitched snoring or rattling sounds caused by secretions in the larger airways. These may be seen in chronic lung diseases and possibly pneumonia.

rib fracture   any break in a rib.

ribs   twelve pairs of bones that help form the thoracic cavity

right   referring to the patient's right.

right of way   permission to travel through traffic without delay.

rigidity   abnormal sense of firmness in the abdomen on palpation indication disease or trauma within.

rigor mortis body stiffness or rigidity that occurs in dead bodies.

rip tides strong currents that run parallel to the beach between the shore and underwater sandbars until they find a deeper opening and turn to head out to sea where they dump the contents into an undertow.

risk the chance of injury, damage, or loss.

route how the medication is administered.

routes of entry the way that hazardous materials can enter the body.

rule of nines method of determining the body surface area (BSA) burned based on dividing the adult body into areas of approximately 9 percent each.

rule of palm method of estimating the body surface area (BSA) burned based on the principle that a patient's palm is equal to approximately 1 percent of his BSA.

run data information about the call itself, such as the unit and crew members responding, the date and time of the call, and the name of the ambulance service.

run report written documentation of the call and patient encounter. Also called a prehospital care report.

S

sacral spine vertebrae that form the posterior pelvis.

sacral vertebrae fused vertebrae that help to form the pelvis.

sacrum or sacral vertebrae fused vertebrae that help to form the pelvis.

safety glass type of glass that, when struck, will break into small pieces. Also called tempered glass.

Safety Officer command staff officer who ensures that the incident safety considerations are recognized and has the power to stop activity or remove people immediately from hazardous situation.

SAMPLE a mnemonic used in obtaining a patient history. The letters stand for Signs and symptoms, Allergies, Medications, Past pertinent medical history, Last oral intake, and Events leading to the injury or illness.

saturated filled, as hemoglobin with oxygen.

scapulae the shoulder blades. Singular scapula.

scene safety an awareness that you must continually assure the safety of yourself, your crew, and your patient. This is done by teamwork, observation, and communication between members of a crew.

scene size-up initial evaluation of several scene factors, including confirming the exact location, nature, and the seriousness of the incident; the number and condition of victims; and risks versus benefits that will dictate a rescue or a body recovery.

schizophrenia a serious condition that involves unusual or bizarre thoughts, behaviors, and speech. The patient may be very quiet or catatonic in some presentations of the disease.

scoop stretcher a device that separates in two and can be used to "scoop" the patient off the ground. Also called an orthopedic stretcher.

scope of practice a detailed description of the specific care and actions EMTs are allowed to perform.

second stage of labor stage of labor from full dilation of the cervix until delivery of the baby.

secondary devices   devices used to intentionally disrupt rescue and to injure emergency responders after an initial attack has taken place.

secondary drowning syndrome   respiratory distress or apnea that can occur minutes to hours after a near-drowning event because of compromised lung tissue.

secreting   releasing of substances.

seizures   interruptions of normal brain function caused by bursts of abnormal electrical signals in the brain.

self-loading   stretchers that are wheeled up to the ambulance and, once the wheels are securely on the floor of the ambulance, the wheels may be lifted into the ambulance. Also called auto-loading.

Sellick's manuever   technique of applying downward pressure on the cricoid cartilage, used to help visualize the vocal cords and to reduce the potential for vomiting.

Semi-Fowler's   a semi-sitting position.

sensory nerves   portion of the nervous system that carries information from the body back to the central nervous system.

septic shock   type of shock caused by severe infections that abnormally dilate the blood vessels.

shock   see hypoperfusion.

short backboard   a flat rigid device primarily used to stabilize the spine of a seated patient during extrication from a vehicle.

side effects   any action of a drug other than the desired action.

sign   something that the EMT can see or observe or has a value that can be recorded.

simple access   means of getting into a vehicle that does not require specialized training, tools, or equipment.

simple radiological device   device that disperses radioactive particles without explosion.

singular command   method of command used for incidents that are smaller in scope that do not involve outside agencies and often occur within a single jurisdiction.

sinoatrial node   beginning of the cardiac conduction pathway, located at the top of the heart near the right atrium.

sirens   audible warning devices used on an emergency vehicle.

six rights   memory aid to remember all things you must check when administering a medication to the patient. These include: right medication, right dose, right route, right patient, right time, and right documentation.

skeletal muscle   see voluntary muscle.

SLUDGEM   acronym for the common signs and symptoms of exposure to nerve agents based on organophosphate pesticides: salivation, lacrimation, urination, defecation, gastrointestinal motility, emesis, and miosis.

small intestine   organ that digests solid foods and absorbs nutrients through the intestinal wall. The small intestine has three segments: duodenum, jejunum, and ileum.

small-volume nebulizer (SVN)   method of continuously administering a vaporized medication, as opposed to the inhaler that provides a one-time dose.

smooth muscle   see involuntary muscle.

smooth-muscle relaxant a medication that relaxes smooth muscles, for example, as nitroglycerin relaxes the muscle in blood vessels and permits an increased blood flow.

snoring intermittent low-pitched sounds heard during inhalation. Often indicative of partial upper airway obstruction caused by the tongue and associated soft tissue.

SOAP acronym for Subjective, Objective, Assessment, and Plan. A method of documentation in which each letter stands for a specific portion of the narrative.

soft palate tissue designed to lift up when a person swallows, closing off the oropharynx from the nasopharynx.

source initial location of the hazardous material or cause of a burn.

span of control the number of organizational elements or people that may be directly managed by another person. Effective span of control may vary from three to seven, although a ratio of one to five reporting elements is commonly recommended.

sperm male sex cell. Male counterpart to the ovum.

spinal column a series of vertebrae that are stacked one on top of the other to form the column.

spinal cord central nervous system (CNS) pathway responsible for transmitting sensory input from the body to the brain and for conducting motor impulses from the brain to the body muscles and organs.

spleen organ that filters the blood, including the removal of old blood cells. The spleen also creates white blood cells.

spontaneous abortion when the embryo or fetus delivers naturally before it is able to survive on its own. Also called a miscarriage.

spontaneous pneumothorax condition where a pneumothorax develops without a traumatic cause.

sprain injury caused by the stretching and/or tearing of the ligaments and tendons that support the joint.

stages of labor divisions of the labor process.

staging area location or locations at an incident where incoming resources report.

stair chair a chair-style device used to move patients up and down stairs in a sitting position.

stale air air that remains in the alveoli increasing carbon dioxide levels in the lungs.

standard of care a modified scope of practice specifically designed to meet the needs of a specific area or region.

standard precautions Centers for Disease Control and Prevention (CDC) guidelines and practices based on the awareness that all patients are potentially infectious regardless of diagnosis or presumed infection. Also called universal precautions.

standing orders a written order issued by a Medical Director that authorizes EMTs and others to perform particular skills in certain situations without medical direction contact.

status asthmaticus prolonged, life-threatening asthma attack, often not responding to the patient's own medications.

status epilepticus multiple seizures without a period of consciousness between them, or one continuous seizure lasting 10 minutes or more.

step chocks wooden blocks or other supportive materials placed in a stair-step pattern to assist in stabilizing a vehicle.

sterilization controlled process that, like disinfection, requires its own specific equipment and is usually done under controlled circumstances. In sterilization, all organisms on the piece of equipment are killed.

sternum the breastbone.

Stokes basket a metal or plastic basket designed to move patients over uneven terrain. Also called a basket stretcher.

stoma a permanent surgical opening in the anterior aspect of the trachea through which the patient breathes.

stomach organ that receives food from the esophagus.

strain injury caused when a muscle is pulled or torn, causing severe pain.

strainer a partial obstruction that filters, or strains, the water such as downed trees or wire mesh; causes an unequal force on the two sides.

stress any event or situation that places extraordinary demands on a person's mental or emotional resources.

stridor a harsh high-pitched sound that can occur during inhalation or exhalation. Indicative of partial upper airway obstruction.

stroke condition that occurs when the blood supply to an area of the brain is interrupted.

stroke volume amount of blood ejected into the aorta with each heart beat.

stylet moldable wire that can be inserted into an endotracheal tube to facilitate tube placement.

subcutaneous emphysema crackling sensation caused by air just underneath the skin.

subcutaneous layer the deepest layer of the skin. It is fatty tissue and provides shock absorption and insulation for the body.

subdural hematoma collection of blood between the dura mater and the arachnoid membrane.

subjective information that is not first hand or that is subject to interpretation.

sublingual beneath the tongue.

sudden infant death syndrome (SIDS) the sudden death of healthy infants in the first year of life.

suicide taking of one's own life.

superficial burns burns that affect the outermost layer of skin, the epidermis.

superior toward the head (e.g., the chest is superior to the abdomen). Opposite of inferior.

supine lying on the back. Opposite of prone.

supine hypotensive syndrome a condition that occurs when the pregnant patient lies flat and the fetus compresses the inferior vena cava. This compression reduces blood flow back to the heart and causes significant hypotension (low blood pressure).

Supply Unit team that receives supplies and equipment from staging and issues them to the operational units as requested.

suspensions solid medication mixed in a fluid. Must be shaken before giving.

sympathetic nervous system part of the nervous system that activates the "fight or flight" response.

symptom something that is experienced and described by the patient as it pertains to his chief complaint.

syncope fainting.

systemic vascular resistance an indicator of the diameter of the blood vessels.

systolic the pressure created when the left ventricle contracts and forces blood out into the arteries.

T

tablets small disk-like compressed form of medication.

tachycardia a pulse rate greater than 100 beats per minute.

tagged placed in a triage category with a triage tag affixed.

tarsals the ankle bones.

technical rescue incidents rescue situations requiring specialized training and equipment.

technician level level of training that is designed for responders who will be capable of hazard recognition, equipment use, techniques necessary to perform, and supervision of a technical rescue incident.

temperature regulation the body's ability to maintain a stable core temperature.

temporal bones bones that form part of the side of the skull. There is a right and a left temporal bone.

temporomandibular joint the movable joint formed between the mandible and the temporal bone, also called the TM joint.

tenderness pain that is elicited through palpation.

tendons tissues that connect muscle to the skeleton.

tension pneumothorax buildup of air under pressure within the thorax. The resulting compression of the lung severely reduces the effectiveness of respirations.

teratogenic causing an increased risk that a developing embryo will have physical defects.

terrorism an illegal act that is dangerous to human life, which is against the laws of the United States or any political subdivision, with intent to intimidate or coerce a government or civilian population in the furtherance of a political or social agenda.

testicles external gland producing the sperm.

thermal (heat) burn type of burn most commonly caused by exposure to fire, steam, hot objects, and hot liquids.

third stage of labor stage of labor from the birth of the baby until delivery of the placenta.

thoracic cavity the area that lies inferior to the clavicles and superior to the diaphragm.

thoracic vertebrae the twelve vertebrae that help form the thoracic cage. A pair of ribs is attached to each thoracic vertebra.

thyroid cartilage prominence in the anterior neck. Also called the Adam's apple.

tibia   the medial and larger bone of the lower leg.

tidal volume   the amount of air moved in and out with each breath.

timeline or sequential   method of narration that tells the story of the call as it happened in a step by step, chronological narrative.

tourniquets   method designed to stop all blood flow past the point at which it is applied.

toxins   poisonous substances produced by animals or plants.

trachea   the structure that connects the pharynx to the lungs. Also called the windpipe.

tracheal deviation   displacement of the trachea laterally from the midline.

tracheostomy tube   tube placed through a surgical opening in the neck to provide an airway.

trade name   the medication name a pharmaceutical company gives to a drug. It could also be referred to as a brand name.

tragus   the projection of skin-covered cartilage in front of the meatus of the external ear.

transdermal   through or by way of the skin.

transient ischemic attack (TIA)   also called mini-stroke, this condition presents as a stroke but signs and symptoms resolve usually within 24 hours.

transmissibility   the ease with which an agent or disease can spread from person to person.

Transportation Group   team responsible for obtaining resources to ensure that all patients are transported to the appropriate hospital.

traumatic asphyxia   condition where a severe blunt force or weight is placed upon the chest forcing blood from the right atrium up into the circulation of the head and neck.

Treatment Group   team that will establish a treatment area where patients can be treated and collected.

Trendelenburg position   a position in which the patient's feet and legs are higher than the head. Also called shock position.

trending   the comparing of multiple sets of vital signs over a period of time in order to reveal a trend in the patient's condition.

triage   the process of sorting patients based on the severity or their injuries and prioritizing them for treatment and transport.

Triage Group   team responsible for the sorting and tagging of all patients according to the seriousness and extent of injuries.

tricuspid valve   a structure between the right atrium and right ventricle that opens and closes to permit the flow of a fluid in only one direction.

triggers   allergies, respiratory infections, exercise, or emotion that may cause bronchoconstriction.

trimester   division of the pregnancy period, usually 13 weeks, or about one-third of the pregnancy.

tripod position   position that may be assumed during respiratory distress to facilitate breathing. The patient usually sits or may stand or crouch, leaning forward with hands placed on the bed, chair, table, or knees.

twisting force   the force caused by a twisting or turning motion.

two-thumb-encircling-hands method   chest compression method which is recommended in CPR for newborns.

U

ulna the medial bone of the forearm.

ultrasound examination technique that uses sound to produce a visual image.

umbilical cord structure that connects the fetus to the placenta.

undertow currents that occur when water is trapped behind sandbars and finds an opening to pull water and anything in the water out to sea.

unified command method of command that is a team effort allowing all agencies with a jurisdictional responsibility for the incident, either geographical or functional, to play a part in the management of the incident.

unit team assigned a specific task.

United States Pharmacopoeia (USP) government listing of all medications.

unity of command the principle that each individual in an organization has only one supervisor. The principle of unity of command should not be confused with a unified command.

ureters transport urine from the kidneys to the bladder.

urethra transports urine from the bladder to be excreted outside the body.

urgent moves a category of patient moves performed when the patient's condition is serious or is deteriorating and the patient must be moved promptly for treatment and/or transportation.

uterus the muscular abdominal organ in which the fetus develops. Also called the womb.

V

vagina the birth canal. The tubular structure leading from the uterus to the outer body.

valeculla space between the tongue and epiglottis.

vapor pressure the pressure exerted by a chemical against the atmosphere.

vas deferens carries the sperm from the testicles to the urethra.

vector borne spread by vectors, or carriers, such as animals, insects, or persons who have the disease.

veins blood vessels that return blood to the heart.

vena cava either of two major veins that carry oxygen-poor blood from the body to the right atrium. The superior vena cava carries blood from the head; the inferior vena cava carries blood from the lower body. Plural venae cavae.

ventral referring to the front of the body. Synonym for anterior.

ventricles the two lower chambers of the heart. There is a right ventricle (which sends oxygen-poor blood to the lungs) and a left ventricle (which sends oxygen-rich blood to the body).

ventricular fibrillation (VF or v-fib) one of the most common electrical rhythms associated with sudden cardiac arrest in which the ventricles of the heart contract spontaneously and in an uncoordinated manner, thus preventing the heart from circulating any meaningful amount of blood.

ventriculoperitoneal (VP) shunt a device that drains excess cerebral spinal fluid from the brain to the abdomen.

venules the smallest kind of vein.

vertebrae   the 33 bones of the spinal column. Singular vertebra.

vest-type extrication device   a rigid vest-type device primarily used to stabilize the spine of a seated patient during extrication from a vehicle.

virulence   the power of infection once started.

viruses   pathogenic organisms made of nucleic acid inside a protein shell, which must utilize a host cell for growth and reproduction.

visceral pleura   membrane that is attached to the lung surface.

vocal cords   tissue found within the larynx that opens and closes the glottis to produce sound vibrations.

voluntary muscle   muscle that can be consciously controlled. Also called skeletal muscle.

W

warning lights   visual warning devices used on an emergency vehicle.

weapons of mass destruction (WMDs)   variety of explosive, chemical, biological, nuclear, or other devices used by terrorists to strike at government, high-profile, or high-population targets; designed to create a maximum number of casualties.

wheeled stretcher   the most commonly used device for moving patients. Also called cot or gurney.

wheezing   a high-pitched sound that is indicative of lower airway constriction and can be heard during both inspiration and expiration but is more commonly heard during expiration.

white blood cells   cells within the blood that produce substances that help fight infection.

withdrawn   pulling into oneself. Retreating from reality.

work of breathing   effort needed for adequate ventilation.

Z

zygote   cell produced by union of egg and sperm.

Answer Key

CHAPTER 1
Stop, Review, Remember! (pp. 14–15)

Multiple Choice

1. b (p. 9)
2. c (p. 11)
3. d (p. 13)

Fill in the Blank

1. First Responder (p. 13)
2. Department of Transportation (DOT) (pp. 12–13)
3. EMS System (p. 9)
4. EMT-Basic (p. 13)
5. NHTSA (p. 9)

Critical Thinking

1. Student answers will vary depending on their location (pp. 9–12)
2. This is the most basic level of nationally recognized care and the NSC for this level represents approximately 40 hours of training. Emergency Medical responders (formerly First Responders) are most often the first people on the scene of an emergency and are trained to identify potential hazards, identify and treat immediate life threats, and assist other EMS personnel at the scene. These First Responders are trained to function with a minimum of equipment. (p. 13)
3. Student answers will vary depending on their location. (p. 13)

Stop, Review, Remember! (pp. 21–22)

Multiple Choice

1. d (p. 16)
2. a (p. 16)
3. d (p. 17)
4. b (p. 17)
5. c (p. 20)

Matching

1. B (p. 16)
2. C (p. 16)
3. A (p. 17)
4. F (p. 17)
5. E (p. 17)
6. D (p. 17)

Critical Thinking

1. This answer will vary depending on where the student lives. (p. 16)
2. The answer to this question will differ depending on the student. (pp. 18–20)
3. This answer will vary depending on where the student lives. (p. 20)

Chapter Review (pp. 23–27)

Multiple Choice

1. d (pp. 9–12)
2. a (p. 9)
3. c (p. 13)
4. b (p. 18)
5. c (p. 20)
6. d (pp. 9–12)
7. a (p. 13)
8. b (pp. 18–20)
9. c (p. 16)
10. d (p. 16)

Matching

1. B (p. 17)
2. C (p. 17)
3. E (p. 20)
4. A (p. 13)
5. D (p. 16)

Critical Thinking

1. The answer to this question will differ from student to student. (pp. 9–12)
2. The answer to this question will differ from student to student. (p. 11)
3. The job of the EMT-B differs from that of the Advanced-EMT or EMT-P in that the EMT-B can only assist with certain prescribed medications and cannot perform advanced procedures except where allowed by local protocols. Emergency Medical Responders are trained to identify and treat immediate life threats and assist other EMS personnel at the scene. (p. 13)
4. A list of available specialty hospitals might include:
   trauma centers
   pediatric centers
   burn centers
   reattachment centers
   hyperbaric centers
   neurosurgery centers (p. 16)
5. Medical direction can include written protocols, standing orders, direct verbal orders given in person, over the radio or telephone. (pp. 16–17)
6. The Emergency Medical Dispatcher differs from the traditional emergency dispatcher in that they are trained to provide pre-arrival medical care instructions until the EMS units arrive. (p. 17)

Case Studies

#1

1. You must respectfully inform this woman that local protocols do not allow you to puncture her blisters. You can offer her a place to rest and perhaps offer some adhesive bandages or gauze to help relieve some of the discomfort. (p. 16)

2. When in doubt regarding the delivery of the most appropriate patient care you should contact medical direction or your immediate field supervisor for direction. (p. 17)

3. It is always important to document any care that you provide a patient. Good care along with good documentation will minimize the chances of liability should the patient's condition get worse. (p. 19)

#2

1. Your primary concern as you arrive and exit your ambulance will be your safety and the overall safety of the scene. (p. 18)

2. The immediate hazard is one of traffic. You are on a blind curve of a well-traveled highway. You must also be alert for spilled fuel and the potential for fire. You must keep your warning lights on and place flares or reflectors a good distance from the scene in both directions. You must be alert to not use an ignition source anywhere near spilled fluids and call for the fire department for additional assistance. (p. 18)

3. Your personal safety comes before that of anyone else at the scene. It is your duty to remain safe and do what you can to minimize threats to anyone else who may enter the scene, even if it results in delayed care to the patient. (p. 18)

CHAPTER 2

Stop, Review, Remember! (pp. 33–35)

Multiple Choice

1. b (p. 30)
2. d (pp. 31–32)
3. a (p. 32)
4. c (p. 33)
5. a (p. 33)

Matching

1. B (p. 31)
2. D (p. 33)
3. A (p. 33)
4. C (p. 33)

Critical Thinking

1. This answer will differ from student to student. (pp. 30–33)
2. This answer will differ from student to student. (p. 31)
3. This answer will differ from student to student. (p. 31)

Stop, Review, Remember! (pp. 41–42)

Multiple Choice

1. b (p. 37)
2. c (p. 38)
3. d (p. 40)
4. a (pp. 40–41)
5. c (p. 40)

Matching

1. B (p. 37)
2. C (p. 38)
3. A (p. 38)
4. E (p. 40)
5. D (p. 40)

Critical Thinking

1. This answer will differ from student to student. (pp. 36–37)

2. Being proactive regarding the management of stress in your life means that you are doing things in advance to better prepare yourself to handle stress when it appears. This may include eating a balanced diet, exercising regularly and being open and honest about your feelings when your job becomes stressful. (pp. 35–37)

3. Resiliency refers to the ability to recover quickly from the stress caused by illness, change, or misfortune. Being resilient requires that you learn to manage stress before it happens and develop habits that will help you cope when stress becomes acute. (p. 39)

Stop, Review, Remember! (pp. 50–52)

Multiple Choice

1. c (p. 43)
2. a (pp. 44–46)
3. b (p. 44)
4. a (p. 43)
5. c (p. 46)

Critical Thinking

1. In most cases that involve patient care, taking proper BSI means utilizing the appropriate PPE for the situation. PPE such as gloves, masks, and eye protection are all a part of proper BSI precautions. (pp. 43–46)

2. You would want to wear specialized suits and self-contained breathing apparatus (SCBA) prior to entry. (p. 49)

3. When entering a potential crime scene you must begin with being careful where you walk and step. Do not disturb. (p. 50)

4. (pp. 43–46)

Guide to Proper BSI Precautions
Given the different situations below choose the appropriate PPE.

Situation	Gloves	Glasses	Mask	Gown
Minor bleed to the left hand	X	X		
Suctioning a vomiting patient	X	X	X	
Assisting with a birth	X	X	X	X
Cleaning a bloody backboard	X	X		
Taking a blood pressure on a medical patient	X			
Major bleed of the lower leg with spurting blood	X	X		
Cleaning the back of the ambulance after a call	X			

Chapter Review (pp. 53–55)

Multiple Choice

1. b (p. 30)
2. c (p. 40)
3. b (p. 32)
4. d (p. 50)
5. a (pp. 40–41)

Critical Thinking

1. The answer to this question will differ depending on the student. (pp. 35–37)
2. The answer to this question will differ depending on the student. (pp. 35–37)
3. The answer to this question will differ depending on the student. (pp. 37–39)

Case Studies

#1

1. It is not a bad idea to engage Will in a conversation about the call so long as he does not reveal any information that might identify the patient. Be sensitive to the fact that talking about it is healthy but Will may not feel comfortable at this time. When appropriate, encourage Will to talk about the event with a supervisor or peer counselor. (pp. 30–41)
2. Many people who have experienced a stressful event will become quiet and somewhat distant in their behavior. They may not have a normal appetite and may want to be alone. They also may get angry easily and lash out for little or no reason. (pp. 30–41)
3. The most important thing you can do is be a good listener when he is willing to talk. Do not judge him or criticize him for anything relating to the incident. (pp. 30–41)

#2

1. You might be having trouble sleeping and are probably not eating well. You also may not be exercising. You may become easily angered and this leads to others seeing you with a negative attitude. (pp. 30–41)
2. At some point you will not be able to cope and may end up experiencing an emotional and/or physical breakdown. (pp. 30–41)
3. This begins with working a reasonable number of hours. You can't work every shift, at least not for long. Be sure to eat as healthy as you can and get plenty of sleep and exercise regularly, even if it's only a nice long walk. (pp. 30–41)

CHAPTER 3

Stop, Review, Remember! (pp. 62–63)

Multiple Choice

1. a (p. 57)
2. b (p. 58)
3. c (p. 61)
4. c (p. 58)
5. a (p. 61)

Matching

1. F (p. 57)
2. G (p. 58)
3. E (p. 58)
4. B (p. 58)
5. C (p. 58)
6. D (p. 61)
7. A (p. 61)

Critical Thinking

1. The answer to this question will differ depending on the system in which you will be working. (pp. 57–58)
2. A legal duty to provide care is determined by law and applies to most EMTs who work for a provider agency regardless if it is volunteer or paid. An ethical duty may apply to the EMT who is "off duty" and comes upon someone who is injured. The EMT also has an ethical duty to always do what is best for the patient and not let personal desires interfere with that care. (pp. 58–61)
3. Good Samaritan laws exist in some form in all 50 states and are designed to encourage the passerby to stop and render care. These laws minimize the exposure to liability for acts and omissions while providing care at the scene of an emergency so long as the caregiver is not being compensated. (p. 61)

Stop, Review, Remember! (pp. 71–73)

Multiple Choice

1. d (p. 64)
2. a (p. 65)
3. c (pp. 65–66)
4. b (p. 67)
5. a (p. 69)
6. c (p. 67)

Matching

1. F (p. 64)
2. G (p. 64)
3. A (p. 65)
4. B (p. 65)
5. D (p. 67)
6. C (p. 69)
7. E (p. 70)

Critical Thinking

1. A responsive and competent adult may provide consent in verbal form by simply saying yes to your request to provide care. Consent can also be nonverbal if you have asked for permission and their actions indicate they want you to help, even though they have not stated so verbally. (p. 64)
2. In situations where a patient's mental status is altered either by injury, illness, or substance it may be difficult to determine if they are legally competent to refuse care. (p. 65)
3. It is best to contact medical direction as soon as possible and when practical initiate care until the DNR can be confirmed. (p. 71)

Stop, Review, Remember! (pp. 77–79)

Multiple Choice

1. b (p. 73)
2. c (p. 74)
3. c (p. 74)
4. d (p. 75)
5. a (p. 74)

Matching

1. G (p. 73)
2. F (p. 73)
3. B (p. 73)
4. D (p. 74)

5. C (p. 74)
6. E (p. 74)
7. A (p. 74)

Critical Thinking

1. The term "assault" refers to the threat to use force against another person. The term "battery" refers to the actual carrying out of that threat. (p. 73)
2. There are many examples of how an EMT may be accused of negligence. A couple examples include performing skills that are clearly outside the scope of care for an EMT or abandoning a patient before someone of equal or higher training takes over. (pp. 73–74)
3. After providing the appropriate care for the patient you should advise the medical personnel at the hospital of your findings. You should immediately document all of your findings including the care that you provided. You must then contact your immediate supervisor or law enforcement officer to report your findings. The specific steps may vary in your system. Follow local laws and protocols. (p. 75)

Chapter Review   (pp. 80–82)

Multiple Choice

1. b (p. 57)
2. b (pp. 70–71)
3. c (p. 64)
4. a (p. 67)
5. a (p. 75)

6. c (p. 65)
7. a (p. 76)
8. c (p. 76)
9. d (p. 58)
10. b (p. 73)

Critical Thinking

1. It may become necessary to use force to restrain a patient if they pose a risk to themselves or anyone else attempting to care for them. While it is not your duty to forcibly restrain patients, it may become unavoidable if the patient suddenly becomes violent. If you are able, it is more appropriate to retreat and call for law enforcement. (p. 73)
2. The answer to this question will vary depending on the laws in your state. (p. 74)
3. Your care should not change simply by the fact that the patient is a potential organ donor. You will want to advise the receiving hospital of this fact in case the patient dies and the family wishes to donate the organs. (p. 76)

Case Studies

#1

1. Your legal obligation to stop and render care will depend on the state where you reside. Ask your instructor for how the laws in your state pertain to this scenario. (p. 74)
2. The legal ramifications of not stopping to render care will depend on the state where you reside. Research the information or ask your instructor for how the laws in your state pertain to this scenario. (p. 74)
3. In most states, the fact that you began care established a legal duty to stay at the scene and continue to provide care to the best of your ability. You could be accused of

abandonment if you leave the patient before someone of equal or higher training takes over. Ask your instructor how the laws of your state pertain to this situation. (pp. 67–69)

#2

1. If in doubt you should contact medical direction for advice. (pp. 70–71)
2. A DNR order can appear in many forms including a formal signed document and written orders on a patient's chart. Most states recognize medical alert jewelry as an acceptable form of a legal DNR order. Check with your instructor regarding your state. (pp. 69–71)
3. It is probably best to continue to ventilate the patient until it can be confirmed that a valid DNR does exist. (pp. 69–71)

CHAPTER 4

Stop, Review, Remember!   (pp. 89–92)

Multiple Choice

1. a (p. 87)
2. c (p. 86)
3. d (p. 87)
4. b (p. 86)

5. c (p. 86)
6. b (p. 85)
7. b (p. 88)

Labeling   (p. 85)

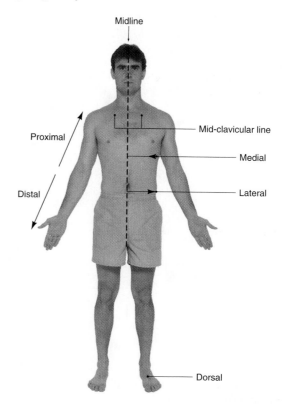

Fill in the Blank

1. proximal/distal (p. 86)
2. prone (p. 87)
3. midclavicular (p. 86)

4. midaxillary/medial/lateral (p. 85)
5. bilateral (p. 85)

Critical Thinking

1. A laceration on the posterior surface of the left arm just proximal to the wrist. (pp. 85–86)
2. A laceration on the posterior surface of the leg just distal to the knee (pp. 85–86)
3. Pain in the lower right quadrant radiating to the umbilicus. (pp. 87–88)
4. Bruising on the right side of the forehead superior to the right eye. (pp. 85–86)
5. A puncture wound to the plantar surface of the left foot. (p. 86)

Stop, Review, Remember! (pp. 103–105)

Multiple Choice

1. c (p. 94)
2. d (pp. 96–97)
3. c (p. 94)
4. b (p. 101)
5. b (p. 94)

Fill in the Blank

1. alveoli (p. 94)
2. nasopharynx (p. 92)
3. arteries (p. 98)
4. capillaries (p. 98)
5. atria/ventricles (pp. 97–98)
6. radial (p. 100)

Labeling (p. 97)

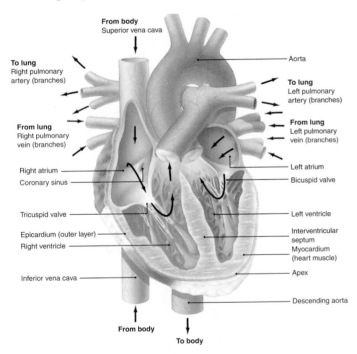

From body
Superior vena cava

To lung
Right pulmonary artery (branches)

Aorta

To lung
Left pulmonary artery (branches)

From lung
Right pulmonary vein (branches)

From lung
Left pulmonary vein (branches)

Right atrium
Coronary sinus

Tricuspid valve

Epicardium (outer layer)
Right ventricle

Inferior vena cava

Left atrium
Bicuspid valve

Left ventricle

Interventricular septum
Myocardium (heart muscle)

Apex

Descending aorta

From body

To body

Critical Thinking

1. Very slow or fast breathing/shallow breathing/irregular breathing/restlessness, anxiety, sleepiness/poor skin color. (p. 95)

2. Perfusion is the process of getting oxygenated blood to all of the tissues of the body and removing waste products. Hypoperfusion is when perfusion is not adequate, that is not reaching all of the tissues of the body with oxygen and failing to remove waste products. (p. 101)
3. Tongues take up proportionately more space in the mouth/all structures are smaller and more easily obstructed/trachea is narrower/trachea is softer and more flexible/cricoid cartilage is less developed. (pp. 95–96)

Stop, Review, Remember! (pp. 120–121)

Multiple Choice

1. c (p. 118)
2. d (p. 112)
3. d (p. 117)
4. a (p. 115)
5. b (p. 115)
6. d (p. 111)
7. a (p. 109)

Fill in the Blank

1. radius/ulna (p. 105)
2. floating (p. 108)
3. hinge (pp. 108–109)
4. cervical (p. 111)
5. involuntary/smooth (p. 112)
6. central/peripheral (p. 112)

Critical Thinking

1. Give the body shape/protect internal organs/provide the ability to move (p. 105)
2. Right upper quadrant, liver/left upper quadrant, spleen/right lower quadrant, appendix/left lower quadrant, colon (p. 117)

Chapter Review (pp. 122–125)

Multiple Choice

1. c (p. 100)
2. b (p. 87)
3. d (p. 86)
4. c (p. 92)
5. a (p. 97)
6. a (p. 85)
7. d (p. 108)
8. d (p. 115)
9. c (p. 117)
10. a (p. 112)

Matching

1. K (p. 106)
2. A (p. 106)
3. E (p. 106)
4. O (p. 106)
5. B (p. 106)
6. C (p. 106)
7. M (p. 106)
8. H (p. 106)
9. N (p. 106)
10. I (p. 106)
11. L (p. 106)
12. J (p. 106)
13. G (p. 106)
14. D (p. 106)
15. F (p. 106)

Labeling   (p. 117)

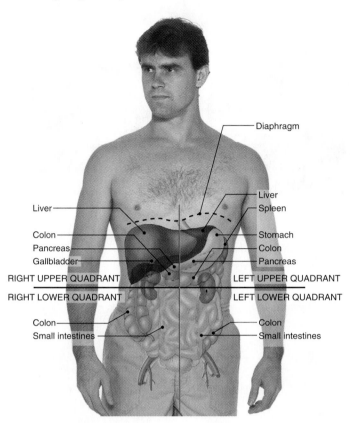

- Diaphragm
- Liver
- Spleen
- Liver
- Colon
- Stomach
- Pancreas
- Colon
- Gallbladder
- Pancreas
- RIGHT UPPER QUADRANT
- LEFT UPPER QUADRANT
- RIGHT LOWER QUADRANT
- LEFT LOWER QUADRANT
- Colon
- Colon
- Small intestines
- Small intestines

Ordering

1. 9, 6, 8, 10, 5, 7, 2, 12, 1, 3, 4, 11 (pp. 96–97)

Critical Thinking

1. The patient has pain in his upper right abdominal quadrant. (pp. 85–88)
2. The patient has a deformity of his distal radius and ulna. (pp. 85–88)
3. The patient has a laceration on the posterior surface of his hand (across the knuckles). (pp. 85–88)

Case Study

1. The trauma that caused injuries to the ribs could also cause trauma to the lungs. Depending on the force involved deeper injury could cause damage to the heart and large blood vessels in the chest cavity. Injury to the lower rib cage could also damage abdominal organs (discussed in question #2) (pp. 108, 117)
2. The liver is the most notable organ in this region. The gallbladder, stomach, colon, and intestines could also be involved. (p. 117)
3. Yes, both could be extremely serious causing problems with breathing and internal bleeding from the liver injury. (p. 117)

CHAPTER 5

Stop, Review, Remember! (pp. 137–138)

Multiple Choice

1. d (pp. 128–129)
2. c (p. 132)
3. d (p. 136)
4. c (p. 131)
5. a (p. 128)
6. a (p. 129)

Matching

1. C (p. 134)
2. B (p. 135)
3. A (p. 135)
4. E (pp. 131–132)
5. D (p. 131)
6. F (p. 136)

Critical Thinking

1. The power grip involves assuring as much of your palm and fingers are in contact with the object being lifted, and that your hands are placed about 10 inches apart.
   The power lift involves placing your feet a comfortable width apart, distributing the weight evenly on both feet, and keeping your back in a locked-in position. (p. 128)
2. Most significantly, you could injure your back. Back injuries in a profession that requires lifting can be career ending. Back injuries are often lingering, causing chronic pain and disability. (pp. 128–130)
3. Your patient could be seriously injured if the stretcher fell from an elevated position or if the patient were thrown from the stretcher. This would almost certainly cause a lawsuit. Your patient may also experience anxiety from awkward, rough, or unsafe moves whether or not injury was caused. If the patient had a problem such as a heart attack, his condition could be worsened by this anxiety. (pp. 127–130)

Stop, Review, Remember! (pp. 146–147)

Multiple Choice

1. a (p. 139)
2. b (p. 139)
3. b (p. 139)
4. b (p. 140)
5. b (p. 141)
6. c (p. 141)
7. b (p. 145)
8. d (p. 139)
9. a (p. 139)

Fill in the Blank

1. right, left (p. 145)
2. emergent (p. 139)
3. prone (p. 141)
4. comfort (p. 144)
5. long, axis (p. 139)

Critical Thinking

1. An emergency move is used when there is an immediate threat to life (for example, car on fire, hazardous materials). An urgent move is performed when the patient must be moved due to a medical condition requiring immediate action. An example is a critical patient who would be harmed by the time it would take to perform spinal immobilization.

Nonemergency moves are done in every situation when it isn't emergent or urgent. It is done with full spinal precautions. A stable patient with neck pain in a safe environment would be an example of a nonemergency move. (pp. 139–141)

2. Emergent moves involve immediate life threats from hazards, or to access a patient who is extremely critical. Urgent moves are performed when the patient's condition is serious enough to warrant immediate action without full spinal immobilization. (pp. 139–141)

Chapter Review (pp. 148–152)

Multiple Choice

1. b (p. 128)	6. c (p. 128)
2. a (p. 135)	7. b (p. 139)
3. b (p. 131)	8. c (p. 134)
4. a (p. 148)	9. d (p. 129)
5. b (p. 135)	10. a (p. 141)

Matching

1. A (p. 141)	4. B (p. 145)
2. D (p. 144)	5. E (p. 145)
3. C (p. 145)	

Labeling

1a. supine (p. 145)
1b. prone (p. 145)
1c. laterally recumbent (p. 145)

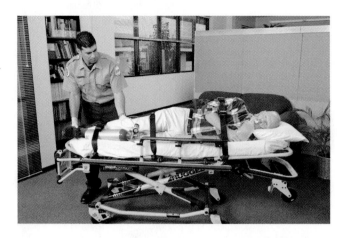

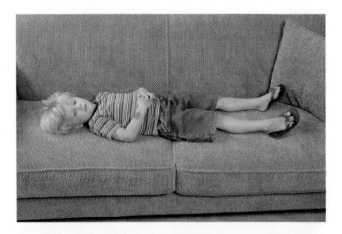

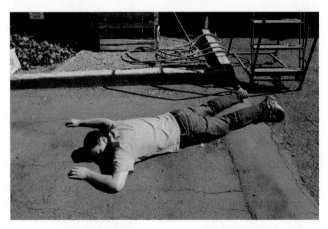

2d. This device is not illustrated in the text. Ask instructor.
2e. stair chair (p. 133)
2f. flexible stretcher (p. 134)
2g. scoop stretcher (p. 136)

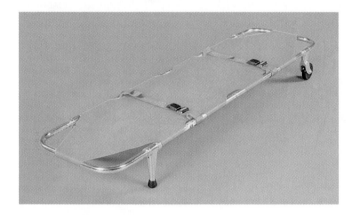

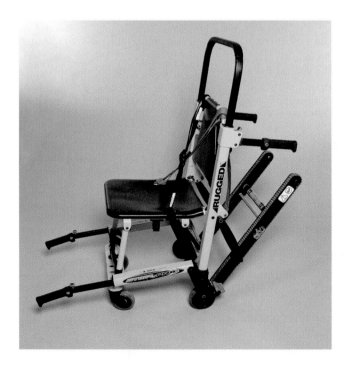

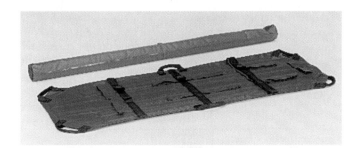

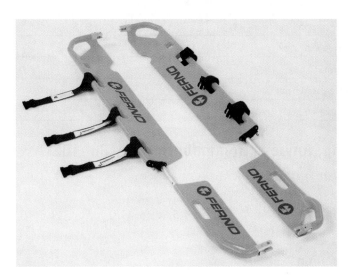

Case Studies

#1

1. d (p. 139)
2. b (p. 139)

#2

1. The patient would be carried on the long backboard. CPR would be discontinued for brief times of movement. CPR would be performed, then movement would begin again. Alternate movement with CPR. (pp. 139–145)
2. Stopping CPR for any amount of time reduces the chances of survival—but is sometimes necessary or we wouldn't be able to ever move a patient. Minimize your movement times—and do CPR walking alongside the stretcher when possible. (pp. 139–145)
3. Some equipment may be carried on the stretcher (strapped in or in specially designed carriers). One member of the three-person crew can carry the bag not strapped to the stretcher as he assists the crew carrying the stretcher. If necessary, one rescuer can reenter the residence quickly after the patient has been loaded in the rig. If the police or other rescuers show up they can assist in this as well. (pp. 139–145)

#3

1. Depending on the location of the patient, you will need significant help in lifting (6-8 people at a minimum). (pp. 127–130)
2. Depending on the weight limit of your stretcher, you may need a special (Bariatric) stretcher designed to hold this weight. This may cause additional issues such as moving the patient through small doorways, and so on. If the patient must be transported down stairs, you may need special Reeves stretchers or stair chairs. (pp. 127–130)

CHAPTER 6

1. d (p. 9)
   Objective 1-1.1
2. a (pp. 9–12)
   Objective 1-1.1
3. b (p. 12)
   Objective 1-1.5
4. c (p. 13)
   Objective 1-1.2
5. c (p. 13)
   Objective 1-1.2
6. b (p. 16)
   Objective 1-1.6
7. a (p. 17)
   Objective 1-1.6
8. d (p. 18)
   Objective 1-1.3 & 1-1.4
9. c (p. 20)
   Objective: 1-1.5
10. d (p. 20)
    Objective: 1-1.5
11. a (p. 32)
    Objective: 1-2.4
12. b (p. 33)
    Objective: Not specific to DOT objectives. See chapter 2.
13. c (p. 32)
    Objective: 1-2.1 & 1-2.5
14. a (p. 35)
    Objective: 1-2.6
15. d (pp. 35–37)
    Objective 1-2.6
16. a (pp. 40–41)
    Objective 1-2.3
17. d (p. 40)
    Objective 1-2.2
18. d (p. 43)
    Objective 1-2.8
19. b (p. 43)
    Objective 1-2.10
20. c (pp. 43–44)
    Objective: 1-2.9 & 1-2.10
21. b (p. 46)
    Objective: 1-2.8, 1-2.9, & 1-2. 10
22. c (p. 47)
    Objective: Not specific to DOT objectives. See Chapter 2.
23. d (p. 49)
    Objective 1-2.10
24. a (p. 50)
    Objective: 1-2.7
25. b (pp. 52–53)
    Objective: 1-2.6
26. b (p. 57)
    Objective: 1-3.1
27. d (p. 58)
    Objective 1-3.1
28. c (p. 60)
    Objective: Not specific to DOT objectives. See Chapter 3.
29. a (p. 61)
    Objective: 1-3.8
30. d (p. 61)
    Objective: 1-3.7
31. d (p. 64)
    Objective: 1-3.3
32. d (pp. 64–67)
    Objective: 1-3.3
33. b (pp. 66–67)
    Objective: 1-3.5
34. b (p. 67)
    Objective: 1-3.6
35. a (p. 67)
    Objective: 1-3.6
36. c (pp. 67–69)
    Objective: 1-3.7
37. a (p. 71)
    Objective: 1-3.2
38. d (p. 73)
    Objective: 1-3.7
39. a (p. 74)
    Objective: 1-3.7
40. d (p. 75)
    Objective: 1-3.9
41. b (p. 84)
    Objective: 1-4.1
42. c (p. 85)
    Objective: 1-4.1

43. a (p. 86)
Objective: 1-4.1
44. d (p. 87)
Objective: Not specific to
DOT objectives.
45. c (pp. 92–93)
Objective: 1-4.2
46. b (p. 94)
Objective: 1-4.2
47. c (p. 95)
Objective: 1-4.2
48. a (p. 96)
Objective: 1-4.2
49. d (p. 96)
Objective: 1-4.2
50. b (p. 100)
Objective: 1-4.2
51. d (p. 100)
Objective: 1-4.2
52. e (p. 101)
Objective: 1-4.2
53. b (p. 100)
Objective: 1-4.2
54. b (p. 105)
Objective: 1-4.2
55. c (p. 108)
Objective: 1-4.2
56. a (p. 109)
Objective 1-4.2
57. d (p. 111)
Objective: 1-4.2
58. a (p. 112)
Objective: 1-4.2
59. c (p. 112)
Objective: 1-4.2

60. b (p. 112)
Objective: 1-4.2
61. d (p. 112)
Objective: Not specific to
DOT objectives.
62. a (p. 112)
Objective: Not specific to
DOT objectives.
63. b (p. 115)
Objective: Not specific to
DOT objectives.
64. d (p. 117)
Objective: 1-4.2
65. c (p. 117)
Objective: Not specific to
DOT objectives.
66. c (p. 118)
Objective: Not specific to
DOT objectives.
67. d (p. 128)
Objective: Not specific to
DOT objectives.
68. d (pp. 131–136)
Objective: 1-6.2
69. c (p. 131)
Objective: 1-6.4
70. c (p. 135)
Objective: 1-6.12
71. a (p. 136)
Objective: 1-6.10
72. a (p. 139)
Objective: 1-6.10
73. d (p. 144)
Objective: 1-6.11

CHAPTER 7
Stop, Review, Remember! (pp. 175–176)
Multiple Choice

1. d (pp. 166–167)
2. a (pp. 166–167)
3. b (p. 174)

4. a (pp. 172–173)
5. c (p. 172)

Critical Thinking

1. Several things to look for in both responsive and
unresponsive patients include:
   a. adequate chest rise and fall (tidal volume)
   b. adequate rate
   c. ability to speak in full sentences
   d. good skin signs (pp. 166–167)
2. When a patient is in respiratory distress the body is still
attempting to compensate by increasing the rate and
volume of breathing. When failure sets in these
compensatory mechanisms begin to fail and breathing rate
and volume decrease and the mental status decreases as
well. (pp. 167–168)

3. You must attempt to create an airway using all the BLS
airway techniques such as insertion of an OPA and/or NPA
and of course the jaw thrust. If these alone do not create an
open airway you must provide slight extension until a patent
airway can be established. (p. 181)
4. (pp. 167–168)

Sign	Distress	Failure
Increased respiratory rate	X	
Decreased respiratory rate		X
Altered mental status	X	X
Use of accessory muscles	X	X
Tripod position		
Nasal flaring	X	
Decreased heart rate		
Increased heart rate		

Stop, Review, Remember! (pp. 186–188)
Multiple Choice

1. c (p. 176)
2. a (p. 177)
3. b (p. 181)

4. d (p. 186)
5. c (p. 178)

Matching

1. E (p. 176)
2. D (pp. 177–178)
3. B (references your training in CPR class]
4. A (p. 181)
5. C (p. 186)

Critical Thinking

1. Whenever you are manually ventilating a patient, regardless
of how good of an airway you may have, there is a strong
likelihood that some air will enter the patient's stomach.
This increases the chances that the patient may vomit. Have
suction ready to help minimize the chances of aspiration.
(p. 176)
2. These airway adjuncts are designed to "assist" the EMT in
maintaining a patent airway and do not guarantee an open
airway when inserted. You must constantly reassess the
airway and maintain manual support of the airway (head tilt
or jaw thrust) when appropriate. (p. 181)
3. NPAs are contraindicated in patients with significant facial
trauma since this may be an indication of a skull fracture.
There is a possibility that an NPA inserted into a patient
with a skull fracture could result in the device entering the
skull and causing damage and infection. (p. 186)

Stop, Review, Remember! (pp. 198–200)
Multiple Choice

1. b (p. 188)
2. c (pp. 189–190)
3. d (p. 188)

4. a (p. 194)
5. d (p. 191)

Critical Thinking

1. This patient's respirations are inadequate for two reasons. They are below the acceptable rate and tidal volume. You must provide assisted ventilations with an appropriate device such as a BVM with supplemental oxygen. You can squeeze the bag whenever the patient attempts to breathe, enhancing his breath. You must also add additional breaths to bring his rate up to the minimum 12 per minute necessary. (pp. 188–189)

2. The ideal device will be a pediatric size BVM. The correct size BVM will minimize the chances that you will over inflate the patient causing a build up of air in the stomach. (p. 191)

3. You must ensure that you have both the proper size mask to ensure a good seal. The head needs only to be extended slightly to ensure an open airway. (pp. 195–196)

4. (pp. 188–195)

Situation	Mouth to Mask	2-rescuer BVM	Demand Valve	1-rescuer BVM
You are alone and off duty with an unresponsive nonbreathing infant.	✔			
You, your partner, and a firefighter are ventilating a patient as you carry him down a flight of stairs on a portable stretcher.		✔	✔	✔
You and a firefighter are ventilating an adult male in the back of an ambulance.		✔	✔	✔
You are alone in the back of an ambulance and ventilating an 8-year-old near-drowning victim.				✔
You are ventilating a 20-year-old male who is the third patient from an accidental carbon monoxide poisoning.			✔	✔

Stop, Review, Remember! (pp. 213–214)

Multiple Choice

1. b (p. 200)
2. c (p. 204)
3. d (p. 202)
4. a (p. 210)
5. c (p. 208)

Matching

1. E (p. 197)
2. C (p. 181)
3. D (p. 208)
4. A (p. 210)
5. B (p. 191)

Critical Thinking

1. Medical oxygen is 100% oxygen while the air that we breathe is approximately 21% oxygen. (p. 200)

2. For a patient who is not getting enough oxygen due to inadequate rate or volume, increasing the concentration of oxygen will compensate for the decrease in rate and/or volume. (p. 200)

3. The nonrebreather mask does not create an air tight seal around the face, therefore it allows room air to enter the mask and mix with the oxygen. When the air mixes with the oxygen it lowers the overall concentration. (p. 208)

Chapter Review (pp. 216–218)

Multiple Choice

1. c (p. 167)
2. b (p. 165)
3. a (p. 166)
4. a (p. 173)
5. a (p. 178)
6. b (p. 177)
7. c (p. 189)
8. c (p. 173)
9. d (p. 176)
10. c (p. 208)

Critical Thinking

1. The best way to determine if the flow rate on a nonrebreather mask is appropriate is when the reservoir bag is able to refill completely between breaths. (p. 210)

2. Passive oxygen delivery devices such as a nonrebreather mask or cannula require that the patient be breathing adequately in order to be effective. They simply increase the concentration of available oxygen that must be breathed in by the patient to provide benefit. In contrast a demand valve or BVM are used to breathe for a patient who is either not breathing or breathing inadequately. (p. 208)

3. Due to the fact that a nonrebreather mask in not air tight, it will always allow some ambient air in around the seal. For this reason, a NRB mask is not capable of providing a breathable oxygen concentration of 100%. In a best case a properly fitted nonrebreather mask may deliver a breathable concentration of approximately 95% oxygen. (p. 208)

Case Studies

#1

1. Your first priority will be to clear this man's airway and begin providing assisted ventilations with supplemental oxygen. Due to the MOI you must do so while maintaining appropriate spinal precautions. (pp. 171–174)

2. The best way to address his airway and breathing problems is to have someone manually stabilize his head while suctioning his airway and then inserting an airway adjunct. You will then need to assist his breathing with manual ventilations. (p. 176)

3. The most appropriate device is most likely going to be a BVM, however a pocket mask with supplemental O_2 or a demand valve could also be used. (pp. 189–190)

#2

1. If you can rule out the possibility of trauma you can use the head-tilt chin-lift maneuver to open her airway. (p. 172)

2. Yes, assisted ventilations are most likely needed since her tidal volume is so poor. A BVM is the most appropriate device for this patient; however a pocket mask with supplemental O_2 or a demand valve could also be used. (p. 189)

3. Assuming she continues to need assisted ventilations you will keep her in the supine position. If her respirations improve you can move her to the recovery position. (pp. 72–73)

CHAPTER 8

1. c (p. 163)
   Objective: Not specific to DOT objectives.
2. a (p. 166)
   Objective: 2-1.1
3. d (p. 164)
   Objective: 2-1.1
4. c (p. 166)
   Objective: 2-1.2
5. a (p. 166)
   Objective: 2-1.2
6. c (p. 166)
   Objective: 2-1.2
7. b (p. 167)
   Objective: 2-1.3
8. d (p. 168)
   Objective: 2-1.3
9. a (p. 171)
   Objective: 2-1.4
10. b (p. 172)
    Objective: 2-1.4
11. c (p. 173)
    Objective: 2-1.5
12. d (p. 176)
    Objective: 2-1.8
13. b (p. 176)
    Objective: 2-1.7
14. c (p. 178)
    Objective: 2-1.8
15. a (p. 178)
    Objective: 2-1.8
16. b (p. 178)
    Objective: 2-1.8
17. d (pp. 178-179)
    Objective: 2-1.8
18. a (p. 178)
    Objective: 2-1.8
19. d (p. 181)
    Objective: Not specific to DOT objectives.
20. c (p. 181)
    Objective: 2-1.17
21. d (p. 197)
    Objective: 2-1.12
22. a (p. 190)
    Objective: 1-2.10
23. d (p. 189)
    Objective: 2-1.12
24. d (p. 190)
    Objective: 2-1.9
25. c (p. 191)
    Objective: 2-1.11
26. c (p. 194)
    Objective: 2-1.17
27. c (p. 194)
    Objective: 2-1.15
28. a (p. 176)
    Objective: 2-1.14
29. b (p. 197)
    Objective: 2-1.12
30. c (pp. 202–203)
    Objective: 2-1.19
31. a (p. 203)
    Objective: 2-1.19
32. b (p. 204)
    Objective: 2-1.19
33. c (p. 208)
    Objective: 2-1.21
34. c (p. 208)
    Objective: 2-1.22
35. d (p. 208)
    Objective: 2-1.20
36. d (p. 208)
    Objective: 2-1.20
37. c (p. 208)
    Objective: Not specific to DOT objectives.
38. b (p. 210)
    Objective: 2-1.22
39. c (p. 210)
    Objective: 2-1.22
40. a (p. 210)
    Objective: 2-1.22
41. b (p. 212)
    Objective: 2-1.22
42. a (p. 176)
    Objective: 2-1.8
43. b (p. 192)
    Objective: 2-1.12
44. c (p. 174)
    Objective: Not specific to DOT objectives.
45. b (p. 191)
    Objective: 2-1.11
46. a (p. 200)
    Objective: 2-1.2
47. c (p. 204)
    Objective: 2-1.19
48. d (pp. 166–167)
    Objective: 2-1.2
49. a (p. 163)
    Objective: Not specific to DOT objectives.
50. a (pp. 166–167)
    Objective: Not specific to DOT objectives.

CHAPTER 9

Stop, Review, Remember! (pp. 236–237)

Multiple Choice

1. d (pp. 227–228)
2. d (pp. 233–235)
3. c (pp. 227–228)
4. b (p. 228)
5. a (p. 230)
6. b (p. 232)

Fill in the Blank

1. Hazardous chemicals can burn, explode, be toxic for inhalation, and pose many other dangers. Call the Fire Department and/or Hazardous Materials Team (pp. 231–233, 234–235)
2. Intoxicated persons can exhibit unpredictable behaviors. In this case yelling is a possible sign of agitation or aggression. Call for police. (pp. 231–233, 235)
3. The vehicle on its side is unstable and must be stabilized to keep it from falling on others or further injuring persons inside. Call for Fire Department and additional ambulances depending on the number of patients. (pp. 231–233, 234–235)
4. A high-angle rescue team may be necessary. You may also need a Stokes basket for transport and additional personnel for lifting and moving over distances. (pp. 231–233, 234–235)

Critical Thinking

1. The dispatcher may be the first to observe something is wrong. Loud voices, things breaking, evasiveness in answering questions will alert personnel to danger in person or over the phone. (pp. 231–233)
2. All EMS personnel are less likely to remember after focusing on details of the call. Since it may take time for the resources to get to the scene the earlier the better. It also helps the call go more smoothly when the needed resources are present. (pp. 233–234)

Stop, Review, Remember! (pp. 245–246)

Multiple Choice

1. d (pp. 241–242)
2. a (p. 242)
3. c (p. 231)
4. b (pp. 239–240)
5. d (pp. 238–239)

Matching

1. S (pp. 240, 244)
2. S (pp. 240, 244)
3. N (pp. 240, 244)
4. S (pp. 240, 244)
5. S (pp. 240, 244)
6. S (pp. 240, 244)
7. N (pp. 240, 244)

Critical Thinking

1. No it does not. It increases the likelihood but it can't guarantee injury. Since we can't X-ray in the field MOI is a significant indicator of potential injury. If the injury is possible from the MOI we consider it present until proven otherwise by tests at the hospital. (pp. 239–240)

2. The type of weapon, the path the weapon or projectile took once entering the skin, the length and width of the object and the angle of the object as it entered the body are several of the factors involved in determining the damage. (p. 243)

Chapter Review (pp. 247–249)

Multiple Choice

1. b (pp. 240, 244)
2. c (p. 242)
3. b (pp. 242–243)
4. b (p. 244)
5. b (p. 243)
6. b (p. 240)

Listing

1. Scene safety (pp. 227–228)
2. Body substance isolation determination (pp. 227–228)
3. Determine the need for additional resources (pp. 227–228)
4. Number of patients (pp. 227–228)
5. Mechanism of injury/nature of illness (pp. 227–228)

Critical Thinking

1. The fact that you have observed significant damage will cause you to have a high index of suspicion for injury. It does not guarantee injury but makes it more likely. You should be alert to developing shock during vital signs. The damage to the vehicle (for example, bent steering wheel) would cause you to check the chest for injury. (pp. 240–242)
2. Blunt trauma is when something strikes the body but does not enter the body. Penetrating trauma causes something to enter the body and sometimes remain inside. (p. 243)
3. (pp. 242–243)
   1. Distance the patient fell
   2. Part of the patient that struck the ground/surface
   3. If anything broke the fall
   4. Surface that the patient landed on
4. You would require gloves and face protection (because of the possibility of spattering blood when the patient talks). If the bleeding is profuse or spraying significantly clothing protection may also be required. (pp. 228–230)

Case Study

1. It appears that the patient may have fallen and suffered an injury to his head—but the fall is only one possibility. He may have an altered mental status caused by intoxication or any number of medical conditions. Spinal precautions and airway care may be necessary. (pp. 238–240, 242–243)
2. Gloves and eye protection because of the blood around his head. (p. 228)
3. You don't know. Remember that all patients with an altered mental status have a medical problem (for example, diabetes, stroke) until proven otherwise. Never assume a patient is "just drunk." (pp. 238–240)
4. You may need ALS if the patient is unresponsive or has an altered mental status. You may also need additional lifting assistance. (p. 234)

CHAPTER 10

Stop, Review, Remember! (pp. 260–261)

Multiple Choice

1. a (pp. 252–253)
2. c (p. 257)
3. d (pp. 257–259)
4. b (p. 259)
5. b (p. 257)

Fill in the Blank

1. sign (p. 252)
2. symptom (p. 253)
3. pupils (p. 254)
4. baseline (p. 254)
5. breathing (p. 257)

Critical Thinking

1. It is important for trending purposes so that we can determine if a patient's condition is changing over time and how quickly it is changing. (pp. 254–255)
2. A sign is something that you as the EMT can see such as a bruise or pale skin. A symptom is something the patient describes such as pain or nausea. (pp. 252–253)
3. Baseline is the name given to the very first set of vital signs taken on a patient. It is the basis for which all subsequent vital signs will be compared in order to spot a trend in the patient's condition. (p. 254)

Stop, Review, Remember! (pp. 272–274)

Multiple Choice

1. b (p. 264)
2. d (p. 263)
3. c (p. 271)
4. b (p. 271)
5. a (pp. 254–255)

Matching

1. F (p. 266)
2. D (p. 262)
3. G (p. 264)
4. B (p. 266)
5. H (p. 266)
6. A (p. 262)
7. E (p. 266)
8. C (p. 264)

Critical Thinking

1. When a patient's blood pressure drops as in the case of shock, the pulses furthest from the heart will become difficult if not impossible to feel. Therefore it is important to confirm the absence or presence of a pulse at one of the central pulse points (carotid or femoral) before beginning CPR. (p. 263)
2. While not all patients know what their blood pressure is normally, many do. Asking a patient if they know what his BP is normally, before taking it may provide you with some idea as to what can be expected. (p. 271)
3. The systolic pressure is the pressure in the arteries as the heart beats. The diastolic pressure is the pressure that remains in the arteries between beats as the heart rests momentarily. (p. 266)

Stop, Review, Remember! (pp. 282–283)

Multiple Choice

1. b (p. 274)
2. c (p. 275)
3. a (p. 279)
4. d (p. 279)
5. a (p. 280)

Fill in the Blank

1. temperature (p. 274)
2. oral mucosa (p. 274)
3. on the inside of the eyelid and the white of the eye (p. 274)
4. jaundice (p. 274)
5. diaphoretic (p. 275)

Matching

1. C (p. 274)
2. D (p. 274)
3. E (p. 274)
4. A (p. 274)
5. B (p. 275)

Critical Thinking

1. The skin of the face, fingers, and toes for capillary refill, conjunctiva around eyes, mucus membranes of mouth. (pp. 274, 276)
2. Pale – shock
   Cyanotic – hypoxia from respiratory distress or shock
   Flushed – Heat exhaustion
   Jaundice – Poor liver function (p. 274)
3. The recommended method for assessing a patient's skin signs for temperature and moisture is to pull the glove off the back of one hand and lay the exposed skin of your hand against the patient's forehead or face. This will allow you to feel the temperature and moisture status of the patient's skin. The normal characteristic for temperature and moisture is warm and dry. (p. 275)

Stop, Review, Remember! (pp. 289–290)

Multiple Choice

1. a (p. 284)
2. b (p. 284)
3. c (p. 285)
4. d (p. 287)
5. a (pp. 285–286)

Matching

1. A (p. 287)
2. B (p. 288)
3. C, D, E (p. 288)
4. F, G (p. 288)
5. H (p. 288)
6. I (p. 288)

Critical Thinking

1. One good technique for investigating the existence of a prior medical condition is to ask about medications. A patient may deny the existence of a medical problem but tell you they take insulin and a pill for high blood pressure. They don't always see existing medical conditions as "problems" since they have lived with them so long. (p. 287)
2. Is your pain sharp or dull? Is your pain steady or does it come and go? Have you ever felt this pain before? What did it feel like the first time you experienced it? (pp. 287–288)

Chapter Review (pp. 292–296)

Multiple Choice

1. b (pp. 253–254)
2. c (p. 254)
3. d (p. 255)
4. a (p. 257)
5. d (p. 262)
6. b (p. 262)
7. a (p. 264)
8. c (p. 274)
9. d (p. 275)
10. b (p. 278)
11. a (p. 276)
12. c (p. 271)
13. d (p. 256)
14. c (p. 266)
15. c (p. 252)

Labeling (p. 262)

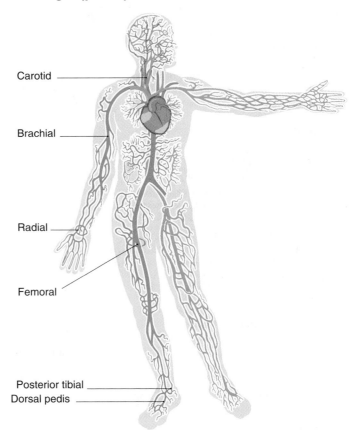

Carotid

Brachial

Radial

Femoral

Posterior tibial
Dorsal pedis

Critical Thinking

1. Time is essential when differentiating multiple sets of vital signs from the same patient. Recording time allows you to compare one set of vitals from another according to when they were taken and spot trends in the condition of the patient based on changes. (pp. 254–255)
2. As the time of the sample you are taking decreases so does the accuracy of the minute rate. The most accurate way to measure heart rate and breathing would be to count for a full minute. Short samples are especially inaccurate when the rhythm is irregular, therefore you must use a longer sample in these cases. (p. 264)
3. An auscultated blood pressure is taken by listening with a stethoscope. A palpated pressure is taken by feeling the pulse in the wrist. The palpated method is used when the environment is too noisy to allow for the use of a

stethoscope or when time is critical and you have several patients. (pp. 269, 271)

4. To properly assess skin color in dark skinned patients you will have to observe alternative areas such as the conjunctiva, nail beds, and the inside of the mouth (mucus membranes). These areas should be pink and moist or show adequate capillary refill. (p. 274)

5. When perfusion is poor the pupils will begin to react more sluggishly and eventually will become fixed (nonreactive) and dilated. (p. 278)

Case Studies

#1

1. Based on the woman's baseline vital signs alone, she has several of the signs of shock such as pale skin, rapid heart rate, and increased respiratory rate. (pp. 256–258, 264–266, 274–275, 277–279)

2. Based on this patient's history and presentation she should be considered unstable, therefore vitals should be taken every 5 minutes. (p. 280)

3. One way to determine what her vitals are normally would be to ask the patient herself. Another would be to ask her caretaker. (p. 271)

#2

1. (p. 285)
   S- Pain in his right elbow and shoulder with no obvious signs of trauma.
   A- Allergy to bee stings
   M- Blood pressure pill and prescription for an epi-pen.
   P- History of reaction to bee stings and high blood pressure.
   L- Breakfast 30 minutes ago.
   E- Heading out to mow the lawn.

2. Due to his altered mental status and potential for bee sting this man should be treated as an unstable patient. (pp. 291–292)

CHAPTER 11

Stop, Review, Remember! (pp. 304–305)

Multiple Choice

1. b (pp. 298–299)
2. c (p. 302)
3. d (p. 302)
4. b (p. 302)
5. c (p. 299)

Fill in the Blank

1. scene size-up (p. 298)
2. immediate life threats (p. 299)
3. general impression (p. 299)
4. general impression (pp. 299–300)
5. event (pp. 301–302)
6. verbal (p. 302)

Critical Thinking

1. The purpose of the initial assessment is to identify and care for any immediate life threats to the patient. You should not feel compelled to always complete an entire assessment if an immediate life threat exists. Your time and effort must be spent dealing with the life threat and not performing less important tasks. (p. 299)

2. Your general impression may include different elements depending on where you work and how you are taught. Every general impression should include the elements of approximate age, gender, and level of distress. (p. 300)

3. A person who is A&O x 2 is able to tell you who they are and where they are, but unable to tell you the time of day accurately. (p. 302)

Stop, Review, Remember! (pp. 311–312)

Multiple Choice

1. c (p. 306)
2. a (p. 307)
3. d (p. 308)
4. b (p. 309)
5. c (p. 307)

Matching

1. B (p. 306)
2. A (p. 299)
3. E (p. 306)
4. C (p. 308)
5. D (p. 308)

Critical Thinking

1. The assessment of the airway of a responsive patient is as simple as asking them a question or two and observing his ability to speak. If he is responsive and able to speak, it can be concluded that his airway is patent. For the unresponsive patient you must place your ear next to their nose and mouth and watch the chest for rise and fall. If you see, hear, and feel evidence of breathing the airway is clear. If you do not see evidence of breathing, you must provide two slow breaths and see the chest rise and fall with each breath. (p. 306)

2. The adequacy of breathing is determined by two factors: the depth of breathing (tidal volume) and the rate. A patient who is breathing adequately will be breathing at least 10 to 12 times each minute and you will see obvious chest rise and fall with each breath. (p. 307)

3. It is safe to say that most patients who are experiencing a medical or traumatic emergency will benefit from supplemental oxygen. You must assess their level of distress, mental status, and vital signs to determine just how much you should give. (pp. 307–308)

Chapter Review (pp. 313–315)

Multiple Choice

1. c (p. 299)
2. a (p. 300)
3. d (p. 299)
4. a (p. 302)
5. b (p. 301)

Critical Thinking

1. Obstructed Airway – Without a clear airway a patient will be unable to breathe and may die within minutes.
   No Breathing – A patient may have a patent airway but still not be breathing. Without an adequate supply of oxygen death will soon follow.

No Pulse – It is safe to assume that if the patient has no pulse, breathing has also stopped. With adequate circulation a patient will experience brain death within minutes. Severe Bleeding – The body must have an adequate supply of blood volume in order to maintain a blood pressure and adequate perfusion. Without it the patient will go into shock and death will soon follow. (p. 299)

2. Student opinion only. (pp. 299, 306)
3. One of the main reasons for forming a general impression with each patient is to establish as early as possible the need for immediate care and/or transport. You are trying to quickly categorize the patient as either "bog sick" or "little sick" so that you can act accordingly. (p. 306)
4. One of your goals is to be a fact finder and remain as objective as possible during your assessment of the patient. By using the patient's own words and descriptions we remain true to this concept.

Case Studies

#1

1. You can call out to the patient and attempt to get him to respond verbally. If he responds, then you know he at least has an open airway, is breathing, and has a pulse. You can also attempt to visualize the patient from outside the vehicle and see if he is breathing or not. (pp. 299, 301)
2. If he is responsive, then about the only element you will not be able to easily assess is severe bleeding. If he is unresponsive, then assessing both pulse and bleeding become very difficult simply by observation. (pp. 308–309)

#2

1. You should begin by kneeling beside the patient and observing for adequate chest rise and fall to confirm the patient has an airway and is breathing. You can do this initially without moving the patient. You can simply observe the patient for obvious bleeding. (pp. 306–309)
2. If you are unable to confirm an open airway and breathing you will have to carefully roll the patient onto their back and open the airway. (p. 307)
3. You must assess the pulse at the carotid artery in the neck before assuming she is in cardiac arrest. As blood pressure falls the pulses furthest from the heart become weak and difficult to feel. (p. 308)

CHAPTER 12
Stop, Review, Remember! (pp. 322–323)

Multiple Choice

1. b (p. 320)
2. a (p. 318)
3. b (pp. 320–321)
4. d (p. 321)
5. a (p. 319)

Critical Thinking

1. Medical:
A patient who is having difficulty breathing; a patient with an altered mental status.

Trauma:
A patient who fell and injured a hip; a patient who was caught under a collapsed structure. (p. 317)
2. How old is the patient? How far did he fall? What caused the fall? What type of surface did he land on? How did he land? Did he lose consciousness? (p. 320)
3. (pp. 320–321)
   1. significant
   2. nonsignificant
   3. significant
   4. significant
   5. nonsignificant

Stop, Review, Remember! (pp. 336–337)

Multiple Choice

1. c (p. 324)
2. a (p. 324)
3. c (p. 327)
4. d (p. 321)
5. a (p. 335)

Matching

1. E (p. 327)
2. C (p. 327)
3. D (p. 327)
4. A (p. 327)
5. B (p. 327)

Critical Thinking

1. The focused trauma assessment is indicated for patients who have not sustained a significant mechanism of injury and it focuses on the site of injury. A rapid trauma assessment is indicated for patients suffering a significant MOI and involves a rapid and systematic head-to-toe assessment of the body. (p. 324)
2. The indication for a rapid trauma assessment is the presence of significant MOI. The focused assessment is used for patients who have not sustained a significant MOI. (p. 324)
3. Uncontrolled bleeding should be controlled immediately upon discovery. When you discover evidence of bleeding, stop your assessment and do what is necessary to control the bleeding. Then resume your assessment. (p. 327)
4. If the mechanism was indeed isolated to the patient's leg, then a focused medical assessment of the injured extremity is indicated. Manually stabilize the leg, then assess CSM before attempting to splint. Once the leg is properly immobilized reassess CSM. (p. 330)
5. (pp. 324–325, 330)
   1. rapid medical assessment
   2. focused trauma assessment
   3. focused medical assessment
   4. rapid trauma assessment
   5. rapid medical assessment

Chapter Review (pp. 338–341)

Multiple Choice

1. a (pp. 321, 324)
2. c (p. 330)
3. d (pp. 331–332)
4. b (p. 327)
5. d (p. 335)
6. b (p. 320)
7. d (p. 321)
8. a (p. 325)
9. c (p. 327)
10. b (p. 330)

Critical Thinking

1. The focus of both the assessment and care of the trauma patient centers around the MOI and any obvious injuries. In most instances, the trauma patient will benefit from rapid transport. Then assessment and care of the medical patient centers on the chief complaint and a thorough medical history. In most instances, immediate transport is less of a priority for medical patients. (p. 317)

2. It is not enough to simply know that someone was in a vehicle collision or has fallen from a height; you must investigate further once on scene. You will want to find out more about the forces involved and how they impacted the patient. This will provide insight into potential injuries that may not be readily apparent. (pp. 319–320)

3. The rapid trauma assessment is indicated for patients who have suffered a significant MOI and involves a rapid, systematic head-to-toe exam. The focused assessment is indicated for patients who have NOT suffered a significant MOI and centers on the site of injury. (pp. 324–325, 330–331)

4. The purpose of the detailed physical exam is to identify any signs or symptoms that may have been missed during the rapid or focused assessments. It is typically conducted during transport to the hospital and when patient condition allows. (pp. 331–332)

Case Studies

#1

1. You will examine the outside of the vehicle to assess the amount of damage and intrusion into the passenger compartment. If possible, you will also want to determine if the patient was wearing a seat belt of any kind and if the car had air bags that had deployed. (pp. 319–322)

2. Due to the significant MOI, the most appropriate assessment path is the rapid trauma assessment. (pp. 324–325)

3. Based on the fact that the patient is unresponsive you must determine that she has an open airway and that she is breathing adequately. This must be accomplished while maintaining spinal precautions. You must immediately control any external bleeding and maintain a high index of suspicion for internal bleeding. (pp. 326–329)

#2

1. You will want to confirm that the cause of the fall was "mechanical" in nature. In other words, she tripped and did not fall as a result of some underlying medical problem such as a seizure. You will also want to determine if she hit her head or lost consciousness. Ask her to describe exactly how she fell and what hit the ground first. (pp. 321, 330)

2. It appears that this patient did NOT sustain a significant MOI, therefore the most appropriate assessment path would be a focused trauma assessment. (pp. 321, 330)

CHAPTER 13

Stop, Review, Remember! (pp. 347–348)

Multiple Choice

1. b (p. 302)
2. a (p. 344)
3. b (p. 299)

Ordering

1. Rapid medical assessment
2. Baseline vitals
3. SAMPLE history
4. Transport

Critical Thinking

1. The trauma assessment is used to assess patients who have suffered some type of injury involving either a significant or nonsignificant MOI and includes an assessment for DCAP-BTLS. The medical assessment is used for patients with an illness or nontraumatic complaint and in most cases is focused on the patient's chief complaint. (pp. 343–344)

2. Since you have no way of knowing whether this patient has suffered an MOI or not, you must assume the worst and maintain spinal precautions while we care for him. After ensuring that the scene is safe you will begin with an initial assessment and initiate supplemental oxygen. If the initial assessment is intact, then you will move on to the rapid medical assessment and attempt to get a SAMPLE history from bystanders. You will then obtain a baseline set of vitals and initiate transport, completing a more detailed physical exam while en route to the hospital. (pp. 346–347)

3. Yes. Since we do not know the exact cause of this man's condition we must assume that he has suffered some sort of trauma and maintain spinal precautions throughout our care and transport. (p. 347)

Stop, Review, Remember! (pp. 358–360)

Multiple Choice

1. a (p. 351)
2. b (p. 346)
3. b (p. 350)

4. a (p. 355)
5. c (p. 358)

Matching

1. C (p. 349)
2. A (p. 349)
3. E (p. 349)

4. D (p. 350)
5. F (p. 350)
6. B (p. 354)

Critical Thinking

1. The indications for a rapid medical assessment are:
   No evidence of trauma
   Unresponsive/altered mental status (pp. 346–347)

2. Findings you might expect to see while assessing the neck of a medical patient are:
   ✳ Stoma
   ✳ Jugular vein distention
   ✳ Tracheal deviation
   ✳ Accessory muscle use
   ✳ Medical jewelry
   ✳ Scars (p. 349)
3. Findings you might expect to see while assessing the abdomen of a medical patient are:
   ✳ Distention
   ✳ Tenderness
   ✳ Rigidity
   ✳ Guarding
   ✳ Scars
   ✳ Referred pain
   ✳ Pulsating mass (p. 350)

Chapter Review (pp. 361–363)

Multiple Choice

1. c (p. 358)
2. b (p. 346)
3. b (p. 354)
4. a (p. 346)
5. c (p. 352)
6. d (p. 355)
7. a (p. 352)
8. d (p. 350)
9. b (p. 350)
10. b (p. 350)

Ordering

Responsive patient: (p. 346)
1. focused history
2. focused physical exam
3. baseline vitals
4. transport

Unresponsive patient: (p. 346)
1. rapid medical assessment
2. baseline vitals
3. focused history
4. transport

Critical Thinking

1. Trauma:
   A patient involved in a vehicle collision, patient who fell from the roof of a house, and a patient who suffered an injury to the leg playing soccer.
   Medical:
   A patient who was having chest pain, a patient who was having an asthma attack and a patient with a sudden onset of abdominal pain. (p. 343)
2. The medical patient is assessed based on his chief complaint with care focusing on the signs and symptoms he is presenting with at the time. A thorough history of both the present illness and past medical problems is important. In contrast, the trauma patient is assessed and cared for primarily based on the MOI. (p. 345)
3. The mental status of a medical patient will determine which assessment path (rapid vs. focused) is most appropriate. It is also important to continuously monitor the airway and breathing status of an unresponsive patient since he cannot speak, therefore letting you know he is breathing. (pp. 345–346)
4. The objective of the ongoing assessment is to reevaluate the ABCs to ensure that no life-threatening conditions develop. It also includes an assessment of vital signs and interventions. (p. 358)

Case Studies

#1

1. Noisy respirations are a strong indication of a partially obstructed airway. In this case the gurgling may be an indication of fluid build up in the oropharynx. (pp. 355–358)
2. Changes in the patient's airway status requires that you abandon the less important detailed physical exam and manage the airway immediately. This patient may need suctioning. (pp. 360–361)

#2

1. Since this man is responsive and able to answer questions the most appropriate assessment path is the focused medical assessment. (p. 346)
2.
   O – What were you doing when the pain began?
      Has this ever happened before?
   P - Does anything you do make the pain worse?
      Does anything you do make the pain better?
   Q - Can you describe your pain for me?
      Is the pain sharp or dull? Is it steady or does it come and go?
   R - Can you point with one finger where the pain is the most?
      Does the pain radiate anywhere else?
   S - On a scale of 1 to 10, how would you rate your pain right now?
      On a scale of 1 to 10, what was your pain when it first began?
   T - When did the pain first begin? Has it gotten better or worse since it first began?
      (pp. 354–355)

CHAPTER 14

Stop, Review, Remember! (pp. 368–369)

Multiple Choice

1. a (p. 366)
2. d (p. 366)
3. c (p. 366)
4. b (pp. 366–367)
5. c (p. 367)

Fill in the Blank

1. 5 (p. 372)
2. initial, vital, chief complaint, interventions, transport (p. 366)
3. trending (p. 366)

Critical Thinking

1. The initial assessment is comprised primarily of the ABCs which are critical to the well being of your patient. It is not enough to simply assess the ABCs at the beginning of your assessment and not again. A patient's condition can and will change and you must be able to recognize and care for any immediate life threats as they arise. (p. 365)

2. (pp. 369–371)
   * **Recheck of the initial assessment** – You will want to verify that the ABCs are all intact and normal.
   * **Recheck vital signs** – You will take additional sets of vital signs and compare them to the baseline set looking for changes and trends.
   * **Repeat assessment of chief complaint or injuries** – You will want to determine if the signs and symptoms of the chief complaint are changing for better or worse.
   * **Check effectiveness of interventions** – You will be determining if your interventions are having any effect on the patient and the signs and symptoms.
   * **Confirm care and transport priority** – Based on your reassessment you may need to change the transport priority of the patient.

3. Trending refers to the changes in a patient's condition over time. It is our desire that a patient's condition will get better with time, but this is not always the case. Establishing a thorough assessment and baseline vital signs as early as possible will enable you to compare subsequent assessments and determine if the patient's condition is staying the same or changing one way or the other. A patient who is getting worse is considered unstable and in need of immediate transport. (p. 366)

Chapter Review (pp. 374–376)

Multiple Choice

1. b (pp. 369–370)
2. b (p. 372)
3. c (pp. 372–373)
4. a (p. 372)
5. d (pp. 369–371)

Critical Thinking

1. Trending involves the tracking of a patient's condition with the idea of spotting changes (trends) in their condition and adjusting care to address these changes. (p. 366)
2. The reassessment of the ABCs is the most critical component of the ongoing assessment simply because of the importance of an adequate airway, breathing, and circulation. (pp. 369–371)

Case Studies

#1

1. Since the chief complaint is respiratory distress your ongoing assessment will focus on her respiratory status. You will need to assess for adequacy of both rate and tidal volume. (pp. 369–371)
2. At the very least you should have her on supplemental oxygen and may need to turn up the flow rate some. If her rate and/or tidal volume become inadequate you may need to consider ventilating with a BVM. (pp. 369–371)

#2

1. Given this man's history it is likely that he has had another stroke. As with any patient with an altered mental status you must be concerned with a patent airway and adequate breathing. (pp. 369–373)

2. This patient will require continuous monitoring. Due to his altered mental status he is considered unstable and therefore his vital signs should be taken every five minutes. (pp. 372–373)
3. Given his altered mental status and the absence of injury, this man should be transported in the recovery position. (p. 371)

CHAPTER 15
Stop, Review, Remember! (pp. 386–387)
Multiple Choice

1. b (p. 385)
2. b (p. 382)
3. d (p. 383)
4. c (p. 383)
5. a (p. 380)
6. a (p, 379)

Matching

1. B (p. 382)
2. A (p. 382)
3. A (p. 382)
4. C (p. 382)

Critical Thinking

1. Depending on the resources available and what methods are routinely used by the patient you may try writing questions on paper, enlisting a friend or relative to use sign language and translate or the patient may read lips. (pp. 381–382)
2. A portable radio is small and designed to be carried on one's person. A mobile radio is mounted in a vehicle such as the ambulance. Base station radios are in a building such as the dispatch center or hospital. (p. 382)

Stop, Review, Remember! (pp. 393–394)
Multiple Choice

1. c (pp. 387–388)
2. c (pp. 387–388)
3. b (p. 389)
4. c (p. 390)
5. d (p. 391–392)

Critical Thinking

1. (pp. 387–388)
   * Identify your unit (ambulance identifier) and your level of certification—in this case EMT.
   * Your estimated time of arrival (ETA)
   * The patient's age and sex
   * The patient's chief complaint
   * A brief, pertinent history of the present illness or injury
   * Relevant past medical history
   * Vital signs including mental status
   * Pertinent findings of your examination
   * The care you have provided
   * The patient's response to your care
2. The hand-off can focus on changes in the patient's condition that have occurred since the radio report if the receiver is familiar with the information.
   The hand-off is done in person, the call-in is done via radio. (pp. 391–392)

3. A hurried and incomplete radio report may imply hurried and incomplete patient care. This reflects on you and your agency. The disorganization in the report may cause hospital personnel to feel they have to check the care you provided—even if the care was excellent. (pp. 387–389)

Chapter Review (pp. 395–398)

Multiple Choice

1. b (pp. 384–385)
2. c (pp. 381–382)
3. d (p. 381)
4. b (p. 383)
5. b (p. 382)

Critical Thinking

1. Get down at the patient's level. Speak to the patient clearly and make sure that there are no barriers to her understanding what you say (hearing, language, etc.) Listen to her to determine why she won't go. You will then be able to address some of her fears. (p. 380)
2. The dispatcher records these events either on paper or in a computer system. These are used for documentation, research, quality improvement, and in the event of a lawsuit. (p. 385)
3. Not listening or looking at the patient implied disrespect, carelessness, or indifference (or all of these). You would likely feel like the provider didn't care. This is not only rude and inconsiderate, it raises the potential for liability. (p. 380)
4. You would confirm the order by repeating it back to the physician and waiting for acknowledgment back from the physician. You would say: "Confirming you would like me to assist the patient with one spray of nitroglycerin sublingually and to give the patient 4 baby aspirins which is 324 mg to chew. Over." (p. 390)
5. (p. 390)
   * You would ask for an order for a medication
   * You would tell the physician if the patient had used the medication already
   * You would verify that the patient was not allergic to the medication
   * You would explain the signs and symptoms (indications) for the medication.
   * You would realize that vital signs have additional relevance in this situation.
6. (pp. 384–385)
   * Information transmitted over the radio may be heard on scanners and violate the patient's privacy.
   * Radio information should be limited to what is pertinent to allow others to use the radio frequency.
7. Most would expect quality clinical care with time spent to reassure and comfort the patient. (p. 380)
   Radio Report #1 (pp. 387–388)
   8, 2, 5, 6, 3, 1, 4, 9, 7
   Radio Report #2 (pp. 387–388)
   6, 4, 9, 7, 2, 8, 1, 3, 10, 5

Case Study

1. Yes, as long as the son is calm and reliable. If not you may wish to find another person who will be calmer (for example, a trusted neighbor). If the son and father don't get along it may be an issue—in any language. (pp. 380–382)

2. You can assure accuracy by taking your time. Determine if the answers you receive match other factors such as injuries, level of distress of the patient, and mechanism of injury. (pp. 380–382)
3. Your assessment will likely be slower because of the time it will take to have everything said and interpreted twice. This time is worthwhile when it leads to accurate assessment and care. In serious trauma you may need to expedite transport and communicate on the move. (pp. 380–382)

CHAPTER 16

Stop, Review, Remember! (pp. 408–410)

Multiple Choice

1. d (p. 401)
2. b (p. 404)
3. b (p. 405)
4. b (p. 405)
5. a (p. 405)
6. d (p. 405)

Labeling

1. S (p. 405)
2. O (p. 405)
3. O (p. 405)
4. S (p. 405)
5. S (p. 405)
6. O (p. 405)

Fill in the Blank   (pp. 404–406)

	TIME	RESP	PULSE	B.P.	LEVEL OF CONSCIOUSNESS	R PUPILS L	SKIN
V I T A L S I G N S	1117	Rate: 22 ☐ Regular ☐ Shallow ☒ Labored	Rate: 94 ☒ Regular ☐ Irregular	122 / 74	☐ Alert ☐ Voice ☐ Pain ☐ Unresp.	☒ Normal ☐ Dilated ☐ Constricted ☐ Sluggish ☐ No-Reaction	☐ Unremarkable ☒ Cool ☐ Warm ☒ Moist ☐ Dry / ☐ Pale ☐ Cyanotic ☐ Flushed ☐ Jaundiced
	1122	Rate: 20 ☐ Regular ☐ Shallow ☒ Labored	Rate: 88 ☒ Regular ☐ Irregular	108 / 70	☐ Alert ☐ Voice ☐ Pain ☐ Unresp.	☒ Normal ☐ Dilated ☐ Constricted ☐ Sluggish ☐ No-Reaction	☐ Unremarkable ☒ Cool ☐ Warm ☐ Moist ☒ Dry / ☐ Pale ☐ Cyanotic ☐ Flushed ☐ Jaundiced
		Rate: ☐ Regular ☐ Shallow ☐ Labored	Rate: ☐ Regular ☐ Irregular	/	☐ Alert ☐ Voice ☐ Pain ☐ Unresp.	☐ Normal ☐ Dilated ☐ Constricted ☐ Sluggish ☐ No-Reaction	☐ Unremarkable ☐ Cool ☐ Warm ☐ Moist ☐ Dry / ☐ Pale ☐ Cyanotic ☐ Flushed ☐ Jaundiced

Critical Thinking

1. Documentation can help minimize liability but only if it is done in conjunction with high quality, patient-centered prehospital care. (p. 404)

Stop, Review, Remember! (pp. 415–417)

Multiple Choice

1. c (p. 410)
2. a (p. 410)
3. c (p. 411)
4. b (pp. 412–413)
5. b (p. 411)
6. b (p. 411)
7. a (pp. 412–413)
8. b (p. 413)
9. b (p. 404)
10. a (pp. 413–414)

Critical Thinking

1. Since the form has already been left at the hospital and likely sent to other agencies, simply crossing out and correcting the error is not enough. Follow your local rules for sending amended copies to agencies that have received copies of the original. (p. 411)

2. Make It Right (pp. 411–412)
   a. Cross out the "1" with a single line and initial it.
   b. Place a single line through the sentence, note the patient's allergies and initial it.
   c. Cross out "increased" with a single line and write in "decreased." Initial it.
   d. Place a single line through the numbers in the BP, write in the correct numbers and initial it.
   e. Write the word "breath" above and between "equal sounds" add the ^ symbol and initial it.

Chapter Review (pp. 418–419)

Multiple Choice

1. a (p. 410)
2. b (p. 413)
3. b (p. 411)
4. d (p. 405)
5. c (p. 411)

Critical Thinking

1. The report could be used for reference in the emergency department, referenced in other units in the hospital where the patient stays, for prehospital research, in quality improvement. (p. 401)
2. Document that the patient vomited en route and that you couldn't obtain a second set of vitals because of a short transport time and the fact that you were providing airway care to the patient. Never make false statements on any report for any reason. (p. 411)
3. Because there are many patients and often not enough EMTs for each, there will be minimal time for documentation. Because of this it is acceptable to make brief, but important notes on triage tags instead of filling out a full report for each patient. Full documentation may be required after the call is completed. (pp. 413–414)
4.
   a. C (p. 411)
   b. O (p. 411)
   c. C (p. 411)
   d. O (p. 411)
   e. C (p. 411)

Case Study

1. It is difficult for us to tell exactly how you would feel. The purpose of this question is to place you in the position of a patient to see how things like confidentiality can be very personal. Your feelings may have ranged from hurt, insulted, angry—or others. You may have done nothing, spoke to the EMTs about it or made a complaint to their agency's leadership. In any case it certainly shows the importance of confidentiality. (p. 410)
2. This breach of patient confidentiality is very severe and unprofessional. There are obviously many factors ranging from where the complaint is filed to the allegations themselves. Suffice it to say that a violation of HIPAA statutes could result in a Federal complaint with substantial fines. Personnel issues such as retraining, suspension, or dismissal could also occur. (p. 410)

CHAPTER 17

1. a (pp. 227–228)
   Objective: 3-1.5
2. c (pp. 228–229)
   3-1.2
3. d (p. 230)
   Objective: 3-1.3
4. b (p. 232)
   Objective: 3-1.1
5. b (pp. 233–234)
   Objective: 3-1.6
6. d (p. 227)
   Objective: There are no DOT objectives specific to this question.
7. b (p. 253)
   Objective: 1-5.24
8. a (p. 252)
   Objective: 1-5.24
9. d (pp. 253–254)
   Objective: 1-5.1
10. c (p. 254)
    Objective: 1-5.1
11. a (p. 257)
    Objective: 1-5.3
12. c (p. 257)
    Objective: 1-5.2
13. d (p. 257)
    Objective: 1-5.2
14. a (pp. 257–258)
    Objective: 1-5.3
15. c (p. 258)
    Objective: 1-5.4
16. d (p. 259)
    Objective: 1-5.4
17. c (p. 262)
    Objective: 1-5.5
18. d (p. 263)
    Objective: 1-5.5
19. a (p. 263)
    Objective: 1-5.5
20. c (p. 264)
    Objective: 1-5.6
21. c (p. 266)
    Objective: 1-5.19
22. d (p. 266)
    Objective: 1-5.20
23. b (p. 266)
    Objective: 1-5.22
24. c (p. 274)
    Objective: 1-5.10
25. c (p. 274)
    Objective: 1-5.9
26. a (p. 279)
    Objective: 1-5.18
27. c (p. 285)
    Objective 1-5.23
28. b (p. 288)
    Objective: There are no DOT objectives specific to this question.
29. c (p. 301)
    Objective: 3-2.2
30. a (p. 299)
    Objective: 3-2.1
31. b (p. 319)
    Objective: 3-3.2
32. a (pp. 320–321)
    Objective: 3-3.1
33. c (pp. 330–331)
    Objective: 3-3.6
34. b (p. 325)
    Objective: 3-3.4
35. c (p. 287)
    Objective: 3-3.7
36. b (p. 372)
    Objective: 3-6.3
37. d (p. 344)
    Objective: 3-4.4
38. d (p. 286)
    Objective: 1-5.23
39. b (p. 288)
    Objective: 1-5.23
40. a (p. 254)
    Objecitve: 3-6.3
41. d (pp. 380–381)
    Objective: 3-7.7
42. c (p. 382)
    Objective: There are no DOT objectives specific to this question.
43. d (p. 383)
    Objective: There are no DOT objectives specific to this question.
44. b (p. 405)
    Objective: 3-8.1
45. a (p. 406)
    Objective: 3-8.3
46. c (p. 410)
    Objective: 3-8.5
47. d (p. 411)
    Objective: 3-8.5
48. a (pp. 380–382)
    Objective: There are no DOT objectives specific to this question.
49. c (p. 411)
    Objective: 3-8.5
50. d (pp. 412–413)
    Objective: 3-8.4
51. d (pp. 257–258)
    Objective: 1-5.3
52. d (p. 259)
    Objective: 1-5.4
53. a (p. 274)
    Objective: 1-5.9
54. c (p. 280)
    Objective: There are no DOT objectives specific to this question.

55. c (p. 302)
   Objective: 3-2.2
56. a (p. 310)
   Objective: 3-2.19
57. c (p. 318)
   Objective: 3-4.1

58. b (p. 318)
   Objective: 3-4.2
59. c (p. 327)
   Objective: 1-5.24
60. a (pp. 381–382)
   Objective: 3-7.5

CHAPTER 18

Stop, Review, Remember! (pp. 431–433)

Multiple Choice

1. c (p. 430)
2. d (p. 431)
3. c (p. 431)

4. a (p. 429)
5. a (p. 431)

Matching

1. B (p. 430)
2. A (p. 430)
3. E (p. 431)

4. D (p. 430)
5. C (p. 431)

Critical Thinking

1. A metered-dose inhaler (sometimes simply called an inhaler) dispenses individual bursts of medication as a fine powder. A nebulizer dispenses a continuous vapor containing the medication through a mouthpiece or oxygen mask. (p. 431)
2. The only difference is in name. Nitrostat is a brand name for nitroglycerin. (p. 503)
3. Disagree. The route of any medication is specific. In the case of nitroglycerin it is absorbed through the tissues under the tongue. This area is richly supplied with blood vessels to absorb the medication as it dissolves. Chewing or swallowing the medication would be ineffective. (pp. 430–431)
4. (p. 430, drug reference)
   1. trade name for nitroglycerin
   2. chemical name for albuterol
   3. generic for activated charcoal
   4. generic for nitroglycerin
   5. trade name for albuterol
   6. trade name for glucose
   7. trade name for activated charcoal
   8. generic for epinephrine

Stop, Review, Remember! (pp. 441–442)

Multiple Choice

1. c (p. 440)
2. a (p. 440)
3. d (p. 434)

4. b (p. 437)
5. a (p. 438)

Matching

1. C (p. 431)
2. D (p. 431)
3. B (p. 431)
4. E (p. 431)

5. F (p. 431)
6. B (p. 431)
7. A (p. 431)
8. F (p. 431)

Critical Thinking

1. In most cases nitroglycerin is not carried on ambulances unless EMT-Intermediates (Advanced EMTs) or paramedics are part of the crew. You will use your patient's nitroglycerin. Always follow your local protocols. (pp. 436–437)
2. The doctor most likely believes he is talking to a paramedic. Explain to the physician that the only epinephrine available to you is 1:1,000 via auto-injector for subcutaneous injection. This underscores the need for repeating and understanding a medication order. (pp. 434–435)
3. The inhaler contains fine powder for inhalation. The fine powder must get into the patient's lungs to cause the desired effect—opening up constricted bronchioles. (p. 438)

Chapter Review (pp. 443–445)

Multiple Choice

1. b (p. 434)
2. d (p. 435)
3. c (p. 438)

4. d (p. 435)
5. d (p. 435)

Matching

1. B (p. 434)
2. F (p. 434)
3. E (p. 434)

4. A (p. 434)
5. D (p. 434)
6. C (p. 434)

Critical Thinking

1. A side effect is something negative that happens after a medication has been administered. A contraindication is a reason a medication should not be given. (p. 434)
2. Assess the patient to determine if there has been any change in his chest pain. You will also perform a full set of vital signs. Pay attention to the patient's pulse and blood pressure. An increased pulse and/or decreased blood pressure can indicate hypotension, a side effect of nitroglycerin. (pp. 436–437)
3. No, you are only allowed to use the patient's own medication. (p. 435)
4. Right patient: Is the medication prescribed for this patient?
   Right medication: Is this the medication prescribed for this condition?
   Right route: How is this medication administered?
   Right dose: How much of the medication do you take?
   Right time: Is this the condition the medication is prescribed for?
   Right documentation: Is the patient's condition, vital signs pre- and post-medication and reaction to the medication documented? (p. 435)

Case Study

1. We are treating a 67-year-old male patient who developed chest pain while mowing the lawn about 10 minutes ago. His chest pain is rated as 5 out of 10 now, it was 8 out of 10. His vital signs are pulse 96 strong and regular, respirations 20 and labored, BP 124/86, his skin is pale, cool

and sweaty. He has prescribed nitroglycerin. He has taken one nitroglycerin tablet so far. He also takes aspirin and Lipitor. We would like permission to assist him with a second nitroglycerin en route to the hospital. (pp. 436–437)

2. The most common side effects include hypotension and headache. (pp. 436–437)

CHAPTER 19
Stop, Review, Remember! (pp. 449–450)
Multiple Choice

1. d (p. 448)
2. b (p. 448)
3. c (p. 449)

Fill in the Blank

1. oropharynx (p. 448)
2. alveoli (p. 448)
3. epiglottis (p. 448)
4. parietal, visceral (p. 448)
5. dead space (p. 448)

Critical Thinking

1. Air passes through the mouth and nose through the oropharynx and nasopharynx into the larynx. Air passes the epiglottis and enters the trachea through the vocal cords. Air travels from the trachea through the main stem bronchi and into increasingly smaller passage called bronchioles until air reaches the alveoli where gas exchange takes place. (p. 448)

2. The respiratory system obtains air from the environment, filters and warms it through the nose and mouth, and delivers it to the alveoli for exchange of gases. Oxygen is transferred to the cells while carbon dioxide is removed. (p. 448)

Stop, Review, Remember! (pp. 459–460)
Multiple Choice

1. c (p. 453)
2. d (p. 452)
3. d (p. 453)
4. c (pp. 456–457)
5. a (p. 456)
6. b (p. 456)

Fill in the Blank

1. Onset, provocation, quality, radiation, severity, time (p. 454)
2. Describe (p. 454)
3. Tripod (p. 451)
4. Rate, depth (p. 451)
5. Nonrebreather mask (p. 452)

Critical Thinking

1. This can provide a significant amount of information for the current problem. For example if a patient is complaining of respiratory distress and he has a history of emphysema and have prescribed medications, this is very pertinent. (pp. 452–453)

2. The history generally provides the most information about a medical patient's condition. The onset of the symptoms, the description of the pain or distress, and the past history generally provides the most valuable information. (p. 452)

Stop, Review, Remember! (pp. 470–471)
Multiple Choice

1. b (p. 466)
2. a (p. 465)
3. b (p. 453)

Fill in the Blank

1. Small-volume nebulizer (p. 468)
2. Medical direction (p. 464)
3. Spacer (spacer device or aerochamber) (p. 466)
4. Sitting (p. 461)
5. Prescribed (p. 465)

Critical Thinking

1. Right patient, dose, medication, route, time, documentation (p. 465)

2. You should administer oxygen to every patient with respiratory distress. A true hypoxic drive is rare. It is even rarer to "knock out" the patient's respiratory drive, especially in the relatively short time we in EMS are with the patient. Give oxygen to patients who need it. (p. 457)

Chapter Review (pp. 472–477)
Multiple Choice

1. d (p. 456)
2. c (p. 451–452)
3. c (p. 464)
4. a (p. 448)
5. c (p. 461)
6. b (p. 465)
7. c (pp. 447, 454)
8. c (p. 472)
9. d (p. 466)
10. c (p. 454)

Matching #1

1. D (p. 458)
2. E (p. 457)
3. F (p. 458)
4. C (p. 458)
5. B (p. 350)
6. A (p. 349)

Matching #2

1. C (p. 452)
2. A (p. 452)
3. B (p. 452)
4. B (p. 452)
5. B (p. 452)
6. A (p. 452)
7. A (p. 452)
8. A (p. 452)
9. A (p. 452)
10. A (p. 452)

Critical Thinking

1. Remember that breathing requires adequate rate AND depth. If breathing is very slow or very fast and shallow, the patient is moving so little air that it is not enough to support life (inadequate breathing). Ventilation with a BVM or pocket face mask is necessary. (p. 452)

2. Yes. Patients who are sleepy and cannot be aroused, in the tripod position, diaphoretic, or using accessory muscles are in significant distress. Be observant. This can all be determined before you reach the patient. It is also known as the "general impression." (p. 451)

3. Increasing the heart rate is one of the body's ways to compensate for hypoxia. (NOTE: Infants and children often

exhibit a slowed heart rate.) Because the body is short of oxygen, it tries to move more blood to increase oxygen distribution. The sweaty skin (often pale and cool) is a sign that the body is in significant distress and the nervous system is taking drastic actions to survive. (pp. 451–453)

Case Studies

#1

1. Marie is breathing adequately based on her mental status, ability to speak long, full sentences and skin color. Obtaining an actual respiratory rate will also help confirm this decision. (p. 453)
2. Marie would likely be a candidate for a nasal cannula. Her distress isn't severe and this level of supplemental oxygen may be sufficient. If your protocols require it, a higher level of oxygen could be administered. (p. 461)
3. If the husband falls, he could become a patient. We must prevent that. Our responsibility is not only to treat the patient, but we must also remain aware of the scene and control it. He is probably concerned about his wife and wants to help. Reassure him and tell him that you are helping Marie. Try to get him to sit down while you care for his wife. Speak to him throughout the call. Call for the nursing staff if necessary to help him around. (p. 451)
4. Marie has distress. It may be minimal, but it is distress. Complete a thorough assessment and begin transport. After giving the report to the hospital, you can ask medical direction if they believe it would benefit the patient to use the inhaler. Often we believe the patient's distress is "minor" and don't help out where we can. If we have the ability to ease even minor distress we should consider doing so. (p. 465)

#2

1. a (pp. 453–455)
2. b (p. 465)

#3

1. d (p. 461)
2. b (pp. 451–452)
3. a (p. 374)

CHAPTER 20

Stop, Review, Remember! (pp. 490–491)

Multiple Choice

1. c (p. 485)
2. b (p. 481)
3. b (p. 479)
4. a (pp. 448–449)
5. d (p. 490)

Fill in the Blank

1. Perfusion (p. 481)
2. Atria (p. 481)
3. Automaticity (p. 481)
4. Arteries, veins (p. 483)
5. CPR, advanced care (p. 486)
6. angina and congestive heart failure (CHF) (p. 487)

Critical Thinking

1. You can evaluate a patient's perfusion status by assessing his mental status, vital signs, capillary refill, and skin signs. (p. 481)
2. When the heart becomes damaged from an MI its ability to pump blood is compromised. This decrease in the heart's ability to pump blood is what leads to the signs and symptoms of cardiac compromise. (pp. 488–489)
3. When a patient experiences an MI a portion of the heart muscle (myocardium) is damaged. Angina results when blood flow to a portion of the heart is diminished but not cut off completely. (pp. 488–490)

Stop, Review, Remember! (pp. 499–501)

Multiple Choice

1. b (p. 495)
2. b (p. 494)
3. c (p. 492)
4. a (p. 495)
5. d (p. 496)

Signs and Symptoms Activity

List as many signs and symptoms as you can for the following medical conditions: (pp. 489–490, 492, 501)

Condition	Signs	Symptoms	Treatment
CHF	Pedal edema Sacral edema Jugular vein distention when sitting	Shortness of breath which may increase when lying down May have chest pain or discomfort	Take appropriate BSI precautions. Perform an appropriate initial assessment. Administer supplemental oxygen. Obtain a thorough SAMPLE history, utilizing the OPQRST assessment mnemonic. Obtain a baseline set of vital signs. Perform an appropriate focused physical exam. Assist with the administration of the patient's prescribed nitroglycerin (follow local protocol).

Condition	Signs	Symptoms	Treatment
			Perform regular ongoing assessments and adjust your care as appropriate. Transport as soon as practical and consider the need for an ALS backup or intercept.
MI ANGINA	Fainting Vomiting	Chest, back, arm, or jaw pain not relieved by rest With angina, often relieved by rest Shortness of breath Nausea Dizziness Weakness Abdominal pain Fatique Indigestion	Take appropriate BSI precautions. Perform an appropriate initial assessment Administer supplemental oxygen. Obtain a thorough SAMPLE history, utilizing the OPQRST assessment mnemonic. Obtain a baseline set of vital signs. Perform an appropriate focused physical exam. Assist with the administration of the patient's prescribed nitroglycerin (follow local protocol). Perform regular ongoing assessments and adjust your care as appropriate. Transport as soon as practical and consider the need for an ALS backup or intercept.

Condition	Signs	Symptoms	Treatment
`			Take appropriate BSI precautions. Perform an appropriate initial assessment. Administer supplemental oxygen. Obtain a thorough SAMPLE history, utilizing the OPQRST assessment mnemonic. Obtain a baseline set of vital signs. Perform an appropriate focused physical exam. Assist with the administration of the patient's prescribed nitroglycerin (follow local protocol). Perform regular ongoing assessments and adjust your care as appropriate. Transport as soon as practical and consider the need for an ALS backup or intercept.

Critical Thinking

1. Edema is caused by an accumulation of fluids within the tissues. The fluid is backing up into the tissues as a result of a decrease in efficiency of the heart. Edema develops in the ankles in patients who are sitting for a long period of time as gravity pulls the fluid to the lowest part of the body. It accumulates in the sacral area of patients who are bed ridden. (p. 492)

2. Cardiac arrest occurs when the heart stops pumping blood effectively. Myocardial infarction is when a portion of the heart dies due to lack of sufficient blood and oxygen. Most patients suffering an MI remain responsive and if they receive proper care in time will go on to survive the event. (pp. 489, 492)

3.

S – Can you describe the feeling that you are having?
A – Do you have any allergies to medications that you know of?
M – Are you currently taking any medications?
P – Do you have any past medical history such as lung or heart problems, seizures, or diabetes?
L – When and what did you last eat?
E – What were the events that led up to you calling for an ambulance? (pp. 494–496)

Stop, Review, Remember! (pp. 506–507)

Multiple Choice

1. c (p. 200)
2. c (p. 486)
3. d (p. 505)
4. b (p. 503)
5. a (p. 505)

Fill in the Blank

1. The following criteria must be met before you may assist a patient with administering their nitroglycerin:
   a. Prescription (p. 503)
   b. Expired (p. 503)
   c. 24 (p. 503)
   d. Systolic, 100 (p. 503)

Critical Thinking

1. Nitroglycerin is a vasodilator, that is to say that it causes the blood vessels in the heart to dilate thereby increasing the blood supply to the heart muscle. (p. 503)
2. Because nitro is a potent vasodilator the patient must have a blood pressure above 100 mmHg systolic prior to administration. This will minimize the chances that the patient may have an unacceptable drop in blood pressure. Another contraindication is if the patient has taken Viagra or other similar erectile dysfunction medication. These medications also cause the blood vessels to dilate and when taken in conjunction with nitro may cause a severe drop in blood pressure. (p. 503)
3. Providing supplemental oxygen to patients presenting with cardiac compromise will increase the percentage of available oxygen and therefore compensate somewhat for the decrease caused by the compromise of the circulatory system. (p. 200)

Stop, Review, Remember! (pp. 510–511)

Multiple Choice

1. d (p. 508)
2. c (p. 486)
3. a (p. 508)
4. d (p. 509)
5. a (p. 509)

Fill in the Blank

1. Blood thinner (p. 506)
2. Third (p. 486)
3. Ventricular fibrillation (p. 508)
4. Trauma (p. 510)

Critical Thinking

1. The fact that the software takes all the guesswork out of operating the device. There is no need to have to interpret a heart rhythm, the device does it all. (pp. 508–509)
2. Research has shown us that the longer a patient who is in VF goes without a shock, the less their chances of survival. It is estimated that for every minute following collapse without a shock, there is a 10 percent less chance of survival. (p. 509)
3. AEDs use adhesive electrode pads that are clearly labeled as to the proper location and once placed they are used to analyze the rhythm and deliver the shocks. AEDs also interpret the patient's rhythm automatically with little or no input or training on behalf of the rescuer. (p. 509)

Chapter Review (pp. 522–525)

Multiple Choice

1. c (p. 485)
2. a (p. 490)
3. d (p. 505)
4. b (p. 492)
5. b (p. 496)
6. c (p. 517)
7. b (p. 514)
8. a (p. 516)
9. d (p. 516)
10. c (p. 514)

Critical Thinking

1. A heart attack (MI) occurs when a portion of the heart muscle dies due to an insufficient supply of well oxygenated blood. In the majority of cases the heart attack patient remains responsive and complains of chest pain or discomfort. In the case of cardiac arrest, the heart has stopped pumping blood effectively and the patient becomes unresponsive with no pulses and no breathing. Death will soon follow. (pp. 488–489, 492)
2. As an EMT you will play an important part in the first three links in the chain. You may be the one calling 9-1-1 and you will be expected to perform CPR and attach an AED if one is available. (pp. 485–487)
3. Once the AED is turned on and the pads are properly placed, the fully automatic AED will analyze and deliver shocks as necessary without any further input from the operator. At a minimum the semi-automatic AED requires the operator to press a button to initiate a shock and some require that a button be pressed to initiate the analyze phase as well. (p. 512)
4. The software that runs the AED will recognize ventricular fibrillation and rapid ventricular tachycardia as shockable rhythms. (pp. 512–513)
5. In most states, medical direction is required for the implementation of an AED program. The medical director must approve the policies, procedures, protocols, and training that are a part of every AED program. In addition, the medical director must review all cases where an AED has been used. (p. 519)

Case Studies

#1

1. You must continue to ventilate this man at a rate of at least 12 per minute. You should use a BVM with supplemental oxygen and constantly monitor his pulse. (pp. 512–514, 516)

2. You must immediately begin CPR and attach the AED as soon as possible. Once the AED is attached you must stop compressions and initiate the analyze phase of the AED. (pp. 512–514, 516)

3. The AED will pause for 60 seconds while you assess the patient and resume CPR if indicated. Now is the time to get the patient on the stretcher and prepare for transport. (pp. 512–514, 516)

#2

1. The first thing is to place this man on high flow oxygen by non rebreather mask and call for ALS back up if available. You need to complete a thorough SAMPLE history including OPQRST. (pp. 501–503)

2. Based on his presentation and history, this man appears to be a candidate for nitro. You have already confirmed that his systolic pressure is adequate, you must now confirm that the medication is indeed his and that it has not expired. You must then confirm that he has not taken any erectile dysfunction medications within the past 24 hours. (pp. 503–505)

CHAPTER 21

Stop, Review, Remember! (pp. 533–534)

Multiple Choice

1. b (p. 530)
2. d (p. 531)
3. c (p. 531)
4. a (p. 532)
5. c (p. 372)

Glasgow Coma Score Activity

1. GCS 13 (p. 532)
2. GCS 8 (p. 532)
3. GCS 3 (p. 532)

Critical Thinking

1. (p. 528)
   * Trauma to the head
   * Stroke
   * Hypoglycemia
   * Hyperglycemia
   * Poisoning
   * Seizures
   * Low blood pressure

2. Patients with a sudden and unexplained change in mental status should be considered a high priority of care and transport. In most cases a patient with a decreased level of responsiveness is at greater risk for airway complications because he is less able to manage his own airway. (p. 527)

3. Due to his decreased ability to manage his own airway, the most appropriate position of the patient with altered mental status who does not have a suspected spinal injury is the recovery position. (p. 531)

Stop, Review, Remember! (pp. 543–544)

Multiple Choice

1. a (p. 536)
2. d (p. 535)
3. c (p. 535)
4. b (p. 539)
5. c (p. 539)

Matching

1. D (p. 534)
2. E (p. 534)
3. B (p. 535)
4. A (p. 536)
5. C (p. 541)

Critical Thinking

1. Without an adequate supply of insulin, glucose will remain in the blood stream and continue to increase in concentration causing hyperglycemia. Insulin acts as the "bridge" that allows glucose to cross over from the blood to the tissues and cells where it can be used for energy. (p. 534)

2. If left untreated, hyperglycemia can develop into a condition know as a diabetic coma. If left untreated, hypoglycemia can develop into a condition known as insulin shock. (pp. 535–536)

3. Some of the questions you would want to ask a known or suspected diabetic patient are: Have you taken your insulin today? If so, when? Have you eaten today? If so, what and when did you last eat? When was the last time you tested your glucose? What was it at that time? (p. 538)

Chapter Review (pp. 554–557)

Multiple Choice

1. c (p. 549)
2. a (p. 546)
3. d (p. 544)
4. b (p. 551)
5. a (p. 552)
6. c (p. 534)
7. a (p. 536)
8. d (p. 548)
9. b (p. 549)
10. d (p. 546)

Critical Thinking

1. Seizures are uncontrolled electrical activity in the brain and can cause anything from isolated muscle spasms to an altered mental status. In more extreme forms of seizures the patient may experience full body muscle contractions known as convulsions. (pp. 544–546)

2. Patients who experience convulsions during a seizure may experience either a partial or complete airway obstruction during the event. If the seizure lasts an extended period of time or the patient experiences one seizure after another (status epilepticus) there is a danger of brain damage due to hypoxia. Patients who do not gain an open airway following the seizure or who have repeated seizures need high-flow, high-concentration oxygen and immediate transport. (p. 546)

3. An ischemic stroke is one caused by a blockage of an artery feeding the brain. The area beyond the blockage becomes ischemic (deprived of blood) and therefore dies. A hemorrhagic stroke is caused when a vessel within the brain ruptures depriving the area beyond the rupture of valuable blood and oxygen. (p. 549)

Case Studies

#1

1. Since you already know that the man is diabetic you will want to try and determine if the man has taken his insulin today and if so, when. You will also want to know if he has had anything at all to eat and if so, what and when. (p. 538)
2. Based on the fact that he is a diabetic, that he has taken his insulin and that he has had nothing to eat, he is very likely suffering an episode of hypoglycemia. (p. 536)
3. Begin by establishing a baseline set of vitals, then you can provide him with oral glucose. Provide glucose or a similar substance only if he is able to swallow and is capable of managing his own airway. Provide supplemental oxygen and transport. (p. 538)

#2

1. Facial droop, arm drift, and the presence of abnormal speech. (p. 551)
2. Based on the fact that she is unable to move her right hand and that there is obvious droop to the right side of her mouth, it is most likely that the stroke has occurred to the left side of her brain. (p. 549)
3. Following your initial assessment you should place this patient on supplemental oxygen by nonrebreather mask. As long as she remains alert you can place her on the stretcher in a semi-Fowler's position. You must complete a focused medical assessment and continue to monitor her breathing status for adequacy of rate and tidal volume as you transport. (p. 552)

CHAPTER 22

Stop, Review, Remember! (pp. 563–565)

Multiple Choice

1. b (p. 559)
2. c (pp. 559–560)
3. a (pp. 561–562)
4. d (p. 562)
5. a (p. 562)

Fill in the Blank

1. Allergic reactions (p. 559)
2. allergens (p. 559)
3. mild reactions (p. 561)
4. anaphylaxis (p. 560)
5. anaphylactic shock (p. 562)

Critical Thinking

1. Allergens are substances foreign to the body that can cause an exaggerated response by the body's immune system resulting in a medical emergency. (p. 559)
2. A mild reaction usually involves some localized swelling at the site of injury but does not involve a systemic reaction. A severe reaction (anaphylaxis) is characterized by swelling to the face, neck, throat, tongue, hands, and/or feet as well as tightness in the chest and difficulty breathing. If not treated promptly, anaphylaxis can be life threatening. (pp. 561–562)
3. There are two primary mechanisms at work during an anaphylactic reaction. The exaggerated immune response is causing the blood vessels to dilate while causing the airway passages to constrict. As the blood vessels dilate it is causing the blood pressure to drop, which decreases the perfusion to the brain and other vital organs. As if this wasn't enough, the body is struggling to bring in an adequate supply of oxygen because the air passages are progressively getting smaller. (p. 562)

Chapter Review (pp. 574–576)

Multiple Choice

1. d (p. 565)
2. b (pp. 565–566)
3. c (p. 565)
4. d (p. 570)
5. a (pp. 572–573)
6. b (pp. 562–563)
7. c (p. 562)
8. b (p. 570)
9. a (p. 562)
10. b (pp. 562–563)

Critical Thinking

1. The care for a patient with a mild reaction must include a thorough history and physical to ensure that the patient has not experienced a severe reaction in the past. Often a cool gauze or ice pack will help with the pain, swelling, and itching. The patient must be observed for and informed of the signs of a severe reaction before being allowed to go about his way assuming he does not want to be transported. A patient with signs of a severe reaction must receive high-flow, high-concentration oxygen and rapid transport. The use of an Epi-pen may be indicated if allowed by local protocols. (pp. 565–568)
2. Epinephrine acts on the blood vessels by causing them to constrict, thus helping to maintain an adequate blood pressure. It acts on the airways causing them to dilate and making it easier for the patient to breathe. (pp. 568–573)
3. Immediately following the administration of epinephrine the patient should be closely observed for indications of improvement in their condition. If the patient responds well to the medication, he will become more responsive and breathing will be easier. It should be noted that epinephrine is rather short acting (several minutes) and transport should not be delayed even if the patient is showing signs of improvement. (pp. 568–573)

Case Studies

#1

1. Your first concern for this woman given her history and presentation will be to ensure that she has a clear airway and adequate breathing. (pp. 565–568)
2. Given that her rate is only 10 per minute and shallow, this woman will need high-flow, high-concentration oxygen via nonrebreather mask at a minimum. You must watch her respiratory status carefully and if her rate drops anywhere below 10 per minute you will have to assist her with manual ventilations using a BVM. (pp. 565–568)
3. Questions such as, does she have any known history of allergic reactions in the past? If so, to what? Does she have an Epi-pen prescribed to her and if so, where is it? Did anyone see by what she may have been bit/stung? Does she have any past pertinent medical history? (pp. 565–566)

#2

1. You will want to assess his respiratory status for adequate rate and tidal volume as well as his mental status and any signs of shock. (pp. 561–562)
2. Based on his presentation and the fact that it has been nearly 30 minutes since he was stung, it appears that this boy is only experiencing a mild allergic reaction. He has no signs of respiratory distress, shock, or altered mental status. (pp. 561–562)
3. There is no reason why you shouldn't transport this child since the parents are insisting. You must follow local protocol in this instance. To be on the safe side it would be appropriate to transport the child with one parent in the ambulance and ask that the other parent follow behind in their car. You can provide supplemental oxygen for the child if they will tolerate it and closely monitor for signs of shock or respiratory distress during transport. (pp. 565–568, 573)

CHAPTER 23
Stop, Review, Remember! (pp. 581–582)

Multiple Choice

1. b (p. 579)
2. a (p. 579)
3. d (p. 579)
4. c (p. 579)
5. a (p. 579)

Matching

1. B (p. 579)
2. B (p. 579)
3. E (p. 580)
4. A (p. 579)
5. D (p. 580)
6. E (p. 580)

Critical Thinking

1. Hyperthermia is when the body retains more heat than it gives off. Hypothermia is when the body gives off more heat than it retains. Hyperthermia is an emergency involving abnormally high body temperature. Hypothermia is an abnormally low body temperature. (p. 579)
2. The patient could be moved to the shade, and clothing removed. The patient may be sprayed with water and/or fanned. All help to reduce body temperature. (p. 580)

Stop, Review, Remember! (pp. 588–589)

Multiple Choice

1. d (p. 582)
2. c (p. 588)
3. b (p. 583)
4. d (pp. 583–584)
5. c (p. 583)
6. a (p. 585)

Fill in the Blank

1. generalized and localized (p. 582)
2. Frostbite (p. 586)
3. loses, retains/gains (p. 582)
4. Conduction (p. 579)

Critical Thinking

1. Hypothermia involves lowering of the body temperature and involves the whole body. Local cold injury, sometimes called frostbite or frostnip, involves an individual area or areas. (p. 582)
2. Active rewarming uses hot packs or another warm device to rewarm the patient. Passive rewarming uses blankets to maintain warmth and provide slower, more gentle rewarming. (p. 585)
3. **Shivering:** Early – present, Late – absent
   Breathing: Early – rapid, Late – slow, shallow eventually absent
   Pulse/Circulatory: Early – rapid, Late – slow, becoming difficult to palpate, may be irregular. Eventually absent.
   Skin: Early – red, Late – pale, becoming cyanotic (blue and/or gray) then hard (pp. 583–584)

Stop, Review, Remember! (pp. 594–595)

Multiple Choice

1. c (p. 592)
2. b (p. 593)
3. c (p. 588)
4. a (p. 586)
5. c (p. 585)

Fill in the Blank

1. late (p. 583–584)
2. early (p. 583–584)
3. late (p. 583–584)
4. late (p. 583–584)
5. early (p. 583–584)
6. late (p. 583–584)
7. late (p. 583–584)
8. early (p. 583–584)

Critical Thinking

1. Skin temperature is the biggest difference between serious and minor heat emergencies. Skin condition (dry or moist) is not as important. (pp. 592–593)
2. Patients with minor heat emergencies may be given sips of water if they have a gag reflex and are not nauseous. When the patient develops hot skin, liquids are no longer given and the patient is actively cooled. (pp. 592–593)

Stop, Review, Remember! (pp. 602–603)

Multiple Choice

1. a (p. 596)
2. d (p. 600)
3. c (p. 597)
4. a (pp. 596–597)
5. a (p. 597)

Fill in the Blank

1. −5 degrees (p. 583)
2. −10 degrees (p. 583)
3. −33 degrees (p. 583)
4. −33 degrees (p. 583)

Critical Thinking

1. High humidity (moisture in the air) reduces the body's ability to lose heat through perspiration/evaporation. (p. 590)
2. Only when the amount of water present in the stomach hinders ventilation or chest expansion. Compression on the stomach can cause aspiration of water into the lungs and be fatal. (p. 597)

3. Anaphylaxis is a life-threatening reaction that involves shock and bronchoconstriction. If left untreated, death is quite possible. (p. 598)

Chapter Review (pp. 604–606)

Multiple Choice

1. a (p. 590)
2. b (p. 587)
3. a (p. 583)
4. b (p. 596)

5. a (p. 582)
6. a (p. 585)
7. b (p. 585)

Critical Thinking

1. In a setting where there will be a delay in getting a patient to medical care (for example, storms, wilderness) you may actively rewarm a local cold injury. This would be done by warm (not hot) water. (p. 588)
2. Geriatric age, pediatric age, medications, certain medical conditions (heart disease, diabetes, fever, fatigue, obesity, dehydration) (p. 582)
3. Radiation – body heat is lost to nearby objects with which the body isn't in contact.
   Conduction – body heat is transferred to an object with which the body is in contact.
   Convection – body heat is lost to surrounding air that becomes warmer, rises, and is replaced with cooler air (pp. 579–580)

Case Studies

1. This is a deep local cold injury. The foot is white and hard. The toes feel stiff and he has lost sensation. (pp. 586–587)
2. Thom should be immediately removed from the cold to protect him from generalized hypothermia and prevent further damage to the foot. Remove wet clothes and cover the foot with warm materials. Splint the extremity. Do not rub the foot or break blisters. (pp. 587–588)
3. Thom's foot could be actively rewarmed because of the extended transport time. Be careful not to thaw the foot only to freeze it again during transport. (p. 588)

CHAPTER 24
Stop, Review, Remember! (pp. 614–615)

Multiple Choice

1. c (p. 611)
2. a (p. 610)
3. b (p. 609)
4. a (p. 611)

5. b (p. 609)
6. b (p. 612)
7. b (p. 610)

Short Answer

1. A behavioral emergency is defined as a situation where a patient's behavior becomes intolerable, dangerous, or bizarre enough to cause concern of family, bystanders, or the patient. (p. 608)
2. Hypoglycemia, seizure, stroke, medication overdose, intoxication, head injury (and many more) (p. 609)

3. 1) single, widowed, or divorced; 2) depressed; 3) abuse of alcohol or other substances; 4) those who appear to have formed a detailed suicide plan (for example, giving away possessions, purchasing or gathering items to use in the suicide attempt); 5) those who have experienced a prior suicide of a loved one (especially a same-sex parent); 6) those who have prior suicide attempts (p. 611)

Critical Thinking

1. a. A medical history of diabetes or seizures may be uncovered.
   b. The patient may be on medications that can cause the problem if stopped or taken in excess.
   c. The patient may have a history of psychiatric problems.
   d. Vital signs may show signs of medical or traumatic conditions. (pp. 609–610)
2. While some patients may end up requiring restraint there are a wide variety of interpersonal techniques that can calm patients and help prevent the need for restraint. This is always the goal (along with safety). We disagree with the statement. (pp. 612–614)

Stop, Review, Remember! (pp. 623–624)

Multiple Choice

1. d (pp. 616–617)
2. c (p. 610)
3. c (p. 622)

4. d (p. 616)
5. c (p. 609)
6. b (p. 616)

Short Answer

1. A person of a legal age to make legal decisions who is oriented and capable of making a rational decision (p. 619)
2. Unusual or bizarre behavior indicating a lack of touch with reality (p. 611)
3. Gauze or commercial restraints that are of a material that is not rigid and less likely to harm the patient (p. 620)

Critical Thinking

1. 1) place an oxygen mask on his face 2) protect your face and clothing from the sputum and saliva. (p. 620)
2. There are several reasons. First, it is a good people-care thing to do. The patient may have some part of him that does recognize the reality. Secondly, the patient must know what you are doing. By explaining, the patient may be less anxious and combative and if he chooses to cooperate he can. (p. 620)
3. Positional asphyxia as it applies to EMS is the death of a patient while restrained. It can be prevented by restraining a patient face up, by not hog-tying or hobbling a patient, and through constant monitoring of the patient's respirations and mental status. (pp. 620–623)

Chapter Review (pp. 625–627)

Multiple Choice

1. a (p. 622)
2. b (p. 611)
3. b (pp 608–609)

4. a (p. 620)
5. c (pp. 620–623)

Matching

1. E (p. 611)
2. C (p. 611)
3. B (p. 610)
4. A (p. 610)
5. F (p. 610)
6. D (p. 611)

Critical Thinking

1. The exact words will be up to you. Everyone may say something a little differently. Respect that the patient is in distress and don't downplay the situation. An example may be: "I can help take care of you and will treat you well. I can see you have a lot going on and I want to help." (pp. 618–619)
2. The history and physical exam will be the key. Determine if the patient is up to date on medications, has eaten, and use a blood glucose monitor if you are allowed to do so. Observe the patient for signs of hypoglycemia such as diaphoresis. (pp. 616–617)
3. No. Let the police enter first. Explain to the parent why you are waiting. Take the time to be sure you are in a safe position and to obtain a history of the events today. (p. 608)

Case Study

1. Conduct a mental status examination. Attempt to identify the patient's medical history. Identify any medications that the patient may be taking. (pp. 616–617)
2. Delusions are false beliefs such as being a famous or religious figure. (p. 610)
3. Warning signs of escalation include a change in voice or speech, pacing, violent hand movements, or other increased patient activity. (p. 619)
4. A firm but respectful attitude is often successful in this situation. Patients in crisis often respond positively to structures. (p. 620)

CHAPTER 25

Stop, Review, Remember! (pp. 637–638)

Multiple Choice

1. b (p. 630)
2. d (p. 630)
3. c (p. 632)
4. c (p. 631)
5. d (pp. 631–632)
6. a (p. 635)

Fill in the Blank

1. 1 (p. 632)
2. 3 (p. 632)
3. 2 (p. 632)
4. 2 (p. 632)
5. 2 (p. 632)
6. 1 (p. 632)

Critical Thinking

1. How long have you been pregnant?
   Are you having contractions or pain?
   How far apart are the contractions?
   How long does each contraction last?
   Have you observed any bleeding or discharge? Do you think your water broke? Have you felt a gush of fluid?
   Do you feel pressure in the vaginal area or the need to move your bowels?
   Do you feel the need to push? (p. 631)

2. Remain calm and reassure the mother, expose and examine the mother, drape the mother, obtain and open the OB kit, call for additional assistance if necessary. (p. 631)

Stop, Review, Remember! (pp. 651–652)

Multiple Choice

1. c (p. 647)
2. d (p. 647)
3. c (p. 644)
4. d (p. 648)
5. a (p. 640)

Short Answer

1. You should call for additional help because you may soon have three patients. (p. 646)
2. At 32 weeks the baby is premature. You will have to prepare for possible resuscitation (call for additional help) and promptly transport to a hospital capable of treating premature infants. (pp. 646–647)
3. Anticipate delivery problems. If the patient's physician was going to do a C-section, you should move the patient to the ambulance and transport promptly. (pp. 644–645)
4. Without prenatal care and check-ups you don't know if there are any developmental problems, multiple fetuses, or in some cases even the number of weeks gestation. While most births happen uneventfully, unfortunately there is no medical confirmation of this. Transport is a priority if there is time. ALS back-up may be required. (p. 633)

Critical Thinking

1. appearance—the color of the baby; pulse—obtain a pulse rate; grimace—response to irritation; activity—is the baby moving; are the limbs moving?; respirations—what is the respiratory rate? (p. 642)
2. (p. 640)

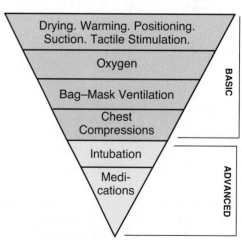

Stop, Review, Remember! (pp. 654–655)

Multiple Choice

1. a (pp. 652–653)
2. b (p. 653)
3. a (p. 653)
4. a (p. 653)
5. b (p. 652)
6. a (p. 653)
7. a (p. 647)
8. c (pp. 652–653)

Short Answer

1. Place an absorbent pad at the vaginal opening. Do not pack the vagina or place anything in the vagina. Administer oxygen, treat for shock, and transport promptly. (pp. 652–653)
2. Yes. It often is. While trauma may cause external bleeding, vaginal bleeding is usually the result of some sort of internal bleeding from the pelvis or female reproductive organ. Ectopic pregnancy is an example of this. (pp. 652–653)
3. When a sexual assault has occurred, it was a violent act that may cause trauma to other parts of the body including the head, neck, torso genitalia, extremities—almost anywhere. A full assessment with a compassionate approach is prudent. (p. 653)

Critical Thinking

1. No, you do not have the right to stop her. The patient will be very upset and will want to clean herself. She may feel that this is a priority and that she might not even want to press charges—or at least that is what she feels now. Some time later, however, she may wish to press charges. If she does and she washed evidence away it will be more difficult. So while we do not have the right to stop them from cleaning, you should try to explain the value of the evidence and attempt to convince them to delay washing slightly for evidence collection—whether or not charges are pressed. (p. 653)
2. The actual care for wounds (lacerations, bruising, bleeding control, and impaled objects) is the same as described in the trauma module of this text. The emotional needs of the patient will likely require much more care than a wound to an extremity. (p. 653)

Chapter Review (pp. 656–658)

Multiple Choice

1. a (p. 635)
2. b (p. 630)
3. c (p. 643)
4. a (p. 639)
5. c (pp. 645–646)

Matching

1. D (p. 647)
2. E (p. 644)
3. I (p. 649)
4. C (p. 646)
5. B (p. 646)
6. A (p. 644)
7. F (p. 645)
8. H (p. 648)

Critical Thinking

1. Many mothers have prenatal care. Prenatal care includes regular visits to an obstetrician and ultrasounds to determine the number of infants and in some cases birth defects. Prenatal care will usually mean that the mother will be aware of her estimated due date. Obtaining this information in the history is crucial to determine whether additional resources will be needed, if the baby will be premature or possibly require resuscitation. (p. 633)
2. Newborns have a greater surface area than adults, do not have the fat layers for insulation, and have minimal temperature regulation abilities, and they are born wet that can cause evaporation and significant cooling. (p. 639)

3. (p. 634)
   1. gloves, face protection, gown: BSI
   2. drapes: to cover the mother
   3. clamps or ties: clamping the umbilical cord
   4. scissors to cut the umbilical cord
   (also may answer bag for the placenta, absorbent pads to place under the mother, bulb syringes for suction of the newborn, towels to dry the newborn)

Case Study

1. Maria could be expecting twins or triplets, or experiencing premature labor. The baby may also have developmental problems or positioning that could complicate delivery and subsequent care. (pp. 633–634, 646)
2. Call for additional resources. Call for an engine company or another ambulance. Remember that you will be carrying two (or more) patients down the stairs—not just one. (p. 646)
3. The patient may appear to be unusually large although this isn't a reliable sign. If a first baby is born and the mother's abdomen still is large or if contractions begin again relatively quickly and before you would expect the placenta to deliver, it could be a second child. (p. 646)
4. As mentioned earlier lifting assistance and a second ambulance in the event resuscitation of the newborn is needed. Multiple births would increase the personnel needed because you will not have three patients. (p. 646)

CHAPTER 26

1. d   Objective: 4-1.2 (p. 430)
2. a   Objective: There are no DOT objectives specific to this question. (p. 430)
3. c   Objective: 4-1.5 (pp. 430–431)
4. b   Objective: There are no DOT objectives specific to this question. (p. 434)
5. c   Objective: There are no DOT objectives specific to this question. (p. 434)
6. d   Objective: There are no DOT objectives specific to this question. (p. 434)
7. a   Objective: 4-1.3 (p. 436)
8. c   Objective: 4-1.4 (p. 438)
9. d   Objective: 4-2.7 (p. 453)
10. d   Objective: There are no DOT objectives specific to this question. (p. 455)
11. c   Objective: There are no DOT objectives specific to this question. (p. 456)
12. d   Objective: 4-2.2 (p. 452)
13. a   Objective: 4-2.5 (p. 468)
14. c   Objective: 4-3.1 (p. 481)
15. b   Objective: 4-3.13 (p. 486)
16. a   Objective: There are no DOT objectives specific to this question. (p. 487)
17. c   Objective: There are no DOT objectives specific to this question. (p. 488)
18. b   Objective: There are no DOT objectives specific to this question. (p. 489)
19. a   Objective: There are no DOT objectives specific to this question. (p. 492)

20. d   Objective: 4-3.31 (p. 503)
21. d   Objective: There are no DOT objectives specific to this question. (p. 528)
22. b   Objective: 4-4.1 (p. 536)
23. b   Objective: 4-4.1 (p. 540)
24. c   Objective: There are no DOT objectives specific to this question. (p. 544)
25. c   Objective: There are no DOT objectives specific to this question. (p. 548)
26. a   Objective: There are no DOT objectives specific to this question. (p. 549)
27. d   Objective: There are no DOT objectives specific to this question. (p. 551)
28. c   Objective: 4-4.3 (p. 554)
29. a   Objective: 4-5.1 (pp. 562–563)
30. d   Objective: 4-5.5 (p. 571)
31. b   Objective: There are no DOT objectives specific to this question. (p. 579)
32. c   Objective: 4-7.1 (p. 580)
33. c   Objective: 4-7.2 (p. 582)
34. d   Objective: 4-7.3 (p. 585)
35. b   Objective: 4-7.3 (p. 585)
36. a   Objective: 4-7.3 (p. 587)
37. c   Objective: 4-7.4 (p. 592)
38. b   Objective: 4-7.5 (pp. 592–593)
39. a   Objective: 4-7.8 (p. 600)
40. a   Objective: 4-8.2 (p. 609)
41. b   Objective: There are no DOT objectives specific to this question. (pp. 610-611)
42. d   Objective: 4-8.8 (pp. 612–613)
43. c   Objective: 4-8.8 (p. 616)
44. b   Objective: 4-9.4 (p. 632)
45. c   Objective: There are no DOT objectives specific to this question. (p. 630)
46. b   Objective: 4-9.13 (p. 640)
47. d   Objective: 4-9.18 (p. 648)
48. c   Objective: 4-3.12 (pp. 508–509)
49. b   Objective: 4-3.4 (p. 510)
50. a   Objective: 4-3.25 (p. 513)
      a. 1 shock
      b. 3 shocks
      c. 6 shocks
      d. 9 shocks

CHAPTER 27

Stop, Review, Remember! (pp. 673–675)

Multiple Choice

1. c (p. 668)
2. a (p. 669)
3. b (p. 670)
4. c (p. 672)
5. d (p. 672)

Fill in the Blank

1. Trauma (p. 667)
2. well oxygenated (p. 668)
3. mental status (p. 668)
4. hypoperfusion (p. 668)
5. chest (p. 670)

Critical Thinking

1. The mechanism of injury is one of the first indicators for possible internal injury and bleeding. When the mechanism of injury is significant enough and involves areas such as the chest, abdomen, and pelvis you must maintain a high index of suspicion for internal bleeding. (pp. 670–672)
2. Internal bleeding occurs deep within the body and is concealed from view by the skin. For this reason a patient can lose a significant amount of blood without realizing it and thus may die before they can receive the necessary care. (pp. 670–671)
3. Anxiety, anxiousness, confusion, altered mental status, increasing pulse rate, increased respiratory rate, decreasing BP, pale, cool and clammy skin, history of significant MOI. (p. 672)

Chapter Review   (pp. 683–687)

Multiple Choice

1. c (p. 675)
2. a (p. 680)
3. b (p. 679)
4. c (p. 682)
5. a (p. 682)
6. d (p. 670)
7. b (p. 672)
8. d (p. 672)
9. a (p. 675)
10. b (p. 678)

Matching

1. F (p. 678)
2. C (p. 672)
3. A (p. 672)
4. E (p. 672)
5. D (p. 672)
6. B (p. 678)

Critical Thinking

1. When a patient loses enough blood, the blood pressure drops and can no longer perfuse the tissues with an adequate supply of well-oxygenated blood. In addition the waste products from the cells cannot be adequately removed. This causes a decrease in cell function which in turn causes the affected organ systems to fail resulting in the death of the patient. (p. 682)
2. The body is capable of compensating well for the loss of blood up to a point. During the compensatory phase the increase in pulse rate and redistribution of fluids into the core can maintain a normal blood pressure for some time. Late in the process when so much blood is lost that the body can no longer compensate, a major drop in blood pressure occurs. (p. 678)
3. The signs and symptoms of internal bleeding and those of shock are essentially the same. With internal bleeding you may have additional signs such as blood in the vomit or in the stool. (pp. 672, 675)

Case Studies

#1

1. The fact that this man suffered blunt trauma to the chest and now is showing signs and symptoms of shock is a strong indication that he may be bleeding internally. (pp. 670–672)
2. You will want to get this man to a supine position, place him on high-flow, high-concentration oxygen and get a baseline

set of vital signs. You will also want to maintain a comfortable body temperature and transport him immediately. (p. 670)

3. Based on his deteriorating condition, this man should be considered unstable and therefore should receive ongoing assessments every 5 minutes. (p. 680)

#2

1. This boy has a clear history of trauma as well as obvious signs of injury (abrasions) to his left abdomen. His pulse is rapid and weak and his breathing rate is elevated. He is nauseous and vomiting. (pp. 670–672)

2. The fact that this boy has what is likely a normal BP for his age and that his skin still appears normal are signs that his body is still in the compensatory state of shock. (pp. 678-679)

3. In the upper left abdomen is part of the liver, the spleen, the pancreas, and the stomach. The lower left quadrant contains mostly small intestines. (pp. 116–117)

CHAPTER 28
Stop, Review, Remember! (pp. 696–697)

Multiple Choice

1. b (p. 691)
2. a (p. 693)
3. c (p. 691)
4. d (p. 694)
5. c (p. 694)

Fill in the Blank

1. Perfusion (p. 690)
2. Vital signs (p. 691)
3. clammy (p. 691)
4. left ventricle (p. 691)
5. internal (p. 696)

Critical Thinking

1. Perfusion is directly related to blood pressure. Assuming all other factors (breathing and heart rate) are functioning properly, a person with a good blood pressure will be perfusing well. (p. 691)

2. A patient who is not perfusing well will have signs and symptoms of shock that include an altered mental status, increased pulse rate, increased breathing rate, and eventually a dropping blood pressure. (p. 691)

3. Being able to assess external blood loss is similar to evaluating the mechanism of injury for a trauma patient. It will provide valuable information as to the amount of blood loss and therefore allow you to make a better determination regarding the severity of the patient's condition. (p. 694)

Stop, Review, Remember! (pp. 606–607)

Multiple Choice

1. a (p. 698)
2. c (p. 698)
3. b (p. 699)
4. d (p. 699)
5. c (p. 699)

Fill in the Blank

1. arteries (p. 698)
2. capillaries (p. 699)
3. dark (pp. 698–699)
4. elevating (pp. 699–700)
5. bone (pp. 700–701)

Critical Thinking

1. Bleeding from arteries is often more difficult to control because the pressure in arteries is much greater than that of veins or capillaries. This pressure makes it difficult for an adequate clot to form at the injury site. The control of arterial bleeding often requires the combination of direct pressure, elevation, and a pressure point. (p. 698)

2. A pressure point is used to help control bleeding that is not easily managed by direct pressure and elevation alone. By placing manual pressure over an artery proximal to the injury site and squeezing it against an underlying bone, blood flow at the injury site can be reduced. This reduction in blood flow at the injury site will increase the likelihood that a clot will form and stop the bleeding. (pp. 700–701)

3. Anytime you are placing a bandage completely around a limb (circumferentially) there is the possibility of creating a tourniquet effect and cutting off all blood flow past the bandage. This is especially true when applying pressure bandages. Be sure to assess circulation, sensation, and motor function before and after application of a pressure bandage. Consider loosening the bandage if circulation is lost following application. (pp. 702–703)

Chapter Review (pp. 713–716)

Multiple Choice

1. d (p. 698)
2. b (pp. 700–701)
3. c (p. 703)
4. d (p. 710)
5. d (p. 712)
6. a (p. 694)
7. c (p. 694)
8. a (pp. 698–699)
9. b (p. 699)
10. c (p. 701)

Matching

1. F (p. 693)
2. C (p. 693)
3. E (p. 693)
4. A (p. 693)
5. G (p. 694)
6. B (p. 699)
7. D (pp. 700–701)

Critical Thinking

1. Large wounds have the potential to cause arterial, venous, and capillary bleeding. In most cases you will want to treat for the worst and assume there is arterial bleeding even if the blood appears dark or is not spurting. Providing direct pressure, elevation, and pressure points should easily control most external bleeding. (pp. 698–699)

2. Arteries are under higher pressure than veins or capillaries. Because of the pressure inside the arteries, arterial bleeding can be difficult to control. (p. 698)

3. **Pale, clammy skin:** caused when the circulation to the skin is redirected to the vital organs in the core of the body. **Increased pulse rate:** results as the heart tries to maintain an adequate blood pressure by increasing the rate. **Decreasing**

BP: Results when the blood loss exceeds the body's ability to compensate. **Increased respiratory rate:** It is the body's attempt to compensate for poor perfusion. **Altered mental status:** Occurs as a result of poor perfusion. (p. 712)

Case Studies

#1

1. Your priority of care for Monique is to control the bleeding as soon as possible. You must expose the wound and attempt to control the bleeding as appropriate. (pp. 703–705)
2. Based on the presentation of her hand it appears that she has arterial, venous, and capillary bleeding going on. The best way to manage this injury is to place medium size trauma dressings on both sides of the hand and put finger tip pressure on the spurting wound on her palm. Keep the hand elevated as best you can and apply a pressure dressing as appropriate. (p. 698–699)
3. You must keep her lying flat and elevate her legs 18 to 24 inches if possible. You must also provide her with supplemental oxygen by nonrebreather mask and transport as soon as possible monitoring her body temperature along the way. (p. 713)

#2

1. As you attempt to stop the bleeding from this man's wound you must consider the possibility of a skull fracture and use only the amount of pressure necessary to control the bleeding. You must also consider the need for spinal stabilization. (p. 705)
2. You will use sterile dressings and direct pressure for this wound. If possible you may use roller gauze or cravats to secure the dressings to the wound. (p. 699)
3. You will keep the patient lying down with his head slightly elevated to minimize the pressure at the site of injury. Place him on supplemental oxygen and monitor for signs of shock during transport. (p. 705)

CHAPTER 29

Stop, Review, Remember! (pp. 727–728)

Multiple Choice

1. a (p. 719)
2. d (p. 719)
3. c (p. 720)
4. a (p. 720)
5. c (p. 723)

Matching

1. B (p. 719)
2. C (p. 719)
3. A (p. 719)
4. G (p. 724)
5. E (p. 720)
6. D (p. 720)
7. F (p. 721)
8. H (p. 721)

Critical Thinking

1. The skin serves as protection from injury for the underlying structures as well as protection from infection. It helps regulate temperature and houses the sensory nerves that allow us to feel hot, cold, and pain. It also serves as an important fluid barrier that keeps moisture in. (p. 719)
2. The primary reason closed injuries have a greater potential for being life threatening is because they are hidden and not easily detected. (p. 720)
3. A contusion, also known as a bruise, is often seen as a reddish purple discoloration of the skin most often caused by blunt trauma. A hematoma is a swelling beneath the skin seen as a raised area or bump caused by an accumulation of fluid beneath the skin. Hematomas are also most often caused by blunt trauma. (p. 721)

Stop, Review, Remember! (pp. 731–732)

Multiple Choice

1. c (p. 724)
2. b (p. 725)
3. a (pp. 732–734)
4. c (p. 730)
5. d (p. 729)

Matching

1. E (p. 730)
2. A (p. 730)
3. I (p. 730)
4. D (p. 730)
5. G (p. 730)
6. C (p. 730)
7. B (p. 730)
8. F (p. 730)
9. H (p. 730)

Stop, Review, Remember! (pp. 737–738)

Multiple Choice

1. d (p. 734)
2. a (p. 735)
3. c (p. 733)
4. b (p. 736)
5. d (pp. 733–734)

Matching

1. C (p. 734)
2. B (p. 732)
3. A (p. 726)

Critical Thinking

1. An impaled object creates a challenge because in most instances it must be left in its place for transport. It also has caused damage and bleeding to internal soft tissue and organs that cannot be treated by the EMT. Impaled objects that interfere with the patient's airway or with attempts to resuscitate the patient should be removed in order to allow for proper care. (pp. 732–734)
2. Damage to major blood vessels in the neck can result in significant blood loss. An open wound to the neck can result in an air embolism entering one of the large vessels of the neck resulting in possible death. It can also affect the airway and make it difficult for the patient to breathe adequately. (p. 736)
3. An amputation of the hand should be managed by first controlling any active bleeding at the injury site with direct pressure, elevation, and pressure point. You must then place the amputated part in a plastic bag, then place the bag with the part on several ice packs to cool the part. (pp. 735–736)

Chapter Review (pp. 747–749)

Multiple Choice

1. b (p. 739)
2. b (pp. 739–740)
3. c (p. 742)
4. a (pp. 740–742)
5. d (p. 742)
6. a (p. 719)
7. c (p. 719)
8. d (p. 721)
9. b (p. 724)
10. a (p. 724)

Fill in the Blank

1. bleeding, infection (p. 739)
2. dressing (p. 739)
3. Adhesive (p. 739)
4. Occlusive (p. 740)
5. bandage (p. 740)
6. position of function (p. 743)

Critical Thinking

1. A dressing, which is typically sterile, is designed to be placed directly onto a wound and covered on all sides. A dressing absorbs blood and helps in the formation of a clot at the injury site. A bandage is designed to secure a dressing in place and can be tied in such a way as to hold pressure against the wound over the dressing. (pp. 739–740)
2. The proper application of dressings and bandages is an important skill that all EMTs must learn. First and foremost this skill aids in minimizing external blood loss and secondly it aids in minimizing infection of the wound. (p. 739)
3. A pressure dressing is different from other types of dressings in that its main purpose is to maintain pressure over a bleeding wound in an attempt to control the bleeding. Other dressings and bandages are applied to wounds where the bleeding has already been controlled and the main purpose is to minimize infection. (pp. 745–746)

Case Studies

#1

1. Given that the mechanism of injury was a fall from a 12-foot height, and the fact that this man is conscious and breathing, your top priority should be maintaining spinal precautions. He should be quickly secured to a long board, given supplemental oxygen, and monitored for signs of shock or any change in breathing during transport. (pp. 729–730)
2. This man has clearly sustained blunt trauma as a result of the fall from 12 feet up. He has high potential for spinal injuries as well as internal injuries to the abdomen due to the fall onto the bucket. (pp. 729–730)

#2

1. Your number one priority will be to minimize the loss of blood while maintaining spinal precautions. Even though he has no obvious injury to the head or torso, the MOI suggests possible spinal injury. (pp. 729–730)
2. Given the severity of the injury you must control the bleeding as quickly as possible. If conventional attempts fail you must apply a tourniquet just above the wound to stop the bleeding. (pp. 745–746)

3. Carefully place the amputated leg into a plastic bag. The common red biohazard bags work well for this type of transport. Transport the limb with the patient, and if possible, place cool packs around the limb to help cool it during transport. (pp. 735–736)

CHAPTER 30

Stop, Review, Remember! (pp. 757–758)

Multiple Choice

1. c (p. 754)
2. a (p. 752)
3. b (p. 754)
4. d (p. 752)
5. a (p. 755)

Fill in the Blank

1. source, depth, severity (p. 751)
2. severity (p. 759)
3. thermal (p. 752)
4. Chemical (p. 752)
5. superficial (p. 754)
6. dermis (p. 754)
7. full thickness (p. 755)

Critical Thinking

1. This answer is student specific and will differ depending on the environment the student works in. (p. 752)
2. This answer is student specific and will differ depending on the environment the student works in. (p. 752)
3. Patients who have experienced a full-thickness burn will have surrounding tissue that has sustained either partial-thickness or superficial burns. For this reason, the areas surrounding the full-thickness burns will likely be very painful. (p. 755)

Stop, Review, Remember! (pp. 771–772)

Multiple Choice

1. d (p. 760)
2. c (pp. 761–762)
3. d (pp. 763–764)
4. a (p. 763)
5. c (p. 760)

Matching

1. C (p. 759)
2. D (p. 759)
3. B (p. 763)
4. E (p. 763)
5. A (p. 763)

Critical Thinking

1. (p. 759)
   ∗ Airway patency and adequacy of breathing
   ∗ Depth of injury
   ∗ Percentage of body surface area (BSA) affected
   ∗ Location of the injury
   ∗ Patient's age
   ∗ Preexisting medical conditions

2. (pp. 759–763)
   * Airway patency and adequacy of breathing – As with any patient, airway and breathing are first and foremost in your assessment. Without an open airway and adequate breathing the patient will quickly die.
   * Depth of injury – the greater the depth of injury the more severe the injury will be from a standpoint of tissue damage and infection.
   * Percentage of body surface area (BSA) affected – The greater the BSA the more severe the burn.
   * Location of the injury – Minor burns can be complicated by location especially if they affect the face, airways, hands, feet, and genitalia.
   * Patient's age – the very old and very young have a much more difficult time recovering from burns.
   * Preexisting medical conditions – a great many medical conditions and medications can complicate the recovery from burns.
3. (pp. 763–764)
   * The source of the burn is still a hazard – You must mitigate the source yourself if appropriate or call for the appropriate resources to do so.
   * Objects on or around the patient may be hot – avoid touching these or wear protective garments when doing so.

Chapter Review (pp. 773–775)

Multiple Choice

1. c (pp. 752–754)
2. a (p. 754)
3. d (p. 754)
4. b (p. 754)
5. c (p. 754)
6. c (p. 755)
7. a (p. 755)
8. a (pp. 767–768)
9. d (pp. 768–769)
10. b (p. 760)

Matching

1. B (p. 752)
2. A (p. 752)
3. E (p. 752)
4. C (p. 752)
5. D (p. 752)

Critical Thinking

1. Once you have confirmed that the burning has stopped and that the ABCs are okay, you must cover both arms with dry sterile dressings. You may want to place sterile gauze between the fingers of each hand before wrapping the entire hand with sterile gauze. (pp. 765–767)
2. Circumferential burns are burns that encircle the entire body area or body part. When this happens the swelling of the tissues either restricts movement as in the case of a circumferential burn to the chest, or it can severely restrict circulation as in the case of an arm, hand, or finger. (pp. 768–769)

Case Studies

#1

1. This boy has burned approximately half of each arm (4.5% x 2 = 9%) and his face (6%) for a total of approximately 15%. (p. 760)

2. You should place sterile dressings between each of his fingers then wrap both hands and forearms with roller bandages. (p. 769)
3. The burns to his face indicate he may have inhaled superheated air or smoke and therefore may experience swelling of his air passages. This will make it difficult for him to breathe and could result in total blockage of his airway. He must be transported immediately in the event his airway begins to swell. (p. 761)

#2

1. Front of one leg = 9% × both legs = 18%
   One half of the anterior torso = 9%
   Total = 27% (p. 760)
2. Entire head = 18%
   Entire right arm = 9%
   Total = 27% (p. 760)
3. Entire back = 18%
   back of one arm (4.5%) × both arms = 9%
   Total = 27% (p. 760)

CHAPTER 31

Stop, Review, Remember! (pp. 786–787)

Multiple Choice

1. a (p. 779)
2. c (p. 780)
3. c (p. 780)
4. d (pp. 783–784)
5. a (p. 783)

Matching

1. D (p. 780)
2. A (p. 780)
3. C (p. 780)
4. E (p. 783)
5. B (p. 780)

Critical Thinking

1. The muscles of the chest wall (intercostal muscles) contract in response to the injury and form a splint of sorts. Late in the injury as the patient's condition worsens and the muscles tire the paradoxical motion may become visible. (p. 780)
2. While both are potentially serious and will require high-flow, high-concentration supplemental oxygen and care for shock, the open chest wound will require the application of an occlusive dressing. (pp. 779, 782)
3. Sealing the dressing on three sides creates a "flutter valve" which allows air to escape during exhalation or when pressure increases while preventing air from entering during inhalation. (p.785)

Stop, Review, Remember! (pp. 791–792)

Multiple Choice

1. d (p. 789)
2. d (p. 789)
3. c (p. 788)
4. c (p. 788)
5. a (p. 789)
6. b (p. 789)
7. b (p. 787)

Matching

1. H (p. 116)
2. A (p. 116)
3. E (p. 116)
4. G (p. 116)
5. F (p. 117)
6. B (p. 116)
7. D (p. 116)
8. C (p. 117)

Critical Thinking

1. Open wounds have the potential to expose abdominal organs. This can result in damage to the organs, infection, and evisceration. These are treated in a specific manner (for example, care for evisceration). Closed wounds have a strong potential for injury as well. This includes internal bleeding. Care for both conditions involves shock. (pp. 789–791)
2. (p. 117)
   a. liver, gallbladder
   b. spleen
   c. appendix, colon, small intestine
   d. colon, small intestine

Chapter Review (pp. 793–795)

Multiple Choice

1. c (p. 784)
2. b (p. 778)
3. a (p. 779)
4. c (p. 779)
5. c (p. 789)
6. b (p. 789)
7. a. (p. 782)

Fill in the Blank

1. tamponade (p. 783)
2. saline (p. 791)
3. retroperitoneal (p. 788)

Critical Thinking

1. The major organ of concern is the liver. This is a solid organ that can cause profuse internal bleeding. The gall bladder and portions of the stomach and duodenum (small intestine) may also be injured. (p. 788)
2. The patient may experience pleuritic chest pain—that is chest pain that is aggravated by breathing. The patient may appear anxious and use accessory muscles to breathe. Auscultation of the chest may reveal unequal breath sounds (diminished on the side of the pneumothorax). The level of the signs and symptoms. (p. 780)
3. The pulse pressure is the difference between the systolic and diastolic pressures. It will narrow (become smaller) in tension pneumothorax—and other conditions that cause shock. (p. 782)

Case Study

1. After the airway opening and suctioning the patient would receive an oral airway (if he didn't have a gag reflex). The patient would require assisted ventilations with a BVM or pocket face mask with supplemental oxygen. The airway would be constantly monitored. (pp. 781–782)
2. Observe and palpate the chest. Remember that the muscles of the chest will create a splint and reduce the "classic"

paradoxical motion. If two or more ribs are broken in two or more places, it is a flail segment. (pp. 779–780)
3. The patient could experience a pneumothorax, tension pneumothorax, hemothorax, and lacerations or damage to great vessels and the heart. (p. 780)

CHAPTER 32

Stop, Review, Remember! (pp. 801–803)

Multiple Choice

1. c (p. 798)
2. b (p. 797)
3. a (p. 799)
4. d (p. 800)
5. a (p. 800)

Labeling (p. 798)

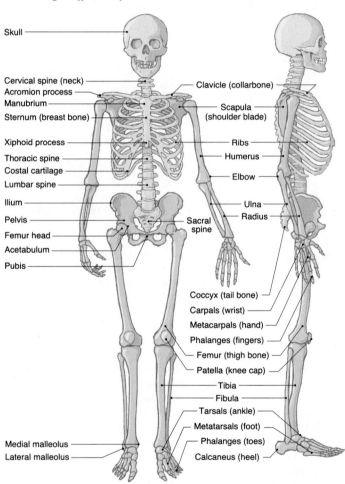

Skull
Cervical spine (neck)
Acromion process
Manubrium
Sternum (breast bone)
Xiphoid process
Thoracic spine
Costal cartilage
Lumbar spine
Ilium
Pelvis
Femur head
Acetabulum
Pubis
Medial malleolus
Lateral malleolus

Clavicle (collarbone)
Scapula (shoulder blade)
Ribs
Humerus
Elbow
Ulna
Radius
Sacral spine
Coccyx (tail bone)
Carpals (wrist)
Metacarpals (hand)
Phalanges (fingers)
Femur (thigh bone)
Patella (knee cap)
Tibia
Fibula
Tarsals (ankle)
Metatarsals (foot)
Phalanges (toes)
Calcaneus (heel)

Critical Thinking

1. A strain is an injury involving a muscle, typically caused when the muscle is stretched beyond normal limitations. A sprain occurs at a joint and results when the joint and the associated supportive tissue (ligaments and tendons) are stretched beyond their normal limitations. (pp. 800–801)
2. The term "suspected fracture" is used to describe an injury to the musculoskeletal system when the MOI as well as signs and symptoms are suggestive of a fracture. (p. 803)

3. Because we cannot determine for certain what type of injury the patient has sustained (fracture, dislocation, sprain, or strain), the appropriate treatment includes caring for the worst possible injury, a fracture. (p. 809)

Stop, Review, Remember! (pp. 808–809)

Multiple Choice

1. b (p. 804)
2. c (p. 804)
3. a (p. 804)
4. d (p. 806)
5. a (p. 800)

Fill in the Blank

1. pain (p. 805)
2. joints (p. 803)
3. closed (p. 803)
4. skin (p. 803)
5. mechanism of injury (p. 804)

Critical Thinking

1. In most cases an injury to a joint will result in the patient being unable to move the joint. This requires that the injured extremity be immobilized in the position that it is found. (pp. 810–812)
2. Assuming that the ABCs are okay, the treatment priorities for an open skeletal injury include controlling the bleeding, keeping the open wound clean, and immobilizing the extremity. (p. 810)
3. An injured extremity with abnormal distal CSM findings may indicate damage to the blood vessels or nerves that feed the extremity. Abnormal findings might include the absence of a pulse, the presence of numbness and tingling, and weakness or the inability to move the distal extremity appropriately. (pp. 806–807)

Stop, Review, Remember! (pp. 828–830)

Multiple Choice

1. d (p. 810)
2. a (p. 818)
3. c (p. 811)
4. b (pp. 821–824)
5. d (p. 812)

Fill in the Blank

1. fracture (p. 810)
2. elevated (pp. 809–810)
3. movement (p. 810)
4. manual stabilization (p. 810)
5. position of function (p. 812)

Critical Thinking

1. The most common signs and symptoms of a closed skeletal injury include: pain, tenderness, deformity, swelling, discoloration, crepitation, and the inability to move the joint. (p. 805)
2. The objective is to immobilize the knee in the position that it is found. This can be accomplished by placing adequate support beneath the knee and either securing a rigid splint on either side to form a triangle or securing the ankle of the

injured extremity to the uninjured extremity. In either case it is best to place the patient on a carrying device such as a long board for easy transport. (p. 811)
3. Immobilizing the joints adjacent to the suspected fracture site help ensure that the bones at the injury site remain immobile and therefore minimize pain and additional soft tissue damage and swelling. (pp. 810–811)

Chapter Review (pp. 831–833)

Multiple Choice

1. c (p. 812)
2. a (p. 813)
3. b (pp. 813–814)
4. b (p. 819)
5. d (pp. 818–819)
6. c (p. 817)
7. d (p. 818)
8. a (pp. 811–812)
9. c (p. 828)
10. a (p. 828)

Matching

1. E (p. 817–818)
2. A (p. 817–818)
3. D (p. 817–818)
4. C (p. 817–818)
5. B (p. 817–818)
6. F (p. 817–818)

Critical Thinking

1. The most common signs and symptoms of an open skeletal injury include; pain, tenderness, open wound, external bleeding, deformity, swelling, and crepitation. (p. 805)
2. A shoulder injury can be easily immobilized by using a sling and swathe. If properly placed, the sling can immobilize the elbow and the swathe immobilizes the shoulder joint. (p. 817)
3. In most cases you will discover a difference in push/pull strength or grip strength from side to side as you assess motor function. This is typically attributed to pain in the injured extremity. (pp. 806–807)

Case Studies

#1

1. With the ABCs addressed your next priority will be to maintain manual stabilization of the head while you package this man in full spinal precautions on a long board. You will also want to provide supplemental oxygen as you package him. (pp. 809–810)
2. Due to the significant MOI, you will most likely immobilize the extremities as a package when you secure the patient to the long board. Given his mental status and the MOI, he is a high priority for rapid transport. (p. 811)
3. While this man may be a candidate for a traction splint, it will not be your top priority. He needs to be packaged on a long board and transported immediately. If you have enough resources at the scene or in transport you might apply a traction splint to his left leg. (pp. 809–810)

#2

1. Since her ABCs are okay and there is no need for spinal precautions your attention should be focused on properly immobilizing the injured arm. As always, pay attention to any changes in her condition that would indicate the need for spinal precautions. (pp. 804–805)

2. You can carefully attempt to align the arm and place it in a splint. Be sure to monitor the status of circulation, sensation, and motor function throughout the process. Regardless, if circulation returns or not you will transport this patient as soon as practical. (p. 811)

3. One way to immobilize this injury will be to place it in a 3-sided cardboard splint that extends from the wrist to just past the elbow. Secure this splint in place with lots of padding and then place the arm in a sling and swathe. (p. 819)

CHAPTER 33
Stop, Review, Remember! (pp. 838–839)

Multiple Choice

1. d (p. 836)   4. c (p. 836)
2. a (p. 837)   5. c (p. 837)
3. d (p. 836)

Matching

1. E (p. 837)   5. F (p. 837)
2. D (p. 837)   6. C (p. 837)
3. A (p. 837)   7. B (p. 837)
4. A (p. 837)   8. E (p. 837)

Critical Thinking

1. A vault is technically defined as a container. The brain is contained within the skull or cranial vault. (p. 835)
2. Blood beneath the dura would be called a subdural hematoma where "sub" means below and hematoma meaning accumulation of blood. (p. 836)

Stop, Review, Remember! (pp. 845–847)

Multiple Choice

1. c (p. 843)   5. d (p. 838)
2. d (p. 843)   6. b (pp. 841–842)
3. a (p. 843)   7. b (p. 842)
4. c (p. 838)

Labeling (p. 836)

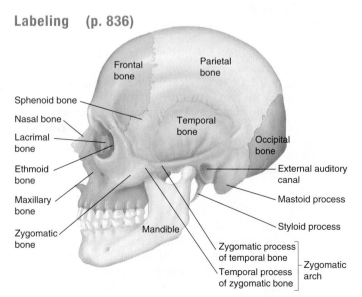

Critical Thinking

1. Herniation presents with specific signs and symptoms including those in Cushing's Triad. In both conditions, an altered mental status is likely but with herniation abnormal posturing and pupillary changes may also be seen. (pp. 840–843)
2. No, these signs and symptoms are most likely caused by some other injury. Remember that you can't lose enough blood into the head to cause shock—a condition that this patient appears to be developing. Based on the mechanism of injury, injury to the chest, abdomen or pelvis is a more likely cause of the patient's current condition. The head injury may still be serious—but it likely isn't causing the vitals you see. (pp. 842–843)

Stop, Review, Remember! (pp. 854–855)

Multiple Choice

1. b (p. 848)   5. c (pp. 948–850)
2. d (p. 848)   6. b (p. 853)
3. c (pp. 848–849) 7. a (p. 847)
4. b (p. 851)

Fill in the Blank

1. 13 (p. 850)   4. 3 (p. 850)
2. 6 (p. 850)   5. 8 (p. 850)
3. 15 (p. 850)

Critical Thinking

1. Your protocols will require you to take the distance to each hospital into consideration. The ability to control the patient's airway, whether you need to ventilate the patient and your ability to ventilate adequately as well as his Glasgow Coma Score are additional considerations. External factors such as weather conditions and transport times (early morning or during commuting times, for example) will also play a part. (p. 850)
2. Probably not. The vital signs indicate developing shock (increased pulse, increased respirations, agitation, cool, clammy skin). Look for possible trauma to the chest, abdomen, and/or pelvis to account for this patient's presentation. (pp. 850–851)

Chapter Review (pp. 856–858)

Multiple Choice

1. a (p. 836)   5. d (p. 850)
2. d (p. 837)   6. b (p. 848)
3. b (p. 843)   7. b (p. 850)
4. a (p. 842)

Labeling   (p. 837)

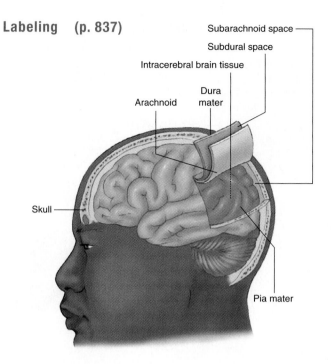

Critical Thinking

1. No. Any patient with indications of a head injury should be encouraged to seek hospital assessment and care of his injury. While concussions may present as with a patient with an altered mental status who gets better, the nature of head injuries is that a patient may sometimes get better—and then experience problems later from bleeding or swelling. (pp. 841–842)
2. Mental status is thought of as the most significant indicator of head injury. The brain works best under certain conditions. Any alteration in oxygen levels, pressure, glucose, or pH quickly results in a change in mental status. A patient with an altered mental status is considered serious—period. (pp. 847–848)

Case Study

1. The patient's clammy skin, altered mental status, and vomiting are all indications of problems. Together they are a giant red flag waving at you that you are dealing with a high priority, unstable patient who requires your help. (p. 842)
2. The patient is having some sort of intracranial bleeding— either from old trauma he doesn't recall or possibly spontaneous rupture of a vessel or vessels around or within the brain. (p. 842)
3. Promptly transport to a facility capable of handling this emergency (a trauma center), if available. Call for ALS assistance if necessary. The patient will require airway maintenance due to the vomiting. Since the patient has signs of herniation including posturing, decreasing GCS, unresponsiveness, and fixed pupils you should ventilate the patient at 20/minute. (pp. 852–853)

CHAPTER 34

Stop, Review, Remember!   (pp. 868–870)

Multiple Choice

1. a (p. 861)
2. d (p. 861)
3. a (p. 862)

4. b (p. 862)
5. d (p. 862)

Labeling   (p. 862)

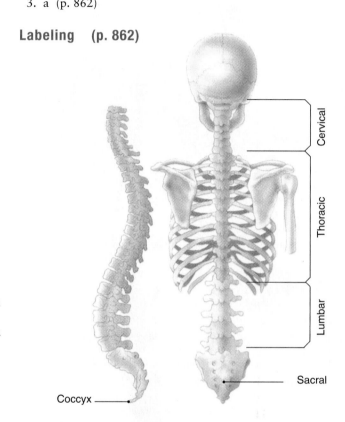

Critical Thinking

1. Evaluation of the mechanism of injury plays an important role in determining the most appropriate care for the suspected spinal injury patient. Unlike suspected fractures where pain is the primary indicator for injury, the presence or absence of pain alone is unreliable in predicting spinal injury. If the MOI is consistent with a potential spinal injury then you must provide the appropriate care, despite the absence of pain or neurological deficit. (pp. 863–867)
2. The central nervous system consists of the brain and spinal cord and is responsible for the control of all basic body functions. The peripheral nervous system consists of an elaborate network of motor and sensory fibers that connect the central nervous system to the rest of the body. (p. 861)
3. While it may be impossible to assess and care for a suspected spinal injury patient without moving them at all, it is essential to keep movement to a minimum. Inappropriate movement of a patient with suspected spinal injury could make the injury worse increasing the potential for permanent damage to the spinal cord and paralysis. (p. 862)

Stop, Review, Remember! (pp. 890–892)

Multiple Choice

1. b (p. 871)
2. c (p. 871)
3. b (p. 872)

4. a (p. 873)
5. d (p. 880)

Labeling (pp. 864–866)

FLEXION INJURY

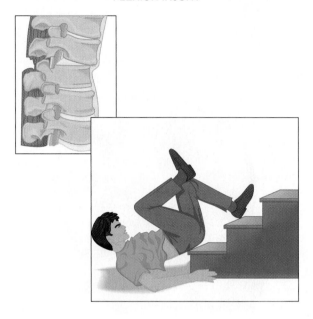

DISTRACTION INJURY

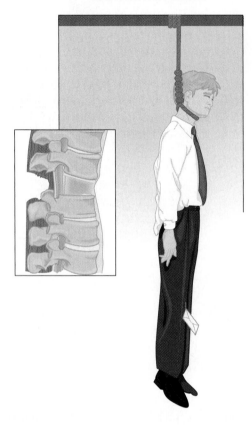

EXTENSION INJURY

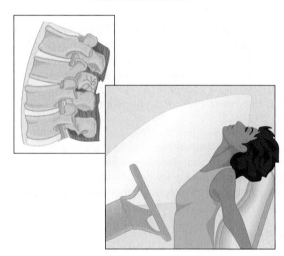

COMPRESSION INJURY

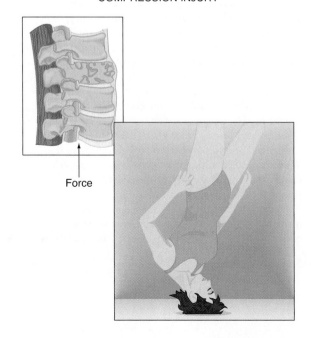

Force

Critical Thinking

1. Your first clue that a patient may have suffered a spinal injury is the mechanism of injury. After assessing the MOI you can then assess for pain along the spine or numbness and/or tingling in any of the extremities. (pp. 867–868)
2. All factors relating to the MOI can help you determine the likelihood of a spinal injury such as the force involved, the surface the patient struck, loss of consciousness, and obvious external trauma. When the MOI is unknown you must assume the worst and treat for suspected spinal injury. (pp. 870–871)
3. It is important to minimize movement of the head and neck of a suspected spinal injury patient. For this reason you must make every attempt to use the chin-lift technique when opening and maintaining the airway of these patients. (p. 871)

Chapter Review   (pp. 900–904)

Multiple Choice

1. c (p. 861)	9. d (p. 881)
2. d (p. 861)	10. b (p. 875)
3. a (pp. 863–864)	11. a (p. 892)
4. d (p. 864)	12. d (p. 896)
5. c (p. 864)	13. a (p. 880)
6. a (pp. 867–868)	14. b (p. 882)
7. c (p. 868)	15. d (p. 873)
8. b (pp. 879–881)	

Fill in the Blank

1. spinal cord (p. 861)	5. lumbar (p. 862)
2. peripheral (p. 861)	6. below (p. 862)
3. cervical spine (p. 862)	7. compression (p. 864)
4. 12 (p. 862)	8. 3rd (p. 868)

Critical Thinking

1. Rapid extrication is necessary when the patient has life threatening problems relating to the ABCs that cannot be easily managed while he remains in the vehicle. It is also indicated when hazards at the scene threaten either the patient or the rescuers. (p. 892)
2. During rapid extrication the priorities of proper spinal immobilization and the need for movement must be balanced. An emphasis is placed on manual stabilization of the head, neck, and spine to accommodate rapid movement of the patient. (pp. 893–894)
3. First and foremost your priority is to ensure that the ABCs are all okay. You must do this while maintaining manual stabilization of the head. In most cases it is better to leave the helmet and shoulder pads in place in order to keep the head properly aligned. If you remove the helmet and not the pads, the head will fall into a hyperextended position. If you remove the helmet you must remove the shoulder pads as well in order to keep the spine in a neutral alignment. (p. 898)

Case Studies

#1

1. Due to the obvious mechanism of injury and wound to the head, this man is definitely a candidate for spinal immobilization. The absence of pain is not justification for clearing this man's spine at the scene. (pp. 863–867)
2. It will be important to know this man's mental status by asking if he lost consciousness and determining if he is A&O ×4. You will also want to determine if he was wearing a seat belt and if the vehicle had an airbag that deployed. (pp. 870–872)
3. Given that the man is standing when you find him, the best approach will be to get him onto a backboard from the standing position. Once he is secured to the board you can control the bleeding from open wounds and complete a more detailed physical exam. You will also want to start him on supplemental oxygen. (p. 882)

4. Given that this man is found in the standing position, the long backboard would be most appropriate for taking full spinal precautions. You must begin by placing an appropriate size cervical collar. (p. 882)

#2

1. Your first priority for this patient will be to establish an open airway and begin artificial ventilations. (pp. 872–873)
2. Yes, you must roll this patient onto his back in order to manage his airway and begin to stabilize his spine. One of you must hold manual stabilization of the head while the other gently rolls the patient onto his back. (pp. 872–873)
3. Yes, you must remove the helmet in order to gain proper access to the airway and to ventilate this patient. Both rescuers hold the head stable. The rescuer at the top of the patient holds the helmet while the other rescuer places her hands beneath the helmet at the base of the skull. Then the first rescuer pulls the straps and slips the helmet off while the second rescuer slides her hands up to maintain control of the head. Once the helmet is removed the first rescuer takes over control of the head. (p. 896)
4. This patient should have a cervical collar placed and be properly secured to a long backboard. (pp. 872–873)

CHAPTER 35

1.	d	Objective: 5-1.1 (p. 691)
2.	b	Objective: 5-1.1 (p. 693)
3.	a	Objective: 5-1.1 (p. 693)
4.	d	Objective: Not specific to DOT Objectives. (pp. 696–696)
5.	a	Objective: 5-1.1 (p. 696)
6.	c	Objective: 5-1.2 (p. 698)
7.	d	Objective: 5-1.3 (p. 699)
8.	d	Objective: 5-1.3 (pp. 700–701)
9.	a	Objective: 5-1.3 (pp. 699–700)
10.	c	Objective: 5-1.3 (pp. 708–710)
11.	b	Objective: 5-1.3 (p. 710)
12.	a	Objective: 5-1.9 (p. 668)
13.	c	Objective: 5-1.9 (p. 672)
14.	b	Objective: 5-1.9 (p. 672)
15.	b	Objective: 5-1.10 (p. 672)
16.	a	Objective: 5-2.1 (p. 719)
17.	c	Objective: 5-2.2 (p. 719)
18.	b	Objective: 5-2.4 (p. 720)
19.	d	Objective: 5-2.4 (pp. 720–722)
20.	c	Objective: 5-2.5 (p. 723)
21.	b	Objective: 5-2.6 (p. 724)
22.	a	Objective: 5-2.7 (p. 734)
23.	d	Objective: 5-2.7 (pp. 734–736)
24.	b	Objective: 5-2.21 (p. 739)
25.	c	Objective: Not specific to DOT Objectives. (pp. 742–743)
26.	b	Objective: Not specific to DOT Objectives. (p. 752)
27.	b	Objective: 5-2.11 (p. 754)
28.	d	Objective: 5-2.15 (p. 754)
29.	c	Objective: 5-2.18, 5-2.19, 5-2.20 (p. 759)
30.	c	Objective: Not specific to DOT Objectives. (p. 760)
31.	b	Objective: Not specific to DOT Objectives. (p. 760)

32. d   Objective: Not specific to DOT Objectives. (p. 760)
33. c   Objective: Not specific to DOT Objectives. (p. 761)
34. d   Objective: Not specific to DOT Objectives. (p. 763)
35. b   Objective: 5-2.28 (p. 767)
36. a   Objective: 5-2.29 (p. 768)
37. d   Objective: 5-2.20 (pp. 754–755)
38. a   Objective: Not specific to DOT Objectives. (p. 778)
39. c   Objective: 5-2.10 (p. 778)
40. b   Objective: Not specific to DOT Objectives. (p. 779)
41. d   Objective: Not specific to DOT Objectives. (p. 780)
42. c   Objective: Not specific to DOT Objectives. (p. 780)
43. d   Objective: 5-2.9 (p. 784)
44. a   Objective: Not specific to DOT Objectives. (p. 788)
45. a   Objective: Not specific to DOT Objectives. (p. 789)
46. c   Objective: 5-2.10 (pp. 789–791)
47. c   Objective: Not specific to DOT Objectives. (p. 798)
48. d   Objective: Not specific to DOT Objectives. (p. 799)
49. d   Objective: Not specific to DOT Objectives. (p. 800)
50. c   Objective: 5-3.8 (p. 805)
51. b   Objective: 5-3.8 (p. 805)
52. a   Objective: 5-3.8 (p. 806)
53. b   Objective: 5-3.5 (p. 810)
54. c   Objective: 5-3.6 (p. 811)
55. d   Objective: 5-3.6 (p. 814)
56. a   Objective: Not specific to DOT Objectives. (p. 817)
57. d   Objective: 5-3.8 (pp. 809–810)
58. c   Objective: 5-4.3 (p. 835)
59. b   Objective: 5-4.3 (p. 835)
60. a   Objective: 5-4.1 (p. 836)
61. c   Objective: 5-4.1 (p. 837)
62. d   Objective: Not specific to DOT Objectives. (p. 840)
63. b   Objective: Not specific to DOT Objectives. (p 841)
64. c   Objective: Not specific to DOT Objectives. (p. 842)
65. b   Objective: Not specific to DOT Objectives. (p. 842)
66. b   Objective: Not specific to DOT Objectives.
        (pp. 847–848)
67. b   Objective: 5-4.11 (p. 853)
68. b   Objective: 5-4.11 (p. 853)
69. a   Objective: 5-4.11 (p. 861)
70. d   Objective: 5-4.11 (p. 862)
71. d   Objective: 5-4.4 (p. 864)
72. d   Objective: 5-4.1 (p. 863)
73. a   Objective: 5-4.3 (p. 873)
74. c   Objective: 5-4.3 (p. 889)
75. b   Objective: 5-4.17 (p. 892)
76. a   Objective: 5-4.20 (p. 896)

CHAPTER 36
Stop, Review, Remember! (pp. 922–923)
Multiple Choice

1. b (p. 918)
2. a (p. 919)
3. d (p. 919)
4. c (p. 920)
5. b (p. 921)

Fill in the Blank

1. airway, breathing (p. 919)
2. 100% oxygen (p. 929)
3. central perfusion (p. 921)
4. decompensates (p. 922)

Critical Thinking

1. The school-age child is able to recall and retell what they have seen or experienced but may not understand what it means. Speaking to the adolescent respectfully and nonjudgmentally will improve your ability to obtain an accurate history. (pp. 918–919)
2. In both cases, look for how the infant or child interacts with his environment and family members. Does he make eye contact or respond to a parent's voice? Listen for loud respiratory noises such as wheezing or grunting. Watch for retractions, nasal flaring, and respiratory rate. (pp. 920–921)
3. The head and tongue are proportionally larger. The trachea is thin and flexible. The nose does not have much supporting cartilage, so nasal flaring is an early sign of respiratory distress. See also Table 36-2 for a more comprehensive listing. (p. 919)

Stop, Review, Remember! (pp. 932–933)
Multiple Choice

1. a (p. 929)
2. d (p. 931)
3. b (p. 936)
4. c (p. 931)
5. b (p. 929)

Critical Thinking

1. Watch and feel for chest expansion. Look for nasal flaring. Note the strength of the cry and listen for the inhalations. (p. 924)
2. Allow a family member to hold the child. Allow the child to examine your stethoscope. Allow the child to hold a favorite toy. (p. 927)
3. (pp. 929–930)
   a. Nasal cannula with low flow (1/2-1 lpm) 100% oxygen
   b. Nonrebreather mask with 100% oxygen
   c. Assisted artificial ventilation
   d. 100% oxygen via nonrebreather mask

Stop, Review, Remember! (pp. 941–942)
Multiple Choice

1. b (p. 937)
2. b (p. 938)
3. b (pp. 938–939)
4. c (p. 940)

Fill in the Blank

1. shock (p. 931)
2. tongue (p. 920)
3. airway, immobilization (p. 935)
4. febrile (p. 936)

Critical Thinking

1. Children have smaller stores of glucose in their bodies, and less fat to insulate them. Hypothermia increases glucose consumption, resulting in decreased blood sugar. (p. 936)
2. Remember to report objectively, identifying specific things you saw or heard, not what you think might have happened. Do not delay transport to accuse or confront a suspected negligent or abusive caregiver. (p. 939)

3. Exposure to the care of children in all settings, getting as much practice as possible with assessing the infant and child, and becoming familiar with the equipment used in their care, will improve provider confidence. (pp. 940-941)

Chapter Review (pp. 943–945)

Multiple Choice

1. b (p. 917)
2. c (p. 924)
3. c (p. 927)
4. a (p. 929)
5. c (p. 931)

Matching

1. F (p. 921)
2. B (p. 921)
3. C (p. 921)
4. E (p. 924)
5. A (p. 938)
6. D (p. 922)

Critical Thinking

1. Children of different ages will respond differently to their environment, caregivers, and strangers. Understanding these differences can give you important clues that will aid with your assessment and interventions. (pp. 915–916)
2. Recognizing respiratory failure and intervening appropriately and quickly can help prevent respiratory failure. (p. 924)
3. Blunt trauma most commonly caused by motor vehicle crashes. (p. 934)
4. An obstructed airway or inadequate respirations are the most common cause of cardiac arrest. Opening the airway and providing 100% oxygen by the appropriate means is the best way to avoid cardiac arrest in these patients. (p. 921)

CHAPTER 37

Stop, Review, Remember! (pp. 953–954)

Multiple Choice

1. b (p. 952)
2. d (p. 950)
3. c (p. 951)

Fill in the Blank

1. Decreased cardiac output, heart failure, changes in the blood vessels including atherosclerosis and aneurysm, high blood pressure, syncope (p. 950)
2. Lung tissue becomes less elastic, hypoxia can develop unchecked for some time, less able to fight respiratory infection (pp. 948–949)
3. Osteoporosis, shrinking of discs in the spine, changes in posture and balance, falls (p. 951)
4. Slowed digestion, decreased taste sensation, dentures make eating difficult (pp. 951–952)
5. Decreased sensory perception, decreased reaction time, changes in balance and coordination (pp. 950–951)

Critical Thinking

1. Elderly patients are not able to compensate for shock as efficiently because they can't constrict blood vessels or elevate the heart rate in the same manner a younger patient can. (p. 950)
2. The skin and underlying connective tissues are not as resilient as that of a younger patient. Shock may be more likely as the body can't compensate for fluid loss. Additionally the potential for infection is greater because of reduced response from the immune system. (p. 952)

Stop, Review, Remember! (pp. 961–963)

Multiple Choice

1. c (p. 955)
2. c (p. 957)
3. a (p. 958)
4. b (p. 949)
5. a (p. 955)
6. a (p. 955)

Fill in the Blank

1. less (p. 949)
2. less (p. 950)
3. more (p. 949)
4. more (p. 957)
5. more (p. 952)
6. less (p. 952)
7. less (p. 949)

Critical Thinking

1. Get down to the patient's level, speak slowly and clearly, ask one question at a time, and allow the patient time to formulate a response and answer. Of course the amount of time you can realistically take depends on the patient's condition. Serious patients should be promptly moved to the ambulance for transport. Obtain additional information en route. (pp. 958–959)
2. Elderly patients may have alterations in their sensations of pain. The injury may in fact feel very painful to this patient. In some other cases dementia may cause the patient to yell out because he doesn't understand what is happening. (pp. 959–960)

Chapter Review (pp. 964–965)

Multiple Choice

1. a (pp. 948–949)
2. a (p. 950)
3. c (p. 951)
4. a (p. 956)
5. a (p. 956)
6. a (p. 951)
7. a (p. 951)

Critical Thinking

1. The risk of burns and falls can be reduced by taking safety measures in the home, such as reducing the temperature of the hot water heater, using nonskid rugs and wearing shoes with nonslip soles, and installing hand-holds in the shower. (p. 957)
2. The fact that the patient seems to call for nonemergent reasons may be from loneliness. This is one indicator. Talk of all her friends dying, a depressed effect, isolation, recent changes in independence or dependence on medical equipment, incontinence of other quality of life issues may be triggers for the depression. (p. 955)

Case Study

1. A complaint of fatigue should cause you to consider the possibility of a cardiac problem. Remember that women and elderly patients may not present with chest pain. Also check her medications to rule out overdose—either accidental or intentional. Finally, because of her history of TIA (mini-strokes) you should still consider stroke a possibility. (pp. 948–957)

2. The cardiac problem can be assessed by asking about fatigue, chest discomfort, or heaviness, if the patient is having any trouble breathing (including sleeping on more pillows at night or having trouble breathing on exertion). Examine her ankles for fluid accumulation. For her medications check the bottles or other containers to see if the remaining dose matches what should be left. Further evaluation for stroke will be difficult. The patient should be transported anyway as altered mental status is a serious finding.

   Take note: It was determined that the patient's daughter set out medications in a plastic container with four compartments for each day. Instead of taking the medications from the compartments vertically, she took three doses horizontally (morning meds for three days) resulting in tripling her anti-anxiety medication dose for the day. She was transported, treated, and released. Her daughter is keeping a closer eye on the medications. You need to remember to always ask about the a patient's medication regimens. (pp. 957–961)

CHAPTER 38

1. c   Objective: 6-1.2 (p. 917)
2. b   Objective: 6-1.1 (p. 918)
3. a   Objective: 6-1.10 (p. 924)
4. a   Objective: There are no DOT objectives specific to this question. (p. 919)
5. d   Objective: 6-1.9 (p. 922)
6. a   Objective: 6-1.8 (p. 921)
7. c   Objective: 6-1.5 (p. 924)
8. b   Objective: 6-1.2 (p. 925)
9. c   Objective: 6-1.7 (p. 925)
10. a   Objective: 6-1.7 (p. 925)
11. a   Objective: 6-1.7 (p. 925)
12. d   Objective: 6-1.7 (p. 926)
13. b   Objective: 6-1.6 (p. 926)
14. c   Objective: 6-1.7 (p. 927)
15. d   Objective: 6-1.7 (p. 928)
16. d   Objective: 6-1.8 (pp. 930–931)
17. c   Objective: 6-1.8 (p. 931)
18. a   Objective: There are no DOT objectives specific to this question. (pp. 919–922)
19. c   Objective: 6-1.13 (p. 934)
20. b   Objective: 6-1.13 (p. 934)
21. d   Objective: 6-1.2 (p. 936)
22. c   Objective: 6-1.16 (pp. 938–939)
23. a   Objective: There are no DOT objectives specific to this question. (p. 940)
24. d   Objective: There are no DOT objectives specific to this question (p. 946)

25. b   Objective: There are no DOT objectives specific to this question. (p. 940)
26. d   Objective: There are no DOT objectives specific to this question. (pp. 948–952)
27. c   Objective: There are no DOT objectives specific to this question. (p. 947)
28. d   Objective: There are no DOT objectives specific to this question. (p. 950)
29. a   Objective: There are no DOT objectives specific to this question. (p. 950)
30. c   Objective: There are no DOT objectives specific to this question. (pp. 950–951)
31. d   Objective: There are no DOT objectives specific to this question. (p. 957)
32. b   Objective: There are no DOT objectives specific to this question. (p. 955)
33. d   Objective: There are no DOT objectives specific to this question. (p. 951)
34. d   Objective: There are no DOT objectives specific to this question. (pp. 951–952)
35. a   Objective: There are no DOT objectives specific to this question. (p. 952)
36. d   Objective: There are no DOT objectives specific to this question. (pp. 950–951)
37. d   Objective: There are no DOT objectives specific to this question. (p. 954)
38. a   Objective: There are no DOT objectives specific to this question. (p. 955)
39. c   Objective: There are no DOT objectives specific to this question. (pp. 955–956)
40. d   Objective: There are no DOT objectives specific to this question. (pp. 955–956)
41. d   Objective: There are no DOT objectives specific to this question. (p. 956)
42. a   Objective: There are no DOT objectives specific to this question. (p. 957)
43. c   Objective: There are no DOT objectives specific to this question. (p. 957)
44. d   Objective: There are no DOT objectives specific to this question. (pp. 957–958)
45. b   Objective: There are no DOT objectives specific to this question. (p. 958)
46. d   Objective: There are no DOT objectives specific to this question. (p. 958)
47. c   Objective: There are no DOT objectives specific to this question. (p. 959)
48. b   Objective: There are no DOT objectives specific to this question. (p. 959)
49. d   Objective: There are no DOT objectives specific to this question. (p. 963)
50. d   Objective: There are no DOT objectives specific to this question. (p. 953)
51. b   Objective: 6-1.11 (p. 936)
52. a   Objective: 6-1.7 (p. 924)
53. c   Objective: 6-1.13 (pp. 922, 934–935)
54. d.   Objective: There are no DOT objectives specific to this question. (pp. 950, 957)
55. d   Objective: There are no DOT objectives related to this question. (pp. 950, 957)

CHAPTER 39
Stop, Review, Remember! (pp. 988–989)
Multiple Choice

1. c (p. 976)
2. b (p. 985)
3. a (p. 983)

4. a (p. 987)
5. b (pp. 983–985)

Matching

1. E (pp. 985–986)
2. C (pp. 983–984)
3. A (pp. 983–985)
4. F (pp. 997–1001)
5. F (pp. 997–1001)

6. D (pp. 994–995)
7. F (pp. 997–1001)
8. B (pp. 986–987)
9. E (pp. 985–986)

Critical Thinking

1. You would find other means to deal with the airway problem. This may include finger sweeps initially followed by manual suction devices or getting a portable unit from another ambulance. Not having suction can cause the patient to aspirate and worsen his condition. Most likely this occurred because the unit wasn't checked or wasn't checked thoroughly at the beginning of the shift. (pp. 976, 979, 998)
2. These pieces of information allow the dispatcher to get the call out to the ambulance quickly and give the ability to get the caller back on the line in the event he is disconnected. (pp. 986–987)

Chapter Review (pp. 1002–1003)
Multiple Choice

1. a (p. 993)
2. a (p. 998)
3. b (p. 989)
4. c (p. 1001)

5. a (p. 989)
6. b (p. 995)
7. a (p. 989)
8. a (p. 995)

Critical Thinking

1. Disinfection kills most organisms on a surface. Sterilization is designed to kill all microorganisms including those spore-forming organisms that are very difficult to kill. (p. 998)
2. You disinfect the surface of the backboard. (p. 1001)

Case Study

1. Every experienced EMT will acknowledge that a serious call involving a child gets his pulse going. If that pulse affects important decisions such as driving safely, you and your crew may never make it to the patient. Drive safely **every time** you activate the lights and sirens regardless of the type of call. (p. 989)
2. Choosing your route to the scene is important to assure a safe and minimal response time. Considerations include choosing a direct route, time of day and traffic, construction or other delays, avoiding one-way streets, and others. (p. 990)

3. In short you will need to balance prompt transportation to the hospital with providing a safe and practical working environment in the back of the moving ambulance. You should avoid sudden stops, sharp turns, swerving, and other actions that could both throw the crew around as well as prevent care of the patient for those times. Careful attention to traffic conditions, road surfaces, and vehicle motion will accomplish this goal. (p. 995)

CHAPTER 40
Stop, Review, Remember! (pp. 1007–1008)
Multiple Choice

1. a (p. 1006)
2. a (p. 1006)
3. c (p. 1006)

4. d (p. 1006)
5. c (p. 1006)

Fill in the Blank

1. National Interagency Incident Management System (p. 1006)
2. Incident Command System (p. 1006)
3. Incident Management System (p. 1006)
4. Multiple Casualty Incidents (p. 1004)
5. Incident Commander (pp. 1004–1005)

Critical Thinking

1. This list should include but not be limited to manufacturing facilities, major traffic intersections, and chemical/ petro-chemical storage facilities. This discussion should raise the awareness of the potential for the need of a working local IMS. (p. 1004)
2. There is a great risk of personal injury or death to all involved when a freelancer enters the scene. This person is not part of the chain of command and is not aware of the procedures. (p. 1006)

Stop, Review, Remember! (pp. 1010–1011)
Multiple Choice

1. c (p. 1008)
2. d (p. 1008)

3. c (p. 1008)
4. b (p. 1008)

Matching

1. B (p. 1009)
2. A (p. 1009)
3. E (p. 1009)

4. C (p. 1009)
5. D (p. 1009)

Critical Thinking

1. All responders have donned PPE. Safety of the crew and of the victims is being taken into account during the operation. (pp. 1008–1009)
2. Refer the media to the Public Information Officer or Incident Commander. (p. 1009)

Stop, Review, Remember! (pp. 1014–1015)

Multiple Choice

1. b (p. 1011)
2. a (p. 1013)
3. c (p. 1012)
4. a (p. 1012)

Matching

1. B (p. 1012)
2. A (p. 1012)
3. D (p. 1011)
4. C (p. 1011)

Critical Thinking

1. This list would be customized to the area. (p. 1011)
2. This would be customized to the area. (p. 1011)

Stop, Review, Remember! (pp. 1018–1019)

Multiple Choice

1. c (p. 1015)
2. b (p. 1015)

Matching

1. B (p. 1017)
2. A (p. 1017)
3. E (p. 1017)
4. D (p. 1017)
5. C (p. 1017)

Critical Thinking

1. In order to prevent chaos, the incident must be resolved with a single vision. (p. 1018)
2. The command post often serves as a site for the media to gather and by-standers to loiter. (p. 1017)
3. To determine scene safety, exact location, additional resources *(for example, fire department, power company, law enforcement)*, the number of patients, and mechanism of injury/nature of illness. (p. 1015)

Stop, Review, Remember! (pp. 1023–1024)

Multiple Choice

1. a (p. 1022)
2. c (p. 1020)
3. d (p. 1020)
4. a (p. 1021)
5. a (p. 1022)
6. b (p. 1022)
7. a (p. 1022)
8. a (p. 1021)

Critical Thinking

1. Documentation is required on all patients receiving emergency care. (p. 1020)
2. Answers will vary. (pp. 1021–1022)

Chapter Review (pp. 1025–1027)

Multiple Choice

1. c (p. 1008)
2. d (p. 1008)
3. c (pp. 1008–1009)
4. b (p. 1008)
5. d (p. 1016)
6. a (pp. 1017–1018)
7. a (p. 1016)
8. b (p. 1018)
9. a (p. 1009)
10. b (p. 1009)

11. b (p. 1016)
12. c (p. 1017)
13. d (p. 1009)
14. c (p. 1012)
15. b (p. 1011)
16. c (p. 1013)
17. a (p. 1016)

Critical Thinking

1. Answers will vary. (pp. 1004–1005)
2. Answers will vary. (pp. 1015–1022)
3. Answers will vary. (pp. 1015–1022)

Case Study

1. We arrived on scene to find a 15-passenger van vs. pickup truck, the driver of the truck was DOA, the van was overturned. There were a total of 10 passengers in the van, four were walking wounded, three red tagged, one yellow tagged, and two black tagged. The six remaining passengers are either pinned or entrapped in the van. The fire department has begun extrication procedures. They estimate that it will take 10 to 15 minutes to free the remaining patients. There is a helicopter on the way to transport two of the most critical patients and you have two more units en route to transport the remaining patients. (p. 1020)

CHAPTER 41

Stop, Review, Remember! (pp. 1034–1035)

Multiple Choice

1. b (p. 1032)
2. a (p. 1029)
3. d (p. 1033)
4. c (p. 1031)
5. a (p. 1033)

Fill in the Blank

1. 2 (p. 1033)
2. 1 (p. 1032)
3. 5 (p. 1034)
4. 3 (p. 1033)
5. 4 (p. 1033)

Critical Thinking

1. Do the best for the most, effectively manage the limited resources, and avoid relocating the disaster. (pp. 1031–1032)
2. A multicasualty incident is one in which the event cannot be handled by normal responding units, but it can be handled by a single system's resources. A Mass-Casualty Incident on the other hand will require the resources of multiple jurisdictions, or even an entire region. (p. 1030)

Stop, Review, Remember! (pp. 1040–1041)

Multiple Choice

1. d (p. 1038)
2. b (p. 1037)
3. a (p. 1036)
4. c (p. 1035)
5. b (p. 1036)

Fill in the Blank

1. French, To Sort (p. 1036)
2. Few, Many (p. 1038)
3. Secondary (p. 1039)
4. Minor, Green (p. 1036)

Critical Thinking

1. The START triage system is designed for adult MCI patients, whereas JumpSTART is specific to children and infants. JumpSTART also focuses more on the respiratory status of the patient than the START system does. (pp. 1036–1038)
2. A patient who is unable to maintain an airway following the assistance of the triaging EMT should be tagged black. A patient who cannot maintain an airway will unfortunately require more time and effort than can be afforded during the initial triage period. (pp. 1036–1038)

Chapter Review (pp. 1042–1044)

Multiple Choice

1. b (pp. 1036–1038)
2. d (p. 1029)
3. d (p. 1038)
4. c (p. 1036)
5. c (p. 1036)
6. a (p. 1039)
7. b (p. 1009)
8. b (p. 1039)
9. b (pp. 1036–1038)
10. b (p. 1036)

Fill in the Blank

A. red (p. 1036)
B. green (p. 1036)
C. red (p. 1036)
D. black (p. 1036)
E. red (p. 1036)
F. yellow (p. 1036)
G. green (p. 1036)
H. red (p. 1036)
I. yellow (p. 1036)
J. yellow (p. 1036)

Critical Thinking

1. Open the child's airway and check for spontaneous breathing. If there is none, give five rescue breaths and reevaluate for spontaneous breathing. If the child starts to breathe on her own, she would receive a red tag and if she doesn't, she should receive a black tag. You would then move on to the next patient. (pp. 1038–1039)
2. In a situation where the numerous "walking wounded" start to disrupt a scene (or simply leave) due to boredom or perceived lack of care, a good solution is to call in buses from local transit companies or schools. The noncritical patients can then be loaded onto the buses and not only be removed from the scene, but also delivered to the most appropriate receiving facilities. (p. 1032)
3. It will most likely take longer to triage the patients on the bus because, due to crowded conditions, some patients will have to be moved following evaluation before other patients can be reached. (p. 1039)

Case Study

1. Determine scene safety. There are many hazards in this type of situation; two damaged vehicles, a dust-obscured roadway, darkness of night, potential for hazardous cargo on the truck, etc. (pp. 1032–1034)

2. You would follow four of the five. You would obviously determine scene safety, size-up the scene, and send the incident information to dispatch by calling 9-1-1. As an off-duty EMT in your personal vehicle, you would forego setting up the medical setting. Following the phone call to dispatch, you would begin triage. (pp. 1032–1034)
3. The vehicle that is nearest to you that appears safe to approach. Be mindful of fires, dripping fluids, and unstable positioning. (pp. 1036–1037)

CHAPTER 42
Stop, Review, Remember! (pp. 1053–1053)

Multiple Choice

1. b (p. 1046)
2. a (p. 1048)
3. c (pp. 1048–1049)
4. b (p. 1050)

Matching

1. C (pp. 1048–1049)
2. B (p. 1048)
3. A (p. 1049)
4. D (p. 1049)

Critical Thinking

1. This will vary from community to community, for example, take into consideration gas and chemical plants. (pp. 1046–1050)
2. This answer will vary from community to community. (pp. 1046–1050)
3. This answer will vary from community to community. (pp. 1046–1050)

Stop, Review, Remember! (pp. 1060–1061)

Multiple Choice

1. c (p. 1053)
2. b (p. 1058)
3. a (p. 1059)
4. c (p. 1058)
5. b (p. 1056)
6. b (p. 1055)
7. a (p. 1055)
8. a (p. 1058)
9. b (p. 1056)
10. a (pp. 1055–1056)
11. a (p. 1058)
12. a (p. 1056)
13. b (p. 1059)

Matching

1. I (p. 1056)
2. H (p. 1056)
3. G (p. 1056)
4. F (p. 1057)
5. E (p. 1058)
6. D (p. 1058)
7. C (p. 1058)
8. B (p. 1059)
9. A (p. 1059)

Critical Thinking

1. The ERG was developed for use by firefighters, police, and other emergency services personnel who may be the first to arrive at the scene of a transportation incident involving

dangerous goods and hazardous materials. It provides the names, procedures, physical behavior, medical issues, and evacuation distances for certain chemicals. (p. 1053)

2. Isolate the scene, restrict or reroute traffic, and conduct evacuation, if necessary. (p. 1054)

Stop, Review, Remember! (pp. 1068–1069)

Multiple Choice

1. a (p. 1065)
2. c (p. 1065)
3. a (pp. 1056–1059)
4. a (p. 1063)
5. d (p. 1064)

Matching

1. C (p. 1062)
2. A (pp. 1062–1063)
3. B (p. 1063)
4. E (p. 1063)
5. D (p. 1063)
6. H (p. 1063)
7. F (p. 1063)
8. G (p. 1064)

Critical Thinking

1. To prevent cross contamination (p. 1066)
2. What are the hazardous properties of the substance, what is the concentration, in what form is the substance, what are the chemical and physical characteristics of the substance, how is the substance contained, what pathways of exposure exist, and what was the duration of exposure? (pp. 1064–1065)

Chapter Review (pp. 1070–1072)

Multiple Choice

1. d (p. 1066)
2. b (pp. 1066–1067)
3. d (p. 1062)
4. a (p. 1066)
5. c (pp. 1066–1067)
6. d (pp. 1056–1059)
7. d (p. 1059)
8. a (p. 1056)
9. b (p. 1059)
10. d (p. 1067)
11. d (p. 1059)

Critical Thinking

1. An *acute exposure* is the exposure to a hazardous substance over a short period of time or at a high dose. A *chronic exposure* is the exposure to a hazardous substance over a long period of time. (p. 1065)
2. (pp. 1063–1064)
   * Absorption (through the skin or eye): When a chemical contacts the skin absorption through the skin can occur. This is called *dermal* exposure.
   * Injection: The most familiar example of injection is that of needle stick, in which the skin is punctured with a needles so that a substance can enter the body.
   * Ingestion: If a patient eats a substance that contains a harmful material, that substance enters our bodies by means of our digestive system.
   * Inhalation: It is also possible to be contaminated by toxic substances when a patient breathes them into his lungs.

Case Study

1. Safety is the primary responsibility of the EMT when responding to a hazardous materials incident. Using the

ERG will allow you to identify potentially hazardous materials prior to entering the scene. (pp. 1054–1056)

2. First remove yourself, other rescuers, any freed victims that can be safely accessed, and all bystanders to a 1500' safety perimeter. Call the HazMat team and deny further access. (pp. 1054–1056)

CHAPTER 43
Stop, Review, Remember! (pp. 1078–1079)

Multiple Choice

1. a (p. 1074)
2. a (p. 1077)
3. b (p. 1076)

Fill in the Blank

1. Number of vehicles (p. 1076)
2. Size of vehicles (p. 1063)
3. Whether an incident can be handled by BLS or ALS (p. 1063)
4. Integrity of vehicle (p. 1063)
5. Stability of vehicle (p. 1063)
6. Number of victims at scene (p. 1063)

Critical Thinking

1. These will be area-specific answers. (pp. 1075–1077)
2. This answer should include a list of rescue squads and fire departments and their rescue capabilities. (pp. 1075–1077)

Stop, Review, Remember! (pp. 1085–1086)

Multiple Choice

1. b (p. 1084)
2. a (p. 1083)
3. c (p. 1082)

Labeling   (pp. 1083–1084)

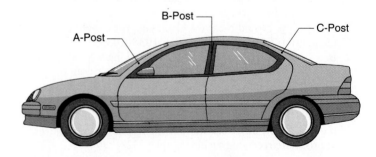

Critical Thinking

1. There are hazards from the vehicle such as sharp metal, glass, fuel and fluids from the vehicle, fire, traffic moving around the vehicle, rescue equipment being used on the vehicle, and utility hazards, i.e., power and gas lines. (pp. 1081–1082)
2. Preparing for the rescue, sizing up the situation, recognizing and managing hazards, stabilizing the vehicle prior to entering, gaining access to the patient, providing initial

patient assessment and a rapid trauma exam, disentangling the patient, immobilizing and extricating the patient from the vehicle, providing a detailed exam, ongoing assessment, treatment and transport, terminating the rescue (p. 1080)

Stop, Review, Remember! (pp. 1090–1091)

Multiple Choice

1. c (p. 1089)
2. a (p. 1089)
3. c (p. 1089)
4. c (p. 1087)
5. a (p. 1089)

Fill in the Blank

1. Area-specific response. (p. 1089)
2. Area-specific response. (p. 1087)
3. Area-specific response. (p. 1089)

Critical Thinking

1. Cold water will drop body temperature 25 times faster than air, cold water and clothing can cause frostbite to extremities. The treatment for victim should focus on gradual re-warming, minimal movement, and treating for shock. (p. 1088)
2. This will be localized to the specific area. (pp. 1086–1089)
3. This will be localized to the specific area. (pp. 1086–1089)

Stop, Review, Remember! (pp. 1096–1097)

Multiple Choice

1. d (p. 1094)
2. a (p. 1089)
3. c (p. 1095)
4. b (p. 1092)

Fill in the Blank

1. a. Carbon dioxide
   b. Carbon monoxide
   c. Hydrogen sulfide
   d. Methane (p. 1095)
2. a. high angle
   b. low angle (p. 1093)

Critical Thinking

1. This would be location specific. (pp. 1094–1095)
2. This would be location specific. (pp. 1094–1095)
3. This would be location specific. (pp. 1093–1094)
4. A trench is an excavation that is over 8 feet deep, has intersection, or is compromised by weather related events and is an unsafe environment for the EMT. (pp. 1092, 1094)

Chapter Review (pp. 1099–1102)

Multiple Choice

1. b (pp. 1094–1095)
2. c (pp. 1075–1077)
3. a (pp. 1081–1082)
4. d (pp. 1086–1089)
5. a (p. 1089)
6. c (p. 1089)
7. c (p. 1085)
8. a (p. 1092)

Labeling   (pp. 1084–1084)

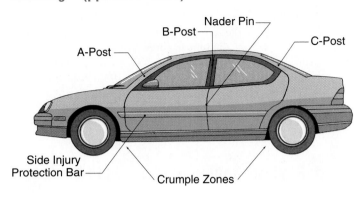

Critical Thinking

1. We radioed for the rescue truck to respond to our location and gave an exact location and condition of the victim. We got on the PA and called to the man to stay were he was, help was on the way. We donned our personal floatation devices and grabbed our throw bags. We threw the man a rope bag and after several attempts he grabbed the rope. The rescue truck arrived shortly and a group of swift water rescue technicians rescued the man from the river and transferred the patient to us. The patient was suffering from hypothermia even though it was a summer rain storm that sent the river out of its banks. The force of the water had battered the man against debris in the tree that he had hung onto, lacerating his legs and causing several soft tissue injuries. The wounds were dressed and the patient placed in a warm ambulance and treated for shock with oxygen. We remembered the awareness standards and the dangers of swift water. The rescue truck had the training and equipment required to retrieve the person. We did our part in reporting conditions, calling for resources, and making ourselves available to treat the rescued person. (pp. 1087–1088)
2. You should get a description of the victims included clothing and supplies that they might have. Prevent the victim's friends from attempting to search for their friends and becoming lost also. (pp. 1086, 1089)

Case Study

1. The second building is unsafe to enter. (pp. 1092–1093)

CHAPTER 44
Stop, Review, Remember! (pp. 1108–1109)

Multiple Choice

1. a (p. 1105)
2. b (pp. 1105–1106)
3. c (p. 1106)

Matching

1. C (p. 1107)
2. F (p. 1107)
3. A (p. 1107)
4. G (p. 1107)
5. B (p. 1107)
6. D (p. 1107)
7. E (p. 1107)

Critical Thinking

1. This will be a community-specific list. (p. 1105)
2. When sizing up the scene, do not park in a location closest to the event. Take the time to survey the scene, look for suspicious packages for example, back packs, packages, or things that look out of place. These are often hidden in trash cans, bushes, or shrubbery or in planted vehicles. If you identify a secondary device, immediately move to a safe distance, notify dispatch or the incident commander to have the bomb squad neutralize the device. (p. 1106)

Stop, Review, Remember! (pp. 1114–1115)

Multiple Choice

1. b (p. 1111)
2. d (pp. 1111–1112)
3. a (p. 111)

Fill in the Blank

1. S L U D G E M is an acronym for the following: (p. 1113)
   Salivation
   Lacrimation
   Urination
   Defecation
   GI Motility
   Emesis
   Miosis or constricted pupils
2. List at least 3 things to do when responding to a terrorist attack. Your answers may include: (p. 1107)
   1. Ask your dispatch center for a weather report.
   2. Look for situations in which the response is being funneled into an area that will bottleneck.
   3. Immediate contact with law enforcement for coordination.
   4. Identify a rally point to meet and regroup in the event of a secondary device.
   5. Identify safe staging areas for other EMS, fire, and police units to respond to.
   6. Approach the scene uphill and upwind.
   7. Make sure you have a quick unimpeded exit route.

Critical Thinking

1. The best way for the EMT to guard against radiation exposure is to follow the rules of time, distance, shielding, and quantity. (pp. 1110–1111)
2. Blistering, red, discolored, or irritated skin or any signs of symptoms of SLUDGEM. (p. 1113)

Chapter Review (pp. 1119–1121)

Multiple Choice

1. a (pp. 1116–1117)
2. d (p. 1111)
3. c (p. 1111)
4. d (p. 1111)
5. d (p. 1111)
6. c (p. 1112)
7. d (p. 1105)
8. d (p. 1062)
9. c (p. 1105)
10. c (p. 1113)
11. c (p. 1113)

Matching

1. B (p. 1105)
2. C (p. 1106)
3. A (p. 1109)
4. E (p. 1109)
5. D (p. 1109)
6. G (p. 1109)
7. H (p. 1110)
8. F (p. 1110)
9. J (p. 1110)
10. I (p. 1110)

Critical Thinking

1. Answers will vary. (p. 1105)
2. Bacteria, virus, and toxins. Biological agents enter the body through one of four common routes of entry: Inhalation, ingestion, dermal, or vector borne. They can be introduced in the air, community water sources, on broken skin wounds and through animals and insects.
   There are no signs during the incubation period, immediately after exposure to a biological agent. The agent multiplies and overwhelms the host. At the end of this period the victim will present with signs and symptoms of the illness. For a bacteria or virus which produce infection this period is measured in days. For a toxin, the timeframe is much shorter. When compared to chemical weapons, the ill effects from biological weapons would be delayed. Therefore it is more difficult to detect a biological agent. (pp. 1111–1113)

Case Study

1. Answers will vary. (p. 1105)
2. Answers will vary. (pp. 1105–1107)
3. Answers will vary. (pp. 1105–1107)

CHAPTER 45

1. c   Objective: 7-1.2 (p. 979)
2. d   Objective: There are no DOT objectives specific to this question. (p. 983)
3. a   Objective: 7-1.7 (pp. 986–987)
4. a   Objective: 7-1.6 (p. 989)
5. a   Objective: There are no DOT objectives specific to this question. (p. 1006)
6. c   Objective: There are no DOT objectives specific to this question. (p. 1006)
7. b   Objective: There are no DOT objectives specific to this question. (p. 1009)
8. c   Objectives: There are no DOT objectives specific to this question. (p. 1009)
9. d   Objective: There are no DOT objectives specific to this question. (p. 1008)
10. a   Objective: 7-3.7 (p. 1004)
11. b   Objective: 7-3.7 (p. 1030)
12. c   Objective: 7-3.11 (p.1012)
13. a   Objective: There are no DOT objectives specific to this question. (p. 1013)
14. a   Objective: 7-3.11 (p. 1016)
15. b   Objective: There are no DOT objectives specific to this question. (p. 1046)
16. c   Objective: There are no DOT objectives specific to this question. (p. 1048)
17. a   Objective: There are no DOT objectives specific to this question. (pp. 1048–1049)

18. d   Objective: There are no DOT objectives specific to this question. (p. 1049)

19. b   Objective: There are no DOT objectives specific to this question. (p. 1050)

20. a   Objective: There are no DOT objectives specific to this question. (p. 1050)

21. b   Objective: There are no DOT objectives specific to this question. (p. 1048)

22. a   Objective: There are no DOT objectives specific to this question. (p. 1053)

23. b   Objective: 7-3.1 (pp. 1062–1063)

24. d   Objective: There are no DOT objectives specific to this question. (p. 1057)

25. c   Objective: There are no DOT objectives specific to this question. (p. 1059)

26. c   Objective: There are no DOT objectives specific to this question. (p. 1063)

27. d   Objective: There are no DOT objectives specific to this question. (p. 1074)

28. c   Objective: 7-2.4 (p. 1075)

29. a   Objective: 7-2.3 (p. 1082)

30. d   Objective: 7-2.6 (p. 1082)

31. c   Objective: There are no DOT objectives specific to this question. (p. 1089)

32. b   Objective: There are no DOT objectives specific to this question. (p. 1091)

33. a   Objective: There are no DOT objectives specific to this question. (pp. 1092–1093)

34. d   Objective: There are no DOT objectives specific to this question. (pp. 1092–1093)

35. b   Objective: There are no DOT objectives specific to this question. (p. 1105)

36. a   Objective: There are no DOT objectives specific to this question. (pp. 1105–1106)

37. d   Objective: There are no DOT objectives specific to this question. (p. 1110)

38. b   Objective: There are no DOT objectives specific to this question. (p. 1110)

39. a   Objective: There are no DOT objectives specific to this question. (p. 1111)

40. c   Objective: 7-3.7 (p. 1029)

41. b   Objective: 7-3.11 (p. 1031)

42. d   Objective: 7-3.8 (p. 1032)

43. a   Objective: 7-3.9 (p. 1036)

44. a   Objective: 7-3.9 (p. 1036)

45. c   Objective: 7-3.9 (p. 1036)

46. a   Objective: 7-3.9 (pp. 1038–1039)

47. b   Objective: 7-3.9 (p. 1040)

48. d   Objective: 7-3.11 (p. 1008)

49. b   Objective: 7-3.11 (p. 1009)

50. a   Objective: 7-3.11 (p. 1017)

51. d   Objective: 7-1.2 (p. 976)

52. b   Objective: 7-1.9 (p. 994)

53. a   Objective: 7-1.14 (p. 998)

54. c   Objective: 7-3.11 (p. 1006)

55. a   Objective: 7-3.11 (p. 1006)

56. d   Objective: 7-3.8 (p. 1031)

57. c   Objective: 7-3.2 (p. 1050)

58. c   Objective: 7-2.2 (pp. 1080–1084)

59. c   Objective: (pp. 1105–1107)

60. b   Objective: There are no DOT objectives specific to this question. (p. 1110)

CHAPTER 46

Stop, Review, Remember! (pp. 1126–1127)

Multiple Choice

1. b (pp. 1133–1135)
2. c (p. 1135)
3. b (p. 1135)
4. d (p. 1136)
5. a (p. 1133)

Fill in the Blank

1. turbinates (p. 1133)
2. trachea (p. 1133)
3. hypopharynx (p. 1133)
4. laryngopharynx (p. 1133)
5. bronchus (p. 1135)

Critical Thinking

1. The conchae (or turbinates) are very vascular and can bleed easily when overstimulated. (p. 1133)
2. The first tracheal ring is anatomically different from the others in that it is the only complete ring. (p. 1133)
3. The upward insertion will irritate the conchae, causing pain and bleeding. The appropriate technique is to insert the airway straight back. (p. 1133)

Stop, Review, Remember! (pp. 1145–1146)

Multiple Choice

1. b (p. 1144)
2. c (p. 1140)
3. b (p. 1140)
4. a (p. 1138)
5. b (p. 1143)

Fill in the Blank

1. laryngoscope (p. 1138)
2. cricoid cartilage (p. 1144)
3. backward, upward, rightward pressure (p. 1144)
4. intubating (p. 1138)
5. stylet (p. 1140)

Critical Thinking

1. The curved blade id designed to fit into the vallecula. When the blade is inserted into the vallecula it indirectly moves the epiglottis away from the glottic opening, allowing you to see the glottic opening. The straight blade is designed to slide under the epiglottis and directly lift the epiglottis away from the glottic opening. Because the straight blade directly manipulates the epiglottis, it is the ideal choice when managing a pediatric airway. (pp. 1138–1139)
2. If the stylet is advanced beyond the distal end of the ET tube, it could cause trauma to the tissue of the airway. (pp. 1140–1141)

Stop, Review, Remember! (pp. 1156–1157)

Multiple Choice

1. d (pp. 1149–1150)
2. c (p. 1148)
3. d (pp. 1139, 1146, 1148)
4. a (p. 1146)
5. d (p. 1139, 1146, 1148)

Fill in the Blank

1. pulse oximetry (p. 1155)
2. two (p. 1152)
3. pneumothorax (p. 1152)
4. capnometer or capnographer (p. 1153)
5. blindly (p. 1146)

Critical Thinking

1. The potential for carbon monoxide toxicity is high during a structure fire and, due to carbon monoxide's affinity to hemoglobin, the pulse oximeter is most likely overestimating the true arterial hemoglobin oxygen saturation. (p. 1155)
2. The Esophageal Tracheal CombiTube (ETC) is a dual-lumen airway with a ventilation port in each lumen. When inserted, one tube will naturally enter the esophagus and the other will settle in the trachea, negating the need for visualization. Since either lumen can be used for ventilation, the EMT must simply determine which one is seated in the patient's trachea. (pp. 1145–1148)

Chapter Review (pp. 1158–1161)

Multiple Choice

1. c (pp. 1145–1148)
2. a (p. 1152)
3. a (p. 1143)
4. b (p. 1152)
5. d (p. 1148)

Matching

1. F (p. 1144)
2. B (p. 1138)
3. E (p. 1140)
4. G (p. 1138)
5. C (p. 1143)
6. A (pp. 1152–1153)
7. D (p. 1146)

Critical Thinking

1. "Rescue airways" are airway devices used when endotracheal intubation fails. Pharyngotracheal Airways, Laryngeal Mask Airways, and CombiTube are all examples of "rescue airways." (p. 1146)
2. Although it can be a helpful diagnostic tool, capnography can be unreliable and may reveal both false-positive and false-negative readings. It shouldn't be the sole factor used to determine proper tube placement or proper ventilation. (p. 1153)
3. You should first watch for chest rise and fall during ventilation. Then auscultate epigastric sounds (to immediately rule out an esophageal intubation in time to prevent vomiting) and conclude by auscultating lung sounds. Remember that lung sounds present on the right side but absent or diminished on the left indicate that the airway device may be advanced too deeply into one of the right mainstem bronchi. (p. 1152)

Case Studies

#1

1. No. Since the patient's anatomy was such that nothing could be seen beyond his hard palate, neither Sellick's nor BURP maneuvers would help to visualize the vocal cords. (p. 1144)

2. As an advocate for every patient's care and dignity, it was very appropriate to have the curtains closed on the photographer since it didn't take away from the care that the patient was receiving. Since most media outlets monitor emergency radio transmissions, there is always the potential for reporters, news crews, or photographers to arrive on scene. (p. 19)
3. The EMT should resort to a "rescue airway" once the maximum number of intubation attempts (per local protocol) are made. In this case, either a Pharyngeotracheal Airway, Laryngeal Mask Airway, or a CombiTube would be appropriate. (p. 1146)

#2

1. a (p. 1138)
2. c (p. 1140)
3. d (p. 1155)

CHAPTER 47

Chapter Review (pp. 1172–1173)

Critical Thinking

1. Answers will vary. (pp. 1162–1172)
2. Answers will vary. (pp. 1162–1172)
3. Answers will vary. (pp. 1162–1172)
4. Answers will vary. (pp. 1162–1172)
5. Answers will vary. (pp. 1162–1172)
6. Answers will vary. (pp. 1162–1172)
7. Answers will vary. (pp. 1162–1172)

CHAPTER 48

1. c Objective: 8-1.1 (p. 1132)
2. c Objective: 8-1.1 (p. 1133)
3. a Objective: 8-1.4 (p. 1133)
4. b Objective: 8-1.1 (p. 1133)
5. c Objective: 8-1.1 (p. 1133)
6. b Objective: 8-1.1 (p. 1134)
7. a Objective: 8-1.4 (p. 1133)
8. c Objective: 8-1.2 (p. 1135)
9. d Objective: 8-1.2 (p. 1135)
10. a Objective: 8-1.1 (p. 1136)
11. a Objective: 8-1.1 (p. 1135)
12. d Objective: There are no DOT objectives specific to this question. (p. 1140)
13. b Objective: 8-1.7 (p. 1144)
14. a Objective: There are no DOT objectives specific to this question. (p. 1144)
15. b Objective: 8-1.9 (p. 1138)
16. a Objective: 8-1.17 (pp. 1138–1139)
17. c Objective: 8-1.13 (p. 1139)
18. c Objective: 8-1.13 (p. 1140)
19. d Objective: 8-1.9 (p. 1138)
20. a Objective: 8-1.9 (p. 1138)
21. a Objective: 8-1.15 (p. 1140)
22. c Objective: 8-1.14 (p. 1140)
23. a Objective: 8-1.17 (p. 1143)
24. b Objective: 8-1.17 (p. 1143)
25. d Objective: 8-1.17 (p. 1143)
26. a Objective: 8-1.19 (p. 1144)
27. c Objective: 8-1.21 (p. 1144)
28. a Objective: 8-1.4 (p. 1145)

29. b   Objective: 8-1.4 (p. 1146)
30. b   Objective: 8-1.4 (p. 1146)
31. c   Objective: There is no DOT objective specific to this question. (p. 1148)
32. d   Objective: 8-1.6 (pp. 1149–1150)
33. a   Objective: 8-1.6 (p. 1150)
34. b   Objective: 8-1.6 (p. 1150)
35. b   Objective: 8-1.6 (p. 1150)
36. a   Objective: 8-1.6 (p. 1150)
37. d   Objective: 8-1.6 (p. 1150)
38. c   Objective: 8-1.19 (p. 1152)
39. b   Objective: 8.1-20 (p. 1152)
40. c   Objective: 8-1.18 (p. 1152)
41. c   Objective: 8-1.18 (p. 1152)
42. a   Objective: 8-1.19 (p. 1155)
43. c   Objective: 8-1.19 (p. 1155)
44. d   Objective: 8-1.19 (p. 1155)
45. b   Objective: 8-1.19 (p. 1152)
46. c   Objective: 8-1.19 (pp. 1152–1153)
47. d   Objective: 8-1.19 (p. 1153)
48. a   Objective: 8-1.19 (p. 1154)
49. b   Objective: 8-1.19 (pp. 1152–1153)
50. c   Objective: 8-1.19 (pp. 1154–1155)

APPENDIX A

Module 1

1. a   Objective: 1-1.2 (p. 13)
2. d   Objective: 1-1.2 (p. 13)
3. c   Objective: 1-1.1 (p. 11)
4. a   Objective: There is no DOT objective specific to this question. (p. 33)
5. b   Objective: 1-2.9 (pp. 44–45)
6. b   Objective: 1-3.3 (p. 64)
7. a   Objective: 1-3.4 (pp. 65–66)
8. a   Objective: 1-3.7 (p. 73)
9. a   Objective: 1-4.2 (p. 101)
10. b   Objective: 1-4.2 (p. 107)
11. d   Objective: 1-4.2 (p. 96)
12. a   Objective: 1-4.2 (pp. 96–97)
13. c   Objective: There is no DOT objective specific to this question. (p. 115)
14. b   Objective: 1-6.11 (p. 139)
15. a   Objective: 1-6.11 (p. 128)

Module 2

16. d   Objective: 2-1.1 (p. 94)
17. c   Objective: 2-1.3 (p. 168)
18. b   Objective: 2-1.3 (p. 168)
19. c   Objective: 2-1.2 (p. 166)
20. b   Objective: 2-1.9 (p. 190)
21. d   Objective: 2-1.4 (p. 172)
22. c   Objective: 2-1.7 (p. 172)
23. c   Objective: 2-1.8 (p. 178)
24. a   Objective: 2-1.8 (p. 178)
25. c   Objective: 2-1.8 (p. 178)
26. b   Objective: 2-1.8 (pp. 178–179)
27. c   Objective: 2-1.8 (p. 181)
28. c   Objective: There is no DOT objective specific to this question. (p. 181)

29. c   Objective: 2-1.17 (p. 182)
30. c   Objective: 2-1.12 (p. 191)
31. b   Objective: 2-1.12 (p. 191)
32. c   Objective: 2-1.12 (p. 197)

Module 3

33. a   Objective: 3-1.3 (p. 230)
34. b   Objective: 3-1.6 (pp. 233–234)
35. a   Objective: 1-5.24 (p. 253)
36. c   Objective: 1-5.24 (p. 252)
37. d   Objective: 1-5.1 (p. 254)
38. b   Objective: 1-5.2 (p. 257)
39. a   Objective: 1-5.3 (p. 257)
40. d   Objective: 1-5.5 (pp. 262–263)
41. c   Objective: 1-5.19 (p. 266)
42. a   Objective: 1-5.20 (p. 266)
43. c   Objective: 1-5.9 (p. 274)
44. a   Objective: 1-5.18 (p. 277)
45. b   Objective: 3-3.2 (p. 319)
46. a   Objective: 3-3.4 (p. 325)
47. c   Objective: 3-4.4 (p. 346)
48. a   Objective: There is no DOT objective specific to this question. (p. 382)
49. b   Objective: 3-8.3 (p. 406)

Module 4

50. a   Objective: There is no DOT objective specific to this question. (p. 430)
51. d   Objective: 4-1.5 (pp. 430–431)
52. d   Objective: There is no DOT objective specific to this question (p. 434)
53. a   Objective: 4-1.3 (p. 430)
54. b   Objective: There is no DOT objective specific to this question. (pp. 436–437)
55. c   Objective: 4-1.3 (p. 437)
56. b   Objective: There is no DOT objective specific to this question. (p. 438)
57. b   Objective: There is no DOT objective specific to this question. (p. 448)
58. a   Objective: 4-2.5 (p. 468)
59. d   Objective: 4-2.7 (p. 455)
60. b   Objective: 4-2.2 (p. 455)
61. c   Objective: 4-2.2 (p. 458)
62. a   Objective: There is no DOT objective specific to this question. (p. 466)
63. c   Objective: There is no DOT objective specific to this question. (p. 488)
64. a   Objective: 4-3.31 (p. 503)
65. a   Objective: 4-3.1 (p. 481)
66. b   Objective: 4-3.12 (p. 508)
67. a   Objective: There is no DOT objective specific to this question. (p. 513)
68. a   Objective: 4-4.1 (pp. 534–535)
69. d   Objective: There is no DOT objective specific to this question. (p. 549)
70. c   Objective: 4-5.1 (p. 562)
71. a   Objective: 4-7.1 (pp. 579–580)
72. a   Objective: 4-7.8 (p. 600)
73. c   Objective: There is no DOT objective specific to this question. (p. 616)
74. b   Objective: 4-9.13 (pp. 639–640)

Module 5

75. b Objective: 5-1.1 (p. 691)
76. d Objective: There is no DOT objective specific to this question. (pp. 694–696)
77. c Objective: 5-1.2 (p. 98)
78. a Objective: 5-1.3 (pp. 699–705)
79. a Objective: 5-1.9 (p. 668)
80. b Objective: 5-1.10, 5-2.2 (p. 672)
81. d Objective: 5-2.4, 5-2.4 (p. 720)
82. b Objective: 5-2.5 (pp. 722–724)
83. a Objective: 5-2.21 (p. 739)
84. b Objective: 5-2.15 (p. 754)
85. d Objective: There is no DOT objective specific to this question. (p. 760)
86. c Objective: There is no DOT objective specific to this question. (p. 761)
87. d Objective: There is no DOT objective specific to this question. (p. 763)
88. b Objective: 5-2.28 (pp. 767–768)
89. b Objective: 5-2.29 (p. 768)
90. a Objective: 5-2.20 (p. 770)
91. a Objective: There is no DOT objective specific to this question. (p. 778)
92. c Objective: 5-2.10 (p. 778)
93. a Objective: There is no DOT objective specific to this question. (p. 779)
94. a Objective: There is no DOT objective specific to this question. (p. 780)
95. a Objective: There is no DOT objective specific to this question. (p. 789)
96. a Objective: There is no DOT objective specific to this question. (p. 799)
97. b Objective: There is no DOT objective specific to this question. (p. 800)
98. c Objective: 5-3.8 (pp. 804–806)
99. b Objective: 5-3.8 (p. 805)
100. b Objective: 5-3.5 (p. 810)
101. a Objective: 5-3.6 (p. 811)
102. d Objective: 5-3.6 (p. 814)
103. a Objective: There is no DOT objective specific to this question. (p. 817)
104. d Objective: 5-3.8 (p. 809–810)
105. b Objective: 5-4.3 (p. 835)
106. b Objective: 5-4.3 (p. 835)
107. d Objective: 5-4.11 (p. 852)
108. b Objective: 5-4.3 (p. 862)
109. a Objective: 5-4.9; 5-4.14 (p. 872)
110. b Objective: 5-4.17 (p. 882)

Module 6

111. a Objective: 6-1.10 (p. 924)
112. b Objective: There is no DOT objective specific to this question. (p. 920)
113. c Objective: 6-1.5 (p. 924)
114. a Objective: 6-1.7; 6-1.6 (p. 925)
115. c Objective: 6-1.7 (p. 927)
116. b Objective: 6-1.13 (p. 934)
117. d Objective: 6-1.2 (p. 936)
118. c Objective: There is no DOT objective related to this question. (p. 940)
119. b Objective: There is no DOT objective related to this item. (p. 946)
120. a Objective: There is no DOT objective related to this item. (p. 948)
121. a Objective: There is no DOT objective related to this item. (p. 950)
122. d Objective: There is no DOT objective related to this item. (pp. 950–951)
123. c Objective: There is no DOT objective related to this item. (p. 959)

Module 7

124. a Objective: There is no DOT objective specific to this question. (p. 1006)
125. b Objective: There is no DOT objective specific to this question. (p. 1046)
126. c Objective: There is no DOT objective specific to this question. (p. 1048)
127. b Objective: There is no DOT objective specific to this question. (pp. 1048–1049)
128. d Objective: There is no DOT objective specific to this question. (p. 1049)
129. b Objective: There is no DOT objective specific to this question. (p. 1050)
130. a Objective: There is no DOT objective specific to this question. (p. 1050)
131. b Objective: There is no DOT objective specific to this question. (p. 1048)
132. a Objective: There is no DOT objective specific to this question. (p. 1053)
133. b Objective: 7-3.1 (pp. 1062–1063)
134. d Objective: There is no DOT objective specific to this question. (p. 1057)
135. c Objective: There is no DOT objective specific to this question. (p. 1059)
136. d Objective: There is no DOT objective specific to this question. (p. 1074)
137. c Objective: There is no DOT objective specific to this question. (p. 1075)
138. a Objective: There is no DOT objective specific to this question. (p.1082)
139. a Objective: There is no DOT objective specific to this question. (p. 1082)
140. c Objective: There is no DOT objective specific to this question. (p. 1089)
141. b Objective: There is no DOT objective specific to this question. (p. 1091)
142. a Objective: There is no DOT objective specific to this question. (p. 1092–1093)

Module 8

143. c Objective: 8-1.4 (p. 1133)
144. a Objective: 8-1.4 (p. 1133)
145. a Objective: There is no DOT objective specific to this question. (p. 1144)
146. c Objective: 8-1.13 (p. 1140)
147. b Objective: 8-1.17 (p. 1143)
148. d Objective: 8-1.6 (pp. 1149–1150)
149. c Objective: 8-1.19 (p. 1152)
150. c Objective: 8-1.19 (pp. 1152–1153)

✳ INDEX